W9-BFH-548

Basic & Clinical Endocrinology

seventh edition

Edited by

Francis S. Greenspan, MD, FACP
Clinical Professor of Medicine and Radiology
Chief, Thyroid Clinic
Division of Endocrinology, Department of Medicine
University of California, San Francisco

David G. Gardner, MD
Professor of Medicine
Department of Medicine and Diabetes Center
University of California, San Francisco

Lange Medical Books/McGraw-Hill
Medical Publishing Division

New York   Chicago   San Francisco   Lisbon   London   Madrid
Mexico City   Milan   New Delhi   San Juan
Seoul   Singapore   Sydney   Toronto

Basic & Clinical Endocrinology, Seventh Edition

3 4 5 6 7 8 9 0 DOC DOC 0 9 8 7 6 5

ISBN: 0-07-140297-7

ISSN: 0891-2068

Notice

Medicine is an ever-changing science. As new research and clinical experience broaden our knowledge, changes in treatment and drug therapy are required. The authors and the publisher of this work have checked with sources believed to be reliable in their efforts to provide information that is complete and generally in accord with the standards accepted at the time of publication. However, in view of the possibility of human error or changes in medical sciences, neither the authors nor the publisher nor any other party who has been involved in the preparation or publication of this work warrants that the information contained herein is in every respect accurate or complete, and they disclaim all responsibility for any errors or omissions or for the results obtained from use of the information contained in this work. Readers are encouraged to confirm the information contained herein with other sources. For example and in particular, readers are advised to check the product information sheet included in the package of each drug they plan to administer to be certain that the information contained in this work is accurate and that changes have not been made in the recommended dose or in the contraindications for administration. This recommendation is of particular importance in connection with new or infrequently used drugs.

This book was set in Times Roman by Pine Tree Composition, Inc.
The editors were Shelley Reinhardt, Peter J. Boyle, and Jim Ransom.
The production supervisor was Catherine H. Saggese.
The illustration manager was Charissa Baker.
The index was prepared by Kathrin Unger.
R.R. Donnelley was printer and binder.

This book is printed on acid-free paper.

The seventh edition of *Basic & Clinical Endocrinology* is dedicated to the memories of Dr. John Karam and Dr. Ralph Ribeiro—outstanding clinicians, teachers, and scientists who contributed enormously to the success of earlier editions.

Contents

8. Metabolic Bone Disease 295

Dolores Shoback, MD, Robert Marcus, MD, & Daniel Bikle, MD, PhD

9. Glucocorticoids & Adrenal Androgens 362

David C. Aron, MD, MS, James W. Findling, MD, & J. Blake Tyrrell, MD

10. Endocrine Hypertension 414

Burl R. Don, MD, Morris Schambelan, MD, & Joan C. Lo, MD

20. Obesity & Overweight 794
Marc K. Hellerstein, MD, PhD, & Elizabeth J. Parks, PhD

21. Humoral Manifestations of Malignancy 814
Dolores Shoback, MD, & Janet Funk, MD

22. Multiple Endocrine Neoplasia 829
David G. Gardner, MD

23. Geriatric Endocrinology 842
Susan L. Greenspan, MD, & Neil M. Resnick, MD

24. Endocrine Emergencies 867
David G. Gardner, MD, & Francis S. Greenspan, MD

25. AIDS Endocrinopathies 893
Grace Lee, MD, & Carl Grunfeld, MD, PhD

Authors

David C. Aron, MD, MS
Professor of Medicine and Epidemiology and Biostatistics, Case Western Reserve University School of Medicine; Director, Center for Quality Improvement Research, Education Office, Louis Stokes Cleveland Department of Veterans Affairs Medical Center, Cleveland, Ohio
david.aron@med.va.gov
Hypothalamus & Pituitary Gland; Glucocorticoids & Adrenal Androgens

John D. Baxter, MD
Professor of Medicine, Diabetes Center, University of California, San Francisco
jbaxter918@aol.com
Introduction to Endocrinology

Daniel Bikle, MD, PhD
Professor of Medicine, Veterans Affairs Medical Center and University of California, San Francisco; Co-Director, Special Diagnostic and Treatment Unit, Veterans Affairs Medical Center, San Francisco
doctor@itsa.ucsf.edu
Metabolic Bone Disease

Glenn D. Braunstein, MD
Professor of Medicine, David Geffen School of Medicine at the University of California, Los Angeles; Chairman, Department of Medicine, Cedars-Sinai Medical Center, Los Angeles
braunstein@cshs.org
Testes

Marcelle I. Cedars, MD
Professor and Director, Division of Reproductive Endocrinology, Department of Obstetrics, Gynecology, & Reproductive Sciences, University of California, San Francisco
cedarsm@obgyn.ucsf.edu
Female Reproductive Endocrinology & Infertility

Orlo H. Clark, MD
Professor and Vice-Chairman, Department of Surgery, University of California, San Francisco; Chief, Department of Surgery, University of California, San Francisco/Mt. Zion Medical Center
clarko@surgery.ucsf.edu
Endocrine Surgery

Felix A. Conte, MD
Professor of Pediatrics Emeritus, University of California, San Francisco
Abnormalities of Sexual Determination & Differentiation

Burl R. Don, MD
Associate Professor of Medicine, Division of Nephrology, University of California, Davis Medical Center
br.don@ucdmc.ucdavis.edu
Endocrine Hypertension

James W. Findling, MD
Clinical Professor of Medicine, Medical College of Wisconsin; Director, Endocrine-Diabetes Center, St. Luke's Medical Center, Milwaukee, Wisconsin
james.findling@aurora.org
Hypothalamus & Pituitary Gland; Glucocorticoids & Adrenal Androgens

Paul A. Fitzgerald, MD
Clinical Professor of Medicine, Department of Medicine, Division of Endocrinology, University of California, San Francisco
paulf@itsa.ucsf.edu
Adrenal Medulla

Janet L. Funk, MD
Assistant Professor of Medicine, University of Arizona, Tucson
jfunk@u.arizona.edu
Humoral Manifestations of Malignancy

David G. Gardner, MD
Professor of Medicine, Department of Medicine and Diabetes Center, University of California, San Francisco
gardner@itsa.ucsf.edu
Mechanisms of Hormone Action; Multiple Endocrine Neoplasia; Endocrine Emergencies

Michael S. German, MD
Associate Professor, Department of Medicine, Division of Endocrinology, University of California, San Francisco
mgerman@biochem.ucsf.edu
Pancreatic Hormones & Diabetes Mellitus

Alan Goldfien, MD
Professor Emeritus, Departments of Medicine, Obstetrics and Gynecology and Reproductive Sciences, and the Cardiovascular Research Institute, University of California, San Francisco
agold@itsa.ucsf.edu
Adrenal Medulla

Francis S. Greenspan, MD, FACP
Clinical Professor of Medicine and Radiology; Chief, Thyroid Clinic, Division of Endocrinology, Department of Medicine, University of California, San Francisco
n520@itsa.ucsf.edu
The Thyroid Gland; Endocrine Emergencies

Susan L. Greenspan, MD
Professor of Medicine, University of Pittsburgh School of Medicine; Director, Osteoporosis Prevention and Treatment Center, Divisions of Endocrinology and Metabolism and Geriatric Medicine, University of Pittsburgh Medical Center Health Sytem, Pittsburgh, Pennsylvania
greenspans@msx.dept-med.pitt.edu
Geriatric Endocrinology

Melvin M. Grumbach, MD, D.M. Hon. causa (University of Geneva, Switzerland), D. Hon. causa (University René Descartes, Paris 5)
Edward B. Shaw Professor of Pediatrics and Chairman Emeritus, Department of Pediatrics, University of California, San Francisco
grumbac@itsa.ucsf.edu
Abnormalities of Sexual Determination & Differentiation

Carl Grunfeld, MD, PhD
Professor of Medicine, University of California, San Francisco; Chief, Metabolism and Endocrine Sections, Veterans Affairs Medical Center, San Francisco
AIDS Endocrinopathies

Marc K. Hellerstein, MD, PhD
Professor of Endocrinology, Metabolism and Nutrition, Department of Medicine, University of California, San Francisco; Doris Howes Calloway Professor of Human Nutrition, Department of Nutritional Sciences, University of California, Berkeley
march@nature.berkeley.edu
Obesity & Overweight

Juan Carlos Jaume, MD
Assistant Professor, University of California, San Francisco
med123@itsa.ucsf.edu
Endocrine Autoimmunity

John P. Kane, MD, PhD
Professor of Medicine, Biochemistry and Biophysics, and Associate Director, Cardiovascular Research Institute; Director, Lipid Clinic, University of California, San Francisco
Disorders of Lipoprotein Metabolism

John H. Karam, MD[†]
Professor of Medicine Emeritus, University of California, San Francisco
Pancreatic Hormones & Diabetes Mellitus; Hypoglycemic Disorders

John L. Kitzmiller, MD
Director, Regional Diabetes and Pregnancy Program, Good Samaritan Hospital, San Jose, California
Pancreatic Hormones & Diabetes Mellitus: Diabetes Mellitus & Pregnancy

Geeta Lal, MD, MSc, FRCS(C)
Clinical Fellow—Endocrine Surgical Oncology, Department of Surgery, University of California, San Francisco/Mt. Zion Medical Center
lalg@surgery.ucsf.edu
Endocrine Surgery

Dan I. Lebovic, MD, MA
Assistant Professor of Obstetrics and Gynecology, Division of Reproductive Endocrinology and Infertility, University of Michigan, Ann Arbor
lebovic@umich.edu
The Endocrinology of Pregnancy

[†]Deceased

Grace Lee, MD
Clinical Endocrine Fellow, Department of Medicine,
University of California, San Francisco
galee@itsa.ucsf.edu
AIDS Endocrinopathies

Vishwanath R. Lingappa, MD, PhD
Professor of Physiology and Medicine, University of
California, San Francisco
vrl@itsa.ucsf.edu
Hormone Synthesis & Release

Joan C. Lo, MD
Assistant Professor of Medicine, University of Cali-
fornia, San Francisco; Division of Endocrinology,
San Francisco General Hospital, California
jlo@itsa.ucsf.edu
Endocrine Hypertension

Mary J. Malloy, MD
Clinical Professor of Medicine and Pediatrics; Direc-
tor, Pediatric Lipid Clinic and Co-Director,
Adult Lipid Clinic, University of California,
San Francisco
Disorders of Lipoprotein Metabolism

Robert Marcus, MD
Professor Emeritus, Stanford University, Stanford,
California; Medical Advisor, Eli Lilly & Com-
pany, Indianapolis, Indiana
rmarcuse@lilly.com
Mineral Metabolism & Metabolic Bone Disease

Umesh Masharani, MB, BS; MRCP(UK)
Associate Clinical Professor of Medicine, Department of Endocrinology and Metabolism, University of California, San Francisco
ubm@itsa.ucsf.edu
*Pancreatic Hormones & Diabetes Mellitus;
Hypoglycemic Disorders*

Synthia H. Mellon, PhD
Professor, Department of Obstetrics, Gynecology
and Reproductive Sciences, Center for Reproductive Sciences, Metabolic Research Unit, University of California, San Francisco
mellon@cgl.ucsf.edu
Hormone Synthesis & Release

Robert A. Nissenson, PhD
Professor of Medicine and Physiology, University of
California, San Francisco; Senior Research Career
Scientist, Department of Veterans' Affairs Med-
ical Center, San Francisco
chicago@itsa.ucsf.edu
Mechanisms of Hormone Action

Elizabeth J. Parks, PhD
Assistant Professor, Department of Food Science and
Nutrition, University of Minnesota, Twin Cities,
St. Paul
eparks@umn.edu
Obesity & Overweight

Neil M. Resnick, MD
Professor of Medicine, Chief of Gerontology and
Geriatric Medicine, and Director, University of
Pittsburgh Institute on Aging, University of Pitts-
burgh School of Medicine and University of
Pittsburgh Medical Center Health System, Penn-
sylvania
Geriatric Endocrinology

Ralff C. J. Ribeiro, MD, PhD [†]
Associate Professor, Department of Pharmaceutical
Sciences, University of Brasilia, Brazil
Introduction to Endocrinology

Mitchell Rosen, MD
Clinical Fellow, Division of Reproductive Endocrinology and Infertility, University of California, San Francisco
rosenm@obgyn.ucsf.edu
Female Reproductive Endocrinology & Infertility

Morris Schambelan, MD
Professor of Medicine, University of California, San
Francisco; Chief, Division of Edocrinology, Pro-
gram Director, General Clinical Research Center,
San Francisco General Hospital
morrie@sfghgcrc.ucsf.edu
Endocrine Hypertension

[†]Deceased

Dolores Shoback, MD
Professor of Medicine, University of California, San Francisco; Staff Physician, San Francisco Veterans Affairs Medical Center
dolores@itsa.ucsf.edu
Metabolic Bone Disease; Humoral Manifestations of Malignancy

Dennis Styne, MD
Professor, Department of Pediatrics, University of California, Davis, Medical Center, Sacramento
dmstyne@ucdavis.edu
Growth; Puberty

Robert N. Taylor, MD, PhD
Professor of Obstetrics, Gynecology, & Reproductive Sciences, Department of Obstetrics and Gynecology and Reproductive Sciences, University of California, San Francisco
taylorr@obgyn.ucsf.edu
The Endocrinology of Pregnancy

J. Blake Tyrrell, MD
Clinical Professor of Medicine; Chief, Endocrine Clinic, Division of Endocrinology and Metabolism, University of California, San Francisco
Hypothalamus & Pituitary Gland; Glucocorticoids & Adrenal Androgens

Paul Webb, PhD
Associate Researcher, Diabetes Center, University of California, San Francisco
webbp@itsa.ucsf.edu
Introduction to Endocrinology

Preface

Endocrinology is an expanding science, with new concepts and ideas appearing in the literature almost daily. Thus, it is imperative to have available a reliable source of information that keeps abreast of this mass of new knowledge. *Basic & Clinical Endocrinology* is just that type of resource. In this seventh edition, internationally recognized and outstanding specialists in each area of endocrinology have reviewed the new pathophysiologic concepts and treatments in their individual fields to bring the text up to date. The Introduction (Chapter 1) provides an excellent overview of the field. The basics of hormone synthesis, release, and action, as well as the important area of endocrine autoimmunity, are reviewed and updated. Chapters discussing each of the endocrine organs and their hormones and diseases have been revised. The endocrine aspects of metabolic bone disease, growth, sexual differentiation, pregnancy, obesity, lipoproteins, and AIDS, as well as the special problems of geriatric patients and endocrine emergencies, have all been brought up to current practice standards.

In this edition there are several new chapters. There is a new and comprehensive review of female reproductive endocrinology and infertility, emphasizing the physiology of the female reproductive system and the management of female endocrine problems and infertility. The new chapter on the adrenal medulla includes a scholarly review of the diagnosis and management of pheochromocytomas. A new chapter on endocrine surgery reviews the indications for and results of operation in patients with endocrine diseases.

In these times of information overload, a concise, authoritative, and readable text dealing with the function and malfunction of the human endocrine system is of extraordinary value. We believe it will be especially helpful to clinicians dealing with endocrine problems in patients, to researchers who wish to review a particular area of hormonal physiology, to medical students, residents, and endocrinology fellows training in this field, and to nurses responsible for patient care. We are proud to continue the tradition of excellence established in previous editions of this text.

Francis S. Greenspan, MD, FACP
David G. Gardner, MD

San Francisco
June 2003

Introduction to Endocrinology

John D. Baxter, MD, Ralff C.J. Ribeiro, MD, PhD, & Paul Webb, PhD

1,25 OHD$_3$	1,25-hydroxycholecalciferol
25, OHD$_3$	25-hydroxycholecalciferol
ACTH	Adrenocorticotropic hormone; corticotrophin
ADH	Antidiuretic hormone
ADP	Adenosine diphosphate
ANP	Atrial natriuretic peptide
AP1	Activating protein 1
ATP	Adenosine triphosphate
cAMP	Cyclic adenosine monophosphate
CAR	Constitutive androstane receptor
CBG	Corticosteroid-binding globulin; transcortin
CCK	Cholecystokinin
CG	Chorionic gonadotropin
cGMP	Guanosine 3′,5′-cyclic monophosphate
CGRH	Calcitonin gene-related hormone
COMT	Catechol-*O*-methyltransferase
CRH	Corticotropin-releasing hormone
CS	Chorionic somatomammotropin, placental lactogen
EGF	Epidermal growth factor
ELISA	Enzyme-linked immunosorbent assay
ER	Estrogen receptor
ERE	Estrogen response element
ERK	Extracellular signal-repeated kinase
ERR	Estrogen-related receptor
FGF	Fibroblast growth factor
FSH	Follicle-stimulating hormone
GABA	Gamma-aminobutyric acid
GH	Growth hormone
GHRH	Growth hormone-releasing hormone
GnRH	Gonadotropin-releasing hormone
GPR	G protein-coupled receptor
HRE	Hormone response element
IGF-I	Insulin-like growth factor-1
IGF-II	Insulin-like growth factor-2
JAK	Janus kinase
LDL	Low-density lipoprotein
LH	Luteinizing hormone
LXR	Liver X receptor
MAO	Monoamine oxidase
MAP	Mitogen-activated protein (kinase)
MCR	Melanocortin receptor
MEN	Multiple endocrine neoplasia
MODY	Maturity-onset diabetes of the young
MRI	Magnetic resonance imaging
mRNA	Messenger RNA
MSH	Melanocyte-stimulating hormone
NF-κB	nuclear factor kappa B
PAS	Period gene, Aryl hydrocarbon receptor nuclear translocator, and Single-minded
PCR	Polymerase chain reaction
PDGF	Platelet-derived growth factor
PPAR	Peroxisomal-proliferator activated receptor
PRL	Prolactin
PTH	Parathyroid hormone
RFLP	Restriction fragment length polymorphism
RTH	Resistance to thyroid hormone
SHBG	Sex hormone-binding globulin
SHP	Short heterodimer partner
SP	Specificity protein
STAT	Signal transducer and activator of transcription
TBG	Thyroid hormone-binding globulin
T$_4$	L-thyroxine
TGF	Transforming growth factor
TNF	Tumor necrosis factor
TR	Thyroid hormone receptor
TRH	Thyrotropin-releasing hormone
TSH	Thyroid-stimulating hormone, thyrotropin
T$_3$	L-3,5,3-triiodothyronine
VIP	Vasoactive intestinal pepetide
VMA	Vanillylmandelic acid

■ THE ENDOCRINE SYSTEM

The endocrine and nervous systems are the major controllers of the flow of information between different cells and tissues (Figure 1–1). The term "endocrine" denotes internal secretion of biologically active substances—in contrast to "exocrine," which denotes secretion outside the body, eg, through sweat glands or ducts that lead into the gastrointestinal tract. The endocrine system uses internal secretion of hormones into the circulation to convey information

to target cells that express cognate receptors. This system of internal hormone secretion is subject to complex regulatory mechanisms that govern receptor activity and hormone synthesis, release, transport, metabolism, and delivery to the interior of the target cells. The endocrine system also has complex relationships with the nervous and immune systems and exerts widespread effects upon development, growth, and metabolism. This chapter provides a broad overview of the field of endocrinology, including basic science facts and principles that are important for the diagnosis of endocrine disorders and the management of patients.

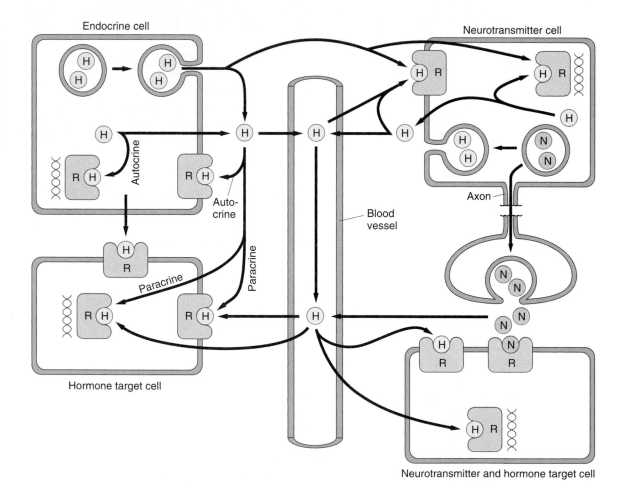

Figure 1–1. Actions of hormones and neurotransmitters. Endocrine and neurotransmitter cells synthesize hormones and release them by specialized secretory pathways of diffusion. The hormones act on the producer cell (autocrine) or on neighboring target cells, including neurotransmitter cells, without entering the circulation (juxtacrine and paracrine). They may go to the target cell through the circulation (hormonal). Neurotransmitter cells release neurotransmitters from nerve terminals. The same neurotransmitters can be released to act as hormones through the synaptic junctions or directly by the cell. (H, hormone; R, receptor; N, neurotransmitter.)

HORMONES: ENDOCRINE, PARACRINE, & AUTOCRINE ACTIONS

The endocrine system uses hormones to convey information between different tissues (Figure 1–1). Hormones are released by endocrine glands and transported through the bloodstream to tissues where they bind to specific receptor molecules and regulate target tissue function (Chapter 3). Some hormones (eg insulin, growth hormone, prolactin, leptin, catecholamines) bind cell surface receptors. Other hormones (eg, steroids, thyroid hormone) bind to intracellular receptors that act in the nucleus. Receptors have bifunctional properties of both recognition (ie, ability to distinguish the hormone from all other molecules to which they are exposed) and signal activation. The hormone acts as an allosteric effector that alters receptor conformation, and this conformational alteration transmits the binding information into postreceptor events that influence cellular function.

In addition to this traditional view, hormones can also act locally by binding to receptors that are expressed by cells that are close to the site of release. When hormones act on neighboring non-hormone-producing cells, the action is called "paracrine," as illustrated by actions of sex steroids in the ovary, angiotensin II in the kidney, and platelet-derived growth factor in the vascular wall. As a variant of this mechanism, peptide hormones can remain in the membrane of one cell and interact with a receptor on a juxtaposed cell. This is seen, for example, with hematopoietic growth factors and is termed "juxtacrine" regulation. When hormone is released and acts on receptors located on the same cell, the action is referred to as "autocrine." Autocrine actions may be important in promoting unregulated growth of cancer cells. Hormones can also act inside the cell without being released, ie, an "intracrine" effect. For example, insulin can inhibit its own release from pancreatic islet B cells and somatostatin can inhibit its own release from pancreatic D cells (Chapter 17).

CHEMICAL COMPOSITION OF HORMONES

Hormones derive from the major classes of biologic molecules (Figures 1–2 and 1–3; see also Chapter 2). Thus, hormones can be proteins (including glycopro-

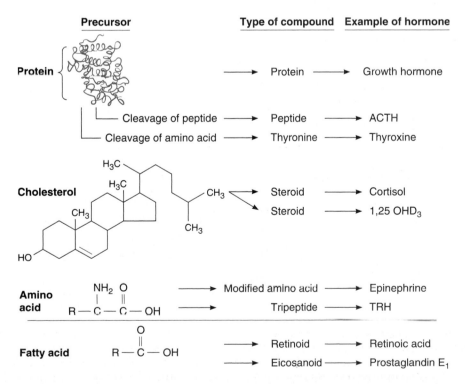

Figure 1–2. Precursors of hormones. Shown are representations of the sources of the major hormones, with examples of different hormones that reflect each chemical type.

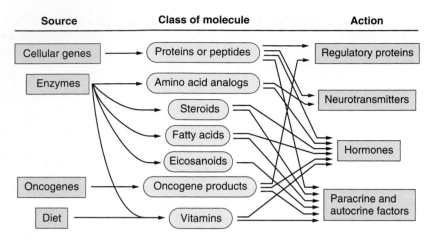

Figure 1–3. Relations between the source, class, and actions of various molecules involved in the endocrine system. These molecules are or become hormones, eicosanoids, oncogene products, and vitamins. Normal genes encode proteins that are regulatory proteins, neurotransmitters, hormones, and paracrine or autocrine factors (or polypeptides from which these are derived). Normal genes also encode enzymes which generate amino acid analogs that can be neurotransmitters, hormones, and autocrine or paracrine factors; steroids that can be hormones or autocrine or paracrine factors; or eicosanoids that can be autocrine or paracrine factors. Oncogenes encode proteins that can be regulatory proteins, hormones, or autocrine or paracrine factors. Vitamin D can be obtained from the diet or synthesized by the body. It can act as a hormone or as an autocrine or paracrine factor.

teins), peptides or peptide derivatives, amino acid analogs, or lipids. Polypeptide hormones are direct translation products of specific mRNAs, cleavage products of larger precursor proteins, or modified peptides. Catecholamines and thyroid hormones are amino acid derivatives. Steroid hormones and vitamin D are derived from cholesterol. Retinoids are derived from carotenoids in the diet that are modified by the body. Eicosanoids are derived from fatty acids.

New hormones are still being discovered. Classically, the field of endocrinology has progressed from discovery of hormones that mediate physiologic effects to identification of receptors. With the advent of molecular biology and large-scale genomic sequencing, it has become possible to identify a receptor based on sequence homology before the hormone is identified. This approach shifts endocrinology into reverse and gives rise to a search for new hormones and their signaling pathways. For example, many orphan nuclear receptors (with no known ligands) were identified on the basis of sequence similarities with other nuclear receptors, and new hormones that interact with many of these orphan receptors were subsequently identified. Similarly, genes encoding proteins with homology to known cell surface receptors

have been cloned in recent years. This suggests that a number of ligands or hormones that act upon cell surface receptors are yet to be discovered. Urotensin II, a vasoactive somatostatin-like peptide, was shown to bind tightly to a previously orphaned G protein-coupled receptor, GPR14, in cardiovascular tissues.

■ RELATIONSHIPS BETWEEN HORMONES & OTHER SIGNALING MOLECULES

Endocrine hormones are part of a large complement of small intercellular signaling molecules. The following sections review parallels and overlaps between the endocrine system and other signaling systems.

NEUROTRANSMITTERS & HORMONES

Traditionally, the endocrine system is distinguished from the nervous system by the fact that endocrine signals are released systemically whereas the nervous system is directly connected to target tissues through neurons (Figure 1–1). Hormones are widely distributed, and reliance is placed on the receptor to distinguish the hormone from other molecules and then to generate responses in specific cells (Figure 1–1). By contrast, the neurotransmitter is synthesized in the cell body of the neuron and travels down the axon, where it is stored in synaptic vesicles, released upon depolarization, and binds specific receptors on the postsynaptic neuron. Here, specificity of response is dependent on targeted local release of signaling molecules.

While there are differences between the endocrine and nervous systems, there are also similarities. Neurotransmitter actions involve ligand-receptor interactions that resemble those of the endocrine system. Indeed, the same molecule can be both a neurotransmitter and a hormone (Figure 1–1). Catecholamines are neurotransmitters when released by nerve terminals and hormones when released by the adrenal medulla. Furthermore, catecholamines utilize the same types of adrenergic receptors and the same postreceptor intracellular signaling pathways in the central nervous system and the peripheral tissues.

Other molecules behave as hormones and neurotransmitters. Thyrotropin-releasing hormone (TRH) is a hormone when it is produced by the hypothalamus, but it has diverse neurotransmitter actions in the central nervous system. Dopamine, corticotropin-releasing hormone (CRH), calcitonin gene-related hormone (CGRH), somatostatin, gonadotropin-releasing hormone (GnRH), vasoactive intestinal peptide (VIP), gastrin, secretin, cholecystokinin, and steroids (neurosteroids) and their receptors are also found in various parts of the brain.

There is also overlap between the function of endocrine glands and the nervous system. For example, the hypothalamus contains specialized neurons that secrete hormones into the circulation. This is reviewed below in the section on neuroendocrinology and is discussed also in Chapter 5.

VITAMINS & HORMONES

Vitamins (Figure 1–3) are essential substances required in small quantities from the diet. They are utilized by the body as cofactors and regulators of cellular functions. Although this definition is acceptable, the body produces molecules that have been described as "vitamins," and vitamins have actions that resemble hormones. For example, vitamin D is produced in individuals who are exposed to sunlight, and supplementation is required only when there is inadequate exposure to sunlight (Chapter 8). Furthermore, the active product of vitamin D is a derivative of the ingested vitamin. Vitamins can also act by mechanisms that resemble hormones. For example, vitamin D and the retinoids (retinoic acid, 9-*cis*-retinoic acid, and others) act through nuclear receptors belonging to the same family as the steroids and thyroid hormone (see Chapter 3).

ONCOGENES & HORMONES

Oncogenes are mutated versions of normal genes that promote cancer (see Chapter 21 and Figure 1–3). Oncogenes were originally identified in oncogenic viruses that captured genes from their host's genome. The chicken erythroleukemia virus contains two cooperating oncogenes that are homologs of hormone receptors: v-*erbA* (viral erbA), which is similar to the thyroid hormone receptor (sometimes designated as c-*erbA*, cellular erbA); and v-*erbB*, which is similar to the epidermal growth factor (EGF) receptor (c-*erbB*). Oncogenes were subsequently identified in the genomes of cancer cells.

In many cases, oncogenes are analogs of the genes encoding hormones, hormone receptors, or factors that are downstream of the hormone receptor. Typically, the oncogene codes for a mutated version of its normal cellular counterpart which is not subject to the usual regulatory controls. Thus, v-erbA does not bind thyroid hormone and acts constitutively as a transcriptional repressor. The mechanisms of action of oncogene products are described in Chapters 3 and 21.

THE IMMUNE SYSTEM & HORMONES

Interrelationships between the endocrine and immune systems are illustrated in Figure 1–4. Many immune signaling events resemble events of endocrine signaling. Thus, antigen recognition and the mechanisms that in-

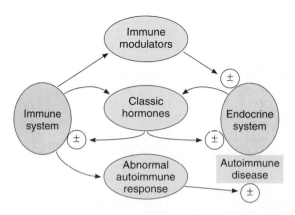

Figure 1–4. Interrelations between the endocrine and immune systems. The plus or minus signs indicate that the influences can be stimulatory or inhibitory.

hibit the recognition of self-antigens involve ligand-receptor interactions similar to those used by hormones (see Chapter 3). Moreover, immunologically competent cells release peptide signaling molecules that resemble endocrine hormones in their actions. These include cytokines (eg, interleukins, interferons, tumor necrosis factor [TNF], and plasminogen activator) that bind to receptors on target cells and stimulate growth, mediate cytotoxicity, or suppress antibody production by B cells, and lymphokines that attract macrophages and neutrophils to an area of infection. In some cases, immune cells produce peptides that have been traditionally considered as hormones (eg, corticotropin [ACTH], prolactin [PRL], and gonadotropin-releasing hormone [GnRH]). The roles of these immune cell-produced classic hormones are not yet clear, though GnRH appears to play a role in lymphocyte homing.

There is extensive cross-talk between the endocrine and immune systems. Substances released by immune cells can affect the function of the endocrine system. For example, TNF can influence the release and metabolism of thyroid hormones (see Chapter 7). Moreover, endocrine hormones regulate the actions of the immune system. Finally, autoimmune-induced disorders of the endocrine glands comprise a major component of endocrine practice. These include autoimmune destruction of glands, as is seen in type 1 diabetes mellitus (Chapter 17) and the most common form of Addison's disease (Chapter 9); and autoimmune stimulation, as is seen in the most common form of hyperthyroidism (Chapter 7).

EICOSANOIDS: PROSTAGLANDINS & RELATED COMPOUNDS

Eicosanoids (including prostaglandins, prostacyclins, leukotrienes, and thromboxanes; Figures 1–2 and 1–3) are derived from polyunsaturated fatty acids with 18-, 20-, or 22-carbon skeletons. Arachidonic acid (*cis*-5,8,11,14-eicosatetraenoic acid) is the most abundant eicosanoid precursor in humans. Eicosanoids are produced by most cells, released with little storage, cleared rapidly from the circulation, and thought to act in a paracrine or autocrine fashion. They have mechanisms of action similar to those of hormones and act through both cell surface receptors and nuclear receptors.

There is cross-talk between eicosanoids and endocrine systems. Eicosanoids regulate hormone release and actions. For example, prostaglandin E (PGE) inhibits growth hormone (GH) and prolactin (PRL) release from the pituitary. Eicosanoid synthesis is also frequently stimulated by hormones, and in these instances eicosanoids act as downstream mediators of hormone action.

■ MECHANISMS OF HORMONE ACTION

The mechanisms of hormone action are discussed in greater detail in Chapter 3.

HORMONE RECEPTORS

Hormones bind specifically to hormone receptors with high affinity and promote allosteric changes within the receptor molecule that translate the signal into biologic activities. The receptors can be expressed on the cell surface or within the cell. Whereas traditionally it was thought that the unliganded receptors are inactive—and only become activated upon hormone binding—there are now many examples (eg, with some nuclear receptors) of unliganded receptors that are active in the absence of hormone, and ligand binding reverses this effect and promotes a different activity of the receptor. The various receptor types are discussed separately in following paragraphs and in more detail in Chapter 3.

Cell Surface Receptors

Cell surface receptors have ligand recognition domains that are exposed on the outer surface of the cell membrane, one or more membrane-spanning domains, and a ligand-regulated cytoplasmic effector domain. This organization allows the cell to sense extracellular events and to pass this information to the intracellular environment.

The cell surface receptors can be divided into four types.

(1) Seven-transmembrane domain receptors—also known as G-protein coupled receptors—mediate actions of catecholamines, prostaglandins, ACTH, glucagon, parathyroid hormone (PTH), thyroid-stimulating hormone (TSH), luteinizing hormone (LH), and others (Chapter 3). They contain a surface-exposed amino terminal domain followed by seven transmembrane domains that span the lipid bilayer and a hydrophilic carboxyl terminal domain that lies in the cytoplasm. These receptors are coupled to the guanylyl nucleotide binding "G proteins." Binding of ligand to the receptor activates G proteins, which in turn act on effectors such as adenylyl cyclase and phospholipase C and in that way initiate production of second messengers with resultant influences on cell organization, enzymatic activities, and transcription.

(2) Receptors with intrinsic ligand-regulated enzymatic activities mediate the actions of growth factors, atrial natriuretic peptide (ANP), and TGFβ. Each con-

tains an amino terminal surface exposed ligand-binding domain, a single membrane-spanning domain, and a carboxyl terminal catalytic domain. Growth factor receptors, including those for insulin and EGF, possess tyrosine kinase activity. Ligand binding results in dimerization, activation of tyrosine kinase, and autophosphorylation. These events lead to recruitment of additional factors that trigger second messenger cascades such as the MAP kinase phosphorylation pathway and activation of the pI3-kinase-protein kinase B-Akt system. The ANP receptors are monomers with ligand-regulated guanylyl cyclase activity, which generates the second messenger cGMP. The TGFβ receptor forms heterodimers upon ligand binding and contains ligand-dependent serine-threonine kinase activity.

(3) Cytokine receptors are part of a large class of receptors that also mediate the actions of growth hormone (GH) and leptin. Like growth factor receptors, this class contains a surface-exposed amino terminal domain that binds ligand, a single membrane-spanning domain, and a carboxyl terminal effector domain. They also function as dimers. However, cytokine receptors do not possess intrinsic enzymatic activity. Instead, liganded receptors associate with cytoplasmic tyrosine kinases (such as the Janus kinases; JAKs) that mediate downstream signaling events such as activation of associated transcription factors (signal transducers and activators of transcription; STATs) and cross-talk with kinase cascades.

(4) Ligand-regulated transporters can bind ligands such as acetylcholine and respond by opening the channel for ion flow. In this case, the ion flux acts as the second messenger.

Other cell surface molecules resemble "receptors" but transport hormones into cells for degradation. Examples include the type C (clearance) ANP receptor and those for low-density lipoprotein (LDL), mannose 6-phosphate, and transferrin. Each of these proteins shares a short cytoplasmic domain with no known signal transduction function. Since most of these receptors are engaged in internalization by endocytosis and degradation of ligands, they are often called "transporters" rather than receptors.

Nuclear Receptors

Nuclear receptors mediate actions of steroid hormones, vitamin D, thyroid hormones, retinoids, fatty acids, bile acids, eicosanoids, xenobiotics, and other molecules. As described above, new nuclear receptor ligands are still being identified and new ligand specificities are being uncovered. Recent examples are the discoveries that the receptor HNF-4A binds tightly to 14-chain and 18-chain fatty acids and that the vitamin D receptor binds bile acids.

Nuclear receptors control gene expression by binding to either DNA response elements in the promoters of target genes or to other transcription factors. They then recruit large corepressor and coactivator complexes that modulate gene expression by modifying chromatin or contacting the basal transcription machinery. The DNA elements are specific sequences, usually a repeated hexanucleotide separated by a variable number of nucleotides aligned either as a direct repeat, a palindrome, or a reverse palindrome. These elements are termed hormone response elements (HREs). Nuclear receptor-protein interactions modulate the activities of heterologous DNA-bound transcription factors such as AP1, SP1, and NF-κB.

Nuclear receptors have similar structures and functions. Each is composed of three domains that can act somewhat independently. The amino terminal domain is the most variable and mediates effects on transcription. The DNA-binding domain is well conserved and mediates HRE recognition and dimerization and contributes to modulation of heterologous transcription factor activity. The carboxyl terminal domain is also well conserved and mediates ligand binding, dimerization, and effects on transcription. The genomic sequence of several organisms is now available, and this permits an estimate of the numbers of nuclear receptor genes based on sequence homology. The human genome contains 48 distinct nuclear receptor genes all of which were previously identified by alternative approaches.

While nuclear receptors exhibit similar organization, there are subclasses that differ in details of their actions. Unliganded steroid receptors form inactive cytoplasmic complexes with heat shock proteins. Ligand binding promotes dissociation from the heat shock protein complex and formation of active receptor homodimers that translocate to the nucleus where they recruit coactivators. By contrast, unliganded thyroid hormone, retinoid, vitamin D, and peroxisomal proliferator-activated receptors bind tightly to chromatin, usually as heterodimers with the retinoid X receptor. Here, ligand promotes dissociation of corepressors and subsequent recruitment of coactivators with a resulting shift from repression to activation of gene expression at positively regulated genes. Other nuclear receptors exhibit variations on the standard structural organization. Steroidogenic factor-1, for example, contains a large hinge domain between the DNA-binding and putative ligand-binding functions, and this region has second messenger-regulated transcriptional activation properties. SHP (short heterodimer partner) consists of an isolated ligand-binding domain that represses the activity of other nuclear receptors and may work in the same way as a cofactor. Other nuclear receptors function as monomers.

Given that there are many transcription factors, it is surprising that there is only a single nuclear hormone receptor family. The aryl hydrocarbon receptor is a widely distributed transcription factor that binds xenobiotics, including man-made chemicals such as dioxin. This receptor is a member of a family of proteins that differ from nuclear receptors but also bind DNA. Although no endogenous ligand is known to bind these receptors, it is possible that natural ligands for the aryl hydrocarbon receptor and other nonclassic nuclear receptors will be identified. There are also complex interrelations between membrane receptors, nuclear receptors, and their ligands. Nuclear receptor ligands can exert rapid effects on the cell membrane. Some of these ligands interact with specialized membrane receptors. Thus, progesterone can antagonize the action of oxytocin by direct and highly selective binding to G protein-coupled membrane oxytocin receptors. However, in other cases, classic nuclear receptors (including estrogen, androgen, and progesterone receptors) interact with proteins at the inner surface of the cell membrane such as the tyrosine kinase Src and the p85 subunit of pI3-kinase, and initiate second messenger cascades. The estrogen receptor (ER) may also be able to interact with the cell membrane directly. In either case, the fact that a single ligand can influence events within the nucleus and at the membrane raises the possibility that these diverse events could exert concerted effects upon cellular function. Finally, nuclear receptors can be activated by second messenger signaling systems in the absence of the ligand. For example, the progesterone receptor can be activated by dopamine through phosphorylation.

HORMONE EFFECTS ON RECEPTOR ACTIVITY

The traditional view of hormone receptor action is that the receptor is inactive in the absence of hormone and that hormone activates the receptor. In this sense, the receptor is often described as an "on-off" switch. However, this simple model does not always account for the full spectrum of hormone effects on receptor activity. As mentioned above, some nuclear receptors are active in the absence of ligand. Thyroid hormone and retinoic acid receptors bind to DNA in the absence of ligand and actively repress transcription of nearby genes. Ligand promotes release of corepressors and recruitment of coactivators and, consequently, promotes simultaneous relief of inhibition and further activation of transcription. The unliganded thyroid hormone receptor can also activate negatively regulated genes, including that of TSH. Here, ligand reverses the activation that is obtained with the unliganded receptor and suppresses transcription below basal levels. Thus, thyroid hormone

and retinoic acids are more properly described as altering the spectrum of receptor activities rather than turning the receptor on or off in the traditional sense. Other receptors can be active in the absence of ligand and either inactive or less active in the presence of ligand. Examples from the nuclear receptor family include constitutive androstane receptor (CAR) and the estrogen-related receptors (ERRs). Among cell surface receptors, the melanocortin receptors (MCRs) may be either stimulated by agonists or inhibited by natural antagonists.

Even if a hormone does promote a true transition from an inactive receptor state to an active state, it need not always elicit maximal agonist responses. Different peptides that bind to the growth factor receptors can show qualitatively different effects on downstream signaling events. ER activity and cofactor binding is dependent on the DNA sequence of the hormone response element or upon whether receptor acts through classic DNA binding sites or through heterologous transcription factors, such as AP1 (see sections on partial agonist and mixed agonist-antagonist activity, below).

■ CLASSES OF HORMONE ACTION

Hormones and hormone analogs can be classified using two criteria (Figure 1–5) . The first utilizes the receptor through which ligand acts. The second utilizes the activity the ligand elicits (agonist, antagonist, etc). Thus, a compound that produces estrogenic effects on breast through ER is an ER agonist. Conversely, a compound that binds to the ER and blocks binding of estrogens but does not allow the receptor to adopt a functionally active state is said to be an ER antagonist.

CLASSIFICATION OF HORMONE ACTION BY RECEPTOR TYPE

Traditionally, hormones were classified according to effects. Glucocorticoids were named for carbohydrate-regulating activities, mineralocorticoids for salt-regulating activities, and pituitary hormones for various tropisms. This nomenclature can pose problems. The effects of a particular hormone that are recognized first might represent a subset of its primary effects. For example, glucocorticoids, named for their glucose-regulating activities, also have widespread anti-inflammatory effects and can influence abdominal fat deposition. Furthermore, several different hormones exert the same

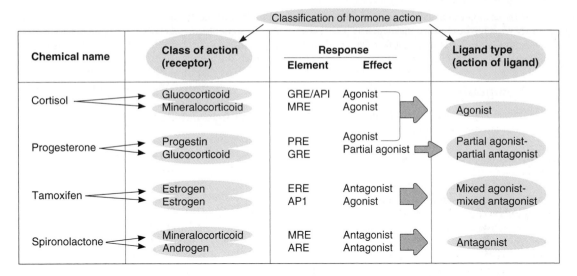

Chemical name	Class of action (receptor)	Response		Ligand type (action of ligand)
		Element	Effect	
Cortisol	Glucocorticoid Mineralocorticoid	GRE/API MRE	Agonist Agonist	Agonist
Progesterone	Progestin Glucocorticoid	PRE GRE	Agonist Partial agonist	Partial agonist- partial antagonist
Tamoxifen	Estrogen Estrogen	ERE AP1	Antagonist Agonist	Mixed agonist- mixed antagonist
Spironolactone	Mineralocorticoid Androgen	MRE ARE	Antagonist Antagonist	Antagonist

Classification of hormone action

Figure 1–5. Classification of actions of ligands that interact with hormone receptors. Shown are examples of different types of ligands with classification of the type of ligand and the receptors through which they interact. (GRE, glucocorticoid response element; AP1, activating protein 1; MRE, mineralocorticoid response element; PRE, progesterone response element; ERE, estrogen response element; ARE, androgen response element.)

effects through the same receptor (Figures 1–5 and 1–6). For example, both the "glucocorticoid" cortisol and the "mineralocorticoid" aldosterone regulate mineral metabolism by interactions with mineralocorticoid receptors. Two hormones can also have the same effect through interactions with different receptors. Both glucocorticoids and insulin promote glycogen deposition. Finally, the same hormone can act through more than one receptor with different physiologic consequences. Prostaglandins and progesterone can act through distinct cell surface and nuclear receptors.

Other hormones were named for the endocrine gland (eg, parathyroid hormone). This classification

can also be confusing since most glands produce multiple hormones and some hormones are made in more than one site. For example, progesterone is made in both the placenta and the ovaries.

One way to avoid confusion is by utilizing the receptor for classifying hormone action (Figure 1–5). This method of classification was used by pharmacologists even before receptors were proved to exist. For example, the classification of catecholamine actions through the α- and β-adrenergic receptors is familiar to clinicians and scientists. This receptor-based method of classification has the advantage that it acknowledges the spectrum of receptor-mediated actions while preserving the historical name. By this system, most actions of cortisol are mediated through glucocorticoid receptors, but cortisol actions through mineralocorticoid receptors are termed a mineralocorticoid action of cortisol.

CLASSIFICATION OF HORMONE ACTION BY LIGAND TYPE

Classification of ligands as agonists, partial agonists-partial antagonists, antagonists, or inactive compounds has been widely utilized. Classification of mixed agonist-antagonist compounds and inverse agonists accounts for new information about mechanisms of action of various ligands whose properties do not fit the other categories. The effects of these compounds vary

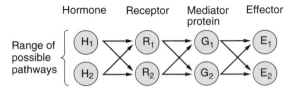

Figure 1–6. Possible pathways of transmission of hormonal signals. Each hormone can work through one or more receptors; each hormone-receptor complex can work through one or more mediator proteins; and each mediating protein or enzyme activated by hormone-receptor complexes can affect one or more effector functions.

in different tissues as well as with respect to the factors that interact with hormone-responsive genes. Thus, the same compound in one tissue or context can act differently in another context.

Inactive Compounds

Inactive compounds are those that do not bind to receptors and have neither agonist nor antagonist activity.

Agonists

An agonist binds to a receptor and transforms binding into a response. Most naturally produced ligands are agonists. However, synthetic hormone analogs may have more potent activity than the natural hormone. Examples include synthetic glucocorticoids such as prednisone, dexamethasone, and triamcinolone that are used to suppress inflammatory and immunologic responses (Chapter 9). It should be noted that some agonists can exert so-called inverse agonist effects—ie, they inhibit activity of active unliganded receptors.

Antagonists

An antagonist binds a receptor but does not transform binding into a response. The antagonist usually competes for agonist binding and thereby prevents agonist actions, defining the term antagonist. The body produces nuclear receptor antagonists, but these usually circulate at levels too low to be effective. For example, progesterone can act as a mineralocorticoid or glucocorticoid receptor antagonist but interacts with each of these receptors with low affinity. Normal progesterone concentrations are too low for the steroid to occupy substantial numbers of either receptor. However, synthetic nuclear receptor hormone antagonists are clinically useful. Examples include the antiestrogens tamoxifen and raloxifene and the antiprogestin and antiglucocorticoid mifepristone (RU 486). In contrast, there are examples of natural high-affinity antagonists for cell surface receptors. The melanocortin 4 receptor (MC4R), which is expressed in hypothalamus and regulates feeding behavior, binds α-MSH, a natural agonist, and agouti-related peptide, a natural antagonist. The balance of α-MSH and agouti-related peptide is affected by hormones such as leptin and factors related to feeding and energy storage, such as fasting behavior. This balance, in turn, dictates the direction of MC4R activity.

Most hormone antagonists compete with the agonist for the hormone binding site and are referred to as competitive antagonists. However, it should be possible to identify other types of antagonists. Noncompetitive antagonists of hormone response could prevent the allosteric alteration that signals ligand binding or could block interactions with downstream cofactors that mediate the signal. For example, efforts are being made to develop drugs that mimic the peptide interactions between nuclear receptors and their downstream coactivators.

Partial Agonist-Partial Antagonists

Partial agonists or partial antagonists bind to receptors and yield a response that is less than that of a full agonist at saturating ligand concentrations. A partial agonist will block binding of a full agonist and suppress receptor activity to the level induced by the partial agonist alone, thereby justifying its "partial antagonist" designation. Some of these compounds are naturally produced, although—as in the case of antagonists—the occupancy of receptors has not been shown to be important in normal circumstances. However, many plant estrogens (phytoestrogens), such as genistein, may behave as partial ER agonists; it has been speculated that this property is related to the apparent protective effect of these compounds on breast cancer incidence.

Mixed Agonists-Antagonists

These compounds act in different ways through the same receptor type depending on the context (which cells, which promoter, etc). As an example, the estrogen "antagonists" tamoxifen and raloxifene act mostly as antagonists in breast but have estrogen agonist actions in bone and uterus. This property has been exploited clinically, since the effects on both breast and bone are useful.

Ligands with Reverse Pharmacology

This classification has been used to describe ligands that exert agonist effects which are completely distinct from those of the native ligand. For example, when estradiol binds to ERβ there is little or no effect at genes with AP1 sites, whereas tamoxifen and raloxifene show potent stimulatory effects at these sites.

MECHANISMS OF LIGAND ACTION

The mechanisms of agonist and antagonist hormone action are addressed in Chapter 3. Although there are exceptions, as discussed earlier, unliganded receptors are commonly in an inactive conformational state. When agonists bind to these receptors, they induce conformational changes that transduce postbinding information into responses. These changes result in alterations of the complement of receptor associated proteins, alterations in receptor enzymatic activity, or modifications of the receptor (such as phosphorylation and ubiquitination).

REGULATION OF HORMONE RESPONSIVENESS

Hormone response depends on the presence of a response system and the availability of hormone. A common mechanism for ensuring specificity of hormone receptor action is to restrict receptor expression. However, even in the absence of effects that restrict receptor expression to particular contexts, hormone responsiveness of a particular tissue or cell type to a particular hormone is not fixed (Figure 1–7). As discussed in a later section on disorders of the endocrine system, alteration of responsiveness to hormones is a major factor in disease. The best-known example is type 2 diabetes mellitus, where insulin resistance plays a prominent role. The factors that regulate overall hormone responsiveness are reviewed in the next sections.

HORMONE RESPONSES CAN BE SELF-LIMITING

Continuous hormone stimulation does not always result in a continuous response. Instead, hormone responses are often self-limiting. Chronic stimulation of cells with peptide hormones can decrease the amounts of receptor that are expressed on the cell surface. Immediate postreceptor signaling events can also exert feedback inhibition of hormone response by decreasing receptor activity. For example, phosphorylation of the β-adrenergic receptor can foster interactions with a protein (arrestin) that locks the receptor in an unresponsive state (Chapter 3). While acute cell surface signaling events are rarely regulated at the transcriptional level, hormone stimulation usually results in induction of genes that mediate the response to the original signal (feed forward) and genes that limit the original signal (feed back). The duration of membrane signaling events can have important functional consequences for cell fate. Acute stimulation of MAP kinase cascades in nerve cells can enhance cellular proliferation, whereas chronic stimulation inhibits cellular proliferation and promotes differentiation.

Nuclear receptor responses can also be self-limiting. Ligands often exert transient effects on gene transcription that peak a few hours after the initial signal and then diminish. In some cases, this may be due to ligand-induced degradation of the receptor. Alternatively, enzymatic activities in the fully assembled nuclear receptor coactivator complex can inhibit the receptor-coactivator interaction.

Finally, far downstream effects of hormone action can feed back and influence the response to the original hormone. One example is the effect of insulin on blood sugar levels, which in turn influence insulin action. Hormone response can also be influenced by counter-regulatory hormones. For example, in stress, the rise in glucocorticoids mitigates the deleterious effects of other hormones (Chapter 9). Occasionally, these effects can feed back to enhance the primary hormone response.

DIFFERENT SIGNALS INFLUENCE HORMONE RESPONSIVENESS

Hormone response networks are subject to multiple regulatory inputs, including endocrine, paracrine, autocrine, and juxtacrine signals; central nervous system inputs; and cell-cell contacts. Different hormones and other signals can interact in different ways (Figure 1–6). In some cases, different hormones bind the same receptor. Thus, insulin and the insulin-like growth factors (IGFs) both bind the IGF receptor, and glucocorticoids and mineralocorticoids bind to each other's receptors. More commonly, different signals interact downstream or upstream of the receptor. In general, these interactions can be classified into four groups:

(1) Cell surface signals stimulate common or interacting second-messenger systems that modulate activi-

Figure 1–7. Regulation of hormone responsiveness by homologous hormone-receptor complexes can occur at multiple loci. Shown are feedback loops that regulate responsiveness through effects on the receptor, effector, or response limbs in any of the elements of the response network. The plus or minus signs indicate that the influences can be stimulatory or inhibitory.

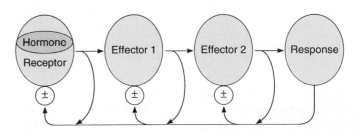

ties of the homologous receptor or other receptors or downstream signal transduction systems or alter expression of genes that encode cell surface receptors or their signal transduction proteins.

(2) Nuclear receptors modulate each others' expression or activities by direct interactions (such as heterodimerization) or by interactions through common cofactors (such as shared coactivators or corepressors). Alternatively, nuclear receptor activities can converge at the level of the same response element, gene, or heterologous transcription factor complexes.

(3) Cell surface receptors activate second-messenger cascades that lead to phosphorylation of the nuclear receptors themselves, their coactivators and corepressors, or transcription factors that cooperate with the nuclear receptors.

(4) Nuclear receptors regulate expression of genes that encode cell surface receptors or components of their downstream signaling pathways.

Together, these schemes for cross-talk allow for wide scope in combinatorial interactions between signaling systems. Combinatorial interactions between signaling systems represents a critical component of endocrine control and can be synergistic, additive, or antagonistic. Figure 1–8 illustrates a hypothetical synergistic hormone response between different receptors. The response to individual hormones is small, but the combination produces a response that is greater than additive. Combinatorial interactions could modulate behavior of an entire response network or particular hormone responses. For example, signal transduction events that lead to phosphorylation of nuclear receptors can potentiate nuclear receptor activity in a wide variety of contexts. However, signal transduction events that lead to

phosphorylation of a transcription factor which cooperates with nuclear receptors might only selectively amplify hormone responses in the context of a limited number of promoters.

■ MODULATION OF HORMONE LEVELS

Hormone response is regulated by hormone concentration. This in turn is governed by hormone production, efficiency of delivery, and metabolism. In many cases, hormones and their actions have short half-lives. Thus, response can be rapidly initiated or terminated by modulating hormone concentration. The following sections review the processes that determine hormone concentration, delivery, and intracellular levels.

HORMONE SYNTHESIS

Details of synthesis of individual hormones are provided in Chapter 2 and in the individual chapters devoted to them. Protein hormone production often does not require special machinery. Thus, growth hormone, prolactin, and PTH are produced similarly to other secreted proteins. However, some peptide hormones (eg, insulin, ACTH, CRH, and glucagon) are produced by cleavage of a larger protein. In these cases, peptide production may be dependent on specific proteases. Other hormones with unique structures are generated by specialized enzymes. Thyroid hormone is produced by iodination and coupling of tyrosine residues contained in a large protein, thyroglobulin, whereas catecholamine production involves modifications of phenylalanine. Steroid hormones are produced from cholesterol in a series of reactions that involve cleavage of the cholesterol side chain residues to yield pregnenolone, followed by a variety of modifications that include hydroxylations, more cleavage reactions, and modification of the ring structures.

REGULATION OF HORMONE PRODUCTION

Hormone production can be regulated at the level of transcription, at the level of posttranscriptional mechanisms that modulate messenger RNA levels or translation efficiency, and at the level of release. Transcriptional regulation can be seen, for example, at polypeptide hormone genes or enzymes involved in steroid synthesis. Control of hormone release can be

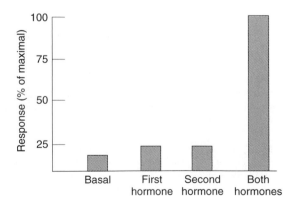

Figure 1–8. Schematic representation of a synergistic hormone response. Note that in this case neither hormone has a major effect alone.

seen in cases in which secretagogues stimulate the release of stored peptide hormones. Finally, hormone production can be augmented by the effects of tropic hormones or growth factors on endocrine cells, which increases the number and size of cells that are actively producing the hormone.

There are a number of patterns of regulation of hormone release (Figure 1-9) . Many hormones are linked to the hypothalamic-pituitary axis (discussed in the section on neuroendocrinology, below). Here, hormones that are produced in the hypothalamus and pituitary (ACTH, TSH, etc) enhance production of hormones in peripheral glands (cortisol, thyroid hormone, etc). Production of hypothalamic and pituitary hormones is subject to negative regulation by peripheral hormones

in classic feedback loops. Other systems are more freestanding. Parathyroid hormone (PTH) increases plasma Ca^{2+} concentration, and this exerts a dominant feedback inhibition on the release of PTH by binding Ca^{2+} sensor receptors in the membrane of PTH-producing cells (Chapter 8). Insulin production leads to decreased glucose levels, and this effect leads to cessation of the stimulus to release more insulin. Hormone release can be triggered by inputs from the nervous system. Hormone production is regulated by all types of regulatory molecules, including tropic hormones and counterregulatory hormones (discussed below), traditional growth factors, eicosanoids, and ions.

HORMONE TRANSPORT IN THE CIRCULATION

Most peptide hormones circulate at low concentrations and are not bound to other proteins. Exceptions include growth hormone, which binds to a protein identical to the hormone-binding portion of the growth hormone receptor; IGF-I and IGF-II, which bind to a variety of IGF-binding proteins (Chapter 6); and vasopressin and oxytocin, which are bound to neurophysins (Chapter 5). By contrast, circulating steroids, thyroid hormones, and vitamin D are bound to plasma proteins (Figure 1–10). The major plasma binding proteins are CBG, which binds cortisol and progesterone (Chapter 9); SHBG, which binds testosterone and estradiol (Chapters 12 and 13); thyroid hormone-binding globulin (TBG) (Chapter 7); and vitamin D-binding protein (Chapter 8). Hormone binding to plasma proteins occurs through noncovalent interactions and increases the half-life of the hormone in the circulation.

The free hormone is that which is not bound by plasma proteins. This fraction is available for receptor binding, dictates feedback inhibition of hormone release, is that which is cleared from the circulation, and correlates best with clinical states of hormone excess and deficiency. Thus, for some clinical tests (discussed later) the best measurement is the free hormone.

Generally, transport proteins bind most soluble circulating hormone, such that the free hormone is a small portion of the total. In general, the binding capacity of transport proteins barely exceeds the normal concentrations of the hormone in plasma. Thus, modest decreases in transport protein levels or modest elevations of hormone concentrations can lead to large increases in free active hormone. Thus, whereas the presence of low or high levels of hormone transport proteins generally does not itself lead to clinical abnormalities, these changes can influence interpretation of laboratory tests. One likely role of transport proteins is to facilitate even delivery of hormones across target tissues (Figure

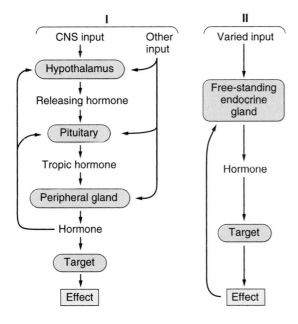

Figure 1–9. The two major types of control of endocrine gland function. **I:** The hypothalamic-pituitary-target gland systems involve central nervous system regulation of releasing hormones from the hypothalamus that stimulate the pituitary to release tropic hormones which act on peripheral glands to release hormones. These hormones can be regulated by other factors. The hormones from the peripheral glands exert feedback control on the hypothalamus and pituitary. **II:** Free-standing endocrine glands (eg, parathyroid and islet cells) release hormones that stimulate a target tissue to produce an effect (eg, a rise in serum calcium or a fall in blood sugar) which in turn modifies the function of the gland.

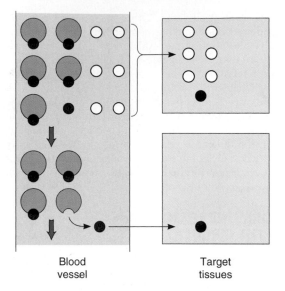

Figure 1–10. Role of plasma binding in delivery of hormones to peripheral tissues. Shown are examples with a hormone that is bound (solid circles) to a plasma protein (large circles) and a hormone that is not bound (open circles). With the bound hormone, only the free fraction is available for tissue uptake. As the free fraction is taken up, additional hormone dissociates from the plasma-binding protein as the blood moves to more distal portions of the tissue and becomes available for tissue uptake. In contrast, all of the hormone that does not bind to plasma proteins is available for uptake by the proximal part of the tissue.

1–10). Thus, a free hormone might be completely sequestered in the proximal portions of the liver as the blood flows through the tissue. By contrast, if the hormone were bound to transport proteins, free hormone would be sequestered in proximal portions of the liver, and additional hormone would be released from the bound fraction as the blood moves distally, making the hormone available for these regions. Differences in the uniformity of hormone delivery probably explain why deletion of the plasma vitamin D-binding protein affects vitamin D action.

TRANSPORT OF HORMONES ACROSS THE MEMBRANE

Nuclear receptor ligands are hydrophobic and are often presumed to enter and exit the cells by traversing the lipid bilayer. However, in some cases influx and efflux varies in different tissues and cell types, as has been demonstrated for thyroid hormones, pointing toward active import and export mechanisms. Specific differences in transport in target cells may regulate hormone concentration and action.

METABOLISM & ELIMINATION OF HORMONES

Metabolism can degrade the hormones and hormone precursors to inactive forms or lead to the generation of more active products (Figure 1–11). These processes affect the plasma levels of the hormone and can have regulatory roles.

Peptide Hormones

Peptide hormones have short half-lives in the circulation (a few minutes), as seen with ACTH, insulin, glucagon, PTH, and the releasing hormones. The glycosylated glycoprotein hormones are more stable; CG has a half-life of several hours. The major mechanism for hormone degradation is through binding to cell surface receptors and nonreceptor hormone-binding sites, with subsequent uptake (internalization) and degradation. An important source for these enzymes is the lysosome, which fuses with endocytotic vesicles to expose its enzymes and its acid environment to the internalized hormone-receptor complex.

Steroid & Thyroid Hormones & Vitamin D

The hydrophobic steroid hormones and the D vitamins are filtered and reabsorbed by the kidney. For instance, 1% of the cortisol that is produced daily appears in the urine (Chapter 9). These compounds are ordinarily metabolized to water-soluble, inactive forms that are more effectively eliminated. Metabolic inactivation generally involves reduction and conjugation to glucuronide and sulfate groups.

Intracellular degradation of ligands provides a means both for eliminating the hormones and for exerting tissue-selective control of hormone levels. For example, cortisol would completely occupy the mineralocorticoid receptor in the kidney if it were not inactivated by 11β-hydroxysteroid dehydrogenase. This process allows aldosterone, which is not affected by the enzyme, to act as the major mineralocorticoid in this tissue. Thyroid hormones are degraded to inactive forms by at least three different deiodinases whose levels vary in different tissues (see Chapter 7). Deaminations and decarboxylations of the alanine side chains as well as conjugations with glucuronic acid and sulfate groups are also involved in degrading thyroid hormones.

Metabolism of prohormones to active forms also plays an important role. Testosterone is reduced to dihydrotestosterone in target tissues. 3,5,3′,5′-Tetraiodo-L-thyronine (thyroxine; T_4) is the major form of thy-

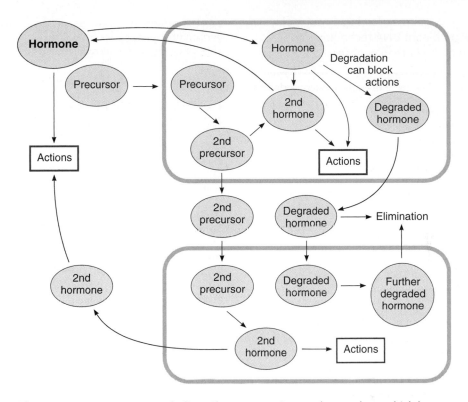

Figure 1–11. Hormone metabolism. Shown are various pathways along which hormones are metabolized and the effects on those pathways with production of additional precursors; with production of more active hormones for local or systemic actions; with selective degradation of hormones to prevent local actions; and with degradation to inactive forms that are eliminated.

roid hormone released from the gland, but T_4 becomes deiodinated to the more active 3,5,3'-triiodo-L-thyronine (triiodothyronine; T_3) in peripheral tissues. The major active form of vitamin D is generated by sequential hydroxylation reactions that occur in the liver and kidney.

Finally, hormones can be produced locally in target tissues. Thus, testosterone can be produced from androstenedione and dehydroepiandrosterone, and estradiol can be produced from testosterone. These mechanisms can provide for high local concentrations of hormones, thereby providing additional control of the hormone response.

Catecholamines & Eicosanoids

Metabolism of catecholamines is discussed in Chapter 11. These compounds have a very short half-life of about 2 minutes. Catecholamines are degraded by two principal routes: catechol-*O*-methyltransferase (COMT) and monoamine oxidase (MAO). Measurement of some of the metabolites—normetanephrine, metanephrine, and vanillylmandelic acid (VMA)—can be useful in evaluating possible catecholamine overproduction. Prostaglandins are also rapidly metabolized—within seconds—by widely distributed enzymes, particularly through oxidation of the 15-hydroxyl group that renders the prostaglandin molecule inactive.

■ RECOMBINANT DNA, GENOMICS, PROTEOMICS, & ENDOCRINOLOGY

The cloning of endocrine system genes has had an enormous impact on endocrinology. This impact will increase with the information provided from sequencing of the human genome. Some contributions of recombinant DNA technology are listed in Table 1–1.

Table 1-1. Impact on endocrinology of molecular biology, recombinant DNA technology, and sequencing of the human genome.

Information about all aspects of endocrinology, including:
  Production and regulation of hormones
  Mechanisms of hormone action
  Actions of hormones
  Mechanisms of disease
  Novel gene products
Diagnosis of endocrine diseases:
  Information gained from studies using the technology
  Reagents from recombinant products (eg, polypeptide hormones)
  DNA analysis, including sequences
Treatment of endocrine diseases:
  Information gained from studies using the technology
  Production of hormones and hormone analogs used for therapy (growth hormone, insulin, growth factors, etc)
  Materials for determination of three-dimensional structures of drug targets (eg, renin, growth hormone receptor, nuclear receptors, polypeptides, signaling molecules such as Ras)
  Technology for gene therapy

Recombinant DNA makes possible the production of therapeutic agents such as GH and insulin and of diagnostic materials such as polypeptide hormones. More importantly, it has provided information about the function of the endocrine system in health and disease. Elucidation of mechanisms that regulate gene expression has provided insights into mechanisms of hormone action (see Chapter 3) and regulation of the entire system, as detailed in subsequent chapters of this book.

Recent research has emphasized larger-scale approaches to understanding of basic biological phenomena. These are loosely termed genomics and proteomics for their emphasis upon the genome and its expression pattern (genomics) and protein expression and function (proteomics), respectively. These approaches capture larger overall pictures of the behavior of cellular signaling pathways rather than focusing on particular genes or proteins.

SEQUENCING OF THE HUMAN GENOME

Completion of the human genome sequence will have an enormous impact on endocrinology. It is now clear that there are about 30,000 genes in humans and that further diversity is generated by alternative RNA processing or alternative promoter usage. The data tell us conclusively, for example, that there are 48 nuclear receptors in humans (discussed earlier) as opposed to previous estimates, which ranged up to 600. Readily available sequence data facilitate studies of gene regulation or of sequences that become altered in disease. Comparison of sequence data from different species will provide clues about altered regulation of endocrine signaling pathways in evolution.

GENOMICS & PATTERNS OF TRANSCRIPTION

In addition to understanding the structure of the genome, genomics can be applied to larger-scale understanding of genome transcription. Most studies use so-called microarray technologies in which small glass or silicon slides are imprinted with cDNAs or oligonucleotides corresponding to a few selected (less than 100) or many (over 20,000) genes. The microarrays are probed with labeled cDNA corresponding to RNA from a given cell line or tissue by conventional DNA hybridization approaches. The information can be used to identify individual genes—or gene families—that may be essential for particular endocrine responses and will help elucidate the functional linkages between different genes that might identify new targets for drug discovery. The technology can also be used to understand the way a particular signal influences the overall patterns of expression of related clusters of genes (cell cycle, metabolic pathways, stress response, etc), which can be of great predictive value. For example, malignancy and hormone responsiveness of breast tumors can be typed according to the overall expression profile of their genes. Coexpression of ER and the cell surface receptor HER2/neu, coupled with amplification of the gene for the coactivator protein AIB1, is predictive of tamoxifen resistance in breast tumors. Other patterns of gene expression in breast tumors may suggest whether more or less aggressive therapies are appropriate. It is likely that analysis of transcription patterns in different tumors will become part of standard clinical diagnosis for tumor biopsies in the future and dictate treatment strategies.

PROTEOMICS

Ultimately, understanding of biologic responses will require a complete understanding of patterns of protein expression, their interconnections, and their activity. To some extent, protein expression patterns can be inferred from the pattern of transcription. However, gene expression studies do not assess the role of factors that govern translation rates or protein stability. Moreover, gene expression studies do not elucidate the functional connections between proteins or alterations in protein activity (which can be influenced by subcellular localization, secondary modifications, etc). For example, regulation of enzymatic activity, protein localization, and stabilization are particularly important in rapid response to peptide hormone signals.

Proteomics covers large-scale approaches that capture the expression patterns and activity states of proteins in a given context. Large-scale yeast two hybrid assays can be used to obtain descriptions of potential protein-protein interactions between many different gene products. Large scale mass spectroscopy of cellular protein preparations can identify the proteins that are expressed in a given context. When this technique is coupled with fractionation of proteins in subcellular compartments—or fractionation according to the biochemical properties of proteins or their particular protein-protein interactions—it is possible to begin to gain insight into the ways in which protein expression and activity bring about changes in endocrine signaling pathways. For example, it may be possible to observe accumulation, down-regulation, or nuclear translocation of subsets of proteins in response to a particular signal. Targeted analysis of proteins in signaling pathways (eg, banks of phosphoprotein-specific antibodies for molecules participating in the insulin or ERK signaling pathways) can also be applied to detect the alterations in activity of subsets of response pathways in given contexts. Like functional genomics, the results of these approaches can identify individual proteins that may be important for a particular endocrine signal or may give an overall picture of the pattern of protein activity alteration in a given endocrine signal.

MOLECULAR BASIS OF GENETIC ENDOCRINE DISEASE

Many endocrine diseases have a strong genetic component. This applies to rare inherited syndromes that are often the result of a single monogenic mutation, such as defects in steroid biosynthesis (Chapters 9, 12, 13, 14, and 15); and mutations in hormone genes, such as GH (Chapter 6). Analysis of inherited monogenic diseases has been greatly facilitated by linkage maps of every human chromosome and by human DNA sequence data, which helps track a particular disease-causing allele through affected families. More common diseases also have genetic components, usually thought to result from the interplay of common variant proteins (polygenic disease). This applies to hypertension (Chapter 10) and type 2 diabetes mellitus (Chapter 17). The genetic basis of polygenic diseases is often less clear than that of monogenic diseases. This is because particular genetic variants may be associated with—but neither necessary nor sufficient for—a disease state. Accordingly, large studies of affected populations are required to achieve sufficient statistical power to elucidate the contributions of individual genes. Future linkage studies of polygenic diseases may be facilitated in two ways:

first, by the realization that much human genetic variation is actually relatively common; and second, by our understanding that long stretches of human DNA exist in so-called haplotype blocks. These long stretches of chromosomal DNA are areas in which very little recombination occurs. Relatively few common haplotypes may exist within each block, and understanding how haplotype blocks are inherited within populations may help to highlight the areas of the genome that contribute to the risk of particular diseases.

The mechanisms underlying genetic disease are discussed in the chapters that follow. Components of the endocrine system can be affected by a wide range of genetic defects. Single nucleotide substitutions alter the coding sequence or create a translational frame shift or premature stop codon. Examples can be seen with loss of mutated polypeptide hormones such as insulin or growth hormone; transcription factors such as Pit-1, which regulates GH expression; or hormone receptors, as in the testicular feminization syndrome (Chapter 14). Point mutations can also lead to gain of function; a point mutation in the mineralocorticoid receptor increases its binding to progesterone and leads to a rare syndrome of pregnancy-associated hypertension. Simple mutations can also affect noncoding sequences that play a role in gene regulation. Larger deletions of all or parts of genes usually result in a complete loss of function, as with deletions of polypeptide genes such as growth hormone (Chapter 6), hormone receptors, or enzymes involved in hormone synthesis. The latter can be observed in congenital adrenal hyperplasia (Chapters 9, 13, 14, and 15). Amplifications of genes, particularly in cancer, can lead to increased gene activity. There can also be insertions or rearrangements between genes. The latter may lead to profound alterations in cell function. For example, rearrangement of growth factor genes can place them under control of a different gene promoter in some malignancies (Chapter 21). It is also observed in a form of glucocorticoid-remediable hypertension where the enzyme that promotes production of aldosterone is placed under the regulatory control of another gene that is regulated by ACTH (Chapter 10).

■ EVOLUTION OF THE ENDOCRINE SYSTEM

Consideration of the evolution of the endocrine system can help us understand endocrine signaling. Any account of the evolution of the endocrine system must explain the origin of signaling molecules, how the signal came to convey specific information, and how signal transduction proteins arose. At a more complex level, we must explain diversity of signaling pathways, development of endocrine organs, and complex regulatory networks. Speculations about the evolution of endocrine signals are outlined in the following sections. A schematic representation of events in evolution of the endocrine system is provided in Figure 1–12.

THE ORIGINS OF REGULATORY CHEMICALS & THE METABOLIC CODE

The interaction of hormones with cellular receptors leads to intracellular communication events such as generation of cAMP, phosphorylation, and effects on gene expression or ion transport. In higher organisms, the responses are governed by endocrine, paracrine, juxtacrine, or autocrine signals, whereas similar responses are governed by extracellular signals in bacteria. The common thread is that the cell perceives extracellular signals and utilizes intracellular control networks to respond to the signal. It is likely that the endocrine system had its origins in these types of bacterial signaling systems.

Bacterial regulatory chemicals are typically modified analogs of essential molecules, as noted by Tomkins over 25 years ago in an article entitled "The Metabolic Code." Tomkins suggested that it would have been impossible for essential molecules to acquire signaling properties in the course of evolution. Thus, ATP func-

tions as an essential mediator of energy balance and would have been unlikely to acquire signaling properties because large variations in ATP concentration would adversely affect cellular function. However, by-products of ATP metabolism could acquire signaling functions. For example, cAMP or related molecules may have been originally generated as by-products of ATP metabolism, such as "idling" of ATP hydrolysis to ADP. Thus, cAMP generation could act as a signal for the idling reaction—and, in turn, for the cellular condition that leads to the idling reaction.

Proteins transduce regulatory signals and must recognize the signaling molecule and initiate appropriate biologic responses. How could such a multifunctional protein evolve? Proteins consist of a limited number of discrete folded structures or domains, and recombination events can splice diverse domains together and create new functional units. In this regard, the response limb for cAMP in bacteria is a transcription factor whose activity is affected by cAMP binding. This could have arisen, for example, by combining a cAMP-binding protein with a DNA-binding protein. If the new hybrid protein could regulate gene expression—even relatively nonspecifically—then a novel regulatory circuit would have arisen, and if resultant changes in gene expression were favorable to cell survival under the original conditions that led to cAMP generation, then the novel regulatory circuit would become fixed in evolution.

Once molecules like cAMP acquire the capacity to function as a signaling molecule, mechanisms would evolve to generate cAMP more efficiently and ultimately, cAMP could acquire the capacity to become produced and regulated independently of ATP production or hydrolysis, thereby giving the organism flexibility to use the same regulatory system in metabolic control. Indeed, Tomkins referred to cAMP as a "symbol" that is produced in response to a "signal"—glucose deprivation—by bacteria. The symbol cAMP in turn induces enzymes that metabolize alternative substrates such as lactose to overcome the deficiency of glucose.

EVOLUTION OF HORMONES & RECEPTORS

Many hormones are by-products of metabolic reactions that acquired the capacity to symbolize metabolic states of the cell, as described above for cAMP. Thus, peptides are specific breakdown products of larger proteins; steroids are derived from cholesterol and catecholamines; and thyroid hormones are derived from amino acids. Other nuclear receptor ligands are by-products of bile acids and fatty acids. The regulatory roles of these by-products suggest that nuclear receptors

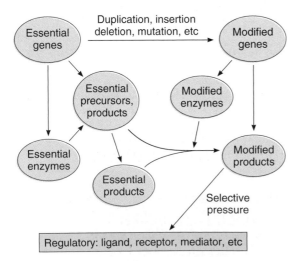

Figure 1–12. Steps in the evolution of the endocrine system, with duplications and mutations of genes that encode essential enzymes and other products that result in new genes that encode products involved in endocrine control.

may have first evolved as nutritional sensors and provides support for the generality of the metabolic code.

Primitive endocrine signaling probably arose in early multicellular organisms, where one cell would sense changes in the environment and release signaling molecules, where they would elicit responses in neighboring cells (ie, paracrine signaling). Eventually, this type of signal would permit specialization of cell types that produce the signal or respond to the signal with an appropriate biologic response that would ensure the survival of both cells. Once the primordial hormones—the precursors to today's hormones—were generated, modifications could create additional properties such as specific mechanisms to regulate production, secretion pathways, increased specificity for receptor binding, bioavailability (including binding to transport proteins), and degradation and clearance.

Hormone receptors probably arose by recombining essential functional proteins, as described above for cAMP signaling. In this regard, it is noteworthy that both cell surface and nuclear receptors are composed of discrete functional domains that could have been linked by gene recombination events and acquired novel emergent properties.

EVOLUTION OF MULTIPLE HORMONE RESPONSE SYSTEMS

Once a prototypical hormone response system is in place, it can be expanded to interpret related signals. The genetic events that lead to expansion of signaling capacity would probably resemble those described in the section on genetic disease, ie, gene duplications, rearrangements, recombinations, and specific mutations. The duplications would create related gene families, and subsequent mutational and other events would generate diversity. Novel patterns of gene expression could be created by alteration of the promoter regions of genes, thereby permitting further generation of specialized functions. The peptide hormone genes for GH, PRL, and placental lactogen (chorionic somatomammotropin; CS) genes comprise one family that arose from gene duplication. The glycoprotein hormones share the same α subunit and have different β subunits (albeit with significant homology). An example of a family of genes involved in hormone synthesis are some of those encoding proteins involved in steroid hormone biosynthesis. Examples of receptor families are the seven-transmembrane receptors and nuclear receptors. Indeed, x-ray crystal studies of nuclear receptor family ligand-binding domains reveal that each possesses a similar fold despite wide variations in primary sequence. This suggests that the basic function of the pri-

mordial ligand-binding domain has been preserved despite sequence alterations that generate new ligand specificities.

EVOLUTION OF ENDOCRINE GLANDS

Endocrine glands must have evolved from the specialization that resulted in organ systems with a need to carry fluids between them. By default, the primitive cell that released a substance acting in a paracrine way became an endocrine cell. This provided a means for delivery of substances more generally than with the nervous systems, which developed axons to deliver a paracrine signal.

INTEGRATIVE NETWORKS

Hormones do not usually regulate a single function and instead elicit coordinated responses in a range of cell types. Furthermore, different hormones play complementary or counterbalancing roles. How might these complex circuits evolve? Once a hormone regulates a given response—eg, glucose metabolism—there would be selective advantages in acquiring the capacity to regulate complementary regulatory processes. Thus, glucocorticoids regulate glucose metabolism and increase glucose production and glycogen storage in response to an "anxiety" stimulus in preparation for starvation, but they have also incorporated complementary actions on lipid and amino acid metabolism. Such networks, once established, would be relatively stable but could become modified and expanded. Hormones with counterbalancing actions could then develop in an analogous fashion.

■ ENDOCRINE & NERVOUS SYSTEM RELATIONSHIPS: NEUROENDOCRINOLOGY

Neuroendocrinology is the subject area that deals with interactions between the nervous and endocrine systems. The actions of both systems and their interactions underlie practically every regulatory mechanism in the body. There are two major mechanisms of neural regulation of endocrine function. The first, neurosecretion, refers to neurons that secrete hormones into the circulation. The hypothalamus contains neurons that secrete hormones into the general circulation or to blood vessels that communicate with the anterior pituitary. This mechanism is discussed in the sections that follow. The second is direct autonomic innervation of endocrine tissues, which couples central nervous system signals to hormone release. Examples of this relationship include innervation of the adrenal medulla, kidney, parathyroid gland, and pancreatic islets and are described in chapters on these organs (see Chapters 8, 10, 11, and 17).

Hormones also affect the nervous system, as described in the section on effects of hormones, below.

Hypothalamic-Pituitary Relationships

The primary neuroendocrine interface is at the hypothalamus and pituitary, which form a unit that controls several peripheral endocrine glands and other physiologic activities (Chapter 5). The hypothalamus contains several nuclei of neuronal cells. It communicates with other brain regions and regulates many brain functions, including temperature, appetite, thirst, sexual behavior, defensive reactions such as rage and fear, and body rhythms. However, the hypothalamus is also an endocrine organ that releases hormones. The ventral hypothalamus supplies axons and nerve endings to form the posterior pituitary. Neurohypophysial neurons in the posterior pituitary release vasopressin (ADH) and oxytocin into the general circulation. Hypophysiotropic neurons of the hypothalamus release hormones into the hypothalamic-pituitary blood vessels, which deliver hormones to the anterior pituitary—a major endocrine organ.

Hypothalamic Hormones

The hypophysiotropic neurons of the hypothalamus produce hormones that are secreted into blood vessels which serve the anterior pituitary and regulate hormone release. Stimulating hormones (releasing hormones) include TRH, GnRH, CRH, GHRH, prolactin-releasing factor, and ADH. Inhibitory hormones include somatostatin and dopamine. Some releasing hormones can regulate multiple hormones. For example, TRH stimulates both TSH and prolactin release. In contrast, more than one releasing hormone can affect a single pituitary hormone. ACTH release is stimulated both by CRH and by ADH.

In addition to specialized hormones, the hypothalamus produces neurotransmitters, including bioactive amines, peptides, and amino acids. The bioactive amines include dopamine, norepinephrine, epinephrine, serotonin, acetylcholine, GABA, and histamine. The neuropeptides include VIP, substance P, neurotensin, components of the renin-angiotensin system, cholecystokinin (CCK), opioid peptides, ANP and related peptides, galanin, endothelin, and neuropeptide Y. The amino acids include glutamate and glycine. Some of these neurotransmitters affect the anterior pituitary. As mentioned above, dopamine regulates prolactin release and has complex influences on somatostatin release (see Chapter 5 and below). VIP stimulates the release of several pituitary hormones, including prolactin, growth hormone, and ACTH. Substance P stimulates prolactin and inhibits CRH-stimulated ACTH release. Neurotensin can affect growth hormone and prolactin release. Little is known about the effects of amino acids on endocrine function.

Regulation of Anterior Pituitary Hormone Release

The anterior pituitary produces endocrine hormones (Chapter 5). It has little innervation, and anterior pituitary hormone release is usually regulated by vascular delivery of hypothalamic and peripheral hormones. There are three main patterns of anterior pituitary hormone release (Figure 1–9).

(1) Spontaneous brain rhythms promote pulsatile hypothalamic and pituitary hormone release, as illustrated by the patterns of luteinizing hormone (LH) and follicle-stimulating hormone (FSH) release under control of GnRH from the hypothalamus. The amplitude and frequency of the pulses are governed by inputs from the central nervous system and intrinsic properties of the cells. Pulses of LH release can be as frequent as every hour during the follicular phase of the menstrual cycle. Release of other pituitary hormones mostly conforms to circadian rhythms (approximately 24-hour periodicity), which are influenced by the sleep-wake cycle.

(2) Peripheral hormones regulate pituitary hormone release through feedback loops. Thus, cortisol, thyroid hormone, and estrogens inhibit release of their tropic hormones—ACTH, TSH, and LH, respectively. Occasionally, target gland hormones exert positive feedback. Contrary to its usual fast-acting negative effect on LH production, estradiol also initiates a preovulatory surge in LH secretion that requires 48–72 hours of sustained estrogen stimulation. Feedback influences can be directed at the pituitary, the hypothalamus, or—and typically—at both.

(3) Intervening factors such as stress, nutritional influences, illnesses, and other hormones affect hormone release. Thus, stress increases the release of ACTH, growth hormone, and prolactin; and systemic illness can suppress the hypothalamic-pituitary-thyroid axis and the release of gonadotropins. Immunomodulators such as interleukin-1 and interleukin-2 and epinephrine increase CRH and ACTH release; and angiotensin II, interleukin-2, cholecystokinin, and oxytocin can stimulate ACTH release.

The regulation of PRL and GH is different from that of other anterior pituitary hormones. GH and PRL are not subject to the same degree of classic feedback regulatory mechanisms as with some other hormones, although IGF-I, which is produced in response to GH, can feed back to inhibit GH release. Specific releasing hormones (prolactin-releasing factor and GHRH, respectively) and inhibitory hormones (dopamine and somatostatin, respectively) regulate PRL and GH production. The inhibitory hormone is more important for PRL release, whereas the stimulatory hormone is dominant for GH release (Chapter 5).

ENDOCRINE ORGANS & HORMONE PRODUCTION

Individual endocrine organs are described in detail in individual chapters. This section summarizes principles of regulation of these endocrine organs and their signaling responses. The tropic anterior pituitary hormones play an essential role in regulation of hormone production by classic endocrine organs. Thus, hormones like ACTH, FSH, LH, and TSH stimulate hormone release in cognate target glands (adrenals, gonads, and thyroid gland), and their release is regulated by feedback loops as described above. The gonads also produce other hormones—inhibin, follistatin, and activin—that regulate tropic hormone release. These regulatory networks tend to control hormone levels within a narrow range, referred to as the set point. (See the chapters on the various glands or systems.)

There are other modes of regulation of hormone release. Hormone production can be regulated through innervation of the endocrine organ. For example, stress-related catecholamine release by the adrenal medulla is regulated by autonomic innervation. Another specialized case is the pineal gland, which lies at the base of the brain and provides an interface free of the blood-brain barrier between the brain, the cerebral circulation, and the cerebrospinal fluid—and, as such, may be described as part of the neuroendocrine system. The gland receives photosensory information through sympathetic innervation that influences production of melatonin, derived from serotonin, which regulates circadian rhythms and can have antireproductive functions, block GnRH-induced LH release, and have other effects on hormone release. Finally, hormone release can be regulated more directly by environmental signals or nutrient levels. Thus, insulin production is intimately linked to blood glucose levels.

It is also becoming clear that many tissues and organs which are not traditionally considered to be endocrine organs do produce endocrine signals. The kidney is the origin of hormones comprising the renin-angiotensin-aldosterone system. Adipose tissue produces leptin, an important mediator of body weight; and resistin, a peptide that may be involved in the pathology of type 2 diabetes. The heart produces natriuretic peptides. It is likely that many more organs will prove to produce endocrine signals.

ACTIONS OF HORMONES

Hormones have widespread effects that are described in subsequent chapters. Some general patterns are summarized in this section.

HORMONE RELEASE

Hormones regulate their own production and release and also that of other hormones. These aspects are described in earlier sections on mechanisms of hormone action, synthesis of hormones, and neuroendocrinology.

FETAL DEVELOPMENT

Hormones exert widespread influences on development. Cretinism resulting from severe hypothyroidism (Chapter 7), dwarfism resulting from growth hormone deficiency (Chapter 6), and inability to develop and survive with a steroid hormone synthesis defect (Chapter 9) illustrate the profound effects of different classes of hormones on development. Hormones influence sexual development, as illustrated by the failure of male sexual development in the androgen-deficient state (Chapter 14).

CELL GROWTH & CANCER

Hormones are important for cell growth. Peptide hormones such as growth hormone, IGF-I, and IGF-II stimulate linear growth and cellular proliferation in other tissues (Chapter 6). Other peptides such as fibroblast growth factor (FGF), platelet-derived growth factor (PDGF), and transforming growth factors α and β (TGFα and TGFβ) are growth factors both in multiple tissues and in endocrine glands. Tropic factors regulate growth of target endocrine glands—eg, ACTH and angiotensin II on the adrenal gland (Chapter 9), TSH on the thyroid gland (Chapter 7), and LH and FSH on the ovary (Chapter 13) and testis (Chapter 12). Thyroid hormones stimulate growth of several tissues (Chapter 7). Steroid hormones can both inhibit and stimulate cell growth. Glucocorticoids inhibit the growth of several cell types and kill some lymphocyte cell types, whereas estradiol and testosterone and dihydrotestosterone stimulate growth of breast and prostate, respectively.

Hormones also influence cancer. Often the hormone influences the growth of the cancer cell in the same way that it influences the growth of the normal progenitor cell. However, deranged hormone signaling pathways can also cause cancer. Many oncogenes are analogs of growth factors or growth factor receptors, as described above in the section on hormones and oncogenes.

HORMONAL EFFECTS ON INTERMEDIARY METABOLISM

Hormones regulate the metabolism of all major classes of macromolecules. Carbohydrate, fat, protein, amino acid, and nucleic acid metabolism are tightly regulated by insulin, glucagon, somatostatin, growth hormone, catecholamines (epinephrine, norepinephrine), thyroid hormones, glucocorticoids, and other hormones. These interactions are coordinated for finely tuned regulation of intermediary metabolism and numerous conditions such as stress or starvation. Insulin is dominant in lowering blood glucose and in stimulating metabolism of glucose and synthesis of fat, proteins, and nucleic acids. By contrast, cortisol, glucagon, catecholamines, and growth hormone elevate blood glucose by diverse mechanisms. However, these hormones differ in their effects on protein, fat, and nucleic acid metabolism. Hormones affect the uptake of glucose, amino acids, nucleosides, and other small molecules. For example, insulin increases glucose uptake by promoting redistribution of glucose transporters to the plasma membrane. Hormones also affect enzymes involved in metabolism, including, among others, those involved in gluconeogenesis, lipolysis, glycogen synthesis, amino acid metabolism and synthesis, and lipid synthesis.

HORMONAL EFFECTS ON MINERAL & WATER METABOLISM

Hormones affect most aspects of mineral metabolism. Vasopressin regulates serum osmolality and water excretion (Chapter 5) and has numerous effects in the cardiovascular and central nervous systems. The mineralocorticoid aldosterone regulates serum sodium and potassium and to some extent chloride and bicarbonate ion concentrations and balance (Chapter 10). Other hormones, including ANP, insulin, glucagon, catecholamines, angiotensin II, and PTH, also regulate ionic balance.

HORMONAL EFFECTS ON CARDIOVASCULAR & RENAL FUNCTION

The renin-angiotensin system, atrial natriuretic peptide, endothelins, catecholamines, steroid hormones, thyroid hormone, prostaglandins, kinins, vasopressin, cytokines, nitric oxide, substance P, and calcitonin generelated hormone and urotensin II can profoundly affect these systems. All of these substances can affect heart rate or contractility and constrictor and dilator mechanisms of arteries and veins (see Chapter 10). The growth factor properties of hormones influence cardiovascular development and muscular hyperplasia and hypertrophy and are involved in pathologic processes leading to hypertensive vascular changes, atherosclerosis, heart failure, and cardiac hypertrophy (see Chapter 10). Hormones influence renal function and blood pressure by regulating renal blood flow, glomerular filtration rate, and the transport of ions, water, and other chemicals. Hormones also regulate active and passive transport processes in kidney through activation, redistribution, and stimulation of the synthesis of channels or by generating energy for active transport. Hormones can have effects on lipoprotein metabolism and on cholesterol transport, and this is particularly true for hormone-bound thyroid receptors, peroxisomal proliferator-activated receptors (PPARs), and LXR nuclear receptors. Drugs that block these steps, such as converting enzyme inhibitors, β-adrenergic blockers, and mineralocorticoid hormone antagonists, are used extensively in therapy (Table 1–2).

Table 1–2. Examples of hormone antagonists used in therapy.

Antagonist to–	Use
Progesterone	Contraceptive, abortifacient
Glucocorticoid	Spontaneous Cushing's syndrome
Mineralocorticoid	Primary and secondary mineralocorticoid excess, hypertension, heart failure
Androgen	Prostate cancer
Estrogen	Breast cancer
GnRH	Prostate cancer
β-Adrenergic receptor	Hypertension, hyperthyroidism
Prostaglandin	Acute and chronic inflammatory disease
Angiotensin II	Hypertension, heart failure

HORMONAL EFFECTS ON SKELETAL FUNCTION

Bone is constantly being deposited and resorbed. This process is under complex hormonal control (Chapter 8). Hormones (eg, IGF-I) control growth and mineralization through influences on both the matrix and mineral phase of bone. Cytokines—particularly tumor necrosis factor (TNF)—play a major role in bone remodeling. Osteoprotegerin, a soluble TNF receptor family member, blocks actions of TNF-related proteins in bone cells and thus serves a protective role in preventing the onset of osteoporosis. Examples of other influences on bone remodeling include the effects of PTH and vitamin D on calcium metabolism and of steroids and thyroid hormone on bone matrix. Estrogens promote accrual of bone matrix and prevent the development of osteoporosis while glucocorticoids and thyroid hormone have the opposite effect.

HORMONAL EFFECTS ON REPRODUCTIVE FUNCTION

Gonadotropins regulate ovarian and testicular function and the secretion of hormones from these organs. Testosterone and dihydrotestosterone regulate the development of male sexual characteristics such as penile, muscle, and prostate growth and deepening of the voice and also affect libido and sexual behavior (Chapters 12 and 14). Female sex steroids regulate functions of female reproductive organs, including the menstrual cycle and ovulation (Chapter 13). Leptin, secreted from adipose tissue, promotes maturation of the reproductive tract and may trigger the onset of puberty.

Pregnancy is regulated, in part, by hormones (Chapter 16). Progesterone is essential for establishing and maintaining pregnancy in humans. It also decreases myometrial sensitivity to oxytocin, leading to suppression of uterine contractile function. Hormones are critical for egg and sperm development, preparation of the uterus for conception and implantation, and development of the fetus. The placenta itself produces a number of hormones, some of which are mostly unique (chorionic somatomammotropin, placental lactogen; CS) and others that are also produced abundantly by other endocrine glands (progesterone and other steroid hormones; Chapters 13 and 16).

HORMONAL EFFECTS ON THE IMMUNE SYSTEM

Endocrine hormones influence the immune system. Glucocorticoids blunt immunologic and inflammatory responses; these actions form the basis for the use of glucocorticoids in therapy to suppress these responses when they are excessive. Sex steroids usually suppress the immune response. Thus, castration results in enlargement of lymph nodes and spleen, more severe graft-versus-host disease, increased skin graft rejection, and stimulation of T lymphocyte mitogen responsiveness in vitro. These effects target mainly cellular immune responses. However, estrogens may stimulate antibody production, and females tend to have higher levels of the major immunoglobulin classes under both basal and stimulated conditions. Females tend to have a higher incidence of autoimmune diseases than males and more active cellular and humoral immune responses. These differences are not observed before puberty. Thyroid hormone, GH, catecholamines, PRL, and other hormones influence immunologic or inflammatory functions, but their roles are still being defined.

Pregnancy, with its associated hormonal changes, can ameliorate autoimmune diseases through unknown mechanisms. Pregnancy tends to suppress the cellular but not the humoral immune responses. This may be critical to prevent maternal rejection of fetal tissues, though susceptibility to a number of viral and fungal diseases is increased. Immunosuppression is most pronounced in the second and third trimesters and rebounds by about 3–6 months postpartum.

HORMONAL EFFECTS ON THE CENTRAL NERVOUS SYSTEM

The endocrine and nervous systems interact in multiple ways (see Chapter 5). Hormones regulate behavioral and cognitive functions such as mood, appetite, learning, memory, and sexual activity. Hormones such as leptin, which controls satiety, have been identified, and new roles for "old" hormones are continuously being identified. Vasopressin increases affiliative behavior in monogamous voles that express brain V1a receptors, whereas low V1a expression correlates with a lack of response to vasopressin and promiscuous behavior.

Hormones also have secondary influences on the central nervous system through effects on general metabolism. There are a number of examples of mental abnormalities associated with hormone excess or deficiency. These include: depressed mental status that can progress to coma with severe hypothyroidism (Chapter 7); psychosis that can occur with glucocorticoid excess; and coma that can occur with hypoglycemia due to insulin excess (Chapter 18). Thus, hormones, neurotransmitters, and the central nervous system interact extensively, producing results that may shape not only development and physiology but also behavior and cognition.

■ SELECTIVE MODULATION

Beneficial effects of hormones are counterbalanced by deleterious effects. Thus, although glucocorticoids suppress excessive inflammatory and immunologic responses, they also cause osteoporosis, physical disfigurement, and other problems. Estrogens reduce bone loss but can increase the risk for breast and uterine cancer. Thyroid hormones might be used to treat obesity if it were not for the fact that these hormones can have deleterious effects on the heart. These considerations point to a need for improved therapies for these classes of actions. A major goal, therefore, is to achieve selective modulation of receptor action—that is, to simultaneously promote desirable effects and inhibit undesirable ones.

Some of the principles outlined in the previous sections on receptor activity and regulation of hormone levels point to several different ways to obtain selective modulation. As described above, some receptor ligands can behave as partial agonists, mixed agonists-antagonists, or inverse agonists. It may be possible to capitalize on these properties. Tamoxifen and raloxifene show estrogen-like effects on bone but inhibit estrogen action in the breast. Thus, both compounds have advantages over estrogens in hormone replacement therapy; they reverse osteoporosis but should not increase breast cancer risk. However, existing selective modulators do not possess ideal selective properties. Tamoxifen increases uterine cancer risk and raloxifene and tamoxifen exacerbate hot flushes and increase the risk of blood clots and stroke.

Better selective modulation may be achieved in several ways. The selective modulation observed for tamoxifen and raloxifene is due to distortion of the receptor's ligand-binding domain, with consequent differences in the way (relative to estradiol) that it binds various cofactors. Improvements in this profile may be forthcoming. The same hormone can interact with more than one receptor, and isoform-specific ligands could show improvements over nonselective counterparts. Thus, adverse thyroid hormone effects on heart rate are mediated by TRα. TRβ-selective agonists might elicit some of the desirable effects of thyroid hormone without deleterious effects on the heart. Localized delivery systems can achieve selective modulation. Limited examples of this concept are the use of inhalation of glucocorticoid receptor agonists for asthma or application of cortisol creams to the skin. It may be possible to utilize tissue-specific uptake or export systems as a means of targeting drugs to particular tissues. Finally, it may be possible to take advantage of tissue selective metabolism to elicit selective responses. Indeed, idealized selective modulators may in the future make use of combinations of these diverse selective properties.

■ DISORDERS OF THE ENDOCRINE SYSTEM

The classic disorders of the endocrine system arise from states of excess or deficiency of hormones. However, resistance to hormones also plays a major role in disease. The endocrinologist is also confronted with specific tumors and other problems such as iatrogenic syndromes. The types of abnormalities that in principle can occur are illustrated in Figure 1–13.

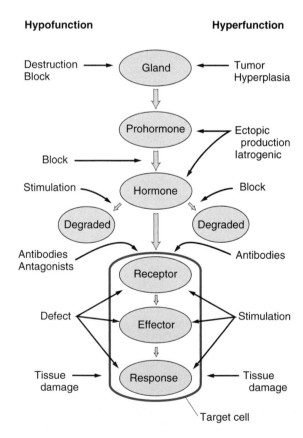

Figure 1–13. Causes of hypofunction and hyperfunction of the endocrine system. (Reproduced, with permission, from Baxter JD in: *Cecil's Textbook of Medicine.* Wyngaarden JB, Smith LH Jr [editors]. Saunders, 1985.)

ENDOCRINE HYPOFUNCTION

Destruction of the Gland

A common mechanism for glandular hypofunction is destruction of the gland through autoimmune disease (Chapter 4). This is seen in type 1 diabetes mellitus (Chapter 17), hypothyroidism (Chapter 7), adrenal insufficiency (Chapter 9), and gonadal failure (Chapters 12 and 13). A polyglandular failure syndrome (Schmidt's syndrome) results from autoimmune destruction of several different endocrine glands in the same patient (Chapter 4). The immunologic damage also results in other abnormalities, including pernicious anemia and vitiligo. Destruction of the pituitary gland is usually due to tumor, ischemia, or autoimmune hypophysitis (Chapter 5). Hypofunction of any of the endocrine glands may result from damage by neoplasms, infection, or hemorrhage.

Extraglandular Disorders

Endocrine hypofunction can be caused by defects outside traditional endocrine glands. In some cases, these are simply due to damage to tissues that produce hormones or convert hormone precursors to active forms. Thus, renal disease can result in defective conversion of $25(OH)D_3$ to $1,25(OH)_2D_3$, with consequent abnormalities in calcium and phosphate balance (Chapter 8). Renal disease can also provoke hyporeninemic hypoaldosteronism (Chapter 10) and anemia by damaging the renin-producing juxtaglomerular cells and the erythropoietin-producing cells.

In some cases, factors that influence hormone degradation or sensitivity can precipitate or aggravate hormone deficiency when there is insufficient reserve in the endocrine gland. For example, glucocorticoid therapy, which reduces insulin sensitivity, increases the need for insulin and can precipitate latent diabetes mellitus or aggravate existing diabetes (Chapter 17). Thyroid hormones increase cortisol metabolism, and treatment of hypothyroidism with thyroid hormone can unmask latent adrenal insufficiency (Chapter 9). Treatment with the anticonvulsant phenytoin can accelerate the degradation of glucocorticoids and increase the need for these hormones (Chapter 9).

Defects in Hormone Biosynthesis

Endocrine hypofunction can be due to defects in hormone synthesis. These can be due to defects in genes that encode hormones, regulate hormone production, or encode hormone-producing enzymes or are involved in hormone metabolism. The 21-hydroxylase deficiency syndrome results in defective cortisol production and is one of the most common genetic diseases (Chap-

ters 9, 14, and 15). Other adrenal gland defects include 11β-hydroxylase, 17-hydroxylase, and 18-hydroxylase deficiency syndromes (Chapters 9, 10, and 14). Dietary iodine deficiency results in deficient thyroid hormone biosynthesis and afflicts millions of people worldwide (Chapter 7). Mutations in genes encoding polypeptide hormones can decrease hormone production or lead to production of defective hormones. Growth deficiency can result from mutations or deletions in the GH gene, defective production of GHRH, or mutations in the gene for the transcription factor Pit-1, which regulates GH synthesis (Chapter 6). A rare form of diabetes mellitus results from a mutation in the insulin gene, with production of abnormal insulin (Chapter 17).

ENDOCRINE HYPERFUNCTION

Hyperfunction of endocrine glands results usually from tumors, hyperplasia, or autoimmune stimulation. Endocrine gland tumors can produce excess hormone. Thus, pituitary tumors can overproduce one of the major classes of pituitary hormones (ACTH, GH, PRL, TSH, LH, and FSH; Chapter 5). This leads to stimulation of other glands, as is seen with cortisol excess due to pituitary ACTH-producing tumors or the rare syndrome of hyperthyroidism due to pituitary TSH-producing tumors. Other examples of tumors in endocrine organs resulting in overproduction of hormones are parathyroid glands, PTH (Chapter 8); thyroid parafollicular cells, calcitonin (Chapter 7); thyroid follicular cells, thyroglobulin or thyroid hormone (Chapter 7); pancreatic islets, insulin, or glucagon (Chapter 17); adrenals, cortisol, aldosterone, deoxycorticosterone, androgens, and other steroids (Chapters 9 and 10); kidney and renin (Chapter 10), or erythropoietin. There are also syndromes of multiple endocrine neoplasia, in which there is a predisposition to develop tumors of several glands (Chapter 22). In contrast, most thyroid gland tumors do not overproduce thyroid hormone (Chapter 7), and it is rare for ovarian or testicular tumors to overproduce steroids or for posterior pituitary tumors to overproduce oxytocin or vasopressin.

There can also be ectopic production of hormones by tumors (Chapter 21). Ectopically produced hormones are usually polypeptide hormones and include ACTH, ADH, and calcitonin. However, other polypeptide hormones such as insulin are rarely if ever expressed ectopically.

Hyperplasia, with increased cellularity and hormone overproduction, can be seen with most endocrine glands. Hyperplasia of the parathyroid glands is seen in renal failure, where depression of serum calcium ion levels stimulates the gland (Chapter 8). Hyperplasia is commonly seen in the adrenal glomerulosa, where it results in aldosterone excess and is a major cause of the syndrome of primary aldosteronism (Chapter 10). Hyperplasia of the adrenal zonae fasciculata and reticularis results in cortisol excess and Cushing's syndrome (Chapter 9) and is almost always due to a pituitary ACTH-producing tumor. The cause of hyperplasia of the adrenal glomerulosa is not known, and the disorder is therefore referred to as idiopathic hyperplasia or idiopathic aldosteronism. Hyperplasia of the thyroid gland is common and may be due to autoimmune stimulation (see below), iodine deficiency with impaired T_4 synthesis and subsequent TSH hypersecretion, or nodular goiter due to genetic biosynthetic abnormalities (Chapter 7). Hyperplasia of the ovaries is very common and results in polycystic ovary syndrome, with abnormalities in ovarian steroid production and insulin resistance; the causes of this syndrome are poorly understood (Chapter 13).

Autoimmune stimulation resulting in hyperfunction is seen most commonly with hyperthyroidism (Chapter 7). In this case, antibodies are produced that bind to and activate the TSH receptor on the gland. Hyperinsulinism due to autoimmune attack on the pancreatic B cells can be seen transiently early in the course of development of type 1 diabetes mellitus (Chapter 17). Otherwise, autoimmune stimulation leading to hyperfunction of endocrine glands is rare.

DEFECTS IN SENSITIVITY TO HORMONES

Genetic and acquired defects in sensitivity to hormones play a crucial role in the pathogenesis of both common and rare disorders. Common disorders include type 2 diabetes mellitus and hypertension. Resistance may be due to a number of different types of defects, eg, in the hormone receptor, in functions distal to the receptor, or in functions extrinsic to the receptor-response pathway.

There are a number of disorders of primary resistance to hormones due to receptor defects. Genetic defects in receptors that cause syndromes of resistance include those for glucocorticoids, thyroid hormones, androgens, vitamin D, leptin, mineralocorticoids, peroxisomal proliferators, PTH, ADH, GH, insulin, and TSH. Defects in hormone response that are due to mutations in postreceptor signaling pathways are less well understood. An exception is the syndrome of pseudohypoparathyroidism, in which mutations occur in the gene encoding the guanylyl nucleotide binding protein that links PTH-receptor binding to activation of adenylyl cyclase (Chapters 3 and 8). Resistance to thyroid hormone is ordinarily due to mutations in the thyroid hormone receptor (TR); however, in a number of cases, defects in the receptor have not been found, and it is thought that the defect may involve postreceptor loci such as receptor association with coregulatory proteins.

Hormone resistance that is due to events distal to the ligand-receptor interaction occurs in type 2 diabetes mellitus, the most common form of that disease (Chapter 17). Weight reduction and diet can normalize these manifestations in some patients, suggesting that the problem is one of impaired adaptation—perhaps due to excessive down-regulation of responsiveness to stimuli. Syndrome X (metabolic syndrome) is characterized by excessive insulin resistance with overlap into type 2 diabetes mellitus, hyperlipidemia with increased triglycerides and cholesterol, and hypertension. This syndrome is commonly observed in obese individuals and accounts for much of the hypertension in Western societies. In hypertension, there are variations in sensitivity to salt, to angiotensin II, to the release of renin in response to various stimuli, and to other effectors. Although mechanisms for the resistance are poorly understood, insights into disorders such as these should come from a better understanding of the physiologic mechanisms that govern sensitivity to hormones. Figure 1–14 is a schematic representation of resistance to hormones at postreceptor loci.

Acquired resistance to hormones can occur when there is frank disease that damages the target tissue and interferes with its ability to respond to the hormone. This can be seen with renal disease and insensitivity to vasopressin and with liver disease and insensitivity to glucagon. It can also occur as a result of excess production of other hormones or substances that promote hormone resistance. Thus, stress responses, hyperglycemia, and states that increase plasma levels of GH, cortisol, or glucagon all lead to insulin resistance that can aggravate or precipitate type 2 diabetes mellitus (Chapter 17). Acquired resistance may also occur in hormone therapy. This is particularly true with GnRH analogs and calcitonin and sometimes occurs with glucocorticoids. In fact, the acquired resistance associated with prolonged exposure to GnRH analogs forms the basis for their use in the treatment of prostate cancer—along with nonsteroidal antiandrogens—to inhibit androgen action. In this clinical context, the GnRH-induced down-regulation of GnRH responsiveness (termed tachyphylaxis) shuts down FSH and LH release with a consequent reduction in testosterone production. Immunologic mechanisms can lead to acquired resistance—as, for example when antibodies are produced to hormones (eg, with insulin or GH therapy) or receptors (eg, insulin receptors; Chapter 17).

The clinical presentations of these syndromes show considerable variations. In classic hormone resistance syndromes, there are elevated or normal hormone levels with clinical manifestations of hormone deficiency and failure of hormonal replacement to correct the disorder. Thus, at worst, the syndromes resemble hormone deficiency states, as is the case with testicular feminization

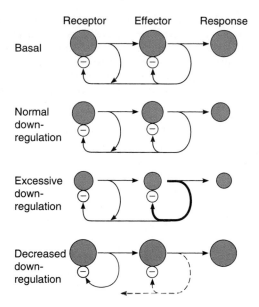

Figure 1–14. Scheme for generation of hyper-responsiveness or hyporesponsiveness to hormones through excessive or impaired down-regulation. The top row indicates the response network before down-regulation occurs. The second row indicates the magnitude of the response network with normal down-regulation. The third row indicates a situation with excessive down-regulation due to a defect in the effector arm of the response with normal receptor function. The sizes of the circles reflect the influence, and the increased size of the arrow reflects the enhanced down-regulation. The fourth row indicates decreased down-regulation at the effector arm of the response. The dotted arrow reflects the decreased down-regulation and the larger response circles, compared with the second panel, reflect the increased response resulting from the decreased down-regulation.

syndrome (androgen insensitivity; Chapter 14), rickets (vitamin D insensitivity; Chapter 8), and nephrogenic diabetes insipidus (ADH insensitivity; Chapter 5). However, there can be wide variations in the clinical presentations. As an example, manifestations due to mutations of the androgen receptor gene can vary from a phenotypic female with a male genotype to mild androgen deficiency with erectile dysfunction in an otherwise normal-appearing male (Chapter 14).

In many cases, secondary hormone hypersecretion largely compensates for the primary defect, and the clinical presentation is more complex. Elevated hormone levels occur because of absence of the usual feedback inhibition of hormone release resulting from tar-get organ resistance. For example, the clinical presentation of the syndrome of resistance to thyroid hormone (Chapter 7) may have features of euthyroidism, hyperthyroidism (tachycardia, poor attention span), and hypothyroidism (poor growth). In this syndrome, the mutation is in the β form of the TR, but the remaining TRβ encoded by the second allele and the TRα encoded by separate genes are normal. The abnormal β gene causes a decrease in the usual pituitary feedback by thyroid hormone, leading to increases in TSH secretion and hypersecretion of thyroid hormone. This increase in thyroid hormone compensates for the defect by binding the normal β and α receptors and, in some cases, the mutated receptors. Thus, thyroid hormone-regulated functions that are normally mediated through the α receptors are hyperstimulated, and functions mediated through the β receptors can be stimulated normally or can be understimulated in cases where a normal complement of β receptors is required for full activity and the elevated hormone levels cannot overcome the defect in the mutated receptors.

Hyperstimulation of the endocrine glands in resistance syndromes sometimes results in overproduction of other hormones. Thus, mutations that reduce the affinity of the glucocorticoid receptor for cortisol result in compensatory ACTH hypersecretion. Whereas the resulting overproduction of cortisol compensates for the primary defect, parallel increases in other steroids such as deoxycorticosterone and testosterone can promote mineralocorticoid hypertension and hirsutism, respectively.

Primary hormone hyperresponsiveness has rarely been encountered. It may occur in low-renin hypertension in humans and in primary aldosteronism with hyperplasia of the zona glomerulosa, a variant of primary aldosteronism. It has also been encountered in a mineralocorticoid receptor defect where the receptor binds progesterone more tightly than with the wild type receptor. Thus, when progesterone levels are elevated in conditions such as in pregnancy, there is overactivation of the receptor and consequent hypertension. Acquired hypersensitivity can be observed, as with catecholamine hypersensitivity in hyperthyroidism and increased sensitivity to insulin with cortisol deficiency.

SYNDROMES OF HORMONE EXCESS DUE TO ADMINISTRATION OF EXOGENOUS HORMONE

Syndromes of hormone excess can result from deliberate or inadvertent administration of exogenous hormones. Deliberate administration of glucocorticoids in therapy to suppress inflammation may lead to Cushing's syndrome. Use of high doses of thyroid hormone to suppress a malignancy in the gland can lead to hyperthyroidism. Androgen excess with suppression of pituitary gonadotropins occurs in athletes who take androgens to improve performance. As an example of inadvertent administration, the authors have observed Cushing's syndrome in a patient who was unaware that she had received glucocorticoids. Outbreaks of hyperthyroidism have occurred with consumption of hamburger meat contaminated by thyroid tissue (Chapter 7). Some nasal sprays have contained substances with mineralocorticoid activity that produces a mineralocorticoid excess state (Chapter 10).

NONENDOCRINE PROBLEMS ASSOCIATED WITH ENDOCRINE DISEASE

Endocrine diseases can cause problems unrelated to the endocrine excess or deficiency states. For example, pituitary tumors can cause increased intracranial pressure or neurologic or ocular problems when they extend outside the sella turcica (Chapter 5). Thyroid tumors or large goiters can cause local problems in the neck (Chapter 7).

■ APPROACH TO THE PATIENT WITH ENDOCRINE DISEASE

Like all other medical specialists, the endocrinologist hopes and tries to prevent diseases and their sequelae or when this is not possible, to detect and treat disease at an early stage. Thus, endocrine diseases are generally most easily recognizable in their more extreme forms, but it is hoped that few patients will progress to that stage. The physician should be aware of subtle early manifestations of endocrine disease and strive for early diagnosis with the aid of laboratory tests. Early diagnosis can also be facilitated by screening for endocrine diseases in certain clinical settings (discussed below).

Several principles should be considered in evaluating endocrine diseases. Symptoms and signs are often vague and attributable to anxiety or depression or to nonendocrine causes. The early presentation of these disorders can be masked even further by compensatory responses. The clinical presentation of a given condition can also differ depending on its chronicity, and a severe deficiency state can present as an acute and severe problem in a patient in whom chronic manifestations of the disorder have not had time to develop. The clinician must decide whether treatment should be instituted immediately, before time-consuming tests leading to definitive diagnosis have been completed. It is sometimes difficult to arrive at a clear diagnosis, and the procedures needed for definitive diagnosis may impose more risk than the disease over a short period of time. In such cases, a decision to follow the patient must be made.

For example, this occurs with ACTH-dependent Cushing's syndrome, where the differentiation between an occult carcinoid tumor and a small pituitary adenoma as the source of ACTH hypersecretion may require invasive procedures (Chapter 9).

In today's environment of cost containment, efficiency of diagnosis is a priority. Although modern tests may involve higher cost, they also allow for greater efficiency of diagnosis. Thus, by combining the most efficient use of tests with a careful history and physical examination and sound clinical judgment, diagnosis and management of endocrine disease should be better, quicker, and cheaper than before.

EVIDENCE-BASED ENDOCRINOLOGY

Evidence-based medicine evolved out of concern that physicians were applying clinical impressions to patient care in some cases without sufficient basis in scientific fact. It was observed, for example, that approaches to given diseases differed in various medical centers and regions around the world. It was noted also that in cases where practice activities were not justified, this frequently led to mistakes in therapy based on inferences drawn from subsequently published data. As an example of this, at one time a number of physicians used fluoride to treat osteoporosis based on the observation that fluoride increased bone density. However, subsequent studies found that fluoride did not decrease the rate of bone fractures. In this instance, the use of bone density proved to be an unacceptable marker for fracture risk. A more recent example is the use of estrogen-progestin combinations to prevent cardiovascular disease. This was based on a number of observational studies suggesting that estrogen deficiency in the postmenopausal setting increases cardiovascular risk. However, more rigorous trials showed that estrogen-progestin combinations failed to decrease cardiovascular risk—and actually seemed to increase risk, at least over the first few years of the trial.

Advocates of evidence-based endocrinology acknowledge that physicians are faced with situations where the evidence is not conclusive and yet diagnostic or therapeutic decisions must be made. Guidelines have thus emerged that rank the importance of the evidence. The hierarchy could range downward from well-done randomized trials to meta-analyses, systematic reviews of observational studies, observational studies, physiologic studies, and unsystematic clinical studies. Thus, there is room for clinical judgment. Recommendations based on evidence-based endocrinology can be found in several sources, including UpToDate, the ACP Journal Club, and the Cochrane Database.

How did physicians make decisions prior to "evidence-based endocrinology"? They based them on the evidence that was available, recommendations of opinion leaders, and their own experience. What is different? First, more recent advances in statistical analyses of data have "raised the bar" concerning the strength of the evidence required to make a recommendation. Second, there has been increased reliance on data related to outcomes. A major result of these changes is that the average physician who reads guidelines from consensus conferences follows treatment plans based on more firmly established evidence.

However, evidence-based endocrinology practiced with higher standards raises additional problems. The rate of scientific progress is accelerating. New methods for diagnosing and treating disease will be developed at a pace much faster than was the rule even a few years ago. It will take many years to prove the efficacy of these developments using today's high standards. For example, recent data from the Pharmaceutical Manufacturers Association states that it takes on average 68 clinical trials, 14 years, and about $500–$800 million to take a drug, once discovered, to approval. These numbers are increasing. This means that it will be many years before many of these developments will be available to most patients, and it may prove impossible to develop many of the newer treatment modalities that will be discovered. How do the opinion leaders deal with this dilemma? They vary in their adherence to established guidelines, often because they are more confident in applying newer modalities. Thus, we can have situations where the leaders in the field are treating patients differently from the generalists who follow the guidelines. Who is right?

Counterbalancing the criticisms outlined earlier justifying the new higher standards are the many examples of treatments that were initiated prior to rigorous proof of efficacy. Examples include the use of histamine H_2 receptor blockers for treating peptic ulcer disease, converting enzyme inhibitors for treating heart failure and hypertension, calcium channel blockers for treating hypertension, and β-adrenergic blockers for treating hypertension. A question that emerges is whether opinion leaders are more often right than not. A related question is whether strict adherence to evidence-based endocrinology, with relegation of clinical judgment-based endocrinology to a secondary position in the decision-making process, is likely to provide better or worse care to the endocrine patient. These important questions remain largely unaddressed as this is written.

HISTORY & PHYSICAL EXAMINATION

A carefully performed history and physical examination can provide information that cannot be obtained from laboratory testing. Some diagnoses, such as hypertension, are based on the physical examination alone. Even when the history and physical are unrevealing, they enable the physician to select appropriate laboratory tests and avoid unnecessary testing. Most specialists have a fund of stories about consultations on extensively studied patients where simply elicited symptoms or signs that were overlooked would have led to early diagnosis. Thus, a history and physical examination should address issues that will lead to the diagnosis and to the plan of approach. These activities should also reveal information about how much tissue damage or physical deformity has occurred; how long the disease has been present; the effect of various manifestations on the patient; and relevant data from the social, family, and personal histories that will facilitate evaluation and management.

Manifestations of endocrine disease that are frequently due to nonendocrine or unknown causes (Table 1–3) include fatigue, malaise, weakness, headache, anorexia, depression, weight gain or loss, bruising, and constipation, among others. Thus, weight loss is a common manifestation of hyperthyroidism, though most weight loss is not caused by hyperthyroidism (Chapter 7). Adrenal insufficiency is a rare disease and an even rarer cause of nausea (Chapter 9).

LABORATORY STUDIES

Laboratory evaluations are critical for making and confirming endocrine diagnoses and for ruling out other causes. However, these tests cannot replace good clinical judgment that incorporates all available information in making clinical decisions. Laboratory tests, in general, measure either the level of the hormone in some body fluid, the effects of the hormone, or the sequelae of the process that contributed to the hormonal abnormality. The tests can be performed under random or basal conditions, precisely defined conditions, or in response to some provocative stimulus. In measuring hormone levels, the sensitivity of the assay refers to the lowest concentration of the hormone that can be accurately detected, and the specificity refers to the extent to which cross-reacting species are scored inappropriately in the assay.

Measurements of Hormone Levels: Basal Levels

Immunologic assays are usually utilized for measurements of hormone levels in body fluids. Most measurements use blood or urine samples. The hormone is measured either directly in the samples or following extraction and purification. Most measurements detect active hormone, though measurement of either a metabolite or precursor of the hormone or a concomitantly released substance sometimes provides the best information. Thus, in assessing vitamin D status, it is usually more informative to measure the precursor hormone, 25(OH)D, even though the final active hor-

Table 1–3. Examples of manifestations of endocrine disease. (The manifestations do not occur in all cases, and the severity can vary markedly.)

Abdominal pain	Addisonian crisis; diabetic ketoacidosis; hyperparathyroidism
Amenorrhea or oligo-menorrhea	Adrenal insufficiency, adrenogenital syndrome, anorexia nervosa, Cushing's syndrome, hyperprolactinemic states, hypopituitarism, hypothyroidism, menopause, ovarian failure, polycystic ovaries, pseudo-hermaphroditic syndromes
Anemia	Adrenal insufficiency, gonadal insufficiency, hypothyroidism, hyperparathyroidism, panhypopituitarism
Anorexia	Addison's disease, diabetic ketoacidosis, hypercalcemia (eg, hyperparathyroidism), hypothyroidism
Constipation	Diabetic neuropathy, hypercalcemia, hypothyroidism, pheochromocytoma
Depression	Adrenal insufficiency, Cushing's syndrome, hypercalcemic states, hypoglycemia, hypothyroidism
Diarrhea	Hyperthyroidism, metastatic carcinoid tumors, metastatic medullary thyroid carcinoma
Fever	Adrenal insufficiency, hyperthyroidism (severe: thyroid storm), hypothalamic disease
Hair changes	Decreased body hair (hypothyroidism, hypopituitarism, thyrotoxicosis); hirsutism (androgen excess states, Cushing's syndrome, acromegaly)
Headache	Hypertensive episodes with pheochromocytoma, hypoglycemia, pituitary tumors
Hypothermia	Hypoglycemia, hypothyroidism
Libido changes	Adrenal insufficiency, Cushing's syndrome, hypercalcemia, hyperprolactinemia, hyperthyroidism, hypokalemia, hypopituitarism, hypothyroidism, poorly controlled diabetes mellitus
Nervousness	Cushing's syndrome, hyperthyroidism
Polyuria	Diabetes insipidus, diabetes mellitus, hypercalcemia, hypokalemia
Skin changes	Acanthosis nigricans (obesity, polycystic ovaries, severe insulin resistance, Cushing's syndrome, acromegaly), acne (androgen excess), hyperpigmentation (adrenal insufficiency, Nelson's syndrome), dry (hypothyroidism), hypopigmentation (panhypopituitarism), striae, plethora, bruising, ecchymoses (Cushing's syndrome), vitiligo (autoimmune thyroid disease, Addison's disease)
Weakness and fatigue	Addison's disease, Cushing's syndrome, diabetes mellitus, hypokalemia (eg, primary aldosteronism, Bartter's syndrome), hypothyroidism, hyperthyroidism, hypercalcemia (eg, hyperparathyroidism, panhypopituitarism, pheochromocytoma)
Weight gain	Central nervous system disease, Cushing's syndrome, hypothyroidism, insulinoma, pituitary tumors
Weight loss	Adrenal insufficiency, anorexia nervosa, cancer of endocrine glands, hyperthyroidism, type 1 diabetes mellitus, panhypopituitarism, pheochromocytoma

mone is $1,25(OH)_2D$ (Chapter 8). In 21-hydroxylase syndrome, the clinical problem is a deficiency of cortisol or aldosterone, but the most sensitive diagnostic measurement is of the plasma 17α-hydroxyprogesterone level, a precursor of cortisol (Chapter 9). In looking for a pheochromocytoma, levels of epinephrine metabolites are sometimes as informative as levels of epinephrine itself (Chapter 11).

Plasma & Urine Assays

Hormone assays only indicate the hormone levels at the time of sampling. For hormones with long half-lives (eg, thyroxine), measurements taken randomly provide an integrated assessment of hormonal status. For hormones with shorter half-lives, such as epinephrine or cortisol, the assay will provide information only for the time of sample collection. Thus, with a pheochromocytoma that episodically releases epinephrine, elevated plasma epinephrine levels would be found only during periods of release and not between them (Chapter 11). Spontaneous Cushing's disease can be associated with an increased number of pulses of cortisol release with normal plasma cortisol levels between pulses (Chapter 9). In early Addison's disease, the number of pulses of cortisol release can be decreased, but occasional releases can result in transient plasma cortisol levels in the normal range (Chapter 9).

Urine assays are generally restricted to measurement of levels of steroid and catecholamine hormones or metabolites and are not useful for polypeptide hormones that are either not cleared or unstable. The collection period can be a random sample or, more often, a 24-hour collection. Interpretations of urinary measurements must account for the fact that urinary levels reflect renal handling of the hormone. Urine measurements were utilized more frequently in the past because larger quantities of the hormone could be obtained. However, with the high sensitivities of today's immunoassays, this advantage is disappearing, and blood measurements are usually preferred. An advantage of urinary assays is that they can provide an integrated assessment of hormonal status. With cortisol, for example, about 1–3% of the hormone released by the adrenal gland appears in the urine, but measurement of the urine cortisol in a 24-hour "urine free cortisol" sample provides an excellent assessment of the integrated cortisol production (Chapter 9). This is important, since cortisol is released episodically, and a random plasma cortisol can be in the normal range in the face of mild to moderate Cushing's disease. Urinary assays are frequently used to document aldosterone excess in primary aldosteronism (Chapter 10) and epinephrine excess in pheochromocytoma (Chapter 11).

Free Hormone Levels

As discussed in an earlier section, many hormones circulate bound to plasma proteins, and the free hormone fraction is generally that which is biologically relevant. Thus, assessment of free hormone levels is more critical than total hormone levels. Tests that measure free hormone levels can utilize equilibrium dialysis, ultrafiltration, competitive binding, and other means. Although such tests are not commonly employed, their use may increase, as evidenced by increasing use of plasma free thyroxine (Chapter 7) and serum ionized Ca^{2+} measurements (Chapter 8).

Immunoassays

Hormone immunoassays utilize animal-derived antibodies with high affinity to the hormone. The antibodies can be polyclonal or monoclonal. In general, a given animal will produce a number of different antibodies to a given antigen, each from a clone of antibody-producing B lymphocytes—thus the term "polyclonal antibodies." This mixture of antibodies can contain some with extremely high affinities for the hormone, and these will provide a high level of sensitivity in a subsequent radioimmunoassay. Monoclonal antibodies are commonly obtained by injecting the antigen into a mouse or rat or by incubating it with cells in vitro. The animal spleen or incubated cells are then immortalized by fus-

ing them to myeloma cells or transforming them with tumor viruses. This produces a number of clones of antibody-producing cells. The clones are then screened with the antigen until a suitable antibody-producing clone is identified. A major disadvantage of monoclonal antibodies is that many of them have a low affinity for the hormone. In addition, each antibody reacts with only one epitope on the antigen, and these antibodies are not as useful for traditional reagent-limiting assays. However, these antibodies are critical for the "sandwich assays" described below.

In traditional assays, the antigen is labeled in order to detect its binding to the antibody; the label must not block binding of the antigen to the antibody. Early immunoassays traditionally utilized radiolabeled hormones as the antigen. Most commonly the radioisotope was iodine, which can be obtained with a very high specific activity. However, the disadvantages with radioactivity in terms of shelf life and escalating expense for disposal have led to increasing use of nonisotopic means to perform immunoassays. For these, the antigen is linked to an enzyme, fluorescent label, chemiluminescent label, or latex particle that can be agglutinated with the antigen. Enzyme-linked immunosorbent assays (ELISAs) that utilize antibody-coated microtiter plates and an enzyme-labeled reporter antibody can be as sensitive as radioimmunoassays.

In practice, measurement of hormone levels by immunoassay involves incubating the plasma or urine sample or an extract with antisera and then measuring the levels of antigen-antibody complexes by one of several means. The classic immunoassays utilize high-affinity antibodies immobilized (at low concentrations to permit maximal sensitivity) on the surface of a test tube, polystyrene bead, or paramagnetic particle. The unknown sample and the antibody are incubated together, and the labeled antigen is added either at zero time or later. A standard curve is prepared using the antibody and a known concentration of hormone. From this curve, the extent of inhibition of the binding of the labeled hormone by the added hormone is plotted, usually as the ratio of bound to free (B:F) hormone as a function of the log of the total hormone concentration. These plots typically provide a sigmoid curve (Figure 1–15). Alternatively, a log-logit plot can be used to linearize the data (Figure 1–15). The hormone level in the sample is determined by relating the B:F value obtained in the sample to the standard curve.

A modification of immunoassays—termed the sandwich technique—utilizes two different monoclonal antibodies that recognize separate portions of the hormone. This aspect limits the technique, as it is difficult to utilize it for small molecules where separable reactive domains cannot be readily identified. The assay is performed by using the first antibody, attached—preferably

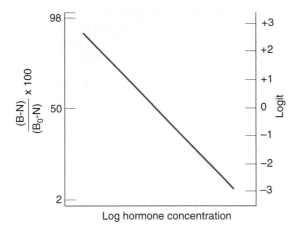

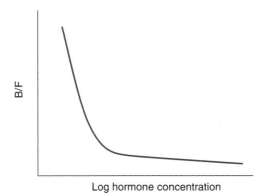

Figure 1–15. Standard curve of hormone radio-immunoassay. (B, counts bound; F, free counts; N, non-specific count; B_0, maximum number of counts bound when only antibody and labeled hormone are incubated.) (Reproduced, with permission, from Vaitukaitis J in: *Hormone Assays in Endocrinology and Metabolism*, 2nd ed. Felig P et al [editors]. McGraw-Hill, 1987.)

in excess relative to the amount of hormone in the sample—to a solid support matrix to adsorb the hormone to be assayed. After removal of the plasma and washing, the second (labeled) antibody is then incubated with the bound hormone–first antibody complex. The amount of binding of the second antibody is proportionate to the concentration of hormone in the sample. Use of two antibodies results in markedly enhanced specificity with a great reduction in background levels, thus improving both specificity and sensitivity of the assay.

Nonimmunologic Assays

Nonimmunologic assays include chemical assays, which take advantage of chemically reactive groups in the molecule; bioassays, which assess the activity of the hormone incubated with cells or tissues in vitro or following injection into an animal; and receptor-binding and other assays, which exploit the high affinity of the hormone for receptors or other molecules such as plasma-binding proteins. These assays are rarely used because immunoassays are sufficiently robust for most applications. For example, immunoassays are superior to receptor assays because antibodies can be obtained that have much higher affinities for hormones than receptors. One example of a receptor assay uses thyroid tumor cells (FRTL-5 cells) that contain TSH receptors to detect antibodies to these receptors in plasma of patients with Graves' disease.

Diagnosis of Genetic Disease

Methods for diagnosis of genetic diseases using DNA analyses are improving rapidly. Thus, DNA can be obtained from peripheral blood cells; the region of interest can be amplified by PCR; and the gene can be sequenced fairly rapidly. The increased availability of these technologic capacities is rapidly supplanting previous methods such as analysis of restriction fragment length polymorphisms (RFLPs) in diagnosis. In cases where the mutation is known, such a procedure can lead to rapid and accurate diagnosis in the general population. This is the case with sickle cell anemia, in which a single mutation in one codon is present in all individuals who have the disease. It is also the case in kindreds with known mutations, such as those with maturity-onset diabetes of the young (MODY) or glucocorticoid remediable aldosteronism or with mutations in the breast cancer susceptibility genes *BRCA1* and *BRCA2*. It is probable that DNA analysis will be increasingly used for identification of affected family members in kindreds with a shared mutation. Thus, people who have inherited the defect can be advised with regard to appropriate follow-up or preventive surgery, and those without the defect can be spared unnecessary anxiety and testing.

It remains true that in some cases other diagnostic measures are easier to perform in screening of the general population. Multiple mutations can lead to the same disease, and screening for any one mutation within a sequence would potentially miss most affected individuals in the population. For example, 21-hydroxylase deficiency is caused by a number of different mutations, and it has been simpler to measure 17-hydroxyprogesterone levels (Chapter 9) than to examine DNA samples for a large number of mutations. Nevertheless, large scale sequencing of key genes that might contribute to a particular disease phenotype can dramatically improve diagnosis. For example, MODY is caused by monogenic defects in a number of genes (including glucokinase or a series of pancreatic transcription factors) that lead to glucose intolerance and diabetes-like symptoms. Many of these patients respond well to glucose-lowering drugs without insulin therapy. Large-scale sequencing of possible MODY genes in patients—along with analysis of other family members—can distinguish the subset of patients with MODY from those with type 1 or type 2 diabetes and alter the preferred treatment regimen.

Indirect Measurements of Hormonal Status

Measurement of the effects of hormones can be even more important than measuring the hormone levels and can provide critical complementary information. Even when hormone levels are known, it is common to obtain at least one index of the effects of the hormone in evaluating an endocrine disease. The blood glucose level is generally more useful than the plasma insulin level in diagnosing and treating diabetes mellitus (Chapter 17). Plasma insulin levels can be high in the face of frank hyperglycemia in type 2 diabetes mellitus, and in type 1 diabetes mellitus insulin levels are a much less reliable index of diabetic status than blood glucose (Chapter 17). Measurement of the serum calcium level is critical for evaluating hyperparathyroidism (Chapter 8). Measurement of plasma renin levels in relation to plasma aldosterone levels (aldosterone:renin ratio) is critical for evaluating primary aldosteronism, in which plasma renin levels are relatively suppressed (Chapter 10). The most common causes of elevated aldosterone levels are dehydration, exercise, diuretic therapy, and other conditions that produce secondary aldosteronism; in these settings, the plasma renin levels tend to be high rather than low (Chapter 9).

Provocative Tests

In many cases, the level of a hormone or parameter affected by a hormone is best interpreted following provocative challenges. For example, with thyroid disease, provocative tests are rarely needed (Chapter 7), whereas with adrenal insufficiency or glucocorticoid excess (Chapter 9), heavy reliance is placed on such tests. With thyroid disease, slow clearance of the hormone results in basal levels of hormone that are highly informative, whereas the pulsatile nature of cortisol release results in fluctuating plasma cortisol levels that need to be measured under more defined conditions. This problem is bypassed in evaluation of adrenal insufficiency by administering an ACTH analog that maximally stimulates the adrenal (Chapter 9). Diagnosis of Cushing's disease reflects a different problem (Chapter 9). Once cortisol hypersecretion has been documented, the cause must be identified. The clinician takes advantage of the

fact that ACTH release by pituitary microadenomas—and, consequently, secretion of cortisol by the adrenal glands—are suppressed by the glucocorticoid dexamethasone to a greater extent than is cortisol release by adrenal tumors or ACTH release by ectopic ACTH-producing tumors. Similarly, GnRH analogs (which stimulate FSH and LH release), TRH (which stimulates both prolactin and TSH release), and insulin hypoglycemia (which stimulates the release of ACTH and GH) can be used to evaluate pituitary reserve (Chapter 5). In evaluating primary aldosteronism, provocative stimuli (diuresis, change in posture, inhibition of converting enzyme) are sometimes used to increase renin release (Chapter 10).

Imaging Studies

Imaging studies are used in diagnosis and follow-up of endocrine diseases. MRI and CT allow visualization of endocrine glands and endocrine tumors at a much greater resolution than in the past. These procedures have been especially useful for evaluation of tumors of the pituitary and adrenals (Chapters 5 and 9). Scanning of the thyroid gland using radioactive iodine has been useful for evaluation of functioning nodules of this gland (Chapter 7). The endocrinologist can also resort to other sophisticated procedures that involve selective sampling from particular sites. For example, selective venous catheterization of the petrosal sinuses can be particularly useful in detecting ACTH hypersecretion in Cushing's disease (Chapter 9), and selective sampling of the renal veins can be helpful in the diagnosis of renovascular hypertension.

Biopsy Procedures

Biopsy procedures are not commonly used for evaluation of endocrine diseases but are occasionally useful to diagnose neoplasia. An exception is the use of fine-needle biopsy of the thyroid gland (Chapter 7), which has had a major impact on evaluation of thyroid nodules.

SCREENING FOR ENDOCRINE DISEASES

Some endocrine diseases are sufficiently common that screening should be part of usual clinical practice. This is true for hypertension and diabetes (Chapter 17). Thus, blood pressure should be measured as part of any physical examination, and when hypertension is present, evaluation for potential causes should be instituted to exclude endocrine disorders (Chapter 10). Thyroid disease has a prevalence of about 3% in women under the age of 60 and an even greater prevalence in both men and women at older ages. The clinical presentations, especially in milder forms, are frequently subtle and missed by the physician. There are no clear recommendations for screening by measuring serum TSH levels, but such recommendations may ultimately emerge given the increasing awareness of the incidence of thyroid disease and of the detrimental sequelae that can result (Chapter 7). Blood glucose levels should be determined in everyone at some interval. Even though hyperparathyroidism and hypercalcemia of malignancy are of much lower incidence than thyroid disease or diabetes mellitus, determinations of serum calcium ion levels can be easily obtained as part of an automated panel of tests (Chapter 8). Finally, clues to endocrine diseases can be obtained from other abnormalities detected in screening, eg, blood counts and serum electrolyte measurements.

CLINICAL INTERPRETATION OF LABORATORY TESTS

Many salient points in interpreting laboratory tests are mentioned in the preceding sections; these and other points can be summarized as follows:

(1) Any result must be interpreted in light of clinical knowledge about the patient based on the history and physical examination.

(2) Basal levels of hormones or peripheral effects of hormones must be interpreted in light of the way the hormone is released and controlled.

(3) Hormone levels must be interpreted in conjunction with information from other tests that reflect the patient's status: serum PTH levels in conjunction with serum calcium levels (Chapter 8), serum aldosterone levels in conjunction with plasma renin levels (Chapters 9 and 10), serum gonadotropin levels in conjunction with serum estradiol (Chapter 13) or testosterone (Chapter 12) levels, etc.

(4) Occasionally, urinary measurements are superior to plasma tests for assaying the integrated release of hormone. With cortisol, salivary levels are used increasingly.

(5) Ranges of normal values vary from one laboratory to the next. The range for the laboratory utilized should be employed.

(6) Laboratory tests must be interpreted with knowledge of the value of the test, including its sensitivity and specificity (discussed earlier). Reported normal ranges for tests cannot be used as absolute reflections of excess or deficiency states and must be interpreted in light of the clinical situation.

(7) Occasionally, extraneous or contaminating substances interfere with laboratory test results. For example, in illness, plasma lipids sometimes interfere with measurement of thyroid hormone-binding capacity (Chapter 7).

(8) Provocative tests are sometimes necessary.

(9) Imaging studies may help with the diagnosis, especially with respect to the source of hormone hypersecretion.

TREATMENT OF ENDOCRINE DISEASES

Treatment of hormone deficiency states ideally requires replacement with the hormone in a manner that mimics the physiologic setting. In many cases, a reasonable approximation of the physiologic status can be achieved by administering the hormone itself or an analog. Thus, treatment of hypothyroidism with thyroxine, adrenal insufficiency with hydrocortisone, and menopausal symptoms with estrogens have proved effective. In other cases, there are problems with replacement therapy. Whereas recombinant GH is available to treat GH deficiency, it must be injected and is expensive. Whereas PTH has recently been approved by the Food and Drug Administration for treatment of osteoporosis, this peptide hormone is short-acting and may be an inefficient way to treat hypoparathyroidism. Thus, most patients with this disorder will probably continue to be treated with high doses of vitamin D and calcium (Chapter 8). Although insulin therapy controls hyperglycemia and prevents ketoacidosis in most patients with diabetes mellitus, long-term complications still occur with most regimens (Chapter 17). This results at least in part from the fact that we do not replace insulin in an ideal manner. When the hormone is injected subcutaneously, it is not delivered first to the liver; the kinetics of the injected hormone do not mimic accurately enough the physiologic release of insulin; and in many cases the delicate balance between normalization of blood glucose and avoidance of hypoglycemia cannot be achieved. For diseases such as type 1 diabetes mellitus, there is a major need for alternative approaches, as might ultimately be achieved through gene transfer, islet transplantation, mechanical pumps linked to glucose sensors, improved versions of insulin, or other means. Diabetes mellitus also illustrates the fact that the control of conditions such as hyperglycemia or hypertension that usually occur in diabetic patients can have a major effect. Indeed, treating high blood pressure in type 2 diabetes is as important as excellent glycemic control.

Since many cases of type 1 diabetes mellitus, Addison's disease, hypothyroidism, and several other endocrine deficiency states result from autoimmune destruction of the gland, there is a clear need to predict the emergence of the condition and to prevent or limit the damage in the first place. It is already clear that measurement of the levels of certain antibodies with type 1 diabetes mellitus, thyroid disease, and other endocrine deficiency states can predict the development of the disorder before there is major destruction of the gland. For hormone excess states, treatment is ordinarily directed at the primary cause, usually a tumor, autoimmune condition, or hyperplasia. Tumors are removed when possible. Improvements in surgical techniques have decreased the mortality and morbidity rates associated with surgical removal of tumors of the endocrine system. In addition, alternative and less invasive approaches are supplanting the need for traditional surgery. For example, laparoscopic surgical techniques are being used for removal of tumors inside the abdomen. We cannot yet cure the autoimmune condition that results in hyperthyroidism, so therapy is directed at reducing the secretions of the thyroid gland by pharmacologic blockade, radioiodine therapy, or surgical removal (Chapter 7). Hormone production may also be blocked by pharmacologic means in many other instances. For example, with prolactin hypersecretion, use of the dopamine receptor agonist bromocriptine is preferred to surgical removal of a small prolactinoma (Chapter 5). Octreotide acetate, a somatostatin analog, is sometimes used to block GH hypersecretion (Chapter 6). Inhibitors of steroid production such as ketoconazole are used as an alternative to surgical removal of the steroid-producing tissue (Chapter 9). Mineralocorticoid receptor antagonists (Table 1–2) are used to treat primary aldosteronism, especially when the disorder is due to hyperplasia.

In many cases, it is necessary to control sequelae of hormone excess by alternative means. Thus, β-adrenergic receptor blockers are useful to control sequelae of hyperthyroidism (Chapter 7), α-adrenergic blockers to control sequelae of pheochromocytoma (Chapter 11), mineralocorticoid antagonists to control blood pressure and hypokalemia in primary aldosteronism (Chapter 10), and inhibitors of cholesterol biosynthesis to treat hypercholesterolemia (Chapter 19). With hypertension, a number of modalities are available to block hormone systems. Examples are angiotensin-converting enzyme inhibitors, which block the renin-angiotensin system; calcium channel or β-adrenergic blockers to inhibit second-messenger signaling; or diuretics to lower blood volume.

■ USES OF HORMONES & SELECTIVE MODULATORS IN THERAPY OF NONENDOCRINE DISEASE

The diverse actions of hormones and hormone antagonists have allowed them to be used extensively in therapy for nonendocrine disease. Hormone action can also be blocked with the use of enzyme inhibitors. Tables 1–2 and 1–4 list examples of hormone and hormone analog agonists (including eicosanoids) and antagonists. The most extensively used agonists are the glucocorticoids that are given to millions of patients to suppress inflammatory and immunologic responses. That the glucocorticoids would have this application came as a great surprise to the medical world. Hench, Kendall, and Reichstein received the Nobel Prize for this discovery about 1 year after cortisone was first used to treat a patient with rheumatoid arthritis. Other examples include the use of estrogen-progesterone combinations for contraception, GnRH analogs such as leuprolide in combination with nonsteroidal antiandrogens to treat prostate cancer, and antiestrogens to treat breast cancer (Table 1–2). Selective ER modulators such as raloxifene are used for treatment of osteoporosis but may also have benefits in reducing breast cancer incidence. It is likely that the numbers of treatments that are based on modulation or selective modulation of endocrine signaling pathways will increase in the future as new pharmaceuticals become available.

Table 1–4. Hormones used in endocrinologic management for purposes other than replacement.

Hormone or Analog	Use	Evaluation
Glucocorticoid	Suppression of inflammatory or immune responses	
Growth hormone	Small stature	Wasting syndromes Osteoporosis
PTH	Osteoporosis	Osteoporosis
IGF-I		Osteoporosis Wasting syndromes
Octreotide acetate	Inhibition of GH release Diarrhea	
Progesterone	Contraception	
Estrogens	Prostate cancer	
Testosterone	Breast cancer	
Prostaglandins	Induce labor, terminate pregnancy, maintain patent ductus arteriosus at surgery	

REFERENCES

General

Alberts B et al: *Molecular Biology of the Cell,* 4th ed. Garland, 2002.

Baxter JD et al: Introduction to the endocrine system. In: *Endocrinology and Metabolism,* 3rd ed. Felig P, Baxter JD, Frohman LA (editors). McGraw-Hill, 1995.

Berg JM, Tymoczko JL, Stryer L: *Biochemistry,* 5th ed. Freeman, 2002.

Frohman L et al: The clinical manifestations of endocrine disease. In: *Endocrinology and Metabolism,* 3rd ed. Felig P, Baxter JD, Frohman LA (editors). McGraw-Hill, 1995.

Habener JF: Genetic control of hormone formation. In: *Williams Textbook of Endocrinology,* 9th ed. Wilson JD et al (editors). Saunders, 1998.

Wilson JD et al: Principles of endocrinology. In: *Williams Textbook of Endocrinology,* 9th ed. Wilson JD et al (editors). Saunders, 1998.

Hormone Actions and Mechanisms

Chang L, Karin M: Mammalian MAP kinase signalling cascades. Nature 2001;410:37. [PMID: 11242034]

Chawla A et al: Nuclear receptors and lipid physiology: opening the X-files. Science 2001;294:1866. [PMID: 11729302]

Glass CK, Rosenfeld MG: The coregulator exchange in transcriptional functions of nuclear receptors. Genes Dev 2000;14: 121. [PMID: 10652267]

Giguere V: Orphan nuclear receptors: from gene to function. Endocr Rev 1999;20:689. [PMID: 10529899]

Kahn CR, Smith RJ, Chin WW: Mechanisms of action of hormones that act at the cell surface. In: *Williams Textbook of Endocrinology,* 9th ed. Wilson JD et al (editors). Saunders, 1998.

McKenna NJ, O'Malley BW: Combinatorial control of gene expression by nuclear receptors and coregulators. Cell 2002; 108:465. [PMID: 11909518]

Ribeiro RC et al: Mechanisms of thyroid hormone action: insights from X-ray crystallographic and functional studies. Recent Prog Horm Res 1998;53:351. [PMID: 9769715]

Re R: The nature of intracrine peptide hormone action. Hypertension 1999;34:534. [PMID: 10523322]

Weatherman RV et al: Nuclear receptor ligands and ligand-binding domains. Annu Rev Biochem 1999;68:559. [PMID: 10872460]

Pharmacology: Agonist and Antagonist Therapy

DeFronzo RA: Pharmacologic therapy for type 2 diabetes mellitus. Ann Intern Med 1999;131:281. [PMID: 10454950]

Gilman AG et al (editors): *Goodman and Gilman's The Pharmacological Basis of Therapeutics,* 9th ed. McGraw-Hill, 1996.

Katzung BG: *Basic and Clinical Pharmacology,* 8th ed. McGraw-Hill, 2000.

McDonnell DP et al: Elucidation of the molecular mechanism of selective estrogen receptor modulators. Am J Cardiol 2002; 90:35F. [PMID: 12106639]

Tyrrell JB: Glucocorticoid therapy. In: *Endocrinology and Metabolism,* 3rd ed. Felig P, Baxter JD, Frohman LA (editors). McGraw-Hill, 1995.

Vance ML, Mauras N: Growth hormone therapy in adults and children. N Engl J Med 1999;341:1206. [PMID: 10519899]

Molecular Biology, Genomics, and Proteomics

Altshuler DM et al: The common PPARgamma Pro12Ala polymorphism is associated with decreased risk of type 2 diabetes. Nat Genet 2000;26:76. [PMID: 10973253]

Gagel RF, Baxter JD: The impact of sequencing of the human genome on endocrinology. In: *Genetics and Endocrinology.* Modern Endocrinology series. Baxter JD, Melmed S, New MI (editors). Lippincott Williams & Wilkins, 2002.

Brown PO, Botstein D: Exploring the new world of the genome with DNA microarrays. Nat Genet 1999;21:33. [PMID: 9915498]

Busch CP, Hegele RA: Genetic determinants of type 2 diabetes mellitus. Clin Genet 2001;50:243. [PMID: 9915498]

Feng X et al: Thyroid hormone regulation of hepatic genes in vivo detected by complementary DNA microarray. Mol Endocrinol 2000;14:947. [PMID: 10894146]

Gardner DG, Gertz BJ: Gene expression and recombinant DNA in endocrinology and metabolism. In: *Endocrinology and Metabolism,* 3rd ed. Felig P, Baxter JD, Frohman LA (editors). McGraw-Hill, 1995.

Ho Y et al: Systematic identification of protein complexes in *Saccharomyces cerevisiae* by mass spectrometry. Nature 2002; 415;180. [PMID: 11805837]

Lifton RP et al: Molecular mechanisms of human hypertension. Cell 2001;104:545. [PMID: 11805837]

Maglich JM et al: Comparison of the complete nuclear receptor sets from the human, *Caenorhabditis elegans* and *Drosophila* genomes. Genome Biol 2001;2:1. [PMID: 11532213]

Richer JK et al: Differential gene regulation by the two progesterone receptor isoforms in human breast cancer cells. J Biol Chem 2002;277:5209. [PMID: 11717311]

Stride A, Hattersley AT: Different genes, different diabetes: lessons of maturity-onset diabetes of the young. Ann Med 2002; 34:207. [PMID: 12087034]

Evolution of the Endocrine System

Baxter JD, Rousseau GG: Glucocorticoids and the metabolic code. In: *Glucocorticoid Hormone Action.* Baxter JD, Rousseau GG (editors). Springer, 1979.

Dasen JS, Rosenfeld MG: Combinatorial codes in signaling and synergy: lessons from pituitary development. Curr Opin Genet Dev 1999;9:566. [PMID: 10508698]

Patthy L: Genome evolution and the evolution of exon-shuffling—a review. Gene 1999;238:103. [PMID: 10570989]

Tomkins GM: The metabolic code. Science 1975;189:760. [PMID: 169670]

Hormone Resistance and Mechanisms of Disease

Brown EM: Physiology and pathophysiology of the extracellular calcium-sensing receptor. Am J Med 1999;106:238. [PMID: 10230755]

Jenkins RC, Ross RJ: Acquired growth hormone resistance in adults. Baillieres Clin Endocrinol Metab 1998;12:315. [PMID: 10083899]

Kahn BB: Type 2 diabetes: when insulin secretion fails to compensate for insulin resistance. Cell 1998;92:593. [PMID: 9506512]

Malloy PJ, Pike JW, Feldman D: The vitamin D receptor and the syndrome of hereditary 1,25-dihydroxyvitamin D-resistant rickets. Endocr Rev 1999;20:156. [PMID: 10204116]

Neves FAR et al: Resistance to glucocorticoid and mineralocorticoid hormones. In: *Genetics and Endocrinology.* Modern Endocrinology series. Baxter JD, Melmed S, New MI (editors). Lippincott Williams and Wilkins, 2002.

New MI et al: Resistance to several steroids in two sisters. J Clin Endocrinol Metab 1999;84:4454. [PMID: 10599702]

Pohlenz J et al: Five new families with resistance to thyroid hormone not caused by mutations in the thyroid hormone receptor beta gene. J Clin Endocrinol Metab 1999;84:3919. [PMID: 10566629]

Shulman GI: Cellular mechanisms of insulin resistance in humans. Am J Cardiol 1999;84:3J. [PMID: 10418851]

Assays as Diagnostic Procedures

Diamandis EP, Christopolos TK: *Immunoassay.* Academic Press, 1996.

Pekary AE, Hershman JM: Hormone assays. In: *Endocrinology and Metabolism,* 3rd ed. Felig P, Baxter JD, Frohman LA (editors). McGraw-Hill, 1995.

Segre GV, Brown EN: Measurement of hormones. In: *Williams Textbook of Endocrinology,* 9th ed. Wilson JD et al (editors). Saunders, 1998.

Hormone Synthesis & Release

2

Vishwanath R. Lingappa, MD, PhD, & Synthia H. Mellon, PhD

ACAT	Acyl-coenzyme A: cholesterol acyl-transferase	**MAO**	Monoamine oxidase
ACTH	Adrenocorticotropic hormone	**M6P**	Mannose-6-phosphate
ATP	Adenosine triphosphate	**NAC**	Nascent chain-associated complex
BIP	Immunoglobulin-binding protein	**NADPH**	Reduced nicotinamide adenine dinucleotide phosphate
CBG	Corticosteroid-binding globulin	**NMDA**	N-Methyl-D-aspartate
COMT	Catechol-O-methyltransferase	**NSF**	N-Ethyl maleimide-sensitive factor
COP	Coat-associated protein	**POMC**	Proopiomelanocortin
DHEA	Dehydroepiandrosterone	**SCP-2**	Sterol carrier protein-2
DHEAS	Dehydroepiandrosterone sulfate	**SHBG**	Sex hormone-binding globulin
EGF	Epidermal growth factor	**SNAP**	Soluble NSF-attachment protein
ER	Endoplasmic reticulum	**SRP**	Signal recognition particle
FSH	Follicle-stimulating hormone	**StAR**	Steroidogenic acute regulator
GABA	Gamma-aminobutyric acid	**TBG**	Thyroid hormone-binding globulin
GDP	Guanosine diphosphate	**TGN**	Trans Golgi network
GTP	Guanosine triphosphate	**TRAM**	Translocating chain-associated membrane protein
HDL	High-density lipoprotein		
HETE	Hydroxyeicosatetraenoic acid	**TSH**	Thyroid-stimulating hormone
HPETE	Hydroxyperoxyeicosatetraenoic acid	**t-SNARE**	Target membrane SNAP receptor
IGF	Insulin-like growth factor	**VMA**	Vanillylmandelic acid
LDL	Low-density lipoprotein	**v-SNARE**	Vesicle membrane SNAP receptor
LH	Luteinizing hormone		

COMPARTMENTATION OF EUKARYOTIC CELLS IN RELATION TO HORMONE SYNTHESIS & RELEASE

A fundamental feature of eukaryotic cells is the presence of a multiplicity of intracellular membrane-delimited compartments. A number of these intracellular compartments are related as components of the **secretory pathway** (discussed further below). The luminal spaces (ie, those within membrane vesicles) of these compartments are generally oxidizing environments, equivalent to the outside world (see Figure 2–1). Across the membrane from the luminal space of these compartments is the cytoplasm, which is a reducing environment with very different protein content and enzyme activities. All hormones start their biosynthesis in the cytoplasm and must be released into the outside world by processes of secretion in order to exert their biologic effects. As we shall see, compartmentation provides both challenges and opportunities for hormone biosynthesis and regulation.

38

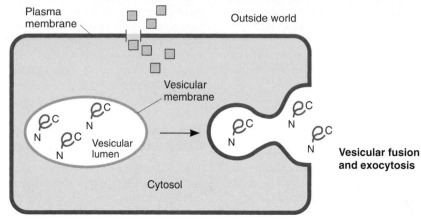

Figure 2–1. Conceptual framework for thinking about vesicular and nonvesicular modes of hormone secretion. Schematic diagram of a cell, indicating that some hormones are transported in vesicles to the cell surface and released in quanta upon fusion of the vesicle with the plasma membrane, while other hormones are transported directly across the plasma membrane either by specific transporters or by diffusion. Vesicular secretion can be regulated separately at the level of synthesis and of release, while control over synthesis is the only known way to regulate hormones released in a nonvesicular manner. Examples of hormones secreted in a vesicle-mediated fashion are most polypeptide hormones and catecholamines. Examples of hormones released in a nonvesicular manner are the eicosanoids, steroids, and thyroid hormones.

OVERVIEW OF HORMONE BIOSYNTHESIS

Any molecule delivered via the bloodstream that can be recognized by a receptor in or on a target cell in a manner that conveys information can, in principle, be used by the body as a hormone. In the course of evolution, an enormous variety of molecules have been utilized as hormones by various organisms. With this diversity of hormone structure comes a corresponding variety in modes of hormone biosynthesis. In this chapter, we shall summarize current concepts of hormone synthesis and release.

Hormones can be divided into two broad classes (Figure 2–1). The first class consists of those that are stored in membrane vesicles. These hormones are released from an endocrine cell by fusion of membrane vesicles with the plasma membrane, typically in response to a stimulus for secretion that may or may not be coupled with the stimulus for hormone synthesis. Hormones of this class are often synthesized and then stored for later release. After release of stored hormone upon fusion of membrane vesicles with the plasma membrane, the "empty" membrane is recycled by a process known as **endocytosis.** The second broad class

of hormones consists of those secreted immediately upon synthesis in a manner not mediated by membrane vesicle fusion. For these hormones, there is typically no distinction between the stimulus for synthesis and the stimulus for release—hence, control over synthesis is the major means known for regulating their secretion.

The **polypeptide hormones** comprise the most prominent example of hormones whose release is vesicle-mediated, and their secretion involves transit through multiple membrane-delimited compartments of the classic secretory pathway (see below). However, the vesicle-mediated pathway is also used for the secretion of a number of nonpolypeptide hormones and neurotransmitters such as catecholamines (eg, dopamine) and γ-aminobutyric acid (GABA). These small molecules do not undergo the full range of intracellular trafficking events involving transport through multiple intracellular compartments that is seen in protein secretion. These nonpolypeptide hormones are either newly synthesized in the cytoplasm or are taken up by specific transporters from outside the cell and pumped back into recycled empty vesicles in preparation for another round of vesicle fusion and secretion. As will be summarized below, great progress has been made in recent years in our understanding of the molecular mechanisms of vesicular traffic involved in biosynthesis and release of both peptide and nonpeptide hormones.

Classes of hormones released by non-vesicle-mediated mechanisms include the **steroids** (**glucocorticoids, androgens, estrogens,** and **mineralocorticoids**—all derived from cholesterol) and the **eicosanoids** (a family of fatty acid-derived signaling molecules that include the **prostaglandins**). Exactly how non-vesicle-mediated release occurs is not as well understood as vesicular secretion. Historically, simple diffusion was assumed to be the mechanism both for release from the hormone-producing cells and for entry into target cells. In recent years, however, specific transporters have been implicated in directing some of these classes of molecules out of the cell. Whether all non-vesicle fusion-mediated secretion will prove to be driven by transporters through specific channels or whether some hormones leave the cell solely by diffusion remains a subject for future investigation.

MEMBRANE VESICLE-MEDIATED HORMONE EXPORT

With the exception of a very small number of proteins synthesized within the mitochondrial matrix and in plants, within chloroplasts, most proteins made in eukaryotic cells are synthesized on ribosomes in the cytoplasm. Proteins that reside in the cytoplasm are not generally released in the absence of cell damage or death. Thus, specialized mechanisms must exist to discriminate between newly synthesized proteins that are destined to be secreted and those that are to remain in the cytoplasm.

The polypeptide hormones are an important subset of secretory proteins, and the classic secretory pathway by which they leave the cell is the best-understood mechanism of hormone export. It appears to be the mechanism used for most but not all polypeptide hormones and can be separated into early and late events. The early events involve getting the newly synthesized secretory protein into the luminal space of the **endoplasmic reticulum (ER),** a membrane-delimited compartment. In the course of those early events, the protein must be properly folded and is often covalently modified, eg, by the addition of carbohydrates. The late events involve transport of the properly synthesized, folded, and modified protein from the ER lumen to the lumen of other membrane-delimited compartments, including the **Golgi apparatus,** and subsequently to **secretory granules** and ultimately, upon fusion of a secretory granule with the plasma membrane, out of the cell. Whereas the early events involve direct transfer of the individual secretory polypeptides across the lipid bi-

layer of the ER membrane, in the later events movement of secretory proteins occurs exclusively by transport within a membrane system—or by budding of membrane vesicles from one compartment and their subsequent fusion with another compartment. Thus, the protein cargo moves from vesicle to vesicle without ever again actually crossing a lipid bilayer directly (Figure 2–1).

Targeting to the Membrane of the Endoplasmic Reticulum

The early events of polypeptide hormone targeting to and translocation across the ER membrane generally occur while the protein is still being synthesized. The mechanism that appears to have evolved as the major pathway of ER membrane translocation in eukaryotes involves a sort of molecular "ZIP code" termed the **signal sequence,** which is found as part of nascent secretory proteins (Figure 2–2). The signal sequence is a sequence of amino acid residues encoded in the mRNA, usually but not always at the 5′ end of the coding region and thus usually occurring at the amino terminal of the encoded protein. Signal sequences typically are composed of three domains, including a stretch of hydrophobic residues. While the hydrophobicity was once thought to relate to interaction with the lipid bilayer, it now seems more likely that it reflects features recognized by other proteins which serve as receptors for signal sequences. Curiously, signal sequences display a substantial heterogeneity from one protein to another. This was once interpreted as meaning that hydrophobicity rather than specific sequence was important for signal sequence function. However, recent findings suggest that even subtle differences in the specific sequence of the hydrophobic domain can have dramatic functional effects due to altered protein-protein interactions (see below).

The signal sequence typically emerges from the ribosome as part of the nascent protein chain and is quickly bound by a cytoplasmic ribonucleoprotein complex composed of six polypeptides and a small RNA, termed **signal recognition particle (SRP),** that serves to target the nascent chain to the membrane of the ER. "Professional" secretory tissues such as endocrine glands often contain a substantial amount of "rough" ER visible under the electron microscope, so-called because of the presence of ribosomes bound to the ER membrane that have been targeted there through the action of SRP.

In molecular terms, SRP serves in two ways to facilitate translocation of nascent secretory proteins across the ER membrane. First, binding of SRP to both the signal sequence and the ribosome slows the rate of chain elongation, thereby increasing the "window of

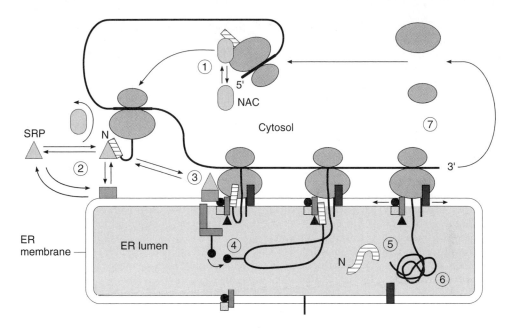

Figure 2–2. Translocation of nascent polypeptide hormones across the ER membrane. Key steps in polypeptide hormone biosynthesis and secretion are indicated by the circled numbers. (1) Ribosomes from the free cytoplasmic pool initiate translation of mRNA encoding secretory proteins. A protein complex termed nascent chain associated complex (NAC) appears to prevent inappropriate or premature targeting of the nascent chain. (2) The initial codons encode a signal sequence that emerges from the ribosome and will serve to target the nascent secretory chain to the ER membrane by virtue of the affinity of a cytosolic particle termed signal recognition particle (SRP) for both the signal sequence and a receptor in the ER membrane. SRP binding displaces NAC from the nascent chain; SRP docking to the ER membrane displaces the nascent chain from SRP. (3) Assembly of a channel across the ER membrane provides a pathway for the nascent growing chain to enter the ER lumen. Translocation involves a ribosome-membrane junction sufficiently "tight" to shield the nascent growing chain from the cytoplasm, thereby preventing the cytoplasm from being secreted into the ER lumen. (4) During translocation, the chain is subject to a host of cotranslational modifications including the addition of carbohydrates which are transferred as a preformed structure composed of 11 carbohydrate residues from lipid carriers to the protein. (5) Translocation-associated events in polypeptide hormone biogenesis usually include cleavage of the signal sequence. (6) As the chain emerges into the ER lumen, folding occurs, governed by molecular chaperones in the ER lumen. (7) After completion of protein synthesis, the ribosome subunits are released back into the free cytosolic pool, the channel disassembles or closes, and the folded chain is localized to the ER lumen.

time" during which the chain can find the cytoplasmic face of the ER while still nascent and thus still able to be translocated into the lumen. Most proteins cannot be translocated after their synthesis has been completed and they have been released from the ribosome. In part this may be because most nascent chains need to be at least partly unfolded for translocation. The cotranslational requirement may also in part reflect a role for the ribosome in opening the channels through which translocation occurs (see below).

Second, when bound to a signal sequence, SRP undergoes conformational changes resulting in high affinity for a receptor on the ER membrane (termed the **SRP receptor**), thereby targeting the nascent chain to the correct subcellular location. It would be inefficient, for example, to target a secretory protein to the mitochondria by accident.

Upon binding the SRP receptor, SRP undergoes another conformational change that releases the signal sequence and the ribosome, allowing the rate of chain elongation to increase and freeing the signal sequence and nascent chain to interact with other proteins in the ER membrane. During the same time, a functional ribosome membrane junction forms by interaction with receptor proteins.

Some of the proteins that comprise both SRP and the SRP receptor are GTP binding proteins, and it appears that cycles of GDP-GTP exchange and GTP hydrolysis serve to ensure the fidelity of targeting and the unidirectionality of several of the early events in translocation, including at least (1) signal recognition by SRP, (2) targeting of the nascent ribosome-signal sequence-SRP complex to the SRP receptor, (3) assembly of the translocation channel, and (4) release of SRP to participate in another round of targeting.

Finally, a non-SRP-mediated pathway of targeting has been described in yeast. Thus, SRP-deficient yeast mutants are viable but grow slowly. Some proteins in these mutants are severely affected by lack of SRP while others appear largely unaffected, presumably because they can target to the ER membrane as efficiently by non-SRP-mediated mechanisms. The full significance of this finding remains to be established. However, it is consistent with the concept that crucial biologic recognition systems have evolved a degree of redundancy in case (for whatever reason) the primary recognition system should fail.

Translocation Across the ER Membrane

Once targeted, the nascent chain must somehow traverse the ER membrane, which is otherwise a barrier to movement of most proteins from the cytosol to the ER lumen. Upon release from SRP, the correctly targeted signal sequence appears to interact with other proteins in the ER membrane to open a channel to the ER lumen. The growing polypeptide chain—but not other proteins or even the ions in the cytosol—has access to the channel. The nascent chain is translocated through this channel into the lumen of the ER, tightly shielded from the cytosol by the ribosome-membrane junction. It appears that there are "gates" at each end of the translocation channel. Recent studies suggest that another form of regulation involves transient opening of the ribosome-membrane junction directed by particular sequences present in some nascent proteins. As a consequence, translocation across the ER membrane is interrupted and specific domains of nascent secretory proteins are exposed to the cytoplasm prior to reestablishment of a tight ribosome-membrane junction and resumption of translocation (see below).

In addition to the GTP hydrolysis-dependent steps of targeting, subsequent steps of translocation also appear to involve ATP hydrolysis. The precise role of the energy requirement of chain translocation—apart from that involving GTP hydrolysis for targeting—remains unclear. Perhaps the energy of ATP hydrolysis is needed to form or maintain the channel in an open conformation, or to actually pull the chain across the membrane, as has been suggested for protein secretion in bacteria. Alternatively, ATP may be hydrolyzed as part of the action of molecular chaperones acting on the chain in the ER lumen, and the actual translocation may even occur by brownian motion without any requirement for ATP hydrolysis.

Major progress has been made in recent years in identifying ER membrane proteins involved in nascent chain translocation across the ER membrane. It appears that at least two membrane protein complexes, the heterodimeric SRP receptor and the heterotrimeric Sec 61p complex, are involved in translocation of essentially every secretory protein. A third membrane protein, termed translocating chain-associated membrane protein (TRAM), is involved in translocation of most but not all secretory proteins. Roles for other accessory proteins in translocation of specific subsets of polypeptides or in more complex modification events associated with translocation of particular proteins have been demonstrated in some cases. Together, the complex of proteins involved in both translocation and modification of newly synthesized secretory proteins is termed the translocon. Recent studies have strongly suggested that the translocon in eukaryotes is an aqueous protein-lined, protein-conducting pore. Yet lipids appear to have at least transient access to the nascent chain during its translocation, perhaps reflecting the dynamic and transient nature of a channel rapidly assembled and disassembled from component subunits. Upon completion of secretory protein synthesis, the ribosomal subunits release from the cytoplasmic side of the ER membrane and the transmembrane channel disassembles or in some other way closes, leaving the newly synthesized secretory protein localized to the luminal space of the ER with no way to return to the cytosol (Figure 2–2).

Co- & Posttranslational Modification of Proteins

During translocation across the ER, subsequently within the ER lumen, and in a variety of later membrane-delimited compartments, newly synthesized proteins may be subject to literally dozens of possible processing events that often vary from protein to protein, tissue to tissue, and species to species. Some of these modifications are covalent—eg, proteolytic removal of the signal sequence, disulfide bond formation, and addition of various moieties to amino acid side chains (eg, carbohydrates). Other modifications are noncovalent, such as proper folding of newly synthesized polypeptides under the supervision of families of proteins termed **molecular chaperones** that are present in the cytosol, ER membrane, and ER lumen. Only a small number of the many possible modifications that are possible actually occur on any given specific protein, and some proteins appear to receive no modifications at all. Furthermore, even for those specific proteins which receive covalent modifications, the modifications are heterogeneous. That is, some copies of the protein receive the full complement of modifications, while other copies receive only some or even no modifications at all. A body of work suggests that these differences are not random or stochastic events but rather may be regulated and of functional significance for hormone action (see below). For the few modifications that have been well studied, it appears that either primary amino acid sequence motifs or secondary or tertiary structural features of a particular newly synthesized protein are recognized by the enzymes that carry out these modifications.

Perhaps the best-understood posttranslational modification is a subset of carbohydrate addition termed N-linked glycosylation (Figure 2–2). This form of glycosylation occurs on selected asparagine residues during translocation of the nascent chain into the ER lumen. The carbohydrate units consist of up to 14 sugars that are assembled in a tree-like structure on lipid transporters called **dolichols.** The entire sugar tree is then transferred en bloc to selected asparagine residues of the nascent protein as it enters the ER lumen (hence the term "N-linked" glycosylation). Subsequently, the individual sugars that comprise the sugar tree are modified, with some removed and others added, in the ER and in more distal compartments of the secretory pathway.

In most cases, the precise functions of the various covalent co- and posttranslational modifications, including N-linked glycosylation, are unknown. However, as will be discussed below, two important roles for N-linked carbohydrates in facilitating proper sorting and traffic of some proteins through the secretory pathway have been discovered. In other cases, changes in carbohydrates have been shown to alter the activity of particular hormones once secreted, either by affecting the affinity of binding to hormone receptors or by altering the clearance from the bloodstream and hence the half-life and effective concentration of the particular hormone in blood. An important frontier of hormone biosynthesis and action is to understand the significance of the observed heterogeneity in modification of hormones and how it is regulated.

Quality Control by the ER

Within the ER lumen, molecular chaperones not only facilitate proper folding of the newly arrived polypep-

tide, they also assess the outcome of folding. Often, as a result of interaction with molecular chaperones, proteins deemed improperly folded are not allowed to leave the ER even though, in at least some cases, those proteins appear sufficiently well folded to be capable of physiologic function in vitro. This "quality control" function appears to be a major role of the ER in the scheme of protein biogenesis. Whether the molecular chaperones that carry out these recognition events for protein folding and quality control also play a role in the actual translocation of proteins into the ER lumen remains controversial. For example, the protein BIP (immunoglobulin-binding protein) has been implicated by some work as a "plug" preventing proteins from leaking back into the cytosol. Other work suggested that BIP may be part of a "molecular ratchet" pulling proteins into the ER lumen via the translocation channel.

In the case of one particular ER molecular chaperone, termed **calnexin,** trimming of the glucose units at the end of the N-linked carbohydrate tree appears to serve as a monitor of the need for further chaperone action for at least some newly synthesized proteins. Calnexin binds these unfolded chains upon trimming of the outer two of the three glucose residues found on the N-linked carbohydrate tree. Like other molecular chaperones, calnexin uses the energy from cycles of ATP hydrolysis to prevent misfolding of the newly synthesized protein. Upon completion of proper folding, the final glucose is trimmed, calnexin is released, and the protein is transported in vesicles out of the ER. If proper folding, as defined by the quality control machinery, is not achieved, glucose may be added back and multiple cycles of calnexin binding, folding, sugar trimming, and release allowed to occur. Calnexin is unusual among the molecular chaperones in that it recognizes the polar carbohydrate moiety. In the case of most other molecular chaperones, hydrophobic interactions seem to be the important determinants of interaction with substrates.

In a number of cases, proteins deemed to be improperly folded by the quality control machinery are not only prevented from leaving the ER, they are rapidly degraded as well. Some data suggest that in the case of some particularly complex secretory and integral membrane polypeptides, rapid degradation in the ER can be a point of regulation of protein biogenesis, multisubunit assembly, and secretion. At least one of the mechanisms of rapid degradation of newly synthesized proteins in the ER involves reverse translocation through the Sec 61p complex, conjugation to the cytoplasmic protein ubiquitin, and subsequent degradation in the cytoplasm by the proteasome.

What keeps the different compartments of the cell "on the same page" with each other in terms of maintaining the correct levels of activity for synthesis, maturation, degradation, etc? The unfolded protein response is a feedback loop, highly conserved from yeast to mammals, that serves as a model for such coordination. Accumulation of unfolded proteins in the ER results in activation of a kinase that signals to the nucleus the need to up-regulate transcription of genes encoding molecular chaperones involved in protein folding, thereby correcting the deficiency of molecular chaperones that resulted in unfolded protein accumulation in the first place. Recent work has implicated this pathway in the degradation of proteins as well. It is likely that many aspects of intracellular coordination between organelles are governed by similar feedback loops yet to be discovered.

The aforementioned summary of protein biogenesis, from synthesis and translocation to degradation or export out of the ER, represents the currently accepted general framework for the early events of the secretory pathway. However, many details relevant to endocrinology may not be fully explained by the simplest version of this paradigm. In particular, the heterogeneity of protein modifications on specific proteins is intriguing. Why does this heterogeneity exist if it is not significant? If significant, how is it achieved and regulated?

Many hormones have been implicated in multiple functions, but often only one major function has been well studied. Might heterogeneity of modification or folding of newly synthesized polypeptide hormones provide a basis for generating subsets of hormone molecules that are responsible for nonclassic hormone actions? Very recently there has been some insight into the regulation of pathways of maturation, which suggests that signal sequences previously thought to be involved only in targeting and translocation, as described above, may also play a role in selecting the precise pathway of maturation achieved by a given nascent chain. The mechanism by which signal sequences do this appears to be altering of the structural organization of the translocation channel through which the nascent protein traverses the ER membrane. This has been demonstrated for signal sequence mutations—but as yet unidentified protein-protein interactions involving the signal sequence could presumably have a similar effect. Thus, two copies of the identical protein traversing translocation channels of different organization could achieve different modifications or different folding and therefore could perform different functions. The precise mechanism by which this process is regulated remains to be fully understood; however, some data suggest that signal peptidase, the multicomponent enzyme which removes the signal sequence from the nascent chain by endoproteolytic cleavage, may be involved.

These findings have led to a provocative new hypothesis which suggests that many chains conventionally viewed as "misfolded" based on their rapid degradation in the ER under normal circumstances may in fact represent alternately folded forms with distinctive functions not wanted by the cell except at particular times—which are extremely transient and therefore hard to detect. Degradation in these cases is therefore not due to misfolding but occurs because the alternately folded forms are not desired at that particular time. Whether this phenomenon is general or is utilized by a few specialized proteins remains to be determined, though some recent data support this hypothesis when applied more generally to polypeptide hormones and their receptors. A protein that can be folded in two different ways both of which are functional is tantamount to being two different proteins—ie, each folded form has a different shape as seen by receptors in the "outside world". Thus, regulated folding of secretory and membrane proteins would have enormous implications for hormones and for the information content of the genome if it proves to be a phenomenon of many proteins.

Post-ER Vesicular Traffic in the Secretory Pathway

Translocation across the ER membrane is the only time that a secretory protein directly crosses a lipid bilayer. All subsequent trafficking steps involve movement within the confines of a membrane compartment (vesicular traffic), ie, the pinching-off of a membrane vesicle containing a cargo of newly synthesized protein from one membrane-delimited compartment and its transfer to another membrane compartment by fusion of the vesicle. Ultimately, vesicles fuse to the plasma membrane (exocytosis) or to the lysosome (lysosomal targeting; Figure 2–3). Concomitantly with traffic of vesicles through the secretory pathway, a recycling of membrane must occur. Both vesicular and tubular pathways of membrane recycling have been proposed (Figure 2–3).

The exact number of membrane subcompartments in the secretory pathway has yet to be determined. Indeed, in some cases the distinction between one compartment and the next may be largely semantic. At the least, all secretory proteins are transported in vesicles from their site of synthesis in the ER to a post-ER "intermediate" compartment from which vesicles deliver them to the Golgi apparatus. The intermediate compartment serves as a kind of recycling center from which proteins that should remain in the ER or which are not competent to progress down the secretory pathway are returned to the ER. Within the Golgi, they are transferred serially from the so-called cis-Golgi network to the medial Golgi stack, to the trans-Golgi stack, and finally to the trans-Golgi network (TGN) membrane cisternae. Each serial compartment is operationally de-

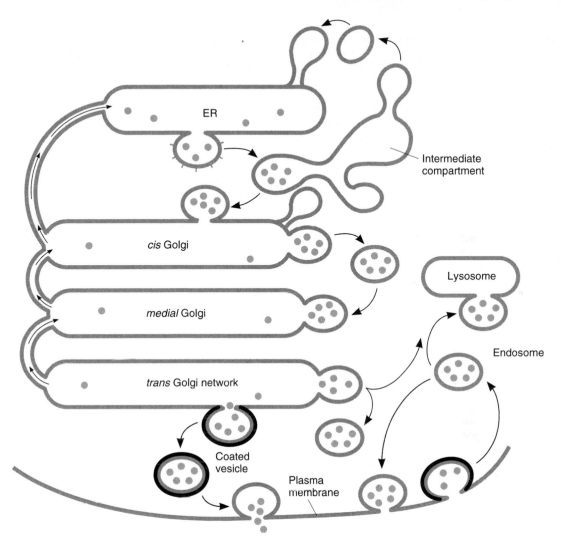

Figure 2–3. Membrane traffic in hormone-secreting cells. Polypeptide hormones travel through a variety of membrane compartments of the secretory pathway, with transport mediated by the fission and fusion of vesicles. Newly synthesized polypeptide hormones exit the ER and travel in vesicles to the intermediate compartment where they are concentrated by a number of different mechanisms, including recycling of "empty" containers back to the ER. Vesicles transport the proteins through the Golgi apparatus to the *trans* Golgi network whence other vesicles transport the proteins to either the regulated or constitutive secretory pathways or to lysosomes for degradation. In addition to forward transport, a pathway of retrograde transport, perhaps largely mediated by tubules rather than vesicles, returns membrane and some proteins to earlier compartments, including the ER and Golgi stacks. Endocytosis is the set of membrane-delimited trafficking pathways whereby hormones bound to receptors at the cell surface are internalized and transported either to the lysosome for degradation or back to the cell surface for re-release. The pathways of endocytosis and biogenesis can overlap in key compartments and share common features of mechanism—eg, the role of "coat" proteins in forming and targeting vesicles from *trans* Golgi network to plasma membrane during protein biogenesis and from plasma membrane to lysosome in endocytosis.

fined by localization of specific enzymes (such as those involved in modifying carbohydrates) to a particular subset of membranes. As more compartment-specific genes are cloned and monospecific antibodies generated to modifying enzymes, it is likely that additional subcompartments will be operationally distinguished within the currently understood secretory pathway. However, not every protein which traverses the secretory pathway receives a modification in any particular compartment as far as is known.

Trafficking of proteins through the vesicular stages of the secretory pathway involves recognition events both in the lumen, such as that described above for calnexin, and in the cytosol. The cytosolic recognition events involve cytoplasmically disposed domains of proteins within the vesicular membrane. Various families of small and large GTP-binding proteins have been implicated in control of these cytosolic recognition processes.

In a manner analogous to the mechanism targeting the nascent secretory protein to the ER membrane described above, cycles of GTP for GDP exchange followed by GTP hydrolysis ensure correct vesicle formation, docking, and fusion to the correct target compartment. Other GTP-binding proteins confer unidirectionality on the membrane fusion event, which is itself mediated by a "fusion machine" assembled from various proteins including some in the cytosol and some that were also involved in vesicle formation and targeting.

Differences in adapter proteins (including some that bind and hydrolyze GTP) and surface receptor proteins termed **v-SNARES** with cognate binding sites (termed **t-SNARES**) on the correct membrane of destination are believed to mediate the correct targeting of vesicles throughout the secretory pathway (Figure 2–4).

In some cases, various "coats" composed of specific proteins form on the outside of membranes, allowing them to be pinched off to form vesicles. A protein called **COP II** is found on vesicles that bud from the ER destined for the intermediate compartment. A protein called **COP I** is found on vesicles that return from the intermediate compartment back to the ER. Vesicles of different sizes, containing different classes of proteins as their cargo and destined for different subcellular fates, are often observed to have different coats or different adapter proteins that mediate assembly of a particular coat, permitting the resulting vesicle to be selectively targeted to the correct membrane destination. The TGN is the last compartment of the Golgi apparatus, from which vesicles are targeted to a variety of locations, including the regulated and constitutive secretory pathways and the lysosome (see below). Phosphatidylinositol transfer proteins greatly stimulate the formation of vesicles from the TGN. These negatively charged phospholipids may play a role in vesicle formation, per-

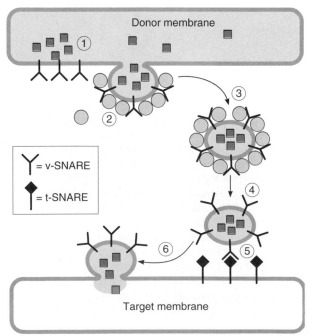

Figure 2–4. SNARE hypothesis for intracellular vesicular traffic. Vesicular traffic requires a means of discrimination on both sides of a membrane so that (1) products destined for one fate can be sorted from those with another, and (2) so that the sorted molecules can be correctly targeted to the correct subsequent membrane compartment. This includes a role for coat proteins that associate with the surface of a compartment to form or pinch off vesicles. (3) Once vesicles have formed—by budding from the so-called donor membrane—their trafficking is governed by recognition events between molecules termed v-SNAREs on their surface with molecules termed t-SNAREs on the surface of the target membrane. Before localization of cargo to the target compartment can be consummated, several events must occur in concert with v-SNARE–t-SNARE interaction, including uncoating (4), docking (5), and fusion (6). These events can be constitutive or regulated simply by placing one or more of them under control of a signal-transduction pathway.

haps by inducing membrane curvature or by recruiting coat proteins and other cytosolic components.

Membrane Trafficking Steps Prior to Sorting of Cargo

Through the TGN, the cargo contained within the vesicles that move from compartment to compartment is nonspecific, meaning that no sorting of content proteins has occurred. Thus, for example, a vesicle leaving the cis Golgi and targeted to the medial Golgi will contain a mixture of newly synthesized proteins including enzymes to be localized within the **lysosome** (an acidic membrane-bound organelle containing various hydrolytic enzymes that are active at low pH), proteins to be secreted continuously, and proteins to be secreted only in response to specific stimuli (ie, hormones). Likewise, the membrane of this vesicle contains various classes of membrane proteins with different destinations (eg, those targeted selectively to the apical plasma membrane and others targeted exclusively to the basolateral plasma membrane). While the cargo delivered to the TGN is nonspecific, the pathway followed by the vesicles is not. A vesicle derived from the cis Golgi must be selectively targeted to the medial Golgi and not the trans stack or back to the ER or to the plasma membrane. A separate pathway of vesicular transport is involved in "recycling" of membrane containers by return from cis Golgi to ER, etc. This recycling pathway is also used to return so-called resident proteins (such as BIP and calnexin) that need to be retained in a particular compartment such as the ER. It appears that at least one of the mechanisms involved is not retention per se but rather efficient *retrieval* of wayward polypeptides from the subsequent compartment. The coats of the intra-Golgi vesicles with nonspecific cargo and involved in recycling also contain a protein COP I. The coats of vesicles involved in ER to intermediate compartment and cis Golgi traffic contain the protein COP II.

Despite the nonspecific nature of their cargo, vesicle recognition events are probably occurring within the lumen of the ER and Golgi stack. For example, it was recently noted that some membrane proteins are concentrated in the intermediate compartment between ER and Golgi, strongly suggesting the occurrence of selective luminal recognition events. Whether this is true for all proteins or only for a subset within the nonspecific cargo remains to be determined.

A large body of evidence, summarized above, supports the notion that transfer from cis to medial to trans Golgi and TGN cisternae involves budding of vesicles from one compartment and their fusion to the next compartment within the Golgi apparatus. However, controversy has emerged as to the relative role of vesicles versus tubules of membranes that may connect one compartment with the next and whether one versus the other mechanism is involved in "forward" transport versus the return of "empty" membrane containers back to their compartment of origin. Recent work suggests that the concept of relatively fixed compartments of the Golgi complex, between which newly synthesized proteins are moved by vesicular traffic, may have to be at least partially revised in favor of a more dynamic "maturational" model in which cisternae progress from cis to medial to trans.

Sorting of Vesicle Cargo at the TGN

Unlike most vesicular transport from ER to TGN, true sorting occurs upon exit from the TGN. Vesicles leaving the TGN are heterogeneous with respect to both their cargo and their destination. Some vesicles are loaded with exclusively lysosomal enzymes and are targeted selectively to an acidic endosomal compartment in a pathway that will lead eventually to the lysosome or to a compartment which becomes a lysosome.

Other vesicles lead to the **regulated secretory pathway,** where the final vesicular fusion event of a secretory granule fusing to the plasma membrane to release the secretory proteins happens only upon specific stimulation. Thus, the stimulus to insulin release via the regulated secretory pathway is hypoglycemia; that of parathyroid hormone release is hypocalcemia; that of renin release includes adrenergic neural stimulation; etc. Some of the vesicles that are released by the regulated secretory pathway first condense their contents into a concentrated precipitate of secretory product and proteoglycans. These vesicles are termed secretory granules (see below). Other regulated secretory vesicles are morphologically distinguishable in that their contents do not undergo concentration. However, they do display stimulus-secretion coupling, the sine qua non of the regulated secretory pathway.

Still other vesicles, including those containing many membrane proteins, enter the **constitutive secretory pathway.** The constitutive pathway differs from the regulated pathway in that nothing prevents the final vesicle from fusing with the plasma membrane as soon as the vesicle has formed and been targeted—ie, no stimulus is required to overcome a preexisting block that prevents vesicle fusion to the plasma membrane in the absence of stimulus.

In addition to segregating content proteins with different subsequent vesicular destinations, the TGN sorting step sets in motion another set of posttranslational modifications. For example, the proteolytic processing of proinsulin to insulin and of pro-opiomelanocortin (POMC) into ACTH and other active peptides is initiated in the TGN and continues in the vesicles targeted to the regulated secretory pathway (see below).

The sorting event that occurs at the TGN is probably mediated by similar interactions on the cytosolic side of the vesicles, as just described for the vesicular transport of nonselective cargo—as well as by additional interactions that specifically connect the sorting event occurring on the luminal side with a particular targeting event on the cytosolic side. The best-defined of these TGN sorting events is that involved in diverting lysosomal enzymes from the common secretory pathway to the lysosome.

Lysosomal Enzyme Sorting

The lysosome is a membrane-delimited organelle in which various hydrolytic enzymes with an acid pH optimum are found. These enzymes—proteases, DNases, RNases, lipases, and the like—are used to break down macromolecules into recyclable building blocks that can be transported to the cytosol or elsewhere for reuse.

The lysosomal hydrolases that ultimately reside within the lysosome start out in the ER lumen, where they are glycosylated along with many other secretory proteins. Once in the cis Golgi, however, lysosomal enzymes are specifically recognized by an *N*-acetylglucosamine (GlcNAc) phosphotransferase, resulting in the addition of a GlcNAc phosphate moiety to the terminal mannose residue of their N-linked carbohydrate tree (exposed upon trimming of the glucose residues discussed above). Unlike the signal sequence, the recognition of lysosomal enzymes by GlcNAc phosphotransferase is not based on binding of a linear sequence of amino acid residues but is rather a function of affinity for a so-called **signal patch** composed of amino acid residues from different parts of the molecule that come together upon three-dimensional folding of the protein. This is an important experimental point since a single linear peptide is easy to define and manipulate, while a targeting-sorting signal composed of disparate parts of a protein is more difficult to analyze.

A subsequent enzyme removes the GlcNAc, exposing mannose 6-phosphate, which specifically binds a luminally disposed domain of the transmembrane mannose 6-phosphate receptor found in the TGN. The cytosolically disposed domain of the transmembrane mannose 6-phosphate receptor binds a specific adapter protein that catalyzes coat formation, vesicle budding, and targeting toward a prelysosomal, early endosomal compartment. Upon fusion with this membrane, the mannose 6-phosphate receptor and the lysosomal enzymes it has bound are exposed to a slightly acidic environment in which mannose 6-phosphate—and therefore the lysosomal enzymes—has much lower affinity for the M6P receptor, resulting in dissociation of lysosomal enzymes from the mannose 6-phosphate receptor. Once dissociation has occurred, the receptor is free

to recycle back to the TGN, leaving the lysosomal enzymes in the endosomal compartment, which can either fuse to late endosomes and ultimately to lysosomes or "mature" into first a late endosome and then into a lysosome. Recent data support the maturational model for the relationship of endosomes to lysosomes.

Note that the presence of an intermediate acidic compartment between TGN and lysosomes allowed recycling of mannose 6-phosphate receptors without subjecting them to the potentially damaging lysosomal environment. While the mannose 6-phosphate receptor pathway provides a framework for understanding one possible way in which sorting occurs, it is likely not to be the only way to sort lysosomal enzymes since patients with I cell disease, in which a mutant GlcNAc phosphotransferase fails to tag lysosomal enzymes, are observed to secrete their lysosomal enzymes from only some tissues (eg, fibroblasts but not liver). In liver and other tissues, lysosomal enzymes are correctly localized to the lysosome despite lack of the M6P tag, suggesting the existence of an alternative pathway for lysosomal enzyme recognition and sorting.

Regulated Secretion

Much of the recent progress in understanding the pathway of regulated secretion by which most hormones are released on specific stimulation comes from work on the molecular events of synaptic transmission, which can be viewed as a specific example of regulated secretion. Synaptic transmission occurs very quickly, placing limits on the number and nature of interactions, including simple diffusion, that can occur between stimulus and secretion. A number of proteins in the synaptic vesicular membrane have been identified and cloned, and functions have been ascribed to most. Many of these proteins are also found in neuroendocrine cells and are not exclusively neuronal proteins.

In both neurons and neuroendocrine cells, regulated secretion is dependent on an elevation of intracellular calcium. However, calcium probably acts at a number of different steps in each, involving both high- and low-affinity calcium receptor proteins. These steps probably include priming or docking of vesicles as well as vesicle fusion itself. They may also include events such as local disassembly of cytoskeletal proteins to allow secretory granules to dock at the plasma membrane. To date, the precise differences between neuronal and neuroendocrine-regulated secretion have not been fully resolved. More importantly, however, it is now recognized that a number of proteins are involved in common in both of these two modes of regulated protein secretion.

Some of the proteins involved probably play a regulatory role but appear not to be required for exocytosis per se, based on studies of transgenic knockout mice and drosophila and *Caenorhabditis elegans* mutations. This group includes the proteins Rab3a, unc-18, synapsin, and synaptotagmin. The latter protein family is believed to comprise the calcium sensors that trigger exocytosis. These conclusions, however, are clouded to some extent by the possibility that multiple genes encoding functionally related products exist and that another gene product is at least partially able to offset the lack of a deleted or mutated gene.

Other proteins are clearly essential components of the universal machinery for vesicular exocytosis. These include gene products specifically cleaved by the clostridial neurotoxins that inhibit regulated secretion from both neurons and neuroendocrine cells. Synaptobrevin, syntaxin, and synaptosome-associated protein 25 are examples of this second group.

Finally, a number of proteins such as N-ethyl maleimide-sensitive factor (NSF) and SNAPs (soluble NSF-attachment proteins) clearly associate with the neurotoxin substrates. Based on this association, synaptobrevin, syntaxin, and synaptosome-associated protein 25 can be viewed as SNAP receptors (SNAREs). Thus, regulated secretion in both neurons (synaptic transmission) and in neuroendocrine cells can be unified under the SNARE hypothesis described earlier for other steps of vesicular transport (Figure 2–4). The novel twist in this hypothesis to accommodate regulated secretion is that the ability of the secretory vesicle v-SNARE to dock with the plasma membrane t-SNARE is dependent on the calcium-signaling step that triggers secretion. In the next few years, this hypothesis is likely to be tested, and if it is fully validated in either neuronal or neuroendocrine systems, a number of unanswered questions can be resolved.

The above general description of regulated secretion is modified to one extent or another in different systems, most likely representing fine-tuned adaptations for homeostasis. For example, in the hypothalamic-pituitary-end organ axis, regulated secretion from the hypothalamus is "pulsatile," with a distinctive amplitude and rate of release of the secretory products. Perturbation of these parameters in the hypothalamus can affect function at every step of the axis. As another example, in the B cells of the pancreatic islets of Langerhans, insulin secretion has a rapid phase and a slower, more delayed phase—both occurring sequentially in response to the secretory stimulus of an elevated blood glucose. The initial rapid phase is believed to exhaust a readily secretable supply of insulin, which is subsequently replenished, giving rise to the slower second phase. From recent work, it appears that glutamate released from mitochondria in the B cell plays an important intracellular signaling role in coordinating the reloading of the "launch bays" for the second phase. Likewise, ATP-sen-

sitive potassium (K^{ATP}) channels are inhibited by intracellular ATP and activated by ADP control exocytosis of insulin in pancreatic B cells. Nutrient oxidation in B cells leads to a rise in the [ATP]-to-[ADP] ratio, which in turn leads to reduced K^{ATP} channel activity and plasma membrane depolarization. This in turn activates voltage-dependent Ca^{2+} channels, which triggers Ca^{2+} entry and exocytosis.

Regulation of Hormone Release After Exocytosis

Upon condensation into secretory granules, the vesicle content exists as a crystalline precipitate and is no longer osmotically active, a property that facilitates their storage in the regulated secretory pathway. Upon fusion of such a secretory granule to the plasma membrane, the insoluble content must dissolve into the extracellular medium. It appears that the ionic composition of the extracellular fluid can significantly influence the rate of phase transition of the insoluble proteoglycan matrix and hence dissolution and effective release of secretory products. This phenomenon is likely to be an important point of regulation in systems where pulse frequency and amplitude of secretion are important properties (eg, release of neurotransmitters).

POMC Processing & Secretion

There has been considerable progress in understanding the nature of the sorting signal on an individual hormone that accounts for how those molecules are segregated in the TGN from lysosomal, constitutive secretory, and other pathways. In the case of POMC, a specific conformational motif responsible for sorting to the regulated secretory pathway has been identified. It is composed of a 13-amino-acid amphipathic loop close to the amino terminal of the polypeptide and appears to be stabilized by a disulfide bridge. This feature is presumably recognized in the lumen by transmembrane receptors whose cytoplasmic tails recognize adaptin-type proteins responsible for coat assembly, vesicle formation, and proper targeting to the appropriate domain of the plasma membrane.

During this transport process, the vesicles "mature" into secretory granules. Key features of this maturation step include proteolysis (eg, in the case of POMC, where a small peptide, ACTH, will be released from the much larger precursor) and concentration. The concentration step is such that often the regulated secretory cargo forms crystalline arrays of precipitated protein within the granule lumen. Upon stimulation, when the granule fuses to the plasma membrane, the exocytosed product is diluted and dissolves into the bloodstream.

Endocytosis & Recycling

In addition to transport and correct localization of newly synthesized hormones and receptors, vesicular membrane trafficking events are involved in important responses to hormones. In parallel with the pathway of membrane vesicles from ER to plasma membrane is a pathway that leads from the plasma membrane back to various compartments, including the TGN and perhaps even the ER. In part this represents the need to recycle membrane. Note that the volume of regulated secretion in endocrine cells is such that the entire intracellular membrane system would be consumed and localized to the plasma membrane literally in minutes if there were no way to recycle the "empty" membrane containers after use. Not only is there such a pathway, but it probably operates in reverse between each forward compartment (ie, from plasma membrane to TGN, from TGN to trans Golgi, from trans to medial Golgi, from medial to cis Golgi, from cis Golgi to intermediate compartment, and from intermediate compartment to ER).

However, endocytosis is not simply a means of recovering "empty" containers. It provides a means for the cell to take up valuable nutrients and to "sample" the environment. Such is the case for endocytosis of low-density lipoproteins via LDL receptors that are internalized as coated vesicles from coated pits on the plasma membrane of hepatocytes.

Finally, of particular interest for endocrinology, endocytosis provides a means of responding to hormones and other signals. Endocytosis of a vesicle from the plasma membrane places hormone receptors in a protected space where they can no longer be activated by external hormone. This is one (of several) molecular bases of receptor down-regulation and tachyphylaxis to drugs.

Whereas some receptors enter the coated pits only when bound to ligand (eg, EGF receptor), others enter constantly whether ligand-bound or not. In some cases, both ligand and receptor are targeted from the endosome to the lysosomes and degraded (eg, EGF and its receptor). In other cases, dissociation of ligand from receptor in an intermediate acidic compartment allows the receptor to be recycled and only the cargo to be sent to the lysosome (eg, LDL receptor).

One difference from the biosynthetic flow of membranes is that different machinery is involved in vesicle formation from the plasma membrane, which is much more rigid than intracellular membrane compartments by virtue of having cytoskeletal elements bound on the inside and extracellular matrix bound on the outside. Thus, the microtubule-associated protein **dynamin** has recently been implicated in driving vesicular invagination, constriction, and pinching off from the plasma membrane.

Recently, noncoated invaginations termed **caveolae** have been noted to occur at the plasma membrane and have been implicated in such hormone-related events as translocation of the insulin-sensitive isoform of the glucose transporter to the cell surface upon insulin stimulation. As mentioned earlier, a complicating issue in vesicular dynamics is whether different gene products can at least partially perform each other's function, thus obscuring the consequences of knockout experiments to assess the role of a particular protein in trafficking events. A better understanding of these features of membrane vesicular dynamics is likely to emerge in the coming years. Some of the differences in pathways defined by the presence or absence of a particular protein may prove to be largely semantic owing to complementary functional activity of another protein despite morphologic, structural, or antigenic differences. In other cases, differences in protein composition may reflect important mechanistic differences in the pathways of vesicular traffic. The importance of recent progress is that such differences in trafficking pathways are no longer the subject of speculation but rather are being detected and studied and the genes associated with them cloned and their expression manipulated.

Secretion of Catecholamines, GABA, & Other Nonpolypeptide Neurotransmitters

Nonpolypeptide products that are released by fusion of vesicles such as catecholamines, acetylcholine, and GABA represent a variation on the theme of recycling through the endocytotic pathway. The vesicles containing these neurotransmitters are loaded with their product by transporters that engage in direct uptake from the cytosol. Loaded vesicles fuse with the plasma membrane in a regulated fashion coupled with a stimulus and usually mediated by a rise in intracellular free calcium. Subsequently, the membrane container is reendocytosed, reloaded, and subjected to another cycle of triggered fusion and content release, as with other forms of stimulus-coupled secretion. Several members of a related family of transporters involved in uptake of these small molecules from the cytosol have been identified.

Secretion of Thyroid Hormone

Thyroid hormone is an example of a hormone whose biogenesis involves a hybrid of vesicular and nonvesicular trafficking. It is synthesized initially as a large polypeptide precursor, termed **thyroglobulin,** which is assembled into a dimer, iodinated, and modified in the classic secretory pathway before constitutive exocytosis across the apical plasma membrane. Iodinated thy-

roglobulin is stored outside of the cell in the thyroid follicle lumen and is termed **colloid.** Upon appropriate stimulation by thyroid-stimulating hormone (TSH), colloid is taken up by endocytosis and transported across the cell in vesicles that fuse to the basolateral plasma membrane. This variant of endocytosis, in which a product is taken up and delivered from one side of a cell to the other in a polarized fashion, is termed **transcytosis.** During transcytosis, the thyroglobulin is degraded by proteases to release active thyroid hormone. Remarkably, out of approximately 6600 amino acid residues comprising the thyroglobulin dimer, six pairs of iodinated, modified tyrosines are released as thyroid hormone, containing either three or four iodines (T_3 or T_4). Thyroid hormone released from the large polypeptide precursor during transcytosis is able to cross the vesicular membrane and the plasma membrane directly and hence is released immediately upon synthesis in a non-vesicle-mediated manner.

Relevance of Membrane Traffic to Disease

Given the complexities of hormone biogenesis and the many gene products involved in synthesis, maturation, and trafficking of hormones, it should not be surprising that defects in membrane trafficking are prominent among those genetic diseases whose molecular basis is well understood. Thus, a common genetic disease, cystic fibrosis, is due to mutations in a membrane protein. As a result of this mutation, this protein is unable to leave the ER despite the fact that it remains functional. Presumably, this is a case in which the ER quality control machinery acts as a "double-edged sword": Preventing export from the ER of a slightly misfolded protein causes a much more severe disease due to a complete lack of the protein at its proper location, the plasma membrane. Similarly, α_1-antiprotease deficiency, which results in emphysema, is due to a trafficking defect in which the misfolded protein fails to leave the ER.

In most cases, our understanding of acquired disorders, including degenerative diseases, does not extend to the relative importance of disorders of trafficking. However, proteins that undergo complex trafficking pathways, including growth factors and hormone receptors, are central to many of these disorders, suggesting that important connections are yet to be discovered.

An emerging principle of cellular pathophysiology seems to be that for the most important pathways, cells have evolved backup systems that can to some extent maintain crucial functions. Thus, yeasts lacking SRP are sick and have substantial defects in translocation across the ER but survive thanks to non-SRP-mediated backup

systems. Thus, patients with I cell disease have correct lysosomal localization of lysosomal enzymes in some tissues even though all tissues lack the GlcNAc phosphotransferase necessary to generate the ligand for the M6P receptor. Two consequences of this principle are that important trafficking defects are apt to be acquired rather than inherited and that identification of these lesions will prove extremely difficult and will require a more intimate understanding of the complex regulation of normal trafficking in the absence of disease.

HORMONE EXPORT NOT MEDIATED BY MEMBRANE VESICLES

1. Steroid Hormones

Steroid hormones are mainly synthesized in the adrenals, gonads, and placenta. Recent experiments indicate that steroids are synthesized in the nervous system as well, and other tissues may also synthesize steroid hormones in much smaller quantities. The overall pathway for the synthesis of all steroid hormones is similar (Figure 2–5). Tissue-specific, cell-specific, and even subcellular compartment-specific differences in the expression of particular steroidogenic enzymes regulate the particular pattern of steroid hormone synthesized.

Chemistry

All steroids are derived from pregnenolone (Figure 2–5). Pregnenolone, naturally occurring progestins, glucocorticoids, and mineralocorticoids contain 21 carbons and are referred to as C-21 steroids. Androgens and estrogens have two less carbons, and are therefore C-19 steroids. The different rings of the steroid structure are designated A–D, and the numbering of each carbon atom is useful in understanding how the different steroid-synthesizing enzymes modify the steroids at particular locations. All steroids have the basic cyclopentanoperhydrophenanthrene ring (four-ring) structure, and all have a single unsaturated carbon-carbon double bond except for the estrogens, in which the A ring is aromatized. Pregnenolone and other steroids called Δ^5 steroids have this double bond between carbons 5 and 6, while progesterone, glucocorticoids, mineralocorticoids, and androgens are called Δ^4 steroids and have this double bond between carbons 4 and 5.

Steroids are given both chemical and trivial names. As the chemical names are often cumbersome, trivial names are commonly used. For example, the chemical name for progesterone is pregn-4-ene-3,20-dione, cortisol is $11\beta,17\alpha,21$-trihydroxypregn-4-ene-3,20-dione, etc. Chemical names are given in a particular order: hydroxyl groups, aldehyde groups, core ring structure, and aldehydes or ketones. The core ring structure is

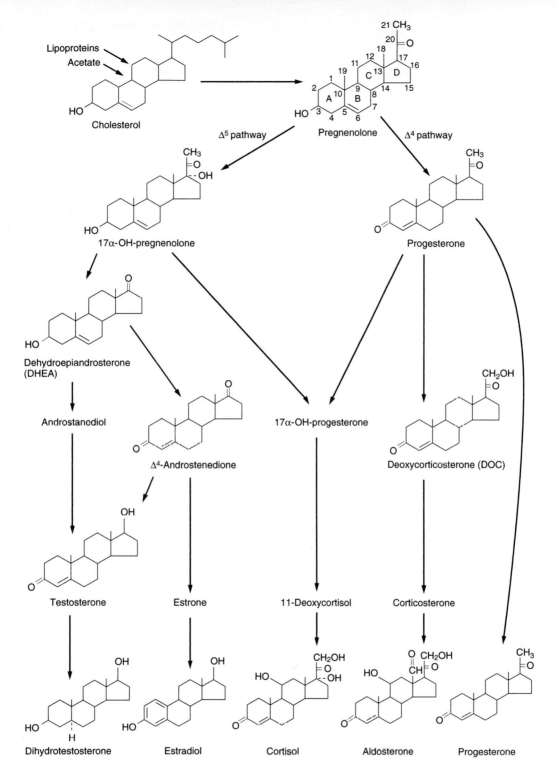

Figure 2–5. Pathways of synthesis of the major classes of steroid hormones. Cholesterol is derived from acetate by synthesis or from lipoprotein particles. The numbering of the steroid molecule is shown for pregnenolone. The major pathways thought to be used are shown. (See also Figures 9–4, 12–2, 13–4, and 14–13.)

given a name based on the number of carbons it contains. Thus, C-27 steroids are cholestanes, C-21 steroids are pregnanes, C-19 steroids are androstanes, and C-18 steroids are estranes. Like all chemical names, a saturated structure is given the suffix *-ane* while an unsaturated structure is given the suffix *-ene.*

In addition to the trivial names for the steroid hormones, steroids may be given a letter abbreviation. These are the names of the steroids as they were originally identified by chromatography by the chemists who first isolated and characterized them about 50 years ago. Therefore, cortisol may be called compound F; cortisone, compound E; corticosterone, compound B, etc. The trivial names and systematic names of some natural and synthetic steroids are listed in Table 2–1. (See also Chapters 9, 10, 12, and 13.)

Cholesterol Synthesis & Uptake

All steroid hormones are synthesized from the precursor cholesterol. There are three sources of cholesterol for use in steroid hormone synthesis: de novo synthesis from acetate, pools of cholesteryl esters in steroidogenic tissues, and dietary sources. About 80% of the cholesterol used for steroid hormone synthesis comes from dietary cholesterol, transported in human plasma as low-density lipoprotein (LDL) particles. In rats and other species, cholesterol is transported as high-density lipoprotein (HDL) particles. Uptake of LDL cholesterol is enhanced by ACTH treatment, which increases the activity of LDL receptors and uptake of LDL cholesterol. The majority of LDL cholesterol uptake is by receptor-mediated endocytosis via coated pits, and less

Table 2–1. Trivial and chemical names of some natural and synthetic steroids.

Trivial Name	(Other Names)	Chemical Name
Aldosterone	Electrocortin	11β,21-Dihydroxy-3,20-dioxo-4-pregnen-18-al
Corticosterone	Compound B	11β,21-Dihydroxy-4-pregnene-3,20-dione
Cortisol	Hydrocortisone, compound F	11β,17α,21-Trihydroxy-4-pregnene-3,20-dione
Cortisone	Compound E	17α,21-Dihydroxy-4-pregnene-3,11,20-trione
Dehydroepiandrosterone	Prasterone, DHEA	3β-Hydroxy-5-androsten-17-one
11-Deoxycorticosterone	DOC	21-Hydrox-4-pregnene-3,20-dione
11-Deoxy-17-hydroxycorticosterone	11-Deoxycortisol, cortexolone, compound S	17α,21-Dihydroxy-4-pregnene-3,20-dione
Estradiol		1,3,5(10)-Estratriene-3,17β-diol
Pregnenolone		3β-Hydroxy-5-pregnen-20-one
Progesterone		4-Pregnene-3,20-dione
Testosterone		17β-Hydroxy-4-androsten-3-one
Allopregnanolone	3α,5α-Tetrahydroprogesterone, THP	5α-Pregnan-3α-ol-20-one
Dexamethasone		9α-Fluoro-11β,17α,21-trihydroxy-16α-methylpregna-1,4-diene-3,20-dione
Betamethasone		9α-Fluoro-11β,17α,21-trihydroxy-16β-methylpregna-1,4-diene-3,20-dione
Prednisone		17α,21-Dihydroxypregna-1,4-diene-3,11,20-trione
Prednisolone		11β,17α,21-Trihydroxypregna-1,4-diene-3,20-dione
Spironolactone	Aldactone	4,17α-Pregnen-21-carboxylicic acid-17β-ol-3-one-7α-thiol-21,17 γ-lactone, 7-acetate
Triamcinolone		9α-Fluoro-11β,16α,17α,21-tetrahydroxypregna-1,4-diene-3,20-dione

than 10% enters the cell independently of this mechanism. HDL cholesterol uptake, however, occurs by receptor-independent mechanisms.

Intracellular Cholesterol Storage & Transport

Several factors have been identified as being important in cholesterol mobilization within steroidogenic tissues. Cholesterol is esterified to polyunsaturated fatty acids in the endoplasmic reticulum by acyl-CoA:cholesterol acyltransferase (ACAT), and accumulated cholesteryl esters form lipid droplets. These fatty acid esters are hydrolyzed to free cholesterol by cholesteryl esterase (sterol ester hydrolase). Tissue-specific tropic hormones (eg, ACTH, LH, and FSH) stimulate the esterase and inhibit the acyltransferase, resulting in increased accumulation of free cholesterol. Some steroids, such as pregnenolone, testosterone, and estradiol, can be reesterified to form fatty acid esters. Pregnenolone fatty acid esters form biosynthetic intermediates in the synthesis of adrenal steroids, and testosterone and estradiol fatty acid esters can accumulate in target tissues and behave as endogenous long-acting androgens and estrogens.

Steroid Hormone Synthesis

The first step in steroid hormone synthesis, the conversion of cholesterol to pregnenolone, occurs in the mitochondria. However, cholesterol does not enter the mitochondria freely but rather must be carried through the cytoplasm to the inner mitochondrial membrane. Free cholesterol, which would be insoluble free in the aqueous cytoplasm, binds to sterol carrier protein-2 (SCP-2), which plays a major role in its transport to the mitochondria. Once there, cholesterol must traverse the outer mitochondrial membrane and the intermembrane space to reach the inner mitochondrial membrane, where the first steroid hydroxylating enzyme, P450scc, resides. A newly characterized protein, given the name StAR (steroidogenic acute regulator), functions to carry out the rate-limiting step in cholesterol transport across the mitochondrial outer membrane. Since steroids are not stored, their synthesis and its cessation must be exquisitely controlled. A novel mechanism of regulation involving StAR activity has recently come to light. It appears that the nuclear-encoded StAR protein is localized to the mitochondrial matrix—yet it has all of its known enzymatic activity on the outer surface of the outer mitochondrial membrane, a location it maintains only transiently during its import. In this case, compartmentalization is used to provide hair-trigger sensitivity to steroid synthesis through its rapid inactivation by substrate depletion upon StAR localization to the mitochondrial matrix.

Cytochromes P450

Most steroidogenic enzymes are members of the cytochrome P450 group of oxidases. All of these enzymes have molecular masses of about 50 kDa and contain a single heme group. They are called "P450" ("pigment" 450) because they all exhibit a characteristic absorbance at 450 nm upon reduction with carbon monoxide. All the steroidogenic P450s function by the same mechanism. They all reduce atmospheric oxygen with electrons from NADPH. These electrons reach the P450 by one or more protein intermediates. For the mitochondrial P450s, two protein intermediates—adrenodoxin reductase and adrenodoxin—are involved. For the microsomal P450s, one protein intermediate, P450 reductase, is involved (Figure 2–6).

The synthesis of all steroid hormones from cholesterol involves one or more of six distinct cytochromes P450 (Figure 2–6), which are expressed in compartment- and tissue-specific patterns, thereby accounting for the differences in compartment- and tissue-specific steroids (eg, made in mitochondria versus ER and in adrenal versus gonads versus placenta). Many of the steroid hydroxylases have multiple enzymatic activities. Purification of the proteins and cloning of the cDNAs encoding these proteins has rigorously demonstrated that these activities indeed reside within single proteins.

Neurosteroidogenesis

In the brain, the expression of the steroidogenic enzymes is developmentally and regionally regulated, ensuring the regulated synthesis of specific neurosteroids. The enzymes are expressed in both neurons and in neuroglia, suggesting that these two cell types must work together in a coordinated fashion to produce the appropriate neurosteroid. The additional pathways leading to the production of the 3α- and 5α-reduced neurosteroids are shown in Figure 2–6. Neurosteroids such as allopregnanolone, DHEA, and DHEAS function mainly through modulation of neurotransmitter receptors such as GABAA, NMDA, and sigma receptors rather than by binding to intracellular steroid hormone receptors. By binding to these receptors, they augment GABA- and NMDA-mediated ion flux through the receptor channels. Thus, their actions may be quite rapid. Neurosteroids that augment GABA function, such as 3α- and 5α-reduced derivatives of progesterone (allopregnanolone) are potent anxiolytics. Other functions attributed to neurosteroids include stimulation of axonal growth (DHEA), stimulation of dendritic growth (DHEAS), regulation of myelination (progesterone), regulation of neurotransmitter receptor subunit expression, and neuroprotection (DHEA). In addition, recent studies have proposed a role of neurosteroids in pre-

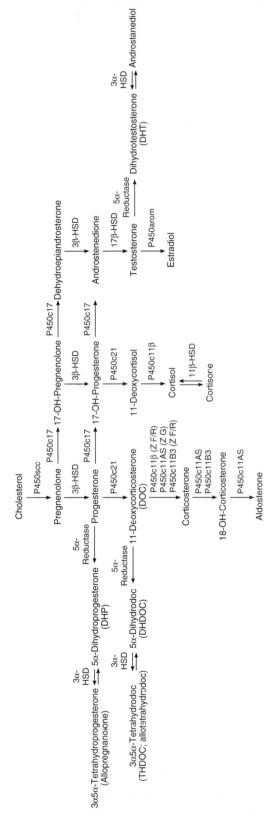

Figure 2–6. Principal steroidogenic pathways in classic endocrine tissues. Other steroids, such as steroid sulfates and lipoidal derivatives, are also produced. The names for each enzyme are shown by each reaction. P450scc, mitochondrial cholesterol side-chain cleavage enzyme, mediates 20α hydroxylation, 22 hydroxylation, and scission of the C20–22 bond; 3β-HSD, a non-P450 enzyme mediates both 3β-hydroxysteroid dehydrogenase and Δ5−Δ4 isomerase activities; P450c21 in the endoplasmic reticulum mediates 21-hydroxylation; P450c11β, mitochondrial 11-hydroxylase in the adrenal fasciculata-reticularis, mediates 11-hydroxylation; P450c11AS, mitochondrial aldosterone synthase in the adrenal glomerulosa, mediates 11-hydroxylation, 18-hydroxylation, and 18-oxidation; P450c11B3, mitochondrial 11,18-hydroxylase in the adrenal fasciculata-reticularis that is expressed in rat adrenals only from day 6 to day 36 after birth; P450c17 in the endoplasmic reticulum mediates both 17α-hydroxylation and scission of the C17,20 bond; 17β-HSD, also called 17-ketosteroid reductase or 17KSR, a non-P450 enzyme of the endoplasmic reticulum, catalyzes a reversible reaction and produces testosterone, which may be converted to estradiol by P450arom in the endoplasmic reticulum, through aromatization of the A ring of the steroid nucleus. 11β-HSD is a non-P450 enzyme that inactivates cortisol in target organs by conversion to cortisone. 5α-Reductase, a membrane-bound non-P450, exists in at least three isoforms in human beings. It catalyzes a reversible reaction favoring the 3α reduced steroid and converts dihydroprogesterone to the potent neurosteroid allopregnanolone. It also converts 5α-dihydrodeoxycorticosterone to allotetrahydrodeoxycorticosterone and dihydrotestosterone to androstanediol. (Z F/R, zonae fasciculata and reticularis; ZG, zona glomerulosa.)

55

menstrual syndrome (withdrawal from allopregnanolone) and in depression (allopregnanolone).

2. Vitamin D

The active form of vitamin D—1,25-$(OH)_2$-cholecalciferol (1,25-$[OH]_2D_3$)—is derived from vitamin D_3 (cholecalciferol; Chapter 8). Cholecalciferol is obtained either from the diet or from the conversion of 7-dehydrocholesterol (present in the skin) in response to ultraviolet irradiation via a 6,7-cis isomer intermediate (provitamin D). Vitamin D_2 (ergocalciferol), which is present in plants and differs from vitamin D_3 in having a double bond at C_{22} and C_{23}, a methyl group at C_{24}, and several features of the A ring of the molecule, also serves as a precursor of active vitamin D products. The ultimate vitamin D products are a mixture of compounds derived from these two compounds and can vary depending on the dietary intake (Chapter 8). Vitamins D_2 and D_3 are transported, bound to a vitamin D transport protein, to the liver, where the actions of a microsomal cytochrome P450c25 convert them to 25-hydroxy derivatives—25-OH-cholecalciferol (25-$[OH]D_3$) for vitamin D_3. 25-$(OH)D_3$ then circulates bound to an α-globulin transport protein; in the proximal tubular cells of the kidney, 25-$(OH)D_3$ is converted to 1,25-$(OH)_2D_3$ by the actions of a mitochondrial cytochrome P450c1α (see Chapter 8). This latter step is rate-limiting for overall 1,25-$(OH)_2D_3$ production and is regulated chiefly by PTH and phosphate ions. States of vitamin D deficiency are best assessed by measuring 25-$(OH)D_3$ levels in serum.

3. Eicosanoids

Arachidonic acid is the most important and abundant precursor of the various eicosanoids in humans and is rate-limiting for eicosanoid synthesis (Figure 2–7). Arachidonic acid is formed from linoleic acid (18:2n-6; an essential fatty acid) in most cases through desaturation and elongation to homo-γ linoleic acid (20:5n-3) and subsequent desaturation. Whereas eicosanoids are not stored by cells, arachidonic acid precursor stores are present in membrane lipids, from which it is released in response to various stimuli through actions of phospholipases. Phospholipase A_2 or both phospholipase C and diglyceride lipase catalyze the cleavage of esterified arachidonic acid from the 2 position of glycerophospholipids in the lipid bilayer of the cell (Figure 2–7). The lipid content of the various cells differs, and this results in different patterns of eicosanoid production from different cell types. Phospholipase A_2 activity in vitro can be strongly inhibited by glucocorticoids through the induction of proteins called lipocortins; this may contribute to glucocorticoid suppression of

certain inflammatory reactions, but the importance of this block in humans is not established.

Arachidonic acid can be converted to the endoperoxide prostaglandin H_2, which is the precursor to the prostaglandins, prostacyclins, and thromboxanes, or it can be acted on by other lipoxygenases to form the leukotrienes and other eicosanoids such as HETE. For prostaglandin synthesis, cyclooxygenase (also called endoperoxide synthetase) converts arachidonic acid to the unstable endoperoxide PGG_2, which is rapidly reduced to PGH_2. Cyclooxygenase is widely distributed throughout the body (except for erythrocytes and lymphocytes) and is inhibited by aspirin, indomethacin, and other nonsteroidal anti-inflammatory agents. In some tissues, PGH_2 can be converted to other prostaglandins (eg, PGD_2, PGE_2, PGF [via PGE_2]) in reactions involving prostaglandin synthetases. Similarly, prostacyclin synthetase, which is prevalent in endothelial and smooth muscle cells, fibroblasts, and macrophages, can convert PGH_2 to prostacyclins, and thromboxane synthetase, prevalent in platelets and macrophages, can convert PGH_2 to thromboxanes (eg, thromboxane A_2). Arachidonic acid metabolism by 5-lipoxygenase results in leukotriene production, and metabolism by 12-lipoxygenase results in 12-HPETE (hydroperoxyeicosatetraenoic acid) that is converted to HETE. Arachidonic acid can also be oxygenated by cytochrome P450 monooxygenases to various omega oxidation products and epoxides and derivatives that may have biologic activities.

Historically, it has been believed that prostaglandins, like steroids, simply diffused across membranes. Recently, however, a prostaglandin transporter has been identified, suggesting specific uptake of these products by target tissues.

METABOLISM, TRANSPORT, ELIMINATION, & REGULATION OF HORMONES

Hormones circulate both free and bound to plasma proteins. There are major differences between the various hormones in the extent of their association with the plasma proteins. In general, the binding of hormones to plasma is through noncovalent interactions, although cholesterol is considered to be bound through ester bonds to phosphatidylcholine. However, even in this case, the esterified cholesterol is bound through hydrophobic interactions to the lipoprotein particles.

Metabolism of Polypeptide Hormones

The metabolism a polypeptide hormone undergoes depends on which pool it belongs to. As described earlier, some proteolytic events such as signal sequence cleavage occur very early in biogenesis. Other events such as re-

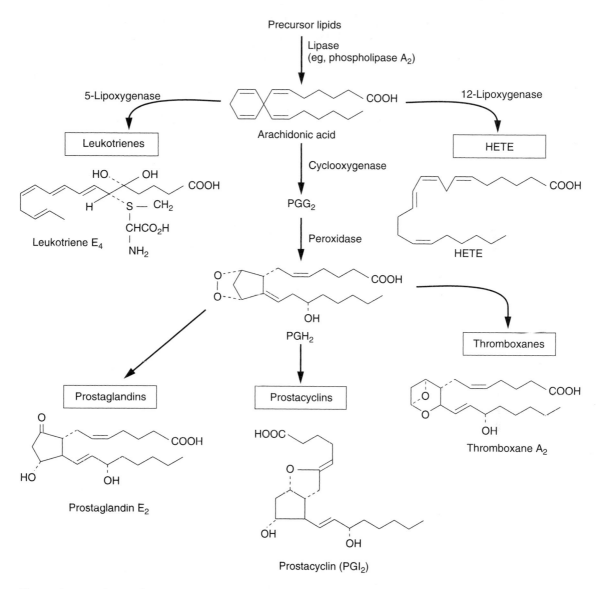

Figure 2-7. Pathways for synthesis of the major classes of eicosanoids: prostaglandins, prostacyclins, thromboxanes, and leukotrienes. All steps in the pathways are not shown. Below each pathway, enclosed by boxes, is a representative compound of the class. (HETE, hydroxyeicosatetraenoic acid; PGG₂, prostaglandin G₂; PGH₂, prostaglandin H₂.)

verse translocation to the cytoplasm for degradation occur only for a particular subset of chains. Secretory granules full of polypeptide hormone that has been stored for too long undergo fusion to lysosomes and degradation. Finally, after secretion, polypeptide hormones have a distinctive half-life in the bloodstream.

Most polypeptide hormones circulate at low concentrations unbound to other proteins, though there are ex-

ceptions. For example, there are several different IGF-I-binding proteins that bind IGF-I. Vasopressin and oxytocin are bound to neurophysins. Growth hormone binds to a protein that is identical to the hormone-binding portion of the growth hormone receptor.

In general, peptide hormones have short half-lives (a few minutes) in the circulation, as seen with ACTH, insulin, glucagon, PTH, and the releasing hormones.

The glycosylated glycoprotein hormones are more stable. Glycosylated chorionic gonadotropin has a half-life of several hours. Although there may be some degradation of the hormone by proteases in the circulation, the major mechanism for hormone degradation is through binding to cell surface receptors for the hormone or through non-receptor cell surface hormone-binding sites, with subsequent uptake into the cell (internalization; see below) and degradation (by enzymes in the cell membrane or inside the cell). A number of specific enzymes mediate these processes, which differ for the various hormones. In addition, several steps may be involved. The first of these may inactivate the hormone, and this can be due—eg, in the case of insulin—to reduction of disulfide bonds in the protein. An important overall source for these enzymes is the lysosome, which may fuse with endocytosed vesicles to expose its enzyme contents and its acid environment to the internalized hormone-receptor complex. An advantage of the short circulating half-lives of some classes of hormones is that the duration of the response can be relatively short. In addition, the persistent presence of significant levels of many classes of hormones that act on the cell surface results in down-regulation of the responsiveness to the hormone that may not be desirable.

Metabolism of Steroid Hormones & Vitamin D

All of the steroid hormones are bound to plasma proteins to some extent, with high-affinity binding to specific globulins and relatively low-affinity and nonspecific binding to proteins such as albumin. The major specific binding proteins are corticosteroid-binding globulin (CBG; transcortin), which binds both cortisol and progesterone; and sex hormone-binding globulin (SHBG), which binds testosterone and estradiol (testosterone more tightly than estradiol). These proteins are present in sufficient concentrations so that over 90% of the total cortisol and about 98% of the testosterone and estradiol are bound. The levels of their binding capacities in some cases exceed only slightly the normal concentrations of the steroid, so that with higher levels a much higher proportion of the hormone can be free. For example, the CBG capacity for cortisol is about 25 μg/dL (690 nmol/L). Aldosterone does not bind to a specific protein, with the result that only about 50% of the plasma aldosterone is bound. Vitamin D circulates mostly bound to vitamin D-binding protein. This protein binds 25-(OH)D_3 more tightly than 1,25-(OH)$_2D_3$ or vitamin D_3.

The hydrophobic steroid hormones and the D vitamins are filtered by the kidney and generally reabsorbed. About 1% of the cortisol produced daily ends up in the urine. Steroid hormones are ordinarily handled by metabolizing them to inactive species and to water-soluble forms that are more effectively eliminated. It is the free steroid fraction that is accessible to metabolic inactivation. The inactivations are accomplished by converting hydroxyl groups to keto groups, reducing double bonds, and conjugating the steroids with glucuronide and sulfate groups. Over 50 different steroid metabolites have been described.

The production of active hormones by metabolism in peripheral tissues, as is seen with androgens, estrogens, and vitamin D, is discussed above in the section on hormone synthesis. In addition, metabolism in peripheral tissues can determine the type of steroid that binds to the receptor. Aldosterone is ordinarily the major mineralocorticoid hormone responsible for the salt-retaining actions of the steroid hormones. This steroid binds to the mineralocorticoid receptor only about ten times more tightly than cortisol, whose total and free concentrations in the circulation are about 1000 times and 100 times (respectively) those of aldosterone; thus, cortisol should ordinarily be the main occupant of the mineralocorticoid receptors. This, in fact, occurs in tissues such as the brain and pituitary, but in the kidney, cortisol is avidly converted to the essentially inactive metabolite cortisone and perhaps other species which do not bind to the mineralocorticoid receptor. Some types of licorice or genetic defects can block the enzyme responsible for the conversion and result in a mineralocorticoid excess state that is due to cortisol (Chapter 10).

Metabolism of Thyroid Hormones

Thyroid hormones circulate bound to plasma proteins such that 0.04% of the T_4 and 0.4% of the T_3 are free. About 68% of the T_4 and 80% of the T_3 are bound by the glycoprotein thyroid hormone-binding globulin (TBG). About 11% of the T_4 and 9% of the T_3 are bound to transthyretin (thyroid hormone-binding prealbumin; TBPA). The remainder is bound to albumin.

The metabolism of thyroid hormones is discussed in Chapter 7. The circulating half-lives of T_4 (7 days) and T_3 (about 1 day) are longer than for most hormones. These differences are due to the higher affinity of T_4 than T_3 for TBG. The hormones are degraded to inactive forms by microsomal deiodinases. The type I 5'-deiodinase is prevalent in most peripheral tissues, including liver and kidney, and is responsible for most of the production of T_3. A type II 5'-deiodinase present in the pituitary and central nervous system is involved in generating T_3 for feedback inhibition of TSH release. The 5'-deiodinases also convert reverse T_3 (3,3',5'-L-triiodothyronine) to 3,3'-T_2 (3,3'-diiodothyronine). 5-Deiodinases act on T_4 to generate reverse T_3 and on T_3 to generate 3,3'-T_2. Deaminations and decarboxylations of the alanine side chains as well as conjugations with glucuronic acid and sulfate groups are also involved in degrading thyroid hormones. (See Chapter 7.)

Metabolism of Catecholamines

The metabolism of the catecholamines is discussed in Chapter 11. These compounds are cleared rapidly, with half-lives of 1–2 minutes. Clearance is primarily by cellular uptake and metabolism, and only about 2–3% of the norepinephrine that enters the circulation is excreted in the urine. Furthermore, a significant amount of the catecholamine metabolites in the circulation reflect catecholamines whose degradation occurred within adrenergic neuron terminals, a point of importance for interpreting clinical data. The catecholamines are degraded by two principal routes, catechol-*O*-methyltransferase (COMT) and monoamine oxidase (MAO). The measurement of some of the metabolites—normetanephrine, metanephrine, and vanillylmandelic acid (VMA)—can be useful in evaluating cases of possible catecholamine overproduction.

Metabolism of Eicosanoids

Prostaglandins are rapidly metabolized within seconds by enzymes that are widely distributed. Prominent in the metabolism is oxidation of the 15-hydroxyl group of the prostaglandin that renders the molecule inactive. Subsequent other reactions involve both oxidations and reductions.

Regulation of Hormone-Binding Proteins in Plasma

The levels of the plasma-binding proteins can vary with both disease states and drug therapy. For example, CBG, SHBG, and TBG levels are increased by estrogens. SHBG levels are increased by thyroid hormones, and SHBG and TBG levels are decreased by androgens.

An understanding of the roles of plasma binding of hormones is just emerging. In general, the hormones are sufficiently soluble to circulate unassociated at levels at which they are highly active. Cholesterol may be an exception if it is considered a hormone. With the steroid and thyroid hormones, deficiency states characterized by genetic defects with very low levels of transport proteins are not associated with clinical abnormalities. The transthyretin gene, which encodes the protein responsible for most of the thyroid hormone binding in the plasma of mice, has been deleted in this species and the animals were phenotypically normal. Thus, there is no evidence that these binding proteins are essential.

In most cases, it is the free hormone that is active; the free levels of the hormone are responsible for the feedback and related regulatory influences that control hormone release (see below). The free levels of hormones are related to their clearance rates. Clinical states correlate best with the free levels of hormones. The latter is a critical consideration in many cases, as with states of adrenal or thyroid hormone excess and deficiency. With these hormones, factors that affect the levels of plasma binding proteins can spuriously elevate or depress the total hormone levels in otherwise normal individuals, or the changes could mask pathologic hormone excess or deficiency states. These considerations are discussed in Chapters 7 and 9. However, transport proteins may greatly facilitate an even delivery of hormones to the target tissues. In a tissue such as the liver, for example, a hormone that is totally free would be completely sequestered as the blood flows through the proximal portions of the tissue, whereas if it were mostly bound, the free hormone would be sequestered in proximal portions and additional hormone would be available for more distal portions through the dissociation of plasma-bound hormone. The latter facilitates more even delivery throughout the tissue. With polypeptide hormones, plasma binding can increase the half-life of the hormone in the circulation; it may also facilitate its delivery into the target tissues.

Overall Regulation of the Endocrine System

The effective concentration of a hormone is determined by the rates of its production, delivery to the target tissue, and degradation. All of these processes are finely regulated to achieve the physiologic level of the hormone. However, the importance of the steps may differ in some cases. By far the most highly regulated process is hormone production. With many classes of hormones, the short half-lives of the hormones provide means of terminating the responses and thus preventing excessive responses. The latter are also blunted by negative regulation of both hormone responsiveness (discussed below) and release, as well as by other factors. For example, in stress, glucocorticoids produced in excess probably blunt the actions of a number of hormones that would otherwise be harmful (Chapter 9). Thus, when the actions and half-lives of the hormones are short, the hormone response can be terminated by simply stopping release of the hormone. An exception is thyroid hormone, with its long half-life. Details of the controls of the individual systems are provided in later chapters.

There are a number of different patterns of regulation of hormone release. Many hormones are linked to the hypothalamic-pituitary axis (discussed in detail in the section on neuroendocrinology; see Chapter 5). These involve both classic feedback loops by hormones that are released by peripheral glands (cortisol, thyroid hormone, etc) and more subtle control, as is seen with GH and PRL. However, many systems are more free-standing. This is illustrated by the parathyroid glands (Chapter 8) and by the pancreatic islets (Chapter 17). With the parathyroid glands, the Ca^{2+} concentration that is increased in the plasma by the hormone exerts a dominant feedback inhibition on the release of PTH. With insulin, depression of glucose levels in response to insulin action results in cessation of the stimulus to release more insulin. In addition, in both cases, the release of the hormone and the overall state of the gland are influenced by numerous other factors.

The stimuli to regulate hormone production include essentially all of the types of regulatory molecules, including hormones such as the tropic hormones and counterregulatory hormones (discussed above), traditional growth factors, eicosanoids, and ions. For example, potassium ion is an important regulator of the adrenal zona glomerulosa. The production of the various eicosanoids is regulated by local factors acting on the cells in which these products are released. For example, tropic stimulation of most endocrine glands results in enhancement of eicosanoid production.

The production of hormones is regulated at multiple levels. First, synthesis of the hormone can be regulated at the level of transcription, as is commonly seen with the polypeptide hormones or the enzymes involved in the synthesis of other hormones such as the steroids. It can also be affected by posttranscriptional mechanisms. Second, release of the hormone stored in secretory granules from tissues that employ the regulated secretory pathway is controlled by secretagogues, as was discussed in the section on hormone synthesis. The secretory cells can store the peptide hormones in sufficient quantity so that the amount released over a short period can exceed the rate of synthesis of the hormone. And third, stimulation of endocrine glands by tropic hormones and other substances such as growth factors can increase the number and size of cells that are actively producing the hormone.

REFERENCES

Aridor M, Balch WE: Integration of endoplasmic reticulum signaling in health and disease. Nat Med 1999;5:745.

Bose H, Lingappa VR, Miller WH: Rapid regulation of steroidogenesis by mitochondrial protein import. Nature 2002;417:87. [PMID: 11986670]

Compagnone NA, Mellon SH: Neurosteroids: Biosynthesis and function of these novel neuromodulators. Front Neuroendocrinol 2000;21:1.

Gerber SH, Sudhof TC: Molecular determinants of regulated exocytosis. Diabetes 2002;51(Suppl 1):S3. [PMID: 11815450]

Gonzalez L, Scheller RH: Regulation of membrane trafficking: structural insights from a rab/effector complex. Cell 1999; 96:755.

Huete-Perez JA et al: Protease trafficking in two primitive eukaryotes is mediated by a prodomain protein motif. J Biol Chem 1999;274:16249.

Huopio H et al: K^{ATP} channels and insulin secretion disorders. Am J Physiol Endocrinol 2002;283:E207. [PMID: 12110524]

Kanai N et al: Identification and characterization of a prostaglandin transporter. Science 1995;268:866.

Kelly RB: Deconstructing membrane traffic. Trends Cell Biol 1999;9:M29.

Lingappa VR, Farey KC: *Physiological Medicine.* McGraw-Hill, 2000.

Lingappa VR et al: Conformational control through translocational regulation: a new view of secretory and membrane protein folding. Bioessays 2002;24:741. [PMID: 12210535]

Maechler P, Wollheim CB: Mitochondrial glutamate acts as a messenger in glucose-induced insulin exocytosis. Nature 1999; 402:685.

Mellon SH, Griffin LD: Neurosteroids: biochemistry and clinical significance. Trends Endocrinol Metab 2002;13:35. [PMID: 11750861]

Miller WL, Mellon SH: Steroidogenesis. In: *Reproductive Medicine: Molecular, Cellular and Genetic Fundamentals,* 2nd ed. Fauser BCJM (editor). Parthenon Press, 2002.

Miller WL: Molecular biology of steroid hormone synthesis. Endocr Rev 1988;9:295.

Miller WL: Steroid hormone biosynthesis and actions in the materno-feto-placental unit. Clin Perinatol 1998;25:799.

Molinari M, Helenius A: Chaperone selection during glycoprotein translation into the endoplasmic reticulum. Science 2000; 288:331. [PMID: 10764645]

Omura T, Morohashi K: Gene regulation of steroidogenesis. J Steroid Biochem Mol Biol 1995;53:19.

Schubert U et al: Rapid degradation of a large fraction of newly synthesized proteins by proteasomes. Nature 2000;404:770. [PMID: 10783891]

Smith SS et al: $GABA_A$ receptor α_4 subunit suppression prevents withdrawal properties of an endogenous steroid. Nature 1998;392:926.

Travers KJ et al: Functional and genomic analyses reveal an essential coordination between the unfolded protein response and ER-associated degradation. Cell 2000;101:249. [PMID: 10847880]

Warren G, Mellman I: Bulk flow redux? Cell 1999;98:125.

Mechanisms of Hormone Action

David G. Gardner, MD, & Robert A. Nissenson, PhD

ACTH	Adrenocorticotropin		**HRE**	Hormone response element
AF-1	Activator function-1		**HSP**	Heat shock protein
AF-2	Activator function-2		**ID**	Receptor-repressor interaction domain
AP-1	Activator protein-1		**IGF**	Insulin-like growth factor
βARK	β-Adrenergic receptor kinase		**IP$_3$**	Inositol 1,4,5-trisphosphate
cAMP	Cyclic adenosine-3′,5′-monophosphate		**IP$_4$**	Inositol 1,3,4,5-tetrakis-phosphate
CARM	Coactivator-associated arginine methyl-transferase		**JAK**	Janus kinase
			LBD	Ligand-binding domain
CBP	CREB-binding protein		**LH**	Luteinizing hormone
cGMP	Cyclic guanosine-3′,5′-monophosphate		**MAPK**	Mitogen-activated protein kinase
CNP	C-type natriuretic peptide		**MEK**	Mitogen-activated protein kinase kinase
CREB	cAMP response element binding protein		**MR**	Mineralocorticoid receptor
DAG	Diacylglycerol		**MSH**	Melanocyte-stimulating hormone
DBD	DNA-binding domain		**N-Cor**	Nuclear receptor corepressor
DRIP	Vitamin D receptor-interacting protein		**NPR**	Natriuretic peptide receptor
EGF	Epidermal growth factor		**NR**	Nuclear receptor
ER	Estrogen receptor		**NRTPK**	Nonreceptor protein tyrosine kinase
ERE	Estrogen response element		**P/CAF**	p300/CBP-associated factor
ERK	Extracellular signal-regulated kinase		**P/CIP**	p300/CBP cointegrator-associated protein
FAD	Flavin adenine dinucleotide			
FGF	Fibroblast growth factor		**PDGF**	Platelet-derived growth factor
FMN	Flavin mononucleotide		**PDK**	Phosphatidyl inositol-3,4,5-triphosphate-dependent kinase
GAP	GTPase-activating protein			
GDP	Guanosine diphosphate		**6-PFK**	6-Phosphofructokinase
GH	Growth hormone		**PI-3K**	Phosphoinositide-3-OH kinase
GLUT 4	Glucose transporter type 4		**PIP$_2$**	Phosphoinositol bisphosphate
GR	Glucocorticoid receptor		**PIP$_3$**	Phosphatidyl inositol-3,4,5-trisphosphate
GRB2	Growth factor receptor-bound protein-2			
GRH	Growth hormone-releasing hormone		**PI(3,4)P$_2$**	Phosphatidyl inositol-3,4,5-bisphosphate
GRIP	Glucocorticoid receptor interacting protein		**PKA**	cAMP-dependent protein kinase
			PKB	Protein kinase B
GSK3	Glycogen synthase kinase-3		**PKC**	Protein kinase C
GTF	General transcription factor		**PKG**	cGMP-dependent protein kinase
GTP	Guanosine triphosphate		**PLC$_β$**	Phospholipase C beta

PLC$_\gamma$	Phospholipase C gamma
PLC$_{PC}$	Phosphatidylcholine-selective phospholipase
POF II	RNA polymerase
PPARγ	Peroxisome proliferator-activated receptor
PR	Progesterone receptor
PTH	Parathyroid hormone
RAR	Retinoic acid receptor
RE	Response element
RSK	Ribosomal S6 kinase
RXR	Retinoid X receptor
SH2	Src homology domain type 2
SIE	sis-inducible element
SMRT	Silencing mediator for RXR and TR
SOS	Son-of-sevenless
SR	Steroid receptor

SRC	Steroid receptor coactivator
SRE	Serum response element
SRF	Serum response factor
STAT	Signal transducers and activators of transcription
SWI/SNF	ATP-dependent chromatin remodeling complex
TBP	TATA-binding protein
TPA	12-*O*-Tetradecanoyl-phorbol 13-acetate
TR	Thyroid hormone receptor
TRAP	Thyroid hormone receptor-associated protein
TRE	TPA response element
TSH	Thyroid-stimulating hormone
V2	Type 2 vasopressin receptor
VDR	Vitamin D receptor

Hormones produce their biologic effects through interaction with high-affinity receptors which are, in turn, linked to one or more effector systems within the cell. These effectors involve many different components of the cell's metabolic machinery, ranging from ion transport at the cell surface to stimulation of the nuclear transcriptional apparatus. Steroids and thyroid hormones exert their effects in the cell nucleus, although regulatory activity in the extranuclear compartment has also been documented. Peptide hormones and neurotransmitters, on the other hand, trigger a plethora of signaling activity in the cytoplasmic and membrane compartments while at the same time exerting parallel effects on the transcriptional apparatus. The discussion that follows will focus on the primary signaling systems employed by selected hormonal agonists and attempt to identify examples where aberrant signaling results in human disease.

RECEPTORS

The biologic activity of individual hormones is dependent upon their interactions with specific high-affinity receptors on the surfaces or in the cytoplasm of target cells. The receptors, in turn, are linked to signaling effector systems responsible for generating the observed biologic response. Receptors therefore convey not only specificity of the response (ie, cells lacking receptors lack responsiveness to the hormone) but also the means for activating the effector mechanism. In general, receptors for the peptide hormones and neurotransmitters are aligned on the cell surface while those for the

steroid hormones, thyroid hormone, and vitamin D are found in the cytoplasmic or nuclear compartments.

Interactions between the hormone ligand and its receptor are governed by the laws of mass action:

$$[H] + [R] \underset{k_{-1}}{\overset{k_{+1}}{\rightleftharpoons}} [HR]$$

where [H] is the hormone concentration, [R] is the receptor concentration, [HR] is the concentration of the hormone-receptor complex, and k_{+1} and k_{-1} are the rate constants for [HR] formation and dissociation respectively. Thus, at equilibrium,

$$k_{+1}[H][R] = k_{-1}[HR]$$

or

$$\frac{[H][R]}{[HR]} = \frac{k_{-1}}{k_{+1}} = K_D$$

where K_D is the equilibrium dissociation constant which defines the affinity of the hormone-receptor interaction (ie, the lower the dissociation constant, the higher the affinity). Assuming that total receptor concentration $R_o = [HR] + [R]$, this equation can be rearranged to give

$$\frac{[HR]}{[H]} = -\left(\frac{[HR]}{K_D}\right) + \frac{R_o}{K_D}$$

This is the Scatchard equation and states that when bound over free ligand (ie, [HR]/[H]) is plotted against bound ligand (ie, [HR]), the slope of the line is defined by $-1/K_D$, the y-intercept by R_o/K_D and the x-intercept by R_o (Figure 3–1). When [HR] = $R_o/2$, [H] = K_D; therefore, the K_D is also the concentration of hormone [H] at which one-half of the available receptors are occupied. Thus, knowledge of bound and free ligand concentrations, which can be determined experimentally, provides information regarding the affinity of the receptor for its ligand and the total concentration of receptor in the preparation.

Agents that bind to receptors with high affinity are classified as either agonists or antagonists based on the

functional outcome of this receptor-ligand interaction. Agonists are ligands that trigger the effector mechanisms and produce biologic effects. Antagonists bind to the receptor but do not activate the effector mechanisms. Since they occupy receptor and block association with the agonist, they antagonize the functional activity of the latter. Partial agonists bind to the receptor but possess limited ability to activate the effector mechanisms. In different circumstances, partial agonists demonstrate variable biologic activity. For example, when employed alone, they may display weak activating activity, whereas their use together with a full agonist may lead to inhibition of function since the latter is displaced from the receptor molecule by a ligand with lower intrinsic activity.

In some systems, receptors are available in a surplus which is severalfold higher than that required to elicit a maximal biologic response. Such spare receptor systems, though they superficially appear redundant, are designed to rectify a mismatch between low circulating ligand levels and a relatively low affinity ligand-receptor interaction. Thus, by increasing the number of available receptors, the system is guaranteed a sufficient number of liganded receptor units to activate downstream effector systems fully, despite operating at sub-saturating levels of ligand.

NEUROTRANSMITTER & PEPTIDE HORMONE RECEPTORS

As mentioned above, neurotransmitter and peptide hormones interact predominantly with receptors scattered on the plasma membrane at the cell surface. These receptors fall into four major groups (Table 3–1). The first includes the so-called serpentine or "seven-transmembrane-domain" receptors. These receptors each contain an amino terminal extracellular domain followed by seven hydrophobic amino acid segments, each of which is believed to span the membrane bilayer (Figure 3–2). The seventh of these, in turn, is followed by a hydrophilic carboxyl terminal domain that resides within the cytoplasmic compartment. As a group, they share a dependence on the G protein transducers (see below) to execute many of their biologic effects. A second group includes the single-transmembrane domain receptors that harbor intrinsic tyrosine kinase activity. This includes the insulin, IGF, and EGF receptors. A third group, which is functionally similar to the second group, is characterized by a large extracellular binding domain followed by a single membrane-spanning segment and a cytoplasmic tail. These receptors do not possess intrinsic tyrosine kinase activity but appear to function through interaction with soluble transducer molecules which do possess such activ-

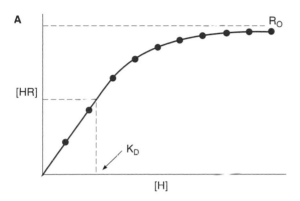

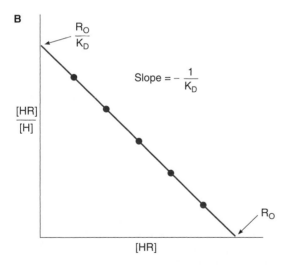

Figure 3–1. Ligand saturation ***(A)*** and Scatchard analysis ***(B)*** of a hypothetical hormone receptor interaction. K_D represents the dissociation constant; R_o the total receptor concentration; [HR] and [H] the bound and free ligand, respectively. Note in ***A*** that the K_D is the concentration [H] at which half of available receptors are occupied.

Table 3–1. Major subdivisions (with examples) of the neurotransmitter-peptide hormone receptor families.[1]

Seven-transmembrane domain
  β-Adrenergic
  PTH
  LH
  TSH
  GRH
  TRH
  ACTH
  MSH
  Glucagon
  Dopamine
  α₂-Adrenergic (–)
  Somatostatin (–)
Single-transmembrane domain
  Growth factor receptors
    Insulin
    IGF
    EGF
    PDGF
  Cytokine receptors
    Growth hormone
    Prolactin
    Erythropoietin
    CSF
  Guanylyl cyclase-linked receptors
    Natriuretic peptides

[1]Receptors have been subdivided based on shared structural and functional similarities. (–) denotes a negative effect on cyclase activity.

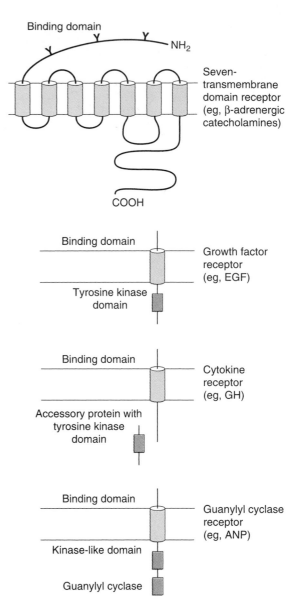

Figure 3–2. Structural schematics of different classes of membrane-associated hormone receptors. Representative ligands are presented in parentheses. (EGF, epidermal growth factor; GH, growth hormone; ANP, atrial natriuretic peptide.)

ity. Prolactin and growth hormone are included in this group. A fourth group, which includes the natriuretic peptide receptors, operates through activation of a particulate guanylyl cyclase and synthesis of cGMP. The cyclase is covalently attached at the carboxyl terminal of the ligand-binding domain and thus represents an intrinsic part of the receptor molecule.

G PROTEIN-COUPLED RECEPTORS

G protein-coupled receptors constitute a large superfamily of molecules capable of responding to ligands of remarkable structural diversity—ranging from photons to large polypeptide hormones. These receptors share overall structural features, most notably seven membrane-spanning regions connected by intracellular and extracellular loops (Figure 3–2). The receptors are oriented such that the amino terminal domain is extracellular, whereas the carboxyl terminal tail is cytoplasmic. The membrane-spanning segments interact with one

another, forming an irregular cylindric bundle around a central cavity within the molecule. G protein-coupled receptors can assume at least two conformations with differing orientations of the membrane-spanning segments relative to one another. One orientation is favored in the absence of an agonist ligand, and in this orientation the receptor does not activate a G protein (inactive conformation). The second orientation is stabilized by the binding of an appropriate agonist ligand, and in this conformation the receptor activates a cognate G protein (active conformation). All G protein-coupled receptors are thought to undergo a similar conformational switch upon agonist binding, producing a structural change in the cytoplasmic domain that promotes G protein activation. Some small agonists like catecholamines are able to enter the cavity formed by the transmembrane segments, thereby directly stabilizing the active receptor conformation. Other agonists, such as large polypeptide hormones, bind primarily to the extracellular domain of their G protein-coupled receptors. This indirectly results in movement of the transmembrane region of the receptor and stabilization of the active receptor conformation.

Heritable mutations in a variety of G protein-coupled receptors are known to be associated with clinical disease. Loss-of-function phenotypes result from mutations that eliminate one or both receptor alleles or that result in the synthesis of signaling-defective receptors. Gain-of-function phenotypes generally result from point mutations that produce receptors which are constitutively active (ie, stably assume the active receptor conformation even in the absence of an agonist ligand). Examples of such G protein-coupled receptor disorders relevant to endocrinology are described below and discussed in greater detail elsewhere in this book.

G PROTEIN TRANSDUCERS

G protein-coupled receptors initiate intracellular signaling by activating one (or in some cases multiple) G proteins. G proteins are a family of heterotrimeric proteins that regulate the activity of effector molecules (eg, enzymes, ion channels) (Table 3–2), resulting ultimately in biologic responses. The identity of a G protein is defined by the nature of its α subunit, which is largely responsible for effector activation. The major G proteins involved in hormone action (and their actions on effectors) are G_s (stimulation of adenylyl cyclase), G_i (inhibition of adenylyl cyclase; regulation of calcium and potassium channels), and $G_{q/11}$ (stimulation of phospholipase Cβ). The β and γ subunits of G proteins are tightly associated with one another and function as a dimer. In some cases, the $\beta\gamma$ subunit dimer also regulates effector function.

G proteins are noncovalently tethered to the plasma membrane and are thus proximate to their cognate receptors and to their effector targets. The basis for specificity in receptor-G protein interactions has not been fully defined. It is likely that specific structural determinants presented by the cytoplasmic loops of the G pro-

Table 3–2. G protein subunits selectively interact with specific receptor and effector mechanisms.

G Protein Subunit	Associated Receptors	Effector
α_s	β-Adrenergic TSH Glucagon	Adenylyl cyclase Ca^{2+} channels K^+ channels
α_i	α_2-Adrenergic Muscarinic (type II)	Adenylyl cyclase Ca^{2+} channels K^+ channels
α_q	α_1-Adrenergic	PLCβ
β/α		Adenylyl cyclase (+ or –) PLC Supports βARK-mediated receptor phosphorylation and desensitization

tein-coupled receptor determine the identity of the G proteins that is activated. It is the nature of the α subunit of the G protein that is critical for receptor recognition. There are about a dozen different G protein α subunits, and hundreds of distinct G protein-coupled receptors. Thus, it is clear that a particular G protein is activated by a large number of different receptors. For example, G_s is activated by receptors for ligands as diverse as β-adrenergic catecholamines and large polypeptide hormones such as LH. LH is thereby able to stimulate adenylyl cyclase and raise intracellular levels of cAMP in cells that express LH receptors (eg, Leydig cells of the testis).

Figure 3–3 is a schematic representation of the molecular events associated with activation of G proteins by G protein-coupled receptors. In the basal, inactive state, the G protein is an intact heterotrimer with guanosine diphosphate (GDP) bound to the α subunit. Agonist binding to a G protein-coupled receptor promotes the physical interaction between the receptor and its cognate G protein. This produces a conformational change in the G protein, resulting in the dissociation of GDP. This in turn allows the binding of GTP (which is present at much higher concentration in cells than is GDP) to the α subunit. Dissociation of the $\beta\gamma$-bound and GTP bound α subunits then occurs, allowing these subunits to activate their effector targets. Dissociation of the hormone-receptor complex also occurs. The duration of activation is determined by the intrinsic GTPase activity of the G protein α subunit. Hydrolysis of GTP to GDP terminates the activity and promotes reassociation of the $\beta\gamma$ subunits, returning the system to the basal state.

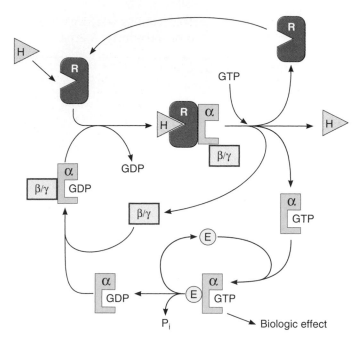

Figure 3–3. G protein-mediated signal transduction. α and β/γ subunits of a representative G protein are depicted. (See text for details.) (R, hormone receptor; H, hormonal ligand; E, effector.)

G PROTEIN DISORDERS

Two bacterial toxins are capable of covalently modifying specific G protein α subunits, thereby altering their functional activity. Cholera toxin is a protein that binds to receptors present on all cells, resulting in the internalization of the enzymatic subunit of the toxin. The toxin enzyme is an ADP-ribosyl transferase that transfers ADP-ribose from NAD to an acceptor site (Arg[201]) on the α subunit of G_s. This covalent modification greatly inhibits the GTPase activity of α_s, enhancing the activation of adenylyl cyclase by extending the duration of the active GTP-bound form of the G protein. Even in the absence of an active G protein-coupled receptor, GDP dissociates (albeit very slowly) from the G protein. Thus, cholera toxin will eventually activate adenylyl cyclase activity even without agonist binding to a G protein-coupled receptor. The result is a large and sustained activation of adenylyl cyclase. When this occurs in intestinal epithelial cells, the massive increase in cAMP results in the increased water and salt secretion characteristic of cholera.

Pertussis toxin is also an ADP-ribosyl transferase. However, in this case, the substrates are the α subunits of different G proteins, most notably G_i and G_o. The ADP-ribose moiety is transferred to a cysteine residue near the carboxyl terminal of the α subunit, a region required for interaction with activated G protein-coupled receptors. Once ADP-ribosylated by pertussis toxin, these G proteins are no longer able to interact with activated receptors and are thus stuck in an inactive (GDP-bound) conformation. Inhibition of receptor-mediated activation of G_i and G_o accounts for many of the clinical manifestations of pertussis infection.

Genetic mutations in G protein α subunits are seen in a number of human diseases. Acquired, activating mutations in α_s can produce a variety of phenotypes depending on the site of expression of the mutant protein. In McCune-Albright syndrome, the mutation occurs in a subset of neural crest cells during embryogenesis. All of the descendants of these cells, including certain osteoblasts, melanocytes, and ovarian or testicular cells, express the mutant protein. The result is a form of genetic mosaicism in which the consequence of unregulated production of cAMP in particular tissues is evident (ie, the progressive bone disorder polyostotic fibrous dysplasia, abnormal skin pigmentation referred to as café au lait spots, gonadotropin-independent precocious puberty). In cells where cAMP is linked to cell proliferation (eg, thyrotropes, somatotropes), a subset of patients with benign tumors have been shown to have acquired activating mutations in α_s. Activating mutations in one of the G_i proteins that is coupled to cell proliferation, α_{i2}, have been reported in a subset of adrenal and ovarian tumors.

Loss-of-function mutations in α_s are associated with the hereditary disorder pseudohypoparathyroidism type Ia (PHP-Ia). This disorder, first described by Fuller Albright, is the first documented example of a human disease attributable to target cell resistance to a hormone. Affected patients display biochemical features of hypoparathyroidism (eg, hypocalcemia, hyperphosphatemia) but have markedly increased circulating levels of parathyroid hormone (PTH) and display target cell resistance to PTH. Many hormone receptors couple to adenylyl cyclase via G_s, yet patients with PHP-Ia generally display only subtle defects in responsiveness to other hormones (eg, TSH, LH). The explanation for this lies in the fascinating genetics of this disorder. In brief, affected patients have one normal and one mutated α_s allele. The mutated allele fails to produce an active form of the protein. Tissues in these patients are expected to express about 50% of the normal level of α_s, a level sufficient to support signaling to adenylyl cyclase. However, in certain tissues, the α_s gene is subject to genetic imprinting such that the paternal allele is expressed poorly or not at all. For individuals harboring inactivating mutations, if it is the paternal allele that is mutated, all cells will express about 50% of the normal level of α_s (derived from the normal maternal allele). However, if the mutation is on the maternal allele, then the cells where paternal imprinting occurs will express low levels or no α_s. One of the major sites of this paternal imprinting is in the proximal renal tubule, an important target tissue for the physiologic actions of PTH. This accounts for the clinical resistance to PTH seen in PHP-Ia and accounts also for the fact that only a subset of patients with haploinsufficiency of α_s are resistant to PTH. Interestingly, essentially all patients with haploinsufficiency of α_s display Albright's hereditary osteodystrophy, a developmental disorder with phenotypic manifestations affecting a variety of tissues. This indicates that even a partial loss of adenylyl cyclase signaling is incompatible with normal development.

EFFECTORS

Numerous effectors have been linked to the G protein-coupled receptors. A number of these are presented in Table 3–2. There are a great many other G proteins—not dealt with here—that are coupled to physical or biochemical stimuli but have very limited involvement in hormone action. As discussed above, adenylyl cyclase, perhaps the best-studied of the group, is activated by G_s (Figure 3–4). This activation results in a transient increase in intracellular cAMP levels. cAMP binds to the inhibitory regulatory subunit of inactive protein kinase A (PKA) and promotes its dissociation from the complex, thereby permitting enhanced activity of the catalytic subunit. The latter phosphorylates a variety of cellular substrates, among them the hepatic phosphorylase kinase that initiates the enzymatic cascade which results

in enhanced glycogenolysis and the nuclear transcription factor CREB (cAMP response element binding protein), which mediates many of the known transcriptional responses to cAMP (and to some extent calcium) in the nuclear compartment. Other transcription factors are also known to be phosphorylated by PKA.

Phospholipase C beta (PLC_β) is a second effector system that has been studied extensively. The enzyme is activated through G_q-mediated transduction of signals generated by a wide array of hormone-receptor complexes, including those for angiotensin II, α-adrenergic agonists, and endothelin. Activation of the enzyme leads to cleavage of phosphoinositol 4,5-bisphosphate in the plasma membrane to generate inositol 1,4,5-trisphosphate (IP_3) and diacylglycerol (Figure 3–5). The former interacts with a specific receptor present on the endoplasmic reticulum membrane to promote release of Ca^{2+} into the cytoplasmic compartment. The increased calcium, in turn, may activate protein kinases, promote secretion, or foster contractile activity. Depletion of intracellular calcium pools by IP_3 results in enhanced uptake of calcium across the plasma membrane (perhaps through generation of IP_4 [1,3,4,5-tetrakisphosphate]), thereby activating a second, albeit indirect, signaling mechanism that serves to increase intracellular calcium levels even further. Diacylglycerol (DAG) functions as an activator of protein kinase C (PKC) within the cell. Several different isoenzymatic forms of PKC (eg, α, β, γ) exist in a given cell type. A number of these are calcium-dependent, a property which, given the IP_3 activity mentioned above, provides the opportunity for a synergistic interaction of the two signaling pathways driven by PLC_β activity. However, not all protein kinase C activity derives from the breakdown of PIP_2 substrate. Metabolism of phosphatidylcholine by PLC_{PC} leads to the generation of phosphocholine and DAG. This latter pathway is believed to be responsible for the more protracted elevations in PKC activity seen following exposure to agonist. Other phospholipases may also be important in hormone-dependent signaling. Phospholipase D employs phosphatidylcholine as a substrate to generate choline and phosphatidic acid. The latter may serve as a precursor for subsequent DAG formation. As with PLC_{PC} above, no IP_3 is generated as a consequence of this reaction. Phospholipase A_2 triggers release of arachidonic acid, a precursor of prostaglandins, leukotrienes, endoperoxides, and thromboxanes, all signaling molecules in their own right. The relative contribution of these other phospholipases to hormone-mediated signal transduction and the role of the idiosyncratic products (phosphocholine, phosphatidic acid, etc) in conveying regulatory information remains an area of active research.

Activation of effectors by G protein-coupled receptors is subject to regulatory mechanisms that prevent overstimulation of cells by an agonist ligand. At the

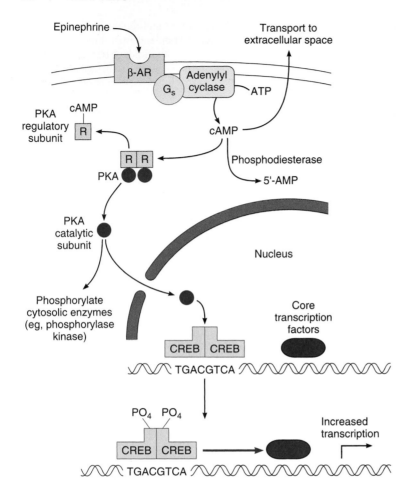

Figure 3–4. β-Adrenergic receptor signaling in the cytoplasmic and nuclear compartments. The cAMP response element binding protein (CREB) is depicted bound to a consensus CRE in the basal state. Phosphorylation of this protein leads to activation of the juxtaposed core transcriptional machinery.

level of the receptor, two regulatory events are known to occur. One is desensitization, wherein initial stimulation of a receptor by its agonists leads to a loss of the ability of the receptor to subsequently elicit G protein activation. This is shown schematically in Figure 3–6 for the β-adrenergic receptor, and a similar regulatory mechanism exists for many G protein-coupled receptors. Agonist binding to the receptor produces G protein activation and results also in activation of a kinase that phosphorylates the cytoplasmic domain of the receptor. By virtue of this phosphorylation, the receptor acquires high affinity for a member of the arrestin family of proteins. The name "arrestin" derives from the observation that the receptor is no longer capable of interacting with a G protein when arrestin is bound. Thus, the phosphorylated receptor becomes uncoupled from its G protein, preventing signaling to the effector. The receptor remains inactive until a phosphatase acts to restore the receptor to its unphosphorylated state. Many G protein-coupled receptors are also susceptible

to agonist-induced down-regulation, resulting in a reduced level of cell surface receptors following exposure of cells to an agonist. This can result from agonist-induced internalization of receptors, followed by trafficking of receptors to lysosomes where degradation occurs. In addition, chronic exposure of cells to an agonist may result in signaling events that suppress the biosynthesis of new receptors, thereby lowering steady state receptor levels. Together, these regulatory events ensure that the cell is protected from excessive stimulation in the presence of sustained high levels of an agonist.

G PROTEIN-COUPLED RECEPTORS & HUMAN DISEASE

Mutations in the genes encoding G protein-coupled receptors are being increasingly recognized as important in the pathogenesis of endocrine disorders. Loss-of-function mutations generally need to be homozygous (or compound heterozygous) in order to result in a significant

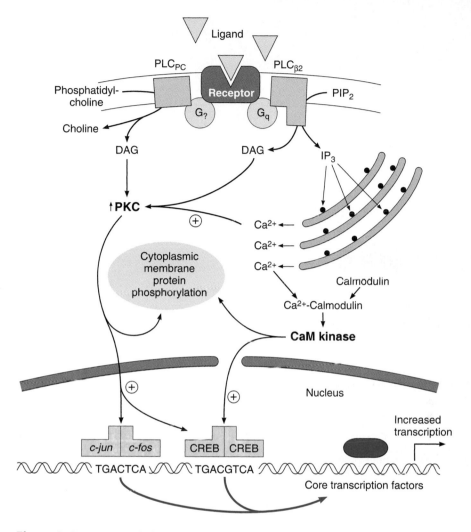

Figure 3–5. PLC$_\beta$-coupled receptor signaling in the cytoplasmic and nuclear compartments. (PLC, phospholipase; PC, phosphatidylcholine; DAG, diacylglycerol; PKC, protein kinase C.)

disease phenotype. This is probably due to the fact that most cells have a complement of receptors which exceeds what is needed for maximal cellular response ("spare receptors"). Thus, a 50% reduction in the amount of a cell surface receptor may have little influence on the ability of a target cell to respond. However, in some situations, haploinsufficiency of a G protein-coupled receptor can produce a clinical phenotype. For instance, heterozygous loss-of-function mutations in the G protein-coupled calcium-sensing receptor results in the dominant disorder familial hypocalciuric hypercalcemia due to mild dysregulation of PTH secretion and renal calcium handling. Homozygous loss of function of the calcium-sensing re-

ceptor results in severe neonatal hyperparathyroidism due to the loss of the ability of plasma calcium to suppress PTH secretion. Syndromes of hormone resistance have also been reported in patients lacking expression of functional G protein-coupled receptors for vasopressin, ACTH, and TSH. Loss of functional expression of the PTH receptor results in Blomstrand chondrodysplasia, a disorder that is lethal due to the inability of PTH-related protein (a PTH receptor agonist) to promote normal cartilage development.

Mutations that render G protein-coupled receptors constitutively-active (in the absence of an agonist ligand) are seen in a number of endocrine disorders. Gen-

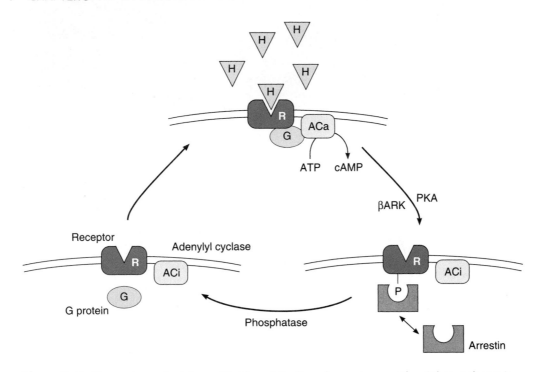

Figure 3–6. Kinase-dependent desensitization of the ligand-receptor complex. Schema shown is that for the β-adrenergic receptor, but similar systems probably exist for other types of G protein-linked receptors. (βARK identifies the β-adrenergic receptor kinase; PKA, protein kinase A; ACa, active adenylyl cyclase; ACi, inactive adenylyl cyclase.)

erally speaking, such mutations produce a disease phenotype resembling that seen with excessive levels of the corresponding hormone agonist. Thus, activating mutations in the TSH produce neonatal thyrotoxicosis, and activating mutations in the LH receptor result in pseudoprecocious puberty or testotoxicosis. Activating mutations in the PTH receptor result in Jansen's metaphysial chondrodysplasia, a disorder characterized by hypercalcemia and increased bone resorption (mimicking the effects of excess PTH on bone) and delayed cartilage differentiation (mimicking the effects of excess PTH-related protein on cartilage). Molecular analysis of G protein-coupled receptors has revealed that point mutations, in addition to producing constitutive activity, can alter the specificity of ligand binding or the ability of the receptor to become desensitized. It is almost certain that such mutations will be found to provide the basis for some perhaps more subtle endocrinopathies.

GROWTH FACTOR RECEPTORS

The growth factor receptors differ from those described above both structurally and functionally. Unlike the G protein-associated receptors, these proteins span the membrane only once and acquire their signaling ability, at least in part, through activation of tyrosine kinase activity, which is intrinsic to the individual receptor molecules. The insulin and IGF receptors fall within this group as do those for the autocrine or paracrine regulators platelet-derived growth factor (PDGF), fibroblast growth factor (FGF), and epidermal growth factor (EGF). Signaling is initiated by the association of ligand (eg, insulin) with the receptor's extracellular domain (Figure 3–7) and subsequent receptor dimerization. This results in phosphorylation of tyrosines both on the receptor itself as well as on nonreceptor substrates. It is assumed that phosphorylation of these substrates results in a cascade of activation events, similar to those described for the G protein-coupled systems, which contribute to perturbations in the intracellular phenotype. The autophosphorylation of the receptor molecules themselves has been studied extensively and provided some intriguing insights into the mechanisms that underlie signal transduction by this group of proteins.

Tyrosine phosphorylation takes place at specific locations in the receptor molecule. Once phosphorylated, these sites associate, in highly specific fashion, with a

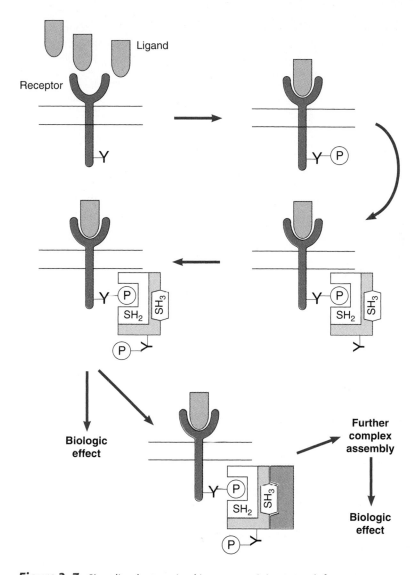

Figure 3–7. Signaling by tyrosine kinase-containing growth factor receptor. Receptors depicted here as monomers for simplicity; typically dimerization of receptors follows association with ligand. Autophosphorylation of one or more critically positioned tyrosine residues in the receptor leads to association with accessory proteins or effectors through SH2 domains present on the latter. In some cases an SH3 domain present on the same protein leads to recruitment of yet other proteins leading to further complex assembly.

variety of accessory proteins that possess independent signaling capability. These include phospholipase Cγ (PLCγ), phosphoinositol (PI) 3′ kinase, GTPase-activating protein (GAP), and growth factor receptor-bound protein-2 (GRB2). These interactions are fostered by the presence of highly conserved type 2 *src* homology (based on sequence homology to the *src* proto-oncogene) domains (SH2) in each of the accessory molecules. Each individual SH2 domain displays specificity for the contextual amino acids surrounding the phosphotyrosine residues in the receptor molecule. In the PDGF receptor, for example, the SH2 domain of PLCγ associates selectively with Tyr^{977} and Tyr^{989} while that of PI 3′ kinase associates with Tyr^{708} and Tyr^{719}. Thus, diversity of response is controlled by contextual sequences around individual phosphotyrosine residues that determine the types of accessory proteins which will be brought into the signaling complex. These protein-protein interactions may provide a means of directly activating the signaling molecule in question, perhaps through a change in steric conformation. Alternatively, they may facilitate the sequestration of these accessory proteins in or near the plasma membrane compartment, in close proximity to key substrates (eg, membrane lipids in the case of PLCγ) or other important regulatory proteins.

While some of these associations trigger immediate signaling events, others (eg, GRB2) may act largely to provide the scaffolding needed to construct a more complex signaling apparatus (Figure 3–8). In the case of GRB2, another accessory protein (son-of-sevenless; SOS) associates with the receptor-GRB2 complex through a type 3 *src* homology (SH3) domain present in the latter. This domain recognizes a sequence of proline-rich amino acids present in the SOS protein. SOS,

in turn, facilitates assembly of the Ras-Raf complex which permits activation of downstream effectors like mitogen-activated protein kinase (MAPK) kinase (MEK). This latter kinase, which possesses both serine-threonine and tyrosine kinase activity, activates the p42 and p44 MAPKs (also called extracellular signal-regulated kinases; ERKs). ERK acts upon a variety of substrates within the cell, including the RSK kinases, which, in turn, phosphorylate the ribosomal S6 protein and thereby stimulates protein synthesis. These phosphorylation reactions (and their amplification in those instances where the MAPK substrate is a kinase itself) often lead to protean changes in the phenotype of the target cells.

The liganded growth factor receptors, including the insulin receptor, may also signal through the phosphoinositide 3-OH kinase (PI-3K). SH2 domains of the p85 regulatory subunit of PI-3K associate with the growth factor receptor through specific phosphotyrosine residues (Tyr^{740} and Tyr^{751} in the PDGF receptor) in a manner similar to that described above for GRB2 (Figure 3–7). This leads to activation of the p110 catalytic subunit of PI-3K and increased production of phos-

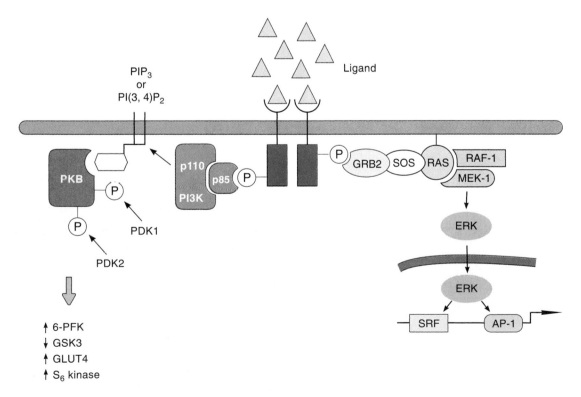

Figure 3–8. Growth factor-dependent pathway. Assembly of the components involved in the *ras/raf*/MEK/MAPK and PI-3 K/PKB signaling mechanisms.

phatidylinositol-3,4,5-trisphosphate (PIP_3) and phosphatidylinositol-3,4-bisphosphate ($PI[3,4]P_2$). These latter molecules sequester protein kinase B (also known as Akt) at the cell membrane through association with the plekstrin homology domains in the amino terminal of the kinase molecule. This in turn leads to phosphorylation of PKB at two separate sites (Thr[308] in the active kinase domain and Ser[473] in the carboxyl terminal tail) by PIP_3-dependent kinases (PDK1 and PDK2). These phosphorylations result in activation of PKB. Downstream targets of activated PKB (eg, following insulin stimulation) include 6-phosphofructo-2-kinase (increased activity), glycogen synthase kinase-3 (decreased activity), the insulin-responsive glucose transporter GLUT 4 (translocation and increased activity) and p70 S6 kinase (increased activity). This leads to increased glycolysis, increased glycogen synthesis, increased glucose transport, and increased protein synthesis, respectively. There is also a growing body of evidence suggesting that PKB may protect cells from programmed cell death through phosphorylation of key proteins in the apoptotic pathway.

It has been reported that G protein-coupled receptors may also activate the Raf-MEK-ERK cascade, though in this case the signal traffics through a non-receptor protein tyrosine kinase (NRPTK such as Src and Fyn) rather than the traditional growth factor receptor-linked tyrosine kinases. The details of the mechanism are incompletely understood, but it appears to require the participation of β-arrestin (see above) as an adaptor molecule linking the G protein receptor to the NRPTK. Interestingly, this implies that β-arrestin, which terminates coupling between the receptor and G protein, actually promotes coupling between the desensitized receptor and downstream effectors traditionally associated with growth factor-dependent activation.

CYTOKINE RECEPTORS

These include the receptors for a variety of cytokines, erythropoietin, colony-stimulating factor, growth hormone, and prolactin. These receptors have a single internal hydrophobic stretch of amino acids, suggesting that they span the membrane but once (Figure 3–9). Interestingly, alternative splicing of the GH receptor gene primary transcript results in a foreshortened "receptor" that lacks the membrane anchor and carboxyl terminal domain of the protein. This "receptor" is secreted and serves to bind GH in the extracellular space (eg, circulating plasma). Unlike the growth factor receptors described above, GH receptors lack a tyrosine kinase domain. Their mechanism of action is not perfectly understood but appears to involve the participation of signaling intermediates, like JAK2, a protein that possesses intrinsic tyrosine kinase activity. The as-

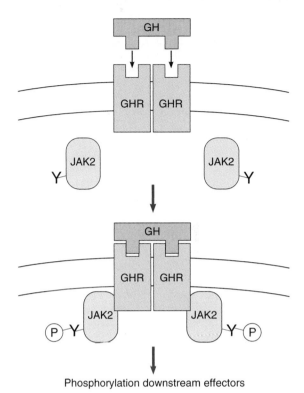

Figure 3–9. Signaling by the growth hormone receptor. Different portions of a single growth hormone molecule associate with homologous regions of two independent growth hormone receptor (GHR) molecules. This is believed to lead to the recruitment of the accessory protein JAK2 and activation of downstream effectors.

sociation of JAK2 with the liganded GH receptor presumably provokes a conformational change in JAK2 and activation of its tyrosine kinase catalytic activity. This, in turn, triggers downstream signaling events, including activation of transcription factors (eg, STAT), and stimulation of MAPK and the S6 kinase (RSK) activity.

GUANYLYL CYCLASE-LINKED RECEPTORS

Activation of guanylyl cyclase-dependent signaling cascades can occur through two independent mechanisms. The first involves activation of the soluble guanylyl cyclase, a heme-containing enzyme that is activated by the gas nitric oxide (NO) generated in the same or neighboring cells. NO is produced by the enzyme nitric oxide synthase. NO synthase exists as three different isozymes in selected body tissues. Constitutive forms of NO synthase are produced in endothelial (NOS-3) and neuronal (NOS-1) cells. The endothelial enzyme possesses binding sites for FAD and FMN as well as calcium and appears to require calcium for optimal activity. Agents like bradykinin and acetylcholine, which interact with receptors on the surface of endothelial cells and increase intracellular calcium levels, trigger an increase in constitutive NO synthase activity with consequent generation of NO and activation of soluble guanylyl cyclase activity in neighboring vascular smooth muscle cells (Figure 3–10). Thus, in this instance, the cGMP-dependent vasodilatory activity of acetylcholine requires sequential waves of signaling activity in two different cell types to realize the ultimate physiologic effect.

The inducible (i) form of NO synthase (NOS-2) is found predominantly in inflammatory cells of the immune system although it has also been reported to be present in smooth muscle cells of the vascular wall. Unlike the endothelial form of NO synthase, expression of iNO synthase is low in the basal state. Treatment of cells with a variety of cytokines triggers an increase in new iNO synthase synthesis (hence, the inducible component of iNO synthase activity), probably through activation of specific cis elements in the iNO synthase promoter. Thus, hormones, cytokines, or growth factors with the capacity for induction of iNO synthase activity may direct at least a portion of their signaling activity through a cGMP-dependent pathway.

A third mechanism for increasing cGMP levels within target cells involves the activation of particulate guanylyl cyclases. From an endocrine standpoint, this involves predominantly the natriuretic peptide receptors (NPR). NPR-A is a single-transmembrane-domain receptor (about 130 kDa) with a large extracellular domain that provides ligand recognition and binding. This is followed by a hydrophobic transmembrane domain and a large intracellular domain which harbors the signaling function. The amino terminal portion of this intracellular region contains a kinase-like ATP-binding domain that is involved in regulating cyclase activity while the carboxyl terminal domain contains the catalytic core of the particulate guanylyl cyclase. It is believed that association of ligand with the extracellular domain leads to a conformational change in the receptor that arrests the tonic inhibitory control of the kinase-like domain and permits activation of guanylyl cyclase activity. NPR-B, the product of a separate gene, has a similar topology and a relatively high level of sequence homology to the NPR-A gene product; however, while NPR-A responds predominantly to the cardiac atrial natriuretic peptide (ANP), NPR-B is activated by the C-type NP (CNP), a peptide found in the central nervous system, endothelium, and reproductive tissues but not in the heart. Thus, segregated expression of the ligand and its cognate receptor convey a high level of response specificity to these two systems despite the fact that they share a common final effector mechanism.

NUCLEAR ACTION OF PEPTIDE HORMONES

Although the initial targets of peptide hormone receptor signaling appear to be confined to the cytoplasm, it is clear that these receptors can also have profound effects on nuclear transcriptional activity. They accomplish this through the same mechanisms they employ to regulate enzymatic activity in the cytoplasmic compartment (eg, through activation of kinases and phosphatases). In this case, however, the ultimate targets are transcription factors that govern the expression of target genes. Examples include hormonal activation of c-*jun* and c-*fos,* nuclear transcription factors which make up the heterodimeric AP-1 complex. This complex has been shown to alter the expression of a wide variety of eukaryotic genes through association with a specific recognition element, termed the phorbol ester (TPA)-response element (TRE), present within the DNA sequence of their respective promoters. Other growth factor receptors that employ the MAPK-dependent signaling mechanism appear to target the serum response factor (SRF) and its associated ternary complex proteins. Posttranslational modification of these transcription factors is believed to amplify the signal that traffics from this complex, when associated with the cognate serum response element (SRE), to the core transcriptional apparatus. cAMP-dependent activation of protein kinase A results in the phosphorylation of a nuclear protein CREB (cAMP response element binding protein) at Ser^{119}, an event which results in enhanced transcriptional activity of closely positioned promoters. The latter requires the participation of an intermediate CREB-binding protein (CBP). CBP is a coactivator molecule that functionally tethers CREB to proteins of the core transcriptional machinery. Interestingly, CBP may also play a similar role in nuclear receptor signaling (see below). Growth hormone is known to induce the phosphorylation of an 84 kDa and a 97 kDa protein in target cells. These proteins have been shown to associate with the sis-inducible element (SIE) in the c-*fos* promoter and to play a role in signaling cytokine activity which traffics through this element. It remains to be demonstrated that these proteins play a similar functional role in mediating GH-dependent effects. Several recent studies have provided evidence suggesting that a number of peptide hormones and growth

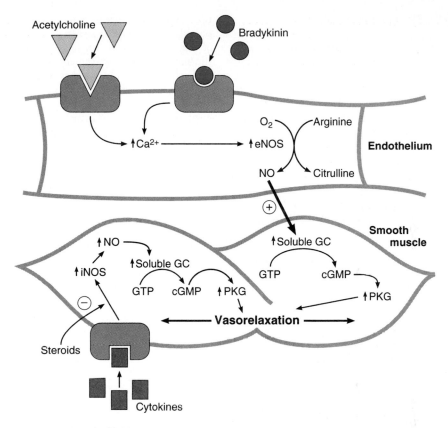

Figure 3-10. Signaling through the endothelial (e) and inducible (i) nitric oxide synthases (NOS) in the vascular wall. Activation of eNOS in the endothelial cell or iNOS in the vascular smooth muscle cell leads to an increase in NO and stimulation of soluble guanylyl cyclase (GC) activity. Subsequent elevations in cGMP activate cGMP-dependent protein kinase (PKG) and promote vasorelaxation.

factors may bind to high-affinity receptors in the cell nucleus. The role these receptors play—if any—in contributing to the signaling profile of these peptides remains undefined.

NUCLEAR RECEPTORS

The nuclear receptors, which include those for the glucocorticoids, mineralocorticoids, androgens, progesterone, estrogens, thyroid hormone, and vitamin D, differ from the receptors of the surface membrane described above in that they are soluble receptors with a proclivity for employing transcriptional regulation as a means of promoting their biologic effects. Thus, though some receptors are compartmentalized in the cytoplasm (eg, glucocorticoid receptor) while others are confined to the nucleus (eg, thyroid hormone receptor),

they all operate within the nuclear chromatin to initiate the signaling cascade. These receptors can be grouped into two major subtypes based on shared structural and functional properties. The first, the steroid receptor family, includes the prototypical glucocorticoid receptor (GR) and the receptors for mineralocorticoids (MR), androgens (AR), and progesterone (PR). The second, the thyroid receptor family, includes the thyroid hormone receptor (TR), estrogen (ER), retinoic acid (RAR and RXR), peroxisome proliferator-activated receptor (PPAR), and vitamin D (VDR) receptors. In addition, there are more than 100 so-called orphan receptors that bear structural homology to members of the extended nuclear receptor family. For most of these the "ligand" is unknown, and their functional roles in the regulation of gene expression have yet to be determined.

STEROID RECEPTOR FAMILY

Steroid receptors (ie, GR, MR, AR, and PR), under basal conditions, exist as cytoplasmic, multimeric complexes that include the heat shock proteins hsp 90, hsp 70, and hsp 56. The estrogen receptor (ER), though demonstrating similar association with heat shock proteins, is largely confined to the nuclear compartment. Association of the steroid ligand with the receptor results in dissociation of the heat shock proteins. This in turn exposes a nuclear translocation signal previously buried in the receptor structure and initiates transport of the receptor to the nucleus, where it associates with the hormone response element (Figure 3–11).

Each of the family members has been cloned and sequenced, and crystallographic structures have been obtained for many of them. Consequently, we know a great deal about their structure and function (Figure 3–12). Each has an extended amino terminal domain of varying length and limited sequence homology to other

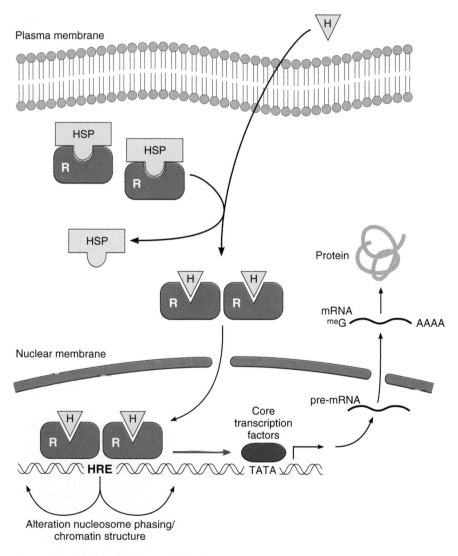

Figure 3–11. Signaling through the steroid receptor complex. Similar mechanisms are employed by members of the TR gene family, though most of the latter are concentrated in the nuclear compartment and are not associated with the heat shock protein complex prior to binding ligand. (^meG, methyl guanosine.)

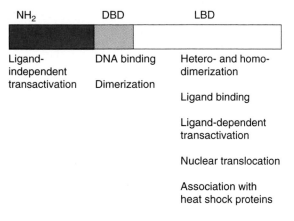

Figure 3–12. Structural schematic of a representative steroid receptor molecule. Separate designations are given to the amino terminal (NH₂), DNA-binding (DBD), and ligand-binding (LBD) domains. Functional activity associated with each of these individual domains, as determined by mutagenesis studies, are indicated below.

family members. In at least some receptors, this region, which has been termed AF-1, is believed to participate in the transactivation function through which the individual receptors promote increased gene transcription. Significant variability in the length of the amino terminal regions of the different receptors suggests potential differences in their respective mechanisms for transcriptional regulation. The amino terminal is followed by a basic region that has a high degree of homology to similarly positioned regions in both the steroid and thyroid receptor gene families. This basic region encodes two zinc finger motifs (Figure 3–13) which have been shown to establish contacts in the major groove of the cognate DNA recognition element (see below). Based on crystallographic data collected for the DNA binding region of the GR, we know that the amino acid sequence lying between the first and second fingers (ie, recognition helix) is responsible for establishing specific contacts with the DNA. The second finger provides the stabilizing contacts that increase the affinity of the receptor for DNA. The DNA binding region also harbors amino acid residues that contribute to the dimerization of monomers contiguously arrayed on the DNA recognition element. Following the basic region is the carboxyl terminal domain of the protein. This domain is responsible for binding of the relevant ligand, receptor dimerization or heterodimerization, and association with the heat shock proteins. It also contributes to the ligand-dependent transactivation function (incorporated in a subdomain termed AF-2) that drives transcriptional activity. Interestingly, in selected cases, nonligands have

been shown to be capable of activating steroid receptors. Dopamine activates the progesterone receptor and increases PR-dependent transcriptional activity, probably through a phosphorylation event, which elicits a conformational change similar to that produced by the association of the receptor with progesterone.

The DNA-binding regions of these receptors contact DNA through a canonical hormone recognition element (HRE) which is described in Table 3–3. Interestingly, each receptor in the individual subfamily binds to the same recognition element with high affinity. Thus, specificity of hormone action must be established either by contextual DNA sequence lying outside the recognition element or by other, nonreceptor DNA-protein interactions positioned in close proximity to the element. Interestingly, the GR, as well as some other nuclear receptors (eg, ER), are capable of binding to DNA sequence lacking the classic HRE. Originally described in the mouse proliferin gene promoter, these composite elements associate with heterologous complexes containing GR, as well as components of the AP-1 transcription factor complex (ie, c-*jun* and c-*fos*), and display unique regulatory activity at the level of contiguously positioned promoters. One such composite element, for example, directs very specific transcriptional effects depending on whether the GR or the MR is included in the complex.

Several steroids, particularly the glucocorticoids and estrogens, have been reported to have independent effects on the stability of target gene transcripts. At this point it is unclear what role the hormone receptors play in this process and whether transcript stabilization is tied mechanistically to the enhancement of transcriptional activity.

THYROID RECEPTOR FAMILY

Included in this group are the TR, RAR, RXR, ER, PPAR, and VDR. They share a high degree of homology to the proto-oncogene c-*erb*A and high affinity for a common DNA recognition site (Table 3–3). With the exception of the ER, they do not associate with the heat shock proteins, and they are constitutively bound to chromatin in the cell nucleus. Specificity of binding for each of the individual receptors is, once again, probably conferred by a contextual sequence surrounding this element, the orientation of the elements (eg, direct repeats or inverted repeats or palindromes), the polarity (ie, 5′ in contrast to 3′ position on two successive repeats), and the number and nature of the spacing nucleotides separating the repeats.

The estrogen receptor binds to its RE as a homodimer, while the VDR, RAR, RXR, and TR prefer binding as heterodimers. The nature of the heterodimeric partners has provided some intriguing insights into the

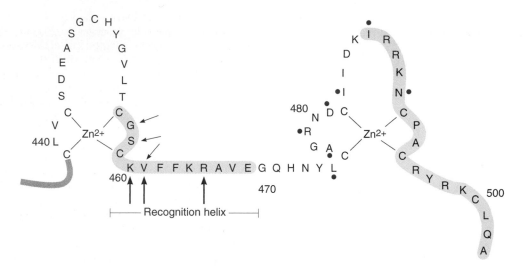

Figure 3–13. Schema of the two zinc fingers, together with coordinated zinc ion, which make up the DNA-binding domain of the glucocorticoid receptor (amino acids are numbered relative to the full length receptor). Shaded regions denote two alpha helical structures which are oriented perpendicularly to one another in the receptor molecule. The first of these, the recognition helix, makes contact with bases in the major groove of the DNA. Large arrows identify amino acids which contact specific bases in the glucocorticoid response element (GRE). Lighter arrows identify amino acids that confer specificity for the GRE; selective substitutions at these positions can shift receptor specificity to other response elements. Dots identify amino acids making specific contacts with the phosphate backbone of DNA. (Modified from Luisi BF et al. Reprinted, with permission, from Nature 1991;352:498. Copyright © 1991 by Macmillan Magazines Ltd.)

biology of these receptors. The most prevalent TR-associated partners appear to be the retinoid X receptors. These latter receptors, which as homodimers form high-affinity associations with 9-*cis*-retinoic acid, also form heterodimeric complexes in the unliganded state with VDR and RAR. In individual cases where it has been examined, heterodimerization with RXR amplifies both the DNA binding and the functional activity of these other receptors. Thus, the ability to form such heterodimeric complexes may add significantly to the flexibility and potency of these hormone receptor systems in regulating gene expression. Interestingly, the positioning (5′ versus 3′) of the participant proteins on the RE is important in determining the functional outcome of the association. In most of those situations linked to transcriptional activation, RXR seems to prefer the upstream (5′) position in the dimeric complex. Thus, diversity of response is engendered by the selection of recognition elements (eg, monomeric versus dimeric versus oligomeric sites) and by the choice and positioning of the dimeric partner (eg, homodimer versus heterodimer) where applicable.

The crystallographic structures of the ligand-binding domains (LBDs) of several members of the thyroid receptor family have been described. These include the dimeric unliganded RXRα, monomeric liganded RARγ, monomeric liganded TRα, dimeric agonist (ie, estradiol)- and antagonist (ie, raloxifene)-liganded ERα, liganded VDR, and liganded PPARγ. Each LBD displays a common folding pattern with 12 alpha helices (numbered by convention H1–H12) and a conserved β turn. Some variability exists in that there is no H2 in RARγ and a short H2′ helix is present in PPARγ, but the overall structural configuration is preserved. The dimeric interface is formed through interaction of amino acids located in helices 7–10, with the strongest influence exerted by H10. These interactions appear to be important for both homo- as well as heterodimeric interactions. Binding of ligand has been shown to occur through what has been termed a "mousetrap" mechanism. In the unliganded state, H12, which contains the carboxyl terminal activation domain AF-2, is displaced away from the ligand-binding pocket (see Figure 3–14). Association of agonist ligand (eg, estradiol in the case of the ER) with the hydrophobic core of the receptor leads to a repositioning of H12 over the ligand-binding cavity, where it stabilizes receptor-ligand interactions and closes the "mousetrap." Binding of an antagonist ligand

Table 3–3. DNA recognition elements for major classes of nuclear hormone receptors.[1]

Element	Recognition Sequence	Receptor
HRE	$\longrightarrow$ $\longleftarrow$ AGAACANNNTGTTCT	Glucocorticoid Mineralocorticoid Progesterone Androgen
ERE	$\longrightarrow$ $\longleftarrow$ AGGTCANNNTGACCT	Estrogen
TRE	$\longleftarrow$ $\longleftarrow$ AGGTCA(N)$_n$AGGTCA	Vitamin D Thyroid hormone Retinoic acids PPAR ligands

[1]Elements represent consensus sequences selected to emphasize the modular nature of the half-sites and their capacity for palindrome generation. Sequences read in the 5′ to 3′ direction. N denotes a spacer nucleoside (either A, G, C, or T). Half-sites are identified by the overlying arrows. The TRE is arrayed as a direct repeat but may also exist as a palindrome or an inverted palindrome. A variable number of spacer nucleotides are positioned between the two direct repeats, depending on the type of hormone receptor. Three, four, and five nucleosides (ie, n = 3, 4, or 5) are preferred for binding of the VDR, TR, or RAR, respectively.

such as raloxifene, which because of its structure engenders steric hindrance in the ligand-binding pocket, prevents closure of H12 into the normal agonist position. Instead, H12 folds into an alternative location between H4 and H3, a conformation that suppresses the activation function of the receptor (see below).

The mechanistic underpinnings of transcriptional regulation by the nuclear receptors have been partially elucidated (Figure 3–15). In the unliganded state, the receptor dimers are associated with a macromolecular complex containing the repressor proteins N-CoR or SMRT, a transcriptional corepressor Sin3, and a histone deacetylase RPD3. N-CoR and SMRT each use two independent IDs (receptor interaction domains) to associate with the nuclear receptors (one repressor: two receptors). Histone acetylation is typically associated with activation of gene transcription (presumably reflecting decompaction of chromatin surrounding the transcriptional unit), so the presence of histone deacetylase activity in the complex promotes a transcriptionally quiescent state. Addition of ligand leads to a change in receptor conformation that no longer favors interaction with the repressor and promotes both ATP-dependent chromatin remodeling and assembly of an activator complex containing p160 coactivator proteins

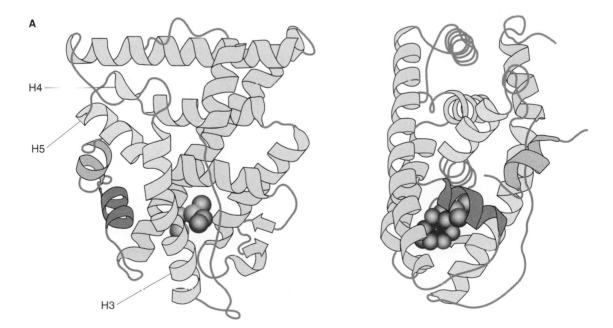

Figure 3–14. Three-dimensional structures for the agonist- and antagonist-occupied ERα LBD. **Panel A:** Orthogonal views of the agonist diethylstilbestrol-ERα LBD-NR Box II peptide complex. Coactivator peptide and LBD are presented as ribbon diagrams. Peptide is colored medium blue, helix (H) 12 (ERα residues 538–546) is colored dark blue. Helices 3, 4, and 5 are colored light blue. Diethylstilbestrol is depicted in a space-filling format.

B

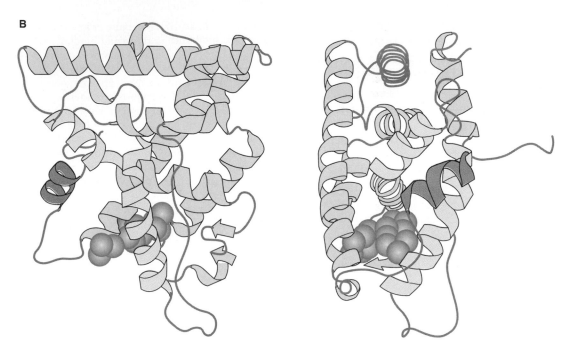

Figure 3–14. ***Panel B:*** Orthogonal views of the antagonist 4-hydroxytamoxifen-ERα LBD complex. Color scheme is the same as in panel A. 4-Hydroxytamoxifen is shown in dark gray in a space-filling format. Note that NR Box II is absent in this structure.

C

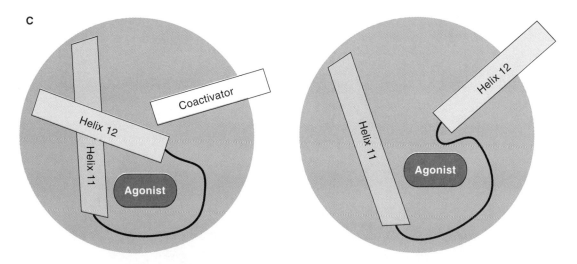

Figure 3–14. ***Panel C:*** Schematic representation of the mechanism underlying agonist-dependent activation of nuclear hormone receptor. In the presence of agonist, helix 12 (the terminal helix in the LBD) folds across the ligand-binding pocket, stabilizing ligand-receptor interaction and promoting a conformation conducive for coactivator association. In the presence of antagonist, steric hindrance precludes folding of helix 12 across the ligand-binding pocket. Instead, it positions itself in the region typically occupied by the coactivator, thereby blocking the activation function of the receptor. (Reprinted, with permission, from Shiau A et al: The structural basis of estrogen receptor/coactivator recognition and the antagonism of this interaction by tamoxifen. Cell 1998;95:927. Copyright © 1998 by Cell Press.)

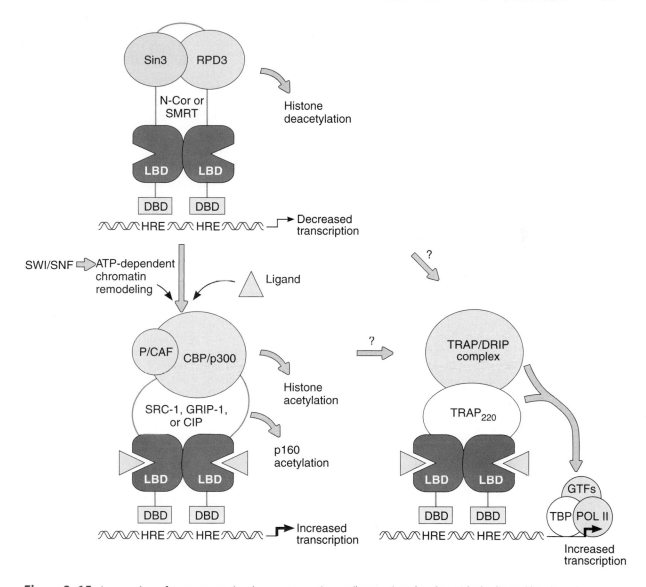

Figure 3–15. Interaction of corepressor (top) versus coactivator (bottom) molecules with the ligand binding domain of a representative nuclear receptor. (See text for details.) The temporal order of p160 versus DRIP/TRAP binding remains undetermined.

(eg, SRC-1, GRIP-1, or P/CIP) and, secondarily, the CREB-binding protein (CBP) and the histone acetylase P/CAF. The net accrual of histone acetylase activity (CBP and P/CIP as well as PCAF possess acetylase activity) leads to acetylation of chromatin proteins (eg, histones) as well as components of the core transcriptional machinery, resulting in chromatin decompaction and a net increase in transcriptional activity. Interaction of

the nuclear receptors with the coactivators in this complex takes place through LXXLL motifs (where L = leucine and X = any amino acid) present in the coactivator proteins. Each coactivator may have several of these motifs, which preferentially associate with different nuclear receptors, other transcription factors, or other coactivators. This allows for a degree of selectivity in terms of which regulatory proteins are incorporated in the complex. Notably, a recent structural analysis showed that a 13-amino-acid peptide, containing an LXXLL motif from the GRIP-1 protein, interacts with TRβ through a hydrophobic cleft generated by helices 3, 4, and 12 (including AF-2) in the receptor protein. This is the same cleft that is occupied by helix 12, which harbors an LXXLL motif, in the raloxifene-bound ERα. This suggests that the antagonist in the latter instance acquires its activation-blocking properties by repositioning helix 12 in a manner that leads to displacement of the coactivator protein from this groove (see above). SRC also interacts with the AF-1 domain, suggesting a potential mechanism for maximizing synergistic activity between AF-1 and AF-2 domains in the receptors.

CBP is thought to function as a pivotal component of the nuclear receptor regulatory complex. While the p160 class of coactivators interact directly with the nuclear receptors, CBP associates primarily with the p160 coactivators, thereby establishing an indirect link to the receptors. As noted above, CBP appears to function as a central integrator of transcriptional regulatory signals from multiple pathways, including the cAMP-dependent activation of the transcription factor CREB. Recent evidence suggests that an additional level of regulatory control may be involved in selectively amplifying nuclear receptor-dependent transcriptional activity. An enzyme called CARM1 (coactivator-associated arginine methyltransferase 1) associates with CBP and methylates the protein. This results in a reduction in CREB-dependent gene activation and, secondarily, an increase in nuclear receptor-dependent gene transcription. This switching mechanism effectively refocuses the transcriptional machinery on expression of nuclear receptor-dependent gene expression.

More recently, another family of coactivator complexes have been identified as playing an important role in nuclear receptor signaling. The human TR-associated protein (TRAP) and vitamin D receptor-interacting protein (DRIP) complexes are the best-characterized to date. These complexes, which contain in the neighborhood of 25 individual proteins, are thought to serve as a functional bridge between the liganded nuclear receptor bound to DNA and the general transcription factors (eg, TBP, TFIIB, RNA polymerase II, and TAFs) involved in formation of the preinitiation complex. The TRAP220 subunit appears to establish the relevant contacts with the nuclear receptors in promoting this assembly. Their role vis-à-vis the p160 coactivators alluded to above remains undefined; however, it has been suggested that they succeed the p160 coactivator complex in binding with liganded nuclear receptors positioned on target gene promoters, establish the requisite structural and functional connections with the core transcriptional machinery, and initiate mRNA

synthesis. It has also been suggested that acetylation of one of the key nuclear receptor (NR) binding motifs (LXXLL) on the SRC coactivator by CBP leads to dissociation of SRC from the nuclear receptors, thereby allowing access for assembly of the TRAP/DRIP complex (Figure 3–15).

While the glucocorticoid receptor is encoded by a single gene, there are two genes for the TR (α and β). TR α1 and TR β1 appear to be the dominant forms of TR in the body. Although considerable overlap exists in their tissue distribution, TR α1 is enriched in skeletal muscle, brown fat, and the central nervous system, while TR β1 is found in the liver, kidney, and central nervous system. They are believed to signal most of the developmental and thermogenic effects of thyroid hormone in the whole animal. TR β2, a splice variant of the TR β gene, is found in the rodent pituitary gland, where it may subserve a specific regulatory function (eg, control of TSH secretion). TR α2, an alternatively spliced product of the TR α gene, lacks the hormone binding domain at the carboxyl terminal of the molecule and thus is not a true thyroid hormone receptor. While under certain experimental conditions TR α2 can block the activity of other members of the TR family, its physiologic role, if one exists, remains undefined. Similar heterogeneity exists in the retinoid receptor family. There are three isoforms for both the RXR and RAR. Collectively, these receptors are thought to play an important role in morphogenesis, but the function of the individual isoforms remains only partially understood.

NONGENOMIC EFFECTS OF THE STEROID HORMONES

While steroids exert most of their biologic activity through direct genomic effects, there are several lines of evidence suggesting that this does not provide a complete picture of steroid hormone action. There are several examples which, for kinetic or experimental reasons, do not fit the classic paradigm associated with a transcriptional regulatory mechanism. Included within this group are the early water imbibition of the uterus associated with estrogen administration, the rapid suppression of ACTH secretion following steroid administration, the modulation of oocyte maturation by progesterone, and regulation of calcium channel function by 1,25-$(OH)_2$ vitamin D. Recent studies have demonstrated the presence of conventional estrogen receptors on the plasma membrane of target cells. The relationship of these receptors to their nuclear counterparts and their role in signaling estrogen-dependent activity (genomic versus nongenomic) is being actively investigated. While we still do not completely understand the mechanisms underlying these nongenomic effects, their potential importance in mediating steroid or thyroid hormone action may, in selected instances, approach that of their more conventional genomic counterparts.

Neurosteroids represent another class of nontraditional hormonal agonists with unique biologic activity. Some of these are native steroids (eg, progesterone), while others are conjugated derivatives or metabolites of the native steroids (eg, dihydroprogesterone). These agonists have been identified in the central nervous system and in some instances shown to have potent biologic activity. It is believed that they operate through interaction with the receptor for γ-aminobutyric acid, a molecule that increases neuronal membrane conductance to chloride ion. This has the net effect of hyperpolarizing the cellular membrane and suppressing neuronal excitability. Interactions that promote receptor activity would be predicted to produce sedative-hypnotic effects in the whole animal, while inhibitory interactions would be expected to lead to a state of central nervous system excitation.

STEROID & THYROID HORMONE RECEPTOR RESISTANCE SYNDROMES

Heritable defects in these receptors have been linked to the pathophysiology of a number of hormone resistance syndromes. These syndromes are characterized by a clinical phenotype suggesting hormone deficiency, by elevated levels of the circulating hormone ligand, and increased (or inappropriately detectable) levels of the relevant trophic regulatory hormone (eg, ACTH, TSH, FSH, or LH). Point mutations in the zinc fingers of the DNA-binding domain as well the ligand-binding domain of the vitamin D receptor leads to a form of vitamin D-dependent rickets (type II) characterized by typical rachitic bone lesions, secondary hyperparathyroidism, and alopecia. It is inherited as an autosomal recessive disorder. Molecular defects scattered along the full length of the androgen receptor, though concentrated in the ligand-binding domain, have been linked to syndromes characterized by varying degrees of androgen resistance ranging from infertility to the full-blown testicular feminization syndrome. Clinical severity, in this case, is thought to be related to the severity of the functional impairment which the mutation imposes on the receptor. Since the androgen receptor is located on the X chromosome, these disorders are inherited in an X-linked fashion. Defects in the glucocorticoid receptor are less common, perhaps reflecting the life-threatening nature of derangements in this system. However, mutations have been identified that impact negatively on receptor function. Clinical presentations in these cases have been dominated by signs and symptoms referable to glucocorticoid deficiency (eg, fatigue, asthenia) and adrenal androgen (eg, hirsutism and sexual precocity) and mineralocorticoid (low renin hypertension) overproduction. This presumably results from defective steroid-mediated suppression of ACTH secretion and adrenal hyperplasia as the former rises in a futile attempt to restore glucocorticoid activity at the periphery. Resistance to thyroid hormone has been linked to a large number of mutations scattered along the full length of the β form of the receptor, although, once again, there is a concentration of mutations in the ligand-binding domain, particularly along the rim of the coactivator binding pocket. No mutations in the α form of the receptor have been linked to a hormone-resistant phenotype. The clinical presentation of thyroid hormone resistance extends from the more typical mild attention deficit syndromes to full-blown hypothyroidism with impaired growth. Different target tissues harboring the mutant receptors display variable sensitivity to thyroid hormone, with some tissues (eg, pituitary) displaying profound resistance and others (eg, heart) responding in a fashion suggesting hyperstimulation with thyroid hormone (ie, thyrotoxicosis). These syndromes are rather unique in that they are inherited as autosomal dominant disorders, presumably reflecting the ability of the mutated receptors to interfere with receptors produced from the normal allele, either by binding to the RE with higher affinity than the wild-type receptors and precluding access of the latter to target genes or by forming inactive heterodimers with the wild-type receptor proteins. Defects in the estrogen receptor are rare, perhaps reflecting the critical role estrogens play in regulating lipoprotein metabolism. However, one male patient has been described who harbors a mutation within the ligand-binding domain of the estrogen receptor. His clinical presentation was characterized by infertility as well as osteopenia, suggesting important roles for estrogens in the maintenance of spermatogenesis as well as bone growth even in male subjects. A syndrome of mineralocorticoid resistance, or pseudohypoaldosteronism, has been described in a number of independent kindreds. Pseudohypoaldosteronism type I is characterized by neonatal renal salt wasting, dehydration, hypotension, hyperkalemia, and hyperchloremic metabolic acidosis despite the presence of elevated aldosterone levels. Heterozygous mutations in the MR are responsible for a milder form of the disease which is inherited in an autosomal dominant pattern. A more severe form of the disease, inherited in an autosomal recessive pattern, appears to be due to loss-of-function mutations in genes encoding subunits of the amiloride-sensitive epithelial sodium channel. Of equivalent interest is the recent identification of an activating mineralocorticoid receptor mutation (Ser_{810}-to-Leu_{810}). This mutation results in severe early-onset hypertension that is markedly exacerbated by pregnancy. The mutation leads to constitutive activation of the

MR and alters the specificity of ligand binding such that traditional MR antagonists, like progesterone, function as partial agonists. This latter property presumably accounts for the dramatic increase in blood pressure during pregnancy.

REFERENCES

G Protein-Coupled Receptors

Caron MG, Lefkowitz RJ: Catecholamine receptors: Structure, function and regulation. Recent Prog Horm Res 1993; 48:277.

Clark AJL, Weber A: Molecular insights into inherited ACTH resistance syndromes. Trends Endocrinol Metab 1994;5:209.

Farfel Z, Bourne HR, Iiri T: The expanding spectrum of G protein diseases. N Engl J Med 1999;340:1012.

Iiri T et al: Rapid GDP release from $G_s\alpha$ in patients with gain and loss of endocrine function. Nature 1994;371:164.

Spiegel AM (editor): *G Proteins, Receptors and Disease.* Humana Press, 1998.

Weinstein LS et al: Endocrine manifestations of stimulatory G protein alpha-subunit mutations and the role of genomic imprinting. Endocr Rev 2001;22:675. [PMID: 11588148]

Effectors

Asaoka Y et al: Protein kinase C, calcium and phospholipid degradation. Trends Biochem Sci 1992;17:414.

Balla T, Catt KJ: Phosphoinositides and calcium signaling. Trends Endocrinol Metab 1994;5:250.

Liscovitch M: Crosstalk among multiple signal-activated phospholipases. Trends Biochem Sci 1992;17:393.

Meyer TE, Habener JF: Cyclic adenosine 3′,5′-monophosphate response element binding protein (CREB) and related transcription-activation deoxyribonucleic acid-binding proteins. Endocr Rev 1993;14:269.

Shikama N, Lyon J, LaThangue NB: The p300/CBP family: integrating signals with transcription factors and chromatin. Trends Cell Biol 1997;7:230.

Sterweis PC, Smrcka AV: Regulation of phospholipase C by G proteins. Trends Biochem Sci 1992;17:502.

Tyrosine Kinase-Coupled and Cytokine Receptors

Carter-Su C, Smit LS: Signaling via JAK tyrosine kinases: Growth hormone receptor as a model system. Recent Prog Horm Res 1998;53:61.

Downward J: Mechanisms and consequences of activation of protein kinase B/Akt. Curr Opin Cell Biol 1998;10:262.

Mussachhio A, Wilmanns M, Saraste M: Structure and function of the SH3 domain. Prog Biophys Molec Biol 1994;61:283.

Nishida E, Gotoh Y: The MAP kinase cascade is essential for diverse signal transduction pathways. Trends Biochem Sci 1993;18:128.

Pazin MJ, Williams LT: Triggering signaling cascades by receptor tyrosine kinases. Trends Biochem Sci 1992;17:374.

Pelech SL, Sanghera JS: Mitogen-activated protein kinases: versatile transducers for cell signaling. Trends Biochem Sci 1992; 17:233.

Roupas P, Herington AC: Postreceptor signaling mechanisms for growth hormone. Trends Endocrinol Metab 1994;5:154.

Guanylyl Cyclase-Linked Receptors

Drewett JG, Garbers DL: The family of guanylyl cyclase receptors and their ligands. Endocr Rev 1994;15:135.

Sessa WC: The nitric oxide synthase family of proteins. J Vasc Res 1994;31:131.

Nuclear Receptors

Freedman LP, Luisi BF: On the mechanism of DNA binding by nuclear hormone receptors: A structural and functional perspective. J Cell Biochem 1993;51:140.

Geller DS et al: Mutations in the mineralocorticoid receptor gene cause autosomal dominant pseudohypoaldosteronism type I. Nat Genet 1998;19:279.

Ito M, Roeder RG: The TRAP/SMCC/Mediator complex and thyroid hormone receptor function. Trends Endocrinol Metab 2001;12:127. [PMID: 11306338]

Lee KC, Kraus WL: Nuclear receptors, coactivators and chromatin: new approaches, new insights. Trends Endocrinol Metab 2001;12:191. [PMID: 11397643]

Moras D, Gronemeyer H: The nuclear receptor ligand binding domain: Structure and function. Curr Opin Cell Biol 1998; 10:384.

Torchia J, Glass C, Rosenfeld MG: Co-activators and co-repressors in the integration of transcriptional responses. Curr Opin Cell Biol 1998;10:373.

Wehling M: Nongenomic actions of steroid hormones. Trends Endocrinol Metab 1994;5:347.

Zhang J, Lazar MA: The mechanism of action of thyroid hormones. Annu Rev Physiol 2000;62:439. [PMID: 10845098]

Endocrine Autoimmunity

4

Juan Carlos Jaume, MD

AADC	Aromatic L-amino decarboxylase	**IL**	Interleukin
ACA	Antibodies recognizing the adrenal cortex	**INF**	Interferon
ADCC	Antibody-dependent cell-mediated cytoxicity	**LFA**	Lymphocyte function-associated antigen
		MHC	Major histocompatibility complex
AICD	Activation-induced cell death	**NK**	Natural killer (cells)
AIRE	Autoimmune regulator gene	**NOD**	Nonobese diabetic (mice)
APECED	Autoimmune polyendocrinopathy-candidiasis-ectodermal dystrophy	**SCA**	Steroid-producing cell antibodies
		SCID	Spontaneous combined immunodeficiency
APS	Autommune polyglandular syndrome		
BB	Bio breeding	**TAP**	Transporter associated with antigen processing
BCR	B cell receptor		
cAMP	Cyclic adenosine monophosphate	**TBI**	Thyrotropin binding inhibition
Ca-SR	Calcium-sensing receptor	**TCR**	T cell receptor
CD	Cluster of differentiation	**TD**	Thymus-dependent
CTLA	Cytotoxic T lymphocyte antigen	**Tg**	Thyroglobulin
DPT	Diabetes Prevention Trial	**TI**	Thymus-independent
FRTL	Fisher rat thyroid cell line	**TNF**	Tumor necrosis factor
GABA	Gamma-aminobutyric acid	**TPO**	Thyroperoxidase
GAD	Glutamic acid decarboxylase	**TSH**	Thyroid-stimulating hormone
HLA	Human leukocyte antigen	**TSH-R**	Thyrotropin receptor
IA-2	Islet cell antigen-2 (tyrosine phosphatase)	**TSI**	Thyroid-stimulating immunoglobulin
		VNTR	Variable number if tandem repeats

Epidemiologic analysis of a large population has reported that about one out of 30 people in the United States (more than 8.5 million individuals) are currently affected by autoimmune diseases. Graves' disease, type 1 diabetes, pernicious anemia, rheumatoid arthritis, chronic thyroiditis (Hashimoto's thyroiditis), and vitiligo are the most prevalent such conditions, accounting for 93% of affected individuals.

These autoimmune diseases have traditionally been looked upon as forming a spectrum. At one end are found organ-specific diseases with organ-specific autoantibodies. Hashimoto's thyroiditis is an example in which a specific lesion affects the thyroid (lymphocytic infiltration, destruction of follicular cells) and autoantibodies are produced with absolute specificity for thyroid proteins. At the other end of the spectrum are the systemic autoimmune diseases, broadly belonging to the class of rheumatologic disorders. Systemic lupus erythematosus is an example of a disease characterized by widespread pathologic changes and a collection of autoantibodies to DNA and other nuclear constituents of all cells. Many organ-specific autoimmune diseases are autoimmune endocrinopathies. Furthermore, autoimmune pathogenesis has been shown to be present in disorders affecting most endocrine glands such as the adrenals (autoimmune Addison's disease), the gonads (autoimmune oophoritis), the pancreas (type 1 diabetes), the pituitary (autoimmune hypophysitis), and the thyroid (autoimmune thyroid disease) (Table 4–1).

85

Table 4–1. Some autoimmune endocrinopathies, antigens, and autoantibodies.

Disease	Gland	Autoantigen	Autoantibody
Autoimmune (lymphocytic) hypophysitis Granulomatous hypophysitis	Pituitary	Pituitary cytosolic protein	Antipituitary
Graves' disease	Thyroid	TSHR, TPO	TSI, TBII, anti-TPO
Hashimoto's thyroiditis	Thyroid	TPO, Tg	Anti-TPO, anti-Tg
Autoimmune (idiopathic) hypoparathyroidism	Parathyroid	Ca-SR	Antiparathyroid
Type 1 diabetes mellitus	Pancreas (β cells)	GAD65, IA-2, insulin	Anti-GAD, anti-IA-2 (ICA), anti-insulin
Type B insulin resistance with acanthosis nigricans (rare)	Adipocytes, muscle cells	Insulin receptor	Insulin receptor blocking
Autoimmune Addison's disease (autoimmune adrenal failure)	Adrenal	21-Hydroxylase 17α-Hydroxylase P450scc	Anti-21-hydroxylase (ACA) Anti-17α-hydroxylase and anti-P450scc (SCA)
Autoimmune oophoritis (premature ovarian failure)	Ovaries	Not yet identified unequivocally, 17α-hydroxylase, P450scc	Also SCA in association with adrenal insufficiency
Autoimmune orchitis Male infertility (some forms)	Testes	Sperm	Antisperm

By far the most common autoimmune endocrine diseases are autoimmune thyroid disease and type 1 diabetes. When the target is the thyroid gland and the clinical manifestation is hypothyroidism (Hashimoto's thyroiditis), the prevalence is about 1%. When the manifestation is hyperthyroidism (Graves' disease), the prevalence is about 0.4%. Both thyroid autoimmune disorders affect women preferentially. When the targets of the autoimmune response are the β cells of the pancreas, the clinical presentation is type 1 diabetes. The prevalence of type 1 diabetes is close to that of Graves' disease (0.2–0.5%); however, it has no gender bias.

Basic immunologic concepts as they apply to clinical autoimmune endocrine diseases as sole entities and as polyglandular failure syndromes are reviewed in this chapter.

■ BASIC IMMUNE COMPONENTS & MECHANISMS

The immune system is constantly confronted with a variety of molecules and recognizes them as either self or foreign. The adaptive immune system has evolved to recognize virtually any foreign molecule, either in exis-

tence or yet to come. The repertoire of immune recognition molecules randomly formed by gene rearrangements is not limited by the genetic information encoded in the genome (Figure 4–1). As a result, an enormously wide array of immune recognition molecules are acquired by the human immune system. By way of illustration, the theoretical diversity of T cell receptors (T cell recognition molecules) by random rearrangements reaches 10^{15}. This mechanism of rearrangement also applies to B cell recognition molecules, ie, immunoglobulins. The random mechanism of gene rearrangement, however, produces immune recognition molecules that react with self components. Potentially dangerous immune cells carrying self-reactive recognition molecules are eliminated (negatively selected) during development of T lymphocytes in the thymus and of B lymphocytes in the bone marrow. It appears that only immune cells which react with foreign antigen strongly and with self antigen very weakly are positively selected and comprise the peripheral immune cell repertoire. This selection mechanism of immune cells is termed "central tolerance." Self-reactive immune cells that skip central tolerance and reach the periphery are managed by other control mechanisms against autoimmunity and are either eliminated, rendered unresponsive, or suppressed ("peripheral tolerance"). Failures in these mechanisms of immunologic

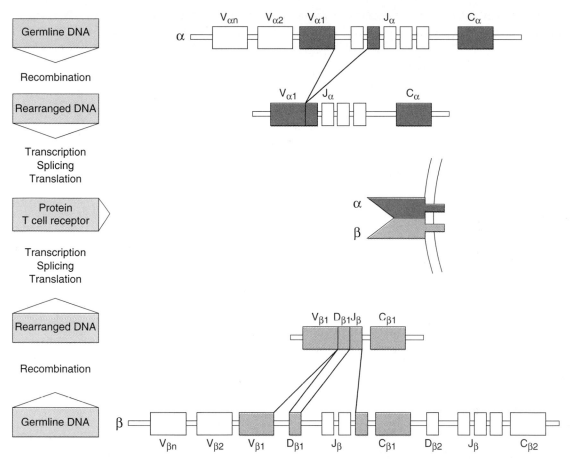

Figure 4–1. Rearrangement of the T cell receptor (TCR) α and β genes to form a functionally diverse receptor. During T cell development, the TCR α and β gene segments rearrange by somatic recombination so that one of the V_α segments pairs with a single J_α segment, and a V_β segment pairs with a single D_β and J_β segment. The C (constant) segments are brought together with the rearranged segments by transcription and splicing to generate the functional mRNA that will be translated into the α and β protein chains that compose the TCR.

regulation, as proposed by Mackay and Burnet in 1964, are central features of the concept of autoimmune disease.

IMMUNE RECOGNITION & RESPONSE

T and B lymphocytes are the fundamental and predominant immune cells. T lymphocyte precursors (pre-T cells) originate in the bone marrow and migrate to the thymus, where they undergo maturation and differentiation. At early stages, they express several T cell surface molecules but still have genomic (not rearranged) configuration of their T cell receptors (TCRs). These now pre-T cells, destined to become T cells with TCR α/β chains (T α/β cells), pass through a critical phase dur-

ing which self-reactive T cells are deleted by negative selection (see T Cell Tolerance, below). Few pre-T cells will express other types of chains on their TCR (T γ/δ cells). T α/β cells differentiate into either mature CD4 or CD8 cells. These now mature lymphocytes migrate to T cell areas of peripheral lymphoid organs and exert their function as helper (TH) or cytotoxic (TC) cells when activated.

B lymphocytes mature and differentiate in the bone marrow and then migrate to the B cell areas of lymphoid organs. Influenced by factors derived from TH cells previously activated by professional antigen-presenting cells (APCs) such as macrophages, some B cells differentiate to become immunoglobulin M (IgM)-producing cells (plasma cells). Most of the other activated

B cells that do not differentiate into plasma cells revert to the resting state to become memory B cells. When memory B cells are further activated, two events occur: isotype switching (immunoglobulin class switching) and hypermutation of the immunoglobulin variable region to further increase diversity and specificity (affinity maturation).

Activation of B cells requires recognition of the antigen as a whole, while T cells require recognition of antigenic peptides bound to major histocompatibility complex (MHC) molecules on the surfaces of professional APCs. Therefore, T cell recognition is said to be MHC-restricted.

The human MHC (human leukocyte antigen; HLA) consists of a linked set of genes encoding major glycoproteins involved in antigen presentation (Figure 4–2). The complex locates to the short arm of chromosome 6 and divides into three separate regions: class I, class II, and class III genes. The class I "classic" region encodes HLA-A, HLA-B, and HLA-C loci; the nonclassic or class I-related region encodes HLA-E, HLA-F, and HLA-G loci and other immunity-related genes such as CD1. The class II region (HLA-D) encodes HLA-DP, HLA-DQ, and HLA-DR loci and other genes related to antigen processing, transport, and presentation such as transporter associated with antigen processing (TAP). The class III region encodes genes for tumor necrosis factors α and β (TNF-α and TNF-β); complement factors C2, C4, and B; and the steroidogenic enzyme 21-hydroxylase. MHC class I (classic) molecules are found on all somatic cells, whereas MHC class I nonclassic antigens are expressed only on some (eg, HLA-F on fetal liver, HLA-G on placental tissues). CD1 molecules are expressed on Langerhans cells, dendritic cells, macrophages, and B cells (all professional APCs). MHC class II molecules are exclu-

sively expressed on these professional APCs. However, virtually all cells except mature erythrocytes can express MHC class II molecules under particular conditions (eg, stimulation with interferon-γ [INF-γ]). As a general rule, MHC class I molecules present peptides derived from endogenous antigens that have access to cytosolic cell compartments (eg, virus) to CD8 Tc cells. On the other hand, MHC class II molecules present peptides derived from antigens internalized by endocytosis into vesicular compartments (eg, bacteria) to CD4 TH cells. MHC class II molecules also bind peptides derived from many membrane-bound self antigens.

Antigen-presenting cells (APCs) process and present antigen in order to activate T cells utilizing MHC-peptide presentation (Figure 4–3). T cells require at least two signals to become activated. The interaction of a TCR expressed on antigen-specific T cells and the antigenic peptide-MHC complex expressed on APCs provides the first signal. The second signal is delivered by the interaction between costimulatory molecules CD80 (B7.1) and CD86 (B7.2) on APCs and CD28 on T cells. These two signals induce proliferation of T cells, production of interleukin-2 (IL-2), and expression of the anti-apoptotic protein Bcl-xL. TH cells and Tc cells are effector cells that require both signals in order to become activated. However, Tc cells also need the "help" provided by TH cells. Until very recently, it was thought that TH and Tc cells needed to interact with the same APC simultaneously and that cytokines (such as IL-2) produced by the TH cell would then act on the Tc cell to facilitate its response. New studies suggest that the interaction between another costimulatory molecule, CD40 ligand (CD154), present on T cells, and CD40, present on APCs, may provide an alternative explanation. It appears that TH cells recognizing antigenic peptides presented by APCs deliver a signal

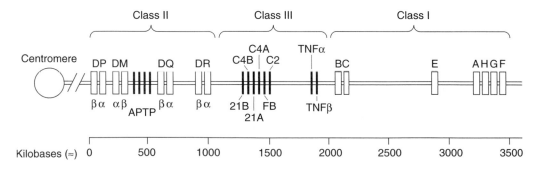

Figure 4–2. Gene organization of the human major histocompatibility complex or human leukocyte antigen (HLA) complex. Regions encoding the three classes of MHC proteins on top. APTP denotes a cluster of genes within the class II region encoding genes related to antigen processing, transport, and presentation. Class III region encodes genes unrelated to class I or class II not involved in antigen presentation (TNF-α and -β, complement factors C2, C4, B, and 21-hydroxylase and others).

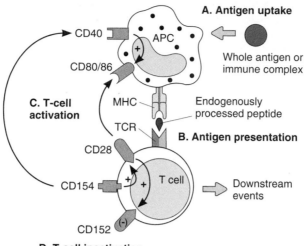

A. Antigen uptake

C. T-cell activation

B. Antigen presentation

D. T-cell inactivation

Figure 4–3. Antigen recognition by T cells. From top to bottom: **A. Antigen uptake:** Incorporation of antigen (via phagocytosis, pinocytosis, or FcR-mediated endocytosis of immune complex). **B. Antigen presentation:** APCs deliver an antigen-specific signal through the MHC-peptide-TCR interaction on T cells (MHC I coupled to CD8 interacts with Tc cells, MHC II coupled to CD4 interacts with TH cells). **C. T-cell activation:** The required second signal is provided via CD80/86 (B7.1; B7.2)-CD28 that induces the expression of CD154 (CD40 L) first and CD152 (CTLA-4) later on. Binding of CD154 on T cells with CD40 on APCs enhances expression of CD80/86. The APC-CD80/86 increased expression and consequent binding of CD28 on T cells perpetuates the activation and proliferation of these effector cells (downstream events). **D. T-cell inactivation:** CD152 (expressed 48–72 hours after T-cell activation) will preferentially bind to CD80/86 on APCs because of its higher affinity, displacing CD28 and in turn suppressing T-cell activity.

through the CD154-CD40 complex that "licenses" APCs to directly stimulate Tc cells (Figure 4–4). Thus, there is no need for simultaneous interactions of TH and Tc cells while encountering the APC. CD154-CD40 interaction also enhances expression of CD80 and CD86 as well as secretion of cytokines (IL-1, -6, -8, -10, and -12 and TNF-α).

Yet another molecule on T cells, the CD28 homolog cytotoxic T lymphocyte antigen 4 (CTLA-4 or CD152), functions to suppress T cell responses (Figure 4–3). CD152 is expressed at low to undetectable levels on resting T cells. It is up-regulated by the ligation of CD28 on T cells with CD80/86 on APCs, or by IL-2. CD152 and CD28 on T cells share the same counter-receptors, namely, CD80/86 on APCs. However, CD152 has a 20-fold higher affinity than CD28 for their ligands.

The integration of all these interactions may be as follows (Figure 4–3): After processing antigen, APCs deliver an antigen-specific first signal through the MHC-peptide-TCR interaction on T cells. A second signal is provided by a costimulatory interaction of the CD80/86-CD28 complex that induces the expression of CD154 first and then CD152. Binding of CD154

on TH cells with CD40 on APCs enhances expression of CD80/86 and licenses APCs for direct activation of Tc cells. Other inflammatory cytokines as well as lipopolysaccharides and viruses may do the same. The increased expression of APC-CD80/86 and consequent binding of CD28 on T cells then perpetuates the activation and proliferation of these effector cells. However, the expression of CD152 48–72 hours after T cell activation will lead to the preferential binding of this molecule to CD80/86 on APCs because of its higher affinity for CD80/86. This may displace CD28 from CD80/86 and, in turn, suppress T cell activity.

Activation and differentiation of B cells often require two signals also. Naive B cells are triggered by antigen but may also require accessory signals that come from activated TH cells. Some antigens can directly activate naive B cells without the need for TH cells (eg, lipopolysaccharides from gram-negative bacteria or polymeric protein structures). The former type of B cell activation (MHC class II-restricted T cell help) is called thymus-dependent (TD). The latter type is called thymus-independent (TI). TH cells also control isotype switching and initiate somatic hypermutation of antibody-variable region genes (see Tolerance, below). In-

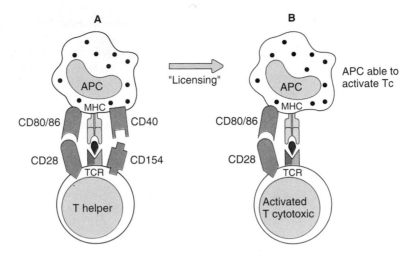

Figure 4–4. Licensed APCs directly activate Tc cells. According to the traditional model, TH cells and Tc cells recognize antigen on the same APC. The APC-activated TH cell produces IL-2, which contributes to the activation of Tc cells while in simultaneous interaction with the same APC. According to the proposed new model *(A)*, APCs are licensed to activate Tc cells by TTH or other stimuli (lipopolysaccharides, INF-γ, viruses). APCs first interact with TH cells. The association of CD154 (CD40 L) on the TTH cell and CD40 on the APC allows (or licenses) the latter to activate TTc cells directly *(B)*. Thus, once licensed, APCs are capable of activating cytotoxic T cells without the need of simultaneous interaction with TTH cells.

teraction between CD154 on TH cells and CD40 on B cells and the cytokines produced by TH cells are essential for isotype switching and formation of germinal centers in peripheral lymphoid organs. The immunoglobulin isotype switching is critical for the generation of functional diversity of a humoral immune response. Somatic hypermutation (point mutations of the variable region genes of immunoglobulins during the course of an immune response) is necessary for the affinity maturation of antibodies.

Overall, the immune response is a combination of effector mechanisms that function to eliminate pathogenic organisms. These effector mechanisms include, as **innate immunity,** phagocytosis (by macrophages, neutrophils, monocytes, and dendritic cells) and cytotoxicity (by natural killer [NK] cells); and as **adaptive immunity,** antibody-dependent complement-mediated cytotoxicity, antibody-dependent cell-mediated cytotoxicity (ADCC), cytotoxicity by T γ/δ cells that recognize heat shock proteins on target cells, and cytotoxicity by CD8 or CD4 Tc cells. CD8 and CD4 Tc cells are activated by the described recognition of specific antigenic peptides bound to class I (for CD8), class II (for CD4) MHC molecules on the APCs and classically by

IL-2 from nearby activated CD4 TH cells. These cells kill the target by either secreting cytotoxins (perforin, granzyme) or by inducing apoptosis through the Fas-FasL interaction (see below).

The specificity of the immune response is crucial if self-reactivity is to be avoided. In order to ensure that lymphocyte responses and the downstream effector mechanisms they control are directed exclusively against foreign antigens and not against "self" components, a number of safety-check barriers must be negotiated before autoreactive lymphocytes can differentiate and proliferate.

TOLERANCE

T Cell Tolerance

T cells developing in the thymus (pre-T cells) are destined to become T α/β cells through rearrangement of the TCR β gene initially, followed by the TCR α gene (Figure 4–5) . If unproductive rearrangements of TCR genes occur (nonfunctional TCR α or β proteins), apoptosis of these pre-T cells follows (Figure 4–5A). If functional rearrangements of TCR α and β proteins occur, cells express TCR α/β dimer and CD3 molecules at low levels on the cell surface. TCR-rearranged cells proliferate 100-fold. Positive and negative selection occurs based on the ability of the rearranged TCR α/β to recognize antigenic peptides in association with self-MHC molecules on thymic epithelial and dendritic cells. Negative selection (**clonal deletion**) appears to take place in the thymus medulla, where pre-T cells bearing TCRs specific for self peptides bound to self-MHC molecules are deleted. At least 97% of developing T cells undergo apoptosis within the thymus ("central tolerance"). Positively selected pre-T cells increase expression of TCR α/β, express either CD4 or CD8, and become mature T cells. These mature T cells exit the thymus and go to the periphery. CD4 T cells are activated in the periphery in an MHC class II-restricted fashion, while CD8 T cells are activated in an MHC class I-restricted fashion.

A differential avidity model in which the fate of T cells is determined by the intrinsic affinity of TCRs for their ligands has been advanced to explain the paradox between positive and negative selection. According to this model, T cells with high avidity for MHC-self peptide complexes would be eliminated (negative selection), whereas T cells with low avidity to MHC-self peptide complexes would be positively selected. If the avidity is close to zero, T cells would not be selected (for lack of effective signal to survive). The biochemical factor or factors that signal survival (low avidity of TCR binding) versus apoptosis (triggered by high avidity interactions) have yet to be found.

Costimulatory interactions between CD28 and CD80/86 and between CD154, CD40, and adhesion molecules, such as lymphocyte function-associated antigen-1 (LFA-1), are also involved in preferential deletion of self-reactive T cells in the medullary region of the thymus. It is known that negative selection is not 100% effective and that some potentially autoreactive T cells do escape to the periphery. Not all self peptides, including those derived from proteins expressed in highly tissue-specific organs such as endocrine glands, would be presented to pre-T cells during their development in the thymus. Therefore, the peripheral immune system must maintain tolerance through complementary control mechanisms.

"Peripheral tolerance" (Figure 4–5B) may be maintained by the induction of unresponsiveness to self antigen (**anergy**) or by the induction of regulatory cells, such as suppressor T cells (**active suppression**). Peripheral **clonal deletion** (apoptosis) of autoreactive T cells that have escaped from the thymus may play an important role in limiting rapidly expanding responses, but there are many examples where autoreactive T cells persist. Some autoreactive T cells may never encounter the self antigen because it may be sequestered from the immune system (**ignorance**). Lastly, **immune deviation**,

whereby noninflammatory TH2 responses suppress an autoreactive inflammatory TH1 response, inducing peripheral tolerance, deserves further discussion (see also Autoimmune Aspects of Thyroid Disease, below). TH1 cells, which regulate cell-mediated responses, secrete interferon-γ (INF-γ) and small amounts of IL-4. In contrast, TH2 cells, which provide help for antibody production, secrete abundant IL-4 and little INF-γ. A prevailing concept in human autoimmunity is that TH1 responses are believed to dominate. It has been shown in animal models that induction of TH2 responses ameliorates TH1 responses. Hence, unbalanced TH1 immune deviation may lead to a breakage of peripheral tolerance. However, evidence to the contrary exists in some endocrinopathies. (See Autoimmune Response in the section on Autoimmune Aspects of Thyroid Disease, below.)

Clonal deletion and **anergy** occur through apoptosis at the site of activation or after passage through the liver. High antigen dose and chronic stimulation induce peripheral elimination of both CD4 and CD8 T cells. Activated T cells express Fas molecules on their surfaces but are resistant to Fas ligand-mediated apoptosis because of the simultaneous expression of Bcl-xL, induced by CD28 ligation during activation (see Immune Recognition and Response, above). Several days after activation, when Bcl-xL has declined, CD4 cells become susceptible to Fas-mediated apoptosis (activation-induced cell death; AICD). A similar mechanism via p75 tumor necrosis factor (TNF) receptor has been shown for CD8 cells. Therefore, autoreactive T cells might be deleted by apoptosis induced by chronic stimulation with self antigens, present abundantly in the periphery. However, autoreactive T cells specific for very rare self antigens may be difficult to eliminate.

Anergy also results from the lack of a second costimulatory signal. When nonhematopoietic cells stimulated by INF-γ present antigen in an MHC class II-restricted fashion (as thyrocytes do in AITD), autoreactive T cells may be rendered unresponsive because of the absence of a CD28-CD80/86-mediated signal (nonhematopoietic cells do not express CD80/86 as professional APCs do). However, even if the two signals are provided, anergy may result from the lack of TH cell-originated cytokines (IL-2, -4, -7, etc). Recently, it has also been shown that in vivo T cell anergy may be induced by CD80/86-CD152 interaction (see also Immune Recognition and Response, above).

T cell **active suppression** is considered to be a major regulatory mechanism of peripheral tolerance; however, its mode of action is still under study. As mentioned above, nonhematopoietic cells stimulated by INF-γ present antigen in an MHC class II-restricted fashion to T cells and render them anergic. These nonhematopoietic cells (nonprofessional APCs) may also present to CD4 T

A

Central T cell tolerence

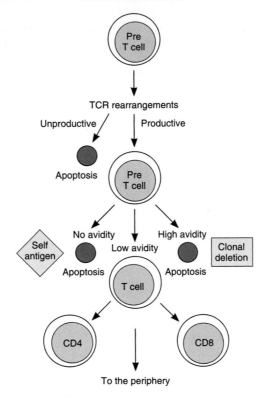

B

Peripheral T cell tolerance

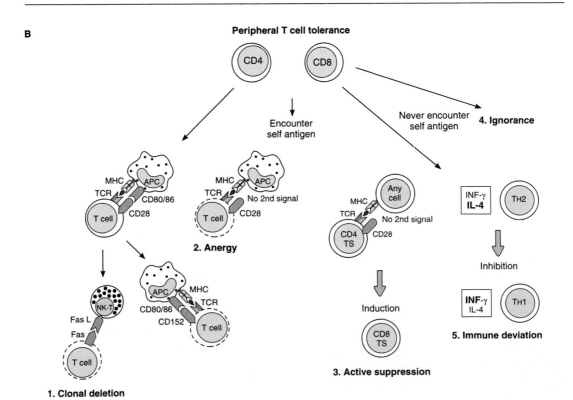

suppressor (TS) cells. Before becoming unresponsive, these cells may induce specific CD8 T suppressor (TS) cells. In turn, these CD8 TS cells may regulate (via T cell suppressor factors or cytotoxicity) antigen-specific autoreactive T cells (see also Figure 4–5B).

B Cell Tolerance

Instead of the thymus, the bone marrow provides the setting for central B cell tolerance. Pre-B cells rearrange their B cell receptor (BCR or membrane-bound immunoglobulin) early in development. The immunoglobulin heavy (H) chain genes rearrange first, followed by light (L) chain gene rearrangement. Unproductive rearrangements and pairings leading to formation of nonfunctional immunoglobulin drive pre-B cells to apoptosis (Figure 4–6A). Functional rearrangements (functional BCRs) allow immature B cell expansion and expression of IgM and CD21 (a marker of functionality). Only one-third of the precursor cells reach this stage. The random rearrangement of the V, D, and J segments of immunoglobulin genes during this period inevitably generates self-recognizing immunoglobulins. Negative selection of autoreactive B cells occurs at the immature B cell stage on the basis of the avidity of the BCR for self antigens. Similar to the T cell **clonal deletion,** immature B cells that strongly bind antigens in the bone marrow are eliminated by apoptosis. Some autoreactive immature B cells, instead of undergoing apoptosis, resume rearrangements of their L chain genes in an attempt to reassemble new κ

or λ genes. This procedure, called **BCR editing,** permanently inactivates the autoreactive immunoglobulin genes. Soluble antigens, presumably because they generate weaker signals through the BCR of immature B cells, do not cause apoptosis but render cells unresponsive to stimuli **(anergy).** These anergic B cells migrate to the periphery, where they express IgD. They may be activated under special circumstances, making anergy less than sufficient as a mechanism of enforcing tolerance. Only immature B cells in the bone marrow with no avidity for antigens (membrane-bound or soluble) become mature B cells with the capacity to express both IgM and IgD. As with T cells, 97% of developing B cells undergo apoptosis within the bone marrow. Also, and as with T cells, **central clonal deletion, anergy,** and **BCR editing** eliminates autoreactive B cells, recognizing bone marrow-derived self antigens.

Peripheral B cell tolerance (Figure 4–6B) is also crucial for protection against autoimmunity. It appears that in the absence of antigen, mature B cells are actively eliminated in the periphery by activated T cells via Fas-FasL and CD40-CD154 interactions. In the presence of specific antigen but without T cell help, antigen recognition by BCRs induces apoptosis or anergy of mature B cells. If antigen and specific T cell help are provided—ie, if antigen bound to the BCR is internalized, processed, and presented in an MHC class II-restricted fashion to a previously activated TH cell specific for the same antigen—two events occur. One, the B cell becomes an IgM-secreting plasma cell, and—in the presence of the appropriate cytokines and after expression of

---

Figure 4–5. **A:** Central T cell tolerance. Mechanisms of central tolerance (at the thymus level) are depicted. From top to bottom, pre-T cells first rearrange their TCR. Unproductive (nonfunctional) rearrangements lead to apoptosis, while productive ones engage pre-T cells in self antigen recognition. Clonal deletion indicates elimination of cells based on their high or no avidity for self antigen (apoptosis). Surviving low-avidity cells reach the periphery as mature CD4 and CD8 cells. **B:** Peripheral T cell tolerance. May be accomplished through any of the five depicted mechanisms. **1. Clonal deletion:** After encountering self antigen in the context of self MHC molecules and simultaneous delivery of a second signal (CD80/86-CD28) by APCs (top left), autoreactive T cells become activated. These activated T cells express Fas molecules on their surface but are resistant to Fas ligand-mediated apoptosis because of the simultaneous expression of Bcl-xL (not shown) induced by CD28 ligation during activation. Several days after activation, when Bcl-xL presence has declined, CD4 cells become susceptible to Fas ligand-mediated apoptosis. Natural killer cells (NK-T) may then accomplish the task of eliminating these autoreactive T cells. **2. Anergy:** Anergy may be induced via CD80/86-CD152 interaction 48–72 hours following activation or may result from the lack of a second costimulatory signal from APCs presenting self antigen (nonprofessional APCs). **3. Active suppression:** Active suppression is thought to occur when nonhematopoietic cells (stimulated by INF-γ) present antigen in an MHC class II restricted fashion to CD4 T suppressor (Ts) cells. Before becoming unresponsive, these cells may induce specific CD8 Ts cells. In turn, these CD8 Ts cells may suppress antigen-specific autoreactive T cells. **4. Ignorance** (top right): Some autoreactive T cells may never encounter self antigen because it may be sequestered from the immune system. Although they may persist in the circulation, they never become activated. **5. Immune deviation:** Under specific circumstances, noninflammatory TH2 responses could suppress inflammatory (autoreactive) TH1 responses (see text).

A
Central B cell tolerance

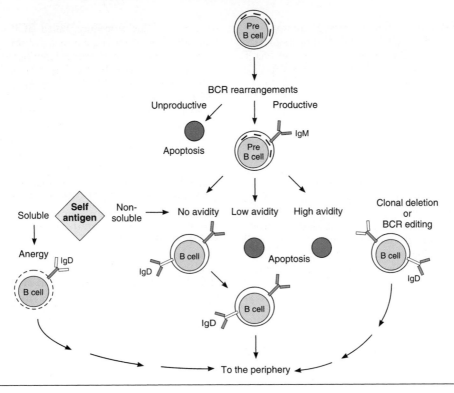

B
Peripheral B cell tolerance

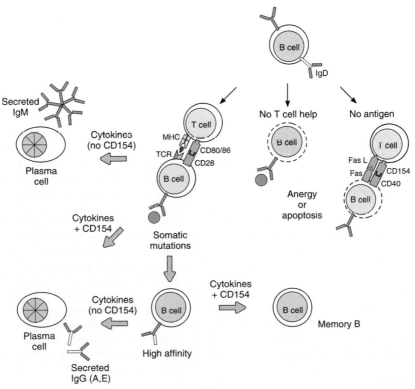

CD40 (for TH cell CD154 interaction)—class switching occurs. Two, further somatic hypermutation of the immunoglobulin variable region genes of such mature B cells, which changes affinity of BCRs for antigens, also occurs in germinal centers (see also Immune Recognition and Response, above). Mutants with low-affinity receptors undergo apoptosis, while enhanced-affinity BCRs are positively selected. In the presence of CD40 ligation of CD154, antigen-stimulated B cells become memory B cells (Figure 4–6B).

The ability of mature B cells to capture very low quantities of antigen via high-affinity BCRs allows them to amplify their antigen-presenting capacity to more than 1000 times that of other professional APCs. This particular property may become critical when developing chronic organ-specific autoimmune diseases in which the source of antigen is limited. Thus, autoreactive B cells that happen to escape the control mechanisms described could amplify and perpetuate autoimmune responses in patients with failing endocrine organs when tissue destruction has left only minute amounts of residual antigen.

■ AUTOIMMUNITY IS MULTIFACTORIAL

Although the breakage of self-tolerance seems to be a central pathogenic step in the development of autoimmune diseases, autoimmunity is a multifactorial event. Specifically, defects in apoptosis-related molecules (Fas-FasL) of thymic dendritic cells have been shown to impair central clonal deletion. Also, in the periphery, similar defects (Fas-FasL, CD152) on T cell-APC molecules may prevent apoptosis of autoreactive T cells. However, it is difficult to consider these general defects as causative of organ-specific disorders. Furthermore, clonal ignorance of T cells cannot be maintained if antigens sequestered from the immune system are released in blood or if cryptic epitopes of antigens that have never been recognized by the immune system are presented to T cells for recognition (after tissue destruction, for example). Defects of active suppression, immune deviation (TH1/TH2 imbalance), and defects in B cell tolerance may all be involved in the pathogenesis of autoimmune diseases. How and why loss of immune self-tolerance occurs is not completely understood. Both genetic and environmental factors appear to be necessary.

GENETIC FACTORS IN AUTOIMMUNITY

Epidemiologic studies demonstrate that susceptibility to most autoimmune diseases has a significant genetic component. In type 1 diabetes, for example, there is a clear association between race and susceptibility to disease—the incidence is approximately 40 times higher in Finland than in Japan. Family studies also demonstrate a strong underlying genetic component. The lifetime risk of developing type 1 diabetes in the United States general population is 0.4%, whereas in relatives of diabetics the risk is substantially higher (4% for parents, 5–7% for siblings, 20% for HLA-identical sibs, 25–40% for monozygotic twins).

The inheritance pattern of autoimmune disorders is complex. These disorders are polygenic, arising from

---

Figure 4–6. ***A:*** Central B cell tolerance. As T cells do in the thymus, B cells rearrange their B cell receptor in the bone marrow. Unproductive rearrangements drive pre-B cells to apoptosis. Functional rearrangements allow expansion and expression of IgM. Next, similar to T cell clonal deletion, immature B cells that strongly bind self antigens in the bone marrow are eliminated by apoptosis. Some autoreactive immature B cells, instead of becoming apoptotic, however, resume rearrangements of their L chain genes, attempting to reassemble new allelic κ or λ genes (BCR editing). Soluble self antigens presumably generate weaker signals through the BCR of immature B cells; they do not cause apoptosis but make cells unresponsive to stimuli (anergy). These anergic B cells migrate to the periphery, expressing IgD, and may be activated under special circumstances. Only immature B cells with no avidity for antigens become mature B cells, expressing both IgM and IgD. These are the predominant cells that make it to the periphery. ***B:*** Peripheral B cell tolerance. In the "absence" of antigen (top right), mature B cells are actively eliminated by activated T cells via Fas-FasL and CD40-CD154 interactions. In the "presence" of specific self antigen but "without T cell help," antigen recognition by BCRs induces apoptosis or anergy on mature B cells. If self antigen and specific autoreactive T cell help are provided, two events develop (center): (1) The B cell becomes an IgM-secreting plasma cell (top left), and, in the presence of the appropriate cytokines after expression of CD40 (for TH cell CD154 interaction), class switching occurs (bottom left). (2) Further somatic hypermutation of the Ig-variable region genes, which changes affinity of BCRs, occurs. Mutants with low-affinity receptors undergo apoptosis, while improved-affinity BCRs are positively selected. In the presence of CD40 ligation of CD154, antigen-stimulated B cells become memory B cells. These two events are the same as in foreign antigen recognition.

several independently segregating genes. The most consistent genetic marker for autoimmune diseases to date is the MHC genotype. Considering again genetic susceptibility to type 1 diabetes, up to 95% of Caucasians developing diabetes express the HLA alleles DR3 or DR4—compared with about 40% of normal individuals. Individuals heterozygous for both DR3 and DR4 have the highest risk. It has been shown that the DQ rather than DR genotype is a more specific marker of susceptibility and that the association of both markers is due to the fact that they are products of closely linked genes. But what is more important than the fact that HLA genes are linked to diabetes is that HLA haplotypes are no longer simply undefined genetic markers. It has been shown that the polymorphisms of the DQ molecules are critical for high-affinity recognition of autoantigens (eg, islet cell antigens) by TCRs. Although the crystal structure of HLA-DQ has not yet been defined, comparisons with HLA-DR structure suggest that the lack of aspartic acid at position 57 (Asp^{57}) on the DQ β chain allows the autoantigen (processed peptide) to fit better in the antigen-binding groove formed by this molecule. To the contrary, the presence of Asp^{57} allows the formation of a salt bridge with a conserved arginine at position 76 on the DQ α chain, preventing the accommodation of the immunogenic peptide recognized by the TCR. Several autoimmune diseases have been linked to HLA-DQβ1 genes, including type 1 diabetes, celiac disease, bullous pemphigoid, autoimmune hepatitis, and premature ovarian failure, and the structure of the DQβ1 molecule may be the reason for the increased susceptibility.

Other candidate genes associated with autoimmune endocrinopathies are discussed further under the single and polyglandular syndromes.

ENVIRONMENTAL FACTORS IN AUTOIMMUNITY

Environmental factors also play a critical role in the pathogenesis of autoimmune disease. The strongest evidence for this statement comes from studies of monozygotic twins, which show that concordance rates for autoimmune disorders are imperfect (never 100%). As mentioned above, in type 1 diabetes, identical twins show less than 50% concordance.

The environmental factors thought to have greatest influence on disease development include infectious agents, diet, and toxins. In type 1 diabetes, viruses have been strongly suspect. Up to 20% of children prenatally infected with rubella develop type 1 diabetes. Children with congenital rubella also have an increased incidence of other autoimmune disorders, including thyroiditis and dysgammaglobulinemia. The mechanisms by which these pathogens may induce autoimmune responses include molecular mimicry and direct tissue injury. The hypothesis of molecular mimicry suggests that immune responses directed at infectious agents can cross-react with self antigens, causing tissue or organ destruction. Support for this concept is found in well-known clinical syndromes, eg, rheumatic fever (immune responses directed against streptococcal M protein seem to cross-react with cardiac myosin, inducing clinical myocarditis). In autoimmune diabetes, the best-studied example of molecular mimicry is the B4 coxsackievirus protein P2-C. Coxsackie B4 virus has also been epidemiologically implicated in the development of type 1 diabetes. There is a striking amino acid sequence similarity between P2-C viral protein and the enzyme glutamic acid decarboxylase (GAD), found in pancreatic β cells (see Autoimmune Aspects of Type 1 Diabetes, below).

The importance of diet in the development of autoimmune diseases remains controversial. An association between early exposure to cow's milk proteins and the risk of type 1 diabetes has been observed in several epidemiologic studies. For example, one study demonstrated that primary immunity to insulin is induced in infancy by oral exposure to cow's milk insulin, but the relevance of this observation is still unknown. On the other hand, selected antigens (from bovine serum albumin to porcine insulin) have been administered orally to mice with a broad spectrum of autoimmune disorders, including nonobese diabetic (NOD) mice, with favorable outcomes. Those data in mice were so compelling that oral tolerance trials in humans have been conducted or are ongoing. Unfortunately, the results of already completed trials in other autoimmune diseases have been disappointing. As examples of ongoing trials in diabetology, the Diabetes Prevention Trial 1 (DPT-1) in the United States and the DIOR study (in recently diagnosed diabetic children and adults) in France are currently attempting to prevent type 1 diabetes in high-risk patients with oral or parenteral insulin. However, another study has shown that oral administration of autoantigen to mice may induce a cytotoxic T lymphocyte response leading to the onset of autoimmune diabetes. This suggests that caution should be used when applying this approach to the treatment of human autoimmune diseases.

■ SINGLE GLAND AUTOIMMUNE SYNDROMES

Organ-specific autoimmune endocrine disorders may present as single entities or may cluster in polyglandular syndromes. Most endocrine glands are susceptible to autoimmune attacks. Some are affected more frequently than others (Table 4–1).

AUTOIMMUNE ASPECTS OF THYROID DISEASE

Autoimmune thyroid disease can present in a polarized fashion with Graves' disease (thyroid hyperfunction) at one end and Hashimoto's thyroiditis (thyroid failure) at the other. This functional subdivision is clinically useful. However, both diseases have a common autoimmune origin.

Genes & Environment

Major susceptibility genes in autoimmune thyroid disease have yet to be identified. Although certain HLA alleles (mainly HLA-DR3 and DQA1*0501) have been shown to be present more frequently in Graves' disease than in the general population, this association has frequently been challenged. In fact, no consistent association has been found between Graves' disease and any known HLA polymorphism. Furthermore, the risk of developing Graves' disease in HLA-identical siblings (7%) is not significantly different from that in control populations. HLA-DR5, -DR3, -DQw7 in Caucasian, -DRw53 in Japanese, and -DR9 in Chinese patients were found to be associated with Hashimoto's thyroiditis. However, genetic linkage between Hashimoto's thyroiditis and a specific HLA locus has not been demonstrated consistently. Overall, the HLA loci are likely to provide less than 5% of the genetic contribution to autoimmune thyroid disease, confirming the relative importance of non-HLA related genes in susceptibility. For example, it has been shown that the inheritance pattern of autoantibodies to thyroperoxidase (TPO) is genetically transmitted. Other candidates are currently under study. However, autoimmune thyroid disease linkage to CTLA-4, HLA, IgH chain, TCR, thyroglobulin (Tg), TPO, and thyrotropin receptor (TSH-R) genes has been excluded.

An important environmental factor influencing the natural history of autoimmune thyroid disease is that of iodine intake (dietary, or present in drugs such as amiodarone, x-ray contrast media). There is considerable evidence that iodine adversely affects both thyroid function and antibody production in those with occult or overt autoimmune thyroid disease.

Autoimmune Response

In Graves' disease, thyrocytes are the differentiated carriers of TSH-Rs and the target cells of autoantibodies and probably the autoimmune response. The development of autoantibodies that functionally stimulate the TSH-R mimicking the action of TSH was the first example of antibody-mediated activities of a hormone receptor in humans. Autoantibodies that may stimulate the calcium-sensing receptor (another G-protein couple receptor) and signal the inhibition of PTH production have been described in autoimmune hypoparathyroidism. Similarly, stimulating antibodies that bind to the adrenocorticotropin (ACTH) receptor may be involved in the pathogenesis of primary pigmented nodular adrenocortical disease (also referred as nodular adrenal dysplasia).

In Graves' disease, antibodies to the TSH-R present with different types of activity. Thyroid-stimulating immunoglobulins (TSIs), the cause of the hyperthyroidism, are most frequently detected by a bioassay that measures cAMP production in a rat thyroid cell line (FRTL5). TSH-blocking autoantibodies which may produce hypothyroidism are identified by their ability to prevent TSH binding to TSH-R. This has allowed development of the TSH-binding inhibition (TBI) assay. No direct immunoassay for the measurement of TSH-R autoantibodies is available yet, and its development may be difficult because TSH-R autoantibodies are present at very low concentrations.

A particular feature of Graves' disease is its early clinical presentation. Unlike other autoimmune endocrinopathies (type 1 diabetes, Hashimoto's thyroiditis, autoimmune Addison's disease), in which much of the target organ has to be destroyed before the disease is manifested, Graves' hyperthyroidism presents with an enlarged and active gland. Minimal lymphocytic infiltration is present when hyperthyroidism (due to the presence of TSH-R-stimulating antibodies) develops. This unique feature may ultimately allow early immune intervention in preference to current ablative therapeutic options.

Another peculiar feature of Graves' disease is the helper T cell response observed in this disease. The activation of antibody-producing B cells by T helper (TH) lymphocytes in Graves' disease is well recognized. At present, a prevailing concept of human autoimmunity suggests that as in acute allograft rejection, "deviation" toward a TH1 response dominates its pathogenesis. Counterdeviation toward TH2 is thought to be a consequence of tolerance induction and has been postulated as a potential therapeutic approach. Graves' disease seems to challenge that concept. Analysis of TSH-R-specific T cell clones from patients with Graves' disease has provided direct evidence for polarization of TH responses; however, instead of TH1 deviation, TH0 and TH2 responses have been observed. As mentioned before, TH1 cells, which regulate cell-mediated responses, secrete mainly IFN-γ and small amounts of IL-4. In contrast, TH2 cells that regulate antibody production (such as TSH-R autoantibodies in Graves' disease) preferentially produce IL-4 and little IFN-γ. T cells expressing both IL-4 and IFN-γ are known as TH0 cells. These experimental results suggest that in Graves' disease TH0-TH2 cell responses appear to be dominant. Hence, in human autoimmunity, Graves' disease appears to be an exception to the usual TH cell pattern.

In Hashimoto's thyroiditis, the hallmark of the humoral immune response is the presence of autoantibodies to TPO. Although the effector mechanism for TPO (or thyroglobulin) autoantibodies is still controversial, under special circumstances (at least in vitro) the autoantibodies are themselves cytotoxic agents or activators of cytotoxic T lymphocytes. Furthermore, in secondary T cell responses, antibodies may play a critical role in antigen processing or presentation to T cells. In short, macrophages internalize (and subsequently process) antigen by phagocytosis and antigen-antibody complex uptake via Fc receptors. B cells have membrane-bound antibodies (B cell receptors; BCRs) which provide a much more powerful system for antigen capture. Indeed, recombinant TPO-specific membrane-bound autoantibody captures antigen and allows presentation efficiently. Antibody binding also modulates antigen processing of immune complexes, enhancing or suppressing the presentation of different T cell peptides. Hence, APCs (internalizing immune complexes through Fc receptors) and B cells (capturing antigen through BCRs) can influence the secondary T cell response that perpetuates autoimmune disease. The potential role of autoantibodies in modulating presentation of T cell determinants in thyroid (and diabetes) autoimmunity is being explored.

Animal Models of Autoimmune Thyroid Disease

The classic immunologic approach to development of an animal model of an autoimmune disease is to immunize the animal with soluble antigen in adjuvant. For autoimmune thyroid disease, the induction of thyroiditis in rabbits using human thyroglobulin (Tg) was one of the earliest attempts to do this—by Rose and coworkers in 1956. In subsequent studies, mice immunized with human or murine Tg developed experimental autoimmune thyroiditis. Immunization with TPO (human or porcine) induces thyroid autoantibodies and, as in the case of Tg, causes thyroiditis to develop in particular MHC strains of mice. However, unlike spontaneous thyroiditis in chickens, none of the immunized mouse models of thyroiditis develop hypothyroidism.

In 1996, Shimojo and coworkers developed a mouse model that clearly mimics some of the major features of Graves' disease. This was achieved by the ingenious approach of immunizing mice with fibroblasts stably transfected with the cDNA for the human TSH-R and syngeneic MHC class II (Figure 4–7). Most of the animals had moderately high TBI activity in their sera, and about 25% were clearly thyrotoxic, with elevated T_4 and T_3 values, detectable TSI activity, and thyroid hypertrophy. For the first time, therefore, an animal model has been established in which a significant number of affected subjects have the immunologic and endocrinologic features of Graves' hyperthyroidism. However, it is not clear that the immune response is confined to the thyroid gland. Nevertheless, this model opens the way to investigation of the pathogenesis of Graves' disease.

AUTOIMMUNE ASPECTS OF TYPE 1 DIABETES

Most type 1 diabetes results from autoimmune destruction of pancreatic β cells in a process that can span several years. This results in glucose intolerance and clinical disease when the majority of β cells have been destroyed. The destruction is marked by circulating antibodies to pancreatic β cells and by massive infiltration of mononuclear lymphocytes into the islets of Langer-

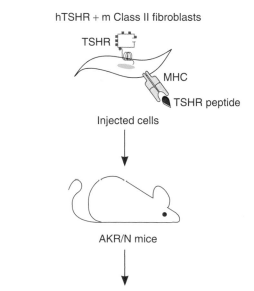

Figure 4–7. Animal model for Graves' disease. This animal model was achieved by injecting AKR/N mice with syngeneic (MHC-identical) fibroblasts dually transfected with mouse MHC class II (H2-k) and human TSH-R cDNA. About 25% of the animals developed endocrinologic (hyperthyroidism) and immunologic (TSI, TBII) features of Graves' disease.

hans where pancreatic β cells remain. The lymphocytes disappear when the β cells are gone. Although insulin is available for replacement therapy, type 1 diabetes remains a chronic disorder of major socioeconomic impact that mainly afflicts the young. Elucidation of the molecular mechanisms underlying this destruction—and the development of methods to prevent autoimmunity—may ultimately lead to effective treatment. Such developments, however, require animal models of type 1 diabetes that closely resemble the disease in humans.

Genes & Environment

The susceptibility to develop type 1 diabetes is associated with certain alleles of the MHC class II locus that have been statistically linked to a variety of autoimmune disorders. The most recent analyses indicate that in Caucasians, HLA-DR3 DQ2 (DQB1*0201) and HLA-DR4 (DRB1*0401), DQ8 (DQB1*0302) haplotypes are most strongly associated with type 1 diabetes. In Asian populations, DRB1*0405 is the major susceptibility haplotype. In contrast, the DR2, DQ6 (DQB1*0602) haplotype is negatively associated with type 1 diabetes. More importantly, susceptibility requires both HLA-DQ β chain alleles to be negative for aspartic acid at position 57 (Asp^{57}) on the amino acid sequence. Studies of different populations have shown a linear relationship between the incidence of type 1 diabetes and the estimated frequency of homozygous absence of Asp^{57}.

Non-HLA candidate genes consistently associated with type 1 diabetes include the "variable number of tandem repeats" (VNTR) polymorphisms in the insulin gene and the CTLA4 gene (CD152). The VNTR polymorphisms are located adjacent to defined regulatory sequences that influence insulin gene expression. Of immunologic importance, CTLA4 gene (see Immune Recognition and Response, above) is the other non-HLA candidate gene consistently found to be associated with type 1 diabetes.

Although environmental factors definitely play a role in the development of type 1 diabetes (eg, Coxsackie B4 virus, mumps virus, rubella virus, Kilham rat virus in the BB-rat; or cow's milk formula exposure), more studies are needed to establish a definite etiologic link.

Autoimmune Response

The autoantibodies associated with β cell destruction can be present up to several years before the clinical onset of disease and are thus excellent markers of disease risk. Furthermore, they have served as important tools to identify human pancreatic β cell autoantigens. In 1990, Baekkeskov and coworkers identified a 64-kDa islet cell protein as the smaller isoform of the GABA-synthesizing enzyme glutamic acid decarboxylase (GAD65). This autoantigen was shown to be recognized by 70–80% of prediabetic and newly diagnosed type 1 diabetic patients' sera. A second component of the 64-kDa antigen was shown to be a putative tyrosine phosphatase, termed IA-2. IA-2 is recognized by 60–70% of prediabetic and newly diagnosed type 1 diabetic patients. Together, GAD65 and IA-2 autoantibodies detect over 90% of individuals who develop type 1 diabetes and can be used to detect individuals at risk several years before the clinical onset of disease.

Although autoantibody responses to GAD65 are not easily detected, there is strong evidence to suggest that GAD65 is an important T cell autoantigen in the nonobese diabetic (NOD) mouse. Thus, GAD65 is the earliest known target of the autoimmune T cell response in the NOD mouse. Administration of the protein in a tolerogenic form prevents disease. In contrast, induction of tolerance to other potential autoantigens in this model (such as carboxypeptidase H and hsp60) does not prevent disease. The NOD mouse does not develop autoimmunity to the IA-2 molecule and thus distinguishes itself from the human disease with regard to this target antigen (see Models, below).

Insulin is a third well-characterized autoantigen in type 1 diabetes. Insulin autoantibodies can be detected in about 50% of newly diagnosed children with type 1 diabetes. Insulin-specific T cell clones can transfer disease in the NOD mouse. Furthermore, administration of whole insulin, insulin B chain, or an insulin peptide epitope in a tolerogenic form can protect against disease in NOD mice. Because animals receiving insulin or insulin B chain continue to have intra-islet insulitis—in contrast to young NOD mice treated with GAD65 in a tolerogenic way—it has been suggested that insulin reactivity is more distal in disease progression. Additional but less well characterized proteins have been implicated as targets of autoantibodies in type 1 diabetes in humans.

Autoantibodies, although they are good markers of disease, do not seem to be directly involved in destruction of pancreatic β cells. Adoptive transfer of diabetes to NOD mice with spontaneous combined immune deficiency lacking T cells (NOD-SCID) can be mediated by T cells alone. Because β cell-deficient NOD mice do not develop disease, it is possible that B lymphocytes function as important APCs in the islet to perpetuate an ongoing autoimmune response and thus are essential for presentation of rare antigens such as GAD65 and I-A2. (See also Autoimmune Response in the section on Autoimmune Aspects of Thyroid Disease, above.)

An important question is whether GAD65, IA-2, and insulin are major target antigens of T cell mediated β cell destruction that results in type 1 diabetes in humans. Proliferative and cytotoxic T cell responses to GAD65 are detected in peripheral blood of newly diagnosed type 1 diabetes patients, but their pathogenicity has not been addressed. Induction of neonatal tolerance to GAD65 specifically prevents diabetes in the NOD mouse model. The role of IA-2 in destructive autoimmunity to the pancreatic β cell in humans is suggested by the high predictive value of IA-2 antibodies for clinical onset of diabetes.

Both GAD65 and IA-2 are neuroendocrine proteins, which are expressed at significant levels in brain and in the β cell. Stiff-man syndrome—a very rare neurologic disorder in humans with a high coincidence of diabetes—is characterized by a strong autoantibody response to GAD65, the titer of which is several orders of magnitude higher than in diabetes. It has been suggested that impairment of γ-aminobutyrate-secreting neurons in stiff-man syndrome is mediated by GAD65 autoantibodies, whereas development of type 1 diabetes is associated with a cellular immune response to GAD65. The low incidence of stiff-man syndrome compared with type 1 diabetes (only one in 10^4 type 1 diabetic patients develops stiff-man syndrome, whereas 40% of stiff-man syndrome patients develop type 1 diabetes) probably reflects in part the protection of GABAergic neurons by the blood-brain barrier and the absence of MHC class II antigen expression in normal neurons. The cellular localization of IA-2 expression in brain is not known, and there are no known disorders of the central nervous system that involve autoimmunity to IA-2.

In the NOD mouse, the destruction of pancreatic β cells requires both the CD4 T helper (TH) cells and CD8 cytotoxic (TC) cells. Whereas TH cells seem to be required for the development of an autoimmune response to the islets and generation of intrasulitis, TC cells are probably the effector cells of β cell destruction. Furthermore, there is evidence that in the CD4 lineage, the TH1 subset is important for development of disease in the NOD mouse. TH1 cells are induced by IL-12 and are biased toward secreting IFN-γ and IL-2. In contrast, there is evidence that the TH2 cytokine IL-4 exerts a dominant-negative effect on diabetes progression in the NOD mouse. In humans, low autoantibody titers associated with type 1 diabetes and high titers associated with a protective haplotype (DR2) suggest that a strong TH2 response can be inhibitory for β cell destruction. A role for TH1 cells in human disease is also suggested by results of cytokine profiles of peripheral human NK cells in identical twins which are discordant for the development of diabetes. This is different from the observed TH responses in Graves' disease. (See Autoimmune Aspects of Thyroid Disease, above.)

Animal Models of Autoimmune Diabetes Mellitus

The nonobese diabetic (NOD) mouse has been invaluable for studies of molecular mechanisms of autoimmunity directed toward the pancreatic β cells and the development of diabetes. It has several features, however, which distinguish it from the human disease. The incidence of diabetes is two to three times higher in female than in male NODs, whereas in humans there is a slight preponderance of type 1 diabetes in males. Furthermore, while the induction of organ-specific autoimmunity and inflammation in humans may be caused by human pathogens or toxins, autoimmunity seems to be the default mechanism in the NOD mouse. Thus, mice in clean, pathogen-free environments have a high incidence of disease, whereas a variety of regimens that stimulate the immune system of the mouse, such as viral infection or injection of complete Freund's adjuvant, prevent disease. To date, more than 125 treatments for successful prevention or delay of diabetes in the NOD mouse (Table 4–2) have been identified, but none have been identified for humans.

The Bio Breeding (BB) rat develops spontaneous T cell-mediated diabetes. The BB-rat disease is significantly distinct from the human disease in that it is accompanied by autoantibodies to lymphocytes and a severe lymphocytopenia, which is essential for development of β cell autoimmunity and diabetes in this model.

While these models of type 1 diabetes have been invaluable for studies of basic immunologic mechanisms associated with pancreatic β cell autoimmunity, other models of type 1 diabetes closer to what occurs in humans are needed if immunoprevention and immunomodulatory techniques are to be tested.

AUTOIMMUNE ASPECTS OF OTHER ENDOCRINOPATHIES

Autoimmune Adrenal Failure

Autoimmune Addison's disease seldom develops as a single gland syndrome. In about 50% of cases, the disease is associated with other glands and organ failures. Anderson and coworkers described the existence of adrenal-specific autoantibodies for the first time in 1963. Using immunofluorescence techniques based on sections of human, bovine, or monkey adrenals, antibodies specifically recognizing the adrenal cortex (ACA) were described. Steroid-producing cell autoantibodies (SCA) reactive with cells of the adrenals, gonads, and placenta were described by Anderson and coworkers in 1968. SCAs are detected predominantly in ACA-posi-

Table 4–2. Some reported therapies for prevention of type I diabetes in the NOD mouse.

Endocrinologic
 Androgen
 Castration
 1,25-Dihydroxyvitamin D therapy
 Gonadectomy
 Insulin or β chain, orally or parenterally or by nasal insufflation
 IGF-1
 Melatonin
 Partial pancreatectomy
 Prolactin
 Somatostatin
 Vitamin E
Immunologic
 Anti-B7.1
 BCG immunization
 Anti-β 7 integrin
 Anti-CD3, -4, -8, -28
 Anti-complement R
 Anti-CTLA-4
 GAD65 or its peptides, orally or parenterally or by intrathymic injection
 INF-α
 Anti-INF-β
 IL-1, -2, -3, -4, -10, -12
 Anti-MHC class I, II
Pharmacologic
 Anesthesia
 Azathioprine
 Cyclosporine
 Dapsone
 Diazoxide
 Lithium
 Monosodium glutamate
 Nicotinamide
 Pentoxifylline
 Probucol
 Tolbutamide
 Troglitazone
Miscellaneous
 Cold exposure
 Elevated temperature
 Immobilization
 Lactate dehydrogenase-elevating virus infection
 Lymphocytic choriomeningitis virus infection
 Mouse hepatitis virus infection
 Mycobacterium infection
 Non–pathogen-free state
 Overcrowding
 Saline (repeated injections)

---

tive patients with Addison's disease who have premature ovarian failure in the context of autoimmune polyglandular syndrome type I (APS-I; see Polyglandular Syndromes, below). Steroid 21-hydroxylase has been identified as a major adrenal autoantigen in ACA-positive patients with Addison's disease. Using a sensitive assay based on the immune precipitation of radiolabeled recombinant 21-hydroxylase, workers in one study reported positive testing for 72% of sera from patients with isolated Addison's disease, 92% of patients with APS-I, 100% of patients with APS-II, and 80% of patients who were positive for ACA by immunofluorescence but did not have clinically overt Addison's disease (apparently healthy blood donors showed 2.5% positivity) (Table 4–3). Another study measured ACA in 808 children with organ-specific autoimmune diseases without adrenal insufficiency. ACAs were detectable in 14. Ten of these ACA-positive children (also positive for 21-hydroxylase antibodies) and 12 ACA-negative children were prospectively followed with adrenocortical function testing and antibodies. Overt Addison's disease developed in 9 (90%) ACA/21-hydroxylase antibody-positive children within 3–121 months, and the one remaining child had subclinical hypoadrenalism throughout a 24 month-observation period. The progression to adrenal failure was not related to ACA titer, sex, adrenal function, type of associated autoimmune disease, or HLA status. Although ACA 21-hydroxylase antibodies appear to be highly predictive in children, in adults the cumulative risk of developing Addison's in patients with organ-specific autoimmune diseases is about 32%.

Steroid 17α-hydroxylase is another adrenal autoantigen. 17α-Hydroxylase antibodies were found in

Table 4–3. Adrenal autoantibodies in different syndromes.

Autoantibodies	Addison's Disease (%)	APS-I[1] (%)	APS-II[2] (%)	ACA(+)[3] (%)
21-Hydroxylase	72	92	100	80
17α-Hydroxylase	5	55	33	20
P450scc	9	45	36	20

[1]APS-I: Autoimmune polyglandular syndrome type I: Autoimmune polyendocrinopathy, candidiasis, and ectodermal dystrophy.
[2]APS-II: Autoimmune polyglandular syndrome type II: Adrenal insufficiency, thyroid disease, and diabetes mellitus.
[3]ACA(+): Adrenal cortex antibody-positive without clinically overt Addison's disease.

5% of patients with isolated Addison's disease, 55% of patients with APS-I, 33% of patients with APS-II, and 20% of sera from patients who were positive for ACA but did not have clinically overt Addison's disease (Table 4–3). Antibodies against another recently described adrenal autoantigen, cytochrome P450 side-chain cleavage enzyme (P450scc), were found to be present in 9% of patients with isolated Addison's disease, 45% of patients with APS-I, 36% of patients with APS-II, and 20% of sera from patients who were positive for ACA but did not have clinically overt Addison's disease (Table 4–3). The prevalence of P450scc antibodies in these groups of patients was always lower than that of 21-hydroxylase antibodies but similar to that of 17α-hydroxylase antibodies. Furthermore, almost all sera that were positive for 17α-hydroxylase or P450scc antibodies were also positive for 21-hydroxylase antibodies. In addition, a comparison of SCAs measured by immunofluorescence with 17α-hydroxylase and P450scc antibody measurements suggested that 17α-hydroxylase and P450scc are the major components of the SCA antigen just as 21-hydroxylase is the major component of ACA antigen.

Overall, immune responses in autoimmune adrenal disease may involve other antigens, but reactivity to the three described, particularly 21-hydroxylase, appears to predominate. Although inhibition of enzymatic activity by these antibodies has been shown in vitro, no clear relationship to the pathogenesis of the clinical syndrome has yet been established.

Autoimmune Oophoritis & Orchitis

An autoimmune origin for premature ovarian failure with concomitant Addison's disease or oophoritis can be based on the following: (1) the presence of autoantibodies to SCA in most cases, (2) the characterization of shared autoantigens between the adrenals and the ovaries (ie, 17α-hydroxylase and P450scc), (3) the histologic features of the ovaries (lymphocyte and plasma cell infiltrate involving steroid-producing cells), and (4) animal models of the syndrome. There is some evidence of autoimmunity in idiopathic premature ovarian failure not associated with Addison's disease (cellular immune abnormalities, presence of various ovarian antibodies in some patients, and associations with type 1 diabetes and myasthenia gravis); however, the absence of histologic confirmation (lack of oophoritis) makes the autoimmune pathogenesis less credible.

Less is known about the autoimmune pathogenesis of human orchitis. Animal models, however, have shown that infectious or traumatic injury to the testes can induce autoimmune responses in this immune-privileged tissue (conferred by **ignorance;** see Tolerance, above).

Autoimmune Hypophysitis

Autoimmune hypophysitis (also called lymphocytic hypophysitis) should be considered in the differential diagnosis of pituitary abnormalities in women (8:1 female:male ratio) during the latter half of pregnancy and in the first 6 months postpartum, as well as in patients with coexisting autoimmune disorders, eg, thyroiditis, adrenalitis, autoimmune hypoparathyroidism, or atrophic gastritis. More than 100 cases have been described since the original report in 1962. Antipituitary antibodies have been detected in a minority of patients. Owing to the lack of markers for the disease, the diagnosis can only be confirmed with histologic examination. Nevertheless, because of the usually transient endocrine and compressive features of this condition, conservative management based on clinical suspicion may prevent the consequences of unnecessary pituitary surgery. Granulomatous hypophysitis—another form of autoimmune hypophysitis—appears to have a similar autoimmune pathogenesis but more commonly affects postmenopausal women.

Autoimmune Hypoparathyroidism

Autoimmune hypoparathyroidism, also called idiopathic hypoparathyroidism, is one of the major components of autoimmune polyglandular failure syndrome type I (APS-I; see next section). It also presents as a sporadic disease, sometimes associated with Hashimoto's thyroiditis in women. The fact that autoimmune hypoparathyroidism presents in association with other autoimmune diseases and the presence of autoantibodies reactive with parathyroid tissue in many affected patients suggest an autoimmune pathogenesis. Parathyroid autoantibodies have been reported to show a complement-dependent cytotoxic effect on cultured bovine parathyroid cells. At least one major parathyroid autoantigen has been identified as the calcium-sensing receptor (Ca-SR). Ca-SR is of great importance in the regulation of parathyroid hormone secretion and renal tubular calcium absorption. This receptor is a member of the seven-membrane spanning domain G protein-coupled receptor family. It is also expressed in thyroid C cells, the pituitary, the hypothalamus, and in other regions of the brain. The relationship of the autoimmune response directed against the receptor to the pathogenesis of the disease is not completely clear. However, stimulation of the Ca-SR with consequent inhibition of PTH synthesis and secretion has been suggested. The prevalence of these antibodies in clinically diagnosed idiopathic hypoparathyroidism was found to be 56% in one study. Measurement of these antibodies may have value in predicting development of autoimmune hypoparathyroidism in patients with autoimmune endocrinopathies who are at risk.

■ AUTOIMMUNE POLYGLANDULAR SYNDROMES

Associations of multiple autoimmune endocrine disorders have been classified in two different syndromes. Autoimmune polyglandular syndrome (APS) type I and type II can be clearly separated clinically (Table 4–4). Some authors have attempted to subdivide APS-II (ie, APS-II and APS-III) on the basis of the association of some autoimmune disorders but not others. However little information is gained by making this subdivision in terms of understanding pathogenesis or prevention of future endocrine failure in patients or their relatives.

AUTOIMMUNE POLYGLANDULAR SYNDROME I (APS-I)

APS-I is an inherited autosomal recessive disorder with 25% incidence among siblings of affected individuals. Also known as APECED, or autoimmune polyendocrinopathy-candidiasis-ectodermal dystrophy, APS-I is characterized by the triad of chronic mucocutaneous candidiasis, autoimmune hypoparathyroidism, and adrenal insufficiency (only two are required in the index case for the diagnosis, and only one in the siblings). Chronic mucocutaneous candidiasis (involving oral mucosa and nails or less frequently the esophagus) is usually first manifested as the initial problem early in life. In most individuals, the development of autoimmune hypoparathyroidism and Addison's disease follows. However, lifelong surveillance is important since decades may elapse between the development of one feature of the disorder and the onset of another. There is no female preponderance in this syndrome, and it is not HLA-associated. APS-I may occur sporadically or in families. The genetic locus responsible for the disease has been mapped to the long arm of chromosome 21 (21q22.3). The haplotype analysis of this region in different populations has shown that APS-I is linked to different mutations of a gene identified as the autoimmune regulator *(AIRE)*. *AIRE* encodes a putative nuclear protein with transcription factor motifs (including two zinc finger motifs). It is expressed in different tissues but particularly in the thymus. The mechanism by which mutations of this putative transcription factor lead to the diverse manifestations of APS-I is still unknown. Other immune response-related genes as well as environmental factors probably play a role in development of the syndrome. Several studies of large cohorts of patients from different ethnic backgrounds have reported the appearance of chronic candidiasis at different sites in all patients. Hypoparathyroidism and Ad-

dison's disease present with similar high frequency (Table 4–4). The occurrence of the diagnostic triad reportedly presents in 57% of patients. Female hypogonadism, presenting as total or partial failure of pubertal development or as adult premature ovarian failure, has been reported in up to 60% of patients. Male hypogonadism is less frequent (14%). Type 1 diabetes is not as frequent as in APS-II but if present usually develops early (under 21 years of age). Autoimmune hypothyroidism (atrophic thyroiditis) is also less frequent than in APS-II; however, thyroid autoantibodies may be present in many euthyroid patients. Other manifestations are described in Table 4–4. Acute autoimmune hepatitis is reportedly less common than chronic hepatitis, which appears to be present in most individuals. Autoantibodies to aromatic *l*-amino acid decarboxylase (AADC) are associated with chronic active autoimmune hepatitis and vitiligo which are found in APS-I. These antibodies, if present, can be helpful in making the diagnosis. Autoantibodies against tryptophan hydroxylase have been associated with gastrointestinal dysfunction in APS-I. Autoantibodies to the H^+-K^+ ATPase and to intrinsic factor are associated with pernicious anemia, and autoantibodies to tyrosinase are associated with vitiligo. Other autoantibodies associated with the single gland disorders that make up this polyglandular syndrome have been discussed above.

AUTOIMMUNE POLYGLANDULAR SYNDROME II (APS-II)

APS-II is the most common of the polyglandular failure syndromes. It affects women in a 3:1 ratio to men. APS-II is diagnosed when at least two of the following are present: adrenal insufficiency, autoimmune thyroid disease (thyroiditis with hypothyroidism or Graves' disease with hyperthyroidism) and type 1 diabetes. Historically, Schmidt (1926) first described the association of Addison's disease and thyroiditis. Carpenter and coworkers in 1964 included type 1 diabetes in the syndrome. Other components of APS-II include the following (Table 4–4): primary hypogonadism, myasthenia gravis, celiac disease, pernicious anemia, alopecia, vitiligo, and serositis. The most frequent association appears to be type 1 diabetes (over 50%) and autoimmune thyroid disease (70% in some series). Adrenal insufficiency may be concurrent, may be delayed in onset for up to 2 decades, or may never be manifested. Some diabetic patients (2–3%) develop celiac disease. Gluten-free diet is usually effective. If the celiac disease is untreated, hypocalcemia (not due to hypoparathyroidism), osteopenia, and occasionally gastrointestinal lymphoma may occur.

Although this syndrome and its components aggregate in families, there is no identifiable pattern of inher-

Table 4–4. Comparison of the different components of autoimmune polyglandular syndromes (APS).

Characteristics	Type I	Type II
Inheritance	Autosomal recessive	Polygenic
Genetic association or linkage	Linked to *AIRE*	Some HLA association
Gender	Equal distribution	Female preponderance
Age at onset	Infancy	Age 20–40
Endocrine disorders		
Addison's disease	60–72%	70%
Hypoparathyroidism	Common (79–96%)	Rare (late onset)
Autoimmune thyroid disease	Less frequent (about 5%)	More frequent (about 70%)
Type 1 diabetes	14% (lifetime)	> 50%
Primary hypogonadism	60% female, 14% male	About 5%
Hypophysitis	Not reported	Reported
Dermatologic		
Chronic mucocutaneous candidiasis	Often at onset (about 100%)	Not reported
Alopecia	Common (about 29%)	Reported
Vitiligo	About 13%	About 5%
Dermatitis herpetiformis	Not reported	Reported
Gastrointestinal		
Celiac disease	None (only steatorrhea)	Present in 2–3%
Autoimmune hepatitis	About 12%	Not reported
Hematologic		
Pernicious anemia	About 13%	As common as in APS-I
Pure red cell hypoplasia	Reported	Not reported
Idiopathic thrombocytopenic purpura	Not reported	Reported
Ectodermal		
Enamel hypoplasia	All reported	Not reported
Nail dystrophy		
Tympanic membrane calcification		
Neurologic		
Myasthenia gravis	None reported	All reported
Stiff-man syndrome		
Parkinson's disease		
Other		
Asplenism	Reported	Not reported
Keratopathy	Reported	Not reported
Progressive myopathy	Reported	Not reported
IgA deficiency	Not reported	Reported
Serositis	Not reported	Reported
Idiopathic heart block	Not reported	Reported
Goodpasture's syndrome	Not reported	Reported

itance. Susceptibility is probably determined by multiple gene loci (HLA being the strongest) that interact with environmental factors. Many of the disorders of APS-II are associated (some genetically linked) with the HLA haplotype identified in single disorders. HLA-A1, B8, DR3 and DR4, DQA1*0501, and DQB1*0201 have all been described as associated with APS II.

MANAGEMENT OF AUTOIMMUNE POLYGLANDULAR SYNDROMES

Hormonal replacement therapy remains the only form of treatment of the autoimmune polyglandular syndromes. The clinical management of these disorders mandates early diagnosis of associated components.

Since the age at onset of associated disorders is clinically unpredictable, long-term follow-up is needed. Endocrine disorders are treated as they develop and are diagnosed. Hormonal treatments for the specific gland failures are described elsewhere in this book. However, specific combinations of endocrine organ failure require specific management. For example, thyroxine replacement can precipitate life-threatening adrenal failure in a patient with untreated Addison's disease. Furthermore, hypoglycemia or decreasing insulin requirements in a patient with type 1 diabetes may be the earliest symptom or sign of adrenal insufficiency. Hypocalcemia, seen in APS-II, is more commonly due to celiac disease than to hypoparathyroidism. Treatment of mucocutaneous candidiasis with ketoconazole in patients with APS-type I may induce adrenal insufficiency in a failing gland (this antifungal medication is a global P450 cytochrome inhibitor). These drugs may also elevate liver enzymes, making the diagnosis of autoimmune hepatitis—requiring treatment with immunosuppressants—more difficult in these patients.

Screening of affected individuals as well as their relatives is the only way of preventing morbidity and mortality. Annual measurement of TSH is recommended as cost-effective in first-degree relatives of patients with type 1 diabetes. Autoantibody measurements may help in the preclinical assessment of several disorders. Electrolytes, calcium and phosphorus levels, thyroid and liver functions, blood smears, and vitamin B_{12} measurements are all recommended in the follow-up of APS-I. For APS-II patients with type 1 diabetes, thyroid disease and celiac disease coexist with sufficient frequency to justify not only TSH measurement but also screening for endomysial antibodies containing transglutaminase antibodies, which are prevalent in celiac disease.

REFERENCES

Blanas E et al: Induction of autoimmune diabetes by oral administration of autoantigen. Science 1996;274:1707. [PMID: 8939860]

Jacobson DL et al: Epidemiology and estimated population burden of selected autoimmune diseases in the United States. Clin Immunol Immunopathol 1997;84:223. [PMID: 9281381]

Janeway CA et al (editors): Immunobiology: The Immune System in Health and Disease, 4th ed. Garland, 1999.

Jaume JC et al: Cellular thyroid peroxidase (TPO), unlike purified TPO and adjuvant, induces antibodies in mice that resemble autoantibodies in human autoimmune thyroid disease. J Clin Endocrinol Metab 1999;84:1651. [PMID: 10323395]

Jaume JC et al: Evidence for genetic transmission of thyroid peroxidase autoantibody epitopic "fingerprints." J Clin Endocrinol Metab 1999;84:1424. [PMID: 10199790]

Jaume JC et al: Thyrotropin receptor autoantibodies in serum are present at much lower levels than thyroid peroxidase autoantibodies: analysis by flow cytometry. J Clin Endocrinol Metab 1997;82:500. [PMID: 9024244]

Jaume JC, Rapoport B, McLachlan SM: Lack of female bias in a mouse model of autoimmune hyperthyroidism (Graves' disease). Autoimmunity 1999;29:269. [PMID: 10433082]

Kita M et al: Regulation and transfer of a murine model of thyrotropin receptor antibody mediated Graves' disease. Endocrinology 1999;140:1392. [PMID: 10067867]

Kwok WW et al: HLA-DQB1 codon 57 is critical for peptide binding and recognition. J Exp Med 1996;1831253. [PMID: 8642268]

Lanzavecchia A: Immunology. Licence to kill. Nature 1998;393:413. [PMID: 9623994]

Rapoport B et al: The thyrotropin (TSH) receptor: interaction with TSH and autoantibodies. Endocr Rev 1998;19:673. [PMID: 9861544]

Roitt IM, Delves PJ: Roitt's Essential Immunology, 10th ed. Blackwell, 2001.

Shimojo N et al: Induction of Graves-like disease in mice by immunization with fibroblasts transfected with the thyrotropin receptor and a class II molecule. Proc Natl Acad Sci USA 1996;93:11074. [PMID: 8855311]

Volpe R (editor): Autoimmune Endocrinopathies. Humana, 1999.

Hypothalamus & Pituitary Gland

5

David C. Aron, MD, MS, James W. Findling, MD, & J. Blake Tyrrell, MD

ACTH	Adrenocorticotropic hormone	**ICSH**	Intersititial (Leydig) cell-stimulating hormone
ADH	Antidiuretic hormone (vasopressin)	**IGF**	Insulin-like growth factor
bFGF	Basic fibroblast growth factor	**LH**	Luteinizing hormone
cAMP	Cyclic adenosine monophosphate	**β-LPH**	β-Lipotropin
CLIP	Corticotropin-like intermediate lobe peptide	**MEN**	Multiple endocrine neoplasia
CRH	Corticotropin-releasing hormone	**MRI**	Magnetic resonance imaging
CRHBP	CRH-binding protein	**MSH**	Melanocyte-stimulating hormone
DI	Diabetes insipidus	**PAS**	Periodic acid-Schiff (histochemical staging reaction)
DIDMOAD	Diabetes insipidus, diabetes mellitus, optic atrophy, deafness (Wolfram's syndrome)	**PIH**	Prolactin-inhibiting hormone
		POMC	Pro-opiomelanocortin
FSH	Follicle-stimulating hormone	**PRL**	Prolactin
GABA	Gamma-aminobutyric acid	**SHBG**	Sex hormone-binding globulin
GAP	GnRH-associated peptide	**SIADH**	Syndrome of inappropriate secretion of antidiuretic hormone
GH	Growth hormone (somatotropin)		
GHBH	Growth hormone-binding protein	**TRH**	Thyrotropin-releasing hormone
GHRH	Growth hormone-releasing hormone	**TSH**	Thyroid-stimulating hormone (thyrotropin)
GnRH	Gonadotropin-releasing hormone		
hCG	Human chorionic gonadotropin	**VIP**	Vasoactive intestinal peptide
hMG	Human menopausal gonadotropin		

The hypothalamus and pituitary gland form a unit which exerts control over the function of several endocrine glands—thyroid, adrenals, and gonads—as well as a wide range of physiologic activities. This unit constitutes a paradigm of neuroendocrinology—brain-endocrine interactions. The actions and interactions of the endocrine and nervous systems whereby the nervous system regulates the endocrine system and endocrine activity modulates the activity of the central nervous system constitute the major regulatory mechanisms for virtually all physiologic activities. The immune system also interacts with both the endocrine and the nervous systems (see Chapter 4). These neuroendocrine interactions are also important in pathogenesis. This chapter will review the normal functions of the pituitary gland, the neuroendocrine control mechanisms of the hypothalamus, and the disorders of those mechanisms.

Nerve cells and endocrine gland cells, which are both involved in cell-to-cell communication, share certain characteristic features—secretion of chemical messengers (neurotransmitters or hormones) and electrical activity. A single chemical messenger—peptide or amine—can be secreted by neurons as a neurotransmitter or neural hormone and by endocrine gland cells as a classic hormone. Examples of such multifunctional chemical messengers are shown in Table 5–1. The cell-to-cell communication may occur by four mechanisms: (1) autocrine communication via messengers that diffuse in the interstitial fluid and act on the cells that secreted them, (2) neural communication via synaptic junctions, (3) paracrine communication via messengers that diffuse in the interstitial fluid to adjacent target cells (without entering the bloodstream), and (4) endocrine communication via circulating hormones (Figure 5–1). The two major mechanisms of neural regulation of endocrine function are direct innervation and neurosecretion (neural secretion of hormones). The adrenal medulla, kidney, parathyroid gland, and pancreatic islets are endocrine tissues that receive direct autonomic innervation (see Chapters 8, 10, 11, and 17). An example of neurosecretory regulation is the hormonal secretion of certain hypothalamic nuclei into the portal hypophysial vessels, which regulate the hormone-secreting cells of the anterior lobe of the pituitary. Another example of neurosecretory regulation is the posterior lobe of the pituitary gland, which is made up of the endings of neurons whose cell bodies reside in hypothalamic nuclei. These neurons secrete vasopressin and oxytocin into the general circulation.

Anatomy & Embryology

The anatomic relationships between the pituitary and the main nuclei of the hypothalamus are shown in Figure 5–2. The posterior lobe of the pituitary (neurohypophysis) is of neural origin, arising embryologically as an evagination of the ventral hypothalamus and the third ventricle. The neurohypophysis consists of the axons and nerve endings of neurons whose cell bodies reside in the supraoptic and paraventricular nuclei of the hypothalamus and supporting tissues. This hypothalamo-neurohypophysial nerve tract contains approximately 100,000 nerve fibers. Repeated swellings along the nerve fibers ranging in thickness from 1 μm to 50 μm constitute the nerve terminals.

The human fetal anterior pituitary anlage is initially recognizable at 4–5 weeks of gestation, and rapid cytologic differentiation leads to a mature hypothalamic-pituitary unit at 20 weeks. The anterior pituitary (adenohypophysis) originates from Rathke's pouch, an ectodermal evagination of the oropharynx, and migrates to join the neurohypophysis. The portion of Rathke's pouch in contact with the neurohypophysis develops less extensively and forms the intermediate lobe. This lobe remains intact in some species, but in humans its cells become interspersed with those of the anterior lobe and develop the capacity to synthesize and secrete pro-opiomelanocortin and adrenocorticotropic hormone (ACTH). Remnants of Rathke's pouch may persist at the boundary of the neurohypophysis, resulting in small colloid cysts. In addition, cells may persist in the lower portion of Rathke's pouch beneath the sphenoid bone, the pharyngeal pituitary. These cells have the potential to secrete hormones and have been reported to undergo adenomatous change.

The pituitary gland itself lies at the base of the skull in a portion of the sphenoid bone called the sella turcica ("Turkish saddle"). The anterior portion, the tuberculum sellae, is flanked by posterior projections of the sphenoid wings, the anterior clinoid processes; the dorsum sellae forms the posterior wall, and its upper corners project into the posterior clinoid processes. The gland is surrounded by dura, and the roof is formed by a reflection of the dura attached to the clinoid processes, the diaphragma sellae. The arachnoid membrane and, therefore, cerebrospinal fluid are prevented

Table 5–1. Neuroendocrine messengers: Substances that function as neurotransmitters, neural hormones, and classic hormones.

	Neurotransmitter (Present in Nerve Endings)	Hormone Secreted by Neurons	Hormone Secreted by Endocrine Cells
Dopamine	+	+	+
Norepinephrine	+	+	+
Epinephrine	+		+
Somatostatin	+	+	+
Gonadotropin-releasing hormone (GnRH)	+	+	+
Thyrotropin-releasing hormone (TRH)	+	+	
Oxytocin	+	+	+
Vasopressin	+	+	+
Vasoactive intestinal peptide	+	+	
Cholecystokinin (CCK)	+		+
Glucagon	+		+
Enkephalins	+		+
Pro-opiomelanocortin derivatives	+		+
Other anterior pituitary hormones	+		+

	GAP JUNCTIONS	SYNAPTIC	PARACRINE	ENDOCRINE
	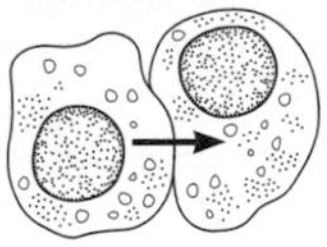	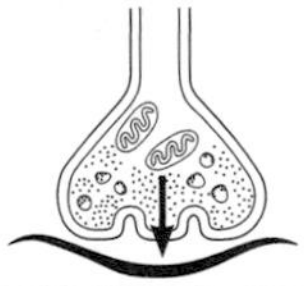	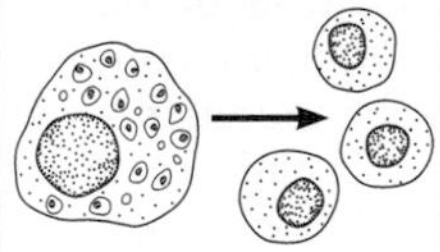	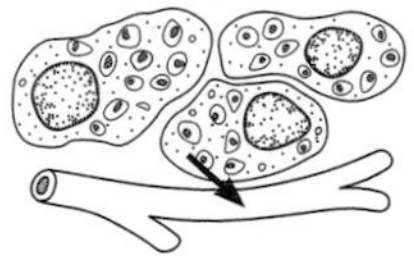
Message transmission	Directly from cell to cell	Across synaptic cleft	By diffusion in interstitial fluid	By circulating body fluids
Local or general	Local	Local	Locally diffuse	General
Specificity depends on	Anatomic location	Anatomic location and receptors	Receptors	Receptors

Figure 5–1. Intercellular communication by chemical mediators.

from entering the sella turcica by the diaphragma sellae. The pituitary stalk and its blood vessels pass through an opening in this diaphragm. The lateral walls of the gland are in direct apposition to the cavernous sinuses and separated from them by dural membranes. The optic chiasm lies 5–10 mm above the diaphragma sellae and anterior to the stalk (Figure 5–3).

The size of the pituitary gland, of which the anterior lobe constitutes two-thirds, varies considerably. It measures approximately $15 \times 10 \times 6$ mm and weighs 500–900 mg; it may double in size during pregnancy. The sella turcica tends to conform to the shape and size of the gland, and for that reason there is considerable variability in its contour.

Blood Supply

The anterior pituitary is the most richly vascularized of all mammalian tissues, receiving 0.8 mL/g/min from a portal circulation connecting the median eminence of the hypothalamus and the anterior pituitary. Arterial blood is supplied from the internal carotid arteries via the superior, middle, and inferior hypophysial arteries. The superior hypophysial arteries form a capillary network in the median eminence of the hypothalamus that recombines in long portal veins draining down the pituitary stalk to the anterior lobe, where they break up into another capillary network and re-form into venous channels. The pituitary stalk and the posterior pituitary are supplied directly from branches of the middle and inferior hypophysial arteries (Figures 5–2 and 5–3).

Venous drainage of the pituitary, the route through which anterior pituitary hormones reach the systemic circulation, is variable, but venous channels eventually drain via the cavernous sinus posteriorly into the supe-rior and inferior petrosal sinuses to the jugular bulb and vein (Figure 5–4). The axons of the neurohypophysis terminate on capillaries that drain via the posterior lobe veins and the cavernous sinuses to the general circulation. The hypophysial-portal system of capillaries allows control of anterior pituitary function by the hypothalamic hypophysiotropic hormones secreted into the portal hypophysial vessels. This provides a short, direct connection to the anterior pituitary from the ventral hypothalamus and the median eminence (Figure 5–5). There may also be retrograde blood flow between the pituitary and hypothalamus, providing a possible means of direct feedback between pituitary hormones and their neuroendocrine control centers.

Pituitary Development & Histology

Anterior pituitary cells were originally classified as acidophils, basophils, and chromophobe cells based on staining with hematoxylin and eosin. Immunocytochemical and electron microscopic techniques now permit classification of cells by their specific secretory products: somatotrophs (growth hormone [GH]-secreting cells), lactotrophs (prolactin [PRL]-secreting cells), thyrotrophs (cells secreting thyroid-stimulating hormone [thyrotropin; TSH]), corticotrophs (cells secreting adrenocorticotropic hormone [corticotropin; ACTH] and related peptides), and gonadotrophs (luteinizing hormone [LH]- and follicle-stimulating hormone [FSH]-secreting cells). The development of the pituitary gland and the emergence of the distinct cell types from common primordial cells is controlled by a limited set of transcription factors, most notably Prop1 and Pit1 (Figure 5–6). The individual hormone-secreting cells emerge in a specific order and from distinct lineages.

see next page

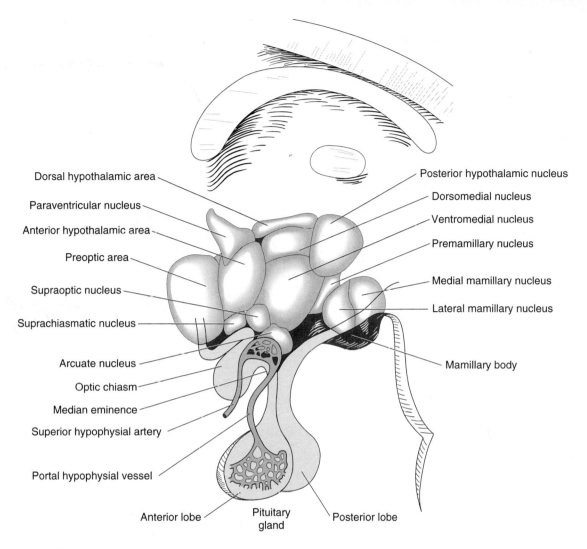

Figure 5–2. The human hypothalamus, with a superimposed diagrammatic representation of the portal hypophysial vessels. (Reproduced, with permission, from Ganong WF: *Review of Medical Physiology,* 15th ed. McGraw-Hill, 1993.)

Abnormalities of pituitary and lineage-specific transcription factors have been associated with the development of hypopituitarism. Although traditionally the pituitary has been conceptualized as a gland with distinct and highly specialized cells that respond to specific hypothalamic and peripheral hormones, it has become clear that local (ie, paracrine) factors also play a role in normal pituitary physiology.

A. SOMATOTROPHS

The GH-secreting cells are acidophilic and usually located in the lateral portions of the anterior lobe. Granule size by electron microscopy is 150–600 nm in di-

ameter. These cells account for about 50% of the adenohypophysial cells.

B. LACTOTROPHS

The PRL-secreting cell is a second but distinct acidophil-staining cell randomly distributed in the anterior pituitary. These cells account for 10–25% of anterior pituitary cells. Granule size averages approximately 550 nm on electron microscopy. There are two types of lactotrophs: sparsely granulated and densely granulated. These cells proliferate during pregnancy as a result of elevated estrogen levels and account for the twofold increase in gland size.

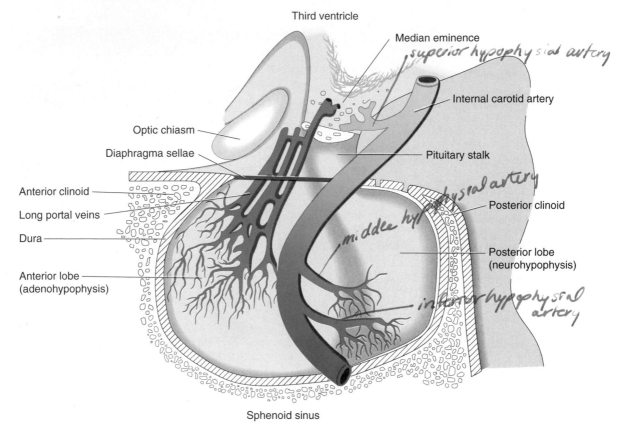

Third ventricle

Median eminence

superior hypophysial artery

Internal carotid artery

Optic chiasm

Diaphragma sellae

Pituitary stalk

Anterior clinoid

Long portal veins

Dura

middle hyphysial artery

Posterior clinoid

Posterior lobe
(neurohypophysis)

Anterior lobe
(adenohypophysis)

inferior hypophysial artery

Sphenoid sinus

Figure 5–3. Anatomic relationships and blood supply of the pituitary gland. (Reproduced, with permission, from Frohman LA: Diseases of the anterior pituitary. In: *Endocrinology and Metabolism,* 3rd ed. Felig P, Baxter JD, Frohman LA (editors). McGraw-Hill, 1995.)

C. THYROTROPHS

These TSH-secreting cells, because of their glycoprotein product, are basophilic and also show a positive reaction with periodic acid-Schiff (PAS) stain. Thyrotrophs are the least common pituitary cell type, making up less than 10% of adenohypophysial cells. The thyrotroph granules are small (50–100 nm); these cells are usually located in the anteromedial and anterolateral portions of the gland. During states of primary thyroid failure, the cells demonstrate marked hypertrophy, increasing overall gland size.

D. CORTICOTROPHS

ACTH and its related peptides (see below) are secreted by basophilic cells that are embryologically of intermediate lobe origin and usually located in the anteromedial portion of the gland. Corticotrophs represent 15–20% of adenohypophysial cells. Electron microscopy shows that these secretory granules are about 360 nm in diameter. In states of glucocorticoid excess, corticotrophs undergo degranulation and a microtubular hyalinization known as Crooke's hyaline degeneration.

E. GONADOTROPHS

LH and FSH originate from basophil-staining cells, whose secretory granules are about 200 nm in diameter. These cells constitute 10–15% of anterior pituitary cells, and they are located throughout the entire anterior lobe. They become hypertrophied and cause the gland to enlarge during states of primary gonadal failure such as menopause, Klinefelter's syndrome, and Turner's syndrome.

F. OTHER CELL TYPES

Some cells, usually chromophobes, contain secretory granules but do not exhibit immunocytochemical staining for the major known anterior pituitary hormones. These cells have been called null cells; they may give rise to (apparently) nonfunctioning adenomas. Some

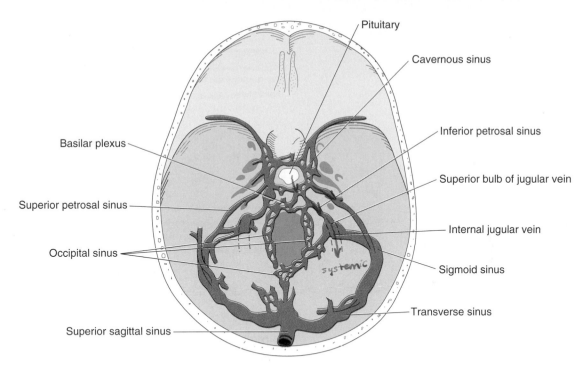

Figure 5–4. Venous drainage of the pituitary gland—the route by which adenohypophysial hormones reach the systemic circulation. (Reproduced, with permission, from Findling JW et al: Selective venous sampling for ACTH in Cushing's syndrome: Differentiation between Cushing's disease and the ectopic ACTH syndrome. Ann Intern Med 1981;94:647.)

may represent undifferentiated primitive secretory cells; others—eg, glia-like or folliculostellate cells—produce one or more of the many paracrine factors that have been described in the pituitary. Mammosomatotrophs contain both GH and PRL; these bihormonal cells are most often seen in pituitary tumors. Human chorionic gonadotropin is also secreted by the anterior pituitary gland, but its cell of origin and physiologic significance are uncertain. The six known major anterior pituitary hormones are listed in Table 5–2.

■ HYPOTHALAMIC HORMONES

The hypothalamic hormones can be divided into those secreted into hypophysial portal blood vessels and those secreted by the neurohypophysis directly into the general circulation. The hypothalamic nuclei, their neurohormones, and their main functions are shown in Table 5–3. The structures of the eight major hypothalamic hormones are shown in Table 5–4.

Hypophysiotropic Hormones

The hypophysiotropic hormones which regulate the secretion of anterior pituitary hormones include growth hormone-releasing hormone (GHRH), somatostatin, dopamine, thyrotropin-releasing hormone (TRH), corticotropin-releasing hormone (CRH), and gonadotropin-releasing hormone (GnRH). The location of the cell bodies of the hypophysiotropic hormone-secreting neurons are depicted in Figure 5–7. Most of the anterior pituitary hormones are controlled by stimulatory hormones, but growth hormone and especially prolactin are also regulated by inhibitory hormones. Some hypophysiotropic hormones are multifunctional. The hormones of the hypothalamus are secreted episodically and not continuously, and in some cases there is an underlying circadian rhythm.

A. GHRH

GHRH stimulates growth hormone (GH) secretion by and is trophic for somatotrophs. GHRH-secreting neurons are located in the arcuate nuclei (Figure 5–2), and axons terminate in the external layer of the median eminence. The major isoform of GHRH is 44 amino acids

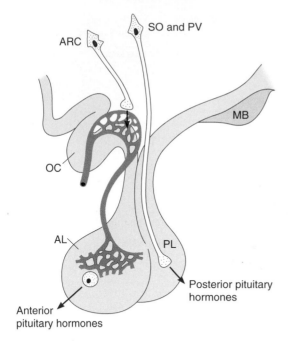

Figure 5–5. Secretion of hypothalamic hormones. The hormones of the posterior lobe (PL) are released into the general circulation from the endings of supraoptic and paraventricular neurons, whereas hypophysiotropic hormones are secreted into the portal hypophysial circulation from the endings of arcuate and other hypothalamic neurons. (AL, anterior lobe; ARC, arcuate and other nuclei; MB, mamillary bodies; OC, optic chiasm; PV, paraventricular nucleus. SO, supraoptic nucleus.)

in length. It was isolated from a pancreatic tumor in a patient with clinical manifestations of growth hormone excess (acromegaly) associated with somatotroph hyperplasia (see below). GHRH is synthesized from a larger precursor of 108 amino acids. Other secretory products derived from this precursor have also been found. Full biologic activity of these releasing factors appears to reside in the 1–29 amino acid sequence of the amino terminal portion of the molecule. Human GHRH is a member of a homologous family of peptides that includes secretin, glucagon, vasoactive intestinal peptide, and others. Like CRH, GHRH has a relatively long half-life (50 minutes).

B. SOMATOSTATIN

Somatostatin inhibits the secretion of GH and TSH. Somatostatin-secreting cells are located in the periventricular region immediately above the optic chiasm

(Figure 5–2) with nerve endings found diffusely in the external layer of the median eminence.

Somatostatin, a tetradecapeptide, has been found not only in the hypothalamus but also in the D cells of the pancreatic islets, the gastrointestinal mucosa, and the C cells (parafollicular cells) of the thyroid. The somatostatin precursor has 116 amino acids. Processing of the carboxyl terminal region of preprosomatostatin results in the generation of the tetradecapeptide somatostatin 14 and an amino terminal extended form containing 28 amino acid residues (somatostatin 28). Somatostatin 14 is the major species in the hypothalamus, while somatostatin 28 is found in the gut. In addition to its profound inhibitory effect on GH secretion, somatostatin also has important inhibitory influences on many other hormones, including insulin, glucagon, gastrin, secretin, and VIP. This inhibitory hypothalamic peptide plays a role in the physiologic secretion of TSH by augmenting the direct inhibitory effect of thyroid hormone on the thyrotrophs; administration of antisomatostatin antibodies results in a rise in circulating TSH level.

C. DOPAMINE

Dopamine, the primary prolactin-inhibitory hormone, is found in the portal circulation and binds to dopamine receptors on lactotrophs. The hypothalamic control of PRL secretion, unlike that of the other pituitary hormones, is predominantly inhibitory. Thus, disruption of the hypothalamic-pituitary connection by stalk section, hypothalamic lesions, or pituitary autotransplantation increases PRL secretion. Dopamine-secreting neurons (tuberoinfundibular dopaminergic system) are located in the arcuate nuclei and their axons terminate in the external layer of the median eminence, primarily in the same area as the GnRH endings (laterally) and to a lesser extent medially (Figure 5–2). The neurotransmitter gamma-aminobutyric acid (GABA) and cholinergic pathways also appear to inhibit PRL release.

D. PROLACTIN-RELEASING FACTORS

The best-studied factor with PRL-releasing activity is thyrotropin-releasing hormone (see below), but there is little evidence for a physiologic role; PRL increase associated with sleep, during stress, and after nipple stimulation or suckling is not accompanied by an increase in TRH or TSH. Another hypothalamic peptide, vasoactive intestinal peptide, stimulates PRL release in humans. Serotonergic pathways may also stimulate PRL secretion, as demonstrated by the increased PRL secretion after the administration of serotonin precursors and by the reduction of secretion following treatment with serotonin antagonists.

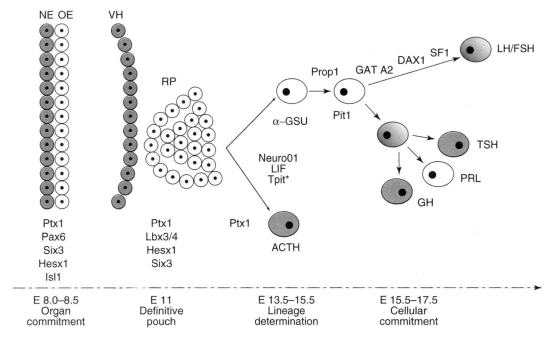

Figure 5–6. Transcription factors involved in the early development of mouse pituitary, including Tpit. *Tpit is expressed on embryonic day E 11.5, followed by expression of POMC cells by E 12.5. DAX1, dosage sensitive sex-reversal-adrenal hypoplasia congenital critical region on the X chromosome 1; GAT A2, GAT A-binding protein 2, zinc-finger transcription factor; α-GSU, α-subunit of pituitary glycoprotein hormones; Hesx1, homeobox gene expressed in embryonic stem cells 1; Isl1, islet 1 transcription factor; LH/FSH, lutenizing hormone/follicle-stimulating hormone; Lhx3/4, L1M-domain transcription factor 314; LIF, leukemia inhibiting factor; NE, neural epithelium; Neuro01, neurogenic basic helix-loop-helix transcription factor 01; OE, oral ectoderm; Pax6, pair-box containing transcription factor 6; Pit1, pituitary transcription factor 1; PRL, prolactin; Prop1, prophet of Pit1; Ptx1, pituitary homeobox 1; RP, Rathke's pouch; SF1, steroidogenic factor 1; Six3, sine oculis-like homeobox transcription factor 3; Tpit, T-box pituitary transcription factor; VH, ventral hypothalamus. (From Asteria C. T-Box and isolated ACTH deficiency. Eur J Endocrinol 2002;146:463.)

E. THYROTROPIN-RELEASING HORMONE (TRH)

TRH, a tripeptide, is the major hypothalamic factor regulating TSH secretion. Human TRH is synthesized from a large precursor of 242 amino acids that contains six copies of TRH. TRH-secreting neurons are located in the medial portions of the paraventricular nuclei (Figure 5–2), and their axons terminate in the medial portion of the external layer of the median eminence.

F. CORTICOTROPIN-RELEASING HORMONE (CRH)

CRH, a 41-amino-acid peptide, stimulates the secretion of adrenocorticotropic hormone (ACTH) and other products of its precursor molecule, pro-opiomelanocortin. The structure of human CRH is identical to that of rat CRH. CRH is synthesized from a precursor of 196 amino acids. CRH has a long plasma half-life (approximately 60 minutes), and both ADH and angiotensin II potentiate CRH-mediated secretion of ACTH. In contrast, oxytocin inhibits CRH-mediated ACTH secretion. CRH-secreting neurons are found in the anterior portion of the paraventricular nuclei just lateral to the TRH-secreting neurons; their nerve endings are found in all parts of the external layer of the median eminence. CRH is also secreted from human placenta. The level of this hormone increases significantly during late pregnancy and delivery. In addition, a specific CRH-binding protein (CRHBP) has been described in both serum and in intracellular locations within a variety of cells. It is likely that CRHBPs modulate the actions of CRH.

Table 5–2. Major adenohypophysial hormones and their cellular sources.[1]

Cellular Source and Histologic Staining	Main Hormone Products	Structure of Hormone	Main Functions
Somatotroph (acidophil)	GH; also known as STH or somatotropin	191 amino acids, 22-kDa protein, mainly nonglycosylated	Stimulates the production of IGF-1 (the mediator of the indirect actions of GH). Also exerts direct actions on growth and metabolism. Modulator of immune function and hemostasis.
Lactotroph or mammotroph (acidophil)	PRL	198 amino acids, 23-kDa protein, mainly nonglycosylated. (Note: most of the decidually produced PRL is glycosylated.)	Stimulation of milk production (protein and lactose synthesis, water excretion, and sodium retention). Inhibits gonadotropin secretion. Immunomodulator.
Corticotroph (small cells with basophil granules with strong PAS positivity, indicating the presence of glycoproteins)	Derivatives of POMC, mainly ACTH and β-LPH	POMC: glycosylated polypeptide of 134 amino acid residues. ACTH: simple peptide of 39 amino acid residues, 4.5 kDa. β-LPH: simple peptide of 91 amino acid residues, 11.2 kDa.	ACTH: stimulation of glucocorticoids and sex steroids in the zona fasciculata and zona reticularis of the adrenal cortex, inducing hyperplasia and hypertrophy of the adrenal cortex. β-LPH: weak lipolytic and opioid actions.
Thyrotroph (large cells with "basophil" granules with PAS positivity)	TSH	Glycoprotein hormone consisting of a shared α (89 amino acid) and a TSH-specific β (112 amino acid) subunit. Total size: 28 kDa.	Stimulation of all aspects of thyroid gland function: hormone synthesis, secretion, hyperplasia, hypertrophy, and vascularization
Gonadotroph (small cells) with "basophil" granules with PAS positivity)	LH: named after its effect in females. It is identical with the ICSH originally described in males	Glycoprotein hormone consisting of a shared α and an LH-specific β (115 amino acid) subunit. Total size: 29 kDa	Females: stimulates steroid hormone synthesis in theca interna cells, lutein cells, and hilar cells; promotes luteinization and maintains the corpus luteum. Males: stimulates steroid hormone production in Leydig cells.
	FSH	Glycoprotein hormone consisting of a shared α and an FSH-specific β (115 amino acid) subunit. Total size: 29 kDa.	Females: targets the granulosa cells to promote follicular development. Stimulates aromatase expression and inhibin secretion. Males: targets the Sertoli cells to promote spermatogenesis and to stimulate inhibin secretion.

[1]Modified from Kacsoh B: *Endocrine Physiology.* McGraw-Hill, 2000.

G. GONADOTROPIN-RELEASING HORMONE (GNRH)

The secretion of luteinizing hormone (LH) and follicle-stimulating hormone (FSH) is controlled by a single stimulatory hypothalamic hormone, gonadotropin-releasing hormone (GnRH). GnRH is a linear decapeptide that stimulates only LH and FSH; it has no effect on other pituitary hormones except in some patients with acromegaly and Cushing's disease (see below). The precursor of GnRH—proGnRH—contains 92 amino acids. ProGnRH also contains the sequence of a 56-amino-acid polypeptide called GnRH-associated peptide (GAP). This secretory product exhibits prolactin-inhibiting activity, but its physiologic role is unknown. GnRH-secreting neurons are located primarily in the preoptic area of the anterior hypothalamus and

Table 5–3. The hypothalamic nuclei and their main functions.[1]

Nucleus	Location	Major Neurohormones or Function
Supraoptic	Anterolateral, above the optic tract	ADH: osmoregulation, regulation of ECF volume Oxytocin: regulation of uterine contractions and milk ejection

Paraventricular	Dorsal anterior periventricular	Magnocellular PVN: ADH, oxytocin: same functions as above
		Parvocellular PVN
		  TRH: regulation of thyroid function
		  CRH: regulation of adrenocortical function, regulation of the sympathetic nervous system and adrenal medulla, regulation of appetite
		  ADH: coexpressed with CRH, regulation of adrenocortical function
		  VIP: prolactin-releasing factor (?)

Suprachiasmatic	Above the optic chiasm, anteroventral periventricular zone	Regulator of circadian rhythms and pineal function ("Zeitgeber" [pacemaker]): VIP, ADH neurons project mainly to the PVN
Arcuate	Medial basal hypothalamus close to the third ventricle	GHRH: stimulation of growth hormone GnRH: regulation of pituitary gonadotropins (FSH and LH) Dopamine: functions as PIH Somatostatin: inhibition of GHRH release Regulation of appetite (neuropeptide Y, agouti-related transcript, α-MSH, cocaine- and amphetamine-related transcript)
Periventricular	Anteroventral	Somatostatin: inhibition of growth hormone secretion by direct pituitary action: most abundant SRIF location
Ventromedial	Ventromedial	GHRH (as above) Somatostatin: inhibition of GHRH release Functions as a satiety center
Dorsomedial	Dorsomedial	Focal point of information processing: receives input from VMN and lateral hypothalamus and projects to the PVN
Lateral hypothalamus	Lateral hypothalamus	Functions as a hunger center (melanin-concentrating hormone, anorexins)
Preoptic area	Preoptic area	Main regulator of ovulation in rodents. Only a few GnRH neurons in primates
Anterior hypothalamus	Anterior hypothalamus	Thermoregulation: "cooling center" Anteroventral third ventricular region: regulation of thirst
Posterior hypothalamus	Posterior hypothalamus	Thermoregulation: "heating center"

[1]Modified from Kacsoh B: *Endocrine Physiology.* McGraw-Hill, 2000.

their nerve terminal are found in the lateral portions of the external layer of the median eminence adjacent to the pituitary stalk (Figure 5–2).

Posterior Pituitary Hormones

The hypothalamo-neurohypophysial system secretes two nonapeptides: antidiuretic hormone (ADH) (also known as arginine vasopressin) and oxytocin. They are synthesized in large cell bodies of neurons (magnocellular neurons) in the supraoptic nuclei and the lateral and superior parts of the paraventricular nuclei (Figures 5–2

and 5–5). The genes encoding these closely related hormones reside on chromosome 20 and probably evolved by duplication and inversion of an ancestral gene. ADH is an important regulator of water balance; it also is a potent vasoconstrictor and plays a role in regulation of cardiovascular function. Oxytocin causes contraction of smooth muscle, especially of the myoepithelial cells that line the ducts of the mammary gland, thus causing milk ejection.

ADH and oxytocin are basic nonapeptides (MW 1084 and 1007, respectively) characterized by a ring structure with a disulfide linkage (see Table 5–4). They

Table 5–4. Hypothalamic hormones.

Hormone	Structure
Posterior pituitary hormones	
Arginine vasopressin	⌐—S————S—⌐ Cys-Tyr-Phe-Gln-Asn-Cys-Pro-Arg-Gly-NH$_2$
Oxytocin	⌐—S————S—⌐ Cys-Tyr-Ile-Gln-Asn-Cys-Pro-Leu-Gly-NH$_2$
Hypophyseotropic hormones	
Thyrotropin-releasing hormone (TRH)	(pyro)Glu-His-Pro-NH$_2$
Gonadotropin-releasing hormone (GnRH)	(pyro)Glu-His-Trp-Ser-Tyr-Gly-Leu-Arg-Pro-Gly-NH$_2$
Somatostatin[1]	⌐—S————————S—⌐ Ala-Gly-Cys-Lys-Asn-Phe-Phe-Trp-Lys-Thr-Phe-Thr-Ser-Cys
Growth hormone–releasing hormone (GHRH)	Tyr-Ala-Asp-Ala-Ile-Phe-Thr-Asn-Ser-Tyr-Arg-Lys-Val-Leu-Gly-Gln-Leu-Ser- Ala-Arg-Lys-Leu-Leu-Gln-Asp-Ile-Met-Ser-Arg-Gln-Gln-Gly-Glu-Ser-Asn-Gln- Glu-Arg-Gly-Ala-Arg-Ala-Arg-Leu-NH$_2$
Prolactin-inhibiting hormone (PIH, dopamine)	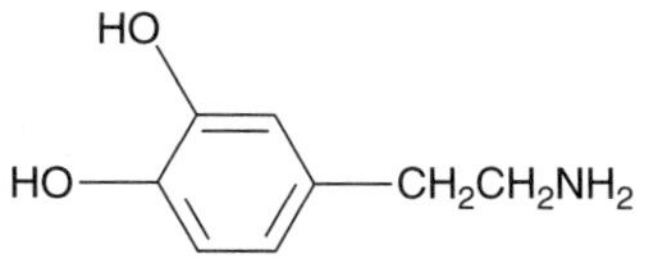
Corticotropin-releasing hormone (CRH)	Ser-Gln-Glu-Pro-Pro-Ile-Ser-Leu-Asp-Leu-Thr-Phe-His-Leu-Leu-Arg-Glu-Val- Leu-Glu-Met-Thr-Lys-Ala-Asp-Gln-Leu-Ala-Gln-Gln-Ala-His-Ser-Asn-Arg-Lys- Leu-Leu-Asp-Ile-Ala-NH$_2$

[1] In addition to the tetradecapeptide shown here (somatostatin 14), an amino terminal extended molecule (somatostatin 28) and a 12-amino-acid form (somatostatin 28 [1–12]) are found in most tissues.

are synthesized by separate cells (ie, there is no cosecretion or synthesis) from prohormones that contain both the peptide and an associated binding peptide or neurophysin specific for the hormone: neurophysin II for ADH and neurophysin I for oxytocin. Since the hormone and neurophysin are synthesized from the same prohormone, defects in gene expression result in deficiency of both products. For example, the Brattleboro rat has a deficiency of ADH and neurophysin II (but not of oxytocin and neurophysin I). Following synthesis and initial processing, secretory granules containing the prohormone migrate by axoplasmic flow (2–3 mm/h) to the nerve endings of the posterior lobe. In the secretory granules, further processing produces the mature nonapeptide and its neurophysin, which are cosecreted in equimolar amounts by exocytosis. Action potentials that reach the nerve endings increase the Ca^{2+} influx and initiate hormone secretion.

Neuroendocrinology: The Hypothalamus as Part of a Larger System

The hypothalamus is involved in many nonendocrine functions such as regulation of body temperature and

food intake and is connected with many other parts of the nervous system. The brain itself is influenced by both direct and indirect hormonal effects. Steroid and thyroid hormones cross the blood-brain barrier and produce specific receptor-mediated actions (see Chapters 7 and 9). Peptides in the general circulation which do not cross the blood-brain barrier elicit their effects indirectly, eg, insulin-mediated changes in blood glucose concentration. In addition, communication between the general circulation and the brain may take place via the circumventricular organs, which are located outside the blood-brain barrier (see below). Moreover, hypothalamic hormones in extrahypothalamic brain function as neurotransmitters or neurohormones. They are also found in other tissues where they function as hormones (endocrine, paracrine, or autocrine). For example, somatostatin-containing neurons are widely distributed in the nervous system. They are also found in the pancreatic islets (D cells), the gastrointestinal mucosa, and the C cells of the thyroid gland (parafollicular cells). Somatostatin is not only secreted into the general circulation as well as locally—it is also secreted into the lumen of the gut, where it may affect gut secretion. A hormone with this activity has

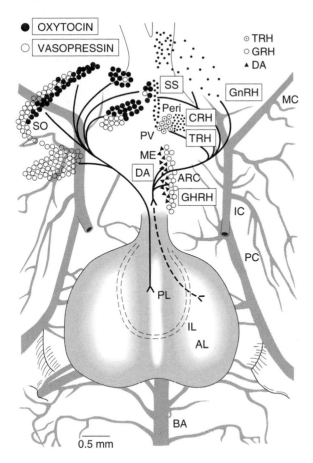

Figure 5–7. Location of cell bodies of hypophysiotropic hormone-secreting neurons projected on a ventral view of the hypothalamus and pituitary of the rat. (AL, anterior lobe; ARC, arcuate nucleus; BA, basilar artery; IC, internal carotid; IL, intermediate lobe; MC, middle cerebral; ME, median eminence; PC, posterior cerebral; Peri, periventricular nucleus; PL, posterior lobe; PVL and PVM, lateral and medial portions of the paraventricular nucleus; SO, supraoptic nucleus.) The names of the hormones are enclosed in the boxes. (SS, somatostatin; DA, dopamine.) (Courtesy of LW Swanson and ET Cunningham Jr.)

been called a "lumone." Hormones common to the brain, pituitary, and gastrointestinal tract include not only TRH and somatostatin but also vasoactive intestinal peptide and peptides derived from pro-opiomelanocortin.

Hypothalamic function is regulated both by hormone-mediated signals—eg, negative feedback—and by neural inputs from a wide variety of sources. These nerve signals are mediated by neurotransmitters including acetylcholine, dopamine, norepinephrine, epinephrine, serotonin, gamma-aminobutyric acid, and opioids. The hypothalamus can be considered a final common pathway by which signals from multiple systems reach the anterior pituitary. For example, cytokines that play a role in the response to infection, such as the interleukins, are also involved in regulation of the hypothalamic-pituitary-adrenal axis. This system of immunoneuroendocrine interactions is important in the organism's response to a variety of stresses.

The hypothalamus also sends signals to other parts of the nervous system. For example, while the major nerve tracts of the magnocellular neurons containing vasopressin and oxytocin terminate in the posterior pituitary, nerve fibers from the paraventricular and supraoptic nuclei project to many other parts of the nervous system. In the brain stem, vasopressinergic neurons are involved in the autonomic regulation of blood pressure. Similar neurons project to the gray matter and are implicated in higher cortical functions. Fibers terminating in the median eminence permit release of ADH into the hypophysial-portal system; delivery of ADH in high concentrations to the anterior pituitary may facilitate its involvement in the regulation of ACTH secretion. Magnocellular neurons also project to the choroid plexus where they may release ADH into the cerebrospinal fluid. In addition to magnocellular neurons, the paraventricular nuclei contain cells with smaller cell bodies—parvicellular neurons. Such neurons are also found in other regions of the nervous system and may contain other peptides such as CRH and TRH.

The Pineal Gland & the Circumventricular Organs

The circumventricular organs are secretory midline brain structures that arise from the ependymal cell lining of the ventricular system (Figure 5–8). These organs are located adjacent to the third ventricle—subfornical organ, subcommissural organ, organum vasculosum of the lamina terminalis, pineal, and part of the median eminence—and at the roof of the fourth ventricle—area postrema (Figure 5–8). The tissues of these organs have relatively large interstitial spaces and have fenestrated capillaries which, being highly permeable, permit diffusion of large molecules from the general circulation; elsewhere in the brain tight capillary endothelial junctions prevent such diffusion—the blood-brain barrier. For example, angiotensin II (see Chapter 10) is involved in the regulation of water intake, blood pressure, and secretion of vasopressin. In addition to its peripheral effects, circulating angiotensin II acts on the

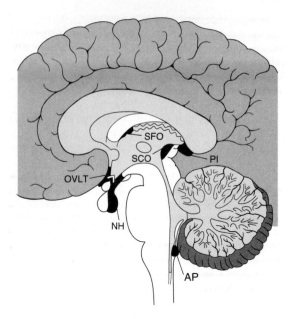

Figure 5–8. Circumventricular organs. The neurohypophysis (NH) and adjacent median eminence, the organum vasculosum of the lamina terminalis (OVLT), the subfornical organ (SFO), and the area postrema (AP) are shown projected on a sagittal section of the human brain. The pineal (PI) and the subcommissural organ (SCO) are also shown but probably do not function as circumventricular organs. (Reproduced, with permission, from Ganong WF: *Review of Medical Physiology,* 15th ed. McGraw-Hill, 1993.)

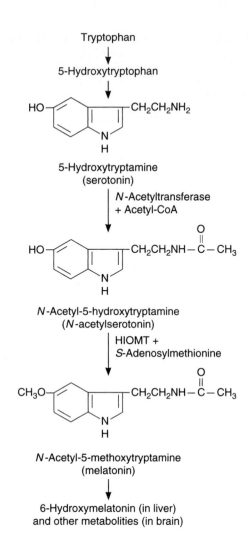

Figure 5–9. Formation and metabolism of melatonin. (HIOMT, hydroxyindole-O-methyltransferase.) (Reproduced, with permission, from Ganong WF. *Review of Medical Physiology,* 15th ed. McGraw-Hill, 1993.)

subfornical organ resulting in an increase in water intake.

The pineal gland, considered by the 17th century French philosopher René Descartes to be the seat of the soul, is located at the roof of the posterior portion of the third ventricle. The pineal gland in humans and other mammals has no direct neural connections with the brain except for sympathetic innervation via the superior cervical ganglion. The pineal gland secretes melatonin, an indole synthesized from serotonin by 5-methoxylation and N-acetylation (Figure 5–9). The pineal releases melatonin into the general circulation and into the cerebrospinal fluid. Melatonin secretion is regulated by the sympathetic nervous system and is increased in response to hypoglycemia and darkness. The pineal also contains other bioactive peptides and amines including TRH, somatostatin, GnRH, and norepinephrine. The physiologic roles of the pineal remain to be elucidated, but they involve regulation of gonadal function and development and chronobiologic rhythms.

The pineal gland may be the site of pineal cell tumors (pinealomas) or germ cell tumors (germinomas). Neurologic signs and symptoms are the predominant clinical manifestations, eg, increased intracranial pressure, visual abnormalities, ataxia, and Parinaud's syndrome—upward gaze palsy, absent pupillary light reflex, paralysis of convergence, and wide based gait. Endocrine manifestations result primarily from deficiency of hypothalamic hormones (diabetes insipidus, hypopituitarism, or disorders of gonadal development). Treatment involves surgical removal or decompression, radiation therapy, and hormone replacement (see below).

■ ANTERIOR PITUITARY HORMONES

The six major anterior pituitary hormones—ACTH, GH, PRL, TSH, LH, and FSH—may be classified into three groups: corticotropin-related peptides (ACTH, LPH, melanocyte-stimulating hormone [MSH], and endorphins); the somatomammotropins (GH and PRL), which are also peptides; and the glycoproteins (LH, FSH, and TSH). The chemical features of these hormones are set forth in Table 5–2.

ACTH & RELATED PEPTIDES

Biosynthesis

ACTH is a 39-amino-acid peptide hormone (MW 4500) processed from a large precursor molecule, pro-opiomelanocortin (POMC) (MW 28,500). Within the corticotroph, a single mRNA directs the synthesis and processing of POMC into smaller biologically active fragments (Figure 5–10) which include β-LPH, α-MSH, β-MSH, β-endorphin, and the amino terminal fragment of pro-opiomelanocortin. Most of these peptides are glycosylated, which accounts for differences in the reporting of molecular weights. These carbohydrate moieties are responsible for the basophilic staining of corticotrophs.

Two of these fragments are contained within the structure of ACTH: α-MSH is identical to $ACTH_{1-13}$, and corticotropin-like intermediate lobe peptide (CLIP) represents $ACTH_{18-39}$ (Figure 5–10). Although these fragments are found in species with developed intermediate lobes (eg, the rat), they are not secreted as separate hormones in humans. β-Lipotropin, a fragment with 91 amino acids (1–91), is secreted by the corticotroph in equimolar quantities with ACTH. Within the β-LPH molecule exists the amino acid sequence for β-MSH (41–58), γ-LPH (1–58), and β-endorphin (61–91).

Function

ACTH stimulates the secretion of glucocorticoids, mineralocorticoids, and androgenic steroids from the adrenal cortex (see Chapters 9 and 10). The amino terminal end (residues 1–18) is responsible for this biologic activity. ACTH binds to receptors on the adrenal cortex and induces steroidogenesis using cAMP.

The hyperpigmentation observed in states of ACTH hypersecretion (eg, Addison's disease, Nelson's syndrome) appears to be primarily due to ACTH binding to the MSH receptor, because α-MSH and β-MSH do not exist as separate hormones in humans.

The physiologic function of β-LPH and its family of peptide hormones, including β-endorphin, is not completely understood. However, both β-LPH and β-endorphin have the same secretory dynamics as ACTH.

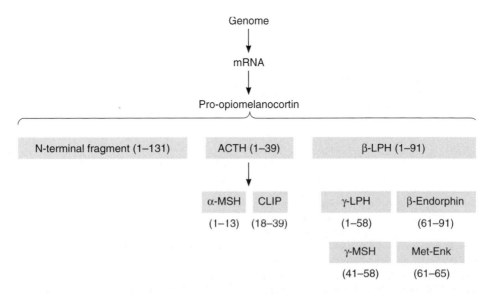

Figure 5–10. The processing of pro-opiomelanocortin (MW 28,500) into its biologically active peptide hormones. Abbreviations are expanded in the text.

Measurement

The development of an immunoradiometric assay using monoclonal antibodies has provided a sensitive and practical clinical ACTH assay for the evaluation of pituitary-adrenal disorders. The basal morning concentration ranges from 9 to 52 pg/mL (2–11 pmol/L). Its short plasma half-life (7–12 minutes) and episodic secretion cause wide and rapid fluctuations both in its plasma concentration and in that of cortisol.

Although β-LPH has a longer half-life than ACTH and is more stable in plasma, its measurement has not been extensively utilized. Current data suggest that the normal concentration of β-LPH is 10–40 pg/mL (1–4 pmol/L).

Secretion

The physiologic secretion of ACTH is mediated through neural influences by means of a complex of hormones, the most important of which is corticotropin-releasing hormone (CRH) (Figure 5–11).

CRH stimulates ACTH in a pulsatile manner: Diurnal rhythmicity causes a peak before awakening and a decline as the day progresses. The diurnal rhythm is a reflection of neural control and provokes concordant diurnal secretion of cortisol from the adrenal cortex (Figure 5–12). This episodic release of ACTH is independent of circulating cortisol levels—ie, the magnitude of an ACTH impulse is not related to preceding plasma cortisol levels. An example is the persistence of diurnal rhythm in patients with primary adrenal failure (Addison's disease). ACTH secretion also increases in response to feeding in both humans and animals.

Many stresses stimulate ACTH, often superseding the normal diurnal rhythmicity. Physical, emotional, and chemical stresses such as pain, trauma, hypoxia, acute hypoglycemia, cold exposure, surgery, depression, and interleukin-1 and vasopressin administration have all been shown to stimulate ACTH and cortisol secretion. The increase in ACTH levels during stress is mediated by vasopressin as well as CRH. Although physiologic cortisol levels do not blunt the ACTH response to stress, exogenous corticosteroids in high doses suppress it.

Negative feedback of cortisol and synthetic glucocorticoids on ACTH secretion occurs at both the hypothalamic and pituitary levels via two mechanisms: "Fast feedback" is sensitive to the rate of change in cortisol levels, while "slow feedback" is sensitive to the absolute cortisol level. The first mechanism is probably nonnuclear; ie, this phenomenon occurs too rapidly to be explained by the influence of corticosteroids on nuclear transcription of the specific mRNA responsible for

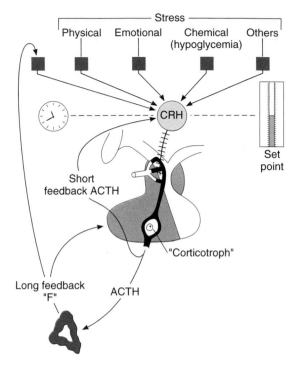

Figure 5–11. The hypothalamic-pituitary-adrenal axis, illustrating negative feedback by cortisol ("F") at the hypothalamic and pituitary levels. A short negative feedback loop of ACTH on the secretion of corticotropin-releasing hormone (CRH) also exists. (Reproduced, with permission, from Gwinup G, Johnson B: Clinical testing of the hypothalamic-pituitary-adrenocortical system in states of hypo- and hypercortisolism. Metabolism 1975;24:777.)

ACTH. "Slow feedback," occurring later, may be explained by a nuclear-mediated mechanism and a subsequent decrease in synthesis of ACTH. This latter form of negative feedback is the type probed by the clinical dexamethasone suppression test. In addition to the negative feedback of corticoids, ACTH also inhibits its own secretion (short loop feedback).

GROWTH HORMONE

Biosynthesis

Growth hormone (GH; somatotropin) is a 191-amino-acid polypeptide hormone (MW 21,500) synthesized and secreted by the somatotrophs of the anterior pituitary. Its larger precursor peptide, preGH (MW 28,000), is also secreted but has no physiologic significance.

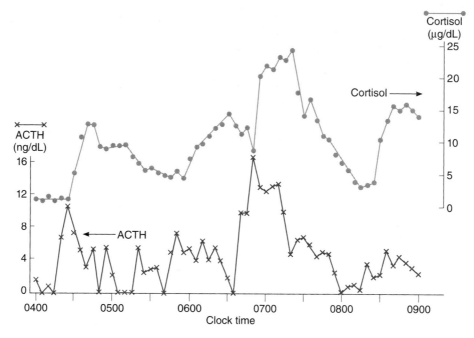

Figure 5–12. The episodic, pulsatile pattern of ACTH secretion and its concordance with cortisol secretion in a healthy human subject during the early morning. (Reproduced, with permission, from Gallagher TF et al: ACTH and cortisol secretory patterns in man. J Clin Endocrinol Metab 1973;36:1058.)

Function

The primary function of growth hormone (somatotropin) is promotion of linear growth. Its basic metabolic effects serve to achieve this result, but most of the growth-promoting effects are mediated by insulin-like growth factor 1 (IGF-I; previously known as somatomedin C). The metabolic and biologic effects of GH and IGF-I are shown in Tables 5–5 and 5–6 (see also Chapter 6).

Growth hormone, via IGF-I, increases protein synthesis by enhancing amino acid uptake and directly accelerating the transcription and translation of mRNA. In addition, GH tends to decrease protein catabolism by mobilizing fat as a more efficient fuel source: It directly causes the release of fatty acids from adipose tissue and enhances their conversion to acetyl-CoA, from which energy is derived. This protein-sparing effect is an important mechanism by which GH promotes growth and development.

GH also affects carbohydrate metabolism. In excess, it decreases carbohydrate utilization and impairs glucose uptake into cells. This GH-induced insulin resistance appears to be due to a postreceptor impairment in insulin action. These events result in glucose intolerance and secondary hyperinsulinism.

Measurement

GH has a plasma half-life of 20–50 minutes. The healthy adult secretes approximately 400 μg/d (18.6 nmol/d); in contrast, young adolescents secrete about 700 μg/d (32.5 nmol/d). There are specific GH-binding proteins in plasma.

The early morning GH concentration in fasting unstressed adults is less than 2 ng/mL (90 pmol/L). There are no significant sex differences.

Concentrations of IGF-I are determined by radioreceptor assays or radioimmunoassays. Determining the levels of these mediators of GH action may result in more accurate assessment of the biologic activity of GH (see Chapter 6). Growth hormone-binding proteins (GHBPs) include a high-affinity GHBP that represents the extracellular portion of the GH receptor and a low-affinity species. About half of circulating GH is bound to GHBPs. Measurement of serum concentrations of the high-affinity GHBP provides an index of GH receptor concentrations.

Table 5–5. Metabolic effects of GH and IGF-1 in vivo.[1]

Function, Parameter Group	Function, Parameter Subgroup	GH	IGF-1
Carbohydrate metabolism	Glucose uptake in extra-hepatic tissues	Decrease[2]	Increase
	Hepatic glucose output	Increase	Decrease
	Hepatic glycogen stores	Increase (jointly with glucocorticoids and insulin)	
	Plasma glucose	Increase	Decrease
	Insulin sensitivity	Decrease	Increase
Lipid metabolism	Lipolysis in adipocytes, plasma free fatty acid levels	Increase	Decrease
	Plasma ketone bodies	Increase	Decrease
Protein metabolism (muscle, connective tissue)	Amino acid uptake	Increase (?)	Increase
	Protein synthesis	Increase (?)	Increase
	Nitrogen excretion	Decrease (?)	Decrease

[1]Modified from Kacsoh B: *Endocrine Physiology*. McGraw-Hill, 2000.
[2]In GH-deficient patients, administration of GH results in a short-lived insulin-like action. During this time, glucose uptake by "peripheral" (extrahepatic) tissues increases.

Table 5–6. Main biologic effect of the GH-IGF-1 axis.[1]

Target, Source	Parameter	Effect
Blood and plasma (liver, bone and bone marrow actions)	IGF-1, acid-labile subunit	Increased by GH only
	IGF-binding protein-3	Increased by both GH and IGF-1
	Alkaline phosphatase (bone-specific)	Increase (mainly IGF-1)
	Fibrinogen	Increase
	Hemoglobin, hematocrit	Increase (mainly IGF-1 action on bone marrow)
Cartilage, bone	Length (before epiphysial closure), width (periosteal and perichondrial growth)	Stimulation (mainly IGF-1)
Visceral organs (liver, spleen, thymus, thyroid), tongue and heart	Growth	Stimulation, organomegaly (both GH and IGF-1)
Renal 25-hydroxyvitamin D 1α–hydroxylase activity	Plasma calcitriol	Increase (mainly GH), promotes positive calcium balance
Kidney	GFR	Increase (IGF-1)
Skin	Hair growth	Stimulation (IGF-1?)
	Sweat glands	Hyperplasia, hypertrophy, hyperfunction (GH?)
	Dermis	Thickening (both GH and IGF-1)

[1]Modified from Kacsoh B: *Endocrine Physiology*. McGraw-Hill, 2000.

Secretion

The secretion of GH is mediated by two hypothalamic hormones: growth hormone-releasing hormone (GHRH) and somatostatin (growth hormone-inhibiting hormone), both of which contribute to the episodic pattern of GH secretion. These hypothalamic influences are tightly regulated by an integrated system of neural, metabolic, and hormonal factors. Table 5–7 summarizes the many factors that affect GH secretion in physiologic, pharmacologic, and pathologic states.

A. GHRH

GHRH binds to specific receptors, stimulating cAMP production by somatotrophs and stimulating both GH synthesis and secretion. The effects of GHRH are partially blocked by somatostatin. The administration of GHRH to normal humans leads to rapid release of GH (within minutes); levels peak at 30 minutes and are sustained for 60–120 minutes.

Other peptide hormones such as ADH, ACTH, and α-MSH may act as GH-releasing factors when present in pharmacologic amounts. Even thyrotropin- and gonadotropin-releasing hormones (TRH and GnRH) often cause GH secretion in patients with acromegaly; however, it is not certain whether any of these effects are mediated by the hypothalamus or represent direct effects on the somatotroph. Regulation of GHRH is primarily under neural control (see below), but there is also short-loop negative feedback by GHRH itself.

B. SOMATOSTATIN

Somatostatin, a tetradecapeptide, is a potent inhibitor of GH secretion. It decreases cAMP production in GH-secreting cells and inhibits both basal and stimulated GH secretion. Somatostatin secretion is increased by elevated levels of GH and IGF-I. Long-acting analogs of somatostatin have been used therapeutically in the management of GH excess and in conditions such as pancreatic and carcinoid tumors that cause diarrhea.

C. GROWTH HORMONE SECRETAGOGUES

Non-GHRH secretagogues act to release GH, not through the GHRH receptor but through an orphan receptor, the growth hormone secretagogue receptor (GHS-R). A number of synthetic secretagogues, both peptides and nonpeptides, have been described. **Ghrelin,** an endogenous ligand for GHS-R, has recently been identified. Its location in the stomach suggests a new mechanism for regulation of GH secretion.

D. NEURAL CONTROL

The neural control of basal GH secretion results in irregular and intermittent release associated with sleep and varying with age. Peak levels occur 1–4 hours after the onset of sleep (during stages 3 and 4) (Figure 5–13).

Table 5–7. Factors affecting growth hormone secretion.[1]

Increase	Decrease[2]
Physiologic	
Sleep	Postprandial hyperglycemia
Exercise	Elevated free fatty acids
Stress (physical or psychologic)	
Postprandial	
Hyperaminoacidemia	
Hypoglycemia (relative)	
Pharmacologic	
Hypoglycemia	Hormones
Absolute: insulin or 2-deoxyglucose	Somatostatin
Relative: postglucagon	Growth hormone
Hormones	Progesterone
GHRH	Glucocorticoids
Peptide (ACTH, α-MSH, vasopressin)	Neurotransmitters, etc
Estrogen	Alpha-adrenergic antagonists (phentolamine)
Neurotransmitters, etc	Beta-adrenergic agonists (isoproterenol)
Alpha-adrenergic agonists (clonidine)	Serotonin agonists (methysergide)
Beta-adrenergic antagonists (propranolol)	Dopamine antagonists (phenothiazines)
Serotonin precursors	
Dopamine agonists (levodopa, apomorphine, bromocriptine)	
GABA agonists (muscimol)	
Potassium infusion	
Pyrogens (pseudomonas endotoxin)	
Pathologic	
Protein depletion and starvation	Obesity
Anorexia nervosa	Acromegaly; dopamine agonists
Ectopic production of GHRH	Hypothyroidism
Chronic renal failure	Hyperthyroidism
Acromegaly	
TRH	
GnRH	

[1]Modified and reproduced, with permission, from Frohman LA: Diseases of the anterior pituitary. In: *Endocrinology and Metabolism,* Felig P et al (editors). McGraw-Hill, 1981.
[2]Suppressive effects of some factors can be demonstrated only in the presence of a stimulus.

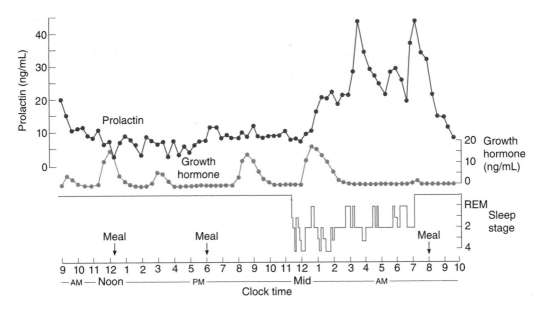

Figure 5–13. Sleep-associated changes in prolactin (PRL) and growth hormone (GH) secretion in humans. Peak levels of GH occur during sleep stages 3 or 4; the increase in PRL is observed 1–2 hours after sleep begins and is not associated with a specific sleep phase. (Reproduced, with permission, from Sassin JF et al: Human prolactin: 24-hour pattern with increased release during sleep. Science 1972;177:1205.)

These nocturnal sleep bursts, which account for nearly 70% of daily GH secretion, are greater in children and tend to decrease with age. Glucose infusion will not suppress this episodic release. Emotional, physical, and chemical stress, including surgery, trauma, exercise, electroshock therapy, and pyrogen administration, provoke GH release; and impairment of secretion, leading to growth failure, has been well documented in children with severe emotional deprivation (see Chapter 6).

E. METABOLIC CONTROL

The metabolic factors affecting GH secretion include all fuel substrates: carbohydrate, protein, and fat. Glucose administration, orally or intravenously, lowers GH in healthy subjects and provides a simple physiologic maneuver useful in the diagnosis of acromegaly (see below). In contrast, hypoglycemia stimulates GH release. This effect depends on intracellular glycopenia, since the administration of 2-deoxyglucose (a glucose analog that causes intracellular glucose deficiency) also increases GH. This response to hypoglycemia depends on both the rate of change in blood glucose and the absolute level attained.

A protein meal or intravenous infusion of amino acids (eg, arginine) causes GH release. Paradoxically, states of protein-calorie malnutrition also increase GH,

possibly as a result of decreased IGF-I production and lack of inhibitory feedback.

Fatty acids suppress GH responses to certain stimuli, including arginine and hypoglycemia. Fasting stimulates GH secretion, possibly as a means of mobilizing fat as an energy source and preventing protein loss.

F. EFFECTS OF OTHER HORMONES

Responses to stimuli are blunted in states of cortisol excess and during hypo- and hyperthyroidism. Estrogen enhances GH secretion in response to stimulation.

G. EFFECTS OF NEUROPHARMACOLOGIC AGENTS

Many neurotransmitters and neuropharmacologic agents affect GH secretion. Biogenic amine agonists and antagonists act at the hypothalamic level and alter GHRH or somatostatin release. Dopaminergic, alpha-adrenergic, and serotonergic agents all stimulate GH release.

Dopamine agonists such as levodopa, apomorphine, and bromocriptine increase GH secretion, whereas dopaminergic antagonists such as phenothiazines inhibit GH. The effect of levodopa, a precursor of both norepinephrine and dopamine, may be mediated by its conversion to norepinephrine, since its effect is blocked by the alpha-adrenergic antagonist phentolamine. Moreover, phentolamine suppresses GH release in response to other stimuli such as hypoglycemia, exercise, and arginine, emphasizing the importance of alpha-adrenergic mechanisms in modulating GH secretion.

Beta-adrenergic agonists inhibit GH, and beta-adrenergic antagonists such as propranolol enhance secretion in response to provocative stimuli.

PROLACTIN

Biosynthesis

Prolactin (PRL) is a 198-amino-acid polypeptide hormone (MW 22,000) synthesized and secreted from the lactotrophs of the anterior pituitary. Despite evolution from an ancestral hormone common to GH and human placental lactogen (hPL), PRL shares only 16% of its residues with the former and 13% with hPL. A precursor molecule (MW 40,000–50,000) is also secreted and may constitute 8–20% of the PRL plasma immunoreactivity in healthy persons and in patients with PRL-secreting pituitary tumors. PRL and GH are structurally related to members of the cytokine-hematopoietin family that include erythropoietin, granulocyte-macrophage colony stimulating factor (GM-CSF), and interleukins IL-2 to IL-7.

Function

PRL stimulates lactation in the postpartum period (see Chapter 16). During pregnancy, PRL secretion increases and, in concert with many other hormones (estrogen, progesterone, hPL, insulin, and cortisol), promotes additional breast development in preparation for milk production. Despite its importance during pregnancy, PRL has not been demonstrated to play a role in the development of normal breast tissue in humans. During pregnancy, estrogen enhances breast development but blunts the effect of PRL on lactation; the decrease in both estrogen and progesterone after parturition allows initiation of lactation. Accordingly, galactorrhea may accompany the discontinuance of oral contraceptives or estrogen therapy. Although basal PRL secretion falls in the postpartum period, lactation is maintained by persistent breast suckling.

PRL levels are very high in the fetus and in newborn infants, declining during the first few months of life.

Although PRL does not appear to play a physiologic role in the regulation of gonadal function, hyperprolactinemia in humans leads to hypogonadism. In women, initially there is a shortening of the luteal phase; subsequently, anovulation, oligomenorrhea or amenorrhea, and infertility occur. In men, PRL excess leads to decreased testosterone synthesis and decreased spermatogenesis, which clinically present as decreased libido, impotence, and infertility. The exact mechanisms of PRL inhibition of gonadal function are un-clear, but the principal one appears to be alteration of hypothalamic-pituitary control of gonadotropin secretion. Basal LH and FSH levels are usually normal; however, their pulsatile secretion is decreased and the mid-cycle LH surge is suppressed in women. Gonadotropin reserve, as assessed with GnRH, is usually normal or even exaggerated. Prolactin also has a role in immunomodulation; extrapituitary synthesis of PRL occurs in T lymphocytes (among other sites), and prolactin receptors are present on T and B lymphocytes and macrophages. PRL modulates and stimulates both immune cell proliferation and survival.

Measurement

The PRL secretory rate is approximately 400 μg/d (18.6 nmol/d). The hormone is cleared by the liver (75%) and the kidney (25%), and its half-time of disappearance from plasma is about 50 minutes.

Basal levels of PRL in adults vary considerably, with a mean of 13 ng/mL (0.6 nmol/L) in women and 5 ng/mL (0.23 nmol/L) in men. The upper range of normal in most laboratories is 15–20 ng/mL (0.7–0.9 nmol/L).

Secretion

The hypothalamic control of PRL secretion is predominantly inhibitory, and dopamine is the most important inhibitory factor. The physiologic, pathologic, and pharmacologic factors influencing PRL secretion are listed in Table 5–8.

A. PROLACTIN-RELEASING FACTORS

TRH is a potent prolactin-releasing factor that evokes release of PRL at a threshold dose similar to that which stimulates release of TSH. An exaggerated response of both TSH and PRL to TRH is observed in primary hypothyroidism, and their responses are blunted in hyperthyroidism. In addition, PRL secretion is also stimulated by vasoactive intestinal peptide and serotonergic pathways.

B. EPISODIC AND SLEEP-RELATED SECRETION

PRL secretion is episodic. An increase is observed 60–90 minutes after sleep begins but—in contrast to GH—is not associated with a specific sleep phase. Peak levels are usually attained between 4 and 7 AM (Figure 5–13). This sleep-associated augmentation of PRL release is not part of a circadian rhythm, like that of ACTH; it is related strictly to the sleeping period regardless of when it occurs during the day.

C. OTHER STIMULI

Stresses, including surgery, exercise, hypoglycemia, and acute myocardial infarction, cause significant elevation

Table 5–8. Factors affecting prolactin secretion.

Increase	Decrease
Physiologic	
Pregnancy	
Nursing	
Nipple stimulation	
Exercise	
Stress (hypoglycemia)	
Sleep	
Seizures	
Neonatal	
Pharmacologic	
TRH	Dopamine agonists (levo-
Estrogen	dopa, apomorphine,
Vasoactive intestinal peptide	bromocriptine, pergolide)
Dopamine antagonists (phe-	GABA
nothiazines, haloperidol,	
risperidone, metoclo-	
pramide, reserpine,	
methyldopa, amox-	
apine, opioids)	
Monoamine oxidase inhibi-	
tors	
Cimetidine (intravenous)	
Verapamil	
Licorice	
Pathologic	
Pituitary tumors	Pseudohypoparathyroidism
Hypothalamic/pituitary	Pituitary destruction or
stalk lesions	removal
Neuraxis irradiation	Lymphocytic hypophysitis
Chest wall lesions	
Spinal cord lesions	
Hypothyroidism	
Chronic renal failure	
Severe liver disease	

of PRL levels. Nipple stimulation in nonpregnant women also increases PRL. This neurogenic reflex may also occur from chest wall injury such as mechanical trauma, burns, surgery, and herpes zoster of thoracic dermatomes. This reflex discharge of PRL is abolished by denervation of the nipple or by spinal cord or brain stem lesions.

D. EFFECTS OF OTHER HORMONES

Many hormones influence PRL release. Estrogens augment basal and stimulated PRL secretion after 2–3 days of use (an effect that is of special clinical importance in patients with PRL-secreting pituitary adenomas); glucocorticoids tend to suppress TRH-induced PRL secre-

tion; and thyroid hormone administration may blunt the PRL response to TRH.

E. EFFECTS OF PHARMACOLOGIC AGENTS

(Table 5–8.) Many pharmacologic agents alter PRL secretion. Dopamine agonists (eg, bromocriptine) decrease secretion, forming the basis for their use in states of PRL excess. Dopamine antagonists (eg, receptor blockers such as phenothiazines and metoclopramide) and dopamine depletors (eg, reserpine) augment PRL release. Serotonin agonists will enhance PRL secretion; serotonin receptor blockers suppress PRL release associated with stress and with nursing.

THYROTROPIN

Biosynthesis

Thyrotropin (thyroid-stimulating hormone, TSH) is a glycoprotein (MW 28,000) composed of two noncovalently linked alpha and beta subunits. The structure of the alpha subunit of TSH is identical to that of the other glycoprotein molecules—FSH, LH, and human chorionic gonadotropin (hCG)—but the beta subunit differs in these glycoproteins and is responsible for their biologic and immunologic specificity. The peptides of these subunits appear to be synthesized separately and united before the carbohydrate groups are attached. The intact molecule is then secreted, as are small amounts of nonlinked subunits.

Function

The beta subunit of TSH attaches to high-affinity receptors in the thyroid, stimulating iodide uptake, hormonogenesis, and release of T_4 and T_3. This occurs through activation of adenylyl cyclase and the generation of cAMP. TSH secretion also causes an increase in gland size and vascularity by promoting mRNA and protein synthesis. (For a more detailed description, see Chapter 7.)

Measurement

TSH circulates unbound in the blood with a half-life of 50–60 minutes. With ultrasensitive immunoradiometric assays for measuring TSH concentration, the normal range is usually 0.5–4.7 μU/mL (0.5–4.7 mU/L). These new assays are helpful in the diagnosis of primary hypothyroidism and hyperthyroidism; however, TSH levels alone cannot be used to evaluate pituitary or hypothalamic hypothyroidism.

The alpha subunit can be detected in about 80% of normals, with a range of 0.5–2 ng/mL. Plasma alpha subunit levels increase after administration of TRH in normal subjects, and basal levels are elevated in primary hypothyroidism, primary hypogonadism, and in patients with TSH-secreting, gonadotropin-secreting, or pure alpha subunit-secreting pituitary adenomas.

Secretion

The secretion of TSH is controlled by both stimulatory (TRH) and inhibitory (somatostatin) influences from the hypothalamus and in addition is modulated by the feedback inhibition of thyroid hormone on the hypothalamic-pituitary axis (Table 7–6 and Figure 7–22).

A. TRH

The response of TSH to TRH is modulated by the circulating concentration of thyroid hormones. Small changes in serum levels (even within the physiologic range) cause substantial alterations in the TSH response to TRH. As shown in Figure 5–14, the administration of T_3 (15 μg) and T_4 (60 μg) to healthy persons for 3–4 weeks suppresses the TSH response to TRH despite only small increases in circulating T_3 and T_4 levels.

Thus, the secretion of TSH is inversely proportionate to the concentration of thyroid hormone.

The set point (the level at which TSH secretion is maintained) is determined by TRH. Deviations from this set point result in appropriate changes in TSH release. Administration of TRH increases TSH within 2 minutes, and this response is blocked by previous T_3 administration; however, larger doses of TRH may overcome this blockade—suggesting that both T_3 and TRH act at the pituitary level to influence TSH secretion. In addition, T_3 and T_4 inhibit mRNA for TRH synthesis in the hypothalamus, indicating that a negative feedback mechanism operates at this level also.

B. SOMATOSTATIN

This inhibitory hypothalamic peptide augments the direct inhibitory effect of thyroid hormone on the thyrotrophs. Infusion of somatostatin blunts the early morning TSH surge and will suppress high levels of TSH in primary hypothyroidism. Octreotide acetate, a somatostatin analog, has been used successfully to inhibit TSH secretion in some patients with TSH-secreting pituitary tumors.

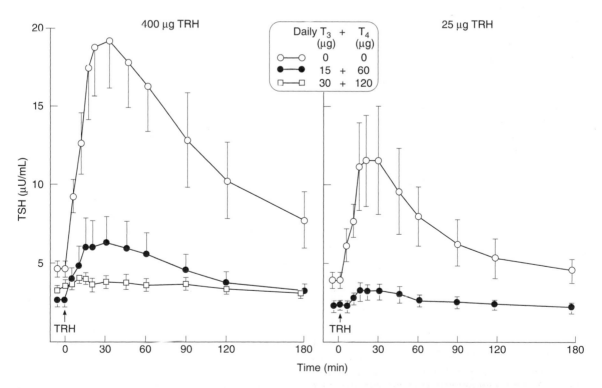

Figure 5–14. Administration of small doses of T_3 (15 μg) and T_4 (60 μg) to healthy subjects inhibits the TSH response to 2 doses (400 μg, left; 25 μg, right) of TRH (protirelin). (Reproduced, with permission, from Snyder PJ, Utiger RD: Inhibition of thyrotropin-releasing hormone by small quantities of thyroid hormones. J Clin Invest 1972;51:2077.)

C. Neural Control

In addition to these hypothalamic influences on TSH secretion, neurally mediated factors may be important. Dopamine physiologically inhibits TSH secretion. Intravenous dopamine administration will decrease TSH in both healthy and hypothyroid subjects as well as blunt the TSH response to TRH. Thus, as expected, dopaminergic agonists such as bromocriptine inhibit TSH secretion and dopaminergic antagonists such as metaclopramide increase TSH secretion in euthyroid subjects. Bromocriptine has also been effective in the management of some TSH-secreting pituitary tumors.

D. Effects of Cortisol and Estrogens

Glucocorticoid excess has been shown to impair the sensitivity of the pituitary to TRH and may lower serum TSH to undetectable levels. However, estrogens increase the sensitivity of the thyrotroph to TRH; women have a greater TSH response to TRH than men do, and pretreatment of men with estradiol will increase their TRH-induced TSH response. (See also Chapter 7 and Table 7–6.)

GONADOTROPINS: LUTEINIZING HORMONE, FOLLICLE-STIMULATING HORMONE

Biosynthesis

Luteinizing hormone (LH) and follicle-stimulating hormone (FSH) are glycoprotein gonadotropins composed of alpha and beta subunits and secreted by the same cell. The specific beta subunit confers on these hormones their unique biologic activity, as it does with TSH and hCG. The biologic activity of hCG, a placental glycoprotein, closely resembles that of LH. Human menopausal gonadotropin (hMG, menotropins)—an altered mixture of pituitary gonadotropins recovered from the urine of postmenopausal women—is a preparation with FSH-like activity. Menotropins and chorionic gonadotropin are used clinically for induction of spermatogenesis or ovulation (see Chapters 12 and 13).

Function

LH and FSH bind to receptors in the ovary and testis and regulate gonadal function by promoting sex steroid production and gametogenesis.

In men, LH stimulates testosterone production from the interstitial cells of the testes (Leydig cells). Maturation of spermatozoa, however, requires both LH and FSH. FSH stimulates testicular growth and enhances the production of an androgen-binding protein by the Sertoli cells, which are a component of the testicular tubule necessary for sustaining the maturing sperm cell. This androgen-binding protein promotes high local concentrations of testosterone within the testis, an essential factor in the development of normal spermatogenesis (see Chapter 12).

In women, LH stimulates estrogen and progesterone production from the ovary. A surge of LH in the mid menstrual cycle is responsible for ovulation, and continued LH secretion subsequently stimulates the corpus luteum to produce progesterone by enhancing the conversion of cholesterol to pregnenolone. Development of the ovarian follicle is largely under FSH control, and the secretion of estrogen from this follicle is dependent on both FSH and LH.

Measurement

The normal levels of LH and FSH vary with the age of the subject (see Appendix). They are low before puberty and elevated in postmenopausal women. A nocturnal rise of LH in boys and the cyclic secretion of FSH and LH in girls usually herald the onset of puberty before clinical signs are apparent. In women, LH and FSH vary during the menstrual cycle; during the initial phase of the cycle (follicular), LH steadily increases, with a midcycle surge that initiates ovulation. FSH, on the other hand, initially rises and then decreases during the later follicular phase until the midcycle surge, which is concordant with LH. Both LH and FSH levels fall steadily after ovulation. (See Chapter 13.)

LH and FSH levels in men are similar to those in women during the follicular phase. The alpha subunit, shared by all the pituitary glycoprotein hormones, can also be measured (see TSH) and will rise following GnRH administration. The normal responses of LH and FSH to GnRH are shown in Table 5–9.

Secretion

The secretion of LH and FSH is controlled by gonadotropin-releasing hormone (GnRH), which maintains basal gonadotropin secretion, generates the phasic release of gonadotropins for ovulation, and determines the onset of puberty. Many other factors are involved in regulation of this axis. For example, activins and follistatins are paracrine factors that exert opposing effects on gonadotrophs. Leptin, a recently described hormone made in adipocytes, is involved in regulation of this axis and may help to explain the suppression of gonadotropin secretion that accompanies caloric restriction.

A. Episodic Secretion

In both males and females, secretion of LH and FSH is episodic, with secretory bursts that occur each hour and are mediated by a concordant episodic release of

Table 5–9. Normal gonadotropin responses (± SD) to GnRH (100 μg).

	Mean Maximum Exchange			
	LH		FSH	
	(μg/L)	(IU/L)	(μg/L)	(IU/L)
Women				
Follicular phase	2.1 ± 0.4	17 ± 3	1.0 ± 0.3	3 ± 1
Around LH peak	20.8 ± 6.2	162 ± 49	2.7 ± 1.0	8 ± 3
Luteal phase	6.3 ± 1.0	49 ± 8	1.0 ± 0.1	3 ± 0.4
Men				
Age 18–40	4.1 ± 0.8	32 ± 6	1.0 ± 0.3	3 ± 1
Age over 65	2.9 ± 0.5	23 ± 4	1.0 ± 0.3	3 ± 1

Conversion factors: For LH (LER 960), 1 ng = 7.8 mIU; for FSH (LER 869), 1 ng = 3 mIU.

GnRH. The amplitude of these secretory surges is greater in patients with primary hypogonadism. The pulsatile nature of GnRH release is critical for sustaining gonadotropin secretion. A continuous, prolonged infusion of GnRH in women evokes an initial increase in LH and FSH followed by prolonged suppression of gonadotropin secretion. This phenomenon may be explained by down-regulation of GnRH receptors on the pituitary gonadotrophs. Consequently, long-acting synthetic analogs of GnRH may be used clinically to suppress LH and FSH secretion in conditions such as precocious puberty.

B. Positive Feedback

Circulating sex steroids affect GnRH secretion and thus LH and FSH secretion by both positive and negative (inhibitory) feedback mechanisms. During the menstrual cycle, estrogens provide a positive influence on GnRH effects on LH and FSH secretion, and the rise in estrogen during the follicular phase is the stimulus for the LH and FSH ovulatory surge. This phenomenon suggests that the secretion of estrogen is to some extent influenced by an intrinsic ovarian cycle. Progesterone amplifies the duration of the LH and FSH surge and augments the effect of estrogen. After this midcycle surge, the developed egg leaves the ovary. Ovulation occurs approximately 10–12 hours after the LH peak and 24–36 hours after the estradiol peak. The remaining follicular cells in the ovary are converted, under the influence of LH, to a progesterone-secreting structure, the corpus luteum. After about 12 days, the corpus luteum involutes, resulting in decreased estrogen and progesterone levels and then uterine bleeding. (See Chapter 13.)

C. Negative Feedback

Negative feedback effects of sex steroids on gonadotropin secretion also occur. In women, primary gonadal failure or menopause results in elevations of LH and FSH, which can be suppressed with long-term, high-dose estrogen therapy. However, a shorter duration of low-dose estrogen may enhance the LH response to GnRH. In men, primary gonadal failure with low circulating testosterone levels is also associated with elevated gonadotropins. However, testosterone is not the sole inhibitor of gonadotropin secretion in men, since selective destruction of the tubules (eg, by cyclophosphamide therapy) results in azoospermia and elevation of only FSH.

Inhibin, a polypeptide (MW 32,000) secreted by the Sertoli cells of the seminiferous tubules, is the major factor that inhibits FSH secretion by negative feedback. Inhibin, which has been purified and sequenced by analysis of its complementary DNA, consists of separate alpha and beta subunits connected by a disulfide bridge. Androgens stimulate inhibin production; this peptide may help to locally regulate spermatogenesis. (See Chapter 12.)

■ ENDOCRINOLOGIC EVALUATION OF THE HYPOTHALAMIC-PITUITARY AXIS

The precise assessment of the hypothalamic-pituitary axis has been made possible by radioimmunoassays of the major anterior pituitary hormones and their specific target gland hormones. In addition, four synthetic hypothalamic hormones—TRH (protirelin), GnRH (gonadorelin), ovine CRH, and human GHRH—which are available commercially, can be used to assess hypothalamic-pituitary reserve.

This section describes the principles involved in testing each pituitary hormone as well as special situations (eg, drugs, obesity) that may interfere with pituitary function or pituitary testing. Specific protocols for performing and interpreting diagnostic procedures are outlined at the end of this section and in Table 5–11. The clinical manifestations of either hypo- or hypersecretion of anterior pituitary hormones are discussed in subsequent sections.

EVALUATION OF ACTH

ACTH deficiency leads to secondary adrenocortical insufficiency, characterized by decreased secretion of cortisol and the adrenal androgens; aldosterone secretion, controlled primarily by the renin-angiotensin axis, is usually maintained. In contrast, excessive ACTH secretion leads to adrenal hyperfunction (Cushing's syndrome, discussed in a later section of this chapter and in Chapter 9).

Plasma ACTH Levels

Basal ACTH measurements are usually unreliable indicators of pituitary function, since its short plasma half-life and episodic secretion result in wide fluctuations in plasma levels (Figure 5–12). Therefore, the interpretation of plasma ACTH levels requires the simultaneous assessment of cortisol secretion by the adrenal cortex. These measurements are of greatest utility in differentiating primary and secondary adrenocortical insufficiency and in establishing the etiology of Cushing's syndrome (see the later section on Cushing's disease and also Chapter 9).

Evaluation of ACTH Deficiency

In evaluating ACTH deficiency, measurement of basal cortisol levels is also generally unreliable. Because plasma cortisol levels are usually low in the late afternoon and evening, reflecting the normal diurnal rhythm, samples drawn at these times are of virtually no value for this diagnosis. Plasma cortisol levels are usually highest in the early morning; however, there is considerable overlap between adrenal insufficiency and normal subjects. A plasma cortisol level less than 5 μg/dL (138 nmol/L) at 8 AM strongly suggests the diagnosis—and the lower the level, the more likely the diagnosis. Conversely, a plasma cortisol greater than 20 μg/dL (552 nmol/L) virtually excludes the diagnosis. Similarly, salivary cortisol levels less than 1.8 ng/mL (5 nmol/L) at 8 AM strongly suggest adrenal insufficiency, while levels in excess of 5.8 ng/mL (16 nmol/L) greatly reduce the probability of the diagnosis. Consequently, the diagnosis of ACTH hyposecretion (secondary adrenal insufficiency) must be established by provocative testing of the reserve capacity of the hypothalamic-pituitary axis.

Adrenal Stimulation

Since adrenal atrophy develops as a consequence of prolonged ACTH deficiency, the initial and most convenient approach to evaluation of the hypothalamic-pituitary-adrenal axis is assessment of the plasma cortisol response to synthetic ACTH (cosyntropin). In normal individuals, injection of cosyntropin (250 μg) causes a rapid increase (within 30 minutes) of cortisol to at least 18–20 μg/dL (496–552 nmol/L), and this response usually correlates with the cortisol response to insulin-induced hypoglycemia. A subnormal cortisol response to ACTH confirms adrenocortical insufficiency. However, a normal response does not directly evaluate the ability of the hypothalamic-pituitary axis to respond to stress (see Chapter 9). Thus, patients withdrawn from long-term glucocorticoid therapy may have an adequate increase in cortisol following exogenous ACTH that precedes complete recovery of the hypothalamic-pituitary-adrenal axis. Therefore, such patients should receive glucocorticoids during periods of stress for at least 1 year after steroids are discontinued, unless the hypothalamic-pituitary axis is shown to be responsive to stress as described below.

The more physiologic dose administered in the 1 μg ACTH test is designed to improve its sensitivity in detection of secondary adrenal insufficiency. The cortisol response to 1 μg of synthetic ACTH correlates better with the cortisol response to insulin-induced hypoglycemia in patients with chronic secondary adrenal insufficiency. However, the results in secondary adrenal insufficiency of recent onset are less reliable. Performance of the 1 μg test is also associated with some technical problems: there are no ready-to-use vials containing 1 μg, and there is controversy about the diagnostic criteria used for the 1 μg test. Even if this latter issue is resolved, clinicians must be wary about comparisons of different cortisol assays (see above). These problems notwithstanding, the low-dose (1 μg) ACTH stimulation test is gaining greater acceptance and may emerge as the diagnostic procedure of choice in suspected secondary adrenal insufficiency.

Pituitary Stimulation

Direct evaluation of pituitary ACTH reserve can be performed by means of insulin-induced hypoglycemia, metyrapone administration, or CRH stimulation. These studies are unnecessary if the cortisol response to rapid ACTH stimulation is subnormal.

A. INSULIN-INDUCED HYPOGLYCEMIA

The stimulus of neuroglycopenia associated with hypoglycemia (blood glucose < 40 mg/dL) evokes a stress-mediated activation of the hypothalamic-pituitary-adrenal axis. Subjects should experience adrenergic symptoms (diaphoresis, tachycardia, weakness, headache) associated with the fall in blood sugar. In normal persons, plasma cortisol increases to more than 18–20 μg/dL (496–552 nmol/L), indicating normal ACTH reserve. Although plasma ACTH also rises, its determination has not proved to be as useful, since pulsatile secretion requires frequent sampling, and the normal response is not well standardized. Although insulin-induced hypoglycemia most reliably predicts ACTH secretory capacity in times of stress, it is rarely performed at present since the procedure requires a physician's presence and is contraindicated in elderly patients, patients with cerebrovascular or cardiovascular disease, and those with seizure disorders. It should be used with caution in patients in whom diminished adrenal reserve is suspected, since severe hypoglycemia may occur; in these patients, the test should always be preceded by the ACTH adrenal stimulation test.

B. METYRAPONE STIMULATION

Metyrapone administration is an alternative method for assessing ACTH secretory reserve. Metyrapone inhibits P450c11 (11β-hydroxylase), the enzyme that catalyzes the final step in cortisol biosynthesis (see Chapter 9). The inhibition of cortisol secretion interrupts negative feedback on the hypothalamic-pituitary axis, resulting in a compensatory increase in ACTH. The increase in ACTH secretion stimulates increased steroid biosynthesis proximal to P450c11, and the increase can be detected as an increase in the precursor steroid (11-deoxycortisol) in plasma. The overnight test is preferred because of its simplicity; it is performed by administering 30 mg/kg of metyrapone orally at midnight. Plasma 11-deoxycortisol is determined the following morning and rises to more than 7 μg/dL (0.2 nmol/L) in healthy individuals. Again the test should be used cautiously in patients with suspected adrenal insufficiency and should be preceded by a rapid ACTH stimulation test (see above). The traditional 3-day metyrapone test should not be used at present because of the risk of precipitating adrenal insufficiency. The overnight metyrapone test is most useful in patients with partial secondary adrenal insufficiency in whom the rapid ACTH stimulation test is normal or borderline and has been shown to correlate well with the response to insulin-induced hypoglycemia. Metyrapone may be obtained directly from the Novartis Pharmaceutical Corporation, East Hanover, New Jersey.

C. CRH STIMULATION

Ovine CRH administered intravenously is used to assess ACTH secretory dynamics. In healthy subjects, CRH (1 μg/kg) provokes a peak ACTH response within 15 minutes and a peak cortisol response within 30–60 minutes. This dose may be associated with mild flushing, occasional shortness of breath, tachycardia, and hypotension. Patients with primary adrenal insufficiency have elevated basal ACTH levels and exaggerated ACTH responses to CRH. Secondary adrenal insufficiency results in an absent ACTH response to CRH in patients with pituitary corticotroph destruction; however, in patients with hypothalamic dysfunction, there is a prolonged and augmented ACTH response to CRH with a delayed peak. Because of overlap between the responses of normal individuals and those

with partial secondary adrenal insufficiency, the CRH test is less useful than the procedures described above.

ACTH Hypersecretion

ACTH hypersecretion is manifested by adrenocortical hyperfunction (Cushing's syndrome). The diagnosis and differential diagnosis of ACTH hypersecretion are outlined in a later section on Cushing's disease and also in Chapter 9.

EVALUATION OF GROWTH HORMONE

The evaluation of GH secretory reserve is important in the assessment of children with short stature and in adults with suspected hypopituitarism. Provocative tests are necessary because basal levels of GH are usually low and therefore do not distinguish between normal and GH-deficient patients. Special attention must be given to the methodology and the laboratory standards of GH measurement. Newer immunometric assays give results that are 30–50% lower than older radioimmunoassays.

Insulin-Induced Hypoglycemia

The most reliable stimulus of GH secretion is insulin-induced hypoglycemia. In normal individuals, GH levels will increase to more than 10 ng/mL (460 pmol/L) after adequate hypoglycemia is achieved. Since 10% of normal individuals fail to respond to hypoglycemia, other stimulatory tests may be necessary.

GHRH-Arginine Test

Both forms of human GHRH (GHRH-40 and GHRH-44) have been used to evaluate GH secretory capacity. A dose of GHRH (1 μg/kg) combined with a 30-minute infusion of arginine (0.5 g/kg to a maximum of 20 g) promptly stimulates GH; the mean peak is 10–15 ng/mL (460–700 pmol/L) at 30–60 minutes in healthy subjects. The results are comparable to those achieved with insulin-induced hypoglycemia.

Tests With Levodopa, Arginine, & Other Stimuli

Stimulation testing with levodopa, arginine infusion alone, propranolol, or glucagon is less reliable in the diagnosis of GH deficiency.

GH Hypersecretion

The evaluation of GH hypersecretion is discussed in the section on acromegaly and is most conveniently assessed by GH suppression testing with oral glucose and measurement of IGF-I levels.

EVALUATION OF PROLACTIN

PRL secretion by the pituitary is the most resistant to local damage, and decreased PRL secretory reserve indicates severe intrinsic pituitary disease.

Prolactin Reserve

The administration of TRH is the simplest and most reliable means of assessing PRL reserve. Although the response of PRL to TRH varies somewhat according to sex and age (Table 5–10), PRL levels usually increase twofold 15–30 minutes after TRH administration. In addition, insulin-induced hypoglycemia will evoke a stress-related increase in PRL.

PRL Hypersecretion

PRL hypersecretion is a common endocrine problem. Its evaluation is discussed in the section on prolactinomas.

EVALUATION OF TSH

Basal Measurements

The laboratory evaluation of TSH secretory reserve begins with an assessment of target gland secretion; thyroid function tests (free thyroxine [FT_4]) should be obtained. Normal thyroid function studies in a clinically euthyroid patient indicate adequate TSH secretion, and no further studies are warranted. Laboratory evidence of hypothyroidism requires measurement of a TSH level. With primary thyroid gland failure, the TSH level will be elevated; low or normal TSH in the presence of hypothyroidism suggests hypothalamic-pituitary dysfunction (see Chapter 7).

TRH Test

Since accurate methods for determining TSH and FT_4 readily establish the diagnosis of hypothyroidism in virtually all patients, the TRH test is rarely indicated today.

EVALUATION OF LH & FSH

Testosterone & Estrogen Levels

The evaluation of gonadotropin function also requires assessment of target gland secretory function, and measurement of gonadal steroids (testosterone in men, estradiol in women) is useful in the diagnosis of hypogonadism. In women, the presence of regular menstrual cycles is strong evidence that the hypothalamic-pituitary-gonadal axis is intact. Estradiol levels rarely fall below 50 pg/mL (180 pmol/L), even during the early follicular phase. A level of less than 30 pg/mL (110 pmol/L) in the presence of oligomenorrhea or amenorrhea is indicative of gonadal failure. In men, serum testosterone (normal range, 300–1000 ng/dL; (10–35 nmol/L) is a sensitive index of gonadal function. (See Chapters 12 and 13.)

LH & FSH Levels

In the presence of gonadal insufficiency, high LH and FSH levels are a sign of primary gonadal failure; low or normal LH and FSH suggest hypothalamic-pituitary dysfunction (hypogonadotropic hypogonadism).

GnRH Test

LH and FSH secretory reserves may be assessed with the use of synthetic GnRH (gonadorelin). Administration of GnRH causes a prompt increase in plasma LH and a lesser and slower increase in FSH (for normal responses, see Table 5–9). However, in most patients the GnRH test provides no more useful information than is obtained by measurement of basal gonadotropin and gonadal steroid levels. Thus, this test is uncommonly performed.

Table 5–10. Normal responses of TSH and prolactin to TRH (500 μg).[1]

	TSH (μU/mL)	(mU/L)
Maximum Δ TSH		
Women and men aged < 40	≥ 6	≥ 6
Men aged 40–79	≥ 2	≥ 2
Time of maximum Δ TSH (min)	≤ 45	
	Prolactin (ng/mL)	(pmol/L)
Basal, men and women	< 15	< 681
Maximum Δ prolactin		
Men aged 20–39	25–49	681–1818
Men aged 40–59	19–50	454–2272
Men aged 60–79	5–90	227–4090
Women aged 20–39	30–120	1383–5454
Women aged 40–59	20–120	909–5454
Women aged 60–79	10–100	454–4545

[1]Reproduced, with permission, from Snyder PJ et al: Diagnostic value of thyrotropin-releasing hormone in pituitary and hypothalamic diseases: Assessment of thyrotropin and prolactin secretion in 100 patients. Ann Intern Med 1974;61:751.

PROBLEMS IN EVALUATION OF THE HYPOTHALAMIC-PITUITARY AXIS

This section briefly outlines some of the disorders and conditions that may cause confusion and lead to misinterpretation of pituitary function tests. The effects of drugs are described in the next section.

Obesity

GH dynamics are impaired in many severely obese patients; all provocative stimuli, including insulin-induced hypoglycemia, arginine, levodopa, and glucagon plus propranolol, often fail to provoke GH secretion. The GH response to GHRH is also impaired in obesity and improves with weight loss.

Diabetes Mellitus

Although glucose normally suppresses GH secretion, most type I diabetic individuals have normal or elevated GH levels that often do not rise further in response to hypoglycemia or arginine. Levodopa will increase GH in some diabetic patients, and even a dopamine infusion (which produces no GH change in nondiabetic subjects, since it does not cross the blood-brain barrier) will stimulate GH in diabetic patients. Despite the increased GH secretion in patients with inadequately controlled diabetes, the GH response to GHRH in insulin-dependent diabetic patients is similar to that of nondiabetic subjects. IGF-I levels are low in insulin-deficient diabetes despite the elevated GH levels.

Uremia

Basal levels of GH, PRL, LH, FSH, TSH, and free cortisol tend to be elevated, for the most part owing to prolongation of their plasma half-life. GH may paradoxically increase following glucose administration and is often hyperresponsive to a hypoglycemic stimulus. Although the administration of TRH (protirelin) has no effect on GH secretion in healthy subjects, the drug may increase GH in patients with chronic renal failure. The response of PRL to TRH is blunted and prolonged. Gonadotropin response to synthetic GnRH usually remains intact. Dexamethasone suppression of cortisol may be impaired.

Starvation & Anorexia Nervosa

GH secretion increases with fasting and malnutrition, and such conditions may cause a paradoxical increase in GH following glucose administration. Severe starvation, such as occurs in patients with anorexia nervosa, may result in low levels of gonadal steroids. LH and FSH responses to GnRH may be intact despite a state of functional hypogonadotropic hypogonadism. Cortisol levels may be increased and fail to suppress adequately with dexamethasone. PRL and TSH dynamics are usually normal despite a marked decrease in circulating total thyroid hormones (see Chapter 7).

Depression

Depression may alter the ability of dexamethasone to suppress plasma cortisol and may elevate cortisol secretion; the response to insulin-induced hypoglycemia usually remains intact. In addition, late-evening salivary cortisol levels usually remain normal and are not elevated as seen in patients with Cushing's syndrome. The ACTH response to CRH is blunted in endogenous depression. Some depressed patients also have abnormal GH dynamics: TRH may increase GH, and hypoglycemia or levodopa may fail to increase GH. These patients may also show blunted TSH responses to TRH.

EFFECTS OF PHARMACOLOGIC AGENTS ON HYPOTHALAMIC-PITUITARY FUNCTION

Glucocorticoid excess impairs the GH response to hypoglycemia, the TSH response to TRH, and the LH response to GnRH. Estrogens tend to augment GH dynamics as well as the PRL and TSH response to TRH. Estrogens increase plasma cortisol secondary to a rise in corticosteroid-binding globulin and may result in inadequate suppression with dexamethasone.

Phenytoin enhances the metabolism of dexamethasone, making studies with this agent difficult to interpret. Phenothiazines may blunt the GH response to hypoglycemia and levodopa and frequently cause hyperprolactinemia. The many other pharmacologic agents that increase PRL secretion are listed in Table 5–8.

Narcotics, including heroin, morphine, and methadone, may all raise PRL levels and suppress GH and cortisol response to hypoglycemia.

In chronic alcoholics, alcohol excess or withdrawal may increase cortisol levels and cause inadequate dexamethasone suppression and an impaired cortisol increase after hypoglycemia.

ENDOCRINE TESTS OF HYPOTHALAMIC-PITUITARY FUNCTION

Methods for performing endocrine tests and their normal responses are summarized in Table 5–11. The indications for and the clinical utility of these procedures are described in the preceding section and will be mentioned again in the section on pituitary and hypothalamic disorders.

Table 5–11. Endocrine tests of hypothalamic-pituitary function.

	Method	Sample Collection	Possible Side Effects; Contraindications	Interpretation
Rapid ACTH stimulation test (cosyntropin test)	Administer synthetic ACTH$_{1-24}$ (cosyntropin), 250 μg intravenously or intramuscularly. The test may be performed at any time of the day or night and does not require fasting. The low-dose test is performed in the same manner except that 1 μg of synthetic ACTH$_{1-24}$ is administered.	Obtain samples for plasma cortisol at 0 and 30 minutes or at 0 and 60 minutes	Rare allergic reactions have been reported.	A normal response is a peak plasma cortisol level > 18–20 μg/dL (496–552 mmol/L)
Insulin hypoglycemia test	Give nothing by mouth after midnight. Start an intravenous infusion with normal saline solution. Regular insulin is given intravenously in a dose sufficient to cause adequate hypoglycemia (blood glucose < 40 mg/dL). The dose is 0.1–0.15 unit/kg (healthy subjects); 0.2–0.3 unit/kg (obese subjects or those with Cushing's syndrome or acromegaly); 0.05 unit/kg (patients with suspected hypopituitarism).	Collect blood for glucose determinations every 15 minutes during the study. Samples of GH and cortisol are obtained at 0, 30, 45, 60, 75, and 90 minutes.	A physician must be in attendance. Symptomatic hypoglycemia (diaphoresis, headache, tachycardia, weakness) is necessary for adequate stimulation and occurs 20–35 minutes after insulin is administered in most patients. If severe central nervous system signs or symptoms occur, intravenous glucose (25–50 mL of 50% glucose) should be given immediately; otherwise, the test can be terminated with a meal or with oral glucose. This test is contraindicated in the elderly or in patients with cardiovascular or cerebrovascular disease and seizure disorders.	Symptomatic hypoglycemia and a fall in blood glucose to less than 40 mg/dL (2.2 mmol/L) will increase GH to a maximal level greater than 10 ng/mL (460 pmol/L); some investigators regard an increment of 6 ng/mL (280 pmol/L) as normal. Plasma cortisol should increase to a peak level of at least 18–20 μg/dL (496–552 mmol/L)
Metyrapone test	Metyrapone is given orally between 11 and 12 PM with a snack to minimize gastrointestinal discomfort. The dose is 30 mg/kg.	Blood for plasma 11-deoxycortisol and cortisol determinations is obtained at 8 AM the morning after metyrapone is given.	Gastrointestinal upset may occur. Adrenal insufficiency may occur. Metyrapone should not be used in sick patients or those in whom primary adrenal insufficiency is suspected.	Serum 11-deoxycortisol should increase to > 7 μg/dL (0.19 μmol/L). Cortisol should be < 10 μg/dL (0.28 μmol/L) in order to ensure adequate inhibition of 11β-hydroxylation.
GHRH-arginine infusion test	The patient should be fasting after midnight. Give GHRH, 1 μg/kg intravenously over 1 minute followed by arginine hydrochloride, 0.5 g/kg intravenously, up to a maximum of 30 g over 30 minutes.	Blood for plasma GH determinations is collected at 0, 30, 60, 90, and 120 minutes	Mild flushing, a metallic taste, or nausea and vomiting may occur. This test is contraindicated in patients with severe liver disease, renal disease, or acidosis.	The lower limit of normal for the peak GH response is 6 ng/mL (280 pmol/L) although most normals reach levels of > 10–15 ng/mL (460–700 pmol/L)

(continued)

Table 5–11. Endocrine tests of hypothalamic-pituitary function. (continued)

	Method	Sample Collection	Possible Side Effects; Contraindications	Interpretation
Glucose growth hormone suppression test	The patient should be fasting after midnight; give glucose, 75–100 g orally.	GH and glucose should be determined at 0, 30 and 60 minutes after glucose administration.	Patients may complain of nausea after the large glucose load.	GH levels are suppressed to less than 2 ng/mL (90 pmol/L) in healthy subjects. Failure of adequate suppression or a paradoxic rise may be seen in acromegaly, starvation, protein-calorie malnutrition, and anorexia nervosa.
TRH test	Fasting is not required, but since nausea may occur, it is preferred. Give protirelin, 500 µg intravenously over 15–30 seconds. The patient should be kept supine, since slight hypertension or hypotension may occur. Protirelin is supplied in vials of 500 µg, although 400 µg will evoke normal responses.	Blood for determination of plasma TSH and PRL is obtained at 0, 30, and 60 minutes. An abbreviated test utilizes samples taken at 0 and 30 minutes only.	No serious complications have been reported. Most patients complain of a sensation of urinary urgency and a metallic taste in the mouth; other symptoms include flushing, palpitations, and nausea. These symptoms occur within 1–2 minutes of the injection and last 5 minutes at most.	Normal TSH and PRL responses to TRH are outlined in Table 5–10.
GnRH test	The patient should be at rest but need not be fasting. Give GnRH (gonadorelin), 100 µg intravenously, over 15 seconds.	Blood samples for LH and FSH determinations are taken at 0, 30, and 60 minutes. Since the FSH response is somewhat delayed, a 90-minute specimen may be necessary.	Side effects are rare, and no contraindications have been reported.	This response is dependent on sex and the time of the menstrual cycle. Table 5–9 illustrates the mean maximal change in LH and FSH after GnRH administration. An increase of LH of 1.3–2.6 µg/L (12–23 IU/L) is considered to be normal; FSH usually responds more slowly and less markedly. FSH may not increase even in healthy subjects.
Clomiphene test	Clomiphene is administered orally. For women, give 100 mg daily for 5 days (being on day 5 of the cycle if the patient is menstruating); for men, give 100 mg daily for 7–10 days.	Blood for LH and FSH determinations is drawn before and after clomiphene is given.	This drug may, of course, stimulate ovulation, and women should be advised accordingly.	In women, LH and FSH levels peak on the fifth day to a level above the normal range. After the fifth day, LH and FSH levels decline. In men, LH should double after 1 week; FSH will also increase, but to a lesser extent.
CRH test	CRH (1 µg/kg) is given intravenously as a bolus injection.	Blood samples for ACTH and cortisol are taken at 0, 15, 30, and 60 minutes.	Flushing often occurs. Transient tachycardia and hypotension have also been reported.	The ACTH response is dependent on the assay utilized and occurs 15 minutes after CRH is administered. The peak cortisol response occurs at 30–60 minutes and is usually greater than 10 µg/dL (276 nmol/L).

NEURORADIOLOGIC EVALUATION

Symptoms of pituitary hormone excess or deficiency, headache, or visual disturbance lead the clinician to consider a hypothalamic-pituitary disorder. In this setting, accurate neuroradiologic assessment of the hypothalamus and pituitary is essential in confirming the existence and defining the extent of hypothalamic-pituitary lesions; however, the diagnosis of such lesions should be based on both endocrine and radiologic criteria. This is because variability of pituitary anatomy in the normal population may lead to false-positive interpretations. Furthermore, patients with pituitary microadenomas may have normal neuroradiologic studies. Imaging studies must be interpreted in light of the fact that 10–20% of the general population harbor nonfunctional and asymptomatic pituitary microadenomas.

Magnetic Resonance Imaging (MRI)

MRI is the current procedure of choice for imaging the hypothalamus and pituitary. It has superseded the use of CT since it allows better definition of normal structures and has better resolution in defining tumors. Arteriography is rarely utilized at present except in patients with intrasellar or parasellar aneurysms.

Imaging is performed in sagittal and coronal planes at 1.5–2 mm intervals. This allows clear definition of hypothalamic and pituitary anatomy and can accurately visualize lesions as small as 3–5 mm. The use of the heavy-metal contrast agent gadolinium allows even more precise differentiation of small pituitary adenomas from normal anterior pituitary tissue and other adjacent structures as shown in Figure 5–15.

A. Normal Anatomy

The normal anterior pituitary is 5–7 mm in height and approximately 10 mm in its lateral dimensions. The superior margin is flat or concave but may be upwardly convex with a height of 10–12 mm in healthy menstruating young women. The floor of the sella turcica is formed by the bony roof of the sphenoid sinus, and its lateral margins are formed by the dural membranes of the cavernous sinuses, which contain the carotid arteries and the third, fourth, and sixth cranial nerves. The posterior pituitary appears on MRI as a high-signal-intensity structure, the "posterior pituitary bright spot," which is absent in patients with diabetes insipidus. The pituitary stalk, which is normally in the midline, is 2–3 mm in diameter and 5–7 mm in length. The pituitary stalk joins the inferior hypothalamus below the third ventricle and posterior to the optic chiasm. All of these normal structures are readily visualized with MRI; the normal pituitary and the pituitary stalk show increased signal intensity with gadolinium.

B. Microadenomas

These lesions, which range from 2 mm to 10 mm in diameter, appear as low-signal-intensity lesions with MRI and do not usually enhance with gadolinium. Adenomas less than 5 mm in diameter may not be visualized and do not usually alter the normal pituitary contour. Lesions greater than 5 mm in diameter create a unilateral convex superior gland margin and usually cause deviation of the pituitary stalk toward the side opposite the adenoma.

MRI scans must be interpreted with caution, since minor abnormalities occur in 10% of patients who have had incidental high-resolution scans but no clinical pituitary disease. These abnormalities may of course represent the clinically insignificant pituitary abnormalities which occur in 10–20% of the general population, and they may also be due to small intrapituitary cysts, which usually occur in the pars intermedia. Artifacts within the sella turcica associated with the bones of the skull base may also result in misinterpretation of imaging studies. Finally, many patients with pituitary microadenomas have normal high-resolution MRI scans. Therefore, despite increased accuracy of neuroradiologic diagnosis, the presence or absence of a small pituitary tumor and the decision concerning its treatment must be based on the entire clinical picture.

C. Macroadenomas

Pituitary adenomas greater than 10 mm in diameter are readily visualized with MRI scans, and the scan will also define the adjacent structures and degree of extension of the lesion. Thus, larger tumors show compression of the normal pituitary and distortion of the pituitary stalk. Adenomas larger than 1.5 cm frequently have suprasellar extension, and MRI scans show compression and upward displacement of the optic chiasm. Less commonly, there is lateral extension and invasion of the cavernous sinus.

D. Other Uses

High-resolution MRI scanning is also a valuable tool in the diagnosis of empty sella syndrome, hypothalamic tumors, and other parasellar lesions.

■ PITUITARY & HYPOTHALAMIC DISORDERS

Hypothalamic-pituitary lesions present with a variety of manifestations, including pituitary hormone hypersecretion and hyposecretion, sellar enlargement, and visual loss. The approach to evaluation should be designed to ensure early diagnosis at a stage when the lesions are amenable to therapy.

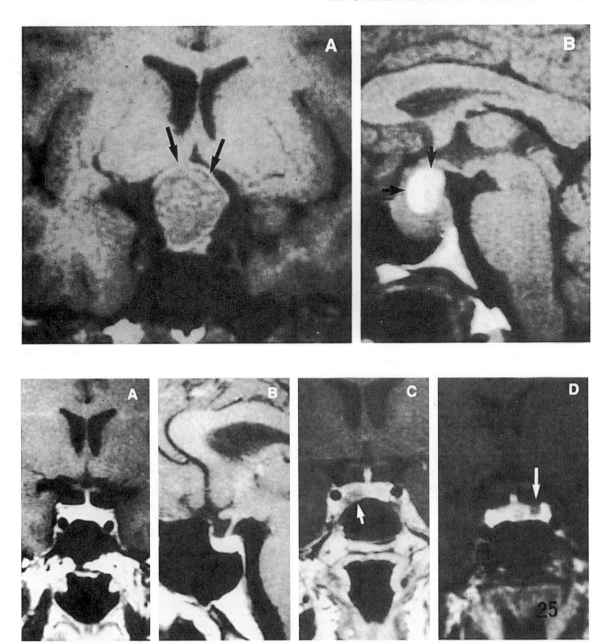

Figure 5–15. Upper Panel: A: The coronal magnetic resonance (MR) image shows a large nonfunctioning pituitary adenoma (arrows) with pronounced suprasellar extension and chiasmal compression. ***B:*** A sagittal MR image of another large pituitary adenoma shows spontaneous hemorrhage within the suprasellar portion of the adenoma (arrows). (Photographs courtesy of David Norman, MD.) (Reproduced, with permission, from West J Med 1995;162:342, 350.) ***Lower Panel:*** Gadolinium-enhanced magnetic resonance images are shown of the pituitary gland. ***A and B:*** Coronal and sagittal images show the normal, uniformly enhancing pituitary stalk and pituitary gland. ***C:*** A pituitary microadenoma appears as a low-intensity lesion in the inferior aspect of the right lobe of the gland (arrow). ***D:*** The pituitary microadenoma appears as a low-intensity lesion between the left lobe of the pituitary and the left cavernous sinus (arrow). (Photographs courtesy of David Norman, MD.)

Etiology & Early Manifestations

In adults, the commonest cause of hypothalamic-pituitary dysfunction is a pituitary adenoma, of which the great majority are hypersecreting. Thus, the earliest symptoms of such tumors are due to endocrinologic abnormalities—hypogonadism is the most frequent manifestation— and these precede sellar enlargement and local manifestations such as headache and visual loss, which are late manifestations seen only in patients with larger tumors or suprasellar extension.

In children, pituitary adenomas are uncommon; the most frequent structural lesions causing hypothalamic-pituitary dysfunction are craniopharyngiomas and other hypothalamic tumors. These also usually manifest as endocrine disturbances (low GH levels, delayed puberty, diabetes insipidus) prior to the development of headache, visual loss, or other central nervous system symptoms.

Common & Later Manifestations

A. PITUITARY HYPERSECRETION

PRL is the hormone most commonly secreted in excess amounts by pituitary adenomas, and it is usually elevated in patients with hypothalamic disorders and pituitary stalk compression as well. Thus, PRL measurement is essential in evaluating patients with suspected pituitary disorders and should be performed in patients presenting with galactorrhea, gonadal dysfunction, secondary gonadotropin deficiency, or enlargement of the sella turcica. Hypersecretion of GH or ACTH leads to the more characteristic syndromes of acromegaly and Cushing's disease (see below).

B. PITUITARY INSUFFICIENCY

Although panhypopituitarism is a classic manifestation of pituitary adenomas, it is present in less than 20% of patients in current large series because of earlier diagnosis of these lesions.

At present, the earliest clinical manifestation of a pituitary adenoma in adults is hypogonadism secondary to elevated levels of PRL, GH, or ACTH and cortisol. The hypogonadism in these patients is due to interference with the secretion of GnRH rather than to destruction of anterior pituitary tissue. Thus, patients with hypogonadism should first be screened with FSH and LH measurements to exclude primary gonadal failure (elevated FSH or LH) and those with hypogonadotropic hypogonadism should have serum PRL levels measured and be examined for clinical evidence of GH or ACTH and cortisol excess.

In children, short stature is the most frequent clinical presentation of hypothalamic-pituitary dysfunction;

in these patients, GH deficiency should be considered. (See Chapter 6.)

TSH or ACTH deficiency is relatively unusual in current series of patients and usually indicates panhypopituitarism. Thus, patients with secondary hypothyroidism or hypoadrenalism should undergo a complete assessment of pituitary function and neuroradiologic studies, since panhypopituitarism and large pituitary tumors are common in this setting. PRL measurement is again essential, since prolactinomas are the most frequent pituitary tumors in adults.

C. ENLARGED SELLA TURCICA

Patients may present with enlargement of the sella turcica, which may be noted on radiographs performed for head trauma or on sinus series. These patients usually have either a pituitary adenoma or empty sella syndrome. Other less common causes include craniopharyngioma, lymphocytic hypophysitis, and carotid artery aneurysm. Evaluation should include clinical assessment of pituitary dysfunction and measurements of PRL and thyroid and adrenal function. Pituitary function is usually normal in the empty sella syndrome; this diagnosis can be confirmed by MRI. Patients with clinical or laboratory evidence of pituitary dysfunction usually have a pituitary adenoma.

D. VISUAL FIELD DEFECTS

Patients presenting with bitemporal hemianopsia or unexplained visual field defects or visual loss should be considered to have a pituitary or hypothalamic disorder until proved otherwise. The initial steps in diagnosis should be neuro-ophthalmologic evaluation and neuroradiologic studies with MRI, which will reveal the tumor if one is present. These patients should also have PRL measurements and be assessed for anterior pituitary insufficiency, which is especially common with large pituitary adenomas.

In addition to causing visual field defects, large pituitary lesions may extend laterally into the cavernous sinus, compromising the function of the third, fourth, or sixth cranial nerve, leading to diplopia.

E. DIABETES INSIPIDUS

Diabetes insipidus is a common manifestation of hypothalamic lesions but is rare in primary pituitary lesions. Diagnostic evaluation is described later. In addition, all patients should undergo radiologic evaluation and assessment of anterior pituitary function.

EMPTY SELLA SYNDROME

Etiology & Incidence

The empty sella syndrome occurs when the subarachnoid space extends into the sella turcica, partially filling it with cerebrospinal fluid. This process causes remodeling and enlargement of the sella turcica and flattening of the pituitary gland.

Primary empty sella syndrome resulting from congenital incompetence of the diaphragma sellae (Figure 5–16) is common, with an incidence in autopsy series ranging from 5% to 23%. It is the most frequent cause of enlarged sella turcica. An empty sella is also commonly seen after pituitary surgery or radiation therapy and may also occur following postpartum pituitary infarction (Sheehan's syndrome). In addition, both PRL-secreting and GH-secreting pituitary adenomas may undergo subclinical hemorrhagic infarction and cause contraction of the overlying suprasellar cistern downward into the sella. Therefore, the presence of an empty sella does not exclude the possibility of a coexisting pituitary tumor.

Clinical Features

A. SYMPTOMS AND SIGNS

Most patients are middle-aged obese women. Many have systemic hypertension; benign intracranial hypertension may also occur. Although 48% of patients complain of headache, this feature may have only initiated the evaluation (ie, skull x-rays), and its relationship to the empty sella is probably coincidental. Serious clinical manifestations are uncommon. Spontaneous cerebrospinal fluid rhinorrhea and visual field impairment may occur rarely.

B. LABORATORY FINDINGS

Tests of anterior pituitary function are almost always normal, though some patients have hyperprolactinemia. Endocrine function studies should be performed to exclude pituitary hormone insufficiency or a hypersecretory pituitary microadenoma.

Diagnosis

The diagnosis of the empty sella syndrome can be readily confirmed by MRI, which demonstrates the herniation of the diaphragma sellae and the presence of cerebrospinal fluid in the sella turcica.

HYPOTHALAMIC DYSFUNCTION

Hypothalamic dysfunction is most often caused by tumors, of which craniopharyngioma is the most common in children, adolescents, and young adults. In older adults, primary central nervous system tumors and those arising from hypothalamic (epidermoid and dermoid tumors) and pineal structures (pinealomas) are more common. Other causes of hypothalamic-pituitary dysfunction are discussed below in the section on hypopituitarism.

Clinical Features

A. CRANIOPHARYNGIOMA

The initial symptoms of craniopharyngioma in children and adolescents are predominantly endocrinologic;

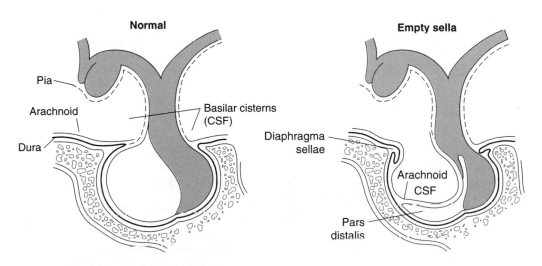

Figure 5–16. Representation of the normal relationship of the meninges to the pituitary gland *(left)* and the findings in the empty sella *(right)* as the arachnoid membrane herniates through the incompetent diaphragma sellae. (Reproduced, with permission, from Jordan RM, Kendall JW, Kerber CW: The primary empty sella syndrome: Analysis of the clinical characteristics, radiographic features, pituitary function, and cerebrospinal fluid adenohypophysial hormone concentrations. Am J Med 1977;62:569.)

however, these manifestations are frequently unrecognized, and at diagnosis over 80% of patients have hypothalamic-pituitary endocrine deficiencies. These endocrine abnormalities may precede presenting symptoms by months or years; GH deficiency is most common, with about 50% of patients having growth retardation and approximately 70% decreased GH responses to stimulation at diagnosis. Gonadotropin deficiency leading to absent or arrested puberty is usual in older children and adolescents; TSH and ACTH deficiencies are less common, and diabetes insipidus is present in about 15%.

Symptoms leading to the diagnosis are, unfortunately, frequently neurologic and due to the mass effect of the expanding tumor. Symptoms of increased intracranial pressure such as headache and vomiting are present in about 40%; decreased visual acuity or visual field defects are the presenting symptoms in another 35%. MRI confirms the tumor in virtually all patients; in 95%, the tumor is suprasellar.

In adults, craniopharyngiomas have similar presentations; ie, the diagnosis is usually reached as a result of investigation of complaints of headache or visual loss. However, endocrine manifestations—especially hypogonadism, diabetes insipidus, or other deficiencies of anterior pituitary hormones—usually precede these late manifestations. MRI readily demonstrates the tumors, which in adults are almost always both intrasellar and suprasellar.

B. OTHER TUMORS

Other hypothalamic or pineal tumors and primary central nervous system tumors involving the hypothalamus have variable presentations in both children and adults. Thus, presentation is with headache, visual loss, symptoms of increased intracranial pressure, growth failure, various degrees of hypopituitarism, or diabetes insipidus. Endocrine deficiencies usually precede neurologic manifestations. Hypothalamic tumors in childhood may present with precocious puberty.

C. OTHER MANIFESTATIONS OF HYPOTHALAMIC DYSFUNCTION

Lesions in the hypothalamus can cause many other abnormalities, including disorders of consciousness, behavior, thirst, appetite, and temperature regulation. These abnormalities are usually accompanied by hypopituitarism and diabetes insipidus.

Somnolence can occur with hypothalamic lesions, as can a variety of changes in emotional behavior. Decreased or absent thirst may occur and predispose these patients to dehydration. When diminished thirst accompanies diabetes insipidus, fluid balance is difficult to control. Hypothalamic dysfunction may also cause increased thirst, leading to polydipsia and polyuria that

may mimic diabetes insipidus. Obesity is common in patients with hypothalamic tumors because of hyperphagia, decreased satiety, and decreased activity. Anorexia and weight loss are unusual manifestations of these tumors.

Temperature regulation can also be disordered in these patients. Sustained or, less commonly, paroxysmal hyperthermia can occur following acute injury due to trauma, hemorrhage, or craniotomy. This problem usually lasts less than 2 weeks. Poikilothermia, the inability to adjust to changes in ambient temperature, can occur in patients with bilateral hypothalamic lesions. These patients most frequently exhibit hypothermia but can also develop hyperthermia during hot weather. A few patients manifest sustained hypothermia due to anterior hypothalamic lesions.

Diagnosis

Patients with suspected hypothalamic tumors should undergo MRI to determine the extent and nature of the tumor. Complete assessment of anterior pituitary function is necessary in these patients, since deficiencies are present in the great majority (see section on hypopituitarism below) and the evaluation will establish the requirements for replacement therapy. PRL levels should also be determined, since most hypothalamic lesions cause hyperprolactinemia either by hypothalamic injury or by damage to the pituitary stalk.

Treatment

Treatment depends upon the type of tumor. Since complete resection of craniopharyngioma is usually not feasible, this tumor is best managed by limited neurosurgical removal of accessible tumor and decompression of cysts, followed by conventional radiotherapy. Patients treated by this method have a recurrence rate of approximately 20%; with surgery alone, the recurrence rate approximates 80%.

Other hypothalamic tumors are usually not completely resectable; however, biopsy is indicated to arrive at a histologic diagnosis.

HYPOPITUITARISM

Hypopituitarism is manifested by diminished or absent secretion of one or more pituitary hormones. The development of signs and symptoms is often slow and insidious, depending on the rate of onset and the magnitude of hypothalamic-pituitary damage—factors that are influenced by the underlying pathogenesis. Hypopituitarism is either a primary event caused by destruction of the anterior pituitary gland or a secondary phenomenon resulting from deficiency of hypothalamic stimulatory factors normally acting on the pituitary.

Treatment and prognosis depend on the extent of hypofunction, the underlying cause, and the location of the lesion in the hypothalamic-pituitary axis.

Etiology

The etiologic considerations in hypopituitarism are diverse. As shown below, a helpful mnemonic device is the phrase "nine I's": Invasive, Infarction, Infiltrative, Injury, Immunologic, Iatrogenic, Infectious, Idiopathic, and Isolated. Most of these lesions may cause pituitary or hypothalamic failure (or both). Establishing the precise cause of hypopituitarism is helpful in determining treatment and prognosis.

A. INVASIVE

Space-occupying lesions cause hypopituitarism by destroying the pituitary gland or hypothalamic nuclei or by disrupting the hypothalamic-hypophysial portal venous system. Large pituitary adenomas cause hypopituitarism by these mechanisms, and pituitary function may improve after their removal. Small pituitary tumors—microadenomas (< 10 mm in diameter)—characteristically seen in the hypersecretory states (excess PRL, GH, ACTH) do not directly cause pituitary insufficiency. Craniopharyngioma, the most common tumor of the hypothalamic-pituitary region in children, frequently impairs pituitary function by its compressive effects. Primary central nervous system tumors, including meningioma, chordoma, optic glioma, epidermoid tumors, and dermoid tumors, may decrease hypothalamic-pituitary secretion by their mass effects. Metastatic lesions to this area are common (especially breast carcinoma) but rarely result in clinically obvious hypopituitarism. Anatomic malformations such as basal encephalocele and parasellar aneurysms cause hypothalamic-pituitary dysfunction and may enlarge the sella turcica and mimic pituitary tumors.

B. INFARCTION

Ischemic damage to the pituitary has long been recognized as a cause of hypopituitarism. In 1914, Simmonds reported pituitary necrosis in a woman with severe puerperal sepsis, and in 1937 Sheehan published his classic description of its occurrence following postpartum hemorrhage and vascular collapse. The mechanism for the ischemia in such cases is not certain. Hypotension along with vasospasm of the hypophysial arteries is currently believed to compromise arterial perfusion of the anterior pituitary. During pregnancy, the pituitary gland may be more sensitive to hypoxemia because of its increased metabolic needs or more susceptible to vasoconstrictive influences because of the hyperestrogenic state. Some degree of hypopituitarism has been reported in 32% of women with severe postpartum hemorrhage. Other investigators have noted that the hypopituitarism does not always correlate with the degree of hemorrhage but that there is good correlation between the pituitary lesion and severe disturbances of the clotting mechanism (as in patients with placenta previa). Ischemic pituitary necrosis has also been reported to occur with greater frequency in patients with diabetes mellitus.

The extent of pituitary damage determines the rapidity of onset as well as the magnitude of pituitary hypofunction. The gland has a great secretory reserve, and more than 75% must be destroyed before clinical manifestations are evident. The initial clinical feature in postpartum necrosis may be failure to lactate after parturition; failure to resume normal menstrual periods is another clue to the diagnosis. However, the clinical features of hypopituitarism are often subtle, and years may pass before pituitary insufficiency is recognized following an ischemic insult.

Spontaneous hemorrhagic infarction of a pituitary tumor (pituitary apoplexy) frequently results in partial or total pituitary insufficiency. Pituitary apoplexy is often a fulminant clinical syndrome manifested by severe headache, visual impairment, ophthalmoplegias, meningismus, and an altered level of consciousness. Pituitary apoplexy is usually associated with a pituitary tumor; it may also be related to diabetes mellitus, radiotherapy, or open heart surgery. Acute pituitary failure with hypotension may result, and rapid mental deterioration, coma, and death may ensue. Emergency treatment with corticosteroids (see Chapter 24) and transsphenoidal decompression of the intrasellar contents may be lifesaving and may prevent permanent visual loss. Most patients who have survived pituitary apoplexy have developed multiple adenohypophysial deficits, but infarction of the tumor in some patients may cure the hypersecretory pituitary adenoma and its accompanying endocrinopathy. Pituitary infarction may also be a subclinical event (silent pituitary apoplexy), resulting in improvement of pituitary hormone hypersecretion without impairing the secretion of other anterior pituitary hormones.

C. INFILTRATIVE

Hypopituitarism may be the initial clinical manifestation of infiltrative disease processes such as sarcoidosis, hemochromatosis, and histiocytosis X.

1. Sarcoidosis—The most common intracranial sites of involvement of sarcoidosis are the hypothalamus and pituitary gland. At one time, the most common endocrine abnormality in patients with sarcoidosis was thought to be diabetes insipidus; however, many of these patients actually have centrally mediated disordered control of thirst that results in polydipsia and polyuria, which in some cases explains the abnormal water metabolism. Deficiencies of multiple anterior pituitary hormones have been well documented in sarcoidosis and are usually secondary to hypothalamic insufficiency. Granulomatous involvement of the hypothalamic-pituitary unit is occasionally extensive, resulting in visual impairment, and therefore may simulate the clinical presentation of a pituitary or hypothalamic tumor.

2. Hemochromatosis—Hypopituitarism, particularly hypogonadotropic hypogonadism, is a prominent manifestation of iron storage disease—either idiopathic hemochromatosis or transfusional iron overload. Hypogonadism occurs in most such cases and is often the initial clinical feature of iron excess; complete iron studies should be obtained in any male patient presenting with unexplained hypogonadotropic hypogonadism. If the diagnosis is established early, hypogonadism in hemochromatosis may be reversible with iron depletion. Pituitary deficiencies of TSH, GH, and ACTH may occur later in the course of the disease and are not reversible by iron chelation therapy.

3. Histiocytosis X—Histiocytosis X, the infiltration of multiple organs by well-differentiated histiocytes, is often heralded by the onset of diabetes insipidus and anterior pituitary hormone deficiencies. Most histologic and biochemical studies have indicated that this infiltrative process involves chiefly the hypothalamus, and hypopituitarism occurs only as a result of hypothalamic damage.

D. Injury

Severe head trauma may cause anterior pituitary insufficiency and diabetes insipidus. Posttraumatic anterior hypopituitarism may be due to injury to the anterior pituitary, the pituitary stalk, or the hypothalamus. Pituitary insufficiency with growth retardation has been described in battered children who suffer closed head trauma with subdural hematoma.

E. Immunologic

Lymphocytic hypophysitis resulting in anterior hypopituitarism is a distinct entity, occurring most often in women during pregnancy or in the postpartum period. It may present as a mass lesion of the sella turcica with visual field disturbances simulating pituitary adenoma. An autoimmune process with extensive infiltration of the gland by lymphocytes and plasma cells destroys the anterior pituitary cells. These morphologic features are similar to those of other autoimmune endocrinopathies, eg, thyroiditis, adrenalitis, and oophoritis. About 50% of patients with lymphocytic hypophysitis have other endocrine autoimmune disease, and circulating pituitary autoantibodies have been found in several cases. It is presently uncertain how this disorder should be diagnosed and treated. It must be considered in the differential diagnosis of women with pituitary gland enlargement and hypopituitarism during pregnancy or the postpartum period.

Lymphocytic hypophysitis may result in isolated hormone deficiencies (especially ACTH or prolactin). Consequently, women with this type of hypopituitarism may continue to menstruate while suffering from secondary hypothyroidism or hypoadrenalism.

F. Iatrogenic

Both surgical and radiation therapy to the pituitary gland may compromise its function. The anterior pituitary is quite resilient during transsphenoidal microsurgery, and despite extensive manipulation during the search for microadenomas, anterior pituitary function is usually preserved. The dose of conventional radiation therapy presently employed to treat pituitary tumors is 4500–5000 cGy and results in a 50–60% incidence of hypothalamic and pituitary insufficiency. Such patients most frequently have modest hyperprolactinemia (PRL 30–100 ng/mL [1.3–4.5 nmol/L]) with GH and gonadotropin failure; TSH and ACTH deficiencies are less common. Heavy particle (proton beam) irradiation for pituitary tumors results in a 20–50% incidence of hypopituitarism. Irradiation of tumors of the head and neck (nasopharyngeal cancer, brain tumors) and prophylactic cranial irradiation in leukemia may also cause hypopituitarism. The clinical onset of pituitary failure in such patients is usually insidious and results from both pituitary and hypothalamic injury.

G. Infectious

Although many infectious diseases, including tuberculosis, syphilis, and mycotic infections, have been implicated as causative agents in pituitary hypofunction, anti-infective drugs have now made them rare causes of hypopituitarism.

H. Idiopathic

In some patients with hypopituitarism, no underlying cause is found. These may be isolated (see below) or multiple deficiencies. Familial forms of hypopituitarism characterized by a small, normal, or enlarged sella turcica have been described. Both autosomal recessive and X-linked recessive inheritance patterns have been reported. A variety of complex congenital disorders may include deficiency of one or more pituitary hormones, eg, Prader-Willi syndrome and septo-optic dysplasia. The pathogenesis of these familial disorders is uncertain.

I. Isolated

Isolated (monotropic) deficiencies of the anterior pituitary hormones have been described. Some of these have been associated with mutations in the genes coding for the specific hormones. Others, particularly GH deficiency, have been associated with mutations in genes necessary for normal pituitary development as noted.

1. GH deficiency—In children, congenital monotropic GH deficiency may be sporadic or familial. These children, who may experience fasting hypoglycemia, have a gradual deceleration in growth velocity after 6–12 months of age. Diagnosis must be based on failure of GH responsiveness to provocative stimuli and the demonstration of normal responsiveness of other anterior pituitary hormones. Monotropic GH deficiency and growth retardation have also been observed in children suffering severe emotional deprivation. This disorder is reversed by placing the child in a supportive psychosocial milieu. A more detailed description of GH deficiency and growth failure is provided in Chapter 6.

2. ACTH deficiency—Monotropic ACTH deficiency is rare and is manifested by the signs and symptoms of adrenocortical insufficiency. Lipotropin (LPH) deficiency has also been noted in such patients. The defect in these patients may be due to primary failure of the corticotrophs to release ACTH and its related peptide hormones or may be secondary to impaired secretion of CRH by the hypothalamus. Most acquired cases of monotropic ACTH deficiency are due to lymphocytic hypophysitis.

3. Gonadotropin deficiency—Isolated deficiency of gonadotropins is not uncommon. Kallman's syndrome, an X-linked dominant disorder with incomplete penetrance, is characterized by an isolated defect in GnRH secretion associated with maldevelopment of the olfactory center with hyposmia or anosmia; a deletion in a gene on the short arm of the X chromosome (Xp22.3) results in decreased expression of the cell adhesion molecule KALIG-1. This in turn interferes with the normal embryonic development and migration of GnRH-secreting neurons. Sporadic cases occur, and other neurologic defects such as color blindness and nerve deafness have been seen. Since anterior pituitary function is otherwise intact, young men with isolated hypogonadotropic hypogonadism develop a eunuchoid appearance, since testosterone deficiency results in failure of epiphysial closure (see Chapter 12). In women, a state of hypogonadotropic hypogonadism manifested by oligomenorrhea or amenorrhea often accompanies weight loss, emotional or physical stress, and athletic training. Anorexia nervosa and marked obesity both result in hypothalamic dysfunction and impaired gonadotropin secretion. Hypothalamic hypogonadism has also been observed in overtrained male athletes. Sickle cell anemia also causes hypogonadotropic hypogonadism due to hypothalamic dysfunction and results in delayed puberty. Clomiphene treatment has been effective in some cases. Isolated gonadotropin deficiency

may also be seen in the polyglandular autoimmune syndrome; this deficiency is related to selective pituitary gonadotrope failure from autoimmune hypophysitis. Other chronic illnesses, eg, poorly controlled diabetes and malnutrition, may result in gonadotropin deficiency. Isolated deficiencies of both LH and FSH without an obvious cause such as those described have been reported but are rare.

4. TSH deficiency—Monotropic TSH deficiency is rare and is caused by a reduction in hypothalamic TRH secretion (tertiary hypothyroidism). Some patients with chronic renal failure appear to have impaired TSH secretion.

5. Prolactin deficiency—PRL deficiency almost always indicates severe intrinsic pituitary damage, and panhypopituitarism is usually present. However, isolated PRL deficiency has been reported after lymphocytic hypophysitis. Deficiencies of TSH and PRL have been noted in patients with pseudohypoparathyroidism.

6. Multiple hormone deficiencies isolated from other pituitary damage—Multiple hormone deficiencies result from abnormal pituitary development related to abnormalities of the genes encoding the transcription factors, PIT-1 and PROP-1.

Clinical Features

The onset of pituitary insufficiency is usually gradual, and the classic course of progressive hypopituitarism is an initial loss of GH and gonadotropin secretion followed by deficiencies of TSH, then ACTH, and finally PRL.

A. SYMPTOMS

Impairment of GH secretion causes decreased growth in children but may be clinically occult in adult patients. GH deficiency is associated with a decreased sense of well-being and a lower health-related quality of life. Hypogonadism, manifested by amenorrhea in women and decreased libido or erectile dysfunction in men, may antedate the clinical appearance of a hypothalamic-pituitary lesion.

Hypothyroidism caused by TSH deficiency generally simulates the clinical changes observed in primary thyroid failure; however, it is usually less severe, and goiter is absent. Cold intolerance, dry skin, mental dullness, bradycardia, constipation, hoarseness, and anemia have all been observed; gross myxedematous changes are uncommon.

ACTH deficiency causes adrenocortical insufficiency, and its clinical features resemble those of primary adrenal failure. Weakness, nausea, vomiting, anorexia, weight loss, fever, and hypotension may occur. Since the zona glomerulosa and the renin-angiotensin system are usually intact, the dehydration and sodium depletion seen in Addison's disease are uncommon. However, these patients are susceptible to hypotension, shock, and cardiovascular collapse since glucocorticoids are necessary to maintain vascular reactivity, especially during stress. Because of their gradual onset, the symptoms of secondary adrenal insufficiency may go undetected for prolonged periods, becoming manifest only during periods of stress. Hypoglycemia aggravated by GH deficiency may occur with fasting and has been the initial presenting feature of some patients with isolated ACTH deficiency. In contrast to the hyperpigmentation that occurs during states of ACTH excess (Addison's disease, Nelson's syndrome), depigmentation and diminished tanning have been described as a result of ACTH insufficiency. In addition, lack of ACTH-stimulated adrenal androgen secretion will cause a decrease in body hair if gonadotropin deficiency is also present.

GH deficiency is associated with decreased muscle mass and increased fat mass, though this may be difficult to discern in any given individual. The only symptom of PRL deficiency is failure of postpartum lactation.

B. SIGNS

Abnormal findings on physical examination may be subtle and require careful observation. Patients with hypopituitarism are not cachectic. A photograph of a cachectic patient with "Simmonds' syndrome" that appeared in some older textbooks of endocrinology caused confusion. That particular patient probably suffered from anorexia nervosa and was found to have a normal pituitary gland at postmortem examination.

Patients with pituitary failure are usually slightly overweight. The skin is fine, pale, and smooth, with fine wrinkling of the face. Body and pubic hair may be deficient or absent, and atrophy of the genitalia may occur. Postural hypotension, bradycardia, decreased muscle strength, and delayed deep tendon reflexes occur in more severe cases. Neuro-ophthalmologic abnormalities depend on the presence of a large intrasellar or parasellar lesion.

C. LABORATORY AND OTHER FINDINGS

These may include anemia (related to thyroid and androgen deficiency and chronic disease), hypoglycemia, hyponatremia (related to hypothyroidism and hypoadrenalism, which cause inappropriate water retention, not sodium loss), and low-voltage bradycardia on electrocardiographic testing. Hyperkalemia, which is common in primary adrenal failure, is not present. Adult

GH deficiency is associated with decreased red blood cell mass, increased LDL cholesterol, and decreased bone mass.

Diagnosis

A. ASSESSMENT OF TARGET GLAND FUNCTION

(Figure 5–17.) If endocrine hypofunction is suspected, pituitary hormone deficiencies must be distinguished from primary failure of the thyroid, adrenals, or gonads. Basal determinations of each anterior pituitary hormone are useful only if compared to target gland secretion. Baseline laboratory studies should include thyroid function tests (free T_4) and determination of serum testosterone levels. Testosterone is a sensitive indicator of hypopituitarism in women as well as in men. In women, a substantial decrease in testosterone is commonly observed in pituitary failure related to hypofunction of the two endocrine glands responsible for its production—the ovary and the adrenal. Adrenocortical reserve should initially be evaluated by a rapid ACTH stimulation test.

B. EVALUATION OF PROLACTIN

Since hyperprolactinemia (discussed later), regardless of its cause, leads to gonadal dysfunction, serum PRL should be measured early in the evaluation of hypogonadism.

C. DIFFERENTIATION OF PRIMARY AND SECONDARY HYPOFUNCTION

Subnormal thyroid function as shown by appropriate tests, a low serum testosterone level, or an impaired cortisol response to the rapid ACTH stimulation test requires measurement of basal levels of specific pituitary hormones. In primary target gland hypofunction (such as polyglandular failure syndrome), TSH, LH, FSH, or ACTH will be elevated. Low or normal values for these pituitary hormones suggest hypothalamic-pituitary dysfunction.

D. STIMULATION TESTS

Provocative endocrine testing may then be employed to confirm the diagnosis and to assess the extent of hypofunction. At present, these tests are not required in most patients.

Treatment

A. ACTH

Treatment of secondary adrenal insufficiency, like that of primary adrenal failure, must include glucocorticoid support (see Chapter 9). Hydrocortisone (20–30 mg/d

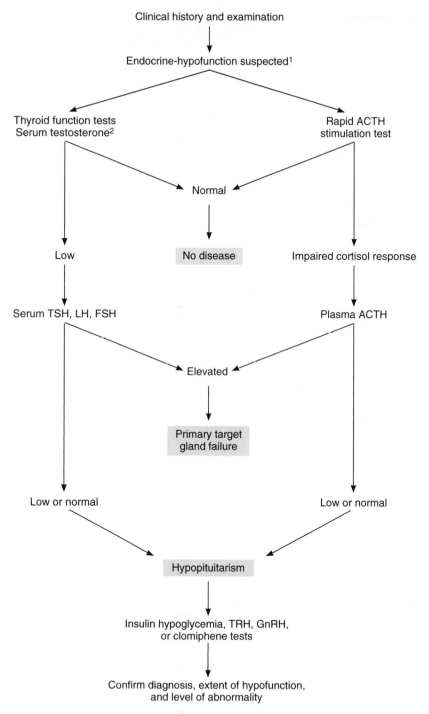

Figure 5–17. Diagnostic evaluation of hypothalamic-pituitary-target gland hypofunction.

orally) or prednisone (5–7.5 mg/d orally) in two or three divided doses provides adequate glucocorticoid replacement for most patients. The minimum effective dosage should be given in order to avoid iatrogenic hypercortisolism. Increased dosage is required during periods of stress such as illness, surgery, or trauma. Patients with only partial ACTH deficiency may need steroid treatment only during stress. A two- to threefold increase in steroid dosage during the stressful situation should be recommended, followed by gradual tapering as the stress resolves. Unlike primary adrenal insufficiency, ACTH deficiency does not usually require mineralocorticoid therapy. Patients with adrenal insufficiency should wear medical alert bracelets so they may receive prompt treatment in case of emergency.

B. TSH

The management of patients with secondary hypothyroidism must be based on clinical grounds and the circulating concentration of serum thyroxine (see Chapter 7). The treatment of secondary and tertiary hypothyroidism is identical to that for primary thyroid failure. Levothyroxine sodium, 0.1–0.15 mg/d orally, is usually adequate. Response to therapy is monitored clinically and with measurement of serum free thyroxine levels, which should be maintained in the mid to upper range of normal. Measurement of TSH levels is obviously of no value in the management of these patients.

Caution: Since thyroid hormone replacement in patients with hypopituitarism may aggravate even partial adrenal insufficiency, the adrenal disorder should be treated first.

C. GONADOTROPINS

The object of treatment of secondary hypogonadism is to replace sex steroids and restore fertility (see Chapters 12 and 13).

1. Estrogens and progesterone—In women, estrogen replacement is essential. Adequate estrogen treatment will maintain secondary sex characteristics (eg, vulvar and vaginal lubrication), prevent osteoporosis, and abolish vasomotor symptoms, with an improvement in sense of well-being. Many estrogen preparations are available, eg, oral estradiol, 1–2 mg daily; conjugated estrogens, 0.3–1.25 mg orally daily; or transdermal estradiol, 0.05–0.1 mg daily. Estrogens should be cycled with a progestin compound (eg, medroxyprogesterone, 5–10 mg orally daily during the last 10 days of estrogen therapy each month) to induce withdrawal bleeding and prevent endometrial hyperplasia.

2. Ovulation induction—Ovulation can often be restored in women with hypothalamic-pituitary dysfunction (see Chapter 13). In patients with gonadal failure of hypothalamic origin, clomiphene citrate may cause a surge of gonadotropin secretion resulting in ovulation. Pulsatile subcutaneous injections of GnRH with an infusion pump can also be used to induce ovulation and fertility in women with hypothalamic dysfunction. Combined treatment with FSH (human menopausal gonadotropins; menotropins) and LH (chorionic gonadotropin) can be utilized to provoke ovulation in women with intrinsic pituitary failure. This form of therapy is expensive, and multiple births are a risk. (See Chapter 13.)

3. Androgens in women—Because of a deficiency of both ovarian and adrenal androgens, some women with hypopituitarism have diminished libido despite adequate estrogen therapy. Although experience is limited, small doses of long-acting androgens (testosterone enanthate, 25–50 mg intramuscularly every 4–8 weeks) may be helpful in restoring sexual activity without causing hirsutism. In addition, some reports have suggested that oral DHEA in doses of 25–50 mg/d may restore plasma testosterone levels to normal. A transdermal delivery system is being evaluated for use in women but is not currently available for routine use.

4. Androgens in men—The treatment of male hypogonadism is discussed in Chapter 12.

Available therapeutic preparations include intramuscular testosterone enanthate or cypionate in doses of 100 mg every week or 200 mg every 2 weeks. Transdermal testosterone patches in doses of 2.5 or 5 mg are also available but require daily application. The most recent product is a testosterone gel in doses of 2.5 or 5 mg which is also applied daily. (See Chapter 12).

5. Spermatogenesis—Spermatogenesis can be achieved in many patients with the combined use of chorionic gonadotropin and menotropins. If pituitary insufficiency is of recent onset, therapy with chorionic gonadotropin alone may restore both fertility and adequate gonadal steroid production. Pulsatile GnRH infusion pumps have also been used to restore fertility in male patients with secondary hypogonadism.

D. GROWTH HORMONE

(See Chapter 6.) Human growth hormone (hGH) produced by recombinant DNA technology is available for use in children with hypopituitarism and for adults with GH deficiency and known pituitary disease. Therapeutic use of human growth hormone in adults with GH deficiency due to other causes, eg, reduced secretion associated with aging, is under investigation. Some studies indicate improvement in body composition, bone density, psychologic well-being, and functional status with GH therapy. However, the long-term benefits and risks remain to be established. In adults, GH is usually administered subcutaneously, once per day in a dosage of 2–5 µg/kg. Monitoring of effectiveness is accomplished by measurement of IGF-I, and the dosage of GH is adjusted accordingly (up to about 10 µg/kg/d). Side effects should be assessed, eg, edema, paresthesias, arrhythmias, and glucose intolerance.

PITUITARY ADENOMAS

Advances in endocrinologic and neuroradiologic research in recent years have allowed earlier recognition and more successful therapy of pituitary adenomas. Prolactinomas are the most common type, accounting for about 60% of primary pituitary tumors; GH hypersecretion occurs in approximately 20% and ACTH excess in 10%. Hypersecretion of TSH, the gonadotropins, or alpha subunits is unusual. Nonfunctional tumors currently represent only 10% of all pituitary adenomas, and some of these may in fact be gonadotropin-secreting or alpha subunit-secreting adenomas.

Early clinical recognition of the endocrine effects of excessive pituitary secretion, especially the observation that PRL excess causes secondary hypogonadism, has led to early diagnosis of pituitary tumors before the appearance of late manifestations such as sellar enlargement, panhypopituitarism, and suprasellar extension with visual impairment.

Pituitary **microadenomas** are defined as intrasellar adenomas less than 1 cm in diameter that present with manifestations of hormonal excess without sellar enlargement or extrasellar extension. Panhypopituitarism does not occur, and such tumors can usually be treated successfully.

Pituitary **macroadenomas** are those larger than 1 cm in diameter and cause generalized sellar enlargement. Tumors 1–2 cm in diameter confined to the sella turcica can usually be successfully treated; however, larger tumors—and especially those with suprasellar, sphenoid sinus, or lateral extensions—are much more difficult to manage. Panhypopituitarism and visual loss increase in frequency with tumor size and suprasellar extension.

Insights into the pathogenesis and biologic behavior of pituitary tumors have been gained from studies of pituitary tumor clonality and somatic mutations. Analyses of allelic X inactivation of specific genes has shown that most pituitary adenomas are monoclonal, a finding most consistent with a somatic mutation model of tumorigenesis; polyclonality of tumors would be expected if tonic stimulation by hypothalamic releasing factors were the mechanism underlying neoplastic transformation. In fact, transgenic animals expressing GHRH have exhibited pituitary hyperplasia but not pituitary adenomas. Recently, an animal model system for ACTH-secreting pituitary tumors has been developed involving transgenic mice. One somatic mutation has been found in 30–40% of growth hormone-secreting tumors (but not in leukocytes from the same patients). Point mutations in the alpha subunit of the GTP binding protein responsible for activation of adenylyl cyclase results in constitutive stimulation of pituitary cell growth and function. In studies of anterior pituitary cell ontogeny, PIT-1 has been identified as a transcription factor important in pituitary differentiation. The restriction of its expression to somatotrophs, lactotrophs, and thyrotrophs may account for the plurihormonal expression seen in some tumors. A pituitary tumor transforming gene *(PTTG)* has also been described.

Treatment

Pituitary adenomas are treated with surgery, irradiation, or drugs to suppress hypersecretion by the adenoma or its growth. The aims of therapy are to correct hypersecretion of anterior pituitary hormones, to preserve normal secretion of other anterior pituitary hormones, and to remove or suppress the adenoma itself. These objectives are currently achievable in most patients with pituitary microadenomas; however, in the case of larger tumors, multiple therapies are frequently required and may be less successful.

A. SURGICAL TREATMENT

The transsphenoidal microsurgical approach to the sella turcica is the procedure of choice; transfrontal craniotomy is required only in the rare patient with massive suprasellar extension of the adenoma. In the transsphenoidal procedure, the surgeon approaches the pituitary from the nasal cavity through the sphenoid sinus, removes the anterior-inferior sellar floor, and incises the dura. The adenoma is selectively removed; normal pituitary tissue is identified and preserved. Success rates approach 90% in patients with microadenomas. Major complications, including postoperative hemorrhage, cerebrospinal fluid leak, meningitis, and visual impairment, occur in less than 5% of patients and are most frequent in patients with large or massive tumors. Transient diabetes insipidus lasting a few days to 1–2 weeks occurs in approximately 15%; permanent diabetes insipidus is rare. A transient form of the syndrome of inappropriate secretion of antidiuretic hormone (SIADH) with symptomatic hyponatremia occurs in 10% of patients within 5–14 days of transsphenoidal pituitary microsurgery. Surgical hypopituitarism is rare in patients with microadenomas but approaches 5–10% in patients with larger tumors. The perioperative management of such patients should include glucocorticoid administration in stress doses (see Chapter 9) and postoperative assessment of daily weight, fluid balance, and electrolyte status. Mild diabetes insipidus is managed by giving fluids orally; in more severe cases—urine output greater than 5–6 L/24 h—ADH therapy in the form of desmopressin acetate should be administered (see section on diabetes insipidus). SIADH is managed by fluid restriction; however, in more severe cases, hypertonic saline may be required. (See section on SIADH.)

B. RADIOTHERAPY

Pituitary irradiation is usually reserved for patients with larger tumors who have had incomplete resection of large pituitary adenomas.

1. Conventional irradiation—Conventional irradiation using high energy sources, in total doses of 4000–5000 cGy given in daily doses of 180–200 cGy, is most commonly employed. The response to radiation therapy is slow, and 5–10 years may be required to achieve the full effect (see section on acromegaly). Treatment is ultimately successful in about 80% of acromegalics but only about 55–60% of patients with Cushing's disease. The response rate in prolactinomas is not precisely known, but tumor progression is prevented in most patients. Morbidity during radiotherapy is minimal, though some patients experience malaise and nausea, and serous otitis media may occur. Hypopituitarism is common, and the incidence increases with time following radiotherapy—about 50–60% at 5–10 years. Rare late complications include damage to the optic nerves and chiasm, seizures, and radionecrosis of brain tissue.

2. Gamma knife radiosurgery—This form of radiotherapy utilizes stereotactic CT-guided cobalt-60 gamma radiation to deliver high radiation doses to a narrowly focused area. Limited experience to date has been obtained in patients with acromegaly and Cushing's disease. (See sections following.)

C. MEDICAL TREATMENT

Medical management of pituitary adenomas became feasible with the availability of bromocriptine, a dopamine agonist that suppresses both prolactin and tumor growth in patients with prolactinomas. Somatostatin analogs are useful in the therapy of acromegaly and TSH-secreting adenomas. Specifics of the use of these and other medications are discussed below.

Posttreatment Follow-Up

Patients undergoing transsphenoidal microsurgery should be reevaluated 4–6 weeks postoperatively to document that complete removal of the adenoma and correction of endocrine hypersecretion have been achieved. Prolactinomas are assessed by basal PRL measurements, GH-secreting tumors by glucose suppression testing and IGF-I levels, and ACTH-secreting adenomas by measurement of urine free cortisol and the response to low-dose dexamethasone suppression (see below). Other anterior pituitary hormones—TSH, ACTH, and LH/FSH—should also be assessed as described above in the section on endocrine evaluation. In patients with successful responses, yearly evaluation should be done to watch for late recurrence; late hypopituitarism does not occur after microsurgery. MRI is not necessary in patients with normal postoperative pituitary function but should be utilized in patients with persistent or recurrent disease.

Follow-up of patients treated by pituitary irradiation is also essential, since the response to therapy may be delayed and the incidence of hypopituitarism increases with time. Yearly endocrinologic assessment of both the hypersecreted hormone and the other pituitary hormones is recommended.

1. Prolactinomas

PRL hypersecretion is the most common endocrine abnormality due to hypothalamic-pituitary disorders, and PRL is the hormone most commonly secreted in excess by pituitary adenomas.

The understanding that PRL hypersecretion causes not only galactorrhea but also gonadal dysfunction and the use of PRL measurements in screening such patients have permitted recognition of these PRL-secreting tumors before the development of sellar enlargement, hypopituitarism, or visual impairment.

Thus, plasma PRL should be measured in patients with galactorrhea, suspected hypothalamic-pituitary dysfunction, or sellar enlargement and in those with unexplained gonadal dysfunction, including amenorrhea, infertility, decreased libido, or impotence (Table 5–12).

Pathology

PRL-secreting pituitary adenomas arise most commonly from the lateral wings of the anterior pituitary, but with progression they fill the sella turcica and com-

Table 5–12. Indications for prolactin measurement.

Galactorrhea
Enlarged sella turcica
Suspected pituitary tumor
Hypogonadotropic hypogonadism
    Unexplained amenorrhea
    Unexplained male hypogonadism or infertility

---

press the normal anterior and posterior lobes. Tumor size varies greatly from microadenomas to large invasive tumors with extrasellar extension. Most patients have microadenomas, ie, tumors less than 1 cm in diameter at diagnosis.

Prolactinomas usually appear chromophobic on routine histologic study, reflecting the inadequacy of the techniques used. The cells are small and uniform, with round or oval nuclei and scanty cytoplasm, and secretory granules are usually not visible with routine stains. The stroma contains a diffuse capillary network.

Electron microscopic examination shows that prolactinoma cells characteristically contain secretory granules that usually range from 100 nm to 500 nm in diameter and are spherical. Larger granules (400–500 nm), which are irregular or crescent-shaped, are less commonly seen. The cells show evidence of secretory activity, with a large Golgi area, nucleolar enlargement, and a prominent endoplasmic reticulum. Immunocytochemical studies of these tumors have confirmed that the secretory granules indeed contain PRL.

Clinical Features

The clinical manifestations of PRL excess are the same regardless of the cause (see below). The classic features are galactorrhea and amenorrhea in women and galactorrhea and decreased libido or impotence in men. Although the sex distribution of prolactinomas is approximately equal, microadenomas are much more common in women, presumably because of earlier recognition of the endocrine consequences of PRL excess.

A. GALACTORRHEA

Galactorrhea occurs in the majority of women with prolactinomas and is much less common in men. It is usually not spontaneous, or may be present only transiently or intermittently; careful breast examination is required in most patients to demonstrate galactorrhea. The absence of galactorrhea despite markedly elevated PRL levels is probably due to concomitant deficiency of the gonadal hormones required to initiate lactation (see Chapter 16).

B. GONADAL DYSFUNCTION

1. In women—Amenorrhea, oligomenorrhea with anovulation, or infertility is present in approximately 90% of women with prolactinomas. These menstrual disorders usually present concurrently with galactorrhea if it is present but may either precede or follow it. The amenorrhea is usually secondary and may follow pregnancy or oral contraceptive use. Primary amenorrhea occurs in the minority of patients who have onset of hyperprolactinemia during adolescence. The necessity of measuring PRL in patients with unexplained primary or secondary amenorrhea is emphasized by several studies showing that hyperprolactinemia occurs in as many as 20% of patients with neither galactorrhea nor other manifestations of pituitary dysfunction. A number of these patients have been shown to have prolactinomas.

Gonadal dysfunction in these women is due to interference with the hypothalamic-pituitary-gonadal axis by the hyperprolactinemia and except in patients with large or invasive adenomas is not due to destruction of the gonadotropin-secreting cells. This has been documented by the return of menstrual function following reduction of PRL levels to normal by drug treatment or surgical removal of the tumor. Although basal gonadotropin levels are frequently within the normal range despite reduction of sex steroid levels in hyperprolactinemic patients, PRL inhibits both the normal pulsatile secretion of LH and FSH and the midcycle LH surge, resulting in anovulation. The positive feedback effect of estrogen on gonadotropin secretion is also inhibited; in fact, patients with hyperprolactinemia are usually estrogen-deficient.

Estrogen deficiency in women with prolactinomas may be accompanied by decreased vaginal lubrication, other symptoms of estrogen deficiency, and osteopenia as assessed by bone densitometry. Other symptoms may include weight gain, fluid retention, and irritability. Hirsutism may also occur, accompanied by elevated plasma levels of dehydroepiandrosterone (DHEA) sulfate. Patients with hyperprolactinemia may also suffer from anxiety and depression. Treatment with dopamine agonists has been shown to improve psychologic distress in such patients.

2. In men—In men, PRL excess may also occasionally cause galactorrhea; however, the usual manifestations are those of hypogonadism. The initial symptom is decreased libido, which may be dismissed by both the patient and physician as due to psychosocial factors; thus, the recognition of prolactinomas in men is frequently delayed, and marked hyperprolactinemia (PRL > 200 ng/mL [9.1 nmol/L]) and sellar enlargement are usual. Unfortunately, prolactinomas in men are often not diagnosed until late manifestations such as headache, visual impairment, or hypopituitarism appear; virtually all such patients have a history of sexual or gonadal dysfunction. Serum testosterone levels are low, and in the presence of normal or subnormal gonadotropin levels, PRL excess should be suspected as well as other causes of hypothalamic-pituitary-gonadal dysfunction (see section on hypopituitarism). Impotence also occurs in hyperprolactinemic males. Its cause is unclear, since testosterone replacement may not reverse it if hyperprolactinemia is not corrected. Male infertility accompanied by reduction in sperm count is a less common initial complaint.

C. TUMOR PROGRESSION

In general, the growth of prolactinomas is slow, and several studies have shown that most microadenomas do not progress.

Differential Diagnosis

The many conditions associated with hyperprolactinemia are listed in Table 5–8. Pregnancy, hypothalamic-pituitary disorders, primary hypothyroidism, and drug ingestion are the most common causes.

Hypothalamic lesions frequently cause PRL hypersecretion by decreasing the secretion of dopamine that tonically inhibits PRL release; the lesions may be accompanied by panhypopituitarism. Similarly, traumatic or surgical section of the pituitary stalk leads to hyperprolactinemia and hypopituitarism. Nonfunctional pituitary macroadenomas frequently cause mild hyperprolactinemia by compression of the pituitary stalk or hypothalamus.

Pregnancy leads to a physiologic increase in PRL secretion; the levels increase as pregnancy continues and may reach 200 ng/mL (9.1 nmol/L) during the third trimester. Following delivery, basal PRL levels gradually fall to normal over several weeks but increase in response to breast feeding. Hyperprolactinemia persisting for 6–12 months or longer following delivery is an indication for evaluation. PRL levels are also high in normal neonates.

Several systemic disorders lead to hyperprolactinemia. Primary hypothyroidism is a common cause, and measurement of thyroid function, and especially TSH, should be part of the evaluation. In primary hypothyroidism, there is hyperplasia of both thyrotrophs and lactotrophs, presumably due to TRH hypersecretion. This may result in significant pituitary gland enlargement, which may be mistaken for a PRL-secreting pituitary tumor. The PRL response to TRH is usually exaggerated in these patients. PRL may also be increased in liver disease, particularly in patients with severe cirrhosis, and in patients with chronic renal failure.

PRL excess and galactorrhea may also be caused by breast disease, nipple stimulation, disease or injury to the chest wall, and spinal cord lesions. These disorders increase PRL secretion by stimulation of afferent neural pathways. Artifactual elevations in prolactin level may be observed in the presence of anti-prolactin antibodies or of macroprolactinemia. In the latter, a high-molecular-weight complex of prolactin molecules maintains immunologic activity but not bioactivity.

The most common cause of hyperprolactinemia is drug ingestion, and a careful history of drug intake must be obtained. Elevated PRL levels, galactorrhea, and amenorrhea may occur following estrogen therapy or oral contraceptive use, but their persistence should suggest prolactinoma. Many other drugs also cause increased PRL secretion and elevated plasma levels (Table 5–8). PRL levels are usually less than 200 ng/mL (9 nmol/L), and the evaluation is primarily by discontinuing the drug or medication and reevaluating the patient after several weeks. In patients in whom drug withdrawal is not feasible, neuroradiologic studies, if normal, will usually exclude prolactinoma.

Diagnosis

A. GENERAL EVALUATION

The evaluation of patients with galactorrhea or unexplained gonadal dysfunction with normal or low plasma gonadotropin levels should first include a history regarding menstrual status, pregnancy, fertility, sexual function, and symptoms of hypothyroidism or hypopituitarism. Current or previous use of medication, drugs, or estrogen therapy should be documented. Basal PRL levels, gonadotropins, thyroid function tests, and TSH levels should be established, as well as serum testosterone in men. Liver and kidney function should be assessed. A pregnancy test should be performed in women with amenorrhea.

Patients with galactorrhea but normal menses may not have hyperprolactinemia and usually do not have prolactinomas. If the PRL level is normal, they may be reassured and followed with sequential PRL measurements. Those with elevated levels require further evaluation as described below.

B. SPECIFIC DIAGNOSIS

When other causes of hyperprolactinemia have been excluded, the most likely cause of persistent hyperprolactinemia is a prolactinoma, especially if there is associated hypogonadism. Since currently available suppression and stimulation tests do not distinguish PRL-secreting tumors from other causes of hyperprolactinemia, the diagnosis must be established by the assessment of both basal PRL levels and neuroradiologic studies. Patients with large tumors and marked hyperprolactinemia usually present little difficulty. With very rare exceptions, basal PRL levels greater than 200 ng/mL (9.1 nmol/L) are virtually diagnostic of prolactinoma. In addition, since there is a general correlation between the PRL elevation and the size of the pituitary adenoma, these patients usually have sellar enlargement and obvious macroadenomas. Similarly, if the basal PRL level is between 100 and 200 ng/mL (4.5 and 9.1 nmol/L), the cause is usually prolactinoma. These patients may have either micro- or macroadenomas; however, with basal levels of PRL greater than 100 ng/mL (4.5 nmol/L), the PRL-secreting tumor is usually radiologically evident, and again the diagnosis is generally straightforward. Patients with mild to moderate hyperprolactinemia (20–100 ng/mL [0.9–4.5 nmol/L]) present the greatest difficulty in diagnosis, since both PRL-secreting microadenomas and the many other conditions causing hyperprolactinemia (Table 5–8) cause PRL hypersecretion of this degree. In such patients, MRI should be performed and will frequently demonstrate a definite pituitary microadenoma. Scans showing only minor or equivocal abnormalities should be interpreted with caution, because of the high incidence of false-positive scans in the normal population (see neuroradiologic evaluation, above). Since the diagnosis cannot be either established or excluded in patients with normal or equivocal neuroradiologic studies, they require further evaluation or serial assessment (see below).

Treatment

Satisfactory control of PRL hypersecretion, cessation of galactorrhea, and return of normal gonadal function can be achieved in most patients with PRL-secreting microadenomas. In patients with hyperprolactinemia, ovulation should not be induced without careful assessment of pituitary anatomy, since pregnancy may cause further expansion of these tumors as discussed below.

Although most microadenomas do not progress, treatment of these patients is recommended to restore normal estrogen levels and fertility and to prevent early osteoporosis secondary to persistent hypogonadism. In addition, medical or surgical therapy is more successful in these patients than in those with larger tumors. Therefore, all patients with PRL-secreting macroadenomas should be treated, because of the risks of further tumor expansion, hypopituitarism, and visual impairment.

Patients with persistent hyperprolactinemia and hypogonadism and normal neuroradiologic studies—ie, those in whom prolactinoma cannot be definitely established—may be managed by observation if hypogonadism is of short duration. However, in patients whose hypogonadism has persisted for more than 6–12 months, dopamine agonists should be used to suppress PRL secretion and restore normal gonadal function. In women with suspected or proved prolactinomas, replacement estrogen therapy is contraindicated because of the risk of tumor growth.

A. SURGICAL TREATMENT

Transsphenoidal microsurgery is the surgical procedure of choice in patients with prolactinomas.

1. Microadenomas—In patients with microadenomas, remission, as measured by restitution of normal PRL levels, normal menses, and cessation of galactor-

rhea, is achieved in 85–90% of cases. Success is most likely in patients with basal PRL levels under 200 ng/mL (9.1 nmol/L) and a duration of amenorrhea of less than 5 years. In these patients, the incidence of surgical complications is less than 2%, and hypopituitarism is a rare complication. Thus, in this group of patients with PRL-secreting microadenomas, PRL hypersecretion can be corrected, gonadal function restored, and secretion of TSH and ACTH preserved. Recurrence rates vary considerably in reported series. In our experience, approximately 85% of patients have had long-term remissions, and 15% have had recurrent hyperprolactinemia.

2. Macroadenomas—Transsphenoidal microsurgery is considerably less successful in restoring normal PRL secretion in patients with macroadenomas; many clinicians would treat these patients with dopamine agonists alone. The surgical outcome is directly related to tumor size and the basal PRL level. Thus, in patients with tumors 1–2 cm in diameter without extrasellar extension and with basal PRL levels under 200 ng/mL (9.1 nmol/L), transsphenoidal surgery is successful in about 80% of cases. In patients with higher basal PRL levels and larger or invasive tumors, the success rate—defined as complete tumor resection and restoration of normal basal PRL secretion—is 25–50%. Although progressive visual loss or pituitary apoplexy are clear indications for surgery, the great majority of these patients should be treated with dopamine agonists.

B. DOPAMINE AGONISTS

Bromocriptine became available in the US more than 20 years ago and was the first effective medical therapy for pituitary adenomas; however, cabergoline is more potent, much longer-acting, and better-tolerated. Cabergoline has therefore become the dopamine agonist of choice in the therapy of prolactinomas.

1. Bromocriptine—Bromocriptine, the first available dopamine agonist, stimulates dopamine receptors and has effects at both the hypothalamic and pituitary levels. It is effective therapy for a PRL-secreting pituitary adenoma and directly inhibits PRL secretion by the tumor. The dosage is 2.5–10 mg/d orally in divided doses. Side effects consisting of dizziness, postural hypotension, nausea, and occasionally vomiting are common at onset of therapy but usually resolve with continuation of the medication. They can usually be avoided by starting with a low dose and gradually increasing the dose over days to weeks until the PRL level is suppressed to the normal range. Most patients tolerate doses of 2.5–10 mg without difficulty; however, in about 10%, persistent postural hypotension and gastrointestinal side effects necessitate discontinuance of therapy.

2. Cabergoline—Cabergoline, a newer nonergot dopamine agonist, is administered once or twice a week and has a better side effect profile than bromocriptine. It is as effective as bromocriptine in reducing macroadenoma size and is more effective in reducing prolactin levels. It has been used successfully in most patients previously intolerant or resistant to bromocriptine. Cabergoline should be started at a dosage of 0.25 mg twice per week and increased if necessary to 0.5 mg twice per week.

a. Microadenomas—In patients with microadenomas, bromocriptine successfully reduces PRL levels to normal in about 80% of cases. About 10% of patients cannot tolerate the drug long-term because of persistent side effects, and another 10% are resistant to the effects of bromocriptine. Cabergoline, now the drug of choice, is successful in about 90% of patients and very few are intolerant or resistant. Correction of hyperprolactinemia allows recovery of normal gonadal function; ovulation and fertility are restored, so that mechanical contraception should be advised if pregnancy is not desired. Bromocriptine induces ovulation in most female patients who wish to become pregnant. There is less current experience with cabergoline. In these patients with microadenomas, the risk of major expansion of adenoma during the pregnancy appears to be less than 5%; however, both the patient and the physician must be aware of this potential complication. Current data do not indicate an increased risk of multiple pregnancy, abortion, or fetal malformations in pregnancies occurring in women taking bromocriptine; however, the patient should be instructed to discontinue bromocriptine at the first missed menstrual period and obtain a pregnancy test.

At present, there is no evidence that dopamine agonists cause permanent resolution of PRL-secreting microadenomas, and virtually all patients have resumption of hyperprolactinemia following discontinuation of therapy even when it has been continued for several years. Although no late toxicity has yet been reported other than the side effects noted above, questions about possible long-term risk and the indicated duration of therapy in such patients with microadenomas are currently unanswered.

b. Macroadenomas—Dopamine agonists are effective in controlling hyperprolactinemia in patients with PRL-secreting macroadenomas even when basal PRL levels are markedly elevated. Dopamine agonists may be used either as initial therapy or to control residual hyperprolactinemia in patients unsuccessfully treated with surgery or radiotherapy. Dopamine agonists should not be used to induce ovulation and pregnancy in women with untreated macroadenomas, since the risk of tumor expansion and visual deficits in the later part of pregnancy is approximately 15–25%. These patients should be treated with surgery prior to induction of ovulation.

Dopamine agonists normalize PRL secretion in about 60–70% of patients with macroadenomas and also reduces tumor size in about the same number. Reduction of tumor size may occur within days to weeks following institution of therapy. The drugs have been used to restore vision in patients with major suprasellar extension and chiasmal compression. Tumor reduction in response to dopamine agonists is sustained only as long as the medication is continued, and reexpansion of the tumor and recurrence of hyperprolactinemia may occur rapidly following discontinuation of therapy.

C. RADIOTHERAPY

Conventional radiation therapy is reserved for patients with PRL-secreting macroadenomas who have persistent hyperprolactinemia and who have not responded to attempts to control their pituitary adenomas with surgery or dopamine agonists. In this group of patients, radiotherapy with 4000–5000 cGy prevents further tumor expansion, though PRL levels usually do not fall into the normal range. Impairment of anterior pituitary function occurs in approximately 50–60% of patients.

Experience with gamma knife radiosurgery in prolactinomas is limited.

Selection of Therapy for Prolactinomas

The selection of therapy for prolactinomas depends on the wishes of the patient, the patient's plans for pregnancy and tolerance of medical therapy, and the availability of a skilled neurosurgeon.

A. MICROADENOMAS

All patients should be treated to prevent the occasional tumor progression, osteopenia, and the other effects of prolonged hypogonadism. Medical therapy with dopamine agonists effectively restores normal gonadal function and fertility, and pregnancy carries only a small risk of tumor expansion. The major disadvantage is the need for chronic therapy. Transsphenoidal adenectomy, either initially or after a trial of dopamine agonist therapy, carries little risk when performed by an experienced neurosurgeon and offers a high probability of long-term remission.

B. MACROADENOMAS

Primary surgical therapy in these patients usually does not result in long-term remission, so medical therapy is the primary therapy of choice, particularly when the patient's prolactin levels are greater than 200 ng/mL (9.1 nmol/L) and the tumor is larger than 2 cm. Although transsphenoidal microsurgery will rapidly decrease tumor size and decompress the pituitary stalk, the optic chiasm, and the cavernous sinuses, there is usually residual tumor and hyperprolactinemia. Thus, these patients will require additional therapy with dopamine agonists. Although tumor growth and prolactin secretion can be controlled by medical therapy in most patients, therapeutic failure can result from drug intolerance, poor compliance, or resistance. Radiation therapy is reserved for postsurgical patients with residual adenomas who are not controlled with dopamine agonists.

2. Acromegaly & Gigantism

GH-secreting pituitary adenomas are second in frequency to prolactinomas and cause the classic clinical syndromes of acromegaly and gigantism.

The characteristic clinical manifestations are the consequence of chronic GH hypersecretion, which in turn leads to excessive generation of IGF-I, the mediator of most of the effects of GH (see Chapter 6). Although overgrowth of bone is the classic feature, GH excess causes a generalized systemic disorder with deleterious effects and an increased mortality rate, though deaths are rarely due to the space-occupying or destructive effects of pituitary adenoma per se.

Acromegaly and gigantism are virtually always secondary to a pituitary adenoma. Ectopic GHRH secretion has been identified as another cause of GH hypersecretion and acromegaly in a few patients with carcinoid or islet cell tumors. Reports of intrapituitary GHRH-secreting gangliocytomas in direct contiguity with GH-secreting somatotroph adenomas and a report of a GHRH-secreting hypothalamic hamartoma in a patient with acromegaly provide a link between ectopic and eutopic GHRH production. Ectopic secretion of GH per se is very rare but has been documented in a few lung tumors.

In adults, GH excess leads to acromegaly, the syndrome characterized by local overgrowth of bone, particularly of the skull and mandible. Linear growth does not occur, because of prior fusion of the epiphyses of long bones. In childhood and adolescence, the onset of chronic GH excess leads to gigantism. Most of these patients have associated hypogonadism, which delays epiphysial closure, and the combination of IGF-I excess and hypogonadism leads to a striking acceleration of linear growth. Most patients with gigantism also have features of acromegaly if GH hypersecretion persists through adolescence and into adulthood.

Pathology

Pituitary adenomas causing acromegaly are usually over 1 cm in diameter when the diagnosis is established.

These tumors arise from the lateral wings of the anterior pituitary; less than 20% are diagnosed as microadenomas.

GH-secreting adenomas are of two histologic types: densely and sparsely granulated. However, there appears to be no difference in the degree of GH secretion or clinical manifestations in these patients. About 15% of GH-secreting tumors also contain lactotrophs, and these tumors thus hypersecrete both GH and PRL.

Etiology & Pathogenesis

Excessive pituitary GH secretion could be secondary to abnormal hypothalamic function, but in most cases it is a primary pituitary disorder. A mutation in the G_s protein leading to excessive cAMP production has been identified in 40% of GH-secreting adenomas. Pituitary adenomas are present in virtually all patients and are usually greater than 1 cm in diameter; hyperplasia alone is rare, and nonadenomatous anterior pituitary tissue does not exhibit somatotroph hyperplasia when examined histologically. In addition, there is a return of normal GH levels and dynamic control of GH secretion following selective removal of the pituitary adenoma.

Pathophysiology

In acromegaly, GH secretion is increased and its dynamic control is abnormal. Secretion remains episodic; however, the number, duration, and amplitude of secretory episodes are increased, and they occur randomly throughout the 24-hour period. The characteristic nocturnal surge is absent, and there are abnormal responses to suppression and stimulation. Thus, glucose suppressibility is lost (see diagnosis, below), and GH stimulation by hypoglycemia is usually absent. TRH and GnRH may cause GH release, whereas these substances do not normally stimulate GH secretion. Dopamine and dopamine agonists such as bromocriptine and apomorphine, which normally stimulate GH secretion, paradoxically cause GH suppression in about 70–80% of patients with acromegaly.

Most of the deleterious effects of chronic GH hypersecretion are caused by its stimulation of excessive amounts of IGF-I (see Chapter 6), and plasma levels of this compound are increased in acromegaly. The growth-promoting effects of IGF-I (DNA, RNA, and protein synthesis) lead to the characteristic proliferation of bone, cartilage, and soft tissues and increase in size of other organs to produce the classic clinical manifestations of acromegaly. The insulin resistance and carbohydrate intolerance seen in acromegaly appear to be direct effects of GH and not due to IGF-I excess.

Clinical Features

The sex incidence of acromegaly is approximately equal; the mean age at diagnosis is approximately 40 years; and the duration of symptoms is usually 5–10 years before the diagnosis is established.

Acromegaly is a chronic disabling and disfiguring disorder with increased late morbidity and mortality if untreated. Although spontaneous remissions have been described, the course is slowly progressive in the great majority of cases—patients once thought to be "burned out" can almost invariably be shown to have continuing clinical manifestations and GH hypersecretion.

A. SYMPTOMS AND SIGNS

Early manifestations (Table 5–13) include soft tissue proliferation, with enlargement of the hands and feet and coarsening of the facial features. This is usually accompanied by increased sweating, heat intolerance, oiliness of the skin, fatigue, and weight gain.

At diagnosis, virtually all patients have classic manifestations; acral and soft tissue changes are always present. Bone and cartilage changes affect chiefly the face and skull (Figure 5–18). These changes include thickening of the calvarium; increased size of the frontal sinuses, which leads to prominence of the supraorbital ridges; enlargement of the nose; and downward and forward growth of the mandible, which leads to prognathism and widely spaced teeth. Soft tissue growth also contributes to the facial appearance, with coarsening of the features and facial and infraorbital puffiness. The hands and feet are predominantly affected by soft tissue growth; they are large, thickened, and bulky, with blunt, spade-like fingers (Figure 5–19) and toes. A bulky, sweaty handshake frequently suggests the diagnosis, and there are increases in ring, glove, and shoe sizes. There is generalized thickening of the skin, with increased oiliness and sweating. Acne, sebaceous cysts, and fibromata mollusca (skin tags and papillomas) are common, as is acanthosis nigricans of the axillae and neck and hypertrichosis in women.

These bony and soft tissue changes are accompanied by systemic manifestations, which include hyperhidrosis, heat intolerance, lethargy, fatigue, and increased sleep requirement. Moderate weight gain usually occurs. Paresthesias, usually due to carpal tunnel compression, occur in 70%; sensorimotor neuropathies occur uncommonly. Bone and cartilage overgrowth leads to arthralgias and in long-standing cases to degenerative arthritis of the spine, hips, and knees. Photophobia of unknown cause occurs in about half of cases and is most troublesome in bright sunlight and during night driving.

GH excess leads to generalized visceromegaly, clinically evident as thyromegaly and enlargement of the

Table 5–13. Clinical manifestations of acromegaly in 100 patients.[1]

Manifestations of GH excess	
Acral enlargement	100[2]
Soft tissue overgrowth	100
Hyperhidrosis	88
Lethargy or fatigue	87
Weight gain	73
Paresthesias	70
Joint pain	69
Photophobia	46
Papillomas	45
Hypertrichosis	33
Goiter	32
Acanthosis nigricans	29
Hypertension	24
Cardiomegaly	16
Renal calculi	11
Disturbance of other endocrine functions	
Hyperinsulinemia	70
Glucose intolerance	50
Irregular or absent menses	60
Decreased libido or impotence	46
Hypothyroidism	13
Galactorrhea	13
Gynecomastia	8
Hypoadrenalism	4
Local manifestations	
Enlarged sella	90
Headache	65
Visual deficit	20

[1]Adapted from Tyrrell JB, Wilson CB: Pituitary syndromes. In: *Surgical Endocrinology: Clinical Syndromes.* Friesen SR (editor). Lippincott, 1978.
[2]Percentage of patients in whom these features were present.

salivary glands. Enlargement of other organs is usually not clinically detectable.

Hypertension occurs in about 25% of patients and cardiomegaly in about 15%. Cardiac enlargement may be secondary to hypertension, atherosclerotic disease, or, rarely, to "acromegalic cardiomyopathy." Renal calculi occur in 11% secondary to the hypercalciuria induced by GH excess.

Other endocrine and metabolic abnormalities are common and may be due either to GH excess or to mechanical effects of the pituitary adenoma. Glucose intolerance and hyperinsulinism occur in 50% and 70%, respectively, owing to GH-induced insulin resistance. Overt clinical diabetes occurs in a minority, and diabetic ketoacidosis is rare. Hypogonadism occurs in 60% of female and 46% of male patients and is of multifactorial origin; tumor growth and compression may impair pituitary gonadotropin secretion, and asso-

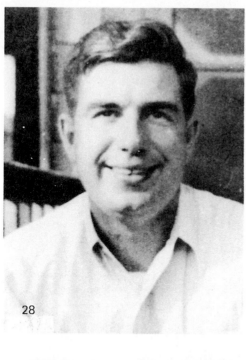
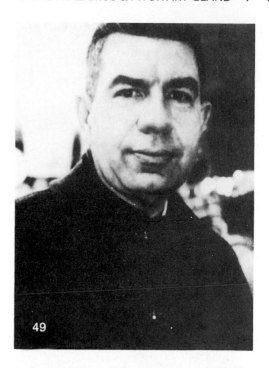
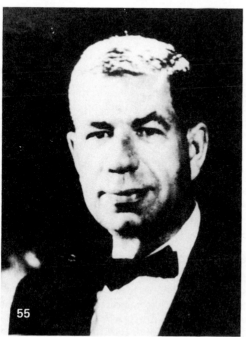
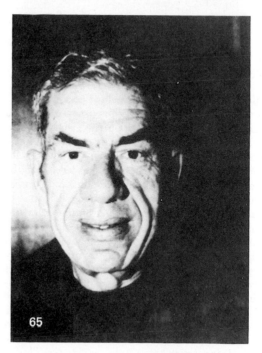

Figure 5–18. Serial photographs of an acromegalic patient at the ages indicated. Note the gradual increase in size of the nose, lips, and skin folds. (Reproduced, with permission, from Reichlin SR: Acromegaly. Med Grand Rounds 1982;1:9.)

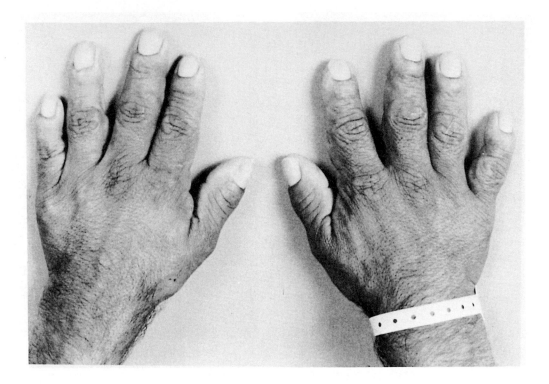

Figure 5-19. Markedly increased soft tissue bulk and blunt fingers in a middle-aged man with acromegaly.

ciated hyperprolactinemia (see below) or the PRL-like effect of excessive GH secretion may impair gonadotropin and gonadal function. In men, low total plasma testosterone levels may be due to GH suppression of sex hormone-binding globulin (SHBG) levels; in these cases, plasma free testosterone levels may be normal, with normal gonadal function. With earlier diagnosis, hypothyroidism and hypoadrenalism due to destruction of the normal anterior pituitary are unusual and are present in only 13% and 4% of patients, respectively. Galactorrhea occurs in about 15% and is usually caused by hyperprolactinemia from a pituitary adenoma with a mixed cell population of somatotrophs and lactotrophs. Gynecomastia of unknown cause occurs in about 10% of men. Although acromegaly may be a component of multiple endocrine neoplasia (MEN) type 1 syndrome, it is distinctly unusual, and concomitant parathyroid hyperfunction or pancreatic islet cell tumors are rare.

When GH hypersecretion is present for many years, late complications occur, including progressive cosmetic deformity and disabling degenerative arthritis. In addition, the mortality rate is increased; after age 45, the death rate in acromegaly from cardiovascular and cerebrovascular atherosclerosis, respiratory diseases, and colon cancer is two to four times that of the normal population. Death rates tend to be higher in patients with hypertension, cardiovascular disease, or clinical diabetes mellitus.

Manifestations of the pituitary adenoma are also common in acromegaly; eg, 65% of patients have headache. Although visual impairment was usually present in older series, it now occurs in only 15–20%, since most patients are now diagnosed because of the manifestations of GH excess.

B. LABORATORY FINDINGS

Postprandial plasma glucose may be elevated, and serum insulin is increased in 70%. Elevated serum phosphorus (due to increased renal tubular resorption of phosphate) and hypercalciuria appear to be due to direct effects of GH or IGF-I.

C. IMAGING STUDIES

Plain films (Figure 5–20) show sellar enlargement in 90% of cases. Thickening of the calvarium, enlargement of the frontal and maxillary sinuses, and enlargement of the jaw can also be seen. Radiographs of the

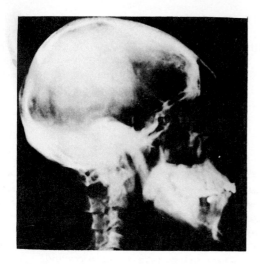
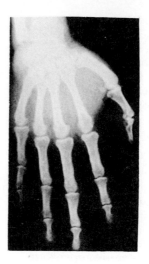
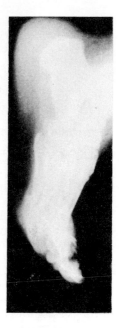

Figure 5–20. Radiologic signs in acromegaly: ***Left:*** Skull with enlarged sella turcica and frontal sinuses, thickening of the calvarium, and enlargement of the mandible. Center: Hand with enlarged sesamoid bone and increased soft tissue shadows. ***Right***: Thickened heel pad. (Reproduced, with permission, from Levin SR: Manifestations and treatment of acromegaly. Calif Med [March] 1972;116:57.)

hand show increased soft tissue bulk, "arrowhead" tufting of the distal phalanges, increased width of intra-articular cartilages, and cystic changes of the carpal bones. Radiographs of the feet show similar changes, and there is increased thickness of the heel pad (normal, < 22 mm).

Diagnosis

Acromegaly is usually clinically obvious and can be readily confirmed by assessment of GH secretion; basal fasting GH levels (normal, 1–5 ng/mL [46–232 pmol/L]) are > 10 ng/mL (465 pmol/L) in over 90% of patients and range from 5 ng/mL (232 pmol/L) to over 500 ng/mL (23,000 pmol/L), with a mean of approximately 50 ng/mL (2300 pmol/L). However, single measurements are not entirely reliable, because GH secretion is episodic in acromegaly and because other conditions may increase GH secretion (see below).

A. GLUCOSE SUPPRESSION

Suppression with oral glucose is the simplest and most specific dynamic test for acromegaly. In healthy subjects, oral administration of 100 g of glucose causes a reduction of the GH level to less than 2 ng/mL (93 pmol/L) at 60 minutes. In acromegaly, GH levels may decrease, increase, or show no change; however, they do

not decrease to less than 2 ng/mL (93 pmol/L), and this lack of response establishes the diagnosis.

Supersensitive GH assays have been developed and are becoming commercially available. With these assays, normal individuals may suppress GH levels to less than 0.1 ng/mL. Thus, the criteria expressed above may need to be adjusted in the near future.

B. IGF-I MEASUREMENT

Measurement of IGF-I (see Chapter 6) is a useful means of establishing the diagnosis of GH hypersecretion. IGF-I results must be interpreted according to the patient's age and sex. IGF-I levels directly reflect GH activity. IGF-I has a long half-life, so that IGF-I levels fluctuate much less than GH levels. IGF-I levels are elevated in virtually all patients with acromegaly (normal ranges vary widely in different laboratories, and some commercial assays are not reliable). Since IGF-I levels decline with age, a level that is in the normal range for a 45-year-old person might be abnormally high in a 65-year-old person (see Appendix).

C. TUMOR LOCALIZATION

Radiographic localization of the pituitary adenoma causing acromegaly is usually straightforward (see Neuroradiologic Evaluation, above). In virtually all patients, tumor location and size can be shown by MRI; 90% have tumors over 1 cm in diameter that are readily visualized. In the rare patient with normal neuroradiologic studies, an extrapituitary ectopic source of GH or GHRH should be considered. If the scans suggest diffuse pituitary enlargement or hyperplasia, ectopic GHRH should also be suspected.

Differential Diagnosis

A. OTHER CAUSES OF GH HYPERSECRETION

The presence of clinical features of GH excess, elevated GH and IGF-I secretion, and abnormal GH dynamics, together with the demonstration of a pituitary tumor by neuroradiologic studies, are diagnostic of acromegaly. However, other conditions associated with GH hypersecretion must be considered in the differential diagnosis. These include anxiety, exercise, acute illness, chronic renal failure, cirrhosis, starvation, protein-calorie malnutrition, anorexia nervosa, and type I (insulin-dependent) diabetes mellitus. Estrogen therapy may increase GH responsiveness to various stimuli. These conditions may be associated with abnormal GH suppressibility by glucose and by abnormal GH responsiveness to TRH; however, patients with these conditions do not have clinical manifestations of GH excess and are thus readily differentiated from patients with acromegaly. In addition, the conditions listed above do not lead to elevation of IGF-I concentrations.

B. ECTOPIC GH OR GHRH SECRETION

These rare patients with acromegaly due to ectopic secretion of GH or GHRH have typical clinical manifestations of acromegaly. This may occur in lung carcinoma, carcinoid tumors, and pancreatic islet cell tumors. These syndromes should be suspected in patients with a known extrapituitary tumor who have GH excess or in those with clinical and biochemical features of acromegaly who have radiologic procedures that show normal pituitary glands or that suggest diffuse pituitary enlargement or hyperplasia.

Treatment

All patients with acromegaly should undergo therapy to halt progression of the disorder and to prevent late complications and excess mortality. The objectives of therapy are removal or destruction of the pituitary tumor, reversal of GH hypersecretion, and maintenance of normal anterior and posterior pituitary function. These objectives are currently attainable in most patients, especially those with smaller tumors and only moderate GH hypersecretion. In patients with large tumors who have marked GH hypersecretion, several therapies are usually required to achieve normal GH secretion.

The criteria for an adequate response to therapy continue to evolve. Until recently, many authors used a basal GH level of 5 ng/mL (232 pmol/L) or less to define remission. However, some of these patients continue to have elevated IGF-I levels, and recent reports describe increased late mortality in patients with GH levels greater than 2.5 ng/mL (116 pmol/L) after therapy. Current guidelines for remission are a fasting GH of 2 ng/mL (93 pmol/L) or less and a glucose-suppressed GH of 2 ng/mL (93 pmol/L) or less accompanied by a normal level of IGF-I.

The initial therapy of choice is transsphenoidal microsurgery because of its high success rate, rapid reduction of GH levels, the low incidence of postoperative hypopituitarism, and the low surgical morbidity rate. Patients with persisting GH hypersecretion after surgery should currently be treated with a sustained-release form of somatostatin analog (octreotide LAR or lanreotide). Radiation therapy should be reserved for those patients with inadequate responses to surgery and medical therapy.

A. SURGICAL TREATMENT

Transsphenoidal selective adenoma removal is the procedure of choice; craniotomy is necessary in the rare patient in whom major suprasellar extension precludes the transsphenoidal approach. Successful reduction of GH levels is achieved in approximately 60–80% of patients. In those with small or moderate-sized tumors (< 2 cm), success is achieved in over 80%, whereas in those with larger tumors and basal GH levels greater than 50 ng/mL (2325 pmol/L)—and particularly in those with major extrasellar extension of the adenoma—successful responses occur in only 30–60%. Recurrence rates in those with a successful initial response are low (about 5% of patients at our institution). Surgical complications (discussed above) occur in less than 2%.

B. MEDICAL TREATMENT

Octreotide acetate, a somatostatin analog was the first effective medical therapy for patients with acromegaly; however, the drug required high doses (100–500 μg) given by subcutaneous injection three times daily. Its use in acromegaly has been superseded by sustained-release somatostatin analogs with activities lasting up to one month. Preparations include octreotide LAR given by injection every four weeks and lanreotide given every two weeks. Octreotide LAR, which is available in the US, normalizes GH and IGF-I levels in 75% of patients; however, tumor reduction occurs in a much smaller percentage. Octreotide LAR has become the therapy of choice for patients with residual GH hypersecretion following surgery. Side effects of this class of agents consist mainly of gastrointestinal symptoms and the development of gallstones. Medical therapy with bromocriptine or other dopamine agonists is successful in only a few patients.

C. RADIOTHERAPY

Conventional supervoltage irradiation in doses of 4500–5000 cGy is successful in 60–80% of patients, though GH levels may not return to normal until years after therapy. Thus, in one series, GH levels were under 10 ng/mL (460 pmol/L) in only 38% of patients at 2 years posttreatment; however, at 5 and 10 years, 73% and 81% had achieved such levels. The incidence of hypopituitarism is appreciable, and in this series hypothyroidism occurred in 19%, hypoadrenalism in 38%, and hypogonadism in approximately 50–60% of patients as a consequence of radiotherapy. Because of the prolonged delay in achieving reduction in GH levels, conventional radiotherapy is generally reserved for patients with persistent GH secretion following pituitary microsurgery and medical therapy. Gamma knife radiosurgery has also been used for tumors confined to the sella. Current series, although limited, suggest remission rates of about 70% at two years following therapy.

Response to Treatment

In patients with successful reduction in GH hypersecretion, there is cessation of bone overgrowth. In addition, these patients experience considerable clinical improvement, including reduction in soft tissue bulk of the extremities, decreased facial puffiness, increased energy, and cessation of hyperhidrosis, heat intolerance, and oily skin. Headache, carpal tunnel syndrome, arthralgias, and photophobia are also reversible with successful therapy. Glucose intolerance and hyperinsulinemia as well as hypercalciuria are also reversed in most cases.

Recent studies have also shown that the excess mortality is reversed if GH levels are normalized.

Posttreatment Follow-Up

Posttreatment assessment includes evaluation of GH secretion, anterior pituitary function, and tumor size. Patients undergoing surgery should be seen 4–6 weeks after the operation for assessment of GH secretion and pituitary function. Those with persistent GH hypersecretion (>2 ng/dL [93 pmol/L]) should receive further therapy with somatostatin analogs. Patients with postoperative GH levels under 2 ng/mL (93 pmol/L) should have follow-up GH and IGF-I determinations at 6-month intervals for 2 years and yearly thereafter to rule out recurrences. Late hypopituitarism after surgery alone does not occur.

Patients treated with radiotherapy should have biannual assessment of GH secretion and annual assessment of anterior pituitary function, since the incidence of late hypopituitarism is appreciable and increases with time following irradiation.

3. ACTH-Secreting Pituitary Adenomas: Cushing's Disease

In 1932, Harvey Cushing documented the presence of small basophilic pituitary adenomas in six of eight patients with clinical features of adrenocortical hyperfunction. Years later, ACTH hypersecretion was identified from such tumors and found to be the cause of bilateral adrenal hyperplasia. Pituitary ACTH hypersecretion (Cushing's disease) is now recognized as the most common cause of spontaneous hypercortisolism (Cushing's syndrome) and must be distinguished from the other forms of adrenocorticosteroid excess—ectopic ACTH syndrome and adrenal tumors (see Chapter 9).

Pathology

ACTH-secreting pituitary tumors exist in virtually all patients with Cushing's disease. These tumors are usually benign microadenomas under 10 mm in diameter; 50% are 5 mm or less in diameter, and microadenomas as small as 1 mm have been described. These tumors in Cushing's disease are either basophilic or chromophobe adenomas and may be found anywhere within the anterior pituitary. Rarely, ACTH-secreting tumors are large, with invasive tendencies, and malignant tumors have rarely been reported.

Histologically, the tumors are composed of compact sheets of uniform, well-granulated cells (granule size, 200–700 nm by electron microscopy) with a sinusoidal arrangement and a high content of ACTH and its related peptides (β-LPH, β-endorphin). A zone of perinuclear hyalinization (Crooke's changes) is frequently observed as a result of exposure of the corticotroph cells to prolonged hypercortisolism. A specific ultrastructural finding in these adenomas is the deposition of bundles of perinuclear microfilaments that encircle the nucleus; these are the ultrastructural equivalent of Crooke's hyaline changes seen on light microscopy. In contrast to the adenoma's cells, ACTH content in the portion of the anterior pituitary not involved with the tumor is decreased.

Diffuse hyperplasia of anterior pituitary corticotrophs or adenomatous hyperplasia, presumed to result from hypersecretion of corticotropin-releasing hormone (CRH), occurs rarely.

The adrenal glands in Cushing's disease are enlarged, weighing 12–24 g (normal, 8–10 g). Microscopic examination shows a thickened cortex due to hyperplasia of both the zona reticularis and zona fasciculata; the zona glomerulosa is normal. In some cases, ACTH-secreting pituitary adenomas cause bilateral nodular hyperplasia; the adrenals show diffuse bilateral cortical hyperplasia and the presence of one or more nodules that vary from microscopic to several centimeters in diameter, with multiple small nodules being the most common.

Pathogenesis

The weight of current evidence is that Cushing's disease is a primary pituitary disorder and that hypothalamic abnormalities are secondary to hypercortisolism. The endocrine abnormalities in Cushing's disease are as follows: (1) hypersecretion of ACTH, with bilateral adrenocortical hyperplasia and hypercortisolism; (2) absent circadian periodicity of ACTH and cortisol secretion; (3) absent responsiveness of ACTH and cortisol to stress (hypoglycemia or surgery); (4) abnormal negative feedback of ACTH secretion by glucocorticoids; and (5) subnormal responsiveness of GH, TSH, and gonadotropins to stimulation.

Evidence that Cushing's disease is a primary pituitary disorder is based on the high frequency of pituitary adenomas, the response to their removal, and the interpretation of hypothalamic abnormalities as being secondary to hypercortisolism. In addition, molecular studies have found that nearly all corticotroph adenomas are monoclonal. These findings suggest that ACTH hypersecretion arises from a spontaneously developing pituitary adenoma and that the resulting hypercortisolism suppresses the normal hypothalamic-pituitary axis and CRH release and thereby abolishes the hypothalamic regulation of circadian variability and stress responsiveness.

Analysis of the response to therapy by pituitary microsurgery sheds some light on the pathogenesis of Cushing's disease. Selective removal of pituitary microadenomas by transsphenoidal microsurgery corrects ACTH hypersecretion and hypercortisolism in most patients. After selective removal of the pituitary adenoma, the following return to normal: the circadian rhythmicity of ACTH and cortisol, the responsiveness of the hypothalamic-pituitary axis to hypoglycemic stress, and the dexamethasone suppressibility of cortisol secretion.

Clinical Features

Cushing's disease presents with the signs and symptoms of hypercortisolism and adrenal androgen excess (see Chapter 9). The onset of these features is usually insidious, developing over months or years. Obesity (with predominantly central fat distribution), hypertension, glucose intolerance, and gonadal dysfunction (amenorrhea or impotence) are common features. Other common manifestations include moon facies, plethora, osteopenia, proximal muscle weakness, easy bruisability, psychologic disturbances, violaceous striae, hirsutism, acne, poor wound healing, and superficial fungal infections. Unlike patients with the classic form of ectopic ACTH syndrome, patients with Cushing's disease rarely have hypokalemia, weight loss, anemia, or hyperpigmentation. Virilization, observed occasionally in patients with adrenal carcinoma, is unusual in Cushing's disease. Clinical symptoms related to the ACTH-secreting primary tumor itself, such as headache or visual impairment, are rare because of the small size of these adenomas.

The usual age range is 20–40 years, but Cushing's disease has been reported in infants and in patients over 70. There is a female:male ratio of approximately 8:1. In contrast, the ectopic ACTH syndrome occurs more commonly in men (male:female ratio of 3:1).

Diagnosis

The initial step in the diagnosis of an ACTH-secreting pituitary adenoma is the documentation of endogenous hypercortisolism, which is confirmed by increased urine free cortisol secretion and abnormal cortisol suppressibility to low-dose dexamethasone. The differentiation of an ACTH-secreting pituitary tumor from other causes of hypercortisolism must be based on biochemical studies, including the measurement of basal plasma ACTH levels and central venous sampling, to detect a central to peripheral gradient of ACTH levels (see Chapter 9). The diagnosis and differential diagnosis of Cushing's syndrome are presented in Chapter 9.

Treatment

Transsphenoidal microsurgery is the procedure of choice in Cushing's disease. A variety of other therapies—operative, radiologic, pharmacologic—are discussed below.

A. Surgical Treatment

Selective transsphenoidal resection of ACTH-secreting pituitary adenomas is the initial treatment of choice. At operation, meticulous exploration of the intrasellar contents by an experienced neurosurgeon is required. The tumor, which is usually found within the anterior lobe tissue, is selectively removed, and normal gland is left intact. If the tumor is too small to locate at surgery, total hypophysectomy may be performed in adult patients who are past the age of reproduction and whose biochemical diagnosis has been confirmed with selective venous ACTH sampling.

In about 85% of patients with microadenomas, selective microsurgery is successful in correcting hypercortisolism. Surgical damage to anterior pituitary function is rare, but most patients develop transient secondary adrenocortical insufficiency requiring postoperative glucocorticoid support until the hypothalamic-pituitary-adrenal axis recovers, usually in 6–18 months. Total hypophysectomy is necessary to correct hypercortisolism in another 10% of patients. In the remaining 5% of patients with microadenomas, selective tumor removal is unsuccessful. By contrast, transsphenoidal surgery is successful in only 25% of the 10–15% of patients with Cushing's disease with pituitary macroadenomas or in those with extrasellar extension of tumor.

Transient diabetes insipidus occurs in about 10% of patients, but other surgical complications (eg, hemorrhage, cerebrospinal fluid rhinorrhea, infection, visual impairment, permanent diabetes insipidus) are rare. Hypopituitarism occurs only in patients who undergo total hypophysectomy.

Before the introduction of pituitary microsurgery, bilateral total adrenalectomy was the preferred treatment of Cushing's disease and may still be employed in patients in whom other therapies are unsuccessful. Total adrenalectomy, which can now be performed laparoscopically, corrects hypercortisolism but produces permanent hypoadrenalism, requiring lifelong glucocorticoid and mineralocorticoid therapy. The ACTH-secreting pituitary adenoma persists and may progress, causing hyperpigmentation and invasive complications (Nelson's syndrome; see below). Persistent hypercortisolism may occasionally follow total adrenalectomy as ACTH hypersecretion stimulates adrenal remnants or congenital rests.

B. Radiotherapy

Conventional radiotherapy of the pituitary is of benefit in patients who have persistent or recurrent disease following pituitary microsurgery. In these patients, reported remission rates are 55–70% at 1–3 years after radiotherapy.

Gamma knife radiosurgery has been reported from one center with remission rates of 75% in adults and 80% in children. However, 55% of the adults developed panhypopituitarism, and each of the children and adolescents were growth hormone-deficient. Therefore, gamma knife radiosurgery may be best suited for postoperative radiotherapy in patients with unsuccessful responses to pituitary microsurgery.

C. Medical Treatment

Drugs that inhibit adrenal cortisol secretion are useful in Cushing's disease, often as adjunctive therapy (see Chapter 9). No drug currently available successfully suppresses pituitary ACTH secretion.

Ketoconazole, an imidazole derivative, has been found to inhibit adrenal steroid biosynthesis. It inhibits the cytochrome P450 enzymes P450scc and P450c11. In daily doses of 600–1200 mg, ketoconazole has been effective in the management of Cushing's syndrome. Hepatotoxicity is common, however, but may be transient. **Metyrapone,** which inhibits P450c11, and **aminoglutethimide,** which inhibits P450scc, have also been utilized to reduce cortisol hypersecretion.

These drugs are expensive; their use is accompanied by increased ACTH levels that may overcome the enzyme inhibition; and they cause gastrointestinal side effects that may limit their effectiveness. More effective control of hypercortisolism with fewer side effects is obtained by combined use of these agents. Adequate data are not available on the long-term use of these drugs as the sole treatment of Cushing's disease. Thus, ketoconazole and aminoglutethimide ordinarily are used while awaiting a response to therapy or in the preparation of patients for surgery.

The adrenolytic drug **mitotane** results in adrenal atrophy predominantly of the zonae fasciculata and reticularis. Remission of hypercortisolism is achieved in approximately 80% of patients with Cushing's disease, but most relapse after therapy is discontinued. Mitotane therapy is limited by the delayed response, which may take weeks or months, and by the frequent side effects, including severe nausea, vomiting, diarrhea, somnolence, and skin rash.

Pharmacologic inhibition of ACTH secretion in Cushing's disease has also been attempted with cyproheptadine and bromocriptine. However, only a very few patients have had successful responses, and the use of these agents is not recommended.

4. Nelson's Syndrome

The clinical appearance of an ACTH-secreting pituitary adenoma following bilateral adrenalectomy as initial therapy for Cushing's disease was first described by Nelson and coworkers in 1958. However, with the evolution of pituitary microsurgery as the initial therapy for Cushing's disease, Nelson's syndrome is now a rare occurrence.

Pathogenesis

It now seems likely that Nelson's syndrome represents the clinical progression of a preexisting adenoma after the restraint of hypercortisolism on ACTH secretion and tumor growth is removed. Thus, following adrenalectomy, the suppressive effect of cortisol is no longer present, ACTH secretion increases, and the pituitary adenoma may progress.

Incidence

Prior to the development of transsphenoidal surgery, when bilateral adrenalectomy was the initial therapy for Cushing's disease, the incidence of Nelson's syndrome ranged from 10% to 78% depending on what criteria were used for diagnosis (see Chapter 9). Approximately 30% of patients adrenalectomized for Cushing's disease developed classic Nelson's syndrome with progressive hyperpigmentation and an obvious ACTH-secreting tumor; another 50% developed evidence of a microadenoma without marked progression; and about 20% never developed a progressive tumor. The reasons for these differences in clinical behavior are uncertain. At present, when adrenalectomy is utilized only in those patients who fail pituitary microsurgery, the incidence of Nelson's syndrome is less than 10%. Nevertheless, continued examination, including plasma ACTH levels and MRI, is required following bilateral adrenalectomy in patients with Cushing's disease.

Clinical Features

The pituitary tumors in patients with classic Nelson's syndrome are among the most aggressive and rapidly growing of all pituitary tumors. These patients present with hyperpigmentation and with manifestations of an expanding intrasellar mass lesion. Visual field defects, headache, cavernous sinus invasion with extraocular muscle palsies, and even malignant changes with local or distant metastases may occur. Pituitary apoplexy may also complicate the course of these tumors.

Diagnosis

Plasma ACTH levels are markedly elevated, usually over 1000 pg/mL (222 pmol/L) and often as high as 10,000 pg/mL (2220 pmol/L). MRI defines the extent of the tumor.

Treatment

Pituitary surgery by the transsphenoidal approach is the initial mode of treatment. Complete resection is usually not possible, because of the large size of these tumors. Conventional radiotherapy is employed postoperatively in patients with residual tumor or extrasellar extension. Experience with gamma knife radiosurgery is limited.

5. Thyrotropin-Secreting Pituitary Adenomas

Thyrotropin-secreting pituitary adenomas are rare tumors manifested as hyperthyroidism with goiter in the presence of elevated TSH. Patients with TSH-secreting tumors are often resistant to routine ablative thyroid therapy, requiring large, often multiple doses of ^{131}I and several operations for control of thyrotoxicosis. Histologically, the tumors are chromophobe adenomas. They are often very large and cause visual impairment, which alerts the physician to a pituitary abnormality. Patients with these tumors do not have extrathyroidal systemic manifestations of Graves' disease such as ophthalmopathy or dermopathy. Pituitary TSH hypersecretion in the absence of a demonstrable pituitary tumor has also been reported to cause hyperthyroidism in a few patients.

The diagnosis is based on findings of hyperthyroidism with elevated serum TSH and alpha subunit, and neuroradiologic studies consistent with pituitary tumor. Differential diagnosis includes those patients with primary hypothyroidism (thyroid failure) who develop major hyperplasia of pituitary thyrotrophs and lactotrophs with sellar enlargement and occasional suprasellar extension.

Treatment should be directed initially at the adenoma via the transsphenoidal microsurgical approach. However, additional therapy is usually required because of the large size of these adenomas.

Somatostatin analogs normalize TSH and T_4 levels in more than 70% of these patients when given subcutaneously in doses similar to those used for the treatment of acromegaly (see above). Shrinkage of the tumor has been observed in about 40% of patients.

If tumor growth and TSH hypersecretion cannot be controlled by surgery and somatostatin analogs, the next step would be to undertake pituitary irradiation. In addition, such patients may also require ablative therapy of the thyroid with either ^{131}I or surgery to control their thyrotoxicosis.

6. Gonadotropin-Secreting Pituitary Adenomas

Although many pituitary adenomas synthesize gonadotropins (especially FSH) and their subunits, only a minority of these patients have elevated serum levels of FSH or LH. The majority of these tumors produce FSH and the alpha subunit, but tumors secreting both FSH and LH and a tumor secreting only LH have been described.

Gonadotropin-secreting pituitary adenomas are usually large chromophobe adenomas presenting with visual impairment. Most patients have hypogonadism and many have panhypopituitarism. Hormonal evaluation reveals elevated FSH in some patients accompanied by normal LH values. Basal levels of the alpha subunit may also be elevated. The presence of elevation of both FSH and LH should suggest primary hypogonadism. TRH stimulation leads to an increase in FSH secretion in 33% and an increase in LH-β in 66% of patients.

Therapy for gonadotropin-secreting adenomas has been directed at surgical removal. Because of their large size, adequate control of the tumor has not been achieved, and radiotherapy is usually required.

7. Alpha Subunit-Secreting Pituitary Adenomas

Excessive quantities of the alpha subunit of the glycoprotein pituitary hormones have been observed in association with the hypersecretion of many anterior pituitary hormones (TSH, GH, PRL, LH, FSH). Recently, however, pure alpha subunit hypersecretion has been identified in several patients with large invasive chromophobe adenomas and partial panhypopituitarism. Thus, the determination of the alpha subunit may be a useful marker in patients with presumed "nonfunctioning" pituitary adenomas.

8. Nonfunctional Pituitary Adenomas

"Nonfunctional" chromophobe adenomas once represented approximately 80% of all primary pituitary tumors; however, with clinical application of radioimmunoassay of anterior pituitary hormones, these tumors currently account for only about 10% of all pituitary adenomas. Thus, the great majority of these chromophobe adenomas have now been documented to be PRL-secreting; a smaller number secrete TSH or the gonadotropins.

Nonfunctional tumors are usually large when the diagnosis is established; headache and visual field defects are the usual presenting symptoms. However, endocrine manifestations are usually present for months to years before the diagnosis is made, with gonadotropin deficiency being the most common initial symptom. Hypothyroidism and hypoadrenalism are also common, but the symptoms are subtle and may be missed.

Evaluation should include MRI and visual field testing; endocrine studies should include assessment of pituitary hormones and end-organ function to determine whether the adenoma is hypersecreting or whether hormonal replacement is needed.

Since these tumors are generally large, both surgery and radiation therapy are usually required to prevent tumor progression or recurrence. In the absence of an endocrine index of tumor hypersecretion such as PRL excess, serial scans at yearly intervals are required to assess the response to therapy and to detect possible recurrence.

■ POSTERIOR PITUITARY

ANTIDIURETIC HORMONE (ADH; VASOPRESSIN)

ADH is metabolized rapidly in the liver and kidney and has a half life of 15–20 minutes. It acts through three receptors, termed V_1, V_2, and V_3 (Table 5–14). The V_1 receptors mediate vascular smooth muscle contraction and stimulate prostaglandin synthesis and liver glycogenolysis. Activation of these receptors increases phosphatidylinositol breakdown, thus causing cellular calcium mobilization. The V_2 receptors, which produce the renal actions of vasopressin, activate G_s proteins and

Table 5–14. ADH receptors in humans.

Receptor Subtype	Second Messenger System	Tissue Distribution	Function
V_1 (V_{1a})	Phospholipase C, phospholipase A_2; diacylglycerol, inositol trisphosphate, Ca^{2+}, arachidonate metabolites	Smooth muscle in the mesenteric artery	Vasoconstriction
V_3 (V_{1b})	Same as V_1	Pituitary gland	Release of ACTH, partly by potentiating the action of CRH
V_2	Adenylyl cyclase	Kidney	Antidiuresis by mobilization of aquaporin 2 in the collecting ducts, stimulation of NaCl reabsorption in the thick ascending limb, stimulation of urea transporter 1-mediated urea reabsorption in the terminal inner medullary collecting ducts

[1]Modified from Kacsoh B: *Endocrine Physiology.* McGraw-Hill, 2000.

stimulate the generation of cAMP (see Chapter 3). The V_3 receptors in the pituitary contribute to ACTH release by potentiating the action of CRH.

Renal Actions

The major renal effect of ADH is to increase the water permeability of the luminal membrane of the collecting duct epithelium via the ADH-sensitive water channels, aquaporin-2 (one of a family of aquaporins). In the absence of ADH, permeability of the epithelium is very low and reabsorption of water decreases, leading to polyuria. When ADH is present, epithelial permeability increases markedly, and water is reabsorbed. This ADH effect is caused by ADH binding to the V_2 receptor. Acutely, ADH mobilizes aquaporin-2 in a manner analogous to insulin's effect on glucose disposal via mobilization of GLUT 4. Water permeability of the luminal membrane is increased by increasing the number of narrow aqueous channels at the luminal surface (radii of about 0.2 nm). Thus, diffusion of water through the membrane is enhanced, as is transcellular flow.

As the collecting ducts traverse the renal medulla, the urine passes regions of ever-increasing osmolality up to a maximum of 1200 mosm/kg of water at the tip of the papilla. In the presence of ADH, collecting duct fluid equilibrates with this hyperosmotic environment, and urine osmolality approaches that of medullary interstitial fluid. Thus, maximal ADH effect results in low urine flow, and urine osmolality may approximate 1200 mosm/kg; with ADH deficiency, urine flow may be as high as 15–20 mL/min, and urine osmolality is less than 100 mosm/kg. The ability to vary urine osmolality over a tenfold range allows maintenance of homeostasis over a wide range of water intake. ADH also stimulates urea absorption in the inner medullary collecting ducts via urea transporters 1.

Cardiovascular & Other Actions

ADH effects on V_1 receptors in peripheral arterioles increase blood pressure. However, these effects are usually blunted by efferent mechanisms such as bradycardia and inhibition of sympathetic nerve activity that result from baroreceptor activation. ADH pressor effects may be important during hypovolemia when plasma ADH levels are very high and maintenance of tissue perfusion is critical. ADH, through V_2 receptors, stimulates release of clotting factor VIII and von Willebrand factor from vascular endothelium. The physiologic significance of these actions in unknown. However, pharmacotherapy with ADH analogs has been useful in treatment of some disorders associated with bleeding diatheses. ADH is also involved in the regulation of the CRH-ACTH-cortisol axis (see above).

OXYTOCIN

Oxytocin primarily affects uterine smooth muscle. It increases both the frequency and the duration of action potentials during uterine contractions. Thus, administration of oxytocin initiates contractions in a quiescent uterus and increases the strength and frequency of muscle contractions in an active uterus. Estrogen enhances the action of oxytocin by reducing the membrane potential of smooth muscle cells, thus lowering the threshold of excitation. Toward the end of pregnancy, as estrogen levels become higher, the membrane potential of uterine smooth muscle cells becomes less negative, rendering the uterus more sensitive to oxytocin. The number of oxytocin receptors in the uterus also increases at this time, and their activation causes cellular calcium to be mobilized through polyphosphatidylinositol hydrolysis.

Actions Affecting the Female Reproductive System

A. PARTURITION

As the fetus enters the birth canal, the lower segment of the uterus, the cervix, and then the vagina are dilated, and this causes reflex release of oxytocin. Strong uterine contractions cause further descent of the fetus, further distention, and further release of oxytocin.

B. LACTATION

Oxytocin is also involved in lactation. Stimulation of the nipple produces a neurohumoral reflex that causes secretion of oxytocin. In turn, oxytocin causes contraction of the myoepithelial cells of the mammary ducts and the ejection of milk.

Other Actions

A number of stimuli that also release ADH such as increased plasma osmolality and hypovolemia cause oxytocin secretion. Since oxytocin is an effective natriuretic agent—particularly at low rates of urine flow—it may be involved in the regulation of sodium balance.

CONTROL OF WATER BALANCE

Water Requirements

Water balance is precisely controlled by an integrated system that balances water intake via thirst mechanism with water output controlled by ADH. The average individual loses 2.5–3 L of water per day (Table 5–15) and must take in that amount in order to maintain balance. Given free access to water, total human body water rarely varies by more than 1–2%. Approximately

Table 5–15. Routes of loss of water in an average adult human.

	mL/24 h
Urine	1500
Skin	600
Lungs	400
Feces	100
	2600

1.2 L of water is taken in food or is provided by oxidative metabolism. The remainder is ingested as water or other fluids.

Concentration of Urine

Renal concentrating mechanisms are essential to the maintenance of water balance in order for the kidney to excrete osmotically active solutes derived from the diet.

The average human excretes 1.5 L of urine per day at an osmolality of approximately 600 mosm/kg of water, ie, twice the concentration of plasma. Without the capacity to concentrate urine, 3 L of water at a concentration of 300 mosm/kg would be excreted and the extra water would have to be ingested. During negative water balance, the urine volume may be reduced to 600 mL/d at a maximum urinary concentration of 1200 mosm/kg. This fourfold capacity (versus plasma) to concentrate the urine is of extreme importance in protection against dehydration and hypovolemia.

Urinary concentration mechanisms can reduce but not completely prevent loss of water in the urine. Even if an individual is maximally concentrating urine, obligatory fluid loss is still considerable. This situation is exacerbated in a warm environment, where many liters of fluid may be lost to maintain a constant temperature via sweating. The only way to bring body fluid levels back to normal is by increasing water intake. It is not surprising that many similarities exist between mechanisms involved in the control of thirst and ADH secretion.

Control of Thirst & ADH Secretion

Cellular and extracellular dehydration are the two major mechanisms involved in the control of thirst and ADH secretion.

A. CELLULAR DEHYDRATION

Cellular dehydration occurs when extracellular fluid osmolality is increased relative to that of intracellular fluids, leading to the efflux of water from cells. When extracellular fluid osmolality increases, all cells, including the hypothalamic osmoreceptors, become dehydrated,

thus providing the signal for secretion of ADH. Hypothalamic osmoreceptor cells that sense the effective plasma-intracellular osmotic gradient contain a unique aquaporin H_2O channel. In the presence of plasma hyperosmolality (usually related to increased serum Na^+), these channels open and allow water migration out of the cell, resulting in a reduction in osmoreceptor cell volume. Stretch-inactivated cation channels become activated, and this in turn leads to depolarization of the cell and subsequently stimulation of ADH secretion and synthesis. In humans, an increase of only 1% in plasma osmolality stimulates thirst, water intake, and simultaneously ADH (Figures 5–21 and 5–22).

The relationship between plasma ADH concentration and plasma osmolality in humans is presented in Figure 5–22. The exquisite sensitivity of ADH release to changing plasma osmolality is obvious.

B. EXTRACELLULAR FLUID DEHYDRATION

Extracellular fluid dehydration—ie, decreased extracellular fluid volume without a change in osmolality—stimulates thirst and ADH secretion. Thus, hemorrhage reduces extracellular fluid volume and results in both thirst and ADH secretion (Figure 5–23). Small

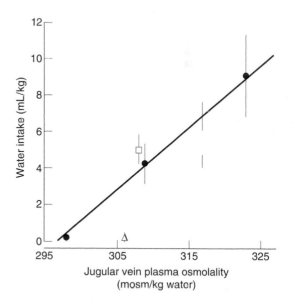

Figure 5–21. Relationship between water intake and jugular vein plasma osmolality. Central osmolality was increased selectively by infusing hypertonic sodium chloride into carotid loops in trained conscious dogs (●). Infusion of hypertonic sucrose was equally effective (□), whereas hypertonic urea (Δ) did not stimulate drinking. (Data from Wood RJ, Rolls BJ, Ramsay DJ: Am J Physiol 1977;323:88.)

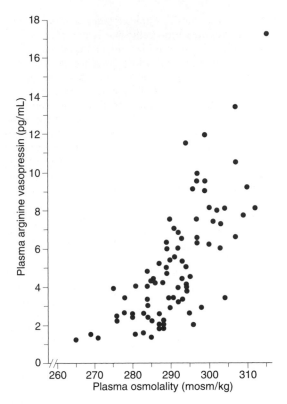

Figure 5–22. Relationship between plasma vasopressin concentration and plasma osmolality in humans during dehydration. (Reproduced, with permission, from Hammer M, Ladefoged J, Olgaard K: Am J Physiol 1980;238:313.)

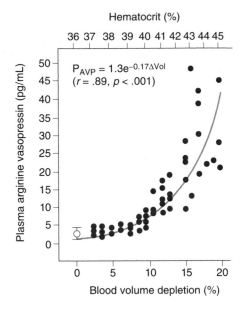

Figure 5–23. Relationship of plasma vasopressin to isosmotic reductions in blood volume in rats. (Reproduced, with permission, from Dunn FL et al: J Clin Invest 1973;52:3212.)

decreases in volume have minimal effects on ADH secretion, but reductions larger than 10% cause a marked stimulation of ADH to values > 100 pg/mL (92.5 pmol/L). These high circulating levels of ADH do not further increase water conservation, since maximum urinary concentration is reached at much lower levels. However, the high levels of ADH may support blood pressure via V_1 receptors.

C. INTERACTION OF OSMOLALITY AND VOLUME

Two major mechanisms are involved in hypovolemic stimulation of thirst and ADH secretion. Moderate reductions in blood volume stimulate low-pressure receptors in the left and right atria and in the pulmonary circulation. With more severe hypovolemia, which reduces blood pressure, the arterial baroreceptors are activated. Responses from these baroreceptor areas in the circulation are then transmitted to magnocellular cells in the hypothalamus. In addition, the renin-angiotensin system may be involved, since hypovolemia

stimulates renin secretion and angiotensin formation. Angiotensin II also stimulates thirst and ADH secretion. The relative roles of the direct baroreceptor input and angiotensin mechanisms in the responses to extracellular dehydration have yet to be determined.

Thus, regulation of water balance involves interaction between osmotic and volume stimuli. In the case of ADH secretion, the fall in extracellular fluid volume sensitizes the release of ADH to a given osmotic stimulus. Thus, for a given increase in plasma osmolality, the increase in plasma ADH will be greater in hypovolemic than in normovolemic states.

In dehydration, increased plasma osmolality results in withdrawal of fluid from cells. Thus, the reduction in total body water is shared equally between intracellular and extracellular fluid compartments. The increase in plasma osmolality and the reduction of extracellular fluid volume act synergistically to stimulate ADH release. In salt depletion, however, plasma ADH concentrations remain constant or even slightly elevated in spite of a fall in plasma osmolality. Hypovolemia in this situation appears to dominate ADH secretory control.

Thirst mechanisms also involve interactions between extracellular fluid volume and osmolality. During periods of dehydration, increased plasma osmolality provides approximately 70% of the increased thirst drive, and the remaining 30% is due to hypovolemia. In salt depletion, the situation is less clear, but the normal or increased drinking that has been observed in experimental animals has been attributed to the associated hypovolemia.

Other factors that affect circulating ADH levels include nausea, pain, and surgery, all of which stimulate ADH secretion. Pregnancy is associated with a reduction in the osmoregulatory threshold for ADH release.

DIABETES INSIPIDUS

Diabetes insipidus is a disorder resulting from deficient ADH action and is characterized by the passage of copious amounts of very dilute urine. This disorder must be distinguished from other polyuric states such as primary polydipsia (see below) and osmotic diuresis. Central (or neurogenic) diabetes insipidus is due to failure of the posterior pituitary to secrete adequate quantities of ADH; nephrogenic diabetes insipidus results when the kidney fails to respond to circulating ADH. The resulting renal concentrating defect leads to the loss of large volumes of dilute urine, ie, free water. This causes cellular and extracellular dehydration, which stimulate thirst and cause polydipsia.

Classification

A. Central Diabetes Insipidus

The major causes of central diabetes insipidus are shown in Table 5–16.

Many of the disorders discussed above in the section on pituitary and hypothalamic disorders which cause hypopituitarism may also cause diabetes insipidus. Primary pituitary adenomas—even those which are large—rarely cause diabetes insipidus, but hypothalamic tumors such as craniopharyngiomas or other primary central nervous system lesions and infiltrative and invasive lesions cause diabetes insipidus more frequently. These lesions cause diabetes insipidus by damage to the pituitary stalk, which interrupts the hypothalamic-neurohypophysial nerve tracts, or by direct

Table 5–16. Causes of central diabetes insipidus.

Hypophysectomy, complete or partial
Surgery to remove suprasellar tumors
Idiopathic
Familial
Tumors and cysts (intra- and suprasellar)
Histiocytosis
Granulomas
Infections
Interruption of blood supply
Autoimmune

damage to the hypothalamic neurons that synthesize ADH. These disorders cause varying degrees of ADH deficiency.

Diabetes insipidus can also be caused by trauma and is common following surgery for hypothalamic or pituitary tumors. Central diabetes insipidus resulting from head trauma frequently follows a triphasic course. The initial phase is followed by a phase of antidiuresis (as ADH is released from damaged axons) and then by persistent diabetes insipidus. How complete the diabetes insipidus is depends upon the extent of the damage. Resection of hypothalamic tumors via craniotomy frequently results in permanent diabetes insipidus, which may be complicated by disorders of thirst. Transsphenoidal pituitary microsurgery causes transient postoperative diabetes insipidus in as many as 20% of patients; however, the diabetes insipidus lasts only a few days and rarely longer than 2–3 weeks.

Familial central diabetes insipidus, which is inherited in both recessive or dominant patterns, is rare and has its onset in infancy. The number of ADH-containing fibers in the supraoptic and paraventricular nuclei, nerve tracts, and posterior pituitary is reduced. Idiopathic diabetes insipidus presents in later childhood or adolescence and in adulthood. It is also associated with a decrease in the number of ADH-containing fibers. As many as 30–40% of these patients have antibodies directed against ADH-secreting hypothalamic neurons. The "posterior pituitary bright spot," which is normally visualized by MRI, is absent in patients with familial or idiopathic diabetes insipidus. An autosomal dominant form of central diabetes insipidus occurs in association with diabetes mellitus, optic atrophy, and deafness (DIDMOAD; Wolfram's syndrome). Diabetes insipidus due to enzymatic destruction of circulating ADH by increased plasma levels of vasopressinase may occur during pregnancy.

B. Nephrogenic Diabetes Insipidus

This group of diseases (Table 5–17) is caused by renal unresponsiveness to the physiologic actions of ADH; thus, ADH levels are normal or elevated. Chronic renal diseases, particularly those affecting the medulla and collecting ducts, can cause nephrogenic diabetes insipidus. Thus, if medullary disease (eg, from pyelonephritis, polycystic disease or medullary cystic disease) prevents formation of a medullary concentration gradient, and urine passing through the collecting duct system cannot become concentrated.

The electrolyte disorders hypokalemia and hypercalcemia reduce urinary concentrating capacity. Many drugs have been implicated in the development of nephrogenic diabetes insipidus. For example, lithium carbonate reduces the sensitivity of the renal tubule to ADH by reducing V_2 receptor density or aquaporin-2

Table 5–17. Causes of nephrogenic diabetes insipidus.

Chronic renal disease: Any renal disease that interferes with collecting duct or medullary function, eg, chronic pyelonephritis
Hypokalemia
Protein starvation
Hypercalcemia
Sickle cell anemia
Sjögren's syndrome
Drugs, eg, lithium, fluoride, methoxyflurane anesthesia, demeclocycline, colchicine, foscarnet, cidofovir
Congenital defect
Familial

---

expression. The ability of demeclocycline to cause nephrogenic diabetes insipidus has been used to advantage in the management of states of ADH excess (see below). Hereditary nephrogenic diabetes insipidus is a rare condition caused by a defect in the response of the renal tubule to ADH, one type is associated with defects in the V_2 receptor gene, which leads to impairment of medullary adenylyl cyclase activity. It is most common in males with a family history of transmission through apparently healthy females, suggesting X-linked inheritance. However, several cases have recently been reported in females. Another form of nephrogenic diabetes insipidus involves a postreceptor defect with abnormalities of the aquaporin-2 gene.

Primary Polydipsia

Primary polydipsia (psychogenic polydipsia, compulsive water drinking) is a disorder of thirst that is either due to psychogenic causes or to altered osmotic and nonosmotic regulation of thirst. It involves greatly increased drinking, usually in excess of 5 L of water per day, leading to dilution of the extracellular fluid, inhibition of vasopressin secretion, and water diuresis.

Differential Diagnosis

It is important to distinguish both types of diabetes insipidus and primary polydipsia from other common causes of polyuria. In general, other forms of polyuria involve osmotic or solute diuresis. For example, in diabetes mellitus, increased excretion of glucose and other solutes requires excretion of increased volumes of water. In osmotic diuresis, the osmolality of the urine tends toward that of plasma. In sharp contrast, the osmolality of the urine in diabetes insipidus and psychogenic polydipsia is very low when compared with that of plasma. Thus, a urine specific gravity less than 1.005 (osmolality < 200 mosm/kg of water) will generally rule out polyuria due to osmotic diuresis. After a careful history has been taken, focusing on patterns of drinking and urination behavior and the family history, a series of investigations should be instituted to distinguish between the two types of diabetes insipidus and primary polydipsia. For unknown reasons patients with idiopathic central diabetes insipidus have a predilection for cold beverages. The physiologic principles are set forth in Table 5–18, and the actual procedures are summarized in Table 5–19.

A. PLASMA AND URINE OSMOLALITY

The first test involves simultaneous estimation of osmolality and sodium in plasma and urine. Since in both forms of diabetes insipidus the primary problem is inappropriate water diuresis, the urine will be less concentrated than plasma, whereas the plasma osmolality may be higher than normal depending upon the state of hydration. In primary polydipsia, however, dilute plasma and hyponatremia are usually associated with the production of dilute urine. The poor sensitivity of these randomly drawn levels necessitates dynamic testing.

Table 5–18. Results of diagnostic studies in various types of polyuria.

	Neurogenic Diabetes Insipidus	Nephrogenic Diabetes Insipidus	Psychogenic Polydipsia
Random plasma osmolality	↑	↑	↓
Random urine osmolality	↓	↓	↓
Urine osmolality during mild water deprivation	No change	No change	↑
Urine osmolality during nicotine or hypertonic saline	No change	No change	↑
Urine osmolality following vasopressin intravenously	↑	No change	↑
Plasma vasopressin	Low	Normal or high	Low

Table 5–19. Differential diagnosis of polyuria.

Procedure	Interpretation
Measure plasma and urine osmolality.	A urine osmolality less than that of plasma is consistent with neurogenic or nephrogenic diabetes insipidus; if both urine and plasma are dilute, that is consistent with psychogenic polydipsia.
Dehydration test: If serum osmolality is less than 295 mosm/kg, allow no fluids for 12–18 hours. Measure body weight, urine flow, urine specific gravity, urine and plasma osmolality every 2 hours. Terminate study if body weight falls more than 3%.	A rise in urine osmolality above that of plasma osmolality indicates psychogenic polydipsia. Urine specific gravity less than 1.005 (or 200 mosm/L) indicates either neurogenic or nephrogenic diabetes insipidus.
Measure serum vasopressin at conclusion of dehydration test.	Normal or high vasopressin level usually indicates nephrogenic diabetes insipidus.
Inject 5 units of aqueous vasopressin or 1 μg vasopressin subcutaneously. Measure urine flow and urine and plasma osmolality.	Rise in urine osmolality above that of plasma osmolality indicates neurogenic diabetes insipidus; failure of urine osmolality to rise indicates nephrogenic diabetes insipidus.

Occasionally, even the tests outlined below do not produce a definitive diagnosis, so that a therapeutic trial of desmopressin may be warranted.

B. WATER DEPRIVATION

The next step is to examine the effect of water deprivation on urine osmolality under supervision. Supervision is necessary both because the patient with primary polydipsia will go to great lengths to obtain water and because the patient with complete diabetes insipidus may become dangerously dehydrated very rapidly. The patient should be weighed and denied access to water and each voided urine sample measured for specific gravity or osmolality (or both). Whereas the healthy individual will soon reduce urine flow to 0.5 mL/min at a concentration greater than that of plasma, the patient with complete diabetes insipidus will maintain a high urine flow at a specific gravity less than 1.005 (200 mosm/kg of water). The test is continued until urinary osmolality plateaus (an hourly increase of < 30 mosm/kg for 3 successive hours). A period of 18 hours is usually ample to

confirm the diagnosis. The test should be terminated if the body weight falls by more than 3%, since serious consequences of dehydration may ensue. Patients with primary polydipsia will always increase urine osmolality to values greater than those of plasma. However, it may be difficult to distinguish these patients from patients with partial central diabetes insipidus.

C. VASOPRESSIN TEST

Once the diagnosis of diabetes insipidus is established, the ADH-insensitive (nephrogenic) disease must be distinguished from the ADH-sensitive (central) form. This is done following water deprivation by injection of aqueous vasopressin or desmopressin acetate. Give 5 units of aqueous vasopressin subcutaneously or 1 μg of desmopressin acetate intravenously, intramuscularly, or subcutaneously, and measure urine osmolality after 1 hour; patients with complete central diabetes insipidus will show an increase of > 50% in urine osmolality, while patients with nephrogenic diabetes insipidus do not respond. Patients with partial central diabetes insipidus show increases of 10–50% after vasopressin administration, whereas patients with primary polydipsia have responses of < 9%. In these cases, measurement of ADH levels is particularly helpful.

D. ADH RADIOIMMUNOASSAYS

Sensitive radioimmunoassays for ADH are available. Random plasma samples are of little value; levels should be measured as part of dynamic testing, either during water deprivation test or with infusions of hyperosmotic saline. Plasma levels should be interpreted based upon nomograms of their relationship to plasma osmolality. Patients with nephrogenic diabetes insipidus have normal or increased levels of vasopressin following water deprivation, allowing a clear distinction to be made from central forms of diabetes insipidus (Figure 5–24). Patients with partial central diabetes insipidus show a smaller than normal increase in plasma vasopressin concentration following dehydration or infusion of hypertonic saline.

Treatment

A. CENTRAL DIABETES INSIPIDUS

Desmopressin acetate, a synthetic analog of vasopressin prepared in aqueous solution containing 100 μg/mL, is administered intranasally as a metered-dose nasal spray that delivers 10 μg (0.1 mL) per spray or via a calibrated plastic catheter in doses of 5–20 μg (0.05–0.2 mL). The frequency of administration varies; patients with mild to moderate diabetes insipidus require one or two doses of 10 μg per 24 hours; Patients with severe diabetes insipidus may require 10–20 μg two or three

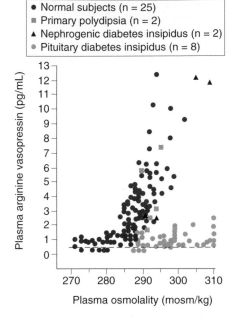

- ● Normal subjects (n = 25)
- ■ Primary polydipsia (n = 2)
- ▲ Nephrogenic diabetes insipidus (n = 2)
- ● Pituitary diabetes insipidus (n = 8)

Figure 5–24. Effect of dehydration on plasma vasopressin concentration in normal subjects and patients with polyuria. Note that patients with neurogenic (pituitary) diabetes insipidus cannot increase plasma vasopressin concentration with dehydration, in contrast to patients with psychogenic polydipsia and nephrogenic diabetes insipidus. (Reproduced, with permission, from Robertson GL et al: J Clin Invest 1973;52:2346.)

times daily. This agent provides excellent control of polyuria and polydipsia in patients with central diabetes insipidus. Serum osmolality and sodium must be monitored at regular intervals (initially every 1–2 weeks, later every 3 months) to be certain that the dose is appropriate. For patients who cannot tolerate intranasal therapy, desmopressin acetate can be given subcutaneously in single doses of 1–2 μg once or twice daily.

More recently, desmopressin acetate has become available in an oral form as tablets containing 0.1 or 0.2 mg. The usual dose ranges from 0.1 mg twice daily to 0.2 mg three times daily. However, many patients do not find this preparation as effective as the nasal spray.

B. Nephrogenic Diabetes Insipidus

The underlying disorder should be treated if possible. It is important to recognize familial disease early, since infants are particularly susceptible to neurologic damage due to dehydration. Diuretics are helpful, along with dietary salt restriction if necessary. Prostaglandin synthesis inhibitors may also be useful. The objective is to maintain the patient in a state of mild sodium depletion and reduce the solute load on the kidney, thus enhancing proximal tubular reabsorption. Reduction in distal tubular flow allows some sodium concentration to take place and minimizes loss of water. Patients with partial sensitivity to vasopressin may be treated with large doses of desmopressin acetate (up to 40 μg/4 h intranasally).

SYNDROME OF INAPPROPRIATE SECRETION OF ANTIDIURETIC HORMONE (SIADH)

A variety of disorders are associated with plasma ADH concentrations that are inappropriately high for the plasma osmolality. Thus, water retention accompanies normal water intake, leading to hyponatremia and hypo-osmolality. The urine is usually more concentrated than plasma but in any case is inappropriately concentrated. Overall sodium balance is essentially normal. It is important to rule out renal and endocrine disorders and drug effects that diminish the kidney's capacity to dilute the urine. The syndrome is termed the syndrome of inappropriate secretion of antidiuretic hormone, or SIADH. The clinical picture can be produced experimentally by giving high doses of vasopressin to a healthy subject receiving normal to high fluid intake. Water restriction in patients suspected of having SIADH will result in plasma osmolality and sodium concentration returning to normal.

The diagnostic criteria for SIADH include (1) hyponatremia with corresponding plasma hypo-osmolality (< 280 mosm/kg); (2) urine less than maximally dilute, ie, inappropriately concentrated (> 100 mosm/kg); (3) euvolemia (including absence of congestive heart failure, cirrhosis, and nephrotic syndrome); and (4) absence of renal, adrenal or thyroid insufficiency. Urinary sodium is usually > 20 mmol/d, probably a consequence of increased atrial natriuretic factor. Dynamic testing and plasma ADH levels are usually unnecessary in diagnosis.

Causes of SIADH

The causes of SIADH are outlined in Table 5–20. A number of malignant neoplasms are associated with ectopic production of vasopressin, leading to high plasma vasopressin levels. Bronchogenic carcinomas are particularly apt to be associated with SIADH. Tumors at other sites such as the pancreas and duodenum have also been shown to produce vasopressin. A number of nonmalignant pulmonary diseases such as tuberculosis and pneumonias are associated with high plasma vasopressin concentrations. Tuberculous lung tissue has

Table 5–20. Conditions associated with SIADH.

Malignant lung disease, particularly bronchogenic carcinoma
Nonmalignant lung disease, eg, tuberculosis
Tumors at other sites (especially lymphoma, sarcoma), eg,
   duodenum, pancreas, brain, prostate, thymus
Central nervous system trauma and infections
Drugs that stimulate vasopressin release, eg, clofibrate,
   chlorpropamide, and other drugs such as thiazides, carba-
   mazepine, phenothiazines, vincristine, cyclophosphamide
   SSRIs (eg, fluoxetine, sertraline)
Endocrine diseases: adrenal insufficiency, myxedema, anterior
   pituitary insufficiency
HIV infection

---

been shown to contain assayable levels of vasopressin. However, it is not known whether all types of lung disease causing SIADH do so by producing ectopic vasopressin or by stimulation of pituitary vasopressin.

Many central nervous system disorders are associated with increased vasopressin secretion, leading to the clinical picture of SIADH. Temporary causes of SIADH include surgical trauma, anesthesia, pain, opiates and anxiety. A number of drugs implicated in vasopressin release are listed in Table 5–20. Endocrine disorders such as adrenal insufficiency, myxedema, and anterior pituitary insufficiency may be associated with increased ADH levels and impaired renal excretion of free water. All of these factors—particularly with fluid loading—can lead to hyponatremia and hypo-osmolality. In fact, the majority of hospitalized patients with euvolemic hyponatremia have inappropriately increased ADH levels. The hyponatremia observed in patients with psychosis may reflect a combination of several factors, including inappropriate ADH release and compulsive water drinking.

Types of Osmoregulatory Defects

Serial measurements of serum ADH in patients with SIADH delineate four patterns of osmoregulatory defects in this syndrome. Type A, found in 20% of patients, is characterized by large irregular changes in plasma ADH completely unrelated to serum osmolality. This erratic and irregular secretion of ADH can be associated with both malignant and nonmalignant disease. Type B is found in about 35% of patients and is associated with secretion of ADH that is excessive but proportionate to osmolality. In these patients, the osmotic control of ADH secretion appears to be either set at a low level or abnormally sensitive to changes in serum osmolality. Type C, found in 35% of patients, is

characterized by a high basal level of ADH that rises even higher with a rise in serum osmolality. Type D, found in only 10% of patients, represents a different type of problem. ADH is normally suppressed in hypovolemic states and rises normally with increase in osmolality. Thus, the SIADH in these patients may be associated with a change in renal sensitivity to serum arginine vasopressin.

Treatment

The treatment of SIADH depends upon the underlying cause. A patient with drug-induced SIADH is treated by withholding the drug. The treatment of SIADH in a patient with bronchogenic carcinoma is more complicated, however, and the prognosis is poor. Treatment aims to return plasma osmolality to normal without causing further expansion of the extracellular fluid compartment, as would occur following infusion of hyperosmotic solutions.

A. FLUID RESTRICTION

The simplest form of treatment is fluid restriction, although in the long term the excessive thirst associated with this treatment may be difficult to manage.

B. DIURETICS

If plasma osmolality is low and rapid correction is required, loop diuretics such as furosemide can be employed. These agents limit free water generation in the loop of Henle and reduce the concentration gradient in the renal medulla, thereby decreasing the effectiveness of vasopressin. Because diuresis is accompanied by significant urinary losses of potassium, calcium, and magnesium, these electrolytes should be replaced by intravenous infusion.

C. OTHER METHODS

In an emergency situation with severe hyponatremia, hypertonic saline, ie, 3% saline, administered intravenously at a rate of 0.1 mL/kg/min, will increase plasma sodium and osmolarity. However, this must be done with caution, since fluid overload may precipitate heart failure or circulatory collapse, and overly rapid correction may lead to central pontine myelinolysis. Drugs (mentioned earlier in this chapter) that reduce the effect of vasopressin on the kidney may be useful. Demeclocycline, 1–2 g/d orally, causes a reversible form of nephrogenic diabetes insipidus, countering the effect of SIADH. However, it is nephrotoxic, and renal function (blood urea nitrogen and serum creatinine) must be monitored carefully. Lithium carbonate has a similar effect, but therapeutic doses are so close to the toxic dose that this drug is rarely useful.

REFERENCES

General

Frohman LA: Disorders of the anterior pituitary. In: *Endocrinology and Metabolism,* 3rd ed. Felig P, Baxter JD, Frohman LA (editors). McGraw-Hill, 1995.

Kacsoh B: *Endocrine Physiology.* McGraw-Hill, 2000.

Krisht AF, Tindall GT: *Pituitary Disorders: Comprehensive Management.* Lippincott Williams & Wilkins, 1999.

Melmed S (editor): *The Pituitary.* Blackwell, 1995.

Molitch ME: Neuroendocrinology. In: *Endocrinology and Metabolism,* 3rd ed. Felig P, Baxter JD, Frohman LA (editors). McGraw-Hill, 1995.

Reeves WB, Bichet DG, Andreoli TE: The posterior pituitary and water metabolism. In: *Williams Textbook of Endocrinology,* 9th ed. Wilson JD et al (editors). Saunders, 1998.

Robertson GL: Posterior pituitary. In: *Endocrinology and Metabolism,* 3rd ed. Felig P, Baxter JD, Frohman LA (editors). McGraw-Hill, 1995.

Robertson GL: The endocrine brain and pituitary gland. In: *Principles and Practice of Endocrinology and Metabolism,* 2nd ed. Becker KL (editor). Lippincott, 1995.

Thorner MO et al: The anterior pituitary. In: *Williams Textbook of Endocrinology,* 9th ed. Wilson JD et al (editors). Saunders, 1998.

Neuroendocrinology

Anderson JR et al: Neurology of the pituitary gland. J Neurol Neurosurg Psychiatry 1999;66:703.

Arzt E et al: Pathophysiological role of the cytokine network in the anterior pituitary gland. Front Neuroendocrinol 1999;20:71.

Arzt E: gp 130 cytokine signaling in the pituitary gland: a paradigm for cytokine-neuro-endocrine pathways. J Clin Invest 2001; 108;1729. [PMID: 11748253]

Asteria C: T-box and isolated ACTH deficiency. Eur J Endocrinol 2002;146:463. [PMID: 11916612]

Barb CR: The brain-pituitary-adipocyte axis: role of leptin in modulating neuroendocrine function. J Anim Sci 1999;77:1249. [PMID: 10340594]

Behan DP et al: Corticotropin-releasing factor-binding protein: A putative peripheral and central modulator of the CRF family of neuropeptides. Ann N Y Acad Sci 1993;697:1.

Ben-Jonathan N, Hnasko R: Dopamine as a prolactin (PRL) inhibitor. Endocr Rev 2001;22:724. [PMID: 11739329]

Brzezinski A: Melatonin in humans. N Engl J Med 1997;336:186. [PMID: 8988899]

Burgess R, Lunyak V, Rosenfeld MG: Signaling and transcriptional control of pituitary development. Curr Opin Gene Develop 2002;12:534. [PMID: 12200158]

Burrows HL et al: Genealogy of the anterior pituitary gland: tracing a family tree. Trends Endocrinol Metab 1999;10:343.

Castro MG, Southgate T, Lowenstein PR: Molecular therapy in a model neuroendocrine disease: developing clinical gene therapy for pituitary tumours. Trends Endocrinol Metab 2001; 12:58. [PMID: 11167123]

Chen C: Growth hormone secretagogue actions on the pituitary gland: multiple receptors for multiple ligands? Clin Exp Pharmacol Physiol 2000;27:323. [PMID: 10831231]

Chesnokova V, Malmed S: Minireview: Neuro-immuno-endocrine modulation of the hypothalamic-pituitary-adrenal (HPA) axis by gp 130 signaling molecules. Endocrinology 2002;143: 1571. [PMID: 11956136]

Chrousos GP: The hypothalamic-pituitary-adrenal axis and immune-mediated inflammation. N Engl J Med 1995;322: 1351.

Clark RG, Robinson ICAF: Up and down the growth hormone cascade. Cytokine Growth Factor Rev 1996;7:65.

Davies T, Marians R, Latif R: The TSH receptor reveals itself. J Clin Invest 2002;110:209. [PMID: 12122107]

Devesa S, Lima L, Tresguerres JAF: Neuroendocrine control of growth hormone secretion. Trends Endocrinol Metab 1992; 3:175.

Dubois PM, El Amraoui A: Embryology of the pituitary gland. Trends Endocrinol Metab 1995;6:1.

Fauquier T et al: Hidden face of the anterior pituitary. Trends Endocrinol Metab 2002;13:304. [PMID: 12163233]

Frohman LA, Kineman RD: Growth hormone-releasing hormone and pituitary development, hyperplasia and tumorigenesis. Trends Endocrinol Metab 2002;13:299. [PMID: 12163232]

Gelato MC: Growth hormone-releasing hormone: Clinical perspectives. Endocrinologist 1994;4:64.

Haugen BR, Ridgway EC: Transcription factor Pit-1 and its clinical implications: From bench to bedside. Endocrinologist 1995;5:132.

Hindmarsh PC, Swift PG: An assessment of growth hormone provocation tests. Arch Dis Child 1995;72:362.

Huhtaniemi IT: The role of mutations affecting gonadotrophin secretion and action in disorders of pubertal development. Best Pract Res Clin Endocrinol Metab 2002;16:123. [PMID: 11987903]

Jansson C et al: Growth hormone (GH) assays: influence of standard preparations, GH isoforms, assay characteristics, and GH-binding protein. Clin Chem 1997;43:950.

Kojima M et al: Ghrelin: discovery of the natural endogenous ligand for the growth hormone secretagogue receptor. Trends Endocrinol Metab 2001;12:118. [PMID: 11306336]

Le Roith D et al: The somatomedin hypothesis. Endocr Rev 2001; 22:53. [PMID: 11159816]

Lowry PJ: The corticotropin-releasing factor-binding protein: From artifact to new ligand(s) and axis. J Endocrinol 1995;144:1.

Moller M, Baeres FM: The anatomy and innervation of the mammalian pineal gland. Cell Tissue Res 2002;309:139. [PMID: 12111544]

Muccioli G et al: Neuroendocrine and peripheral activities of ghrelin: implications in metabolism and obesity. Eur J Pharmacol 2002;440:235. [PMID: 12007539]

Nakazato M et al: A role for ghrelin in the central regulation of feeding. Nature 2001;409:194. [PMID: 11196643]

Orth DN: Corticotropin-releasing hormone in humans. Endocr Rev 1992;13:164.

Perez FM, Rose IC, Schwartz J: Anterior pituitary cells: Getting to know their neighbors. Mol Cell Endocrinol 1995;111:C1.

Reyes-Fuentes A, Velduis JD: Neuroendocrine physiology of the normal male gonadal axis. Endocrinol Metab Clin North Am 1993;22:93.

Richard D, Lin Q, Timofeeva E: The corticotropin-releasing factor family of peptides and CRF receptors: their roles in the regulation of energy balance. Eur J Pharmacol 2002;12:189. [PMID: 12007535]

Savino W et al: Immunoneuroendocrine connectivity: the paradigm of the thymus-hypothalamus/pituitary axis. Neuroimmunomodulation 1999;6:126.

Sheng HZ, Westphal H: Early steps in pituitary organogenesis. Trends Genet 1999;15:236.

Shupnik MA: Thyroid hormone suppression of pituitary hormone gene expression. Rev Endocr Metab Disord 2000;1:35. [PMID: 11704990]

Pituitary Function Testing and Neuroradiology

Aron DC: Hormone screening in the patients with an incidentally discovered pituitary mass: Current practice and factors in clinical decision making. Endocrinologist 1995;5:357.

Chong BW et al: Pituitary gland MR: A comparative study of healthy volunteers and patients with microadenomas. Am J Neuroradiol 1994;15:675.

Cianfarani S et al: Is IGF binding protein-3 assessment helpful in the diagnosis of GH deficiency? Clin Endocrinol (Oxf) 1995;43:43.

Clark PM et al: Defining the normal cortisol response to the short Synacthen test: implications for the investigation of hypothalamic-pituitary disorders. Clin Endocrinol (Oxf) 1998;49:287.

Elster AD: Modern imaging of the pituitary. Radiology 1993;187:1.

Hall WA et al: Pituitary magnetic resonance imaging in normal human volunteers: occult adenomas in the general population. Ann Intern Med 1994;121:817.

Naidich MJ et al: Current approaches to imaging of the sellar region and pituitary. Endocrinol Metab Clin North Am 1999;28:45.

Oelkers W: Comparison of low- and high-dose corticotropin stimulation tests in patients with pituitary disease. J Clin Endocrinol Metab 1998;83:4532.

Tordjman K et at: The role of the low dose (1 μg) adrenocorticotropin test in the evaluation of patients with pituitary disease. J Clin Endocrinol Metab 1995;80:1301.

Pituitary Adenomas: General

Aron DC (editor): Incidentaloma. Endocrinol Metab Clin North Am 2000;29:1.

Asa SL, Ezzat S: The cytogenesis and pathogenesis of pituitary adenomas. Endocr Rev 1998;19:798.

Asa SL: The pathology of pituitary tumors. Endocrinol Metab Clin North Am 1999;28:13.

Castro MG: Gene therapy strategies for the treatment of pituitary tumours. J Mol Endocrinol 1999;22:9.

Clayton RN, Wass JA: Pituitary tumours: recommendations for service provision and guidelines for management of patients. Committee on Endocrinology of the Royal College of Physicians and the Society for Endocrinology, and the Research Unit of the Royal College of Physicians. Eye 1998;12:7.

Donovan LE, Corenblum B: The natural history of the pituitary incidentaloma. Arch Intern Med 1995;155:181.

Fagin JA (editor): Pituitary tumors. Baillieres Clin Endocrinol Metab 1995;9:203.

Farrell WE, Clayton RN: Molecular biology of human pituitary adenomas. Ann Med 1998;30:192.

Farrell WE, Clayton RN: Molecular genetics of pituitary tumours. Trends Endocrinol Metab 1998;9:20.

Freda PU et al: Differential diagnosis of sellar masses. Endocrinol Metab Clin North Am 1999;28:81.

Jackson IM et al: Role of gamma knife therapy in the management of pituitary tumors. Endocrinol Metab Clin North Am 1999;28:133.

King JT Jr, Justice A, Aron DC: Management of incidental pituitary macroadenomas: a cost-effectiveness analysis. J Clin Endocrinol Metab 1997;82:3625.

Kwekkeboom DJ et al: Receptor imaging in the diagnosis and treatment of pituitary tumors. J Endocrinol Invest 1999;22:80.

Laws ER Jr et al: Pituitary surgery. Endocrinol Metab Clin North Am 1999;28:119.

Melmed S: Pathogenesis of pituitary tumors. Endocrinol Metab Clin North Am 1999;28:1.

Mindermann T, Wilson CB: Pediatric pituitary adenomas. Neurosurgery 1995;36:259.

Molitch ME (editor): Advances in diagnosis and treatment of pituitary disease. Endocrinol Metab Clin North Am 1999;28:1.

Molitch ME: Evaluation and treatment of the patient with a pituitary incidentaloma. J Clin Endocrinol Metab 1995;80:3.

Nammour GM et al: Incidental pituitary macroadenomas: a population based study. Am J Med Sci 1997;314:287.

Russell EI, Molitch ME: The pituitary incidentaloma. Ann Intern Med 1990;112:925.

Shimon I et al: Management of pituitary tumors. Ann Intern Med 1998;129:472.

ACTH: Cushing's Disease

Aron DC, Tyrrell JB (editors): Cushing's syndrome. Endocrinol Metab Clin North Am 1994;23:451,925.

Bochicchio D, Losa M, Buchfelder M: Factors influencing the immediate and late outcome of Cushing's disease treated by transsphenoidal surgery: a retrospective study by the European Cushing's Disease Survey Study Group. J Clin Endocrinol Metab 1995;80:3114.

Carney IA, Young WF Jr: Primary pigmented nodular adrenal hyperplasia and its associated conditions. Endocrinologist 1992;2:6.

Dahia PL et al: The molecular pathogenesis of corticotroph tumors. Endocr Rev 1999;20:136.

Danese RD, Aron DC: Principles of epidemiology and their application to the diagnosis of Cushing's syndrome: Rev. Bayes meets Dr. Cushing. Endocrinologist 1994;5:339.

Extabe S, Vazquez IA: Morbidity and mortality in Cushing's disease: An epidemiological approach. Clin Endocrinol (Oxf) 1994;40:479.

Findling JW et al: Newer diagnostic techniques and problems in Cushing's disease. Endocrinol Metab Clin North Am 1999; 28:191.

Helseth A et al: Transgenic mice that develop pituitary tumors: A model for Cushing's disease. Am J Pathol 1992;140:1071.

Lebrethon MC et al: Food-dependent Cushing's syndrome: characterization and functional role of gastric inhibitory polypeptide receptor in the adrenals of three patients. J Clin Endocrinol Metab 1998;83:4515.

Magiakow MA et al: Cushing's syndrome in children and adolescents. N Engl J Med 1994;331:752.

McCane DR el al: Assessment of endocrine function after transsphenoidal surgery for Cushing's disease. Clin Endocrinol (Oxf) 1993;38:79.

Newell-Price J et al: The diagnosis and differential diagnosis of Cushing's syndrome and pseudo-Cushing's states. Endocr Rev 1998;19:647.

Oldfield EH et al: Petrosal sinus sampling with and without corticotropin-releasing hormone for the differential diagnosis of Cushing's syndrome. N Engl J Med 1991;325:897.

Orth DN: Cushing's syndrome. N Engl J Med 1995;332:791.

Raff H, Raff JL, Findling JW: Late-night salivary cortisol as a screening test for Cushing's syndrome. J Clin Endocrinol Metab 1998;83:2681.

Sonino N et al: Medical therapy for Cushing's disease. Endocrinol Metab Clin North Am 1999;28:211.

Stenzel-Poore MP et al: Development of Cushing's syndrome in corticotropin-releasing factor transgenic mice. Endocrinology 1992;130:3378.

Tsigos C, Chrousos OP: Clinical presentation, diagnosis, and treatment of Cushing's syndrome. Curr Opin Endocrinol Diabetes 1995;2:203.

Wajchenberg BL et al: Ectopic adrenocorticotropic hormone syndrome. Endocr Rev 1994;15:752.

Growth Hormone: Acromegaly

Barzilay J, Heatley GJ, Cushing GW: Benign and malignant tumors in patients with acromegaly. Arch Intern Med 1991; 151:1629.

Corpas B, Harman SM, Blackman MR: Human growth hormone and human aging. Endocr Rev 1993;14:20.

de Boer H, Blok GJ, Van der Veen EA: Clinical aspects of growth hormone deficiency in adults. Endocr Rev 1995;16:63.

Ezzat S et al: Octreotide treatment of acromegaly: A randomized multicenter study. Ann Intern Med 1992;117:711.

Fradkin JE: Creutzfeldt-Jakob disease in pituitary growth hormone recipients. Endocrinologist 1993;3:108.

Freda PU et al: Evaluations of disease status with sensitive measures of growth hormone secretion in 60 postoperative patients with acromegaly. J Clin Endocrinol Metab 1998;83:3808.

Ho KY at al: Therapeutic efficacy of the somatostatin analog SMS 2O1-995 (octreotide) in acromegaly: Effects of dose and frequency and long-term safety. Ann Intern Med 1990;112:173.

Melmed S (editor): Acromegaly. Endocrinol Metab Clin North Am 1992;21:483.

Melmed S et al: Clinical Review 75: Recent advances in pathogenesis, diagnosis and management of acromegaly. J Clin Endocrinol Metab 1995;80:3395.

Melmed S et al: Current treatment guidelines for acromegaly. J Clin Endocrinol Metab 1998;83:2646.

Newman CB: Medical therapy for acromegaly. Endocrinol Metab Clin North Am 1999;28:171.

Sacca L, Cittadini A, Fazio S: Growth hormone and the heart. Endocr Rev 1994;15:555.

Terzolo M et al: High prevalence of colonic polyps in patients with acromegaly: influence of sex and age. Arch Intern Med 1994; 154:1272.

Vance ML, Harris AG: Long-term treatment of 189 acromegalic patients with the somatostatin analog octreotide: Results of the international multicenter acromegaly study group. Arch Intern Med 1991;151:1573.

PRL: Prolactinoma

Bevan JS et al: Dopamine agonists and pituitary tumor shrinkage. Endocr Rev 1992;13:220.

Biller BMK et al: Progressive trabecular osteopenia in women with hyperprolactinemic amenorrhea. J Clin Endocrinol Metab 1992;75:692.

Colao A et al: Prolactinomas resistant to standard dopamine agonists respond to chronic cabergoline treatment. J Clin Endocrinol Metab 1997;82:876.

Cunnah D, Besser M: Management of prolactinomas. Clin Endocrinol (Oxf) 1991;34:231.

Davis JRE, Shepard MC, Heath DA: Giant invasive prolactinoma: A case report and review of nine further cases. Q J Med 1990;74:227.

Leite V et al: Characterization of big, big prolactin in patients with hyperprolactinemia. Clin Endocrinol (Oxf) 1992;37:365.

Molitch ME: Diagnosis and treatment of prolactinomas. Adv Intern Med 1999;44:117.

Molitch ME: Medical treatment of prolactinomas. Endocrinol Metab Clin North Am 1999;28:143.

Schlecte J, Walkner L, Kathol M: A longitudinal analysis of premenopausal bone loss in healthy women and women with hyperprolactinemia. J Clin Endocrinol Metab 1092;75:698.

Vance ML et al: Treatment of prolactin-secreting pituitary macroadenomas with the long-acting non-ergot dopamine agonist CV 205-502. Ann Intern Med 1990;112:668.

Verhelst J et al: Cabergoline in the treatment of hyperprolactinemia: a study in 455 patients. J Clin Endocrinol Metab 1999; 84:2518.

Webster J et al: Low recurrence rate after partial hypophysectomy for prolactinoma: The predictive value of dynamic prolactin function tests. Clin Endocrinol (Oxf) 1992;36:35.

Gonadotropins (LH/FSH): Gonadotropin-Secreting Pituitary Tumors

Daneshdoost L et al: Identification of gonadotroph adenomas in men with clinically nonfunctioning adenomas by the luteinizing hormone subunit response to thyrotropin-releasing hormone. J Clin Endocrinol Metab 1993;77:1352.

Daneshdoost L et al: Recognition of gonadotroph adenomas in women. N Engl J Med 1991;324:589.

Katznelson L, Alexander IM, Klibanski A: Clinically nonfunctioning pituitary adenomas. J Clin Endocrinol Metab 1993; 76:1089.

Nobels FRE et al: A comparison between the diagnostic value of gonadotropins, alpha-subunit, and chromogranin-A and their response to thyrotropin-releasing hormone in clinically non-functioning, alpha-subunit secreting, and gonadotroph pituitary adenomas. J Clin Endocrinol Metab 1993;77:784.

Oppenheim OS et al: Prevalence of α-subunit hypersecretion in patients with pituitary tumors: Clinically non-functioning and somatotroph adenomas. J Clin Endocrinol Metab 1990;70:859.

Shomali ME et al: Medical therapy for gonadotroph and thyrotroph tumors. Endocrinol Metab Clin North Am 1999;28:223.

Snyder PJ: Extensive personal experience: gonadotroph adenomas. J Clin Endocrinol Metab 1995;80:1059.

Wilson CB: Endocrine-inactive pituitary adenomas. Clin Neurosurg 1992;38:10.

Young WF et al: Gonadotroph-secreting adenoma of the pituitary gland. Mayo Clin Proc 1996;71:649.

TSH-Secreting Pituitary Tumors

Beck-Peccoz P et al: Thyrotropin-secreting pituitary tumors. Endocr Rev 1996;17:610.

Brucker-Davis F et al: Thyrotropin-secreting pituitary tumors: diagnostic criteria, thyroid hormone sensitivity, and treatment outcome in 25 patients followed at the National Institutes of Health. J Clin Endocrinol Metab 1999;84:476.

Shomali ME et al: Medical therapy for gonadotroph and thyrotroph tumors. Endocrinol Metab Clin North Am 1999;28:223.

Hypopituitarism & Other Hypothalamic-Pituitary Disorders

Burman P, Deijen JB: Quality of life and cognitive function in patients with pituitary insufficiency. Psychother Psychosom 1998;67:154.

Cacciari E et al: Empty sella in children and adolescents with possible hypothalamic-pituitary disorders. J Clin Endocrinol Metab 1994;78:767.

Cohen LE, Radovick S, Wondisford FE: Transcription factors and hypopituitarism. Trends Endocrinol Metab 1999;10:326.

Consensus guidelines for the diagnosis and treatment of adults with growth hormone deficiency: Summary statement of the Growth Hormone Research Society Workshop on Adult Growth Hormone Deficiency. J Clin Endocrinol Metab 1998;83:379.

Constine LS et al: Hypothalamic-pituitary dysfunction after radiation for brain tumors. N Engl J Med 1993;328:87.

Crowley WF Jr, Jameson IL: Gonadotropin-releasing hormone deficiency: Perspectives from clinical investigation. (Clinical Counterpoint.) Endocr Rev 1992;13:635.

De Boer H, Blok G-J, Van der Veen EA: Clinical aspects of growth hormone deficiency in adults. Endocr Rev 1995;16:63.

Freda PU et al: Hypothalamic-pituitary sarcoidosis. Trends Endocrinol Metab 1992;3:321.

Gallardo B et at: The empty sella: Results of treatment in 76 successive cases and high frequency of endocrine and neurological disturbances. Clin Endocrinol (Oxf) 1992;37:529.

Lamberts SW, de Herder WW, van der Lely AJ: Pituitary insufficiency. Lancet 1998;352:127.

Maccagnan P et al: Conservative management of pituitary apoplexy: A prospective study. J Clin Endocrinol Metab 1995;80:2190.

Powrie JK et al: Lymphocytic adenohypophisitis: Magnetic resonance imaging features of two new cases and a review of the literature. Clin Endocrinol (Oxf) 1995;42:315.

Rolih CA: Ober KP: Pituitary apoplexy. Endocrinol Metab Clin North Am 1993;22:291.

Thodou E et al: Lymphocytic hypophysitis: Clinicopathological findings. J Clin Endocrinol Metab 1995;80:2302.

Vance ML: Hypopituitarism. N Engl J Med 1994;330:1651.

Vance ML, Mauras N: Growth hormone therapy in adults and children. N Engl J Med 1999;341:1206.

Posterior Pituitary

Bankir L: Antidiuretic action of vasopressin: quantitative aspects and interaction between V1a and V2 receptor-mediated effects. Cardiovasc Res 2001;51:372. [PMID: 11476728]

Buonocore CM, Robinson AG: The diagnosis and management of diabetes insipidus during medical emergencies. Endocrinol Metab Clin North Am 1993;22:411.

Kamoi K et al: Hyponatremia and osmoregulation of vasopressin secretion in patients with intracranial bleeding. J Clin Endocrinol Metab 1995;80:2906.

Kim JK et al: Osmotic and non-osmotic regulation of arginine vasopressin (AVP) release, mRNA, and promoter activity in small cell lung carcinoma (SCLC) cells. Mol Cell Endocrinol 1996;123:179.

Lee MD, King LS, Agre P: The aquaporin family of water channel proteins in clinical medicine. Medicine (Baltimore) 1997;76:141.

Maghnie M et al: Correlation between magnetic resonance imaging of posterior pituitary and neurohypophyseal function in children with diabetes insipidus. J Clin Endocrinol Metab 1992;74:795.

Nielsen S et al: Physiology and pathophysiology of renal aquaporins. J Am Soc Nephrol 1999;10:647.

Olson BR et al: Isolated hyponatremia after transsphenoidal pituitary surgery. J Clin Endocrinol Metab 1995;80:85.

Robertson GL: Diabetes insipidus. Endocrinol Metab Clin North Am 1995;24:549.

Saito T et al: Acute aquaresis by the nonpeptide arginine vasopressin (AVP) antagonist OPC-31260 improves hyponatremia in patients with syndrome of inappropriate secretion of antidiuretic hormone (SIADH). J Clin Endocrinol Metab 1997;82:1054.

Stricker EM, Huang W, Sved AF: Early osmoregulatory signals in the control of water intake and neurohypophyseal hormone secretion. Physiol Behav 2002;76:415. [PMID: 12117578]

Tang WW et al: Hyponatremia in hospitalized patients with the acquired immunodeficiency syndrome (AIDS) and the AIDS-related complex. Am J Med 1993;94:169.

Thompson CJ, Edwards CR, Baylis PH: Osmotic and non-osmotic regulation of thirst and vasopressin secretion in patients with compulsive water drinking. Clin Endocrinol (Oxf) 1991;35:221.

Ugrumov MV: Magnocellular vasopressin system in ontogenesis: development and regulation. Microsc Res Tech 2002;56:164. [PMID: 11810719]

Verbalis JG: Hyponatremia: Epidemiology, pathophysiology and therapy. Curr Opin Nephrol Hypertens 1993;2:636.

Growth

6

Dennis Styne, MD

ACTH	Adrenocorticotropic hormone		**IGF-I**	Human insulin-like growth factor 1
BMI	Body mass index		**IGF-II**	Human insulin-like growth factor 2
cAMP	Cyclic adenosine monophosphate		**IGFBP**	Insulin-like growth factor binding protein
CRF	Corticotropin-releasing factor		**IUGR**	Intrauterine growth retardation or restriction
DNA	Deoxyribonucleic acid		**LH**	Luteinizing hormone
EGF	Epidermal growth factor		**LS**	Lower segment
EGF-R	Epidermal growth factor receptor		**NCHS**	National Center for Health Statistics
FGF	Fibroblast growth factor		**PDGF**	Platelet-derived growth factor
FGF-R	Fibroblast growth factor receptor		**PTH**	Parathyroid hormone
GH	Growth hormone		**RTA**	Renal tubular acidosis
GHBP	Growth hormone-binding protein		**RWT**	Roche, Wainer, and Thissen method of height prediction
GHRH	Growth hormone-releasing hormone		**SGA**	Small for gestational age
GHRP	Growth hormone-releasing peptide		**TBG**	Thyroid hormone-binding globulin
GnRH	Gonadotropin-releasing hormone		**TRH**	Thyrotropin-releasing hormone
hCG	Human chorionic gonadotropin		**TSH**	Thyroid-stimulating hormone (thyrotropin)
hCS	Human chorionic somatomammotropin		**US**	Upper segment
hGH	Human growth hormone			
IGF	Human insulin-like growth factor (somatomedin)			

Assessment of growth in stature is an essential part of the pediatric examination. Growth is an important index of physical and mental health and of the quality of the child's psychosocial environment; chronic problems in any of these areas may be reflected in a decreased growth rate. We shall consider influences on normal growth, the normal growth pattern, the measurement of growth, and conditions that lead to disorders of growth.

■ NORMAL GROWTH

INTRAUTERINE GROWTH

The growth of a fetus begins with a single fertilized cell and ends with differentiation into more than 200 cell types, length increasing by 5000-fold, surface area by

6×10^6-fold, and weight by 6×10^{12}-fold. Overall, the growth of the fetus is dependent upon the availability of adequate oxygen and nutrition. It is orchestrated by a group of growth factors, all operating according to a basic genetic plan. This genetic plan is especially important early in gestation, whereas the maternal environment is of more importance late in gestation.

The classic definition of intrauterine growth retardation or intrauterine growth restriction (IUGR) is a birth weight below the fifth percentile or below 2500 g for a term baby in the United States, though some suggest that the designation small-for-gestational-age (SGA) be used for infants born weighing less than the tenth percentile and IUGR be reserved for those lower than the third percentile and/or those with demonstrated decrease of intrauterine growth rate. The term symmetric IUGR indicates that the head as well as the body is small, while asymmetric IUGR indicates that the head is relatively spared from the growth failure;

asymmetric IUGR is more common in the developed world, and symmetric IUGR is more common in the developing world. The former group shows "catch-up growth" more frequently than the latter, but 10–30% of IUGR infants remain short as children and adults, in contrast to appropriate-for-gestational-age premature infants, who are smaller at birth but generally experience catch-up growth in the first 2 years.

THE PLACENTA

The placenta acts as an endocrine organ that influences most aspects of fetal growth, including the supply of adequate nutrition and oxygen and regulation of hormones and growth factors. Aberrant delivery or control of any of these factors will affect fetal growth; placental weight is usually directly related to birth weight.

CLASSIC HORMONES OF GROWTH & FETAL GROWTH

The hormones that mediate postnatal growth do not play the same roles in fetal growth. Growth hormone (GH) is present in very high concentrations in the fetus, in contrast to the limited presence of GH receptors. While this discrepancy suggests limited activity of GH in the fetus, GH does play a role in fetal growth that is reflected in their average birth weight 1 SD below the mean that is found in growth hormone-deficient infants. Infants with Laron's syndrome (GH resistance due to reduced or absent GH receptors) have elevated GH and low serum IGF-I levels; they also have decreased birth length and weight. Thyroid hormone deficiency does not directly affect human birth weight, but prolonged gestation is a feature of congenital hypothyroidism, and this factor will itself increase weight. Placental lactogen exerts no effect on birth size in human beings. However, the concentration of placental growth hormone (from the *GHV* gene) is significantly decreased in the serum of a pregnant woman bearing a fetus with intrauterine growth retardation.

GROWTH FACTORS & ONCOGENES IN FETAL GROWTH

Oncogenes may be responsible for neoplastic growth in postnatal life, but expression of these genes is important in the normal development of many fetal organs. Remarkably, the same oncogenes that cause postnatal neoplasia are prevented from causing tumors in the normally differentiating fetus. For example, a mutation in the von Hippel-Lindau gene predisposes to retinal, cerebellar, and spinal hemangioblastomas, renal cell carcinomas, and pheochromocytomas, but the normal *VHL* gene is expressed in all three germ cell layers of the embryo and in the central nervous system, kidneys, testis, and lung of the fetus, suggesting a role in normal fetal development for this gene.

INSULIN-LIKE GROWTH FACTORS, RECEPTORS, & BINDING PROTEINS

IGF-I in the fetus is regulated by metabolic factors rather than undergoing significant influence by GH, as is the case in postnatal life. One explanation is that there are fewer GH receptors in the fetus than after birth. In the human fetus, serum GH falls during later gestation owing to maturation of central nervous system negative control, while serum IGF-I and IGFBP-3 rise during gestation, demonstrating their independence from GH stimulation. Artificial elevation of maternal IGF-I can increase growth in mouse and rat fetuses and overcome the restraint imposed by uterine limitations of litter size.

Studies of knockout mice, which lack various growth factors or binding proteins, indicate a role for IGF-II in growth during early gestation and one for IGF-I during later gestation. Knockout of type 1 IGF receptors leads to a more profound growth failure than is found in IGF-I knockout mice alone, suggesting that factors other than IGF-I (eg, IGF-II) exert effects upon fetal growth through the type 1 receptor.

Study of transgenic mice overexpressing IGF-binding proteins supports the concepts that excess IGFBP-1 stunts fetal growth while excess IGFBP-3 leads to selective organomegaly. For example, overexpression of IGFBP-3 in mice led to organomegaly of the spleen, liver, and heart, though birth weight was not different from that of wild-type mice.

While controversy remains over some of the data regarding IGFs and fetal growth, a summary of the complex IGF system in the fetus, based upon the evidence from various species, appears to apply to the human being: (1) IGFs are detectable in many fetal tissues from the first trimester onward; (2) levels of IGFs in the fetal circulation increase during pregnancy, and at term the levels of IGF-I are directly related to birth weight; (3) in mice, disruption of the *IGF* gene leads to severe growth retardation; (4) at the end of the first trimester, there is a striking increase in IGFBP-1 and IGFBP-2 levels in amniotic fluid; (5) the major binding proteins in the human fetus are IGFBP-1 and IGFBP-2; (6) from as early as 16 weeks, there is an inverse correlation between fetal levels of IGFBP-1 and birth weight; (7) in the mother, circulating levels of IGF-I and IGFBP-1 increase during pregnancy; (8) maternal levels of IGFBP-1 are elevated in severe preeclampsia and intrauterine growth retardation; and (9) fetal levels of IGFBP-1 are elevated in cases of intrauterine growth retardation, especially those associated with specific evidence of reduced uteroplacental blood flow. Levels of IGFBP-1 appear to be a sensitive indicator of the short- or long-term response to reduced fetal nutrition.

INSULIN

While insulin is a major regulatory factor for carbohydrate metabolism, many lines of evidence demonstrate its importance in fetal growth as well. Macrosomia is a well known effect of fetal hyperinsulinism such as found in the infant of the diabetic mother. Errors in the normal pattern of IGF-II gene expression from the paternal chromosome and type 2 IGF receptor for IGF-II from the maternally derived gene may underlie the pathogenesis of Beckwith-Wiedemann syndrome. Affected infants are large and have elevated insulin concentrations. At the other end of the spectrum is the small-for-gestational-age (SGA) infant born to a diabetic mother with vascular disease, or under extremely tight control, or who has eclampsia or preeclampsia; this demonstrates that limited nutrient delivery compromises the growth of the infant.

Just as increased insulin stimulates fetal growth, syndromes of fetal insulin deficiency such as are found in congenital diabetes mellitus, pancreatic dysgenesis, or fetal insulin resistance (eg, leprechaunism) are characterized by intrauterine growth retardation.

EPIDERMAL GROWTH FACTOR

Epidermal growth factor (EGF) is involved with fetal growth, and expression varies with disordered fetal growth. Microvilli purified from the placentas of infants with intrauterine growth retardation (IUGR) have decreased or absent placental epidermal growth factor receptor (EGF-R) phosphorylation and tyrosine kinase activity. Maternal smoking decreases birth weight by an average of 200 g, with the major effect occurring late in pregnancy; the placenta responds to smoking by significant changes in its vascularity, which leads to fetal hypoxia. There are decreased numbers of EGF-Rs and a reduced affinity of these receptors for EGF in the placentas of women who are smokers. Hypertensive patients also have decreased numbers of placental EGF-Rs, which may result in IUGR.

EGF levels in amniotic fluid are normally increased near term but decreased in pregnancies complicated by IUGR—though not, conversely, increased in infants who are large for gestational age. EGF levels in the first urines to be voided by IUGR and macrosomic infants are lower than in control infants.

EGF administered to fetal monkeys results in histologic and biochemical maturation of their lungs, leading to improved air exchange and a diminished requirement for respiratory support. Surfactant apoprotein A concentration and the lecithin:sphingomyelin ratio are both significantly higher in the amniotic fluid of the EGF-treated fetuses. Whereas birth weight is not affected by EGF, adrenal and gut weights, standardized for body weight, are increased significantly. Furthermore, EGF stimulates gut muscle, enzyme maturation, and gut size and content, improving the ability of the infant to absorb nutrients. Lastly, EGF advances the maturation of the fetal adrenal cortex, increasing the expression of 3β-hydroxysteroid dehydrogenase. Since EGF can be absorbed orally, this raises a question about whether EGF could be a useful treatment for premature infants or, postnatally, for causing more rapid maturation of the neonate and improving survival in premature infants.

Fibroblast Growth Factor

Genetically engineered fibroblast growth factor receptor (FGF-R)-deficient mice are severely growth-retarded and die before gastrulation. Aberrant FGF signaling during limb and skeletal development in the human being can lead to dysmorphic syndromes. For example, achondroplasia is due to mutations in the transmembrane domain of the type 3 fibroblast growth factor receptor.

Genetic, Maternal, & Uterine Factors

Maternal factors, often expressed through the uterine environment, exert more influence on birth size than paternal factors. The height of the mother correlates better with fetal size than the height of the father. However, there is a genetic component to length at birth that is not sex specific. Firstborn infants are on the average 100 g heavier than subsequent infants; maternal age over 38 years leads to decreased birth weight; and male infants are heavier than female infants by an average of 150–200 g. Poor maternal nutrition is the most important condition leading to low birth weight and length on a worldwide basis. Chronic maternal disease and eclampsia can also lead to poor fetal growth. Maternal alcohol ingestion has severe adverse effects on fetal length and mental development and predisposes to other physical abnormalities seen in the fetal alcohol syndrome such as microcephaly, mental retardation, midfacial hypoplasia, short palpebral fissures, wide-bridged nose, long philtrum, and narrow vermilion border of the lips; affected infants never recover from this loss of length but attain normal growth rate in the postnatal period. Abuse of other substances and chronic use of some medications (eg, phenytoin) can cause intrauterine growth retardation. Cigarette smoking causes not only retarded intrauterine growth but also decreased postnatal growth for as long as 5 years after parturition. Maternal infection—most commonly toxoplasmosis, rubella, cytomegalovirus infection, herpes simplex infection, and HIV infection—leads to many developmental abnormalities as well as short birth length. In multiple births, the weight of each fetus is usually less than that of the average singleton. Uterine tumors or malformations may decrease fetal growth.

Chromosomal Abnormalities & Malformation Syndromes

Many chromosomal abnormalities that lead to malformation syndromes also cause poor fetal growth. Other malformation syndromes associated with a normal karyotype are characterized by intrauterine growth retardation. In most cases, endocrine abnormalities have not been noted. For further discussion of this extensive subject, the reader is referred to other sources listed in the references at the end of this chapter.

FETAL ORIGINS OF ADULT DISEASE

Many lines of evidence demonstrate long-lasting effects of abnormalities in fetal growth. Inanition during the last two trimesters of pregnancy, which occurred during the famine in Holland during World War II, led to an 8–9% decrease in birth weight; however, female infants born under these conditions later gave birth to normal-sized infants. On the other hand, in the Dutch and Leningrad famines, babies born after early gestational starvation of their mothers but with improved maternal nutrition in late gestation were of normal size at birth. However, the female infants born of normal size after this early gestational maternal starvation themselves gave birth to small babies (IUGR of 300–500 g decrease). In other populations, women with a history of IUGR tend to have IUGR babies themselves, and some studies show that generations of malnutrition must be followed by generations of normal nutrition before there is correction of the birth weight of subsequent babies.

Numerous studies from around the world indicate a relationship between low birth weight or low weight at 1 year of age and chronic disease in adulthood. Birth weight—not prematurity—is inversely related to cardiovascular mortality and the insulin resistance syndrome (syndrome X), which consists of (1) elevation of systolic and diastolic blood pressure, (2) impaired glucose tolerance, and (3) elevated triglycerides among other features. The individuals most affected were those with the largest placentas but smaller birth weights. This is attributed to fetal and neonatal "metabolic programming," in which early adjustments to enhance survival in difficult intrauterine circumstances set the stage for later disorders.

Insulin resistance, which might be the basis for most or all of these complications, may spare nutrients from utilization in muscle, thus leaving them available for the brain, a mechanism which would serve to minimize central nervous system damage in the fetus during periods of malnutrition. Studies of otherwise normal thin children who had a history of IUGR demonstrated insulin resistance before the teenage years, suggesting early metabolic programming. Present-day adults who were born in the Netherlands during the Dutch famine and had the lowest birth weights and the lowest maternal weights (those subjects whose mothers experienced malnutrition during the last two trimesters) show a degree of insulin resistance which is directly related to their degree of IUGR, further documenting the relationship between fetal undernutrition and adult insulin resistance.

On the other hand, large babies born to mothers with diabetes mellitus develop childhood obesity after a period of normal weight between 1 year and 5 years of age. Remarkably, studies of the offspring of Dutch mothers exposed to famine during World War II in the first two trimesters (the time in which birth weight is least affected by maternal starvation) demonstrated a twofold increase in the incidence of obesity at 18 years of age compared with a 40% decrease of the incidence of obesity if the individual was exposed to famine in the last trimester (the time in which birth weight is most negatively impacted by maternal starvation).

POSTNATAL GROWTH

Postnatal growth in stature and weight follows a characteristic pattern in normal children (Figures 6–1 and 6–2). The highest overall growth rate occurs in the fetus, the highest postnatal growth rate just after birth, and a slower growth rate follows in mid childhood (Figures 6–3 and 6–4). There are two periods characterized by brief growth spurts in childhood: the infant-childhood growth spurt between 1½ years and 3 years and the mid childhood growth spurt between 6½ years and 7 years. In addition, there is an "adiposity rebound" of accelerating weight gain and rising BMI in mid childhood after a previous period of relative stability of weight gain. An early adiposity rebound is a risk factor for the development of obesity later in childhood and thereafter.

After another plateau, the striking increase in stature known as the pubertal growth spurt follows, causing a second peak of growth velocity. The final decrease in growth rate then ensues, until the epiphyses of the long bones fuse and growth ceases.

Endocrine Factors

A. GROWTH HORMONE AND INSULIN-LIKE GROWTH FACTORS

As discussed in Chapter 5, somatotropin, or growth hormone (GH), is suppressed by hypothalamic growth hormone release-inhibiting factor (or somatostatin) and

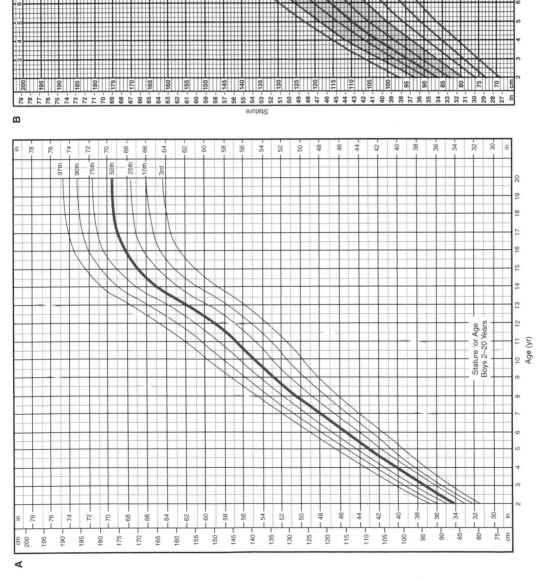

Figure 6–1. A. Chart appropriate for boys in most clinical situations showing the third to the ninth percentiles. (Redrawn from the original developed by the National Center for Health Statistics in collaboration with the National Center for Chronic Disease Prevention and Health Promotion, 2000.) **B.** Growth chart appropriate for boys in the extremes of growth showing standard deviations from the mean. (Redrawn and reprinted with permission of Genentech, Inc. Sources of data: 1976 study of the National Center for Health Statistics [NCHS; Hyattsville, MD]; Hamill PVV et al: Physical growth: National Center for Health Statistics percentiles. Am J Clin Nutr 1979;32:607.)

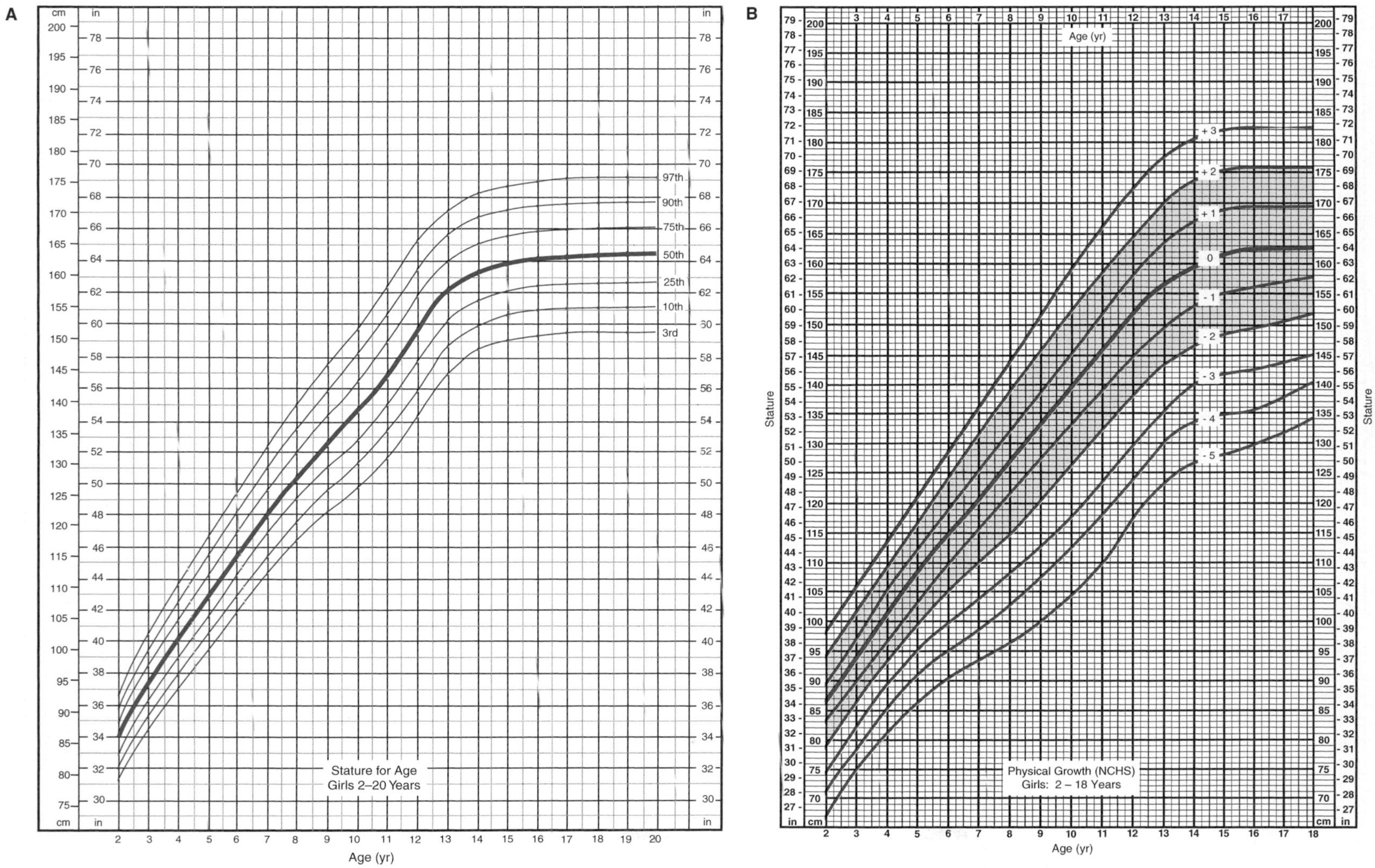

Figure 6–2. A. Growth chart appropriate for girls in most clinical situations showing the third to ninth percentiles. (Redrawn from the original developed by the National Center for Health Statistics in collaboration with the National Center for Chronic Disease Prevention and Health Promotion, 2000.) **B.** Growth chart appropriate for girls in the extremes of growth, showing standard deviations from the mean. (Redrawn and reprinted with permission of Genentech, Inc. Sources of data: 1976 study of the National Center for Health Statistics [NCHS; Hyattsville, MD]; Hamill PVV et al: Physical growth: National Center for Health Statistics percentiles. Am J Clin Nutr 1979;32:607.)

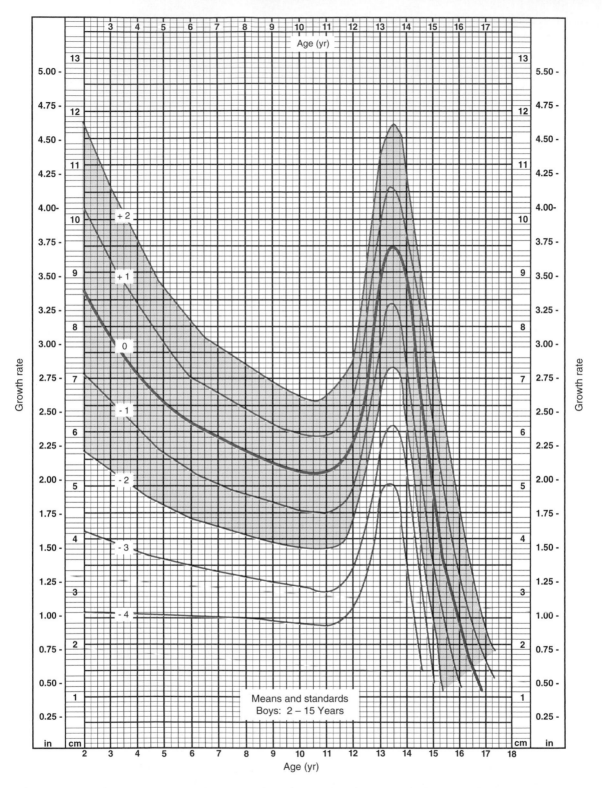

Figures 6–3 and 6–4. Incremental growth charts for boys (Figure 6–3) and girls (Figure 6–4). Height velocity can be compared with the percentiles on the right axis of the charts. (Redrawn with permission from Genetech, Inc.)

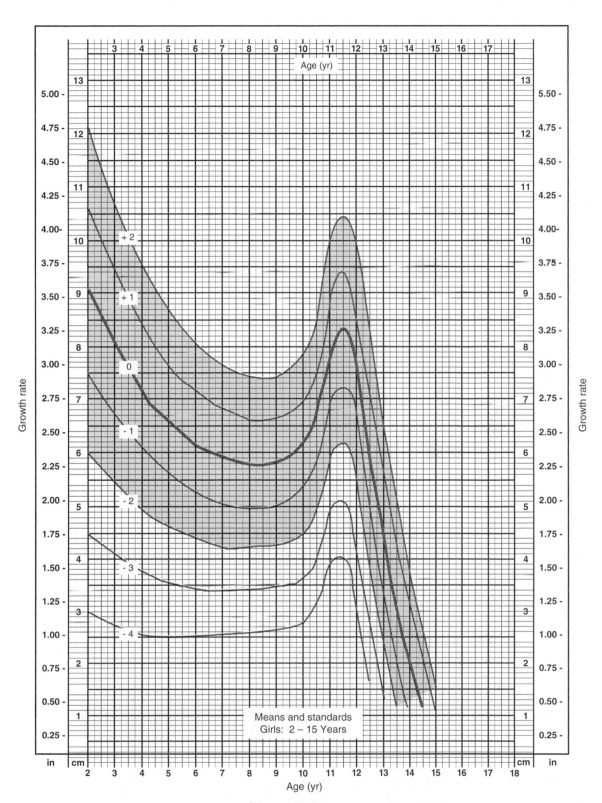

Means and standards
Girls: 2 – 15 Years

stimulated by growth hormone-releasing hormone (GHRH). The gene for GH is located on the long arm of chromosome 17 in a cluster of five genes: *GHN* codes for human GH (a single 191-amino-acid polypeptide chain with a molecular weight of 22 kDa); *GHV* codes for a variant GH produced in the placenta; *CSH1* and *CSH2* code for prolactin; and *CSHP1* codes for a variant prolactin molecule. A 20-kDa variant of pituitary growth hormone accounts for 5–10% of circulating GH.

The effects of growth hormone are mainly mediated by the insulin-like growth factors, but GH also has direct effects such as lipolysis, increased amino acid transport into tissues, and increased protein synthesis in liver. Growth hormone produces insulin resistance and is a diabetogenic substance, increasing blood sugar. GH is secreted in a pulsatile manner, so that serum concentrations are low much of the day but peak during short intervals. Values are higher in the immediate neonatal period, decrease through childhood, and rise again as a result of increased pulse amplitude (but not frequency) during puberty. GH secretion falls again during aging. GH secretion is decreased significantly in obesity but rises in states of starvation.

Growth hormone circulates in plasma bound to a protein, the growth hormone-binding protein (GHBP), with a sequence equivalent to that of the extracellular membrane domain of the growth hormone receptor. The physiology of the GH-binding protein appears to be of great importance in growth. For example, obese patients have lower plasma GH concentrations but higher GHBP levels, while starvation raises GH concentrations and lowers GHBP levels. Patients with abnormalities of the GH receptor (eg, Laron dwarfism) also have the defect reflected in the serum GHBP concentrations; those with decreased numbers of GH receptors have decreased serum GHBP concentrations.

GH exerts its effects on growth mainly through the insulin-like growth factors (IGFs) and their binding proteins. IGF-I and IGF-II have structures similar to that of the proinsulin molecule but differ from insulin in regulation, receptors, and biologic effects. The structure of the insulin-like factors (originally called sulfation factor and then somatomedin), the genes responsible for their production, and information about their physiology have been elucidated. Recombinant IGFs are available for clinical studies.

The single copy gene for prepro-IGF-I is located on the long arm of chromosome 12. Posttranslational processing produces the 70-amino-acid mature form, and alternative splicing mechanisms produce variants of the molecule in different tissues and developmental stages. The IGF-I cell membrane receptor (the type I receptor) resembles the insulin receptor in its structure of two α and two β chains. Binding of IGF-I to type I receptors stimulates tyrosine kinase activity and autophosphorylation of tyrosine residues in the receptor. This leads to cell differentiation or division (or both). IGF-I receptors are down-regulated by increased IGF-I concentrations, while decreased IGF-I concentrations increase IGF-I receptors.

IGF molecules in the circulation are mostly bound to a variety of IGF-binding proteins (IGFBPs); at present, information is available about the molecular weights and other properties of six IGFBPs. IGFBP-1 and IGFBP-3 have been extensively studied. IGFBP-1 is a 25-kDa protein. The serum levels of IGFBP-1 are inversely proportionate to insulin levels; this protein does not appear to be regulated by GH. IFGBP-1 is mainly inhibitory of IGF action. It is present in high concentrations in fetal serum and amnionic fluid. Serum values in blood are inversely proportionate to birth weight.

IGF-I circulates bound to IGFBP-3 and an acid labile subunit in a 150-kDa complex. Serum IGFBP-3 concentrations are directly proportionate to GH concentrations but also to nutritional status—in malnutrition, IGFBP-3 and IGF-I levels fall while GH rises. IGF-I directly regulates IGFBP-3 as well. IGFBP-3 rises with advancing age through childhood, with highest values achieved during puberty; however, the pattern of change of IGF-I at puberty is different from that of IGFBP-3. The molar ratio of IGF-I to IGFBP-3 rises at puberty, suggesting that more IGF-I is free to influence growth during this period.

IGF-I is produced in most tissues and appears to be exported to neighboring cells to act upon them in a paracrine manner or upon the cell of origin in an autocrine manner. Thus, serum IGF-I concentrations may not reflect the most significant actions of this growth factor. The liver is a major site of IGF-I synthesis, and much of the circulating IGF-I probably originates in the liver; serum IGF-I concentrations vary in liver disease with the extent of liver destruction. IGF-I is a progression factor, so that a cell which has been exposed to a competence factor such as platelet-derived growth factor (PDGF) in stage G_0 of the cell cycle and has progressed to G_1 can, with IGF-I exposure in G_1, undergo division in the S phase of the cell cycle. Aside from the stimulatory effects of IGF-I on cartilage growth, IGF-I has stimulatory effects upon hematopoiesis, ovarian steroidogenesis, myoblast proliferation and differentiation, and differentiation of the lens.

IGF-I was in short supply until production by recombinant DNA technology became possible. IGF-I administration in clinical trials increases nitrogen retention and decreases BUN—and, in GH-resistant patients (Laron dwarfs), IGF-I stimulates growth without the presence of GH. Thus, IGF-I may prove useful in treatment of various clinical conditions from pathologic short stature to catabolic states, including the postoperative period and burns.

IGF-II is a 67-amino-acid peptide. The gene for prepro-IGF-II is located on the short arm of chromosome 11, close to the gene for preproinsulin. The type II IGF receptor preferentially binds IGF-II and is identical to the mannose 6-phosphate receptor, a single-chain transmembrane protein. While most of the effects of IGF-II appear mediated by its interaction with the type I receptor, independent actions of IGF-II via the type II receptor are described.

Plasma concentrations of the IGFs vary with age and physiologic condition. IGF-I concentrations are low at term in neonates and remain relatively low in childhood until a peak is reached during puberty, with values rising higher than at any other time in life. Serum IGF-I then decreases to adult levels, values higher than in childhood but lower than in puberty. With advancing age, serum GH and IGF-I decrease. IGF-I concentrations are more highly correlated in monozygotic twins than in same-sex dizygotic twins, indicating a genetic effect upon IGF-I regulation.

GH deficiency leads to lower serum IGF-I and IGF-II concentrations, while GH excess leads to elevated IGF-I but no rise in IGF-II above normal. Because serum IGF-I is lower during states of nutritional deficiency, IGF-I is not a perfect tool in the differential diagnosis of conditions of poor growth, which often include impaired nutritional state. IGF-I suppresses GH secretion, so that patients who lack GH receptors (Laron dwarfs) and are unable to produce IGF-I have elevated GH concentrations but negligible IGF-I concentrations.

B. THYROID HORMONE

As noted above, congenital hypothyroid newborns are of normal length, but if untreated they manifest exceedingly poor growth soon after birth. Infants with untreated congenital hypothyroidism will suffer permanent mental retardation. Acquired hypothyroidism leads to a markedly decreased growth rate but no permanent intellectual defects. Bone age advancement is severely delayed in hypothyroidism, usually more so than in GH deficiency, and epiphysial dysgenesis is seen when calcification of the epiphyses progresses. The normal decrease in the upper to lower segment ratio with age (Figure 6–5) is delayed and therefore elevated, owing to poor limb growth in hypothyroidism.

C. SEX STEROIDS

Gonadal sex steroids exert an important influence on the pubertal growth spurt, while absence of these factors is not of major importance in prepubertal growth.

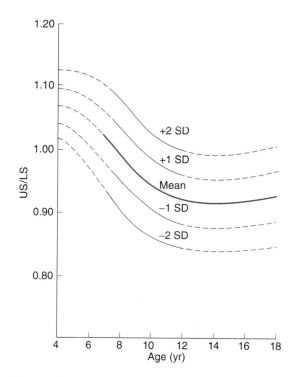

Figure 6–5. Normal upper to lower segment (US:LS) ratios, based on findings in 1015 white children. Values are slightly lower for black children. (Reproduced, with permission, from McKusick V: *Hereditable Disorders of Connective Tissue,* 4th ed. Mosby, 1972.)

Gonadal and adrenal sex steroids in excess can cause a sharp increase in growth rate as well as the premature appearance and progression of secondary sexual features. If unabated, increased sex steroids will cause advancement of skeletal age, premature epiphysial fusion, and short adult stature.

The pubertal rise in gonadal steroids exerts direct and indirect effects upon IGF-I production. Sex steroids directly stimulate the production of IGF-I from cartilage. They also increase GH secretion, which stimulates IGF-I production indirectly. Both actions appear important in the pubertal growth spurt (see Chapter 15).

D. GLUCOCORTICOIDS

Endogenous or exogenous glucocorticoids in excess will quickly stop growth; this effect occurs more quickly than weight gain. The absence of glucocorticoids has little effect on growth if the individual is clinically well in other respects (ie, if hypotension and hypoglycemia are absent).

Other Factors

A. GENETIC FACTORS

Genetic factors influence final height. Correlation is found between midparental height and the child's height; appropriate methods to utilize this phenomenon and determine the target height for a child are presented in Figure 6–6. There is a heritable pattern to birth length, postnatal increase in length, and the intrinsic rate of change in growth. These effects are sex-specific.

B. SOCIOECONOMIC FACTORS

Worldwide, the most common cause of short stature is poverty and its effects. Thus, poor nutrition, poor hygiene, and poor health influence growth both before and after birth. In people of the same ethnic group and in the same geographic location, variations in stature are often attributable to these factors. For example, Japanese individuals born and reared in North America after World War II are generally taller than Japanese-born immigrants to North America. Conversely, when socioeconomic factors are equal, the differences in average height between various ethnic groups are mainly genetic. The new growth charts for children in the United States from the CDC are not ethnicity-specific because it is believed that the major differences between growth in ethnic groups are due to socioeconomic status and nutrition rather than genetic endowments.

C. NUTRITIONAL FACTORS

The influence of malnutrition accounts for much of the socioeconomic discrepancy in height noted above, but malnutrition may occur in the midst of plenty and must always be suspected in disorders of growth. Other factors may be blamed for poor growth when nutritional deficiencies are actually responsible. For example, Sherpas were thought to have short stature mainly because of genetic factors or the effects of great altitude on the slopes of Mount Everest; nutritional supplementation increased stature in this group, however, demonstrating the effects of adequate nutrition. The developed world places a premium on appearance, and women portrayed as beautiful in the media are characteristically thin. Significant numbers of children, chiefly teenagers, voluntarily decrease their caloric intake even if they are not obese; this accounts for some cases of poor growth. Chronic disease, which hampers adequate nutrition, often leads to short stature. For example, bronchopulmonary dysplasia decreases growth to some degree because it increases metabolic demands, shifting nutrient usage from growth; improved nutrition will increase growth in these patients. Feeding problems in infants, resulting from inexperience of parents or poor child-parent interactions (maternal deprivation), may

account for poor growth. Fad diets such as poorly constructed vegan diets that put children at risk for vitamin B_{12} or iron deficiency as well as dietary manipulation for expected benefit, such a low-fat diet, may place children at risk for deficiency of fat-soluble vitamins. Deliberate starvation of children by caregivers is an extreme form of child abuse that may be first discovered because of poor growth.

There are significant endocrine changes associated with malnutrition. Decreased GH receptors or postreceptor defects in GH action, leading to decreased production of IGF-I and decreased concentration of serum IGF-I are notable. The characteristic results of malnutrition are elevation of serum GH and decrease in IGF-I. Remarkably, obesity increases IGF-I concentrations by increasing GH receptors even though GH secretion is suppressed to levels suggesting GH deficiency. IGFBP-1, a suppressor of IGF-I effects, is elevated in obesity.

D. PSYCHOLOGIC FACTORS

Aberrant intrafamilial dynamics, psychologic stress, or psychiatric disease can inhibit growth either by altering endocrine function or by secondary effects on nutrition (psychosocial dwarfism or maternal deprivation). It is essential to differentiate these situations from true disease states.

E. CHRONIC DISEASE

Even aside from the effects of poor nutrition, many chronic systemic diseases interfere with growth. For example, congestive heart failure and asthma, if uncontrolled, are associated with decreased stature; in some cases, final height is in the normal range because growth continues over a longer period of time. Children of mothers with HIV infection are often small at birth and have an increased incidence of poor postnatal growth, delayed bone age development, and reduced IGF-I concentrations; in addition, thyroid dysfunction may develop, further complicating the growth pattern. Infants born of HIV-infected mothers but themselves not infected may exhibit catch-up growth.

Catch-Up Growth

Correction of growth-retarding disorders may be temporarily followed by an abnormally high growth rate as the child approaches normal height for age. This catch-up growth will occur after initiation of therapy for hypothyroidism and GH deficiency, after correction of glucocorticoid excess, and after appropriate treatment of many chronic diseases such as celiac disease. Catch-up growth is usually short-lived and is followed by a more average growth rate.

MEASUREMENT OF GROWTH

Accurate measurement of height is an essential part of the physical examination of children and adolescents. The onset of a chronic disease may often be determined by an inflection point in the growth chart. In other cases, a detailed growth chart will indicate a normal constant growth rate in a child observed to be short for age. If careful growth records are kept, a diagnosis of constitutional delay in growth and adolescence or genetic short stature may be made in such a patient; without previous measurements, the child might be subjected to unnecessary diagnostic testing or months of delay may occur as the child's growth is finally carefully monitored.

Height

The National Center for Health Statistics revised the growth charts for children in the United States (Figures 6–1 and 6–2). The new charts display the third and 97th percentiles rather than the fifth and 95th percentiles, and standard deviations are also available. Charts displaying BMI by age contain data appropriate for the evaluation of obesity and underweight.

But growth charts still leave 6 out of 100 healthy children outside of their boundaries, with 3 out of 100 below the more worrisome (to parents) "lower limits of normal." It is both unnecessary and impractical to evaluate 3% of the population. Instead, the examining physician should determine which short children warrant further evaluation and which ones (and their parents) require only reassurance that the child is healthy. When parents see that their child is below the third percentile and in a section of the chart colored differently from the "normal area," they assume that there is a serious problem. Thus, the format of the chart can dictate parental reaction to height, since all parents want their children to be in the "normal range." Figures 6–1 and 6–2 furnish data necessary to evaluate the height of children at various ages using percentiles or the standard deviation method (SD) used by the WHO. Standard deviation determination is more useful in extremely short children below the second or first percentile.

Pathologic short stature is usually more than 3.5 SD below the mean, whereas the third percentile is only at 2 SD below the mean. However, a diagnosis of pathologic short stature is best not based on a single measurement. Serial measurements are required because they allow determination of growth velocity, which is a more sensitive index of the growth process than a single determination. A very tall child who develops a postnatal growth problem will not fall 3.5 SD below the mean in height for some time but will fall below the mean in growth velocity soon after the onset of the disorder. As

Figures 6–3 and 6–4 demonstrate, growth velocity varies at different ages, but as a rough guide, a growth rate of less than 5 cm per year between age 4 years and the onset of puberty is abnormal. In children under 4 years of age, normal growth velocity changes more strikingly with age. Healthy term newborns tend to be clustered in length measurements around 21 inches (mostly owing to difficulties in obtaining accurate measurements). In the ensuing 24 months or so, the healthy child's height will enter a channel on the growth chart and remain there throughout childhood. Thus, a child with constitutional delay in growth or genetic short stature whose height is at the mean at birth and gradually falls to the tenth percentile at 1 year of age and to the fifth percentile by 2 years of age may in fact be healthy in spite of crossing percentile lines in the journey to a growth channel at the fifth percentile. Although the growth rate may decrease during these years, it should not be less than the fifth percentile for age. A steeper decrease in growth rate may be a sign of disease. When a question of abnormal growth arises, previous measurements are always helpful; every physician treating children should record supine length (under 2 years of age) or standing height (after 2 years of age) as well as weight at every office visit. As the child leaves infancy, height and growth velocity should be determined in relation to the standards for the child's age on a graphic chart with clear indication of the child's position (supine or standing) at measurement.

Patients who cannot be measured in the standing position (eg, because of cerebral palsy) require other approaches: The use of arm span is a possible surrogate for the measurement of height, and there are formulas available for the calculation of height based upon the measurement of upper arm length, tibial length, and knee length (see below).

This discussion presupposes accuracy of measurements, which should be available for children followed by a single physician or group. However, it is reported that screening examinations in the real world fall short of that ideal. Forty-one percent of a presumably normal population screened at a school in England met the criteria for evaluation of abnormal growth (approximately two-thirds grew faster than the normal growth category and one-third were in the slower than normal category), leading to an unreasonable size of a referral population, all due to simple measuring error.

Relation to Midparental Height: The Target Height

There is a positive correlation between midparental height (the average of the heights of both parents) and the stature of a child. One way to use this relationship

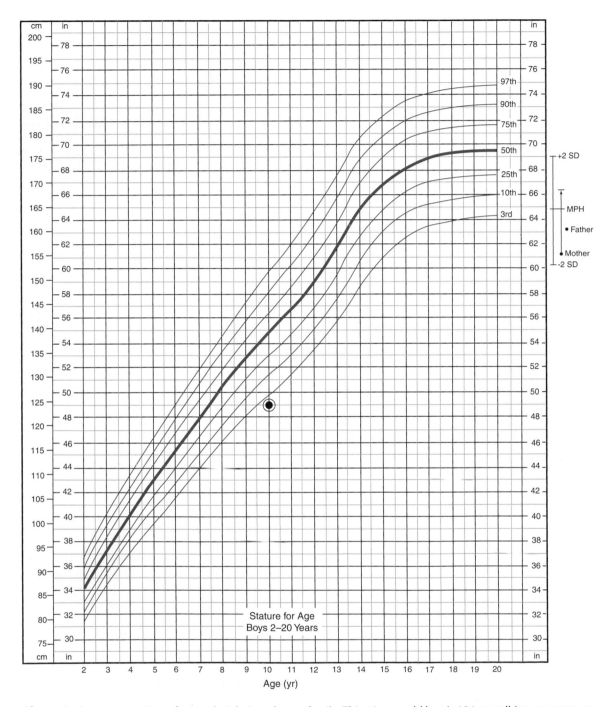

Figure 6–6. Determination of target height in a shorter family. This 10-year-old boy is 124 cm tall (we measure patients in cm), his mother is 61 inches tall (adults recall their heights in inches and feet but, if they are available, their height should be actually measured in centimeters), and the father is 63 inches tall. Five inches are added to the mother's height to convert her height percentile to the equivalent percentile on a boy's chart. (If we were considering a daughter whose height is plotted on a girl's chart, the mother's height would be directly plotted and 5 inches would be subtracted from the father's height to correct his height percentile to the equivalent for an adult

of parents' heights to the expected heights of children within a given family is the calculation of target adult height range using parents' heights and correcting these heights for the sex of the child. For boys, add 5 inches to the mother's height, add the result to the father's height, and divide by 2. This is the target height, and it is expected that sons of these parents will reach a height within 2 SD of this target—or, for simplicity, within 4 inches above and 4 inches below the target height. (Two inches approximates 1 SD for adults.) For girls, subtract 5 inches from the father's height and add the result to the mother's height and divide by 2, leading to the target height for the girl. The range for girls will also be within 4 inches above and below this target. In effect, this corrects the North American growth charts for the particular family being considered. The calculated target height corresponds to the 50th percentile for the family, and the limits of the ± 2 SD approximate the fifth to 95th percentile for the family (see Figures 6–1 and 6–2). This method is useful only in the absence of disease affecting growth, and the prediction is more valid when the parents are of similar rather than of widely different heights. Figures 6–6 and 6–7 demonstrate the calculation of target height and the ranges. When there is a large discrepancy between the heights of the mother and the father, prediction of final height becomes difficult. A child may follow the growth pattern of the shorter parent more closely than the midparental height. Furthermore, a boy may, for example, follow the growth of a short mother rather than a taller father.

A parent who spent the growing years in poverty, with chronic disease, or in an area of political unrest might have a falsely lowered adult height. Of course, the height of an adopted child will have no relationship to the adoptive parents' heights.

Technique of Measurement

Length and height must be measured accurately. Hasty measurements derived from marks made on paper at an infant's foot and head while the infant is squirming on the paper on the examining table are useless. Infants must be measured on a firm horizontal surface with a permanently attached rule, a stationary plate perpendicular to the rule for the head, and a movable perpendicular plate for the feet. One person should hold the head stable while another makes sure the knees are straight and the feet are firm against the movable plate. Children over age 2 are measured standing up. These measurements cannot be accurately performed with the measuring rod that projects above the common weight scale; the rod is too flexible, and the scale footplate will in fact drop lower when the patient stands on it. Instead, height should be measured with the child standing back to the wall with heels at the wall, ankles together, and knees and spine straight against a vertical metal rule permanently attached to the wall or to a wide upright board. Height is measured at the top of the head by a sliding perpendicular plate (or square wooden block). A Harpenden stadiometer is a mechanical measuring device capable of such accurate measurement. Standing height is on the average 1.25 cm less than supine length, and it is essential to record the position of measurement each time; shifting from supine height at 2 years to standing height at 2½ years can falsely suggest an inadequate growth rate over that 6-month period. It is preferable to measure in the metric system, since the smaller gradations make measurements more accurate by eliminating the tendency to round off numbers. Growth is not constant but is characterized by short spurts and periods of slowed growth. The interval between growth measurements should be adequate to allow an accurate evaluation of growth velocity. Appropriate sampling intervals vary with age but should not be less than 3 months in childhood, with a 6-month interval being optimal.

The problem of measuring the growth rate of children with orthopedic deformities or contractures is significant, as these patients may have nutritional or endocrine disorders as well. The measurement of knee height, tibial length, or upper arm length correlates well with standing height ($r = .97$); thus, these measurements may be translated, using special linear regression

---

woman.) Her corrected height and that of the father are plotted at the far right of the chart where adult heights are displayed. The midparental height is calculated by adding the father's height to the corrected mother's height and the sum is divided by two; the result is the target height. The limits of 2 SD above and below the target height are displayed by plotting 2 SD (approximately 4 inches above and below the target height. This process is equivalent to moving the 50th percentile for the United States population to a conceptual 50th percentile for the family under consideration. It is evident that the height of the child, while below the third percentile, is within the bounds of the percentiles described by ± 2 SD from the target height and the child appears to fit within the genetic pattern of the family. The growth velocity and the degree of skeletal maturation are some of the factors necessary to evaluate this analysis in more detail.

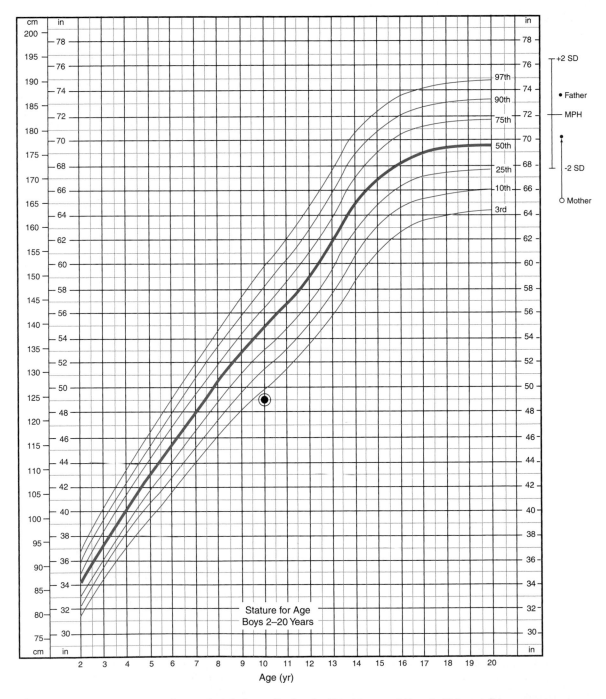

Figure 6–7. Determination of target height in a taller family. This 10-year-old boy is 124 cm tall (we measure patients in centimeters), his mother is 65 inches tall (adults recall their heights in inches and feet but, if they are available, their height should be actually measured in centimeters), and the father is 73.5 inches tall. Five inches are added to the mother's height to convert her height percentile to the equivalent percentile on a boy's chart. (If we were considering a daughter whose height is plotted on a girl's chart, the mother's height would be directly plotted and 5 inches should be subtracted from the father's height to correct his height percentile to the equivalent height

equations, into total height, which is then plotted on standard growth charts. Specialized laser-calibrated devices to measure tibial length ("kneeometry") are reported to be accurate for assessment of short-term growth down to weekly intervals.

In addition to height or length, other significant measurements include (1) the frontal-occipital head circumference; (2) horizontal arm span (between the outspread middle fingertips with the patient standing against a flat backboard); and (3) the upper segment (US) to lower segment (LS) ratio. For the latter, the LS is measured from the top of the symphysis pubis vertically to the floor with the patient standing straight, and the US is determined by subtracting the LS from the standing height measurement noted above. (Normal standard US:LS ratios are shown in Figure 6–5.) Sitting height is used in some clinical studies of growth, but the sitting stadiometer is rarely available.

Height & Growth Rate Summary

In summary, we may consider three criteria for pathologic short stature: (1) height more than 3.5 SD below the mean for chronologic age; (2) growth rate more than 2 SD below the mean for chronologic age; and (3) height more than 2 SD below the target height when corrected for midparental height.

Weight

The measured weight should be plotted for age on standard graphs developed by the National Center for Health Statistics (NCHS), which are available from various companies producing baby food or growth hormone. Variation in the weights of children in the USA due to differing diets or activity regimens makes it difficult to exactly compare percentiles of height with percentiles of weight. Body mass index (BMI) charts displaying percentiles of BMI (weight in kilograms divided by height in meters squared) are widely available and provide an excellent way to assess nutritional status.

SKELETAL (BONE) AGE

Skeletal development is a reflection of physiologic maturation. For example, menarche is better correlated with a bone age of 13 years than with a given chronologic age. Estrogen plays the major role in advancing skeletal maturation. Patients with aromatase deficiency, who cannot convert estrogen from testosterone, and patients with estrogen receptor defects, who cannot respond to estrogen, grow taller well into their twenties without having epiphysial fusion. Bone age indicates remaining growth available to a child and can be used to predict adult height. However, bone age is not a definitive diagnostic test of any disease; it can assist in diagnosis only when considered along with other factors.

Bone age is determined by comparing the appearance and stage of fusion of epiphyses or shapes of bones on the patient's radiograph with an atlas demonstrating normal skeletal maturation for various ages. The Greulich and Pyle atlas of radiographs of the left hand and wrist is most commonly used in the USA, but other methods of skeletal age determination such as Tanner and Whitehouse maturity scoring are preferred in Europe. Any bone age more than 2 SD above or below the mean for chronologic age is out of the normal range. For newborn infants, knee and foot radiographs are compared with an appropriate bone age atlas; for late pubertal children, just before epiphysial fusion, the knee atlas will reveal whether any further growth can be expected or whether the epiphyses are fused.

Height is predicted by determining bone age and height at the time the radiograph was taken and consulting the Bayley-Pinneau tables in the Greulich and Pyle skeletal atlas of the hand. The Roche, Wainer, and Thissen (RWT) method of height prediction uses patient weight and midparental height—in addition to the variables noted above—to calculate predicted height (Table 6–1). Recently, the method was simplified by eliminating the necessity for a bone age assessment in the Khamis-Roche method; results are almost as accurate as the RWT method in white American children. Height prediction by any method becomes more accurate as the child approaches the time of epiphysial fusion.

---

percentile for an adult woman.) Her corrected height and that of the father are plotted at the far right of the chart where adult heights are displayed. The midparental height is calculated by adding the father's height to the corrected mother's height and the sum is divided by 2; the result is the target height. The limits of 2 SD above and below the target height are displayed by plotting 2 SD (which equals approximately 4 inches) above and below the target height. This is equivalent to moving the 50th percentile for the United States population to a conceptual 50th percentile for the family under consideration. It is evident that the height of the child, which is below the third percentile for the United States, is even farther outside the bounds of the percentiles described by ± SD from the target height, and, thus, the child appears to fall far outside the genetic pattern of the family. The growth velocity and the degree of skeletal maturation are some of the other factors necessary to evaluate this analysis in more detail.

Table 6-1. The RWT method for predicting adult stature.[1]

Tables of Multipliers for Boys

Age Yrs. Mos	Recumbent length	Weight	Midparental stature	Skeletal age	Adjustment factor
1 0	0.966	0.199	0.606	-0.673	1.632
1 3	1.032	0.086	0.580	-0.417	-1.841
1 6	1.086	-0.016	0.559	-0.205	-4.852
1 9	1.130	-0.106	0.540	-0.033	-7.528
2 0	1.163	-0.186	0.523	0.104	-9.764
2 3	1.189	-0.256	0.509	0.211	-11.618
2 6	1.207	-0.316	0.496	0.291	-13.114
2 9	1.219	-0.369	0.485	0.349	-14.278
3 0	1.227	-0.413	0.475	0.388	-15.139
3 3	1.230	-0.450	0.466	0.410	-15.729
3 6	1.229	-0.481	0.458	0.419	-16.081
3 9	1.226	-0.505	0.451	0.417	-16.228
4 0	1.221	-0.523	0.444	0.405	-16.201
4 3	1.214	-0.537	0.437	0.387	-16.034
4 6	1.206	-0.546	0.431	0.363	-15.758
4 9	1.197	-0.550	0.424	0.335	-15.400
5 0	1.188	-0.551	0.418	0.303	-14.990
5 3	1.179	-0.548	0.412	0.269	-14.551
5 6	1.169	-0.543	0.406	0.234	-14.106
5 9	1.160	-0.535	0.400	0.198	-13.672
6 0	1.152	-0.524	0.394	0.161	-13.267
6 3	1.143	-0.512	0.389	0.123	-12.901
6 6	1.135	-0.499	0.383	0.085	-12.583
6 9	1.127	-0.484	0.378	0.046	-12.318
7 0	1.120	-0.468	0.373	0.006	-12.107
7 3	1.113	-0.451	0.369	-0.034	-11.948
7 6	1.106	-0.434	0.365	-0.077	-11.834
7 9	1.100	-0.417	0.361	-0.121	-11.756
8 0	1.093	-0.400	0.358	-0.167	-11.701
8 3	1.086	-0.382	0.356	-0.217	-11.652
8 6	1.079	-0.365	0.354	-0.270	-11.592
8 9	1.071	-0.349	0.353	-0.327	-11.498
9 0	1.063	-0.333	0.353	-0.389	-11.349
9 3	1.054	-0.317	0.353	-0.455	-11.118
9 6	1.044	-0.303	0.355	-0.527	-10.779
9 9	1.033	-0.289	0.357	-0.605	-10.306

Tables of Multipliers for Girls

Age Yrs Mos	Recumbent length	Weight	Midparental stature	Skeletal age	Adjustment factor
1 0	1.087	-0.271	0.386	0.434	21.729
1 3	1.112	-0.369	0.367	0.094	20.684
1 6	1.134	-0.455	0.349	-0.172	19.957
1 9	1.153	-0.530	0.332	-0.374	19.463
2 0	1.170	-0.594	0.316	-0.523	19.131
2 3	1.183	-0.648	0.301	-0.625	18.905
2 6	1.195	-0.693	0.287	-0.690	18.740
2 9	1.204	-0.729	0.274	-0.725	18.604
3 0	1.210	-0.757	0.262	-0.736	18.474
3 3	1.215	-0.777	0.251	-0.729	18.337
3 6	1.217	-0.791	0.241	-0.711	18.187
3 9	1.217	-0.798	0.232	-0.684	18.024
4 0	1.215	-0.800	0.224	-0.655	17.855
4 3	1.212	-0.797	0.217	-0.626	17.691
4 6	1.206	-0.789	0.210	-0.600	17.548
4 9	1.199	-0.777	0.205	-0.582	17.444
5 0	1.190	-0.761	0.200	-0.571	17.398
5 3	1.180	-0.742	0.197	-0.572	17.431
5 6	1.168	-0.721	0.193	-0.584	17.567
5 9	1.155	-0.697	0.191	-0.609	17.826
6 0	1.140	-0.671	0.190	-0.647	18.229
6 3	1.124	-0.644	0.189	-0.700	18.796
6 6	1.107	-0.616	0.188	-0.766	19.544
6 9	1.089	-0.587	0.189	-0.845	20.489
7 0	1.069	-0.557	0.189	-0.938	21.642
7 3	1.049	-0.527	0.191	-1.043	23.011
7 6	1.028	-0.498	0.192	-1.158	24.602
7 9	1.006	-0.468	0.194	-1.284	26.416
8 0	0.938	-0.439	0.196	-1.418	28.448
8 3	0.960	-0.411	0.199	-1.558	30.690
8 6	0.937	-0.384	0.202	-1.704	33.129
8 9	0.914	-0.359	0.204	-1.853	35.747
9 0	0.891	-0.334	0.207	-2.003	38.520
9 3	0.868	-0.311	0.210	-2.154	41.421
9 6	0.845	-0.289	0.212	-2.301	44.415
9 9	0.824	-0.269	0.214	-2.444	47.464

(continued)

Age (yr)	(mo)					
10	0	1.021	0.360	-0.276	-0.690	-9.671
10	3	1.008	0.363	-0.263	-0.781	-8.848
10	6	0.993	0.368	-0.252	-0.878	-7.812
10	9	0.977	0.373	-0.241	-0.983	-6.540
11	0	0.960	0.378	-0.231	-1.094	-5.010
11	3	0.942	0.384	-0.222	-1.211	-3.206
11	6	0.923	0.390	-0.213	-1.335	-1.113
11	9	0.902	0.397	-0.206	-1.464	1.273
12	0	0.881	0.403	-0.198	-1.597	3.958
12	3	0.859	0.409	-0.191	-1.735	6.931
12	6	0.837	0.414	-0.184	-1.875	10.181
12	9	0.815	0.413	-0.177	-2.015	13.684
13	0	0.794	0.421	-0.170	-2.156	17.405
13	3	0.773	0.422	-0.163	-2.294	21.297
13	6	0.755	0.422	-0.155	-2.427	25.304
13	9	0.738	0.418	-0.146	-2.553	29.349
14	0	0.724	0.412	-0.136	-2.668	33.345
14	3	0.714	0.401	-0.125	-2.771	37.183
14	6	0.709	0.387	-0.112	-2.856	40.738
14	9	0.709	0.367	-0.098	-2.922	43.869
15	0	0.717	0.342	-0.081	-2.962	46.403
15	3	0.732	0.310	-0.062	-2.973	48.154
15	6	0.756	0.271	-0.040	-2.949	48.898
15	9	0.792	0.223	-0.015	-2.885	48.402
16	0	0.839	0.167	-0.014	-2.776	46.391

The RWT method predicts the height of an individual at 18 years of age; after this age the average age total increase in stature is 0.6 cm for girls and 0.8 cm for boys. *Recumbent length* is measured in cm (add 1.25 cm to the standing height, without shoes, if that is available). Weight is measured in kg. The *midparental height* is calculated by adding the standing height of each paren: in cm (without shoes) and dividing by two; if the parents' heights are unknown, in the USA a height of 174.5 cm can be substituted for the father's height or 162 cm for the mother's height. The skeletal age is determined from an x-ray of the left wrist anc hand comparing it to the Greulich and Pyle atlas.

A prediction is made by:

1. Recording the child's data as noted below.
2. Finding the multipliers from the charts on these pages, making sure the positive and negative signs are retained for the calculations.
3. Multiplying the data by the multipliers, taking note of the positive or negative sign.
4. Adding the products to the adjustment factor, taking note of the sign of the factor; the result is a prediction of the height at 18 years of age.

Age (yr)	(mo)					
10	0	0.803	-0.250	0.216	-2.581	50.525
10	3	0.783	-0.233	0.217	-2.710	53.548
10	6	0.766	-0.217	0.217	-2.829	56.481
10	9	0.749	-0.203	0.217	-2.936	59.267
11	0	0.736	-0.190	0.216	-3.029	61.841
11	3	0.724	-0.179	0.214	-3.108	64.123
11	6	0.716	-0.169	0.211	-3.171	66.093
11	9	0.711	-0.159	0.206	-3.217	67.627
12	0	0.710	-0.151	0.201	-3.245	68.670
12	3	0.713	-0.143	0.193	-3.254	69.140
12	6	0.720	-0.136	0.184	-3.244	68.966
12	9	0.733	-0.129	0.173	-3.214	68.061
13	0	0.752	-0.121	0.160	-3.166	66.339
13	3	0.777	-0.113	0.144	-3.100	63.728
13	6	0.810	-0.105	0.127	-3.015	60.150
13	9	0.850	-0.085	0.106	-2.915	55.533
14	0	0.898	-0.083	0.083	-2.800	49.781

The RWT method predicts the height of an individual at 18 years of age; after this age the average total increase in stature is 0.6 cm for girls and 0.8 cm for boys.

DATA	MULTIPLIERS	PRODUCTS
Recumbent length (cm) _____	× _____	= _____
Weight (kg) _____	× _____	= _____
Midparental stature (cm) _____	× _____	= _____
Skeletal age (years) _____	× _____	= _____
Adjustment factor for age _____		= +/− _____
Predicted height at age 18 years (cm) _____		= _____

[1]Modified and reproduced, with permission, from Roche AF, Wainer H, Thissen D: The RWT method for the prediction of adult stature. Pediatrics 1975;56:1026, as modified in Styne DM: Growth Disorders. Page 99 in: *Handbook of Clinical Endocrinology*. Fitzgerald PA (editor). Jones Medical Publications, 1986.

■ DISORDERS OF GROWTH

SHORT STATURE DUE TO NONENDOCRINE CAUSES

There are many causes of decreased childhood growth and short adult height (Table 6–2). The following discussion covers only the more common conditions, emphasizing those that might be included in an endocrine differential diagnosis. Shorter than average stature need not be considered a disease, since variation in stature is a normal feature of human beings, and a normal child should not be burdened with a misdiagnosis. While the classifications described below may apply to most patients, some will still be resistant to definitive diagnosis.

1. Constitutional Short Stature

Constitutional short stature (constitutional delay in growth and adolescence) is not a disease but rather a variation from normal for the population and is considered a slowing of the pace of development. There is usually a delay in pubertal development as well as a decrease in growth (see Constitutional Delay in Adolescence in Chapter 15). It is characterized by moderate short stature (usually not far below the third percentile), thin habitus, and retardation of bone age. The family history often includes similarly affected members (eg, mother with delayed menarche or father who shaved late and kept growing past his teen years).

All other causes of decreased growth must be considered and ruled out before this diagnosis can be made with confidence. The patient may be considered physiologically (but not mentally) delayed in development. Characteristic growth patterns include normal birth length and height, with a gradual decrease in percentiles of height for age by 2 years; on the contrary, a rapid decrease in percentiles is an ominous sign of pathology. Onset of puberty is usually delayed for chronologic age but normal for skeletal age. Adult height is in the normal range but varies according to parental heights. The final height is often less than the predicted height, because growth is less than expected during puberty.

2. Genetic Short Stature

Short stature may also occur in a familial pattern without retarded bone age or delay in puberty; this is considered "genetic" short stature. Affected children are closer to the mean on the normal population growth charts after correction for midparental height by calculation of the target height (Figures 6–6 and 6–7). Adult height depends on the mother's and father's heights. Patients with the combination of constitutional short stature and genetic short stature are quite noticeably short due to both factors and are the patients most likely to seek evaluation. Boys are brought to consultation more often than girls.

3. Prematurity & Intrauterine Growth Retardation

While the majority show catch-up growth, 30% of IUGR infants may follow a lifelong pattern of short stature. Symmetric IUGR infants are most likely to demonstrate this finding. In comparison, appropriate-for-gestational-age premature infants will usually catch up to the normal range of height and weight by 1–2 years of age. Severe premature infants with birth weights less than 800 g (that are appropriate for gestational age), however, may maintain their growth retardation at least through their third year; only follow-up studies will determine whether this classification of premature infants reaches reduced adult heights. Bone age, age at onset of puberty, and yearly growth rate are normal in IUGR patients, and the patients are characteristically thin. Within this grouping are many distinctive genetic or sporadically occurring syndromes. The most common example is Russell-Silver dwarfism, characterized by small size at birth, triangular facies, a variable degree of asymmetry of extremities, and clinodactyly of the fifth finger. Intrauterine infections with *Toxoplasma gondii,* rubella virus, cytomegalovirus, herpesvirus, and human immunodeficiency virus are noted to cause IUGR. Furthermore, maternal drug usage, either illicit (eg, cocaine), legal but ill-advised (eg, alcohol during pregnancy), or legally prescribed medication (eg, phenytoin) may cause IUGR. Reports of other syndromes in small-for-gestational-age infants can be found in sources listed in the bibliography.

While IUGR is not an endocrine cause of short stature, several studies report increased growth velocity when GH is administered. GH is presently approved for use in intrauterine growth retardation. The effects of final height are known in only a few patients, but the early results suggest a beneficial action.

4. Syndromes of Short Stature

Many syndromes include short stature as a characteristic feature. Some include intrauterine growth retardation and some do not. Common ones are described briefly below. Laurence-Moon, Biedl-Bardet, or Prader-Willi syndrome combine obesity with short stature, as do the endocrine conditions, hypothyroidism, glucocorticoid excess, pseudohypoparathyroidism, and GH deficiency. Moderately obese but otherwise normal children without these conditions tend to have slightly advanced bone age and advanced physiologic matura-

Table 6–2. Causes of abnormalities of growth.

I. CAUSES OF SHORT STATURE

Nonendocrine causes
  Constitutional short stature
  Genetic short stature
  Intrauterine growth retardation
  Syndromes of short stature
    Turner's syndrome and its variants
    Noonan's syndrome (pseudo-Turner's syndrome)
    Prader-Willi syndrome
    Laurence-Moon and Bardet-Biedl syndromes
    Other autosomal abnormalities and dysmorphic
      syndromes
  Chronic disease
    Cardiac disorders
      Left-to-right shunt
      Congestive heart failure
    Pulmonary disorders
      Cystic fibrosis
      Asthma
    Gastrointestinal disorders
      Malabsorption (eg, celiac disease)
      Disorders of swallowing
    Hepatic disorders
    Hematologic disorders
      Sickle cell anemia
      Thalassemia
    Renal disorders
      Renal tubular acidosis
      Chronic uremia
    Immunologic disorders
      Connective tissue disease
      Juvenile rheumatoid arthritis
      Chronic infection
    Central nervous system disorders
    Malnutrition
      Decreased availability of nutrients
      Fad diets
      Voluntary dieting
      Anorexia nervosa
      Anorexia of cancer chemotherapy

Endocrine disorders
  GH deficiency and variants
    Congenital GH deficiency
      With midline defects
      With other pituitary hormone deficiencies
      Isolated GH deficiency
      Pituitary agenesis
    Acquired GH deficiency
      Hypothalamic-pituitary tumors
      Histiocytosis X
      Central nervous system infections
      Head injuries
      GH deficiency following cranial irradiation
      Central nervous system vascular accidents
      Hydrocephalus
      Empty sella syndrome
    Abnormalities of GH action
      Laron's dwarfism
      Pygmies
  Psychosocial dwarfism
  Hypothyroidism
  Glucocorticoid excess (Cushing's syndrome)
    Endogenous
    Exogenous
  Pseudohypoparathyroidism
  Disorders of vitamin D metabolism
  Diabetes mellitus
  Diabetes insipidus, untreated

II. CAUSES OF TALL STATURE

Nonendocrine causes
  Constitutional tall stature
  Genetic tall stature
  Syndromes of tall stature
    Cerebral gigantism
    Marfan's syndrome
    Homocystinuria
    Beckwith-Wiedemann syndrome
    XYY and XYYY syndromes
    Klinefelter's syndrome

Endocrine disorders
  Pituitary gigantism
  Sexual precocity
  Thyrotoxicosis
  Infants of diabetic mothers

tion with increased stature during childhood and early onset of puberty. Thus, short stature in an overweight child must be considered to have an organic cause until proved otherwise.

Turner's Syndrome & Its Variants

While classic Turner's syndrome of 45,XO gonadal dysgenesis (see Chapter 14) is often correctly diagnosed, it is not always appreciated that any phenotypic female with short stature may have a variant of Turner's syndrome. Thus, a karyotype determination should be done for every short girl if no other cause for short stature is found, especially if puberty is delayed (see Chapters 13, 14, and 15).

Noonan's Syndrome (Pseudo-Turner Syndrome)

This syndrome shares several phenotypic characteristics of Turner's syndrome, including short stature, webbed neck, low posterior hairline, and facial resemblance to Turner's syndrome, but the karyotype is 46,XX in the female or 46,XY in the male with Noonan's syndrome, and other features clearly differentiate it from Turner's syndrome—eg, in Turner's syndrome there is characteristically left-sided heart disease and in Noonan's syndrome right-sided heart disease. Noonan's syndrome is an autosomal dominant disorder at gene locus 12q24 (see Chapters 14 and 15).

Prader-Willi Syndrome

This condition is characterized by fetal (poor intrauterine movement) and infantile hypotonia, acromicria (small hands and feet), developmental delay, almond-shaped eyes, and extreme obesity. Glucose intolerance and delayed puberty are characteristic. This syndrome is due to deletion of the small nuclear riboprotein polypeptide N (SNRPN) on paternal chromosome 15 (q11–13), uniparental disomy of maternal chromosome 15, or methylation of this region of chromosome 15 of paternal origin. If a mutation of the same locus is derived from the mother, Angelman's syndrome results (see Chapter 15).

Laurence-Moon Syndrome & Biedl-Bardet Syndrome

Biedl-Bardet syndrome, associated with mutations on chromosome 16 (q21), is characterized by developmental delay, retinitis pigmentosa, polydactyly, and obesity. Laurence-Moon syndrome is characterized by developmental delay, retinitis pigmentosa, delayed puberty, and spastic paraplegia. Both syndromes are associated with poor growth and obesity. They are inherited as autosomal recessive disorders (see Chapter 15).

Autosomal Chromosomal Disorders & Syndromes

Numerous other autosomal chromosomal disorders and syndromes of dysmorphic children with or without mental retardation are characterized by short stature. Often the key to diagnosis is the presence of several major or minor physical abnormalities that indicate the need for karyotype determination. Other abnormalities may include unusual body proportions, such as short extremities, leading to aberrant US:LS ratios, and arm spans quite discrepant from stature. Some conditions, such as trisomy 21 (Down's syndrome), are quite common, while others are rare. Details of these syndromes can be found in the references listed at the end of the chapter.

Skeletal Dysplasias

There are more than 100 known types of genetic skeletal dysplasias (osteochondrodysplasias). Often they are noted at birth because of the presence of short limbs or trunk, but some are only diagnosed after a period of postnatal growth. The most common condition is autosomal dominant achondroplasia. This condition is characterized by short extremities in the proximal regions, a relatively large head with a prominent forehead due to frontal bossing and a depressed nasal bridge, and lumbar lordosis in later life. Intelligence is normal. Mutations of the tyrosine kinase domain of the fibroblast growth factor receptor gene (*FGFR3* gene locus 4p16.3) have been described in this condition. Adult height is decreased, with a mean of 132 cm for males and 123 cm for females. Limb lengthening operations are used to increase stature in a few centers. Children with achondroplasia who have received GH have in some instances demonstrated improved growth; however, one child experienced atlanto-occipital dislocation. The potential for abnormal brain growth and its relationship to aberrant skull shape mandates the caution that GH is not considered established therapy for this condition. Hypochondroplasia is manifested on a continuum from severe short-limbed dwarfism to apparent normal development until puberty, when there is an attenuated or absent pubertal growth spurt, leading to short adult stature. This disorder may be caused by an abnormal allele in the achondroplasia gene.

5. Chronic Disease

Severe chronic disease involving any organ system can cause poor growth in childhood and adolescence. In many cases, there will be adequate physical findings by the time of consultation to permit diagnosis; in some cases, however—most notably celiac disease and regional enteritis—short stature and decreased growth may precede obvious signs of malnutrition or gastrointestinal disease. In some cases, growth is only delayed and may spontaneously improve. In others, growth can be increased by improved nutrition; patients with gastrointestinal disease, kidney disease, or cancer may benefit from nocturnal parenteral nutritional infusions. Cystic fibrosis combines several causes of growth failure: lung disease impairs oxygenation and predisposes to chronic infections, gastrointestinal disease decreases nutrient availability, and late-developing abnormalities of the endocrine pancreas cause diabetes mellitus. Children with cystic fibrosis experience decreased growth rates after one year of age following a normal birth size. The pubertal growth spurt is often decreased in magnitude and delayed in its timing: secondary sexual development may be delayed especially in those with impaired pulmonary function. Study of growth in these patients allowed development of a cystic fibrosis specific growth chart and indicates that a reasonable outcome is an adult height in the 25th percentile. Children with congestive heart failure due to a variety of congenital heart diseases or acquired myocarditis grow poorly unless successfully treated with medications or surgery; patients with cyanotic heart disease experience less deficit in growth.

Celiac disease may present initially with growth failure. Early diagnosis can be made by determination of antigliadin, antiendomysial, or antireticulin antibodies while on a normal wheat-containing diet. These studies may be falsely positive, and a biopsy may still be required for diagnosis. On a gluten-free diet, patients experience catch-up growth which is strongest in the first year of therapy but continues for several more. Adult height may still be impaired, depending upon the duration of the period without treatment. Untreated patients with celiac disease have decreased serum IGF-I concentrations, presumably due to malnutrition while IGF-I concentrations rise with dietary therapy; thus serum IGF-I in this condition, as in many with nutritional deficiencies, is not a reliable indicator of GH secretory status.

Crohn's disease is associated with poor growth and decreased serum IGF-I concentrations. On an elemental diet growth rate increases and with glucocorticoid therapy (moderate doses), growth rate improves even though serum IGF-I decreases.

Patients with chronic hematologic diseases, such as sickle cell anemia or thalassemia, often have poor growth, delayed puberty, and short adult stature. Juvenile rheumatoid arthritis may compromise growth before or after therapy with glucocorticoids. GH treatment is reported to increase the growth rate of these children, but it is too early to draw conclusions about the efficacy and safety of such therapy in juvenile rheumatoid arthritis.

Chronic renal disease is known to interfere with growth. Hypophosphatemic vitamin D-resistant rickets will usually lead to short adult stature, but treatment with 1,25-hydroxyvitamin D_3 (cholecalciferol) and oral phosphate in most cases will lead to increased—if not normal—adult stature. Children with chronic renal failure are reported to have increased growth rate with improved nutrition and GH therapy.

Proximal and distal renal tubular acidosis may both cause short stature. Proximal renal tubular acidosis demonstrates bicarbonate wasting at normal or low plasma bicarbonate concentrations; patients have hypokalemia, alkaline urine pH, severe bicarbonaturia, and, later, acidemia. The condition may be inherited, sporadic, or secondary to many metabolic or medication-induced disorders. Distal renal tubular acidosis is caused by inability to acidify the urine; it may occur in sporadic or familial patterns or be acquired as a result of metabolic disorders or medication therapy. Distal renal tubular acidosis is characterized by hypokalemia, hypercalciuria, and occasional hypocalcemia. The administration of bicarbonate is the primary therapy for proximal renal tubular acidosis, and proper treatment can substantially improve growth rate.

Obstructive sleep apnea is associated with poor growth. The amount of energy expended during sleep in children with sleep apnea appears to limit weight and length gain, a pattern which reverses with the resolution of the obstruction.

Hemoglobin, white blood cell count, erythrocyte sedimentation rate, serum carotene and folate levels, antigliadin, antiendomysial, antireticulin or tissue transglutaminase antibodies, plasma bicarbonate levels, and liver and kidney function should be assessed in short but otherwise apparently healthy children before endocrine screening tests are done. Urinalysis should be performed, with attention to specific gravity (to rule out diabetes insipidus) and ability to acidify urine (to evaluate possible renal tubular acidosis). All short girls without a diagnosis should undergo karyotype analysis to rule out Turner's syndrome. A list of chronic diseases causing short stature is presented in Table 6–2.

6. Malnutrition

Malnutrition (other than that associated with chronic disease) is the most common cause of short stature worldwide. Diagnosis in the developed world is based on historical and physical findings, particularly the dietary history. Food faddism and anorexia nervosa—as well as voluntary dieting can cause poor growth. Infection with parasites such as *Ascaris lumbricoides* or *Giardia lamblia* can decrease growth. Specific nutritional deficiencies can have particular effects upon growth. For example, severe iron deficiency can cause a thin habitus as well as growth retardation. Zinc deficiency can cause anorexia, decreased growth, and delayed puberty, usually in the presence of chronic systemic disease or infection. Children with nutritional deficiencies will characteristically demonstrate failure of weight gain before growth rate decreases, and weight for height will decrease. This is in contrast to many endocrine causes of poor growth, where weight for height remains in the normal or high range. There are no simple laboratory tests for diagnosis of malnutrition, though serum IGF-I concentrations are low in malnutrition, as they are in GH deficiency.

7. Medications

Children with hyperactivity disorders (or those incorrectly diagnosed as such) are frequently managed with chronic dextroamphetamine or methylphenidate administration. In larger doses, these agents can decrease weight gain—probably because of their effects on appetite—and they have been reported to lower growth rate, albeit inconsistently. These drugs must be used in moderation and only in children who definitely respond to them.

Exogenous glucocorticoids are a potent cause of poor growth (see below).

SHORT STATURE DUE TO ENDOCRINE DISORDERS

1. Growth Hormone Deficiency & Its Variants (Table 6–3)

The incidence of GH deficiency is estimated to be between 1:4000 and 1:3500 in Utah and in Scotland, so the disorder should not be considered rare. Using the conservative criteria of height less than the third percentile and growth velocity less than 5 cm per year, the incidence of endocrine disease in 114,881 Utah children was 5%, with a higher incidence in boys than girls by a ratio of over 2.5:1. In this population, 48% of the children with Turner's syndrome or growth hormone deficiency were not diagnosed prior to the careful evaluation afforded by this study.

There may be abnormalities at various levels of the hypothalamic-pituitary GH-IGF-I axis. Most patients with idiopathic GH deficiency apparently lack GHRH. One autopsied GH-deficient patient had an adequate number of pituitary somatotrophs that contained considerable GH stores; the pituitary gland produced growth hormone, but it could not be released. Long-term treatment of such patients with GHRH can cause GH release and improve growth. Patients with pituitary tumors or those rare patients with congenital absence of

Table 6–3. Postulated disorders of hGH release and action.

Site of Defect	Clinical Condition
Hypothalamus	Idiopathic GH deficiency due to decreased GHRH secretion; hypothalamic tumors
Pituitary gland	Dysplasia, trauma, surgery, or tumor of the pituitary gland; gene defect with impaired GH biosynthesis
Sites of IGF production	Laron's dwarfism with high GH and low IGF concentrations (GH receptor defect) Pygmies with normal GH, low IGF-1, and normal IGF-2 concentrations
Cartilage	Glucocorticoid-induced growth failure. Resistance to IGF-1

the pituitary gland lack somatotrophs. Several kindreds have been described that lack various regions of the GH gene responsible for producing GH. Alternatively, gene defects responsible for the embryogenesis of the pituitary gland may cause multiple pituitary deficiencies. Absence of the *PIT1* gene (a pituitary-specific transcription factor) causes deficient GH, TSH, and prolactin synthesis and secretion. Mutations of the *PROP1* gene cause deficiencies of GH, TSH, FSH, LH production, and possibly ACTH.

Congenital Growth Hormone Deficiency

Congenital GH deficiency presents with slightly decreased birth length (−1 SD) but decreased growth rate soon after birth. The disorder is identified by careful measurement in the first year and becomes more obvious by 1–2 years of age. Patients with classic GH deficiency have short stature, obesity with immature facial appearance, immature high-pitched voice, and delay in skeletal maturation. Less severe forms of partial GH deficiency are described with few abnormal characteristics apart from short stature. Growth hormone deficient patients lack the lipolytic effects of growth hormone partially accounting for the pudgy appearance. There is a higher incidence of hyperlipidemia with elevated total cholesterol and LDL in GH deficiency, and longitudinal studies demonstrate elevation of HDL with GH treatment. Males with GH deficiency may have microphallus (penis less than 2 cm in length at birth), especially if the condition is accompanied by gonadotropin-releasing hormone (GnRH) deficiency (Figure 6–8). GH deficiency in the neonate or child can also lead to symptomatic hypoglycemia and seizures; if ACTH deficiency is also present, hypoglycemia is usually more severe. The differential diag-

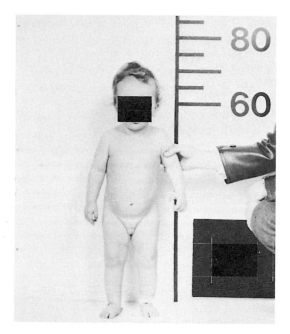

Figure 6–8. A 12-month-old boy with congenital hypopituitarism. He had hypoglycemic seizures at 12 hours of age. At 1 year, he had another hypoglycemic seizure (plasma glucose, 25 mg/dL) associated with an episode of otitis media, and it was noted that his penis was quite small. At 12 months, length was 66.5 cm (–2 SD) and weight was 8.5 kg (–3 SD). The penis was less than 1.5 cm long, and both testes were descended (each 1 cm in diameter). Plasma GH did not rise above 1 ng/mL after arginine and levodopa testing. (No insulin was given because of the history of hypoglycemia.) LH rose very little after administration of GnRH (gonadorelin), 100 µg. Serum thyroxine was low (T_4, 6.6 µg/dL; T_4 index, 1.5), and after administration of 200 µg of protirelin (TRH), serum TSH rose with a delayed peak characteristic of tertiary hypothyroidism. Plasma ACTH rose only to 53 pg/mL after metyrapone. Thus, the patient had multiple defects in the hypothalamic-pituitary axis. He was given six doses of 2000 units each of chorionic gonadotropin (hCG) intramuscularly over 2 weeks, and plasma testosterone rose to 62 ng/dL, indicating normal testicular function. He was then treated with 25 mg of testosterone enanthate every month for 3 months, and his phallus enlarged to 3.5 × 1.2 cm without significant advancement of bone age. With hGH therapy (0.05 mg/kg intramuscularly every other day), he grew at a greater than normal rate for 12 months (catch-up growth), and growth then continued at a normal rate.

nosis of neonatal hypoglycemia in a full-term infant who has not sustained birth trauma must include neonatal hypopituitarism. If microphallus (in a male subject), optic hypoplasia, or some other midline facial or central nervous system defect is noted, the diagnosis of congenital GH deficiency is more likely (see below). Congenital GH deficiency is also statistically correlated with breech delivery. Intelligence is normal in GH deficiency unless repeated or severe hypoglycemia or a significant anatomic defect has compromised brain development. When thyrotropin-releasing hormone (TRH) deficiency is also present, there may be additional signs of hypothyroidism. Secondary or tertiary congenital hypothyroidism is not usually associated with mental retardation as is congenital primary hypothyroidism, but a few cases of isolated TRH deficiency and severe mental retardation have been reported.

Congenital GH deficiency may present with midline anatomic defects. Optic hypoplasia with visual defects ranging from nystagmus to blindness is found with variable hypothalamic deficiency, including diabetes insipidus; about half of patients with optic hypoplasia have absence of the septum pellucidum on CT scan or MRI, leading to the diagnosis of **septo-optic dysplasia.** Septo-optic dysplasia is most often sporadic in occurrence, but families are reported with mutations of the *HESX1* locus (3p21.2–p21.1), a homeobox gene. Cleft palate or other forms of oral dysraphism are associated with GH deficiency in about 7% of cases; thus, such children may need more than nutritional support to improve their growth. An unusual midline defect associated with GH deficiency is described in children with a single maxillary incisor.

Congenital absence of the pituitary, which occurs in an autosomal recessive pattern, leads to severe hypopituitarism, including hypoglycemia and hypopituitarism; affected patients have shallow development or absence of the sella turcica. This defect is quite rare but clinically devastating if treatment is delayed.

Hereditary GH deficiency is described in several kindreds. Recent biochemical techniques have defined various genetic defects of the *GHN* gene (17q22–24) in affected families. Type IA GH deficiency is inherited in an autosomal recessive pattern, and patients have deletions, frameshifts, and nonsense mutations in the GH genome; unlike those with classic sporadic GH deficiency, some of these children are reported with short birth lengths. Patients with absent or abnormal GH genes do initially respond to exogenous hGH administration, but some soon develop high antibody titers that eliminate the effect of therapy; one reported kindred had a heterogeneous response as one sibling continued to grow and did not develop blocking antibodies while the opposite effect occurred in two other siblings in the same family. Patients with high titers of blocking antibodies are reported to benefit from IGF-I therapy in place of GH therapy. Type IB patients have autosomal recessive splice site mutations and incomplete GH deficiency; they are less severely affected. Type II patients have autosomal dominant GH deficiency due to splice site or missense mutations; and type III patients have X-linked GH deficiency often associated with hypogammaglobulinemia. A few patients are described with abnormalities of the *GRF* gene, while others are described with mutant GH molecules.

Acquired Growth Hormone Deficiency

Onset of GH deficiency in late childhood or adolescence, particularly if accompanied by other pituitary hormone deficiencies, is ominous and may be due to a hypothalamic-pituitary tumor. The development of posterior pituitary deficiency in addition to anterior pituitary deficiency makes a tumor even more likely. The empty sella syndrome is more frequently associated with hypothalamic-pituitary abnormalities in childhood than in adulthood; thus, GH deficiency may be found in affected patients.

Some patients, chiefly boys with constitutional delay in growth and adolescence, may have transient GH deficiency on testing before the actual onset of puberty; when serum testosterone concentrations begin to increase in these patients, GH secretion and growth rate also increase. This transient state may incorrectly suggest bona fide GH deficiency but does not require therapy. Conditions that cause acquired GH deficiency—craniopharyngiomas, germinomas, gliomas, histiocytosis X, etc—are described in Chapters 5 and 15. It is remarkable that after craniopharyngioma removal, some patients, mainly obese subjects, continue to grow quite well in spite of the absence of GH secretion. This appears to be caused by hyperinsulinemia.

Cranial irradiation of the hypothalamic-pituitary region to treat head tumors or acute lymphoblastic leukemia may result in GH deficiency approximately 12–18 months later, owing to radiation-induced hypothalamic (or perhaps pituitary) damage. Higher doses of irradiation such as the 24 Gy previously routinely used for the treatment of central nervous system leukemia have greater effect (final height may be as much as 1.7 SD below the mean) than the 18 Gy used more routinely now. Girls treated at an early age with this newer regimen still appear to be at risk for growth failure. All children must be carefully observed for growth failure after irradiation. If these patients receive spinal irradiation, upper body growth may also be impaired, causing a decreased US:LS ratio. Abdominal irradiation for Wilms' tumor may also lead to decreased spinal growth (estimated loss of 10 cm height from megavoltage therapy for treatment at 1 year of age, and

7 cm from treatment at 5 years of age). Others receiving gonadal irradiation (or chemotherapy) have impaired gonadal function and lack onset or progression of puberty and have diminished or absent pubertal growth spurt.

Other Types of Growth Hormone Dysfunction or Deficiency

Other disorders of GH production or action are not manifested in the classic manner of GH deficiency.

Laron's syndrome (primary GH resistance or insensitivity or primary IGF-I deficiency) is due to GH receptor or postreceptor defects in an autosomal recessive pattern. Patients with decreased or absent GH receptors have decreased serum GHBP levels, while those with postreceptor defects have normal GHBP concentrations. Affected children are found throughout the world, including Israel, where the syndrome was first reported, and Ecuador, where several generations of a large kindred were studied in great detail; defects in various kindreds include nonsense mutations, deletions, RNA processing defects, and translational stop codons. Serum GH is elevated, with decreased or absent IGF-I. The growth deficiency does not respond to GH treatment. Patients are short at birth, confirming the importance of IGF-I in fetal growth that was apparent in IGF-I gene knockout experiments in mice. The head circumference and jaw are small, and there is some intellectual impairment. About one-third have hypoglycemia, and half of boys have microphallus. Patients treated with recombinant DNA-derived IGF-I grew at an improved rate but did not respond as well to IGF-I as GH-deficient children do to GH treatment, indicating the direct role of GH in fostering growth above the effect of IGF-I itself.

Other forms of GH resistance are described, but the majority of patients with disorders of the GH axis have abnormalities of GH secretion, not action. Very short, poorly growing children with delayed skeletal maturation, normal GH and IGF-I values, and no signs of organic disease have responded to GH therapy with increased growth rates equal to those of patients with bona fide GH deficiency. These patients may have a variation of constitutional delay in growth or genetic short stature, but a subtle abnormality of GH secretion or action is possible.

A few patients are reported with defects of the IGF-I gene or with deficiency of the IGF-I receptor.

Why do certain normal children, perhaps within a short family, have stature significantly lower than the mean? There is no definite answer to this persistent question, but some patients have decreased serum GHBP concentrations, which suggests a decrease in GH receptors in these children. A minority of short, poorly growing children have definable genetic abnormalities of their GH receptors. It is likely that short stature is the final common pathway of numerous biochemical abnormalities.

With plentiful GH supplies, there is increasing pressure to treat more children—usually boys—who are not severely short and are not growing extremely slowly and do not have greatly delayed bone ages. Some studies suggest that increased final height can be achieved with such treatment, but others do not, and the treatment is not standard and has not proved to be effective.

Pygmies have normal serum GH, low IGF-I, and normal IGF-II concentrations. They will not respond to exogenous GH with improved growth rate or a rise in IGF-I. Thus, they have a congenital inability to produce IGF-I, which has greater importance in stimulating growth than IGF-II. Pygmy children are reported to lack a pubertal growth spurt, suggesting that IGF-I is essential to attain a normal peak growth velocity. Efe pygmies, the shortest of the pygmies, are significantly smaller at birth than neighboring Africans, and their growth is slower throughout childhood, leading to statures displaced progressively below the mean. Presumably, IGF-I therapy would increase growth rates in this population during childhood and puberty, but such therapy has not yet been reported.

Adults who had growth hormone deficiency in childhood or adolescence have decreased bone mass compared with normals even when bone mass is corrected for their smaller size. Many of these patients were treated with GH for various periods, but it appears that GH therapy may not completely reverse the effects of GH deficiency on skeletal density.

Diagnosis of Growth Hormone Deficiency

Because basal values of serum GH are low in normal children and GH-deficient patients alike, the diagnosis of GH deficiency rests upon demonstration of an inadequate rise of serum GH after provocative stimuli or upon some other measure of GH secretion. This process is complicated because different radioimmunoassay systems vary widely in their measurements of GH in the same blood sample (eg, a result on a single sample may be above 10 ng/mL in one assay but only 6 ng/mL in another). The physician must be familiar with the standards of the laboratory being used. Most insurance companies and state agencies will accept inability of GH to rise above 10 ng/mL with stimulation as inadequate and diagnostic of GH deficiency.

Another complicating factor is the state of pubertal development. Prepubertal children secrete less GH than pubertal subjects and, especially as they approach the onset of puberty, may have sufficiently reduced GH secretion to falsely suggest bona fide GH deficiency. This factor is sometimes addressed by administering a dose of estrogen to such subjects before testing. The very concept of GH testing provides a further complication. GH is released in episodic pulses. While a patient who does not secrete GH in response to standard challenges is generally considered to be GH-deficient, a normal GH response to these tests may not rule out GH deficiency. Testing should occur after an overnight fast; carbohydrate or fat ingestion will suppress GH response. Obesity suppresses GH secretion, and a chubby child may falsely appear to have GH deficiency. Because 10% or more of healthy children will not have an adequate rise in GH with one test of GH reserve, at least two methods of assessing GH reserve are necessary before the diagnosis of classic GH deficiency is assigned. Of course, if GH rises above 10 ng/mL in a single test, classic GH deficiency is eliminated. Serum GH values should rise after 10 minutes of vigorous exercise; this is used as a screening test. After an overnight fast, GH levels should rise in response to arginine infusion (0.5 g/kg body weight [up to 20 g] over 30 minutes), oral levodopa (125 mg for up to 15 kg body weight, 250 mg for up to 35 kg, or 500 mg for over 35 kg), or clonidine (0.1–0.15 mg/m² orally). Side effects of levodopa include nausea; those of clonidine include some drop in blood pressure and drowsiness.

GH levels also rise after acute hypoglycemia due to insulin administration; however, this test carries a risk of seizure if the blood glucose level drops excessively. An insulin tolerance test may be performed if a 10–25% dextrose infusion is available for emergency administration in the face of hypoglycemic coma or seizure, if the patient can be continuously observed by a physician, and if the patient has no history of hypoglycemic seizures. The patient must have a normal glucose concentration at the beginning of the test in the morning after an overnight fast (water intake is acceptable). Regular insulin, 0.075–0.1 unit/kg in saline, may be given as an intravenous bolus. In 20–40 minutes, a 50% drop in blood glucose will occur, and a rise in serum GH and cortisol and ACTH should follow. Serum glucose should be monitored, and an intravenous line must be maintained for emergency dextrose infusion in case the patient becomes unconscious or has a hypoglycemic seizure. If dextrose infusion is necessary, it is imperative that blood glucose not be raised far above the normal range, since hyperosmolality has been reported from overzealous glucose replacement; undiluted 50% dextrose should not be used (see Chapter 5).

A family of penta- and hexapeptides called growth hormone-releasing peptides (GHRPs) stimulate GH secretion in normals and in growth hormone-deficient subjects. GHRPs act via ghrelin receptors that are different from the GRF receptors, and their effects are additive to that of GRF. These agents are used in diagnosis and therapy.

Patients who respond to pharmacologic stimuli (eg, levodopa, clonidine, or insulin) but not to physiologic stimuli such as exercise or sleep were said to have neurosecretory dysfunction; these patients have decreased 24-hour secretion of hGH (or integrated concentrations of hGH) compared with healthy subjects, patterns similar to those observed in GH-deficient patients. It is not clear how frequently this condition is encountered.

This long discussion of the interpretation of GH after secretagogue testing brings into question the very standard for the diagnosis of GH deficiency. It is clear that pharmacologic testing cannot always determine which patients truly need GH therapy, and some authorities suggest we abandon such dynamic testing.

Serum IGF-I and IGFBP-3 measurements are alternative methods for evaluating GH adequacy. Serum IGF-I values will be low in most GH-deficient subjects, but, as noted above, some short patients with normal serum IGF-I concentrations may require GH treatment to improve growth rate. In addition, starvation will lower IGF-I values in healthy children and incorrectly suggest GH deficiency. Children with psychosocial dwarfism—who need family therapy or foster home placement rather than GH therapy—have low GH and IGF-I concentrations and may falsely appear to have growth hormone deficiency. Likewise, patients with constitutional delay in adolescence will have low IGF-I values for chronologic age but normal values for skeletal age and may have temporarily decreased GH response to secretagogues. Thus, IGF-I determinations are not infallible in the diagnosis of GH deficiency. They must be interpreted with regard to nutrition, psychosocial status, and skeletal ages. IGFBP-3 is GH-dependent, and if its concentration is low, it is more indicative of GH deficiency than IGF-I determination.

Although pharmacologic tests of GH secretion and serum IGF-I and IGFBP-3 values will usually identify those individuals who have classic GH deficiency, the diagnosis will remain in doubt in some cases. This should not lead to the conclusion that all short children should receive GH therapy. Only about half of very short children (height well below the fifth percentile or > 2.5–3.5 SD below the mean) who grow very slowly (growth velocity below the fifth percentile for age) with delayed bone ages, meticulously studied in research protocols, were shown to benefit from hGH therapy in the absence of classic GH deficiency. However, children meeting less stringent criteria have been treated with GH in controlled trials, producing some increase in growth rate in some but not all studies; it is not yet clear whether this treatment increases adult height. Thus, in the absence of classic GH deficiency, no clearly recognized measurement can predict which short child is likely to respond to GH therapy before it is instituted. The Growth Hormone Research Society produced criteria that attempt to deal with the diagnosis of growth hormone deficiency in childhood in spite of the uncertainty of the methods. These criteria use clinical findings of various conditions associated with growth hormone deficiency, the severity of short stature, and the degree and duration of decreased growth velocity to identify individuals that may have GH deficiency. The guidelines and diagnostic considerations in this chapter include most of the GH Society criteria. (See "Consensus guidelines" reference in the Short Stature section at the end of this chapter for details of the GH Society statement.) A 3- to 6-month therapeutic trial of GH therapy may be necessary. In patients who were diagnosed late, have entered puberty, and appear to have limited time to respond to GH before epiphysial fusion causes the cessation of growth, a GnRH agonist has been used to delay epiphysial fusion in clinical trials.

GH therapy will increase adult height in Turner's syndrome if started early enough; the addition of low-dose oxandrolone will further increase growth rate. Estrogen must be used during the adolescent years only in low doses and only after the normal age of onset of puberty is reached to preserve adult height.

Treatment of Growth Hormone Deficiency

A. Hormonal Replacement

Before 1986, the only available method of treatment for GH deficiency was replacement therapy with human GH (hGH) derived from cadaver donors. In 1985 and thereafter, Creutzfeldt-Jakob disease, a degenerative neurologic disease rare in patients so young, was diagnosed in some patients who had received natural hGH 10–15 years before. Because of the possibility that prions contaminating donor pituitary glands were transmitted to the GH-deficient patients, causing their deaths, natural growth hormone from all sources was removed from distribution. Recombinant growth hormone now accounts for the world's current supply.

Commercial growth hormone is currently available in the 191-amino-acid natural-sequence form (somatropin) and, less commonly, in the 192-amino-acid methionyl form (somatrem). There is no convincing evidence that either form is clinically superior to the other, but somatropin is prescribed more often. GH is now available in virtually unlimited amounts, allowing innovative treatment regimens not previously possible owing to scarce supplies; however, the potential for abuse of GH in athletes or in children of normal size whose parents wish them to be taller than average must now be addressed.

GHRH was isolated, sequenced, and synthesized and is now available for use in diagnosis and treatment. GH-deficient patients demonstrate lower or absent GH secretion after administration of GHRH. However, episodic doses of GHRH can restore GH secretion, IGF-I production, and growth in children with idiopathic GH deficiency. The ability of GHRH administration to cause pituitary GH secretion further supports the concept that idiopathic GH deficiency is primarily a disease of the hypothalamus, not of the pituitary gland.

IGF-I is now produced by recombinant DNA technology. Although no long-term human treatment program has yet been reported, initial studies suggest that IGF-I may be a useful treatment for short stature, particularly in Laron dwarfism (and perhaps for African pygmies, should treatment be desired) where no other treatment is possible. Growth disturbances due to disorders of GH release or action are shown in Table 6–3. GH-deficient children require biosynthetic somatropin (natural sequence GH) or somatrem (methionyl GH) at a dose of 0.3 mg/kg/wk administered in one dose per day six or seven times per week during the period of active growth before epiphysial fusion. A depot preparation that may be given every 2 weeks or every 4 weeks is now available; a larger volume and sometimes multiple injections are required. The increase in growth rate (Figures 6–9, 6–10, and 6–11) is most marked during the first year of therapy. Older children do not respond as well and may require larger doses. Higher doses are approved by the FDA for use in puberty. GH will not increase growth rate without adequate nutrition and euthyroid status. During the roughly 50 years since the first use of GH in children, long-term effects are reported in several series. If only the children most recently treated with recombinant GH are considered, the mean final height was 1.4 SD below the mean, a significant improvement over the −2.9 SD mean height at the start of therapy but not a true normalization of height. With earlier diagnosis and treatment, final height might reach genetic potential.

Antibodies to GH may be present in measurable quantities in the serum of children receiving GH. However, a high titer of blocking antibodies with significant binding capacity is rare except in patients with absence or abnormality of GH genes. Only a few patients are reported to have temporarily ceased growing on somatrem therapy because of antibody formation.

GH exerts anti-insulin effects. Although clinical diabetes is not a likely result of GH therapy, the long-term effects of a small rise in glucose in an otherwise healthy child are unknown. Another potential risk is the rare tendency to develop slipped capital femoral epiphyses in children receiving GH therapy. Recent data have weakened the link between slipped capital femoral epiphyses and GH therapy, but the final import of the relationship is not yet clear. Slipped capital femoral epiphyses, if associated with endocrinopathies, are most common in treated hypothyroid patients (50% one series of 80 episodes of slipped capital femoral epiphyses), followed by treated GH-deficient patients (25% of the series). This condition may occur bilaterally, and prophylactic treatment of the nonaffected side is recommended by several authorities. Pseudotumor cerebri may rarely occur with GH therapy and is usually associated with severe headache. It is reported to reverse after cessation of GH therapy, but if allowed to continue it may impair vision and cause severe complications. Organomegaly and skeletal changes like those found in acromegaly are other theoretical side effects of excessive GH therapy but do not occur with standard doses. Furthermore, several cases of prepubertal gynecomastia are reported with growth hormone therapy.

The discovery of leukemia in young adults previously treated with growth hormone was worrisome, but no cause and effect relationship has been established, and GH treatment is not considered a cause of leukemia. GH does not increase the recurrence rate of tumors existing before therapy. Thus, patients with craniopharyngiomas, for example, may receive GH, if indicated, after the disease is clinically stable without significant worry that the GH will precipitate a recurrence. Clinicians usually wait 1 year after completion of tumor therapy before starting patients on GH therapy, but doing so is not a requirement.

There are numerous studies of GH treatment in idiopathic short stature without classic growth hormone deficiency, but they are rarely controlled studies, and some suffer from methodologic flaws that may account for the variable results. The increased growth rate may be accompanied by advancing bone age, according to some studies, leading to a final height of 1.7 SD below the mean, a result indistinguishable from untreated children with the same conditions. The Lawson Wilkins Pediatric Endocrine Society and the American Academy of Pediatrics both recommend a conservative approach to the treatment of idiopathic short stature with growth hormone.

There are other conditions for which the FDA has approved the use of GH. In the most successful series of children with IUGR treated with GH, the agent increased final height between 2.0 SD and 2.7 SD. Girls with Turner's syndrome treated with GH reach a final height of more than 150 cm, an improvement from the average untreated height which is about 144 cm.

Treatment with GH is approved for chronic renal disease in childhood. GH increases growth rate above the untreated state without excessive advancement in bone age. Prader-Willi syndrome may also be treated with GH to improve growth rate and to increase lean tissue mass and bone density.

Monitoring of growth hormone replacement is mainly accomplished by measuring growth rate and annually assessing bone age advancement. Serum IGF-I

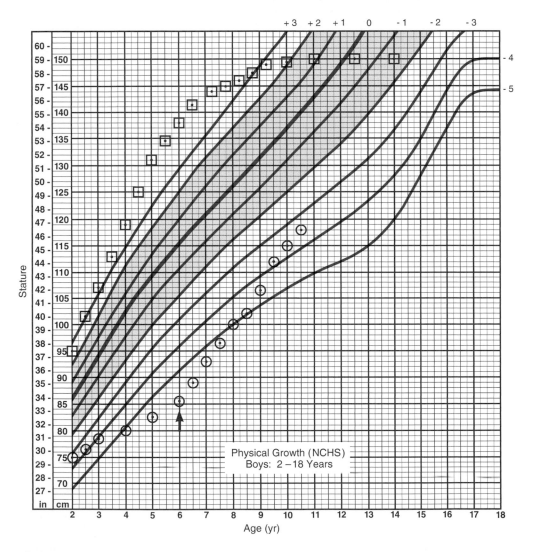

Figure 6–9. Examples of abnormal growth charts. Squares (□) represent the growth pattern of a child (such as patient A in Figure 6–11) with precocious sexual development and early excessive growth leading to premature closure of the epiphyses and cessation of growth. Circles (○) represent growth of a boy (such as patient B in Figure 6–11) with GH deficiency who showed progressively poorer growth until 6 years of age, when he was treated with hGH (arrow), after which catchup growth occurred. The curves describe standard deviations from the mean.

and IGFBP-3 will rise with successful therapy while GHBP will not change appreciably, but these factors are not routinely tested after the start of therapy. Clinical studies are under way to evaluate the utility of titrating the dose of GH to restore serum IGF-I to the high-normal range. Serum bone alkaline phosphatase rises with successful therapy. Urinary hydroxyproline, deoxypyridinolone, and galactosyl-hydroxylysine reflect

growth rate and are used in clinical studies to reflect increased growth rate with therapy.

Growth hormone deficiency is associated with an adverse lipid profile with elevated LDL cholesterol and decreased HDL cholesterol in addition to an increased BMI; GH-deficient adolescents treated with GH develop these findings within a few years after discontinuation of GH therapy. Low-dose GH therapy is now ap-

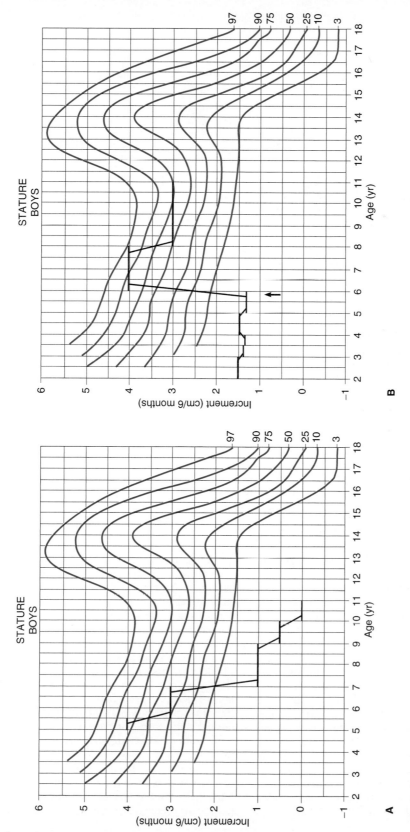

Figure 6–10. Two examples of abnormal growth plotted on a height velocity chart. **A:** The plot is taken from the data recorded as squares in Figure 6–9, describing a patient with precocious puberty, premature epiphysial closure, and cessation of growth. **B:** The plot is taken from the data recorded as circles in Figure 6–9, describing a patient with GH deficiency who was treated with hGH (arrow) at age 6. Initial catch-up growth is noted for 2 years, with a lower (but normal) velocity of growth following. These charts display growth rate over growth intervals rather than 12-month intervals as shown on Figures 6–3 and 6–4.

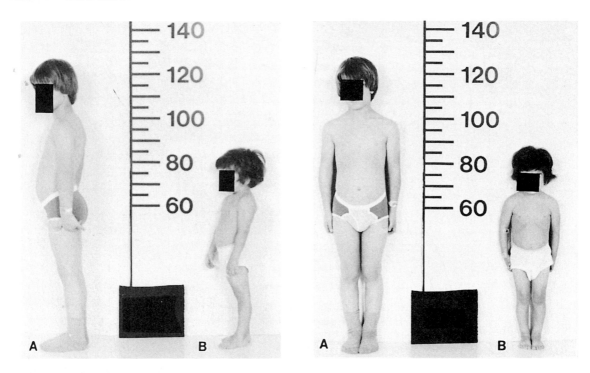

Figure 6–11. Two boys demonstrating extremes of growth. The boy at left in each photograph **(A)** has precocious puberty due to a central nervous system lesion. At 4¹/₂ years, he was 125.1 cm tall, which is 5 SD above the mean. (The mean height for a 4-year-old is 101.5 cm.) His testes measured 2 × 3.5 cm each, his penis 9.8 × 2.8 cm. He was muscular and had acne and a deep voice. His bone age was 10 years, the testosterone level was 480 ng/dL, and the LH rose after 100 μg of GnRH (gonadorelin) to a pubertal response. His brain CT scan revealed a hamartoma of the tuber cinereum. The boy at right **(B)** at 4¹/₂ years was 85 cm tall, which is 4.5 SD below the mean. He had the classic physical and historical characteristics of idiopathic GH deficiency, including early growth failure and a cherubic appearance. His plasma GH values did not rise after provocative testing.

proved for use in adults with childhood-onset growth hormone deficiency and is said to forestall these metabolic changes. One can therefore inform the parents of a child with GH deficiency that the patient may still benefit from GH therapy even after he or she stops growing.

B. Psychologic Management and Outcome

Research into the psychologic outcome of patients with short stature is flawed by lack of consistent methods of investigation and lack of controlled studies, but some results are of interest. Studies vary in concluding whether short stature is harmful to a child's psychologic development or not and whether, by inference, growth hormone is helpful in improving the child's psychologic functioning. Children with growth hormone deficiency are the most extensively studied; earlier investigations suggest that they have more passive personality traits than do healthy children, may have delayed emo-

tional maturity, and suffer from infantilization from parents, teachers, and peers. Many of these children have been held back in school because of their size without regard to their academic abilities. Some patients retain a body image of short stature even after normal height has been achieved with treatment. More recent studies challenge these views and suggest that self-image in children with height below the fifth percentile, who do not have growth hormone deficiency, is closely comparable to a population of children with normal height. These findings may not be representative of the patient population discussed above in that a normal ambulatory population of "short" children may differ from the selected group that seeks medical attention. The data suggest that short stature itself is not cause for grave psychologic concern, and such concerns should not be used to justify growth hormone therapy. Nonetheless, in certain cases depression and suicidal behavior can occur in affected adolescents because of the psychologic stress associated with short stature and delayed development. We cannot avoid the fact that our "heightist" society values physical stature and equates it with the potential for success, a perception that is not lost on the children with short stature and their parents. A supportive environment in which they are not allowed to act younger than their age nor to occupy a "privileged place" in the family is recommended for children with short stature. Psychologic help is indicated in severe cases of depression or maladjustment.

2. Psychosocial Dwarfism (Figure 6–12)

Children with psychosocial dwarfism present with poor growth, potbellied immature appearance, and bizarre eating and drinking habits. Parents may report that the affected child begs for food from neighbors, forages in garbage cans, and drinks from toilet bowls. As a rule, this tragic condition occurs in only one of several children in a family. Careful questioning and observation

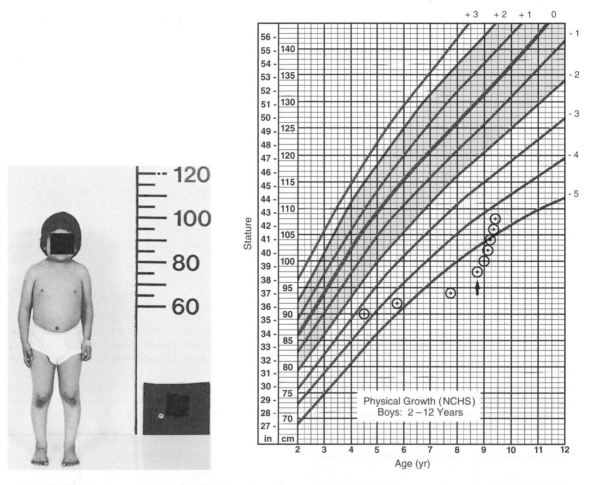

Figure 6–12. Photograph and growth chart of a 9½-year-old boy with psychosocial dwarfism. He had a long history of poor growth (< 3 cm/yr). The social history revealed that he was given less attention and punished more frequently than his seven sibs. He ate from garbage cans and begged for food, though he was not completely deprived of food at home. When the photograph was taken, he was 99 cm tall (–7 SD) and weighed 14.7 kg (–3 SD). His bone age was 5 years, with growth arrest lines visible. Serum thyroxine was 7.8 μg/dL. Peak serum GH varied from nondetectable to 8 ng/mL on different provocative tests between age 6 years and 8½ years. He was placed in a hospital chronic care facility (arrow) for a 6-month period and grew 9 cm, which projects to a yearly growth velocity of 18 cm. On repeat testing, the peak serum GH was 28 ng/mL.

reveal a disordered family structure in which the child is either ignored or severely disciplined. Caloric deprivation or physical battering may or may not be a feature of the history. These children have functional hypopituitarism. Testing will often reveal GH deficiency at first, but after the child is removed from the home, GH function quickly returns to normal. Diagnosis rests upon improvement in behavior or catch-up growth in the hospital or in a foster home. Separation from the family is therapeutic, but the prognosis is guarded. Family psychotherapy may be beneficial, but long-term follow-up is lacking.

Growth disorder due to abnormal parent-child interaction in a younger infant is called maternal deprivation. Caloric deprivation due to parental neglect may be of greater significance in this younger age group. Even in the absence of nutritional restriction or full-blown psychosocial dwarfism, constant negative interactions within a family may inhibit the growth of a child.

It is essential to consider family dynamics in the evaluation of a child with poor growth. It is not appropriate to recommend GH therapy for emotional disorders.

3. Hypothyroidism

Thyroid hormone deficiency decreases postnatal growth rate and skeletal development and, if onset is at or before birth, leads to severe developmental delay unless treatment is rapidly provided. Screening programs for the diagnosis of congenital hypothyroidism have been instituted all over the world, and early treatment following diagnosis in the neonatal period markedly reduces growth failure and has virtually eliminated mental retardation caused by this disorder. Indeed, early treatment of congenital hypothyroidism results in normal growth. Acquired hypothyroidism in older children (eg, due to lymphocytic thyroiditis) may lead to growth failure. Characteristics of hypothyroidism are decreased growth rate and short stature, retarded bone age, and an increased US:LS ratio for chronologic age (Figure 7–33). Patients are apathetic and sluggish and have constipation, bradycardia, coarsening of features and hair, hoarseness, and delayed pubertal development. Intelligence is unaffected in late-onset hypothyroidism, but the apathy and lethargy may make it seem otherwise.

The diagnosis of congenital hypothyroidism is usually made on the basis of neonatal screening studies. In this procedure, currently in use in developed countries throughout the world, a sample of blood is taken from the heel or from the umbilical cord at birth and analyzed for total T_4 or TSH. A total T_4 of under 6 μg/dL or a TSH over 25 mU/L is usually indicative of congenital hypothyroidism, but values differ by state and laboratory. A low total T_4 alone may be associated with low circulating thyroxine-binding globulin (TBG), but the significantly elevated TSH is diagnostic of primary hypothyroidism. The diagnosis may be accompanied by radiologic evidence of retarded bone age in severe congenital hypothyroidism.

In older children, serum TSH is the most reliable diagnostic test. Elevated TSH with decreased free T_4 eliminates the potential confusion resulting from the use of total T_4, which may vary with the level of TBG or other thyroxine-binding proteins. A positive test for serum thyroglobulin antibodies or thyroperoxidase antibodies would lead to the diagnosis of autoimmune thyroid disease (Hashimoto's thyroiditis) as an explanation for the development of hypothyroidism (see Chapter 7). If both FT_4 and TSH are low, the possibility of central hypothyroidism (pituitary or hypothalamic insufficiency) must be considered. This must initiate a search for other hypothalamic-pituitary endocrine deficiencies such as GH deficiency and central nervous system disease (see Chapter 5).

Treatment is by thyroxine replacement. The dose varies from a range of 10–15 μg/kg in infancy to 2–3 μg/kg in older children and teenagers. Suppression of TSH to normal values for age is a useful method of assessing the adequacy of replacement in acquired primary hypothyroidism. However, there are additional considerations in treatment of neonates, and consultation with a pediatric endocrinologist is essential in this age group to ensure optimal central nervous system development.

4. Cushing's Syndrome

Excess glucocorticoids (either exogenous or endogenous) will lead to decreased growth before obesity and other signs of Cushing's syndrome develop. The underlying disease may be bilateral adrenal hyperplasia due to abnormal ACTH-cortisol regulation in Cushing's disease, autonomous adrenal adenomas, or adrenal carcinoma. The appropriate diagnosis may be missed if urinary cortisol and 17-hydroxycorticosteroid determinations are not interpreted on the basis of the child's body size or if inappropriate doses of dexamethasone are used for testing (appropriate doses are 20 μg/kg/d for the low-dose and 80 μg/kg/d for the high-dose dexamethasone suppression test) (see Chapter 9). Furthermore, daily variations in cortisol production necessitate several urinary or plasma cortisol determinations before Cushing's disease can be appropriately diagnosed or ruled out. The high-dose dexamethasone test was positive in 68% of a recent series of children with Cushing's disease. The corticotropin-releasing hormone (CRH) test was positive in 80% of affected patients, whereas

MRI of the pituitary was positive in only 52%. Inferior petrosal sampling (see Chapter 9) was 100% accurate in the diagnosis of Cushing's disease. Transsphenoidal microadenomectomy is the treatment of choice.

Exogenous glucocorticoids used to treat asthma or even overzealous use of topical corticosteroid ointments or creams may suppress growth. These iatrogenic causes of Cushing's syndrome, if resolved early, may allow catch-up growth and so may not affect final height. Thus, an accurate history of prior medications is important in diagnosis. Treatment of the underlying disorder (eg, transsphenoidal microadenomectomy for Cushing's disease) will restore growth rate to normal (catch-up growth may occur initially) if epiphysial fusion has not occurred, but final height will depend upon the length of the period of growth suppression.

5. Pseudohypoparathyroidism

Pseudohypoparathyroidism type 1A is a rare disorder consisting of a characteristic phenotype and chemical signs of hypoparathyroidism (low serum calcium and high serum phosphate), though circulating PTH levels are elevated and target tissues fail to respond to exogenous PTH administration. Children with pseudohypoparathyroidism are short and chubby, with characteristic round facies and short fourth and fifth metacarpals. This constellation of findings is called Albright's hereditary osteodystrophy. Developmental delay is common. The condition is due to a defect in the alpha subunit of the G_s protein transducer (*GNAS1* gene). When imprinted paternally, this results in a defect in the guanylyl nucleotide-sensitive regulatory protein that couples PTH-occupied receptors to adenylyl cyclase. Thus, patients with pseudohypoparathyroidism type 1A have a blunted rise of urinary cAMP in response to administration of PTH. Remarkably, this defect occurs in the same regulatory protein system affected in McCune-Albright syndrome, in which hyperactive endocrine events result (see Chapter 15). A rarer variant of this disorder (pseudohypoparathyroidism type 1B), in which administration of PTH produces a rise in nephrogenous cAMP but fails to induce an increase in phosphate excretion, appears to be due to a defect distal to the receptor-adenylyl cyclase complex. Treatment with high-dose vitamin D or physiologic replacement with 1,25-dihydroxyvitamin D_3 (calcitriol) and exogenous calcium as well as phosphate-binding agents will correct the biochemical defects and control hypocalcemic seizures in patients with pseudohypoparathyroidism.

Two remarkable patients are reported with pseudohypoparathyroidism and premature Leydig cell maturation, both due to abnormalities in the same G protein. The defective protein was shown to be inactive at normal body temperature, leading to defective PTH activity at the level of the kidney and bone. However, it was hyperactive at the cooler temperatures in the scrotum, leading to ligand-independent activation of Leydig cell function.

Children with the pseudohypoparathyroid phenotype of Albright's hereditary osteodystrophy but with normal circulating levels of calcium, phosphate, and PTH have pseudopseudohypoparathyroidism. They require no calcium or vitamin D therapy. (See Chapter 8.)

6. Disorders of Vitamin D Metabolism

Short stature and poor growth are features of rickets in its obvious or more subtle forms. The cause may be vitamin D deficiency due to inadequate oral intake, fat malabsorption, inadequate sunlight exposure, anticonvulsant therapy, or renal or hepatic disease. In addition, there are inherited forms of vitamin D-dependent rickets. Classic findings of vitamin D-deficient rickets include bowing of the legs, chest deformities (rachitic rosary), and characteristic radiographic findings of the extremities associated with decreased serum calcium and phosphate levels and elevated serum alkaline phosphatase levels. There are two forms of hereditary vitamin D-dependent rickets. Type I involves a renal 25OHD 1-hydroxylase deficiency, and type II involves an absent or defective vitamin D receptor. However, the most common type of rickets in the United States is X-linked hypophosphatemic rickets, a dominant genetic disorder affecting renal reabsorption of phosphate. It is associated with short stature, severe and progressive bowing of the legs (but no changes in the wrists or chest), normal or slightly elevated serum calcium, very low serum phosphate, and urinary phosphate wasting. Short stature is linked with rickets in other renal disorders associated with renal phosphate wasting. Examples include Fanconi's syndrome (including cystinosis and other inborn errors of metabolism) and renal tubular acidosis.

When treatment is effective in these disorders (eg, vitamin D for vitamin D deficiency or alkali therapy for appropriate types of renal tubular acidosis), growth rate will improve. Replacement of vitamin D and phosphate is appropriate therapy for vitamin D-resistant rickets. It improves the bowing of the legs and leads to improved growth, though there is a risk of nephrocalcinosis. This necessitates annual renal ultrasound examinations when patients are receiving vitamin D therapy (see Chapter 8).

In the Williams syndrome of elfin facies, supravalvular aortic stenosis, and mental retardation with gregarious personality, patients have intrauterine growth retardation and greatly reduced height in childhood and as adults; this disorder may have infantile hypocalcemia but is no longer considered a disorder of vitamin D since a genetic defect in the elastin gene at 7q11.23 occurs in most affected patients (see Chapters 8 and 15).

7. Diabetes Mellitus

Growth in type 1 diabetes mellitus depends on the efficacy of therapy; well-controlled diabetes mellitus is compatible with normal growth, while poorly controlled diabetes often causes slow growth. Liver and spleen enlargement in a poorly controlled short diabetic child is known as Mauriac's syndrome, rarely seen now owing to improved diabetic care. Another factor that may decrease growth rate in children with diabetes mellitus is the increased incidence of Hashimoto's thyroiditis; yearly thyroid function screening is advisable, especially as the peripubertal period approaches. Growth hormone concentrations are higher in children with diabetes, and this factor may play a role in the development of complications of diabetes mellitus. IGF-I concentrations tend to be normal or low, depending upon glucose control, but judging from the elevated GH noted above, the stimulation of IGF-I production by GH appears to be partially blocked in these children. (See Chapter 17.)

8. Diabetes Insipidus

Polyuria and polydipsia due to inadequate vasopressin (neurogenic diabetes insipidus) or inability of the kidney to respond to vasopressin (nephrogenic diabetes insipidus) leads to poor caloric intake and decreased growth. With appropriate treatment (see Chapter 5), the growth rate should return to normal. Acquired neurogenic diabetes insipidus may herald a hypothalamic-pituitary tumor, and growth failure may be due to associated GH deficiency.

THE DIAGNOSIS OF SHORT STATURE

An initial decision must determine whether a child is pathologically short or simply distressed because height is not as close to the 50th percentile as desired by the patient or the parents. Performing unnecessary tests is expensive and may be a source of long-term concern to the parents—a concern that could have been avoided by appropriate reassurance. Alternatively, missing a diagnosis of pathologic poor growth may cause the patient to lose inches of final height or may allow progression of disease.

If a patient's stature, growth rate, or height adjusted for midparental height is sufficiently decreased to warrant evaluation, an orderly approach to diagnosis will eliminate unnecessary laboratory testing. The medical

history will provide invaluable information regarding intrauterine course and toxin exposure, birth size and the possibility of birth trauma, mental and physical development, symptoms of systemic diseases (Table 6–2), abnormal diet, and family heights and ages at which pubertal maturation occurred. Evaluation of psychosocial factors affecting the family and the relationship of parents and child can be carried out during the history-taking encounter. Often the diagnosis can be made at this point.

On physical examination, present height—measured without shoes on an accurate measuring device—and weight should be plotted and compared with any previous data available. If no past heights are available, a history of lack of change in clothing and shoe sizes or failure to lengthen skirts or pants may reflect poor growth. Questions about how the child's stature compares with that of his or her peers and whether the child's height has always had the same relationship to that of classmates are useful. One of the most important features of the evaluation process is to determine height velocity and compare the child's growth rate with the normal growth rate for age. Adjustment for midparental height is calculated and nutritional status determined. Arm span, head circumference, and US:LS ratio are measured. Physical stigmas of syndromes or systemic diseases are evaluated. Neurologic examination is essential.

If no specific diagnosis emerges from the physical examination, a set of laboratory evaluations may prove useful. Complete blood count, urinalysis, and serum chemistry screening with electrolyte measurements may reveal anemia, abnormalities of hepatic or renal disease (including concentration defects), glucose intolerance, acidosis, calcium disorder, or other electrolyte disturbances. Age-adjusted values must be used, since the normal ranges of serum alkaline phosphatase and phosphorus values are higher in children than in adults. An elevated sedimentation rate, low serum carotene, or positive antigliadin, antiendomysial, antireticulin, or tissue transglutaminase antibody determination may indicate connective tissue disease, Crohn's disease, celiac disease or malabsorption. Serum TSH and free T_4 are important measurements to exclude existing thyroid disease. Skeletal age evaluation will not make a diagnosis; however, if the study shows delayed bone age, the possibility of constitutional delay in growth, hypothyroidism, or GH deficiency must be considered. The tests used for the diagnosis of GH deficiency are detailed above. If serum IGF-I is normal for age, classic GH deficiency or malnutrition is unlikely; if serum IGF-I is low, it must be considered in relation to skeletal age, nutritional status, and general health status before interpretation of the value can be made. Serum IGFBP-3 adds to the evaluation of short stature. Serum gonadotropin and sex steroid determinations are performed if puberty is delayed. Serum prolactin may be elevated in the presence of a hypothalamic disorder. Karyotyping for Turner's syndrome is obtained in any short girl without another diagnosis, especially if puberty is delayed or gonadotropins are elevated. If Turner's syndrome is diagnosed, evaluation of thyroid function and determination of thyroid antibodies is also important. Elevated urinary free cortisol (normal: < 60 μg/m^2/24 h [< 18.7 μmol/m^2/24 h]) signifies Cushing's syndrome. If GH deficiency or impairment is found or if there is another hypothalamic-pituitary defect, an MRI is indicated with particular attention to the hypothalamic-pituitary area to rule out a congenital defect or neoplasm of the area. Ectopic location of the posterior pituitary on MRI is relatively frequent in congenital GH deficiency, as is a decreased pituitary volume.

If no diagnosis is apparent after all of the above have been considered and evaluated, more detailed procedures, such as provocative testing for GH deficiency, are indicated. It must be emphasized that a long and expensive evaluation is not necessary until it is demonstrated that psychologic or nutritional factors are not at fault. Likewise, if a healthy-appearing child presents with borderline short stature, normal growth rate, and short familial stature, a period of observation may be more appropriate than laboratory tests.

TALL STATURE DUE TO NONENDOCRINE CAUSES

1. Constitutional Tall Stature

A subject who has been taller than his or her peers through most of childhood, is growing at a velocity within the normal range with a moderately advanced bone age, and has no signs of the disorders listed below may be considered to be constitutionally advanced. Predicted final height will usually be in the normal adult range for the family.

Exogenous obesity in an otherwise healthy child will usually lead to moderate advancement of bone age, slightly increased growth rate, and tall stature in childhood. Puberty will begin in the early range of normal, and adult stature will conform to genetic influences. Thus, an obese child without endocrine disease should be tall; short stature and obesity are worrisome.

2. Genetic Tall Stature

Children with exceptionally tall parents have a genetic tendency to reach a height above the normal range. The child will be tall for age, will grow at a high normal rate, and the bone age will be close to chronologic age,

leading to a tall height prediction. Some children with tall stature have been noted to have growth hormone secretory patterns similar to those associated with acromegaly—eg, GH levels increase after TRH administration.

Occasionally, children will be concerned about being too tall as adults. These worries are more common in girls and will often be of greater concern to the parents than to the patient. Final height can be limited by promoting early epiphysial closure with estrogen in girls or testosterone in boys but such therapy should not be undertaken without careful consideration of the risks involved. Testosterone therapy decreases HDL cholesterol levels. Acne fulminans may be caused by testosterone therapy and progression may occur, even after therapy has been withdrawn. Estrogen carries the theoretical risk of thrombosis, ovarian cysts, and galactorrhea, but few of these complications are reported. High-dose estrogen therapy is estimated to decrease predicted final height by as much as 4.5–7 cm but only if started 3–4 years before epiphysial fusion. No therapy to limit stature is warranted until a careful assessment of the parents' and the child's expectations and reasons for seeking therapy is performed. Counseling and reassurance are usually more appropriate than endocrine therapy. Height-limiting therapy is extremely rarely invoked in the present era.

3. Syndromes of Tall Stature

Cerebral Gigantism

The sporadic syndrome of rapid growth in infancy, prominent forehead, high-arched palate, sharp chin, and hypertelorism (Sotos' syndrome) is not associated with GH excess. Mentation is usually impaired. The growth rate decreases to normal in later childhood, but stature remains tall.

Marfan's Syndrome

Marfan's syndrome is an autosomal dominant abnormality of connective tissue exhibiting variable penetrance. The disorder is due to mutation of the fibrillin-1 gene, 15q21.1. This condition may be diagnosed by characteristic physical manifestations of tall stature, long thin fingers (arachnodactyly), hyperextension of joints, and superior lens subluxation. Pectus excavatum and scoliosis may be noted. Furthermore, aortic or mitral regurgitation or aortic root dilation may be present, and aortic dissection or rupture may ultimately occur. In patients with this syndrome, arm span exceeds height, and the US:LS ratio is quite low owing to long legs. Aortic root ultrasound and slitlamp ophthalmologic examinations are indicated.

Homocystinuria

Patients with homocystinuria have an autosomal recessive deficiency of cystathionine β-synthase (gene locus 21q22.3) and phenotypes similar to those of patients with Marfan's syndrome. Additional features of homocystinuria include developmental delay, increased incidence of seizures, osteoporosis, inferior lens dislocation, and increased urinary excretion of homocystine with increased plasma homocystine and methionine but low plasma cystine. Thromboembolic phenomena may precipitate a fatal complication. This disease is treated by restricting dietary methionine and, in responsive patients, administering pyridoxine.

BECKWITH-WIEDEMANN SYNDROME

Patients with Beckwith-Wiedemann syndrome demonstrate overweight (> 90th percentile birth weight) in 88%, increased postnatal growth, omphalocele in 80%, macroglossia in 97%, and hypoglycemia due to the hyperinsulinism of pancreatic hyperplasia in 63%. Other reported features include fetal adrenocortical cytomegaly, and large kidneys with medullary dysplasia. The majority of patients occur in a sporadic pattern due to a mutation at 11p15.5, but analysis of some pedigrees suggests the possibility of familial patterns.

XYY Syndrome

Patients with one (47,XYY) or more (48,XYYY) extra Y chromosomes achieve greater than average adult heights. They have normal birth lengths but higher than normal growth rates. Excess GH secretion has not been documented (see Chapter 14).

Klinefelter's Syndrome

Patients with Klinefelter's syndrome (see Chapter 15) tend toward tall stature, but this is not a constant feature.

TALL STATURE DUE TO ENDOCRINE DISORDERS

1. Pituitary Gigantism

Pituitary gigantism is caused by excess GH secretion before the age of epiphysial fusion. The increased growth hormone secretion may be due to somatotroph-secreting tumors, to the constitutive activated GH secretion sometimes found in the McCune-Albright syndrome, or to allelic deletion of the 11q13 locus (a tumor suppressor which is abnormal in tumors of MEN 1 or in spontaneous adenomas); alternatively, it may result from excess secretion of GHRH. Patients—besides growing excessively rapidly—have coarse fea-

tures, large hands and feet with thick fingers and toes, and often frontal bossing and large jaws. Although this condition is quite rare, the findings appear similar to those observed in the more frequent acromegaly (which occurs with GH excess after epiphysial fusion). Thus, glucose intolerance or frank diabetes mellitus, hypogonadism, and thyromegaly are predicted. Treatment is accomplished by surgery (the transsphenoidal approach is used if the tumor is small enough), radiation therapy, or by therapy with a somatostatin analog.

2. Sexual Precocity

Early onset of secretion of estrogens or androgens will lead to abnormally increased height velocity. Because bone age is advanced, there will be the paradox of the tall child who, because of early epiphysial closure, is short as an adult. The conditions include complete and incomplete sexual precocity (including virilizing congenital adrenal hyperplasia) (Figures 6–9, 6–10, and 6–11).

3. Thyrotoxicosis

Excessive thyroid hormone due to endogenous overproduction or overtreatment with exogenous thyroxine will lead to increased growth, advanced bone age, and, if occurring in early life, craniosynostosis. If the condition remains untreated, final height will be reduced.

4. Infants of Diabetic Mothers

Birth weight and size in infants of moderately diabetic mothers will be quite high, though severely diabetic women who have poor control may have babies with intrauterine growth retardation due to placental vascular insufficiency. Severe hypoglycemia and hypocalcemia will be evident in the babies soon after birth. The appearance and size of such babies is so striking that women have been diagnosed with gestational diabetes as a result of giving birth to affected infants. Infants of diabetic mothers have an increased prevalence of obesity by 10 years of age and thereafter.

REFERENCES

Normal Growth

Chard T: Insulin-like growth factors and their binding proteins in normal and abnormal human fetal growth. Growth Regul 1994;4:91.

Himes JH: Minimum time intervals for serial measurements of growth in recumbent length or stature of individual children. Acta Paediatr 1999;88:120.

Juul A et al: Serum levels of insulin-like growth factor (IGF)-binding protein-3 (IGFBP-3) in healthy infants, children, and adolescents: The relation to IGF-I, IGF-II, IGFBP-1, IGFBP-2, age, sex, body mass index, and pubertal maturation. J Clin Endocrinol Metab 1995;80:2534.

Khamis HJ, Roche AF: Predicting adult stature without using skeletal age: The Khamis-Roche method. Pediatrics 1994;94:504.

Le Roith DL, Butler AA: Insulin-like growth factors in pediatric health and disease. J Clin Endocrinol Metab 1999;84:4355.

Pierson M, Deschamps J-P: Growth. In: *Pediatric Endocrinology.* Job J-C, Pierson M (editors). Wiley, 1981.

Reiter EO, Rosenfeld RG: Normal and aberrant growth. In: *Williams Textbook of Endocrinology,* 10th ed. Wilson JD et al (editors). Saunders, 2002.

Roche AF, Wainer H, Thissen D: The RWT method for the prediction of adult stature. Pediatrics 1975;56:1027.

Styne DM: Growth. In: *Handbook of Pediatric Endocrinology.* Williams & Wilkins, 2003. [no pages yet as in press]

Tanner JM, Whitehouse RH: Clinical longitudinal standards for height, weight, height velocity, weight velocity, and stages of puberty. Arch Dis Child 1976;51:170.

Thorner MO: The discovery of growth hormone-releasing hormone. J Clin Endocrinol Metab 1999;84:4671.

Short Stature

August GP, Julius JR, Blethen SL: Adult height in children with growth hormone deficiency who are treated with biosynthetic growth hormone: the National Cooperative Growth Study experience. Pediatrics 1998;102:512.

Buchlis JG et al: Comparison of final heights of growth hormone-treated vs. untreated children with idiopathic growth failure. J Clin Endocrinol Metab 1998;83:1075.

Brown P: Human growth hormone therapy and Creutzfeldt-Jakob disease: A drama in three acts. Pediatrics 1988;81:85.

Byard PJ: The adolescent growth spurt in children with cystic fibrosis. Ann Hum Biol 1994;21:229.

Consensus guidelines for the diagnosis and treatment of growth hormone (GH) deficiency in childhood and adolescence: summary statement of the GH Research Society. GH Research Society. J Clin Endocrinol Metab 2000;85:3990.

De Zegher F et al: Early, discontinuous, high dose growth hormone treatment to normalize height and weight of short children born small for gestational age: results over 6 years. J Clin Endocrinol Metab 1999;84:1558.

Fine RN et al: Growth after recombinant human growth hormone treatment in children with chronic renal failure: report of a multicenter randomized double-blind placebo-controlled study. Genentech Cooperative Study Group. J Pediatr 1994; 124:374.

Guyda HJ: Four decades of growth hormone therapy for short children: what have we achieved? J Clin Endocrinol Metab 1999;84:4307.

Harris DA et al: Somatomedin-C in normal puberty and in true precocious puberty before and after treatment with a potent luteinizing hormone-releasing hormone agonist. J Clin Endocrinol Metab 1985;61:152.

Hintz RL: The role of auxologic and growth factor measurements in the diagnosis of growth hormone deficiency. Pediatrics 1998;102:524.

Kaplan SL: Normal growth. In: *Rudolph's Pediatrics,* 20th ed. Rudolph AM, Hoffman JIE, Rudolph CD (editors). Appleton & Lange, 1996.

Kunwar S, Wilson CB: Pediatric pituitary adenomas. J Clin Endocrinol Metab 1999;84:4385.

Lafferty AR, Chrousos GP: Pituitary tumors in children and adolescents. J Clin Endocrinol Metab 1999;84:4317.

Laron Z: The essential role of IGF-I: lessons from the long-term study and treatment of children and adults with Laron syndrome. J Clin Endocrinol Metab 1999;84:4397.

Levitsky LL: Growth and pubertal pattern in insulin-dependent diabetes mellitus. Semin Adolesc Med 1987;3:233.

Lindsay RM et al: Utah Growth Study: Growth standards and the prevalence of growth hormone deficiency. J Pediatr 1994; 125:29.

Loder RT, Wittenberg B, DeSilva G: Slipped capital femoral epiphysis associated with endocrine disorders. J Pediatr Orthop 1995;15:349.

Magiakou MA et al: Cushing's syndrome in children and adolescents. Presentation, diagnosis, and therapy. N Engl J Med 1994;331:629.

Matarazzo P et al: Growth impairment, IGF I hyposecretion and thyroid dysfunction in children with perinatal HIV-1 infection. Acta Paediatr 1994;83:1029.

Nishi Y et al: Treatment of isolated growth hormone deficiency type IA due to *GH-I* gene deletion with recombinant human insulin-like growth factor I. Acta Paediatr 1993;82:983.

Oberfield SE, Sklar CA: Endocrine sequelae in survivors of childhood cancer. Adolesc Med 2002;13:161.

Ogilvy-Stuart AL et al: Treatment of radiation-induced growth hormone deficiency with growth hormone-releasing hormone. Clin Endocrinol (Oxf) 1997;46:571.

Parks JS et al: Heritable disorders of pituitary development. J Clin Endocrinol Metab 1999;84:4362.

Price DA et al: Efficacy and safety of growth hormone treatment in children with prior craniopharyngioma: an analysis of the Pharmacia and Upjohn International Growth Database (KIGS) from 1988–1996. Horm Res 1998;49:91.

Rose SR et al: Diagnosis of central hypothyroidism in survivors of childhood cancer. J Clin Endocrinol Metab 1999;84:4472.

Rosenbloom AL et al: Growth hormone receptor deficiency in Ecuador. J Clin Endocrinol Metab 1999;84:4436.

Rosenfeld RG, Cohen P: Disorders of growth hormone; insulin-like growth factor secretion and action. In: Sperling MA (editor): *Pediatric Endocrinology.* Saunders, 2002.

Rosenfeld RG et al: Growth hormone therapy of Turner's syndrome: beneficial effect on adult height. J Pediatr 1998; 132:319.

Rosenfeld RG, Rosenbloom AL, Guevara Aguirre J: Growth hormone (GH) insensitivity due to primary GH receptor deficiency. Endocrine Reviews 1994;15:369.

Rosenfeld RL et al: Optimizing estrogen replacement treatment in Turner syndrome. Pediatrics 1998;102:486.

Saenger P: Growth-promoting strategies in Turner's syndrome. J Clin Endocrinol Metab 1999;84:4345.

Saenger P et al: Metabolic consequences of 5-year growth hormone (GH) therapy in children treated with GH for idiopathic short stature. Genentech Collaborative Study Group. J Clin Endocrinol Metab 1998;83:3115.

Smith GC et al: First-trimester growth and the risk of low birth weight. N Engl J Med 1998;339:1817.

Stevenson RD: Use of segmental measures to estimate stature in children with cerebral palsy. Arch Pediatr Adolesc Med 1995; 149:658.

Styne DM et al: Treatment of Cushing's disease in childhood and adolescence by transsphenoidal microadenomectomy. N Engl J Med 1984;310:889.

Tanaka H et al: Effect of growth hormone therapy in children with achondroplasia: growth pattern, hypothalamic-pituitary function, and genotype. Eur J Endocrinol 1998;138:275.

Tanner JM, Davies PS: Clinical longitudinal standards for height and height velocity for North American children. J Pediatr 1985;107:317.

Thomas AG et al: Insulin like growth factor-I, insulin like growth factor binding protein-1, and insulin in childhood Crohn's disease. Gut 1993;34:944.

Thorner M et al: Once daily subcutaneous growth hormone-releasing hormone therapy accelerates growth in growth hormone-deficient children during the first year of therapy. J Clin Endocrinol Metab 1996;81:1189.

Tillmann V et al: The relationship between stature, growth, and short-term changes in height and weight in normal prepubertal children. Pediatr Res 1998;44:882.

Tiulpakov AN et al: Growth in children with craniopharyngioma following surgery. Clin Endocrinol (Oxf) 1998;49:733.

Van Wyk JJ, Smith EP: Insulin-like growth factors and skeletal growth: possibilities for therapeutic intervention. J Clin Endocrinol Metab 1999;84:4349.

Wollmann HA et al: Reference values for height and weight in Prader-Willi syndrome based on 315 patients. Eur J Pediatr 1998;157:634.

Tall Stature

Elliott MR et al: Clinical features and natural history of Beckwith-Wiedemann syndrome: presentation of 74 new cases. Clin Genet 1994;46:168.

Eugster EA, Peskovitz OH: Gigantism. J Clin Endocrinol Metab 1999;84:4379.

Karlberg J, Wit JM: Linear growth in Sotos syndrome. Acta Paediatr Scand 1991;80:956.

The Thyroid Gland

Francis S. Greenspan, MD

CGRP	Calcitonin gene-related peptide
5'-DI	5'-Deiodinase
DIT	Diiodotyrosine
ELISA	Enzyme-linked immunosorbent assay
FMTC	Familial medullary thyroid cancer
FNAB	Fine-needle aspiration biopsy
FT_4	Free thyroxine
FT_4D	Free thyroxine by dialysis
FT_4I	Free thyroxine index
GRTH	Generalized resistance to thyroid hormone
hTG	Human thyroglobulin
hTR	Human thyroid hormone receptor
IP_3	Inositol 1,4,5-trisphosphate
LATS	Long-acting thyroid stimulator (TSH-R Ab [stim])
MIT	Monoiodotyrosine
PBI	Protein-bound iodine
perRTH	Peripheral resistance to thyroid hormones
PIP_2	Phosphatidylinositol 4,5-bisphosphate
PRTH	Pituitary resistance to thyroid hormone
RAIU	Radioactive iodine uptake
RER	Rough endoplasmic reticulum
rhTSH	Recombinant human TSH
RIA	Radioimmunoassay
rT_3	Reverse T_3;3,3',5'-triiodothyronine
RT_4U	Resin T_4 uptake
RXR-DBD	Retinoid X receptor DNA-binding domain

RXR-LBD	Retinoid X receptor ligand-binding domain
T_2	Diiodothyronine
T_3	3,5,3'-Triiodothyronine, liothyronine
T_4	Tetraiodothyronine, levothyroxine
TBG	Thyroxine-binding globulin
TBII	Thyrotropin binding inhibiting immune globulin
TBP	Thyroxine-binding protein
TBPA	Thyroxine-binding prealbumin; transthyretin
Tg	Thyroglobulin
THBR	Thyroid hormone binding ratio
TPO	Thyroperoxidase
TR-DBD	T_3 receptor DNA-binding domain
TRE	Thyroid hormone response element
TRH	Thyrotropin-releasing hormone
TRH-R	Thyrotropin-releasing hormone receptor
TRIAC	Triiodothyroacetic acid
TR-LBD	T_3 receptor ligand-binding domain
TSH	Thyroid-stimulating hormone; thyrotropin
TSH-R	TSH receptor
TSH-R Ab [block]	TSH receptor-blocking antibody
TSH-R Ab [stim]	TSH receptor-stimulating antibody

The thyroid gland is the largest organ specialized for endocrine function in the human body. The major function of the thyroid follicular cells is to secrete a sufficient amount of thyroid hormones, primarily 3,5,3′,5′-l-tetraiodothyronine (T_4), and a lesser quantity of 3,5,3′-l-triiodothyronine (T_3). Thyroid hormones promote normal growth and development and regulate a number of homeostatic functions, including energy and heat production. In addition, the parafollicular cells of the human thyroid gland secrete calcitonin, which is important in calcium homeostasis (Chapter 8).

■ ANATOMY & HISTOLOGY

The thyroid gland originates as an outpouching in the floor of the pharynx, which grows downward anterior to the trachea, bifurcates, and forms a series of cellular cords. These form tiny balls or follicles and develop into the two lateral lobes of the thyroid connected by a thin isthmus. The origin of the gland at the base of the tongue is evident as the foramen cecum. The course of its downward migration is marked by the **thyroglossal duct,** remnants of which may persist in adult life as thyroglossal duct cysts. These are mucus-filled cysts, lined with squamous epithelium, and are usually found in the anterior neck between the thyroid cartilage and the base of the tongue. A remnant of the caudal end of the thyroglossal duct is found in the pyramidal lobe, attached to the isthmus of the gland (Figure 7–1).

The isthmus of the thyroid gland is located just below the cricoid cartilage, midway between the apex of the thyroid cartilage ("Adam's apple") and the suprasternal notch. Each lobe is pear-shaped and measures about 2.5–4 cm in length, 1.5–2 cm in width, and 1–1.5 cm in thickness. The weight of the gland in the normal individual, as determined by ultrasonic examination, varies depending on dietary iodine intake, age, and body weight but in adults is approximately 10–20 g. Upward growth of the thyroid gland is limited by the attachment of the sternothyroid muscle to the thyroid cartilage; however, posterior and downward growth is unhampered, so that thyroid enlargement, or goiter, will frequently extend posteriorly and inferiorly or even substernally.

Transverse section of the neck at the level of the thyroid isthmus shows the relationships of the thyroid gland to the trachea, esophagus, carotid artery, and jugular vein (Figure 7–2). Ultrasonography, CT scans, or MRI reveals these relationships in vivo.

The thyroid gland has a rich blood supply (Figure 7–3). The superior thyroid artery arises from the common or external carotid artery, the inferior thyroid artery from the thyrocervical trunk of the subclavian artery, and the small thyroid ima artery from the brachiocephalic artery at the aortic arch. Venous drainage is via multiple surface veins coalescing into superior, lateral, and inferior thyroid veins. The blood flow to the thyroid gland is about 5 mL/g/min; in hyperthyroidism, the blood flow to the gland is markedly increased, and a whistling sound, or bruit, may be heard over the lower poles of the gland and may even be felt in the same areas as a vibration, or thrill. Other important anatomic considerations include the two pairs of parathyroid glands that usually lie behind the upper and middle thyroid lobes and the recurrent laryngeal nerves, which course along the trachea behind the thyroid gland.

On microscopic examination, the thyroid gland is found to consist of a series of follicles of varying sizes. The follicles contain a pink-staining material (with hematoxylin-eosin stain) called "colloid" and are surrounded by a single layer of thyroid epithelium. Tissue culture studies suggest that each follicle may represent an individual clone of cells. These cells become columnar when stimulated by TSH and flattened when resting (Figure 7–4). The follicle cells synthesize thyroglobulin, which is extruded into the lumen of the follicle. The biosynthesis of T_4 and T_3 occurs within thyroglobulin at the cell-colloid interface. Numerous microvilli project from the surface of the follicle into the lumen; these are involved in endocytosis of thyroglobulin, which is then hydrolyzed in the cell to release thyroid hormones (Figure 7–5).

■ PHYSIOLOGY

STRUCTURE OF THYROID HORMONES

Thyroid hormones are unique in that they contain 59–65% of the trace element iodine. The structures of the thyroid hormones, T_4 and T_3, are shown in Figure 7–6. The iodinated thyronines are derived from iodination of the phenolic rings of tyrosine residues in thyroglobulin to form mono- or diiodotyrosine, which are coupled to form T_3 or T_4 (see below).

IODINE METABOLISM

Iodine* enters the body in food or water in the form of iodide or iodate ion, the iodate ion being converted to iodide in the stomach. In the course of millennia, io-

*In this chapter, the words "iodine" and "iodide" are used interchangeably.

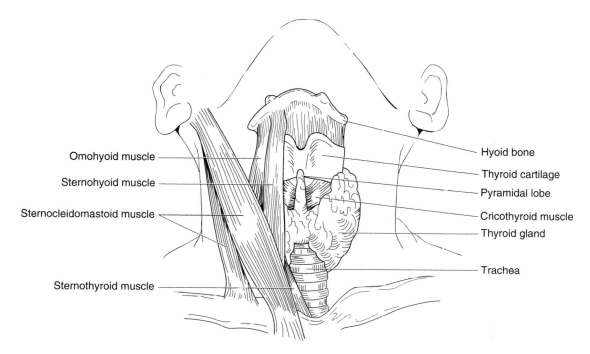

Figure 7–1. Gross anatomy of the human thyroid gland (anterior view).

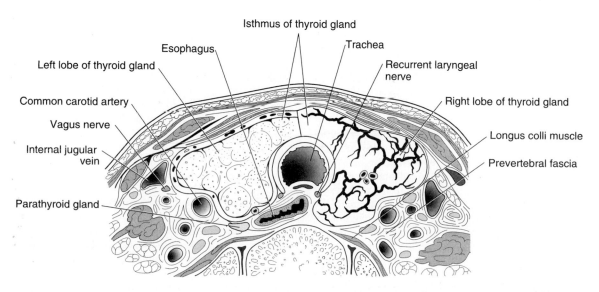

Figure 7–2. Cross section of the neck at the level of T1, showing thyroid relationships. (Reproduced, with permission, from Lindner HH: *Clinical Anatomy*. McGraw-Hill, 1989.)

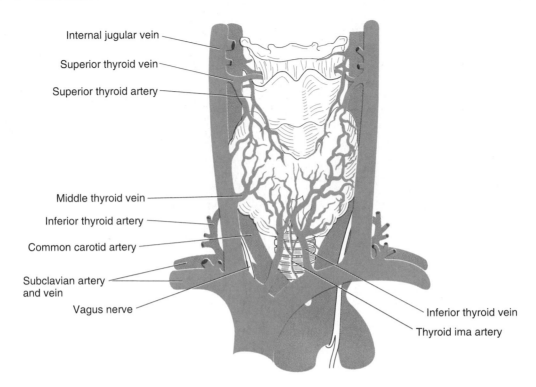

Figure 7–3. Arteries and veins related to the thyroid gland. (Reproduced, with permission, from Lindner HH: *Clinical Anatomy*. McGraw-Hill, 1989.)

dine has been leached from the soil and washed down into the oceans, so that in mountainous and inland areas the supply of iodine may be quite limited, whereas the element is plentiful in coastal areas. The thyroid gland concentrates and traps iodide and synthesizes and stores thyroid hormones in thyroglobulin, which compensates for the scarcity of iodine.

The recommendations of the World Health Organization for optimal daily iodide intake are as follows: for adults, 150 µg; during pregnancy and lactation, 200 µg; for the first year of life, 50 µg; for ages 1–6, 90 µg; and for ages 7–12, 120 µg. If iodide intake is below 50 µg/d, the gland is unable to maintain adequate hormonal secretion, and thyroid hypertrophy (goiter) and hypothyroidism result. In the United States, the average daily iodide intake increased from a range of 100–200 µg/d in the 1960s to 240–740 µg/d in the 1980s. This was largely due to the introduction of iodate as a dough conditioner, though other sources of dietary iodine included iodized salt, vitamin and mineral preparations, iodine-containing medications, and iodinated contrast media. In the 1990s, bromine salts replaced iodine in the baking industry, and iodine intake has fallen considerably, indicating the need for continued monitoring.

An approximation of iodine turnover in subjects on a high-iodine diet is depicted in Figure 7–7. Iodide, like chloride, is rapidly absorbed from the gastrointestinal tract and distributed in extracellular fluids as well as in salivary, gastric, and breast secretions. Although the concentration of inorganic iodide in the extracellular fluid pool will vary directly with iodide intake, extracellular fluid I^- is usually quite low because of the rapid clearance of iodide from extracellular fluid by thyroidal uptake and renal clearance. In the example shown, the basal I^- concentration in extracellular fluid is only 0.6 µg/dL, or a total of 150 µg of I^- in an extracellular pool of 25 L despite a daily oral intake of 500 µg I^-. In the thyroid gland there is active transport of I^- from the serum across the basement membrane of the thyroid cell (see below). The thyroid gland takes up about 115 µg of I^- per 24 hours, or, in this example, about 18% of the available I^-. About 75 µg of I^- is utilized for hormone synthesis and stored in thyroglobulin; the remainder leaks back into the extracellular fluid pool. The thyroid pool of organified iodine is very large, averaging 8–10 mg, and represents a store of hormone and iodinated tyrosines, protecting the organism against a period of iodine lack. From this storage pool, about 75 µg of hormonal iodide is released into the cir-

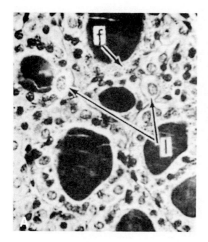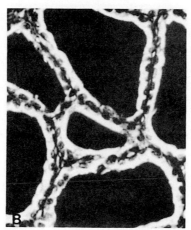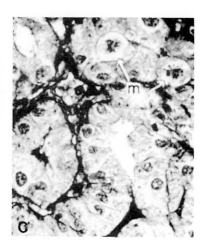

Figure 7–4. **A:** Normal rat thyroid. A single layer of cuboidal epithelial cells surrounds PAS-positive material in the follicular space (colloid). The larger, lighter-staining cells indicated by the arrows (I) are C cells that produce calcitonin. (F, follicular cells.) **B:** Inactive rat thyroid several weeks after hypophysectomy. The follicular lumens are larger and the follicular cells flatter. **C:** Rat thyroid under intensive TSH stimulation. The animal was fed an iodine-deficient diet and injected with propylthiouracil for several weeks. Little colloid is visible. The follicular cells are tall and columnar. Several mitoses (m) are visible. (Reproduced, with permission, from Halmi NS in: *Histology.* Greep RO, Weiss L [editors]. McGraw-Hill, 1973.)

culation daily. This hormonal iodide is mostly bound to serum thyroxine-binding proteins, forming a circulating pool of about 600 μg of hormonal I^- (as T_3 and T_4). From this pool, about 75 μg of I^- as T_3 and T_4 is taken up and metabolized by tissues. About 60 μg of I^- is returned to the iodide pool and about 15 μg of hormonal I^- is conjugated with glucuronide or sulfate in the liver and excreted into the stool. Since most of the dietary iodide is excreted in the urine, a 24-hour urinary iodide excretion is an excellent index of dietary intake. The 24-hour radioactive iodine uptake (RAIU) by the thyroid gland is inversely proportionate to the size of the inorganic iodide pool and directly proportionate to thyroidal activity. Typical RAIU curves are shown in Figure 7–8. In the USA, the 24-hour thyroidal radioiodine uptake has decreased from about 40–50% in the 1960s to about 8–30% in the 1990s because of increased dietary iodide intake.

THYROID HORMONE SYNTHESIS & SECRETION

The synthesis of T_4 and T_3 by the thyroid gland involves six major steps: (1) active transport of I^- across the basement membrane into the thyroid cell (trapping of iodide); (2) oxidation of iodide and iodination of tyrosyl residues in thyroglobulin; (3) coupling of iodoty-

rosine molecules within thyroglobulin to form T_3 and T_4; (4) proteolysis of thyroglobulin, with release of free iodothyronines and iodotyrosines; (5) deiodination of iodotyrosines within the thyroid cell, with conservation and reuse of the liberated iodide; and (6) under certain circumstances, intrathyroidal 5'-deiodination of T_4 to T_3.

Thyroid hormone synthesis involves a unique glycoprotein, thyroglobulin, and an essential enzyme, thyroperoxidase (TPO). This process is summarized in Figure 7–9.

Thyroglobulin

Thyroglobulin is a large glycoprotein molecule containing 5496 amino acids, with a molecular weight of about 660,000 and a sedimentation coefficient of 19S. It contains about 140 tyrosyl residues and about 10% carbohydrate in the form of mannose, *N*-acetylglucosamine, galactose, fucose, sialic acid, and chondroitin sulfate. The 19S thyroglobulin compound is a dimer of two identical 12S subunits, but small amounts of the 12S monomer and a 27S tetramer are often present. The iodine content of the molecule can vary from 0.1% to 1% by weight. In thyroglobulin containing 0.5% iodine (26 atoms of iodine per 660-kDa molecule), there would be 5 molecules of monoiodotyrosine (MIT), 4.5 molecules of diiodotyrosine (DIT), 2.5 molecules of

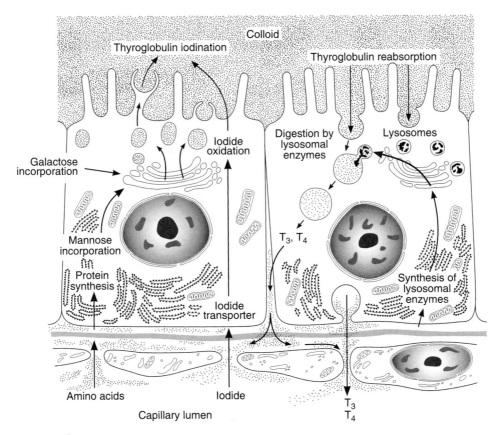

Figure 7–5. Processes of synthesis and iodination of thyroglobulin (left) and its reabsorption and digestion (right). These events occur in the same cell. (Reproduced, with permission, from Junqueira LC, Carneiro J, Kelley R: *Basic Histology*, 7th ed. McGraw-Hill, 1992.)

thyroxine (T_4), and 0.7 molecules of triiodothyronine (T_3). About 75% of the thyroglobulin monomer consists of repetitive domains with no hormonogenic sites. There are four tyrosyl sites for hormonogenesis on the thyroglobulin molecule: One site is located at the amino terminal end of the molecule, and the other three are located in a sequence of 600 amino acids at the carboxyl terminal end. There is a surprising homology between this area of the thyroglobulin molecule and the structure of acetylcholinesterase, suggesting conservation in the evolution of these proteins.

The human thyroglobulin *(hTg)* gene lies on the long arm of chromosome 8 distal to the c-*myc* oncogene. TSH stimulates the transcription of the thyroglobulin gene, and hypophysectomy or T_3 therapy decreases its transcription. The thyroglobulin gene contains about 8500 nucleotides, which encode the prethyroglobulin (pre-Tg) monomer. The pre-thyroglobulin monomer contains a 19-amino-acid signal peptide, followed by a 2750-amino-acid chain that constitutes the thyroglobulin monomer. The mRNA is translated in the rough endoplasmic reticulum, and thyroglobulin chains are glycosylated during transport to the Golgi apparatus (Figure 7–5). In the Golgi apparatus, the thyroglobulin dimers are incorporated into exocytotic vesicles that fuse with the basement membrane and release the thyroglobulin into the follicular lumen. There, at the apical-colloid border, tyrosines within thyroglobulin are iodinated and stored in colloid.

Thyroidal Peroxidase

Thyroidal peroxidase is a membrane-bound glycoprotein with a molecular weight of about 102,000 and a heme compound as the prosthetic group of the enzyme. This enzyme mediates both the oxidation of iodide ions and the incorporation of iodine into tyrosine residues of thyroglobulin. Thyroidal peroxidase is synthesized in the rough endoplasmic reticulum (RER). After insertion into the membrane of RER cisternae, it is trans-

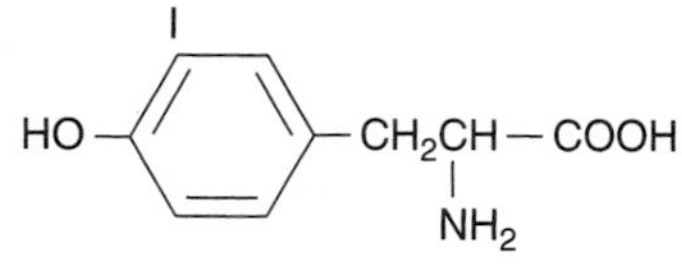

3-Monoiodotyrosine (MIT)

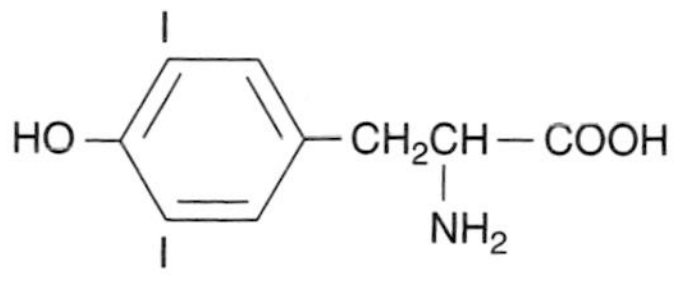

3,5-Diiodotyrosine (DIT)

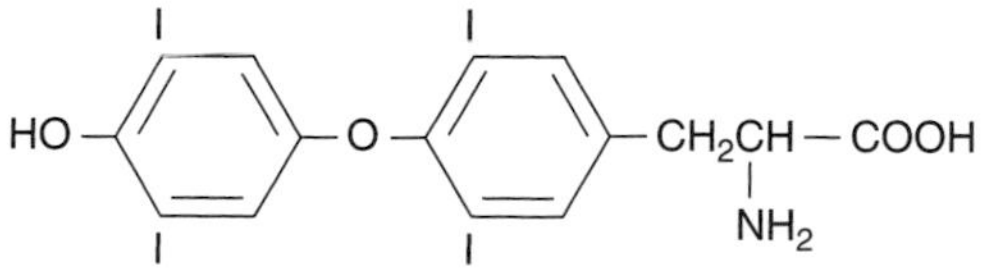

3,5,3′,5′-Tetraiodothyronine (thyroxine [T_4])

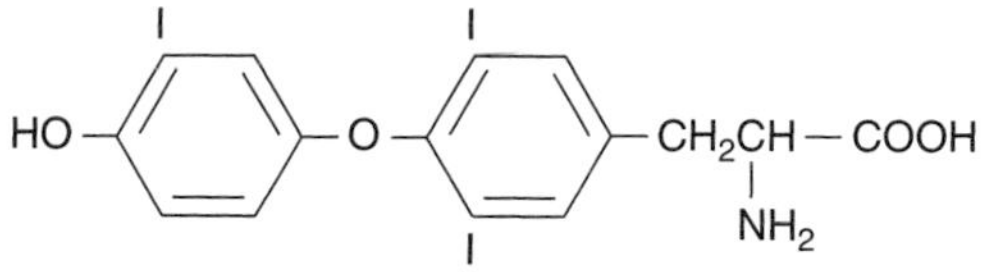

3,5,3′-Triiodothyronine (T_3)

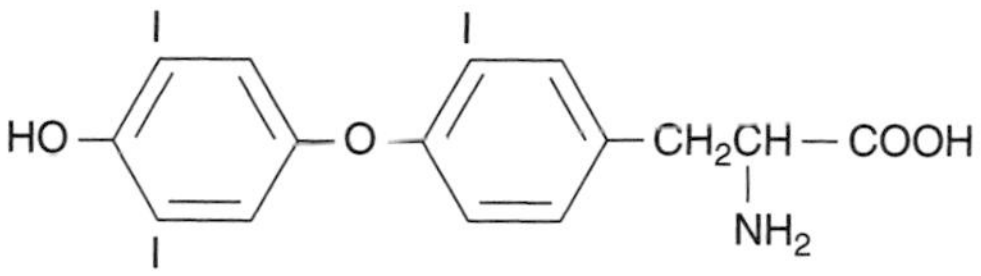

3,3′,5′-Triiodothyronine (reverse T_3 [rT_3])

Figure 7–6. **Structure of thyroid hormones and related compounds.** (Reproduced, with permission, from Murray RK et al: *Harper's Biochemistry,* 24th ed. McGraw-Hill, 1996.)

ferred to the apical cell surface through Golgi elements and exocytic vesicles. Here, at the cell colloid interface, it is available for iodination and hormonogenesis in thyroglobulin. Thyroidal peroxidase biosynthesis is stimulated by TSH.

Iodide Transport (the Iodide Trap)

I^- is transported across the basement membrane of the thyroid cell by an intrinsic membrane protein called the Na^+/I^- symporter (NIS). At the apical border, a second I^- transport protein called pendrin moves iodine into the colloid where it is involved in hormonogenesis (Figure 7–10). The NIS derives its energy from Na^+-K^+ ATPase, which drives the transport process. This active transport system allows the human thyroid gland to maintain a concentration of free iodide 30–40 times that in plasma. The NIS is stimulated by TSH and by the TSH receptor-stimulating antibody found in Graves' disease. It is saturable with large amounts of iodide and inhibited by ions such as ClO_4^-, SCN^-, NO_3^-, and TcO_4^-. Some of these ions have clinical utility. Sodium perchlorate will discharge nonorganified iodide from the NIS and has been used to diagnose organification defects (Figure 7–11) and in the treatment of iodide-induced hyperthyroidism. Sodium pertechnetate Tc99m, which has a 6-hour half-life and a 140-keV gamma emission, is used for rapid visualization of the thyroid gland for size and functioning nodules. Pendrin, encoded by the Pendred syndrome gene *(PDS),* is a transporter of chloride and iodide. Mutations in the *PDS* gene have been found in patients with goiter and congenital deafness (Pendred's syndrome). Although iodide is concentrated by salivary, gastric, and breast tissue, these tissues do not organify or store I^- and are not stimulated by TSH.

Iodination of Tyrosyl in Thyroglobulin

Within the thyroid cell, at the cell-colloid interface, iodide is rapidly oxidized by H_2O_2, catalyzed by thyroperoxidase, and converted to an active intermediate which is incorporated into tyrosyl residues in thyroglobulin. H_2O_2 is probably generated by a dihydronicotinamide adenine dinucleotide phosphate (NADPH) oxidase in the presence of Ca^{2+}; this process is stimulated by TSH. The iodinating intermediate may be iodinium ion (I^+), hypoiodate, or an iodine-free radical. The site of iodination at the apical (colloid) border of the thyroid cell can be demonstrated by autoradiography.

Thyroidal peroxidase will catalyze iodination of tyrosyl molecules in proteins other than thyroglobulin, such as albumin or thyroglobulin fragments. However, no thyroactive hormones are formed in these proteins. The metabolically inactive protein may be released into the circulation, draining thyroidal iodide reserves.

Coupling of Iodotyrosyl Residues in Thyroglobulin

The coupling of iodotyrosyl residues in thyroglobulin is also catalyzed by thyroperoxidase. It is thought that this is an intramolecular mechanism involving three steps: (1) oxidation of iodotyrosyl residues to an activated form by thyroperoxidase; (2) coupling of activated iodotyrosyl residues within the same thyroglobulin molecule to form a quinol ether intermediate; and (3) splitting of the quinol ether to form iodothyronine, with conversion of the alanine side chain of the donor iodotyrosine to dehydroalanine (Figure 7–12). For this process to occur, the dimeric structure of thyroglobulin is essential: Within the thyroglobulin molecule, two

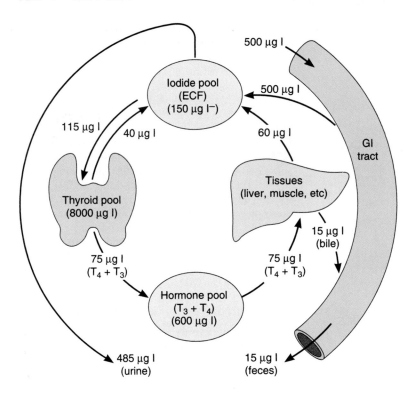

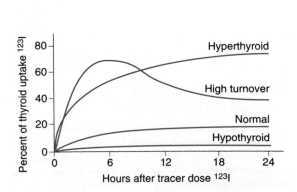

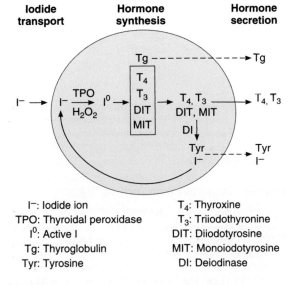

Figure 7–7. Iodine metabolism. The values indicated are representative of those that might be found in a healthy subject ingesting 500 μg of iodine a day. The actual iodine intake varies considerably among different individuals.

Figure 7–8. Typical curves of 24-hour radioiodine uptake in normal subjects and in patients with thyroid disease. A "high-turnover" curve may be seen in patients taking an iodine-deficient diet or with a defect in hormone synthesis.

Figure 7–9. Thyroid hormone synthesis in a thyroid follicle.

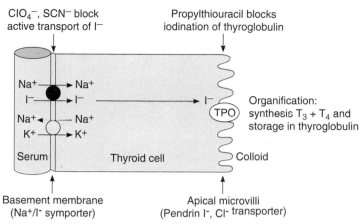

Figure 7–10. The iodide transporter in the thyroid cell. The large solid circle represents the Na⁺/I⁻ symporter actively transporting I⁻ into the cell; the large open circle represents Na⁺-K⁺ ATPase supplying the ion gradient which drives the reaction. I⁻ is transported across the apical membrane by pendrin. Hormone synthesis takes place in the colloid at the colloid-apical membrane, catalyzed by thyroperoxidase (TPO).

molecules of DIT may couple to form T_4, and an MIT and a DIT molecule may couple to form T_3. Thiocarbamide drugs—particularly propylthiouracil, methimazole, and carbimazole—are potent inhibitors of thyroperoxidase and will block thyroid hormone synthesis (Figure 7–13). These drugs are clinically useful in the management of hyperthyroidism.

Proteolysis of Thyroglobulin & Thyroid Hormone Secretion

The pattern of proteolysis of thyroglobulin and secretion of thyroid hormones is illustrated in Figure 7–5. Lysosomal enzymes are synthesized by the rough endoplasmic reticulum and packaged by the Golgi apparatus into lysosomes. These structures, surrounded by membrane, have an acidic interior and are filled with proteolytic enzymes, including proteases, endopeptidases, glycoside hydrolyases, phosphatases, and other enzymes. At the cell-colloid interface, colloid is engulfed into a colloid vesicle by a process of macropinocytosis or micropinocytosis and is absorbed into the thyroid cell. The lysosomes then fuse with the colloid vesicle and hydrolysis of thyroglobulin occurs, releasing T_4, T_3, DIT, MIT, peptide fragments, and amino acids. T_3 and T_4 are released into the circulation, while DIT and MIT are deiodinated and the I⁻ is conserved. Thyroglobulin with a low iodine content is hydrolyzed more rapidly than thyroglobulin with a high iodine content, which may be beneficial in geographic areas where natural iodine intake is low. The mechanism of transport of T_3 and T_4 through the thyroid cell is not known, but it may involve a specific hormone carrier. Thyroid hormone secretion is stimulated by TSH, which activates adenylyl cyclase, and by the cAMP analog Bu_2cAMP, suggesting that it is cAMP-dependent.

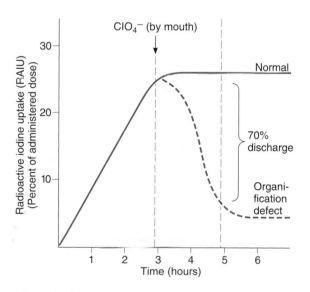

Figure 7–11. Perchlorate discharge of thyroidal inorganic iodine. Two to 3 hours after administration of a tracer dose of radioactive iodide, perchlorate is administered orally, blocking further active transport of iodide into the thyroid cell. In the normal subject (solid line), no significant decrease in radioactivity is detectable over the thyroid gland. In the representative example shown by the dashed line, there is a significant discharge of thyroidal iodide, indicating that iodide organification has been incomplete. (ClO_4^-, perchlorate.)

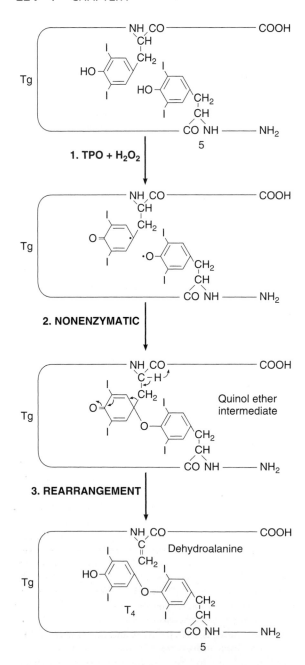

Figure 7–12. Hypothetical coupling scheme for intramolecular formation of T_4 within the thyroglobulin molecule. The major hormonogenic site at tyrosyl residue 5 is indicated. (Reproduced, with permission, from Taurog A: Thyroid hormone synthesis. Thyroid iodine metabolism. In: *Werner and Ingbar's The Thyroid*, 7th ed. Braverman LE, Utiger RD [editors]. Lippincott, 1996.)

Thyroglobulin proteolysis is inhibited by excess iodide (see below) and by lithium, which, as lithium carbonate, is used for the treatment of bipolar disorders. A small amount of unhydrolyzed thyroglobulin is also released from the thyroid cell; this is markedly increased in certain situations such as subacute thyroiditis, hyperthyroidism, or TSH-induced goiter (Figure 7–9). Thyroglobulin (perhaps modified) may also be synthesized and released by certain thyroid malignancies such as papillary or follicular thyroid cancer and may be useful as a marker for metastatic disease.

Intrathyroidal Deiodination

MIT and DIT formed during the synthesis of thyroid hormone are deiodinated by intrathyroidal deiodinase (Figure 7–9). This enzyme is an NADPH-dependent flavoprotein found in mitochondria and microsomes. It acts on MIT and DIT but not on T_3 and T_4. The iodide released is mostly reutilized for hormone synthesis; a small amount leaks out of the thyroid into the body pool (Figure 7–7). The 5′-deiodinase that converts T_4 to T_3 in peripheral tissues is also found in the thyroid gland. In situations of iodide deficiency, the activity of this enzyme may increase the amount of T_3 secreted by the thyroid gland, increasing the metabolic efficiency of hormone synthesis.

ABNORMALITIES IN THYROID HORMONE SYNTHESIS & RELEASE

Inherited Metabolic Defects (Dyshormonogenesis)

Inherited metabolic defects may involve any phase of hormonal biosynthesis. These result in "dyshormonogenesis," or impaired hormonal synthesis. Patients present with thyroid enlargement, or goiter, mild to severe hypothyroidism, low serum T_3 and T_4, and elevated serum TSH. The defects are described in more detail in the section on nontoxic goiter, below.

Effect of Iodide Deficiency on Hormone Biosynthesis

A diet very low in iodine reduces intrathyroidal iodine content, increases the intrathyroidal ratio of MIT to DIT, increases the ratio of T_3 to T_4, decreases the secretion of T_4, and increases serum TSH. In the adult, this results in goiter, with a high iodine uptake and mild to severe hypothyroidism; in the neonate, it may result in cretinism (see below). The adaptations that occur involve the increased synthesis of T_3 relative to T_4 and the increased intrathyroidal 5′-deiodination of T_4 to T_3 to produce a more active hormone mixture.

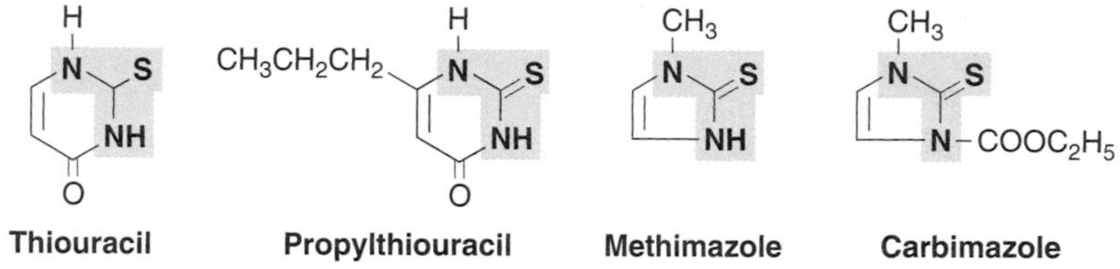

Figure 7–13. Thiocarbamide inhibitors of thyroidal iodide organification.

Thiouracil   Propylthiouracil   Methimazole   Carbimazole

Effect of Iodine Excess on Hormone Biosynthesis

Increasing doses of iodide given to iodide-deficient rats initially induce increased iodide organification and hormone formation until a critical level is reached, whereupon inhibition of organification occurs and hormonogenesis decreases. This **Wolff-Chaikoff effect** (Figure 7–14) is probably due to inhibition of H_2O_2 generation by the high intrathyroidal I^- content. The most striking observation was that the effect is transient and that the normal thyroid gland "escapes" from the I^- effect. This is due to inhibition of the transport of I^- with reduction in intrathyroidal iodide, allowing hormonogenesis to pro-

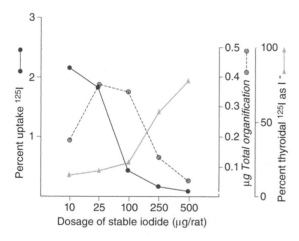

Figure 7–14. The Wolff-Chaikoff block. As increasing doses of iodide are administered to rats, there is an initial increase in iodide organification. At a critical concentration, however, higher doses of iodide given to the animals block iodide organification. The effect of increasing doses of iodide on thyroid hormone synthesis is therefore biphasic. Concomitantly with the increase in the organification block, the intracellular inorganic iodide concentration rises. As the amount of stable iodide injected is increased, there is a decrease in thyroidal uptake of radioactive iodide. (Reproduced, with permission, from DeGroot LJ, Stanbury JB: *The Thyroid and Its Diseases,* 4th ed. Wiley, 1975.)

ceed. If the gland is unable to make this adaptation—as may occur in patients with autoimmune thyroiditis or in some patients with dyshormonogenesis—iodide-induced hypothyroidism will ensue. In some patients, an iodide load will induce hyperthyroidism ("jodbasedow" effect). This may develop in patients with latent Graves' disease, in those with multinodular goiters, or occasionally in those with previously normal thyroid glands.

THYROID HORMONE TRANSPORT

Thyroid hormones are transported in serum bound to carrier proteins. Although only 0.04% of T_4 and 0.4% of T_3 are "free," it is the free fraction that is responsible for hormonal activity (Figure 7–15). There are three major thyroid hormone transport proteins: thyroxine-binding globulin (TBG); thyroxine-binding prealbumin (TBPA), or transthyretin; and albumin (Figure 7–16).

Thyroxine-Binding Globulin (TBG)

TBG, a single 54-kDa polypeptide chain, is synthesized in the liver. It contains four carbohydrate chains, representing 23% of the molecule by weight, and has homology with α_1-antichymotrypsin and α_1-antitrypsin. Normally, there are about ten sialic acid residues per molecule. Pregnancy or estrogen therapy increases the sialic acid content of the molecule, resulting in decreased metabolic clearance and elevated serum levels of TBG. Each molecule of TBG has a single binding site for T_4 or T_3. The serum concentration of TBG is 15–30 $\mu g/mL$, or 280–560 nmol/L. The affinity constant (K_a) for T_4 is 1×10^{10} M^{-1}, and for T_3 it is 5×10^8 M^{-1}. The high affinity for T_3 and T_4 allows TBG to carry about 70% of the circulating thyroid hormones. When fully saturated, TBG can carry about 20 μg of T_4 per deciliter.

Congenital TBG deficiency is an X-linked trait with a frequency of 1:2500 live births. One variant occurs in African Pygmies, Panamanians, African blacks, Micronesians, and Indonesians. Another variant occurs in 40% of Australian aborigines. Despite the low circulating T_4 and T_3 levels, the free hormone levels are normal and the patients are not hypothyroid. Congenital TBG

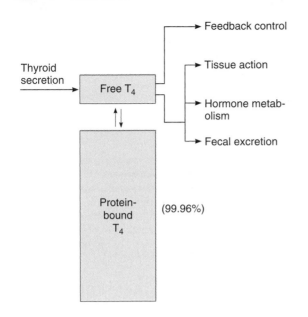

Figure 7–15. Representation of free T_4 (and free T_3) as the biologically active hormone at the level of the pituitary and the peripheral tissues. Most of the thyroid hormones circulating in plasma are protein-bound and have no biologic activity. This pool of bound hormone is in equilibrium with the free hormone pool. (Reproduced, with permission, from DeGroot LJ, Stanbury JB: *The Thyroid and Its Diseases,* 4th ed. Wiley, 1975.)

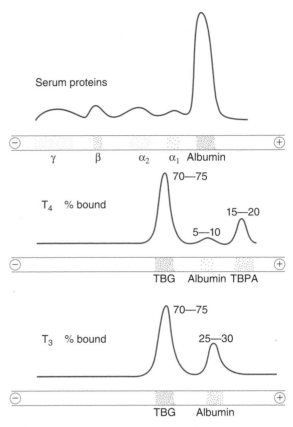

Figure 7–16. Diagrammatic representation of the distribution of radioactive T_4 and T_3 among serum thyroid hormone-binding proteins. **Top:** Paper electrophoretic pattern of serum proteins. **Middle:** Radioactive T_4 was added to serum and was then subjected to paper electrophoresis. The peaks represent the mobility of radioactive T_4 bound to different serum proteins. (TBG, thyroid hormone-binding globulin; TBPA, thyroxine-binding prealbumin.) **Bottom:** Radioactive T_3 was added to serum and subjected to paper electrophoresis. The peaks indicate the relative distribution of protein-bound radioactive T_3. The figures above each peak indicate the relative hormone distribution among the binding proteins in a normal adult. (Reproduced, with permission, from Rosenfield RL et al: *Pediatric Nuclear Medicine.* James AE Jr, Wagner HN Jr, Cooke RE [editors]. Saunders, 1974.)

deficiency is often associated with congenital corticosteroid-binding globulin (CBG) deficiency (Chapter 9). Congenital TBG excess is rare; it presents with elevated total T_4 and T_3 concentrations but normal free hormone levels and normal TSH.

Androgenic steroids and glucocorticoids lower TBG levels, as does major systemic illness as well (Table 7–1). Drugs such as salicylates, phenytoin, phenylbutazone, and diazepam may bind to TBG, displacing T_4 and T_3, in effect producing a low-TBG state. Heparin stimulates lipoprotein lipase, releasing free fatty acids, which displace T_3 and T_4 from TBG. This can occur in vivo and also in vitro, eg, in blood drawn through a heparin Heplock, where even minute quantities of heparin will increase the measured levels of free T_4 and T_3.

Thyroxine-Binding Prealbumin

Transthyretin, or thyroxine-binding prealbumin (TBPA), is a 55-kDa globular polypeptide consisting of four identical subunits, each containing 127 amino acids. It binds about 10% of circulating T_4. Its affinity for T_3 is about tenfold lower than for T_4, so that it mostly carries T_4. The dissociation of T_4 and T_3 from TBPA is rapid, so that TBPA is a source of readily available T_4. There are binding sites on TBPA for retinol-binding protein, but the transport of T_4 is independent of the transport of retinol-binding protein. The concentration of TBPA in serum is 120–240 mg/L, or 2250–4300 nmol/L.

Table 7–1. Factors influencing the concentration of protein-bound thyroid hormones in serum.

A. Increased TBG concentration
  1. Congenital
  2. Hyperestrogenic states: pregnancy, estrogen therapy
  3. Diseases: acute infectious hepatitis, hypothyroidism
B. Decreased TBG concentration
  1. Congenital
  2. Drugs: androgenic steroids, glucocorticoids
  3. Major systemic illness: Protein malnutrition, nephrotic syndrome, cirrhosis, hyperthyroidism
C. Drugs affecting thyroid hormone binding to normal concentrations of binding protein
  1. Phenytoin
  2. Salicylates
  3. Phenylbutazone
  4. Mitotane
  5. Diazepam
  6. FFA released by heparin stimulation of lipoprotein lipase

---

Increased levels of TBPA may be familial and may occur in patients with glucagonoma or pancreatic islet cell carcinoma. These patients have an elevated total T_4 but a normal free T_4. Abnormal TBPA has been described in familial amyloidotic polyneuropathy, associated with a low total T_4 but normal free hormone levels.

Albumin

Albumin has one strong binding site for T_4 and T_3 and several weaker ones. Because of its high concentration in serum, albumin carries about 15% of circulating T_4 and T_3. The rapid dissociation rates of T_4 and T_3 from albumin make this carrier a major source of free hormone to tissues. Hypoalbuminemia, as occurs in nephrosis or in cirrhosis of the liver, is associated with a low total T_4 and T_3, but the free hormone levels are normal.

Familial dysalbuminemic hyperthyroxinemia is an autosomal dominant inherited disorder in which 25% of the albumin exhibits high-affinity T_4 binding, resulting in an elevated total T_4 level but normal free T_4 and euthyroidism. Affinity for T_3 may be elevated but is usually normal.

Kinetics of Thyroid Hormone Binding to Transport Proteins

The kinetics of thyroid hormone binding to the thyroid binding proteins can be expressed by conventional equilibrium equations. Thus, for T_4:

$$(T_4) + (TBG) \underset{\leftarrow}{\overset{\rightarrow}{}} (TBG - T_4)$$

where (T_4) represents free (unbound) hormone, (TBG) is TBG not containing T_4, and $(TBG - T_4)$ is TBG-bound T_4. This can be expressed by the mass action relationship:

$$K_{T4} = \frac{(TBG - T_4)}{(T_4)(TBG)}$$

where K is the equilibrium constant for the interaction. Rearranging:

$$(T_4) = \frac{(TBG - T_4)}{K_{T4}(TBG)}$$

From this equation, it can be seen that T_4 exists in plasma in both free and bound forms, and the free hormone level is inversely proportionate to the free binding sites on TBG and the binding affinity for the hormone. The same relationships exist for the other thyroid hormone-binding proteins.

The effect of a change in the concentration of thyroid hormone-binding protein is shown in Figure 7–17. The levels of free thyroid hormone are normal in states where there are primary or secondary changes in plasma binding, because TSH release is controlled by the free thyroid hormone level and adjusts to normalize it irrespective of how much hormone is bound by the plasma proteins.

There has been much speculation on the role of the thyroid hormone transport proteins. The three major hypotheses are as follows: (1) they form a storage pool of readily available free hormone; (2) they allow the delivery of T_3 and T_4 to all tissues because the tiny free hormone pool is continually replenished as the hormones are absorbed by tissues; and (3) they protect tissues from massive hormone release. Thus, although the transport proteins are not essential for thyroid hormone activity, they may make the system more efficient.

METABOLISM OF THYROID HORMONES

The daily secretion of the normal thyroid gland is about 100 nmol of T_4, about 5 nmol of T_3, and less than 5 nmol of metabolically inactive reverse T_3 (rT_3) (Figure 7–18). Most of the plasma pool of T_3 is derived from peripheral metabolism (5'-deiodination) of T_4. The biologic activity of thyroid hormones is greatly dependent on the location of the iodine atoms (Table 7–2). Deiodination of the *outer ring* of T_4 (5'-deiodination) produces 3,5,3'-triiodothyronine (T_3), which is three to eight times more potent than T_4. On the other hand, deiodination of the *inner ring* of T_4 (5-deiodination) produces 3,3',5'-triiodothyronine (reverse T_3, or

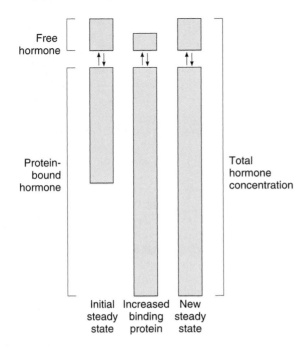

Free hormone

Protein-bound hormone

Total hormone concentration

Initial steady state   Increased binding protein   New steady state

Figure 7–17. The effect of an increase in thyroid hormone-binding protein concentration on the free and protein-bound hormone concentrations. The initial increase in binding protein concentration (as may occur with estrogen administration) increases the amount of bound hormone and transiently decreases the free hormone concentration. There follows a transient increase in thyroid hormone secretion under the stimulus of TSH to replenish the free hormone pool. Another contributing factor is a transient decrease in the metabolic clearance rate of thyroid hormone. A new steady state is attained in which the free hormone secretion, metabolism, and plasma concentration are the same as initially except that the free hormone is now in equilibrium with a larger pool of bound hormone. In subjects receiving thyroid hormone medication, the same daily dose of thyroid hormone is necessary to maintain euthyroidism irrespective of the size of the bound hormone pool.

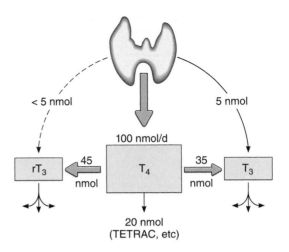

Figure 7–18. Major pathways of thyroxine metabolism in normal adult humans. Rates are expressed in nmol/24 h and are approximations based upon available data. 100 nmol of T_4 is equivalent to approximately 75 µg. (rT_3, reverse T_3; TETRAC, tetraiodothyroacetic acid.) (Reproduced, with permission, from Cavalieri RR, Rapoport B: Impaired peripheral conversion of thyroxine to triiodothyronine. Ann Rev Med 1977;28:5765.)

rT_3), which is metabolically inert. The deiodinative pathways of thyroxine metabolism are presented in Figure 7–19. Monodeiodination of the outer ring of thyroxine is a "step up" process, increasing the metabolic activity of the resultant compound, while monodeiodination of the inner ring is a "step down" or inactivation process. Further deiodination of the molecule abolishes hormonal activity.

At least three enzymes catalyze these monodeiodination reactions: type 1 5'-deiodinase; type 2 5'-deiodi-

nase; and type 3 tyrosyl ring deiodinase, or 5-deiodinase. They differ in tissue localization, substrate specificity, and effect of disease. The properties of these deiodinases are summarized in Table 7–3.

Type 1 5'-deiodinase is the most abundant deiodinase and is found largely in liver and kidney and in lesser quantity in the thyroid gland, skeletal muscle, heart muscle, and other tissues. Molecular cloning of type 1 5'-deiodinase has revealed that it contains selenocysteine and that this is probably the active deiodinating site. The major function of type 1 5'-deiodinase is to provide T_3 to the plasma. It is increased in hyperthyroidism and decreased in hypothyroidism. The increased activity in hyperthyroidism accounts in part for the high T_3 levels in this syndrome. The enzyme is inhibited by propylthiouracil but not methimazole, which explains why propylthiouracil is more effective than methimazole in reducing T_3 levels in severe hyperthyroidism. Inhibition of type 1 5'-deiodinase activity results in impaired conversion of T_4 to T_3. Some conditions associated with decreased conversion of T_4 to T_3 are listed in Table 7–4. Note that only propylthiouracil, amiodarone, and ipodate impair intracellular conversion of T_4 to T_3; the other conditions may modify the ratio of T_4 to T_3 in serum, requiring interpretation of thyroid tests (see below), but they do not change intracellular T_3 production. Dietary deficiency of selenium also impairs conversion of T_4 to T_3. In the presence of

Table 7–2. Chemical structures and biologic activity of thyroid hormones.

Hormone	Common Name	Biologic Activity
L-3,5,3′,5′-Tetraiodothyronine	L-Thyroxine; T_4	100
L-3,5,3′-Triiodothyronine	T_3	300–800
L-3,3′,5′-Triiodothyronine	Reverse T_3; rT_3	< 1
DL-3,3′-Diiodothyronine	3,3′-T_2	< 1–3
DL-3,5-Diiodothyronine	3,5-T_2	7–11
DL-3′,5′-Diiodothyronine	3′5′-T_2	0
L-3,5,3′,5′-Tetraiodothyro-acetic acid	Tetrac	? 10–50
L-3,5,3′-Triiodothyroacetic acid	Triac	? 25–35

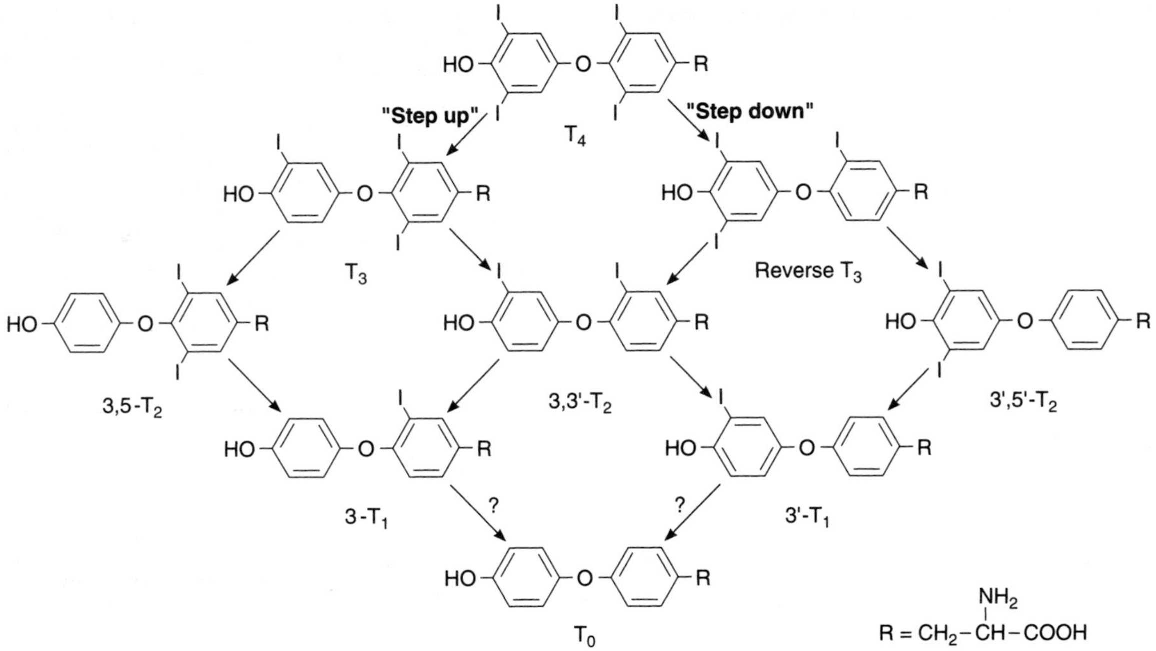

Figure 7–19. The deiodinative pathway of thyroxine metabolism. The monodeiodination of T_4 to T_3 represents a "step up" in biologic potency, whereas the monodeiodination of T_4 to reverse T_3 has the opposite effect. Further deiodination of T_3 essentially abolishes hormonal activity.

Table 7–3. Iodothyronine deiodinases.[1]

Parameter	Type 1 (5′)	Type 2 (5′)	Type 3 (5)
Physiologic role	Provides T_3 to plasma	Provides intracellular T_3	Inactivates T_3 and T_4
Tissue location	Liver, kidney, muscle, thyroid	CNS, pituitary, brown fat, placenta	Placenta, CNS, skin, fetal liver
Substrate	$rT_3 \gg T_4 > T_3$	$T_4 = rT_3$	$T_3 > T_4$
K_m for T_4	1×10^{-6} M	1×10^{-9} M	6×10^{-9} M (T_3), 37×10^{-9} M (T_4)
Deiodination site	Outer and inner ring	Outer ring	Inner ring
Kinetic mechanism	Ping-pong	Sequential	Sequential
Dithiothreitol	Stimulates	Stimulates	Stimulates
K_i for PTU	5×10^{-7} M (sensitive)	4×10^{-3} M (resistant)	$? > 10^{-3}$ M (resistant)
Active site	Selenocysteine	Selenocysteine	Selenocysteine
Ipanoic acid	Inhibits	Inhibits	Inhibits
Hypothyroidism	Decrease	Increase	Decrease
Hyperthyroidism	Increase	Decrease	Increase

[1]Adapted and modified, with permission, from Larsen PR, Ingbar SH. The thyroid gland. In: *Williams Textbook of Endocrinology*, 8th ed. Wilson JW, Foster DW (editors). Saunders, 1992.

Table 7–4. Conditions or factors associated with decreased conversion of T_4 or T_3.

1. Fetal life
2. Caloric restriction
3. Hepatic disease
4. Major systemic illness
5. Drugs:
    Propylthiouracil
    Glucocorticoids
    Propranolol (mild effect)
    Iodinated x-ray contrast agents (iopanoic acid, ipodate sodium)
    Amiodarone
6. Selenium deficiency

iodine deficiency, repletion of selenium causes increased type 1 5′-deiodinase activity, an acceleration of T_4 metabolism, and a worsening of hypothyroidism, since the iodine-deficient gland cannot compensate for the increased T_4 metabolism.

Type 2 5′-deiodinase is found largely in the brain and pituitary gland. It is resistant to propylthiouracil but very sensitive to circulating T_4. The major effect of the enzyme is to maintain a constant level of intracellular T_3 in the central nervous system. Reduction in circulating T_4 results in a rapid increase in the amount of the enzyme in brain and pituitary cells, probably by altering the rate of enzyme degradation and inactivation, maintaining the level of intracellular T_3 and cellular function. High levels of serum T_4 reduce type 2 5′-deiodinase, protecting brain cells from excessive T_3. This may be the mechanism whereby the hypothalamus and pituitary monitor the levels of circulating T_4. Other metabolic products of T_4 metabolism such as rT_3 can also modify the levels of type 2 5′-deiodinase in the brain and the pituitary gland, and alpha-adrenergic compounds stimulate type 2 5′-deiodinase in brown fat. The physiologic significance of these reactions is not clear.

Type 3 5-deiodinase, or tyrosyl ring deiodinase, is found in placental chorionic membranes and glial cells in the central nervous system. It inactivates T_4 by converting it to rT_3 and T_3 by converting it to 3,3′-diiodothyronine ($3,3'\text{-}T_2$) (Figure 7–19). It is elevated in hyperthyroidism and decreased in hypothyroidism. Thus, it may help to protect the fetus and the brain from excess or deficiency of T_4.

Overall, the functions of the deiodinases may be threefold: (1) they may provide a means for local tissue and cellular control of thyroidal activity; (2) they may allow the organism to adapt to changing environmental

states such as iodine deficiency or chronic illness; and (3) they have an important role in the early development of many vertebrates, including amphibia and mammals.

About 80% of T_4 is metabolized by deiodination, 35% to T_3 and 45% to rT_3 (Figure 7–18). The remainder is inactivated mostly by glucuronidation in the liver and secretion into bile, or to a lesser extent by sulfation and deiodination in the liver or kidney. Other metabolic reactions include deamination of the alanine side chain, forming thyroacetic acid derivatives of low biologic activity (Table 7–2); or decarboxylation or cleavage of the ether bridge, forming inactive compounds.

Representative iodothyronine kinetic values are summarized in Table 7–5. The volume of distribution is the quantity of plasma that would contain the equivalent of the total extrathyroidal pool of the compound. Thus, for T_4, the serum concentration is about 100 nmol/L; the volume of distribution is about 10 L; and the body pool is about 1000 nmol. The metabolic clearance rate for T_4 is only about 10% per day (100 nmol), and the half-life of T_4 in plasma is about 7 days. The body pool of T_3 is much smaller and the turnover more rapid, with a plasma half-life of 1 day. The total body pool of rT_3 is about the same size as that of T_3, but rT_3 has a much more rapid turnover, with a plasma half-life of only 0.2 day. The rapid clearance of T_3 and rT_3 is due to lower binding affinity for thyroid binding proteins.

Table 7–5. Representative iodothyronine kinetic values in a euthyroid human.

	T_4	T_3	rT_3
Serum levels			
Total, µg/dL (nmol/L)	8 (103)	0.12 (1.84)	0.04 (0.51)
Free, ng/dL (pmol/L)	1.5 (19)	0.28 (4.3)	0.24 (3.69)
Body pool, µg (nmol)	800 (1023)	46 (70.7)	40 (61.5)
Distribution volume (L)	10	38	98
Metabolic clearance rate (MCR) (L/d)	1	22	90
Production (disposal) rate. MCR X serum concentration, µg/d (nmol/d)	80 (103)	26 (34)	36 (46)
Half-life in plasma ($t_{1/2}$) (days)	7	1	0.2

(**Note:** T_4 µg/dL × 12.87 = nmol/L; T_3 µg/dL × 15.38 = nmol/L)

CONTROL OF THYROID FUNCTION

The growth and function of the thyroid gland and the peripheral effects of thyroid hormones are controlled by at least four mechanisms: (1) the classic hypothalamic-pituitary-thyroid axis (Figure 7–20), in which hypothalamic thyrotropin-releasing hormone (TRH) stimulates the synthesis and release of anterior pituitary thyroid-stimulating hormone (TSH), which in turn stimulates growth and hormone secretion by the thyroid gland; (2) the pituitary and peripheral deiodinases, which modify the effects of T_4 and T_3; (3) autoregulation of hormone synthesis by the thyroid gland itself in relationship to its iodine supply; and (4) stimulation or inhibition of thyroid function by TSH receptor autoantibodies. In addition, the effects of T_3 may be modified by the status of the T_3 receptor (repressor or activation) and potentially by nonthyroidal T_3 receptor agonists or antagonists.

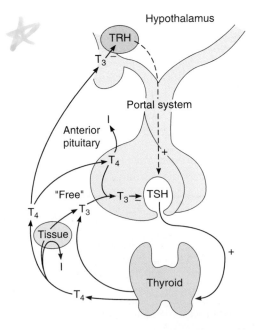

Figure 7–20. The hypothalamic-hypophysial-thyroidal axis. TRH produced in the hypothalamus reaches the thyrotrophs in the anterior pituitary by the hypothalamic-hypophysial-portal system and stimulates the synthesis and release of TSH. In both the hypothalamus and the pituitary, it is primarily T_3 that inhibits TRH and TSH secretion. T_4 undergoes monodeiodination to T_3 in neural and pituitary as well as in peripheral tissues.

Thyrotropin-Releasing Hormone

Thyrotropin-releasing hormone (TRH) is a tripeptide, pyroglutamyl-histidyl-prolineamide, synthesized by neurons in the supraoptic and supraventricular nuclei of the hypothalamus (Figure 7–21). It is stored in the median eminence of the hypothalamus and then transported via the pituitary portal venous system down the pituitary stalk to the anterior pituitary gland, where it controls synthesis and release of TSH. TRH is also found in other portions of the hypothalamus, the brain, and the spinal cord, where it may function as a neurotransmitter. The gene for human preproTRH, located on chromosome 3, contains a 3.3-kb transcription unit that encodes six TRH molecules. The gene also encodes other neuropeptides that may be biologically significant. In the anterior pituitary gland, TRH binds to specific membrane receptors on thyrotrophs and prolactin-secreting cells, stimulating synthesis and release of both TSH and prolactin. Thyroid hormones cause a slow depletion of pituitary TRH receptors, diminishing TRH response; estrogen increases TRH receptors, increasing pituitary sensitivity to TRH.

The response of the pituitary thyrotroph to TRH is bimodal: First, it stimulates release of stored hormone; and second, it stimulates gene activity, which increases hormone synthesis. The TRH receptor (TRH-R) is a member of the seven-transmembrane-spanning, GTP-binding, protein-coupled receptor family (Table 3–1; Figure 3–2). The *TRHR* gene is located on chromosome 8. Large glycoprotein hormones such as TSH and LH bind to the extracellular portions of their receptors, but TRH, a small peptide, binds to the transmembrane helix 3 of the TRH-R. After binding to its receptor on the thyrotroph, TRH activates a G protein, which in turn activates phospholipase c to hydrolyze phosphatidylinositol 4,5-bisphosphate (PIP_2) to inositol 1,4,5-trisphosphate (IP_3). IP_3 stimulates the release of intracellular Ca^{2+}, which causes the first burst response

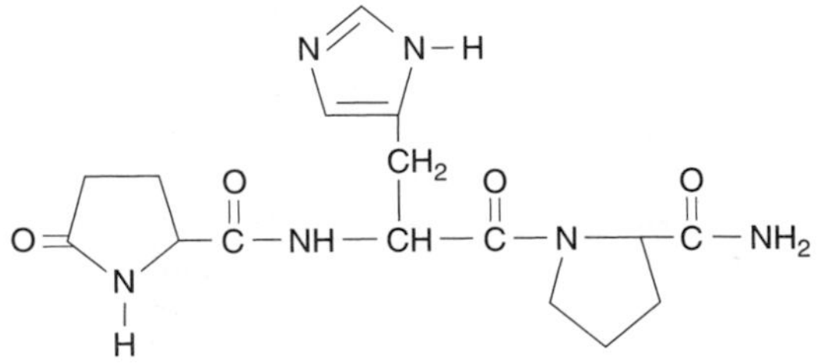

(pyro)Glu-His-Pro-(NH₂)

Figure 7–21. Chemical structure of thyrotropin-releasing hormone (TRH).

of hormone release. Simultaneously, there is generation of 1,2-diacylglycerol, which activates protein kinase C, thought to be responsible for the second and sustained phase of hormone secretion. The increases in intracellular Ca^{2+} and in protein kinase C may be involved in increased transcription of TSH. TRH also stimulates the glycosylation of TSH, which is necessary for full biologic activity of the hormone. Thus, patients with hypothalamic tumors and hypothyroidism may have measurable TSH, which is not glycosylated and is biologically inactive.

Elegant studies in vitro and in vivo demonstrated that T_3 directly inhibits the transcription of prepro-TRH gene and thus the synthesis of TRH in the hypothalamus. Since T_4 is converted to T_3 within peptidergic neurons, it is also an effective inhibitor of TRH synthesis and secretion (Table 7–6).

TRH is rapidly metabolized, with a half-life of intravenously administered hormone of about 5 minutes. Plasma TRH levels in normal subjects are very low, ranging from 25 to 100 pg/mL.

TRH-stimulated TSH secretion occurs in a pulsatile fashion throughout the 24 hours (Figure 7–22). Normal subjects have a mean TSH pulse amplitude of about 0.6 μU/mL and an average frequency of one pulse every 1.8 hours. In addition, normal subjects show a circadian rhythm, with a peak serum TSH at night, usually between midnight and 4 AM. This peak is unrelated to sleep, eating, or the secretion of other pituitary hormones. This rhythm is presumably controlled by a hypothalamic neuronal "pulse generator" driving TRH synthesis in the supraoptic and supraventricular nuclei. In hypothyroid patients, the amplitude of the pulses and the nocturnal surge are much larger than normal, and in patients with hyperthyroidism both the pulses and the nocturnal surge are markedly suppressed.

In experimental animals and in the newborn human, exposure to cold increases TRH and TSH secretion, but this is not noted in the adult human.

Certain hormones and drugs may modify TRH synthesis and release. TRH secretion is stimulated by decreased serum T_4 or T_3 (with decreased intraneuronal T_3), by alpha-adrenergic agonists, and by arginine vasopressin. Conversely, TRH secretion is inhibited by increased serum T_4 or T_3 (with increased intraneuronal T_3) and alpha-adrenergic blockade (Table 7–6).

TRH administered intravenously to humans in a bolus dose of 200–500 μg results in a rapid threefold to fivefold rise in serum TSH, peaking at about 30 minutes and lasting for 2–3 hours (see Figure 5–14). In patients with primary hypothyroidism—in whom basal TSH is elevated—there is an exaggerated response. The response is suppressed in patients with hyperthyroidism, in those who have nodular goiters with au-

Table 7–6. Factors controlling the secretion of thyroid hormones.

1. HYPOTHALAMIC: Synthesis and release of TRH
   Stimulatory:
   Decreased serum T_4 and T_3, and intraneuronal T_3
   Neurogenic: Pulsatile secretion and circadian rhythm
   Exposure to cold (animals and human newborn)
   Alpha-adrenergic catecholamines
   Arginine vasopressin
   Inhibitory:
   Increased serum T_4 and T_3, and intraneuronal T_3
   Alpha-adrenergic blockers
   Hypothalamic tumors
2. ANTERIOR PITUITARY: Synthesis and release of TSH
   Stimulatory:
   TRH
   Decreased serum T_4 and T_3, and intrathyrotrope T_3
   Decreased activity Type 2 5'-deiodinase
   Estrogen: increased TRH binding sites
   Inhibitory:
   Increased serum T_4 and T_3, and intrathyrotrope T_3
   Increased activity Type 2 5'-deiodinase
   Somatostatin
   Dopamine, dopamine agonists: bromocriptine
   Glucocorticoids
   Chronic illness
   Pituitary tumors
3. THYROID: Synthesis and release of thyroid hormones
   Stimulatory:
   TSH
   TSH-R stimulating antibodies
   Inhibitory:
   TSH-R blocking antibodies
   Iodide excess
   Lithium therapy

tonomously functioning nodules, in patients on high-dose thyroxine therapy, and in patients with pituitary hypothyroidism. In a patient with a hypothalamic lesion, a partial TSH response to TRH injection would indicate an intact pituitary. TRH and its dipeptide metabolite cyclo(HisPro) are also found in the islet cells of the pancreas, the gastrointestinal tract, the placenta, the heart, and in the prostate, testes, and ovaries. TRH mRNA in these peripheral tissues is not inhibited by T_3, and the role of TRH in these tissues has not yet been determined.

Thyrotropin

Thyroid-stimulating hormone, or thyrotropin (TSH), is a glycoprotein synthesized and secreted by the thyrotrophs of the anterior pituitary gland. It has a molec-

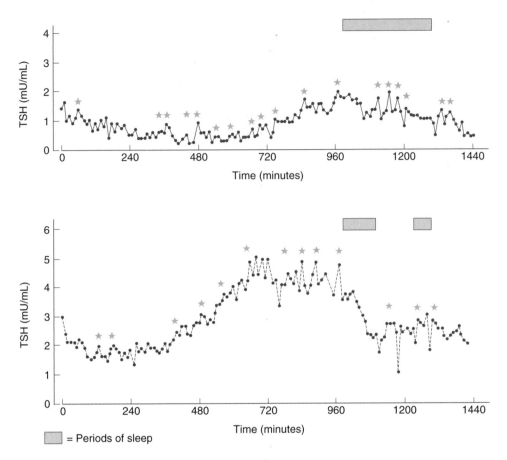

Figure 7–22. Serum TSH in two normal subjects demonstrating spontaneous pulses and the circadian rhythm of TSH secretion. (0 time is 0900; Stars indicate significant pulses.) (Reproduced, with permission, from Greenspan SL et al: Pulsatile secretion of TSH in man. J Clin Endocrinol Metab 1986;63:664. Copyright © 1986 by The Endocrine Society.)

ular weight of about 28,000 and is composed of two noncovalently linked subunits, α and β. The α subunit is common to the two other pituitary glycoproteins, FSH and LH, and also to the placental hormone hCG; the β subunit is different for each glycoprotein hormone and confers specific binding properties and biologic activity. The human α subunit has an apoprotein core of 92 amino acids and contains two oligosaccharide chains; the TSH β subunit has an apoprotein core of 112 amino acids and contains one oligosaccharide chain. The α and β subunit amino acid chains of TSH each form three loops which are intertwined into a knot-like structure called a "cystine knot" (Figure 7–23). Mutations of the amino acids in either chain can result in either decreased or increased TSH activity. Glycosylation takes place in the rough endoplasmic reticulum and the Golgi of the thyrotroph, where glu-

cose, mannose, and fucose residues and terminal sulfate or sialic acid residues are linked to the apoprotein core. The function of these carbohydrate residues is not entirely clear, but it is likely that they enhance TSH biologic activity and modify its metabolic clearance rate. For example, deglycosylated TSH will bind to its receptor, but its biologic activity is markedly decreased and its metabolic clearance rate is markedly increased.

The gene for the human α subunit is located on chromosome 6 and the gene for the human β subunit on chromosome 1. Several kindreds have been reported with a point mutation in the *TSHβ* gene, resulting in a TSH-β subunit that did not combine with the α subunit to produce biologically active TSH. The disorders were autosomal recessive, and the clinical picture was that of nongoitrous hypothyroidism.

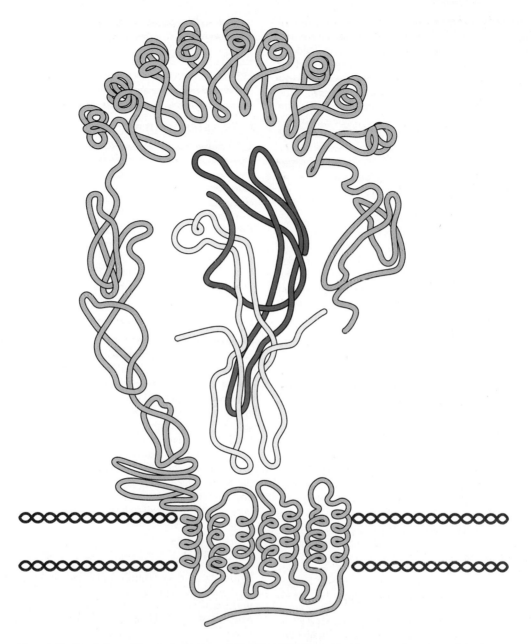

Figure 7–23. Schematic configuration of the TSH-TSHR complex. The central portion of the figure represents the ribbon-like structure of TSH within the TSH receptor. The dark blue line represents the β subunit and the light blue line the α subunit. See also Figure 7–24. (Reproduced, with permission, from Szkudlinski MW et al: Thyroid-stimulating hormone and thyroid-stimulating hormone receptor structure-function relationships. Physiol Rev 2002;82:473.)

TSH is the primary factor controlling thyroid cell growth and thyroid hormone synthesis and secretion. It achieves this effect by binding to a specific **TSH receptor** (TSH-R) on the thyroid cell membrane and activating both the G protein-adenylyl cyclase-cAMP and the phospholipase C signaling systems. The human TSH receptor *(TSH-R)* gene is located on chromosome 14q3. The TSH-R is a single-chain glycoprotein containing 764 amino acids. Like the TRH receptor of the anterior pituitary, the TSH-R in the thyroid follicular cell is a member of the seven-membrane spanning, GTP-binding protein-coupled receptor family. Structurally, it can be divided into two subunits: subunit A, containing 397 amino acids, representing the ectodomain which is involved in ligand binding; and subunit B, which includes the intramembrane and intracellular portion of the receptor involved in activation of thyroid cell growth, thyroid hormone synthesis, and release of the hormone (Figure 7–24). The TSH-R is unique in that it has binding sites not only for TSH but also for TSH receptor-stimulating antibodies (TSH-R Ab [stim]), which are found in patients with autoimmune hyperthyroidism (Graves' disease), and also for autoantibodies that bind to the TSH receptor and block the action of TSH (TSH-R Ab [block]). These latter antibodies are found in patients with severe hypothyroidism due to autoimmune atrophic thyroiditis and in some infants with neonatal hypothyroidism.

Mutations in the TSH-R have been associated with either spontaneous activation of the receptor and clinical hyperthyroidism or with resistance to TSH. Activating mutations involving the B subunit of the TSH-R have been found in solitary autonomous adenomas and in multinodular goiters as well as in rare cases of sporadic familial hyperthyroidism. Resistance to TSH due to mutations in either subunit of the receptor is associated with elevated serum TSH levels and euthyroidism or hypothyroidism.

Effects of TSH on the Thyroid Cell

TSH has many actions on the thyroid cell. Most of its actions are mediated through the G protein-adenylyl cyclase-cAMP system, but activation of the phosphatidylinositol (PIP$_2$) system with increase in intracellular calcium may also be involved. The major actions of TSH include the following:

A. Changes in Thyroid Cell Morphology

TSH rapidly induces pseudopods at the cell-colloid border, accelerating thyroglobulin resorption. Colloid content is diminished. Intracellular colloid droplets are formed and lysosome formation is stimulated, increasing thyroglobulin hydrolysis (Figure 7–5).

B. Cell Growth

Individual thyroid cells increase in size (Figure 7–4); vascularity is increased; and, over a period of time, thyroid enlargement, or goiter, develops.

C. Iodine Metabolism

TSH stimulates all phases of iodide metabolism, from increased iodide uptake and transport to increased iodination of thyroglobulin and increased secretion of thyroid hormones. The increase in cAMP mediates increased iodide transport, while PIP$_2$ hydrolysis and increased intracellular Ca^{2+} stimulate the iodination of thyroglobulin. The TSH effect on iodide transport is biphasic: Initially, it is depressed (iodide efflux); and then, after a lag of several hours, iodide uptake is increased. The efflux of iodide may be due to the rapid increase in hydrolysis of thyroglobulin with release of hormone and leakage of iodide out of the gland.

D. Other Effects of TSH

Other effects include increase in mRNA for thyroglobulin and thyroperoxidase, with an increase in incorporation of I⁻ into MIT, DIT, T$_3$ and T$_4$; and increased lysosomal activity, with increased secretion of T$_4$ and T$_3$ from the gland. There is also increased activity of type 1 5′-deiodinase, conserving intrathyroidal iodine.

TSH has still other effects on the thyroid gland, including stimulation of glucose uptake, oxygen consumption, CO_2 production, and an increase in glucose oxidation via the hexosemonophosphate pathway and the Krebs cycle. There is accelerated turnover of phospholipids and stimulation of synthesis of purine and pyrimidine precursors, with increased synthesis of DNA and RNA.

Serum TSH

Normally, only α subunit and intact TSH are present in the serum. The level of α subunit is about 0.5–2 µg/L; it is elevated in postmenopausal women and in patients with TSH-secreting pituitary tumors (see below). The serum level of TSH is about 0.5–5 mU/L; it is increased in hypothyroidism and decreased in hyperthyroidism, whether endogenous or from excessive oral intake of thyroid hormones. The plasma half-life of TSH is about 30 minutes, and the daily production rate is about 40–150 mU/d.

Control of Pituitary TSH Secretion

The two major factors controlling the synthesis and release of TSH are the level of intrathyrotroph T$_3$, which

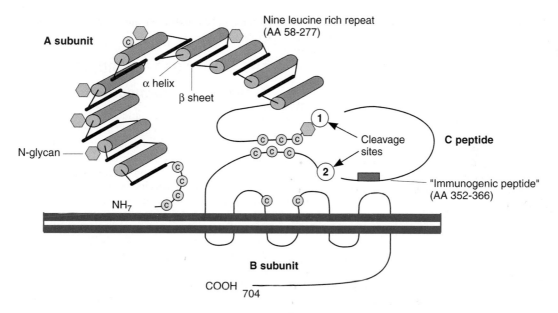

Figure 7–24. Schematic representation of the TSH receptor. The A subunit is the ligand-binding portion of the receptor and the B subunit is the activation portion. The ligands which bind to the receptor include TSH, TSH-stimulating antibody, and TSH-blocking antibody. There are two cleavage sites which allow breakage of the receptor and loss of the A subunit into the serum. (Reproduced, with permission, from Rapoport R et al: The thyrotropin (TSH)-receptor: interaction with TSH and autoantibodies. Endocr Rev 1998;19:673.)

controls mRNA for TSH synthesis and release; and TRH, which controls glycosylation, activation, and release of TSH (Table 7–6).

TSH synthesis and release are inhibited by high serum levels of T_4 and T_3 (hyperthyroidism) and stimulated by low levels of thyroid hormone (hypothyroidism). In addition, certain hormones and drugs inhibit TSH secretion. These include somatostatin, dopamine, dopamine agonists such as bromocriptine, and glucocorticoids. Acute or chronic disease may cause inhibition of TSH secretion during active illness, and there may be a rebound rise in TSH as the patient recovers. The magnitude of these effects is variable; thus, the drugs mentioned above will suppress serum TSH, but it will usually be detectable. In contrast, hyperthyroidism will turn off TSH secretion entirely. These observations are important clinically in interpreting serum TSH levels in patients receiving these medications.

Destructive lesions or tumors of the hypothalamus or anterior pituitary gland may impair TRH and TSH secretion by destruction of secretory cells. This will result in "secondary hypothyroidism" due to pituitary thyrotroph destruction or "tertiary hypothyroidism" due to destruction of TRH-secreting neurons. Differential diagnosis of these lesions is discussed below (see Thyroid Tests).

Other Thyroid Stimulators & Inhibitors

The thyroid follicle has a rich supply of capillaries that carry noradrenergic nerve fibers from the superior cervical ganglion and acetylcholine esterase-positive nerve fibers derived from the vagal nodose and thyroid ganglia. The parafollicular C cells secrete both calcitonin and calcitonin gene-related peptide (CGRP). In experimental animals, these and other neuropeptides modify thyroid blood flow and hormone secretion. In addition, growth factors such as insulin, IGF-I, and EGF and the autocrine actions of prostaglandins and cytokines may modify thyroid cell growth and hormone production. However, it is not yet clear how important these effects are in clinical situations.

Role of Pituitary & Peripheral Deiodinases

Pituitary type 2 5'-deiodinase converts T_4 to T_3 in the brain and pituitary, providing the main source of intracellular T_3. Its increased activity in hypothyroidism helps to maintain cerebral intracellular T_3 in the presence of falling serum T_4 concentrations. In hyperthyroidism, the decrease in its activity helps to prevent overloading of pituitary and neural cells with thyroid hormone. In contrast, type 1 5'-deiodinase is decreased in hypothyroidism, conserving T_4, and increased in hyperthyroidism, accelerating T_4 metabolism (Table 7–3).

Thyroidal Autoregulation

Autoregulation may be defined as the capacity of the thyroid gland to modify its function to adapt to changes in the availability of iodine, independent of pituitary TSH. Thus, humans can maintain normal thyroid hormone secretion with iodide intakes varying from 50 μg to several milligrams per day. Some of the effects of iodide deficiency or excess are discussed above. The major adaptation to low iodide intake is the preferential synthesis of T_3 rather than T_4, increasing the metabolic effectiveness of the secreted hormone. Iodide excess, on the other hand, inhibits many thyroidal functions, including I⁻ transport, cAMP formation, H_2O_2 generation, hormone synthesis and secretion, and the binding of TSH and TSH-R Ab to the TSH receptor. Some of these effects may be mediated by the formation of intrathyroidal iodinated fatty acids. The ability of the normal thyroid to "escape" from these inhibitory effects (Wolff-Chaikoff effect) allows the gland to continue to secrete hormone despite a high dietary iodide intake. It is important to note that this is different from the therapeutic effect of iodide in the treatment of Graves' disease. Here, the high levels of iodide inhibit thyroglobulin endocytosis and lysosomal activity, decreasing thyroid hormone release and lowering circulating hormone levels. In addition, the inhibition of TSH-R Ab [stim] activity reduces the vascularity of the gland, with beneficial consequences during surgery. This effect is also transient, lasting about 10 days to 2 weeks.

Autoimmune Regulation

The ability of B lymphocytes to synthesize TSH receptor antibodies that can either block the action of TSH or mimic TSH activity by binding to different areas on the TSH receptor provides a form of thyroid regulation by the immune system.

Summary

Thus, the synthesis and secretion of thyroid hormones are controlled at three different levels: (1) the level of the hypothalamus, by modifying TRH secretion; (2) the pituitary level, by inhibition or stimulation of TSH secretion; and (3) the level of the thyroid, by autoregulation and blockade or stimulation of the TSH receptor (Table 7–6).

THE ACTION OF THYROID HORMONES

1. The Thyroid Hormone Receptor

Thyroid hormones, T_3 and T_4, circulate in plasma largely bound to protein but in equilibrium with the free hormone. It is the free hormone that is transported, either by passive diffusion or by specific carriers, through the cell membrane, through the cell cytoplasm, to bind to a specific receptor in the cell nucleus. Within the cell, T_4 is converted to T_3 by 5' deiodinase, suggesting that T_4 is a prohormone and T_3 the active form of the hormone. The nuclear receptor for T_3 has been cloned. It is one of a "family" of receptors, all similar to the receptor for the retrovirus that causes erythroblastosis in chickens, v-erbA, and to the nuclear receptors for glucocorticoids, mineralocorticoids, estrogens, progestins, vitamin D_3, and retinoic acid (Figure 3–13).

In the human, there are two genes for the thyroid hormone receptor, alpha and beta. *TRα* is located on chromosome 17 and *TRβ* on chromosome 3. Each gene produces at least two products, TRα 1 and 2 and TRβ 1 and 2. The structure and characteristics of these products are portrayed in Figure 7–25. Each has three domains: a ligand-independent domain at the amino terminal, a centrally located DNA binding area with two cysteine-zinc "fingers," and a ligand-binding domain at the carboxyl terminal (Figures 3–12 and 3–13). Note that TRα2 does not bind T_3 and may actually inhibit T_3 action. The concentration of these receptors in tissue varies with the stage of development and the tissue. For example, the brain contains mostly TRα, the liver mostly TRβ, and cardiac muscle contains both. The binding affinity of T_3 analogs is directly proportionate to the biologic activity of the analog. Point mutations in the ligand-binding domain of the TRβ gene are responsible for the syndrome of generalized resistance to thyroid hormone (GRTH—Refetoff's syndrome; see below).

The thyroid hormone receptors may bind to the specific thyroid hormone response element (TRE) sites on DNA even in the absence of T_3 (Figure 7–26)—unlike the steroid hormone receptors). The TREs are located near—generally upstream with respect to the start of transcription—to the promoters where transcription of specific thyroid hormone-responsive genes is initiated. T_3 binding to the receptors results in stimulation—in some cases inhibition—of the transcription of these genes with consequent changes in the levels of the mRNAs transcribed from them. The changes in mRNA levels alter the levels of the protein product of these

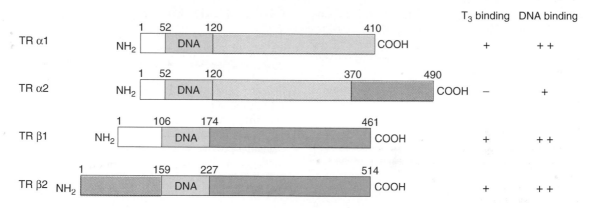

Figure 7–25. Deduced protein structure of the thyroid hormone receptor α and β gene products. The receptor protein has three domains: a DNA-binding domain with a high degree of similarity among the different types of receptors, a carboxyl terminal triiodothyronine (T_3) binding domain, and an amino terminal domain that is not required for full function. The numbers above the structures represent amino acid numbers. The properties of the receptors with respect to their ability to bind T_3 and bind to a T_3-response element of DNA are shown on the right. Identical shading of receptor domains indicates identical amino acid sequences. (TR, thyroid hormone receptor.) (Reproduced, with permission, from Brent GA: The molecular basis of thyroid hormone action. N Engl J Med 1994;331:847.)

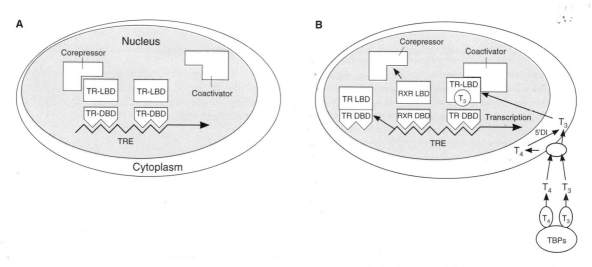

Figure 7–26. Model of the interaction of T_3 with the T_3 receptor. **Panel A, Inactive Phase:** The unliganded T_3 receptor dimer bound to the TRE along with corepressors acts as a suppressor of gene transcription. **Panel B, Active Phase:** T_3 and T_4 circulate bound to thyroid-binding proteins (TBPs). The free hormones are transported into the cell by a specific transport system. Within the cytoplasm, T_4 is converted to T_3 by 5′-deiodinase and T_3 moves into the nucleus. There it binds to the ligand-binding domain of the TR monomer. This promotes disruption of the TR homodimer and heterodimerization with RXR on the TRE, displacement of corepressors, and binding of coactivators. The TR-coactivator complex activates gene transcription, which leads to alteration in protein synthesis and cellular phenotype. (TR-LBD, T_3 receptor ligand-binding domain; TR-DBD, T_3 receptor DNA-binding domain; RXR-LBD, retinoid X receptor ligand-binding domain; RXR-DBD, retinoid X receptor DNA-binding domain; TRE, thyroid hormone response element; TBPs, thyroxine-binding proteins; T_3, triiodothyronine; T_4, tetraiodothyronine, L-thyroxine; 5′DI, 5′-deiodinase.

genes. These proteins then mediate the thyroid hormone response. These receptors often function as heterodimers with other transcription factors such as the retinoid X receptor and the retinoic acid receptor (Figure 7–26).

2. Physiologic Effects of Thyroid Hormones

The transcriptional effects of T_3 characteristically demonstrate a lag time of hours or days to achieve full effect. These genomic actions result in a number of effects, including those on tissue growth, brain maturation, and increased heat production and oxygen consumption, which is due in part to increased activity of Na^+-K^+ ATPase and in part to production of increased beta-adrenergic receptors. Some actions of T_3 are not genomic, such as reduction of pituitary type 2 5'-deiodinase and increase in glucose and amino acid transport. Some specific effects of thyroid hormones are summarized in what follows.

Effects on Fetal Development

The thyroid and the anterior pituitary TSH system begin to function in the human fetus at about 11 weeks. Prior to this time, the fetal thyroid does not concentrate ^{123}I. Because of the high placental content of type 3 5-deiodinase, most maternal T_3 and T_4 are inactivated in the placenta, and very little free hormone reaches the fetal circulation. This small amount of free hormone from the mother may be important for early fetal brain development. However, after 11 weeks of gestation, the fetus is largely dependent on its own thyroidal secretion. Although some fetal growth occurs in the absence of fetal thyroid hormone secretion, brain development and skeletal maturation are markedly impaired, resulting in cretinism (mental retardation and dwarfism).

Effects on Oxygen Consumption, Heat Production, & Free Radical Formation

T_3 increases O_2 consumption and heat production in part by stimulation of Na^+-K^+ ATPase in all tissues except the brain, spleen, and testis. This contributes to the increased basal metabolic rate (O_2 consumption by the whole animal at rest) and the increased sensitivity to heat in hyperthyroidism—and the converse in hypothyroidism. Thyroid hormones also decrease superoxide dismutase levels, resulting in increased superoxide anion free radical formation. This may contribute to the deleterious effects of chronic hyperthyroidism.

Cardiovascular Effects

T_3 stimulates transcription of myosin heavy chain α and inhibits myosin heavy chain β, improving cardiac muscle contractility. T_3 also increases transcription of Ca^{2+} ATPase in the sarcoplasmic reticulum, increasing diastolic tone of the heart; alters isoforms of Na^+-K^+ ATPase genes; and increases beta-adrenergic receptors and the concentration of G proteins. Thus, thyroid hormones have marked positive inotropic and chronotropic effects on the heart. This accounts for the increased cardiac output and marked increase in heart rate in hyperthyroidism and the reverse in hypothyroidism.

Sympathetic Effects

As noted above, thyroid hormones increase the number of beta-adrenergic receptors in heart muscle, skeletal muscle, adipose tissue, and lymphocytes. They also decrease myocardial alpha-adrenergic receptors. In addition, they may amplify catecholamine action at a postreceptor site. Thus, sensitivity to catecholamines is markedly increased in hyperthyroidism, and therapy with beta-adrenergic blocking agents may be very helpful in controlling tachycardia and arrhythmias.

Pulmonary Effects

Thyroid hormones maintain normal hypoxic and hypercapnic drive in the respiratory center. In severe hypothyroidism, hypoventilation occurs, occasionally requiring assisted ventilation.

Hematopoietic Effects

The increased cellular demand for O_2 in hyperthyroidism leads to increased production of erythropoietin and increased erythropoiesis. However, blood volume is usually not increased because of hemodilution and increased red cell turnover. Thyroid hormones increase the 2,3-diphosphoglycerate content of erythrocytes, allowing increased O_2 dissociation from hemoglobin and increasing O_2 availability to tissues. The reverse occurs in hypothyroidism.

Gastrointestinal Effects

Thyroid hormones stimulate gut motility, which can result in increased motility and diarrhea in hyperthyroidism and slowed bowel transit and constipation in hypothyroidism. This may also contribute to the modest weight loss in hyperthyroidism and weight gain in hypothyroidism.

Skeletal Effects

Thyroid hormones stimulate increased bone turnover, increasing bone resorption and, to a lesser degree, bone formation. Thus, chronic hyperthyroidism may result in significant osteopenia and, in severe cases, modest hypercalcemia, hypercalciuria, and increased excretion of urinary hydroxyproline and pyridinium cross-links.

Neuromuscular Effects

Although thyroid hormones stimulate increased synthesis of many structural proteins, in hyperthyroidism there is increased protein turnover and loss of muscle tissue, or myopathy. This may be associated with spontaneous creatinuria. There is also an increase in the speed of muscle contraction and relaxation, noted clinically in the hyperreflexia of hyperthyroidism—or the reverse in hypothyroidism. As noted above, thyroid hormones are essential for normal development and function of the central nervous system, and failure of fetal thyroid function results in severe mental retardation. In the adult, hyperactivity in hyperthyroidism and sluggishness in hypothyroidism can be striking.

Effects on Lipid & Carbohydrate Metabolism

Hyperthyroidism increases hepatic gluconeogenesis and glycogenolysis as well as intestinal glucose absorption. Thus, hyperthyroidism will exacerbate underlying diabetes mellitus. Cholesterol synthesis and degradation are both increased by thyroid hormones. The latter effect is due largely to an increase in the hepatic low-density lipoprotein (LDL) receptors, so that cholesterol levels decline with thyroid overactivity. Lipolysis is also increased, releasing fatty acids and glycerol. Conversely, cholesterol levels are elevated in hypothyroidism.

Endocrine Effects

Thyroid hormones increase the metabolic turnover of many hormones and pharmacologic agents. For example, the half-life of cortisol is about 100 minutes in the normal individual, about 50 minutes in a hyperthyroid patient, and about 150 minutes in a hypothyroid patient. The production rate of cortisol will increase in the hyperthyroid patient with normal adrenal function, thus maintaining a normal circulating hormone level. However, in a patient with adrenal insufficiency, the development of hyperthyroidism or thyroid hormone treatment of hypothyroidism may unmask the adrenal disease. Ovulation may be impaired in both hyperthyroidism and hypothyroidism, resulting in infertility, which will be corrected by restoration of the euthyroid state. Serum prolactin levels are increased in about 40% of patients with hypothyroidism, presumably a manifestation of increased TRH release; this will revert to normal with T_4 therapy. Other endocrine effects will be discussed in appropriate sections elsewhere in this chapter.

PHYSIOLOGIC CHANGES IN THYROID FUNCTION

Thyroid Function in the Fetus

Prior to the development of independent fetal thyroid function, the fetus is dependent on maternal thyroid hormones for early neural development. However, by the 11th week of gestation, the hypophysial portal system has developed, and measurable TSH and TRH are present. At about the same time, the fetal thyroid begins to trap iodine. The secretion of thyroid hormone probably begins in mid gestation (18–20 weeks). TSH increases rapidly to peak levels at 24–28 weeks, and T_4 levels peak at 35–40 weeks. T_3 levels remain low during gestation; T_4 is converted to rT_3 by type 3 5-deiodinase during fetal development. At birth, there is a sudden marked rise in TSH, a rise in T_4, a rise in T_3, and a fall in rT_3. These parameters gradually return to normal over the first month of life.

Thyroid Function in Pregnancy

The striking change in thyroid parameters during pregnancy is the rise in TBG and consequent rise in total T_4 and total T_3 in the serum. The rise in TBG is due to estrogen-induced hepatic glycosylation of TBG with N-acetylgalactosamine, which prolongs the metabolic clearance rate of TBG. There is usually no change in thyroxine-binding prealbumin and little change in albumin. Although total T_4 and T_3 are increased, a new equilibrium develops between free and bound thyronines, and the levels of free T_4 and free T_3 are normal. Other changes in pregnancy include an increase in iodide clearance, which, in areas of low iodine intake, may result in impaired hormone synthesis and a fall in T_4, a rise in TSH, and thyroid enlargement. hCG, which peaks near the end of the first trimester, has a weak TSH agonist activity and may be responsible for the slight thyroid enlargement that occurs at that time. Maternal I^- crosses the placenta and supplies the fetal requirement; in large amounts, I^- can inhibit fetal thyroid function. Maternal TSH-R Ab [stim] and TSH-R Ab [block] can also cross the placenta and may be responsible for thyroid dysfunction in the fetus. As noted above, most maternal T_3 and T_4 are deiodinated by placental type 3 5-deiodinase and do not reach the fetus.

However, antithyroid drugs such as propylthiouracil and methimazole do cross the placenta and in large doses will block fetal thyroid function (Chapter 16).

Changes in Thyroid Function with Aging

Thyroxine turnover is highest in infants and children and gradually falls to adult levels after puberty. The T_4 turnover rate is then stable until after age 60, when it again drops slightly. Thus, replacement doses of levothyroxine will vary with age and other factors, and patients taking the drug must be monitored regularly (see below and Chapter 23).

Effects of Acute & Chronic Illness on Thyroid Function (Euthyroid Sick Syndrome)

Acute or chronic illness may have striking effects on circulating thyroid hormone levels by modifying the peripheral metabolism of T_4 or by interference with T_4 binding to TBG. These effects can be classified as (1) the low T_3 syndrome or (2) the low T_3-T_4 syndrome.

The peripheral metabolism of T_4 is diagrammed in Figure 7–19. Inhibition of outer ring type 1 5'-deiodinase or activation of type 3 5-deiodinase accelerates conversion of T_4 to rT_3 and conversion of T_3 to 3,3'-T_2. These reactions will markedly lower the circulating level of T_3, resulting in the low T_3 syndrome. This occurs physiologically in the fetus and pathologically in circumstances of carbohydrate restriction, as in malnutrition, starvation, anorexia nervosa, and diabetes mellitus, and in patients with hepatic disease or major acute or chronic systemic illnesses (Table 7–4). Drugs that

inhibit type 1 5'-deiodinase also lower the circulating levels of T_3; corticosteroids, amiodarone, and iodinated dyes are the most effective, and propylthiouracil and propranolol are relatively weak. The pathogenesis of the low T_3 syndrome when associated with acute or chronic illness is thought to involve cytokines such as tumor necrosis factor, secreted by inflammatory cells, which inhibit type 1 5'-deiodinase, accelerating inner ring deiodination of T_4.

Serum thyroid hormone levels in the low T_3 syndrome are presented diagrammatically in Figure 7–27. T_3 levels are low; total T_4 levels are normal or slightly elevated; free T_4 (by dialysis) often is slightly elevated; and rT_3 is elevated. TSH is normal. True hypothyroidism can be ruled out by the normal T_4, FT_4, and TSH and by the elevated rT_3.

Patients with the low T_3-T_4 syndrome are usually much sicker, and indeed the mortality rate in this group of patients may approach 50%. Serum T_3 and T_4 levels are both low; FT_4 (by dialysis) is usually normal; and rT_3 is elevated. TSH is usually normal, though it may be low if the patient is receiving dopamine or corticosteroids, which suppress TSH. The pathogenesis of this syndrome is thought to involve the liberation of unsaturated fatty acids, such as oleic acid, from anoxic or injured tissue, which inhibits the binding of T_4 to TBG. The syndrome can be differentiated from true hypothyroidism by the normal levels of free T_4 and TSH.

These abnormalities normalize when the patient recovers. Recovery is frequently accompanied by a transient elevation of the serum TSH that may be misinterpreted as hypothyroidism. In this setting, in the absence of clinically apparent hypothyroidism, it is best to avoid thyroid hormone therapy and to reevalu-

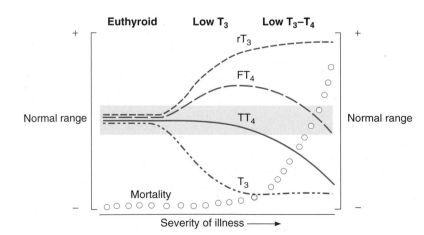

Figure 7–27. A schematic representation of the changes in serum thyroid hormone values with increasing severity of nonthyroidal illness. A rapidly rising mortality rate accompanies the fall in serum total T_4 (TT$_4$) and free T_4 (FT$_4$) values. (Reproduced, with permission, from Nicoloff JT: Abnormal measurements in nonendocrine illness. In: *Medicine for the Practicing Physician*, 2nd ed. Hurst JW [editor]. Butterworth-Heinemann, 1991.)

ate at a later time following recovery. It is possible that intracellular hypothyroidism exists in these patients, but administration of T_3 or T_4 does not benefit the patient and may worsen the situation. Thus, these changes may represent a protective adaptation on the part of the organism to severe illness. For example, one effect would be to reduce oxygen and other metabolic demands.

THYROID AUTOIMMUNITY

Autoimmune mechanisms are involved in the pathogenesis of many thyroid diseases, including the hyperthyroidism, ophthalmopathy, and dermopathy associated with Graves' disease; the nontoxic goiter or atrophic hypothyroidism associated with Hashimoto's thyroiditis; neonatal Graves' disease and some forms of neonatal hypothyroidism; and postpartum hyperthyroidism or hypothyroidism. Thus, it is important that we understand how the immune system works and how thyroid disease develops (see Chapter 4).

Immunologic defense against foreign substances and neoplastic cells involves macrophages that ingest and digest the foreign material and present peptide fragments on the cell surface in association with a class II protein coded by the HLA-DR region of the MHC gene complex. This complex is recognized by a T cell receptor on a CD4 helper T cell, which stimulates the release of cytokines such as interleukin-2 (IL-2). These cytokines amplify the response by inducing T cell activation and division, induction of killer cell activity in CD8 suppressor cells, and stimulation of antibody formation against the foreign antigen by B lymphocytes. Eventually, the activation process is muted by the action of the CD8 suppressor cells.

In 1956, three major observations suggested the possibility that immunologic reactions could develop involving the thyroid gland: (1) Rose and Witebsky produced thyroiditis in one lobe of a rabbit thyroid by immunization of the animal with a suspension of the other lobe in Freund's adjuvant; (2) Roitt and Doniach demonstrated the presence of precipitating human thyroglobulin antibodies in the serum of patients with thyroiditis; and (3) Adams and Purves demonstrated the presence of a long-acting thyroid stimulator (later proved to be an antibody to the TSH receptor) in the serum of patients with Graves' disease. Thus, the concept of autoimmune thyroid disease was born.

There are three major thyroidal autoantigens: thyroglobulin (Tg), thyroperoxidase (TPO), and the TSH receptor (TSH-R). Autoantibodies to these antigens are useful as markers for the presence of autoimmune thyroid disease. However, the pathogenesis of the thyroid disease probably involves lymphocyte sensitization to these and possibly other thyroidal antigens. Thyroid cells have the capacity to ingest antigen (eg, thyroglobulin) and, when stimulated by cytokines such as gamma interferon, will express cell surface class II molecules (eg, HLA-DR4) to present these antigens to T lymphocytes. Whereas the presence of both the antigen and the class II molecule may be required for autoimmune thyroid disease to develop, other unknown factors also are critical. Active inquiry is under way into whether the process is initiated or promoted either by external antigens that lead to antibody and cellular immune responses through cross-reactivity with thyroid gland antigens or by primary or secondary immunologic imbalances—or by both mechanisms. Clues to the pathogenesis may come from understanding the roles of both genetic and environmental factors now known to be associated with autoimmune thyroid disease.

Genetic factors play a large role in the autoimmune process. HLA typing in patients with Graves' disease reveals a high incidence of HLA-B8 and HLA-DR3 in Caucasians, HLA-Bw46 and HLA-B5 in Chinese, and HLA-B17 in blacks. In Caucasians, atrophic thyroiditis has been associated with HLA-B8 and goitrous Hashimoto's thyroiditis with HLA-DR5. These associations are of limited diagnostic or prognostic value but illustrate the genetic predisposition to autoimmune thyroid disease. It has been suggested that a genetically induced antigen-specific defect in suppressor T lymphocytes may be the basis for autoimmune thyroid disease.

Environmental factors may also play a role in the pathogenesis of autoimmune thyroid disease. Viruses infecting human thyroid cell cultures induce the expression of HLA-DR4 on the follicle cell surface, probably as an effect of a cytokine such as alpha interferon. The increased incidence of autoimmune thyroid disease in postpubertal and premenopausal women, as well as the occurrence of postpartum thyroiditis, implies a role for sex hormones in the pathogenesis of autoimmune thyroid disease. The gram-negative bacillus *Yersinia enterocolitica,* which can cause chronic enterocolitis in humans, has a saturable binding site for mammalian thyrotropin as well as antigens that cross-react with human thyroid antigens. It has been postulated that antibodies against *Y. enterocolitica* could cross-react with the TSH-R on the thyroid cell membrane and trigger an episode of Graves' disease. A high iodine intake may result in more highly iodinated thyroglobulin, which is more immunogenic and would favor the development of autoimmune thyroid disease. Therapeutic doses of lithium, used for the treatment of manic-depressive psychoses, can interfere with suppressor cell function and precipitate autoimmune thyroid disease. Thus, there are a number of environmental and genetic factors that could contribute to the development of this disorder.

■ TESTS OF THYROID FUNCTION

The function of the thyroid gland may be evaluated in many different ways: (1) tests of thyroid hormones in blood, (2) evaluation of the hypothalamic-pituitary-thyroid axis, (3) assessment of iodine metabolism, (4) estimation of gland size, (5) thyroid biopsy, (6) observation of the effects of thyroid hormones on peripheral tissues, and (7) measurement of thyroid autoantibodies.

TESTS OF THYROID HORMONES IN BLOOD

The total serum T_4 and total serum T_3 are measured by radioimmunoassay or immunofluorescent assay. If the concentration of serum thyroid hormone binding proteins is normal, these measurements provide a reasonably reliable index of thyroid gland activity. However, changes in serum concentration of thyroid-binding proteins or the presence of drugs that modify the binding of T_4 or T_3 to TBP (Table 7–1) will modify the total T_4 and T_3 but not the amount of free hormone. Thus, further tests must be performed to assess the *free* hormone level that determines biologic activity (Figure 7–15).

Serum free thyroxine (FT_4) can be estimated using the free thyroxine index (FT_4I). This is the product of the total T_4 multiplied by the percentage of free T_4 as estimated by the amount of T_4 which binds to resin or charcoal added to the system. A more precise estimate of free thyroxine is obtained by a two-step chemiluminescent immunoassay in which the thyroxine antibody system is modified to react with the free hormone. The normal range for FT_4 by this assay is 0.7–1.85 ng/dL (9–24 pmol/L). Although the FT_4I or the FT_4 is valid for normal subjects, these assays may not be valid in subjects with dysproteinemias and abnormal thyroxine-binding proteins (TBPs)—or in subjects taking medications modifying TBP (see Table 7–1)—or in subjects with the euthyroid sick syndrome. In these subjects, free thyroxine by equilibrium dialysis (FT_4D) will more accurately reflect the level of free thyroxine. Note that FT_4 does not measure T_3, so that patients receiving high oral doses of T_3 or with T_3 hyperthyroidism (early Graves' disease or toxic nodular goiter), FT_4 may be low despite the hyperthyroid state (T_3 toxicosis). Antiepileptic drugs such as phenytoin and carbamazepine and the antituberculous drug rifampin increase hepatic metabolism of T_4, resulting in a low total T_4, a low free T_4, and a low FT_4I. However, serum T_3 and serum TSH levels are normal, indicating that patients receiving these drugs are euthyroid. As noted above, T_4 and FT_4I may be low in severe illness, but FT_4D and TSH are usually normal,

which will distinguish these very ill patients from patients who are hypothyroid.

At times, FT_4I and FT_4D will be inappropriately elevated. For example, drugs such as iodinated contrast media, amiodarone, glucocorticoids, and propranolol (Table 7–4) inhibit type 1 5′-deiodinase and the conversion of T_4 to T_3 in peripheral tissues, resulting in elevation of total T_4, FT_4I, and FT_4D and depression of T_3. Hyperthyroidism is ruled out by the low T_3 and normal TSH. FT_4I and FT_4D are inappropriately elevated in the rare syndrome of generalized resistance to thyroid hormone (see below). The presence of heparin in serum, even in the tiny amounts that would be found in a patient with a "heparin lock" indwelling intravenous catheter, will cause a spurious increase in FT_4D. This occurs in the test tube, since heparin activates lipoprotein lipase, releasing free fatty acids that displace T_4 from TBG.

Total T_3 can be measured in serum by immunoassay with specific T_3 antisera. The normal range in adults is 70–132 ng/dL (1.1–2 nmol/L). The measurement of total T_3 is most useful in the differential diagnosis of hyperthyroidism, because T_3 is preferentially secreted in early Graves' disease or toxic nodular goiter. For example, the normal ratio of serum T_3 in ng/dL to T_4 in μg/dL is less than 20 (eg, T_3 120 ng/dL, T_4 8 μg/dL: ratio = 15). In hyperthyroidism, this ratio will usually be well over 20, and it will be even higher in T_3 thyrotoxicosis. T_3 levels are often maintained in the normal range in hypothyroidism because TSH stimulation increases the relative secretion of T_3; thus, serum T_3 is not a good test for hypothyroidism.

T_3 is bound to TBG, and the total T_3 concentration in serum will vary with the level of TBG (Table 7–1). Serum free T_3 (FT_3) can be measured by immunoassay or more precisely by equilibrium dialysis; the normal adult FT_3 is 230–420 pg/dL (3.5–6.5 pmol/L).

Reverse T_3 (rT_3) can be measured by radioimmunoassay. The serum concentration of rT_3 in adults is about one-third of the total T_3 concentration, with a range of 25–75 ng/dL (0.39–1.15 nmol/L). RT_3 can be used to differentiate chronic illness from hypothyroidism because rT_3 levels are elevated in chronic illness and low in hypothyroidism. However, this differential diagnosis can be made by determination of TSH (see below), so that it is rarely necessary to measure rT_3.

Thyroglobulin (Tg) can be measured in serum by double antibody radioimmunoassay. The normal range will vary with method and laboratory, but generally the normal range is less than 40 ng/mL (< 40 μg/L) in the euthyroid individual and less than 2 ng/mL (< 2 μg/L) in a totally thyroidectomized individual. The major problem with the test is that endogenous thyroglobulin antibodies interfere with the assay procedure and, depending on the method, may result in spuriously low or spuriously high values. Serum thyroglobulin is elevated in situations of thyroid overactivity such as Graves' disease and toxic multinodular goiter; in subacute or chronic thyroiditis, where it is released as a consequence of tissue damage; and in patients with large goiters, in whom the thyroglobulin level is proportionate to the size of the gland. Serum thyroglobulin determinations have been most useful in the management of patients with papillary or follicular thyroid carcinoma. Following thyroidectomy and ^{131}I therapy, thyroglobulin levels should be very low. In such a patient, serum thyroglobulin greater than 2 ng/dL (> 2 μg/L) indicates the presence of metastatic disease, and a rise in serum thyroglobulin in a patient with known metastases indicates progression of the disease.

EVALUATION OF THE HYPOTHALAMIC-PITUITARY-THYROID AXIS

The hypothalamic-pituitary-thyroid axis is illustrated in Figure 7–20. It has not been clinically feasible to measure TRH in the peripheral circulation in humans. However, very sensitive methods for the measurement of TSH have been developed using monoclonal antibodies against human TSH. The general principle is this: One monoclonal TSH antibody is fixed to a solid matrix to bind serum TSH, and a second monoclonal TSH antibody labeled with isotope or enzyme or fluorescent tag will bind to a separate epitope on the TSH molecule. The quantity of TSH in the serum is thus proportional to the quantity of bound second antibody. The earlier TSH radioimmunoassays, which could detect about 1 μU of TSH/mL, were adequate for the diagnosis of elevated TSH in hypothyroidism but could not detect suppressed TSH levels in hyperthyroidism. The "second generation" of "sensitive" TSH assays, using monoclonal antibodies, can detect about 0.1 μU/mL, and the "third generation" of "supersensitive" assays are sufficiently sensitive to detect about 0.01 μU/mL. This has allowed measurement of TSH well below the normal range of 0.5–5 μU/mL (0.5–5 mU/L) and has enabled the clinician to detect partially and totally suppressed serum TSH levels. The level of FT_4 is inversely related to the logarithm of the TSH concentration (Figure 7–28A). Thus, a small change in FT_4 may result in a large change in TSH. The relationship between TSH and FT_4 in various situations is demonstrated in Figure 7–28A and 7–28B. Serum TSH below 0.1 μU/mL (0.1 mU/L) and an elevated FT_4 or FT_4I is indicative of hyperthyroidism. This may be due to Graves' disease, toxic nodular goiter, or high-dose thyroxine therapy. In the rare case of hyperthyroidism due to a TSH-secreting pituitary tumor, FT_4I or FT_4 will be elevated and TSH will not be suppressed but will actually be normal or slightly elevated. An elevated TSH (> 10 μU/mL; 10 mU/L) and a low FT_4 or FT_4I is diagnostic of hypothyroidism. In patients with hypothyroidism due to a pituitary or hypothalamic tumor (central hypothyroidism), FT_4I or FT_4 will be low and TSH will not be elevated. This diagnosis can be confirmed by demonstrating the failure of serum TSH to increase following an injection of TRH. The TRH test is performed as follows: 200 μg of TRH is administered intravenously. Serum TSH is determined prior to the injection and at 30 and 60 minutes afterward. The absence of a rise in TSH indicates either pituitary insufficiency or suppression. A modest or delayed rise may be seen in patients with hypothalamic disease and hypothyroidism. The test can also be used to differentiate the hyperthyroxinemia of the T_3 resistance syndrome from thyrotoxicosis due to a TSH-secreting pituitary tumor. TRH will produce a rise in TSH in the patient with a thyroid hormone resistance syndrome, whereas TSH-secreting tumors will not respond to TRH. Note that corticosteroids and dopamine inhibit TSH secretion (Table 7–6), which will modify the interpretation of serum TSH levels in patients taking these drugs.

Serum TSH levels reflect the anterior pituitary gland sensing the level of circulating FT_4. High FT_4 levels suppress TSH and low FT_4 levels increase TSH release. Thus, the ultrasensitive measurement of TSH has become the most sensitive, most convenient, and most specific test for the diagnosis of both hyperthyroidism and hypothyroidism. Indeed, a suppressed TSH correlates so well with impaired pituitary response to TRH that the simple measurement of serum TSH has replaced the TRH test in the diagnosis of hyperthyroidism.

IODINE METABOLISM & BIOSYNTHETIC ACTIVITY

Radioactive iodine allows assessment of the turnover of iodine by the thyroid gland in vivo. Iodine-123 is the ideal isotope for this purpose: It has a half-life of 13.3 hours and releases a 28-keV x-ray and a 159-keV gamma photon but no beta emissions. Thus, it is easily measured and causes little tissue damage. It is usually administered orally in a dose of 100–200 μCi, and radioactivity over the thyroid area is measured with a scintillation counter at 4 or 6 hours and again at 24 hours (Figure 7–8). The normal **radioactive iodine uptake** (RAIU) will vary with the iodide intake. In areas of low iodide intake and endemic goiter, the 24-hour RAIU may be as high as 60–90%. In the USA—a country with a relatively high iodide intake—the normal uptake at 6 hours is 5–15% and at 24 hours 8–30%. In thyrotoxicosis due to Graves' disease or toxic nodular goiter, the 24-hour RAIU is markedly el-

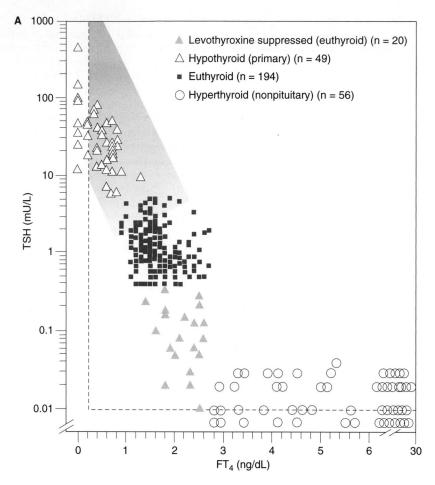

Figure 7–28. A: Relationship between serum free thyroxine by dialysis (FT$_4$) ng/dL and log$_{10}$ TSH in euthyroid, hyperthyroid, hypothyroid, and L-T$_4$-suppressed euthyroid individuals. Note that for each unit change in T$_4$ there is a logarithmic change in TSH.

evated, though if the iodide turnover is very rapid, the 5-hour uptake may be even higher than the 24-hour uptake (Figure 7–8). Thyrotoxicosis with a very low thyroidal RAIU occurs in the following situations: (1) in subacute thyroiditis; (2) during the active phase of Hashimoto's thyroiditis, with release of preformed hormone, causing "spontaneously resolving thyrotoxicosis"; (3) in thyrotoxicosis factitia due to oral ingestion of a large amount of thyroid hormone; (4) as a result of excess iodide intake (eg, amiodarone therapy), inducing thyrotoxicosis in a patient with latent Graves' disease or multinodular goiter, the low uptake being due to the huge iodide pool; (5) in struma ovarii; and (6) in ec-

topic functioning metastatic thyroid carcinoma after total thyroidectomy.

In normal individuals, administration of 75–100 µg of T$_3$ in divided doses daily for 5 days will reduce the 24-hour RAIU by more than 50% (suppression test). Failure of the thyroid to suppress on this treatment indicates autonomous thyroid function, as in Graves' disease, or autonomously functioning thyroid nodules.

The efficiency of the thyroid organification process may be tested with the "perchlorate discharge test." As noted above, KClO$_4$ will displace I$^-$ from the iodide trap. Thus, oral administration of 0.5 g KClO$_4$ to a normal individual will block further uptake of ^{123}I, but not more

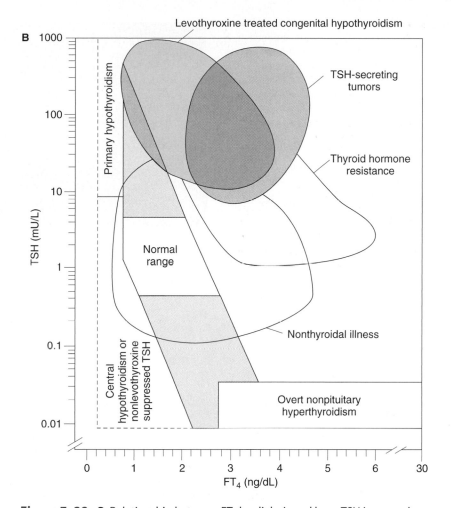

Figure 7–28. B: Relationship between FT$_4$ by dialysis and log$_{10}$ TSH in normal subjects and subjects with various illnesses including primary hypothyroidism, central hypothyroidism and non-levothyroxine-suppressed TSH, levothyroxine-treated congenital hypothyroidism, TSH-secreting tumors, thyroid hormone resistance, nonthyroidal illness, and nonpituitary hyperthyroidism. (Reproduced, with permission, from Kaptein EM: Clinical applications of free thyroxine determinations. Clin Lab Med 1993;13:654.)

than 5% of the previously accumulated radioiodine will be released. Conversely, if there is an organification defect, not only is further uptake blocked but I⁻ diffuses out of the gland or is "discharged." Positive tests are seen in some patients with congenital iodide organification defects, Hashimoto's thyroiditis, Graves' disease after ^{131}I therapy, or patients receiving inhibitors of iodide organification such as methimazole or propylthiouracil. The perchlorate discharge test is rarely used clinically, but it can be very helpful in understanding the pathophysiology of some of the above illnesses (see Figure 7–11).

THYROID IMAGING

1. Radionuclide Imaging

[123]I and technetium Tc 99m pertechnetate (^{99m}Tc as TcO$_4$) are useful for determining the *functional* activity

of the thyroid gland. ^{123}I is administered orally in a dose of 200–300 µCi, and a scan of the thyroid is obtained at 8–24 hours. ^{99m}TcO$_4$ is administered intravenously in a dose of 1–10 mCi, and the scan is obtained at 30–60 minutes. Images can be obtained with either a rectilinear scanner or a gamma camera. The rectilinear scanner moves back and forth over the area of interest; it produces a life-size picture, and special areas, such as nodules, can be marked directly on the scan (Figure 7–29). The gamma camera has a pinhole collimator, and the scan is obtained on a fluorescent screen and recorded on Polaroid film or a computer monitor. The camera has greater resolution, but special areas must be identified with a radioactive marker for clinical correlation (Figure 7–30). Radionuclide scans provide information about both the size and shape of the thyroid gland and the geographic distribution of functional activity in the gland. Functioning thyroid nodules are called "hot" nodules, and nonfunctioning ones are called "cold" nodules. The incidence of malignancy in hot nodules is about 1%, but they may become toxic, producing enough hormone to suppress the rest of the gland and induce thyrotoxicosis. About 16% of surgically removed cold nodules are malignant. Occasionally, a nodule will be hot with ^{99m}TcO$_4$ and cold with ^{123}I, and a few of these nodules have been malignant. For large substernal goiters or for distant metastases from a thyroid cancer, ^{131}I is the preferred isotope because of its long half-life (8 days) and its 0.72 MeV gamma emission.

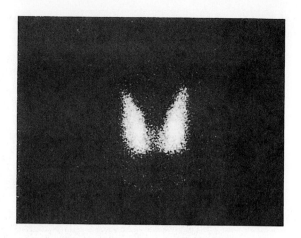

Figure 7–30. Scintiphoto (pinhole collimator) thyroid scan performed 6 hours after the ingestion of 100 µCi of sodium ^{123}1. (Courtesy of RR Cavalieri.)

2. Fluorescent Scanning

The iodine content can be determined and an image of the thyroid gland can be obtained by fluorescent scanning without administration of a radioisotope. An external source of americium-241 is beamed at the thyroid gland, and the resulting emission of 28.5 keV x-ray from iodide ions is recorded, producing an image of the thyroid gland similar to that obtained with ^{123}I (Figure 7–29). The advantage of this procedure is that the patient receives no radioisotope and the gland can be imaged even when it is loaded with iodine—as, for example, after intravenous contrast media. The disadvantage of this study is that it requires specialized equipment that may not be generally available.

THYROID ULTRASONOGRAPHY OR MAGNETIC RESONANCE IMAGING

A rough estimate of thyroid size and nodularity can be obtained from radionuclide scanning, but much better detail can be obtained by thyroid ultrasonography or MRI.

Thyroid ultrasonography is particularly useful for measuring the size of the gland or individual nodules and for evaluating the results of therapy (Figure 7–31). It is useful also for differentiating solid from cystic lesions and to guide the operator to a deep nodule during fine-needle thyroid aspiration biopsy (see below). Thy-

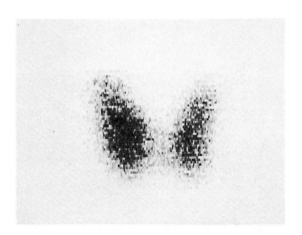

Figure 7–29. Rectilinear sodium ^{123}I scan performed 6 hours after the ingestion of 100 µCi of sodium ^{123}I. (Courtesy of RR Cavalieri.)

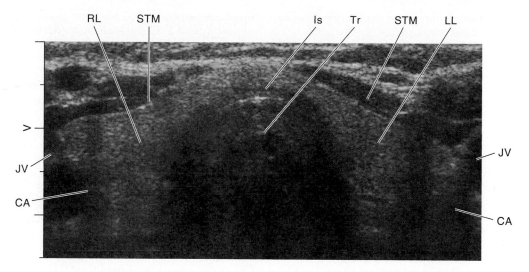

Figure 7–31. Ultrasound of the normal thyroid gland. Tr, trachea; LL, left lobe of thyroid; RL, right lobe of thyroid; Is, isthmus; CA, carotid artery; JV, jugular vein; STM, sternothyroid muscle. (Courtesy of RA Filly.)

roid ultrasonography is limited to thyroid tissue in the neck, ie, it cannot be used for substernal lesions.

MRI provides an excellent image of the thyroid gland, including posterior or substernal extension of a goiter or malignancy. Both transverse and coronal images of the gland can be obtained, and lymph nodes as small as 1 cm can be visualized. MRI is invaluable for the demonstration of tracheal compression from a large goiter, tracheal invasion or local extension of a thyroid malignancy, or metastases to local or mediastinal lymph nodes.

THYROID BIOPSY

Fine-needle aspiration biopsy of a thyroid nodule has proved to be the best method for differentiation of benign from malignant thyroid disease. It is performed as an outpatient procedure and requires no preparation. The skin over the nodule is cleansed with alcohol, and, if desired, a small amount of 1% lidocaine can be injected intracutaneously for local anesthesia. A No. 25 one and one-half-inch needle is then inserted into the nodule and moved in and out until a small amount of bloody material is seen in the hub of the needle; the needle is then removed, and with a syringe the contents of the needle are expressed onto a clean slide. A second clean slide is placed on top of the first slide, and a thin smear is obtained by drawing the slides apart quickly. Alternatively, a 10 mL or 20 mL syringe in an appro-

priate syringe holder can be used with a No. 23 one-inch needle to sample the nodule or to evacuate cystic contents.

The slides are fixed—either dry and stained with Wright's or Giemsa's stain, or fixed in alcohol and stained with Papanicolaou stain. The sensitivity (true-positive results divided by total cases of disease) is about 95%, and the specificity (true-negative results divided by total cases of no disease) is also about 95%. For best results, fine-needle aspiration biopsy requires an adequate tissue sample and a specially trained cytologist to interpret it.

EFFECTS OF THYROID HORMONES ON PERIPHERAL TISSUES

The definitive test of thyroid function would be a test of the effect of thyroid hormones on body tissues. Thyroid hormones increase heat production and oxygen consumption. A measurement of this basal oxygen in the intact organism became one of the first tests of thyroid function, the **basal metabolic rate** (BMR). However, this test is nonspecific and insensitive and is rarely used today. The speed of muscle contraction and relaxation is increased in hyperthyroidism and decreased in hypothyroidism. The contraction and relaxation time of the Achilles tendon has been standardized and measured by an instrument called the **photomotogram.** However, there is considerable overlap between normal subjects and patients with thyroid dysfunction, limiting the usefulness of this procedure.

Cardiac muscle contractility can also be measured as an index of thyroid hormone action. With echocardiography, it is relatively easy to measure such indices as the preejection period (PEP), the time from onset of the QRS complex to the opening of the aortic valve; or the left ventricular ejection time (LVET). These are prolonged in hypothyroidism and shortened in hyperthyroidism. Although these measurements are modified by coexistent cardiac disease, they may be the best objective tests for measuring the peripheral effects of thyroid hormone action.

Thyroid hormones influence the concentration of a number of enzymes and blood constituents. For example, serum cholesterol is usually lowered in hyperthyroidism and elevated in hypothyroidism. Serum creatine kinase and lactic dehydrogenase, probably of skeletal muscle origin, are elevated in hypothyroidism—and indeed, isoenzyme determination may be required to differentiate the enzyme changes occurring in myocardial infarction from those occurring in myxedema.

Sex hormone-binding globulin (SHBG) and angiotensin-converting enzyme are also increased in hyperthyroidism and decreased in hypothyroidism. However, none of these biochemical or enzyme changes are sensitive or specific enough for diagnostic use.

MEASUREMENT OF THYROID AUTOANTIBODIES

Thyroid autoantibodies include (1) thyroglobulin antibody (Tg Ab); (2) thyroperoxidase antibody (TPO Ab), formerly called microsomal antibody; and (3) TSH receptor antibody, either stimulating (TSH-R Ab [stim]) or blocking (TSH-R Ab [block]). Tg Ab and TPO Ab have been measured by hemagglutination, enzyme-linked immunosorbent assay (ELISA), or radioimmunoassay (RIA). The hemagglutination technique is much less sensitive than the ELISA or RIA methods. For example, in the Whickham study of a normal population in northeastern England, TPO antibodies were found in about 8% of young women (aged 18–24) and 13.7% of older women (aged 45–54). In a similar study of normal blood donors and using radioimmunoassay, TPO antibodies were found in 10.6% of younger and in 30.3% of older women. The incidence of positive TPO antibodies in normal men (by hemagglutination) was low—about 2%—and did not increase with age. On the other hand, high Tg Ab and TPO Ab titers by RIA are found in 97% of patients with Graves' disease or Hashimoto's thyroiditis. Thyroglobulin antibodies are often high early in the course of Hashimoto's thyroiditis and decrease with time; TPO antibodies are

usually measurable for the life of the patient. The titers of both Tg and TPO antibodies will decrease with time following institution of T_4 therapy in Hashimoto's thyroiditis or with antithyroid therapy in Graves' disease. A strongly positive test for either of these antibodies is an indication of the presence of autoimmune thyroid disease but is not specific for the type of disease, ie, hyperthyroidism, hypothyroidism, or goiter.

The thyroid receptor stimulating antibody (TSH-R Ab [stim]) is characteristic of Graves' disease (see above). It was originally measured by demonstrating prolonged discharge of radioiodine from the thyroid gland of the mouse after injection of serum from a patient with Graves' disease; it was then called long-acting thyroid stimulator (LATS). This laborious assay has been replaced by a bioassay using human thyroid cells in culture or culture of hamster ovary cells into which the human TSH receptor gene has been introduced. Then, the increase in thyroid cAMP is measured following incubation with serum or IgG. The test is positive in 80–90% of patients with Graves' disease and undetectable in healthy subjects or patients with Hashimoto's thyroiditis (without ophthalmopathy), nontoxic goiter, or toxic nodular goiter. It is most useful for the diagnosis of Graves' disease in patients with euthyroid ophthalmopathy or in predicting neonatal Graves' disease in the newborn of a mother with active or past Graves' disease.

The same type of assay can be used to detect TSH receptor-blocking antibody (TSH-R Ab [block]). In this assay, the increase in cAMP induced by TSH added to a human thyroid cell culture or the culture of hamster ovary cells containing the *TSH-R* gene is blocked by concurrent incubation with the patient's serum. The TSH-binding inhibition assay (TBII) measures the ability of serum IgG to inhibit the binding of labeled TSH to a thyroid cell membrane preparation containing the TSH receptor. This technique is not as satisfactory as the bioassay because there are a variety of nonspecific interfering substances, such as thyroglobulin, which inhibit TSH binding. However, a modification of the TSH-binding inhibition assay using recombinant human TSH receptor has proved to be more reliable. Detection of a TSH receptor-blocking antibody in maternal serum may be very helpful in predicting the occurrence of congenital hypothyroidism in newborns of mothers with autoimmune thyroid disease.

SUMMARY: CLINICAL USE OF THYROID FUNCTION TESTS

The diagnosis of thyroid disease has been greatly simplified by the development of sensitive assays for TSH and free thyroxine. The estimate of free thyroxine, either FT_4I or FT_4, and a sensitive TSH determination are used both for the diagnosis of thyroid disease and for following patients receiving T_4 replacement or antithyroid drug therapy. An elevated TSH and low free thyroxine establish the diagnosis of hypothyroidism, and a suppressed TSH and elevated FT_4 establish the diagnosis of hyperthyroidism.

Other tests are available for special uses. In hypothyroidism, Tg Ab or TPO Ab tests will clarify the cause of the illness, and in hyperthyroidism elevation of free T_3, abnormal radioiodine uptake and scan, and a positive test for TSH-R Ab [stim] may be useful. In patients with nodules or goiter, fine-needle aspiration biopsy will rule out malignancy; radioiodine scan may help to determine function; and thyroid ultrasound or MRI may be helpful in following the size or growth of the goiter. Patients with known thyroid cancer are followed with serial thyroglobulin determinations, and ^{131}I scan or MRI may be useful for detection of metastatic disease.

■ DISORDERS OF THE THYROID

Patients with thyroid disease will usually complain of (1) thyroid enlargement, which may be diffuse or nodular; (2) symptoms of thyroid deficiency, or hypothyroidism; (3) symptoms of thyroid hormone excess, or hyperthyroidism; or (4) complications of a specific form of hyperthyroidism—Graves' disease—which may present with striking prominence of the eyes (exophthalmos) and, rarely, thickening of the skin over the lower legs (thyroid dermopathy).

History

The history should include evaluation of symptoms related to the above complaints, discussed in more detail below. Exposure to ionizing radiation in childhood has been associated with an increased incidence of thyroid disease, including cancer. Iodide ingestion in the form of kelp or iodide-containing cough preparations or intravenous iodide-containing contrast media used in angiography or CT scanning may induce goiter, hypothyroidism, or hyperthyroidism. Lithium carbonate, used in the treatment of manic-depressive psychiatric disorder, can also induce hypothyroidism and goiter or hyperthyroidism. Residence in an area of low dietary iodide is associated with iodine deficiency goiter ("endemic goiter"). Although dietary iodide is generally adequate in developed countries, there are still areas low in natural iodine (ie, developing countries in Africa, Asia, South America, and inland mountainous areas).

Finally, the family history should be explored with particular reference to goiter, hyperthyroidism, hypothyroidism, or thyroid cancer as well as immunologic disorders such as diabetes, rheumatoid disease, pernicious anemia, alopecia, vitiligo, or myasthenia gravis, which may be associated with an increased incidence of autoimmune thyroid disease. Multiple endocrine neoplasia type 2A (Sipple's syndrome) with medullary carcinoma of the thyroid gland is an autosomal dominant condition.

Physical Examination

Physical examination of the thyroid gland is illustrated in Figure 7–32. The thyroid is firmly attached to the anterior trachea midway between the sternal notch and the thyroid cartilage; it is often easy to see and to palpate. The patient should have a glass of water for comfortable swallowing. There are three maneuvers: (1) With a good light coming from behind the examiner, the patient is instructed to swallow a sip of water. Observe the gland as it moves up and down. Enlargement and nodularity can often be noted. (2) Palpate the gland anteriorly. Gently press down with one thumb on one side of the gland to rotate the other lobe forward, and palpate as the patient swallows. (3) Palpate the gland from behind the patient with the middle three fingers on each lobe while the patient swallows. An outline of the gland can be traced on the skin of the neck and measured (Figure 7–32D). Nodules can be measured in a similar way. Thus, changes in the size of the gland or in nodules can easily be followed.

On physical examination, the palpable bulbous portion of each lobe of the normal thyroid gland measures about 2 cm in vertical dimension and about 1 cm in horizontal dimension above the isthmus. An enlarged thyroid gland is called **goiter.** Generalized enlargement is termed diffuse goiter; irregular or lumpy enlargement is called nodular goiter.

HYPOTHYROIDISM

Hypothyroidism is a clinical syndrome resulting from a deficiency of thyroid hormones, which in turn results in a generalized slowing down of metabolic processes. Hypothyroidism in infants and children results in marked slowing of growth and development, with serious permanent consequences including mental retardation. Hypothyroidism with onset in adulthood causes a generalized slowing down of the organism, with deposition of glycosaminoglycans in intracellular spaces, particularly in skin and muscle, producing the clinical picture of **myxedema.** The symptoms of hypothyroidism in adults are largely reversible with therapy.

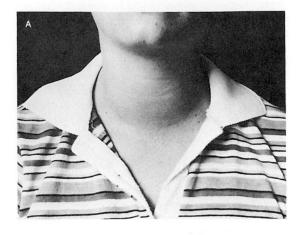

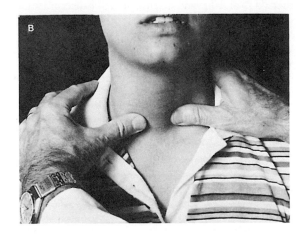

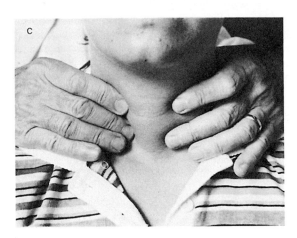

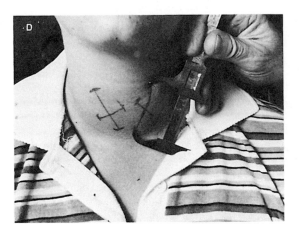

Figure 7–32. Examination of the thyroid gland. **A:** Observe the neck, especially as the patient swallows. **B:** Examine from the front, rotating the gland slightly with one thumb while palpating the other lobe with the other thumb. **C:** Examine from behind, using three fingers and the same technique. **D:** The size of each lobe or of thyroid nodules can be measured by first drawing an outline on the skin.

Etiology & Incidence (Table 7–7)

Hypothyroidism may be classified as (1) primary (thyroid failure), (2) secondary (to pituitary TSH deficit), or (3) tertiary (due to hypothalamic deficiency of TRH)—or may be due to (4) peripheral resistance to the action of thyroid hormones. Hypothyroidism can also be classified as goitrous or nongoitrous, but this classification is probably unsatisfactory, since Hashimoto's thyroiditis (autoimmune thyroiditis) may produce hypothyroidism with or without goiter.

The incidence of various causes of hypothyroidism will vary depending on geographic and environmental factors such as dietary iodide and goitrogen intake, the genetic characteristics of the population, and the age distribution of the population (pediatric or adult). The causes of hypothyroidism, listed in approximate order of frequency in the USA, are presented in Table 7–7. Hashimoto's thyroiditis is probably the most common cause of hypothyroidism. In younger patients, it is more likely to be associated with goiter; in older patients, the gland may be totally destroyed by the immunologic process, and the only trace of the disease

Table 7–7. Etiology of hypothyroidism.

Primary:
1. Hashimoto's thyroiditis:
   a. With goiter.
   b. "Idiopathic" thyroid atrophy, presumably end-stage autoimmune thyroid disease, following either Hashimoto's thyroiditis or Graves' disease.
   c. Neonatal hypothyroidism due to placental transmission of TSH-R blocking antibodies.
2. Radioactive iodine therapy for Graves' disease.
3. Subtotal thyroidectomy for Graves' disease or nodular goiter.
4. Excessive iodide intake (kelp, radiocontrast dyes).
5. Subacute thyroiditis.
6. Rare causes in the USA:
   a. Iodide deficiency.
   b. Other goitrogens such as lithium; antithyroid drug therapy.
   c. Inborn errors of thyroid hormone synthesis.

Secondary: Hypopituitarism due to pituitary adenoma, pituitary ablative therapy, or pituitary destruction.

Tertiary: Hypothalamic dysfunction (rare).

Peripheral resistance to the action of thyroid hormone.

will be a persistently positive test for TPO (thyroperoxidase) autoantibodies. Similarly, the end stage of Graves' disease may be hypothyroidism. This is accelerated by destructive therapy such as administration of radioactive iodine or subtotal thyroidectomy. Thyroid glands involved in autoimmune disease are particularly susceptible to excessive iodide intake (eg, ingestion of kelp tablets, iodide-containing cough preparations, or the antiarrhythmic drug amiodarone) or intravenous administration of iodide-containing radiographic contrast media. The large amounts of iodide block thyroid hormone synthesis, producing hypothyroidism with goiter in the patient with an abnormal thyroid gland; the normal gland usually "escapes" from the iodide block (see above). Although the process may be temporarily reversed by withdrawal of iodide, the underlying disease will often progress, and permanent hypothyroidism will usually supervene. Hypothyroidism may occur during the late phase of subacute thyroiditis; this is usually transient, but it is permanent in about 10% of patients. Iodide deficiency is rarely a cause of hypothyroidism in the USA but may be more common in developing countries. Certain drugs can block hormone synthesis and produce hypothyroidism with goiter; at present, the most common pharmacologic causes of hypothyroidism (other than iodide) are lithium carbonate, used for the treatment of manic-depressive states, and amiodarone. Chronic therapy with the antithyroid drugs propylthiouracil and methimazole will do the same. Inborn errors of thyroid hormone synthesis result in severe hypothyroidism if the block in hormone synthesis is complete, or mild hypothyroidism if the block is partial. Pituitary and hypothalamic deficiencies as causes of hypothyroidism are quite rare and are usually associated with other symptoms and signs of pituitary insufficiency (Chapter 5). Peripheral resistance to thyroid hormones is discussed below.

Pathogenesis

Thyroid hormone deficiency affects every tissue in the body, so that the symptoms are multiple. Pathologically, the most characteristic finding is the accumulation of glycosaminoglycans—mostly hyaluronic acid—in interstitial tissues. Accumulation of this hydrophilic substance and increased capillary permeability to albumin account for the interstitial edema that is particularly evident in the skin, heart muscle, and striated muscle. The accumulation is due not to excessive synthesis but to decreased destruction of glycosaminoglycans.

Clinical Presentations & Findings

A. NEWBORN INFANTS (CRETINISM)

The term cretinism was originally applied to infants—in areas of low iodide intake and endemic goiter—with mental retardation, short stature, a characteristic puffy appearance of the face and hands, and (frequently) deaf mutism and neurologic signs of pyramidal and extrapyramidal tract abnormalities (Figure 7–33). In the USA, neonatal screening programs have revealed that in the white population the incidence of neonatal hypothyroidism is 1:5000, while in the black population the incidence is only 1:32,000. Neonatal hypothyroidism may result from failure of the thyroid to descend during embryonic development from its origin at the base of the tongue to its usual site in the lower anterior neck, which results in an "ectopic thyroid" gland that functions poorly. Placental transfer to the embryo of TSH-R Ab [block] from a mother with Hashimoto's thyroiditis may result in agenesis of the thyroid gland and "athyreotic cretinism." Inherited defects in thyroid hormone biosynthesis induce neonatal hypothyroidism and goiter. Rare causes of neonatal hypothyroidism include administration during pregnancy of iodides, antithyroid drugs, or radioactive iodine for thyrotoxicosis.

The symptoms of hypothyroidism in newborns include respiratory difficulty, cyanosis, jaundice, poor feeding, hoarse cry, umbilical hernia, and marked retar-

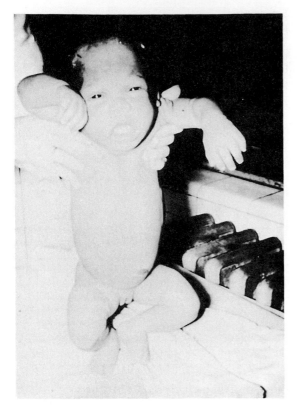

Figure 7–33. A 9-month-old infant with hypothyroidism (cretinism). Note the puffy face, protuberant abdomen, umbilical hernia, and muscle weakness (infant cannot sit up unassisted).

dation of bone maturation. The proximal tibial epiphysis and distal femoral epiphysis are present in almost all full-term infants with a body weight over 2500 g. Absence of these epiphyses strongly suggests hypothyroidism. The introduction of routine screening of newborns for TSH or T_4 has been a major achievement in the early diagnosis of neonatal hypothyroidism. A drop of blood obtained by heel stick 24–48 hours after birth is placed on filter paper and sent to a central laboratory. A serum T_4 under 6 μg/dL or a serum TSH over 25 μU/mL is suggestive of neonatal hypothyroidism. The diagnosis can then be confirmed by radiologic evidence of retarded bone age. Note that euthyroid infants born to hypothyroid mothers inadequately treated during pregnancy may have symptoms of mild mental retardation later in life—emphasizing the importance of maintaining the mother in a euthyroid state throughout pregnancy.

B. CHILDREN

Hypothyroidism in children is characterized by retarded growth and evidence of mental retardation. In the adolescent, precocious puberty may occur, and there may be enlargement of the sella turcica in addition to short stature. This is not due to pituitary tumor but probably to pituitary hypertrophy associated with excessive TSH production.

C. ADULTS

In adults, the common features of hypothyroidism include easy fatigability, coldness, weight gain, constipation, menstrual irregularities, and muscle cramps. Physical findings include a cool, rough, dry skin, puffy face and hands, a hoarse, husky voice, and slow reflexes (Figure 7–34). Reduced conversion of carotene to vitamin A and increased blood levels of carotene may give the skin a yellowish color.

1. Cardiovascular signs—Hypothyroidism is manifested by impaired muscular contraction, bradycardia, and diminished cardiac output. The ECG reveals low voltage of QRS complexes and P and T waves, with improvement in response to therapy. Cardiac enlargement may occur, due in part to interstitial edema, nonspecific myofibrillary swelling, and left ventricular dilation but often due to pericardial effusion (Figure 7–35). The degree of pericardial effusion can easily be determined by echocardiography. Although cardiac output is reduced, congestive heart failure and pulmonary edema are rarely noted. There is controversy about whether myxedema induces coronary artery disease, but coronary artery disease is more common in patients with hypothyroidism, particularly in older patients. In patients with angina pectoris, hypothyroidism may protect the heart from ischemic stress, and replacement therapy may aggravate the angina.

2. Pulmonary function—In the adult, hypothyroidism is characterized by shallow, slow respirations and impaired ventilatory responses to hypercapnia or hypoxia. Respiratory failure is a major problem in patients with myxedema coma.

3. Intestinal peristalsis—Peristalsis is markedly slowed, resulting in chronic constipation and occasionally severe fecal impaction or ileus.

4. Renal function—Renal function is impaired, with decreased glomerular filtration rate and impaired ability to excrete a water load. This predisposes the myxedematous patient to water intoxication if excessive free water is administered.

5. Anemia—There are at least four mechanisms that may contribute to **anemia** in patients with hypothyroidism: (1) impaired hemoglobin synthesis as a result of

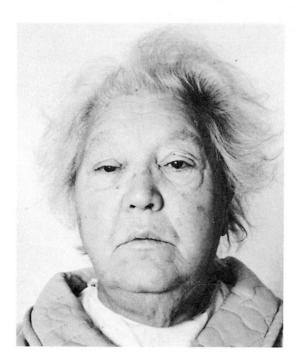

Figure 7–34. Hypothyroidism in adult (myxedema). Note puffy face, puffy eyes, frowsy hair, and dull and apathetic appearance.

thyroxine deficiency; (2) iron deficiency from increased iron loss with menorrhagia, as well as impaired intestinal absorption of iron; (3) folate deficiency from impaired intestinal absorption of folic acid; and (4) pernicious anemia, with vitamin B_{12}-deficient megaloblastic anemia. The pernicious anemia is often part of a spectrum of autoimmune diseases, including myxedema due to chronic thyroiditis associated with thyroid autoantibodies, pernicious anemia associated with parietal cell autoantibodies, diabetes mellitus associated with islet cell autoantibodies, and adrenal insufficiency associated with adrenal autoantibodies (Schmidt's syndrome; see Chapter 4).

6. Neuromuscular system—Many patients complain of symptoms referable to the neuromuscular system, eg, severe muscle cramps, paresthesias, and muscle weakness.

7. Central nervous system symptoms—Symptoms may include chronic fatigue, lethargy, and inability to concentrate. Hypothyroidism impairs the conversion of estrogen precursors to estrogens, resulting in altered FSH and LH secretion and in anovulatory cycles and infertility. This may also be associated with severe menorrhagia. Patients with myxedema are usually quite placid but can be severely depressed or even extremely agitated ("myxedema madness").

Diagnosis

The combination of a low serum FT_4 or FT_4I and an elevated serum TSH is diagnostic of primary hypothyroidism (Figure 7–36). Serum T_3 levels are variable and may be within the normal range. A positive test for thyroid autoantibodies suggests underlying Hashimoto's thyroiditis. In patients with pituitary myxedema, the FT_4I or FT_4 will be low but serum TSH will not be elevated. It may then be necessary to differentiate pituitary from hypothalamic disease, and for this the TRH test is most helpful (see above). Absence of TSH response to TRH indicates pituitary deficiency. A partial or "normal" type response indicates that pituitary function is intact but that a defect exists in hypothalamic secretion of TRH. The patient may be taking thyroid medication (levothyroxine or desiccated thyroid tablets) when first seen. A palpable or enlarged thyroid gland and a positive test for thyroid autoantibodies would suggest underlying Hashimoto's thyroiditis, in which case the medication should be continued. If antibodies are absent, the medication should be withdrawn for 6 weeks and determinations made for FT_4I or FT_4 and for TSH. The 6-week period of withdrawal is necessary because of the long half-life of thyroxine (7 days) and to allow the pituitary gland to recover after a long period of suppression. The pattern of recovery of thyroid function after withdrawal of T_4 is noted in Figure 7–37. In hypothyroid individuals, TSH becomes markedly elevated at 5–6 weeks and T_4 remains subnormal, whereas both are normal after 6 weeks in euthyroid controls.

The clinical picture of fully developed myxedema is usually quite clear, but the symptoms and signs of mild hypothyroidism may be very subtle. Patients with hypothyroidism will at times present with unusual features: neurasthenia with symptoms of muscle cramps, paresthesias, and weakness; refractory anemia; disturbances in reproductive function, including infertility, delayed puberty, or menorrhagia; idiopathic edema or pleuropericardial effusions; retarded growth; obstipation; chronic rhinitis or hoarseness due to edema of nasal mucosa or vocal cords; and severe depression progressing to emotional instability or even frank paranoid psychosis. In the elderly, hypothyroidism may present with apathy and withdrawal, often attributed to senility (Chapter 23). In such cases, the diagnostic studies outlined above will confirm or rule out hypothyroidism as a contributing factor.

Complications

A. MYXEDEMA COMA

Myxedema coma is the end stage of untreated hypothyroidism. (See Chapter 24.) It is characterized by progressive weakness, stupor, hypothermia, hypoventila-

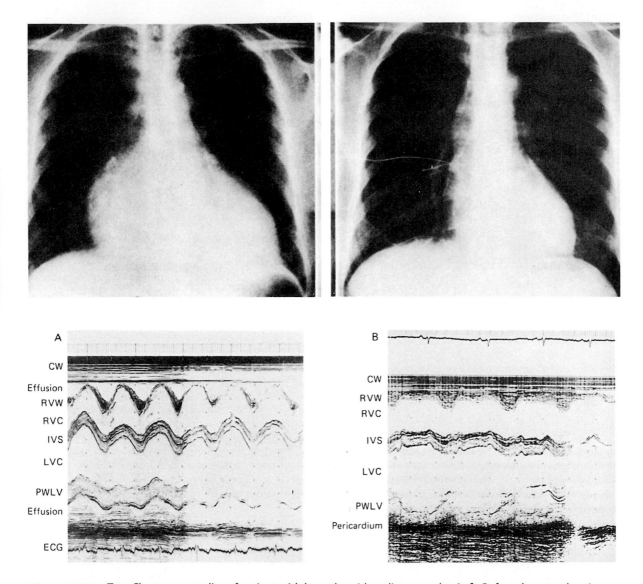

Figure 7–35. ***Top:*** Chest x-ray studies of patient with hypothyroid cardiomyopathy. ***Left:*** Before therapy, showing pronounced cardiomegaly. ***Right:*** Six months after institution of thyroxine therapy, the heart size has returned to normal. (Reproduced, with permission, from Reza MJ, Abbasi AS: Congestive cardiomyopathy in hypothyroidism. West J Med 1975;123:228.) ***Bottom:*** Echocardiogram of a 29-year-old woman with hypothyroidism ***(A)*** before and ***(B)*** after 2 months of therapy with levothyroxine sodium. (CW, chest wall; RVW, right ventricular wall; RVC, right ventricular cavity; IVS, interventricular septum; LVC, left ventricular cavity; PWLV, posterior wall left ventricle.) Note disappearance of pericardial effusion following levothyroxine therapy. (Reproduced, with permission, from Sokolow M, McIlroy MB: *Clinical Cardiology*, 4th ed. McGraw-Hill, 1986.)

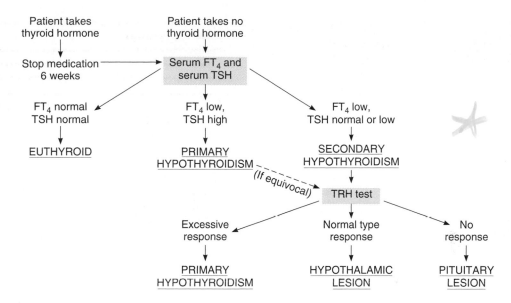

Figure 7–36. Diagnosis of hypothyroidism. Either free thyroxine (FT$_4$) or free thyroxine index (FT$_4$I) may be used with TSH for evaluation.

tion, hypoglycemia, hyponatremia, water intoxication, shock, and death. Although rare now, in the future it may occur more frequently in association with the increasing use of radioiodine for the treatment of Graves' disease, with resulting permanent hypothyroidism. Since it occurs most frequently in older patients with underlying pulmonary and vascular disease, the mortality rate is extremely high.

The patient (or a family member if the patient is comatose) may recall previous thyroid disease, radioiodine therapy, or thyroidectomy. The medical history is of gradual onset of lethargy progressing to stupor or coma. Examination reveals bradycardia and marked hypothermia, with body temperature as low as 24 °C (75 °F). The patient is usually an obese elderly woman with yellowish skin, a hoarse voice, a large tongue, thin hair, puffy eyes, ileus, and slow reflexes. There may be signs of other illnesses such as pneumonia, myocardial infarction, cerebral thrombosis, or gastrointestinal bleeding. Laboratory clues to the diagnosis of myxedema coma include lactescent serum, high serum carotene, elevated serum cholesterol, and increased cerebrospinal fluid protein. Pleural, pericardial, or abdominal effusions with high protein content may be present. Serum tests will reveal a low FT$_4$ and a markedly elevated TSH. Thyroidal radioactive iodine uptake is low, and thyroid autoantibodies are usually strongly positive, indicating underlying chronic thyroiditis. The ECG shows sinus bradycardia and low voltage. If laboratory studies are not readily available, which is frequently the case, the diagnosis must be made clinically.

The pathophysiology of myxedema coma involves three major aspects: (1) CO_2 retention and hypoxia, (2) fluid and electrolyte imbalance, and (3) hypothermia. CO_2 retention and hypoxia are probably due in large part to a marked depression in the ventilatory responses to hypoxia and hypercapnia, though factors such as obesity, heart failure, ileus, immobilization, pneumonia, pleural or peritoneal effusions, central nervous system depression, and weak chest muscles may also contribute. Failure of the myxedema patient to respond to hypoxia or hypercapnia may be due to hypothermia. Impairment of ventilatory drive is often severe, and assisted respiration is almost always necessary in patients with myxedema coma. Thyroid hormone therapy in patients with myxedema corrects the hypothermia and markedly improves the ventilatory response to hypoxia. The major fluid and electrolyte disturbance is water intoxication due to reduced renal perfusion and impaired free water clearance. This presents as hyponatremia and is managed by water restriction. Hypothermia is frequently not recognized, because the ordinary clinical thermometer only goes down to about 34 °C (93 °F); a laboratory type thermometer that registers a broader scale must be used to obtain accurate body temperature readings. Active rewarming of the body is contraindicated, because it may induce vasodilation and vascular collapse. A rise in

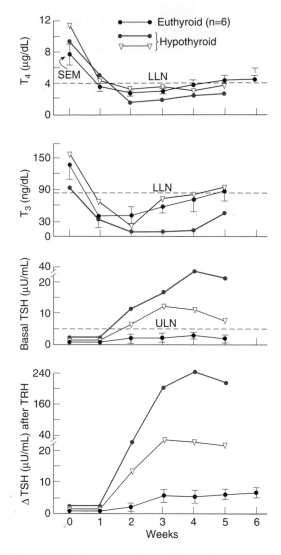

Figure 7–37. Changes in T_4, T_3, TSH, and TRH response following abrupt withdrawal of suppressive thyroxine therapy. Note that in euthyroid individuals the T_4 may not return to normal until 6 weeks after withdrawal of therapy and that serum TSH is never elevated. In hypothyroid patients, TSH may be elevated as early as 2 weeks after withdrawal of therapy, and TRH response is exaggerated. (LLN, lower limit of normal; ULN, upper limit of normal.) (Reproduced, with permission, from Wood LC: Controversial questions in thyroid disease. Workshop in the Thyroid, American Thyroid Association, Nov 1979, as adapted from Vagenakis AG et al: Recovery of pituitary thyrotropic function after withdrawal of prolonged thyroid suppression therapy. N Engl J Med 1975;293:681.)

body temperature is a useful indication of therapeutic effectiveness of thyroxine.

Disorders that may precipitate myxedema coma include heart failure, pneumonia, pulmonary edema, pleural or peritoneal effusions, ileus, excessive fluid administration, or administration of sedative or narcotic drugs to a patient with severe hypothyroidism. Adrenal insufficiency occurs occasionally in association with myxedema coma, but it is relatively rare and usually associated with either pituitary myxedema or concurrent autoimmune adrenal insufficiency (Schmidt's syndrome). Seizures, bleeding episodes, hypocalcemia, or hypercalcemia may be present. It is important to differentiate *pituitary* myxedema from *primary* myxedema. In pituitary myxedema, glucocorticoid replacement is essential. Clinical clues to the presence of pituitary myxedema include the following: a history of amenorrhea or impotence; scanty pubic or axillary hair; and normal serum cholesterol and normal or low TSH levels. CT scan or MRI may reveal an enlarged sella turcica. The treatment of myxedema coma is discussed below.

B. Myxedema and Heart Disease

In the past, treatment of patients with myxedema and heart disease, particularly coronary artery disease, was very difficult, because levothyroxine replacement was frequently associated with exacerbation of angina, heart failure, or myocardial infarction. Now that coronary angioplasty and coronary artery bypass surgery are available, patients with myxedema and coronary artery disease can be treated surgically first, and more rapid thyroxine replacement therapy will then be tolerated.

C. Hypothyroidism and Neuropsychiatric Disease

Hypothyroidism is often associated with depression, which may be quite severe. More rarely, myxedematous patients may become confused, paranoid, or even manic ("myxedema madness"). Screening of psychiatric admissions with FT_4 and TSH is an efficient way to find these patients, who will frequently respond to levothyroxine therapy alone or in combination with psychopharmacologic agents. The effectiveness of levothyroxine therapy in disturbed hypothyroid patients has given rise to the hypothesis that the addition of T_3 or T_4 to psychotherapeutic regimens for depressed patients may be helpful in patients without demonstrable thyroid disease. Further work needs to be done to establish this concept as standard treatment.

Treatment

A. Treatment of Hypothyroidism

Hypothyroidism is treated with levothyroxine (T_4), which is available in pure form and is stable and inexpensive. Intracellularly, levothyroxine is converted to T_3, so that both hormones become available even though only one is administered. Desiccated thyroid is unsatisfactory because of its variable hormone content, and triiodothyronine (as liothyronine) is unsatisfactory because of its rapid absorption, short half-life, and transient effects. The half-life of levothyroxine is about 7 days, so it need be given only once daily. It is well absorbed, and blood levels are easily monitored by following FT_4I or FT_4 and serum TSH levels. There is a rise in T_4 or FT_4I of about 1–2 μg/dL (13–26 nmol/L) and a concomitant fall in TSH of 1–2 μU/mL (1–2 mU/L) beginning about 2 hours and lasting about 8–10 hours after an oral dose of 0.1–0.15 mg of levothyroxine (Figure 7–38). It is best, therefore, to take the daily dose of levothyroxine in the morning to avoid symptoms such as insomnia if the medication is taken at bedtime. In addition, when monitoring serum thyroxine levels, it is important that blood be drawn fasting or before the daily dose of the hormone in order to obtain consistent data.

B. DOSAGE OF LEVOTHYROXINE

Replacement doses of levothyroxine in adults range from 0.05 to 0.2 mg/d, with a mean of 0.125 mg/d. The dose of levothyroxine varies according to the patient's age and body weight (Table 7–8). Young children require a surprisingly high dose of levothyroxine compared with adults. In adults, the mean replacement dose of T_4 is about 1.7 μg/kg/d, or about 0.8 μg/lb/d. In older adults, the replacement dose is lower, about 1.6 μg/kg/d, or about 0.7 μg/lb/d. For TSH suppression in patients with nodular goiters or cancers of the thyroid gland, the average dose of levothyroxine is about 2.2 μg/kg/d (1 μg/lb/d). In younger patients with mild hypothyroidism, one can begin treatment with one-half of the estimated dose requirement for 4–6 weeks and then adjust the final dose based on the FT_4 and TSH. In older patients or patients with severe hypothyroidism, it is best to start with a low dose of

Table 7–8. Replacement doses of levothyroxine.[1]

Age	Dose of Levothyroxine (μg/kg/d)
0–6 mo	10–15
7–11 mo	6–8
1–5 yr	5–6
6–10 yr	4–5
11–20 yr	1–3
Adult	1–2

[1]Adapted and modified, with permission, from Foley TP Jr. Congenital hypothyroidism. In: *Werner and Ingbar's The Thyroid*, 7th ed. Braverman LE, Utiger RD (editors). Lippincott, 1996.

levothyroxine, eg, 0.025 mg daily, and increase the dose at 4- to 6-week intervals based on FT_4 and TSH measurements. Malabsorptive states or concurrent administration of aluminum preparations, cholestyramine, calcium, or iron compounds will modify T_4 absorption. In these patients, levothyroxine should be given before breakfast, when the stomach is empty, and the other compounds taken 2–4 hours later. Levothyroxine has a sufficiently long half-life (7 days) so that if the patient is unable to take medications by mouth for a few days, omitting levothyroxine therapy will not be detrimental. If the patient is being managed by sustained parenteral therapy, the parenteral dose of T_4 is about 75–80% of the usual oral dose.

C. TREATMENT OF MYXEDEMA COMA

Myxedema coma is an acute medical emergency and should be treated in the intensive care unit. Blood gases must be monitored regularly, and the patient usually requires intubation and mechanical ventilation. Associated illnesses such as infections or heart failure must be sought for and appropriately treated. Intravenous fluids should be administered with caution, and excessive free

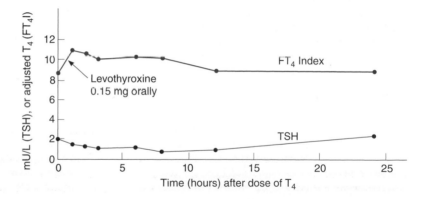

Figure 7–38. Rise in serum free thyroxine index (FT₄I) and fall in serum TSH following an oral dose of 0.15 mg levothyroxine.

water intake must be avoided. Because patients with myxedema coma absorb all drugs poorly, it is imperative to give levothyroxine intravenously. These patients have marked depletion of serum thyroxine with a large number of empty binding sites on thyroxine-binding globulin and therefore should receive an initial loading dose of 300–400 μg of levothyroxine intravenously, followed by 50 μg intravenously daily. The clinical guides to improvement are a rise in body temperature and the return of normal cerebral and respiratory function. If the patient is known to have had normal adrenal function before the onset of coma, adrenal support is probably not necessary. If, however, no data are available, the possibility of concomitant adrenal insufficiency (due to autoimmune adrenal disease or pituitary insufficiency) does exist. In this case, a cosyntropin stimulation test should performed (Chapter 9). Full adrenal support should then be administered, eg, hydrocortisone hemisuccinate, 100 mg intravenously, followed by 50 mg intravenously every 6 hours, tapering the dose over 7 days. Adrenal support can be withdrawn sooner if the pretreatment plasma cortisol is 30 μg/dL or greater or if results of a cosyntropin stimulation test are within normal limits. When giving levothyroxine intravenously in large doses, there is an inherent risk of precipitating angina, heart failure, or arrhythmias in older patients with underlying coronary artery disease. Thus, this type of therapy is not recommended for ambulatory patients with myxedema; in these patients, it is better to start slowly and build up the dose as noted below. (See also Chapter 24.)

D. Myxedema With Heart Disease

In long-standing hypothyroidism or in older patients—particularly those with known cardiovascular disease—it is imperative to start treatment slowly. Levothyroxine is given in a dosage of 0.025 mg/d for 2 weeks, increasing by 0.025 mg every 2 weeks until a daily dose of 0.075 mg is reached. This dose is continued for about 6 weeks. TSH is then measured and the dosage adjusted accordingly. It usually takes about 2 months for a patient to come into equilibrium on full dosage. In these patients, the heart is very sensitive to the level of circulating thyroxine, and if angina pectoris or cardiac arrhythmia develops, it is essential to reduce the dose of thyroxine immediately.

Toxic Effects of Levothyroxine Therapy

There are no reported instances of allergy to pure levothyroxine, though it is possible that a patient may develop an allergy to the coloring dye or some component of the tablet. The major toxic reactions to levothyroxine overdosage are symptoms of hyperthyroidism—particularly cardiac symptoms—and, in postmenopausal women, osteoporosis. The most common thyrotoxic cardiac symptom is arrhythmia, particularly paroxysmal atrial tachycardia or fibrillation. Insomnia, tremor, restlessness, and excessive warmth may also be troublesome. Simply omitting the daily dose of levothyroxine for 3 days and then reducing the dosage will correct the problem.

Increased bone resorption and severe osteoporosis have been associated with long-standing hyperthyroidism and will develop in postmenopausal women chronically overtreated with levothyroxine. This can be prevented by regular monitoring and by maintaining normal serum FT_4 and TSH in patients receiving long-term replacement therapy. In patients receiving TSH-suppressive therapy for nodular goiter or thyroid cancer, if FT_4I or FT_4 is kept in the upper range of normal—even if TSH is suppressed—the adverse effects of T_4 therapy on bone will be minimal (Chapter 23). In addition, concomitant administration of estrogen or bisphosphonate to postmenopausal women receiving high-dose thyroxine therapy will minimize bone resorption.

Course & Prognosis

The course of untreated myxedema is one of slow deterioration, leading eventually to myxedema coma and death. With appropriate treatment, however, the long-term prognosis is excellent. Because of the long half-life (7 days) of thyroxine, it takes time to establish equilibrium on a fixed dose. Therefore, it is important to monitor the FT_4I or FT_4 and the serum TSH every 4–6 weeks until equilibrium is reached. Thereafter, FT_4 and TSH can be monitored once a year. The dose of T_4 must be increased about 25% during pregnancy. Older patients metabolize T_4 more slowly, and the dose will gradually decrease with age (Chapter 23).

The mortality rate of myxedema coma was about 80% at one time. The prognosis has been vastly improved as a result of recognition of the importance of mechanically assisted respiration and the use of intravenous levothyroxine. At present, the outcome probably depends upon how well the underlying disease problems can be managed.

HYPERTHYROIDISM & THYROTOXICOSIS

Thyrotoxicosis is the clinical syndrome that results when tissues are exposed to high levels of circulating thyroid hormone. In most instances, thyrotoxicosis is due to hyperactivity of the thyroid gland, or hyperthyroidism. Occasionally, thyrotoxicosis may be due to other causes such as excessive ingestion of thyroid hormone or excessive secretion of thyroid hormone from ectopic sites. The various forms of thyrotoxicosis are listed in Table 7–9. These syndromes will be discussed individually below.

1. Diffuse Toxic Goiter (Graves' Disease)

Graves' disease is the most common form of thyrotoxicosis and may occur at any age, more commonly in females than in males. The syndrome consists of one or more of the following features: (1) thyrotoxicosis, (2) goiter, (3) ophthalmopathy (exophthalmos), and (4) dermopathy (pretibial myxedema).

Etiology

Graves' disease is currently viewed as an autoimmune disease of unknown cause. There is a strong familial predisposition in that about 15% of patients with Graves' disease have a close relative with the same disorder, and about 50% of relatives of patients with Graves' disease have circulating thyroid autoantibodies. Females are involved about five times more commonly than males. The disease may occur at any age, with a peak incidence in the 20- to 40-year age group. (See section on thyroid autoimmunity, above.)

Pathogenesis

In Graves' disease, T lymphocytes become sensitized to antigens within the thyroid gland and stimulate B lymphocytes to synthesize antibodies to these antigens. (See Chapter 4. See also the section on thyroid autoimmunity, above, and Figure 7–39.) One such antibody is directed against the TSH receptor site in the thyroid cell membrane and has the capacity to stimulate the thyroid cell to increased growth and function (TSH-R Ab [stim]). The presence of this circulating antibody is positively correlated with active disease and with relapse of the disease. There is an underlying genetic predisposi-

Table 7–9. Conditions associated with thyrotoxicosis.

1. Diffuse toxic goiter (Graves' disease)
2. Toxic adenoma (Plummer's disease)
3. Toxic multinodular goiter
4. Subacute thyroiditis
5. Hyperthyroid phase of Hashimoto's thyroiditis
6. Thyrotoxicosis factitia
7. Rare forms of thyrotoxicosis: ovarian struma, metastatic thyroid carcinoma (follicular), hydatidiform mole, "hamburger thyrotoxicosis," TSH-secreting pituitary tumor, pituitary resistance to T_3 and T_4

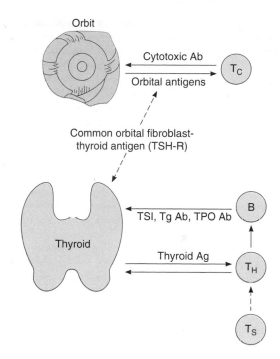

Figure 7–39. One theory of the pathogenesis of Graves' disease. There is a defect in suppressor T lymphocytes (T_s) that allows helper T lymphocytes (T_H) to stimulate B lymphocytes (B) to synthesize thyroid autoantibodies. The thyroid-stimulating immunoglobulin (TSI) is the driving force for thyrotoxicosis. The inflammatory process in the orbital muscles may be due to sensitization of cytotoxic T lymphocytes (T_c), or killer cells, to orbital antigens in association with cytotoxic antibodies. The thyroid and the eye are linked by a common antigen, the TSH-R, found in thyroid follicular cells and orbital fibroblasts. It is not yet clear what triggers this immunologic cascade. (Tg Ab, thyroglobulin antibody; TPO Ab, thyroperoxidase or microsomal antibody; Ag, antigen; Ab, antibody.)

tion, but it is not clear what "triggers" the acute episode. Some factors that may incite the immune response of Graves' disease are (1) pregnancy, particularly the postpartum period; (2) iodide excess, particularly in geographic areas of iodide deficiency, where the lack of iodide may hold latent Graves' disease in check; (3) lithium therapy, perhaps by modifying immune responsiveness; (4) viral or bacterial infections; and (5) glucocorticoid withdrawal. It has been postulated that "stress" may trigger an episode of Graves' disease, but there is no evidence to support this hypothesis. The pathogenesis of ophthalmopathy may involve cytotoxic lymphocytes (killer cells) and cytotoxic antibodies sensitized to a common antigen such as the TSH-R found in orbital fibroblasts, orbital muscle, and thyroid tissue (Figure 7–39). Cytokines from these sensitized lymphocytes would cause inflammation of orbital fibroblasts and orbital myositis, resulting in swollen orbital muscles, proptosis of the globes, and diplopia as well as redness, congestion, and conjunctival and periorbital edema (thyroid ophthalmopathy; Figures 7–40 and 7–41). The pathogenesis of thyroid dermopathy (pretibial myxedema) (Figure 7–42) and the rare subperiosteal inflammation on the phalanges of the hands and feet (thyroid osteopathy) (Figure 7–43) may also involve lymphocyte cytokine stimulation of fibroblasts in these locations.

Many symptoms of thyrotoxicosis suggest a state of catecholamine excess, including tachycardia, tremor, sweating, lid lag, and stare. Circulating levels of epinephrine are normal; thus, in Graves' disease, the body appears to be hyperreactive to catecholamines. This may be due in part to a thyroid hormone-mediated increase in cardiac catecholamine receptors.

Clinical Features

A. SYMPTOMS AND SIGNS

In younger individuals, common manifestations include palpitations, nervousness, easy fatigability, hyperkinesia, diarrhea, excessive sweating, intolerance to heat, and preference for cold. There is often marked weight loss without loss of appetite. Thyroid enlargement, thyrotoxic eye signs (see below), and mild tachycardia commonly occur. Muscle weakness and loss of muscle mass may be so severe that the patient cannot rise from a chair without assistance. In children, rapid growth with accelerated bone maturation occurs. In patients over age 60, cardiovascular and myopathic manifestations predominate; the most common presenting complaints are palpitation, dyspnea on exertion, tremor, nervousness, and weight loss (Chapter 23).

The eye signs of Graves' disease have been classified by Werner as set forth in Table 7–10. This classification is useful in describing the extent of the eye involvement, but it is not helpful in following the progress of the illness since one class does not always progress into the next. The first letters of each class form the mnemonic "NO SPECS." Class 1 involves spasm of the upper lids associated with active thyrotoxicosis and usually resolves spontaneously when the thyrotoxicosis is adequately controlled. Classes 2–6 represent true infiltrative disease involving orbital muscles and orbital tissues (Figures 7–40 and 7–41). Class 2 is characterized by soft tissue involvement with periorbital edema, congestion or redness of the conjunctiva, and swelling of the conjunctiva (chemosis). Class 3 consists of proptosis as measured by the Hertel exophthalmometer. This instrument consists of two prisms with a scale mounted

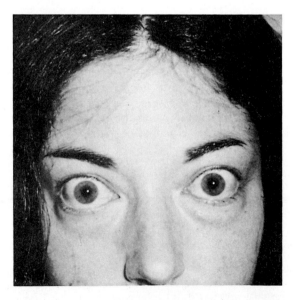 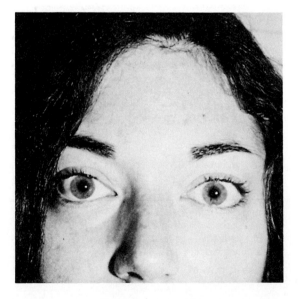

Figure 7–40. Patient with mild ophthalmopathy of Graves' disease. ***Left:*** Before radioactive iodine therapy. Note white sclera visible above and below the iris as well as mild periorbital edema. Classification (Table 7–10): class 1, mild; class 2, mild: class 3, mild. ***Right:*** After radioactive iodine therapy. Marked improvement is noted.

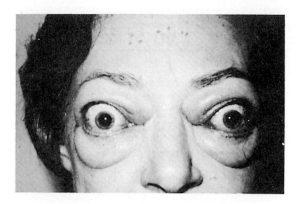

Figure 7–41. Severe ophthalmopathy of Graves' disease. Note marked periorbital edema, injection of corneal blood vessels, and proptosis. There was also striking limitation of upward and lateral eye movements and reduced visual acuity. **Classification** (Table 7–10): class 1, severe; class 2, severe; class 3, severe; class 4, severe; class 5, none; class 6, mild.

on a bar. The prisms are placed on the lateral orbital ridges, and the distance from the orbital ridge to the anterior cornea is measured on the scale (Figure 7–44). The upper limits of normal according to race are listed in the footnote to Table 7–10. Class 4 consists of muscle involvement. The muscle most commonly involved in the infiltrative process is the inferior rectus, limiting upward gaze. The muscle next most commonly involved is the medial rectus, impairing lateral gaze. Class 5 is characterized by corneal involvement (keratitis) and class 6 loss of vision from optic nerve involvement. As noted above, thyroid ophthalmopathy is due to infiltration of the extraocular muscles with lymphocytes and edema fluid in an acute inflammatory reaction. The orbit is a cone enclosed by bone, and swelling of the extraocular muscles within this closed space causes proptosis of the globe and impaired muscle movement, resulting in diplopia. Ocular muscle enlargement can be demonstrated by orbital CT scanning or MRI (Figure 7–45). When muscle swelling occurs posteriorly, toward the apex of the orbital cone, the optic nerve is compressed, which may cause loss of vision.

Thyroid dermopathy consists of thickening of the skin, particularly over the lower tibia, due to accumulation of glycosaminoglycans (Figure 7–42). It is relatively rare, occurring in about 2–3% of patients with Graves' disease. It is usually associated with ophthalmopathy and with a very high serum titer of TSH-R Ab [stim]. The skin is markedly thickened and cannot be picked up between the fingers. Sometimes the dermopathy involves the entire lower leg and may extend

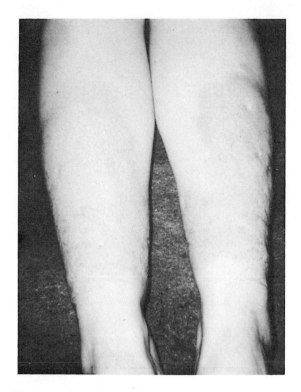

Figure 7–42. Dermopathy of Graves' disease. Marked thickening of the skin is noted, usually over the pretibial area. Thickening will occasionally extend downward over the ankle and the dorsal aspect of the foot but almost never above the knee.

onto the feet. Bony involvement (osteopathy), with subperiosteal bone formation and swelling, is particularly evident in the metacarpal bones (Figure 7–43). This too is a relatively rare finding. A more common finding in Graves' disease is separation of the fingernails from their beds, or onycholysis (Figure 7–46).

B. LABORATORY FINDINGS

The laboratory findings in hyperthyroidism are summarized in Figure 7–47. Essentially, the combination of an elevated FT_4 and a suppressed TSH makes the diagnosis of hyperthyroidism. If eye signs are present, the diagnosis of Graves' disease can be made without further tests. If eye signs are absent and the patient is hyperthyroid with or without a goiter, a radioiodine uptake test should be done. An elevated uptake is diagnostic of Graves' disease or toxic nodular goiter. A low uptake is seen in patients with spontaneously resolving hyperthyroidism, as in subacute thyroiditis or a flare-up of Hashimoto's thyroiditis. Low uptakes will

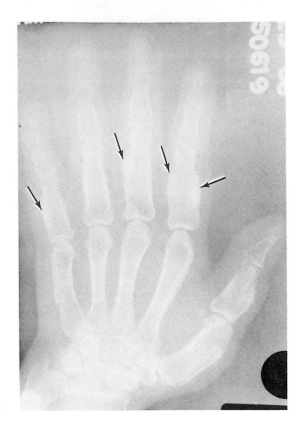

Figure 7–43. X-ray of hand of patient with thyroid osteopathy. Note marked periosteal thickening of the proximal phalanges.

Table 7–10. Classification of eye changes in Graves' disease.[1] "NO SPECS"

Class	Definition
0	*No* signs or symptoms.
1	*Only* signs, no symptoms. (Signs limited to upper lid retraction, stare, lid lag.)
2	*Soft* tissue involvement (symptoms and signs).
3	*Proptosis* (measured with Hertel exophthalmometer).[2]
4	*Extraocular* muscle involvement.
5	*Corneal* involvement.
6	*Sight* loss (optic nerve involvement).

[1]Reproduced, with permission, from Werner SC: Classification of the eye changes of Graves' disease. J Clin Endocrinol Metab 1969;29:782 and 1977;44:203.
[2]Upper limits of normal according to race: 18 mm; white, Asian, 20 mm; black, 22 mm. Increase in proptosis of 3–4 mm is mild involvement; 5–7 mm, moderate involvement; and over 8 mm, severe involvement. Other classes can be similarly graded as mild, moderate, or severe.

also be found in patients who are iodine-loaded or are on T_4 therapy—or, rarely, in association with a struma ovarii. If both FT_4 and TSH are elevated and radioiodine uptake is also elevated, consider a TSH-secreting pituitary tumor or generalized or pituitary resistance syndromes. If FT_4 is normal and TSH is suppressed, check FT_3, which will be elevated in early Graves' disease or in T_3-secreting toxic nodules. Low FT_3 will be found in the euthyroid sick syndrome or in patients receiving corticoids or dopamine.

Thyroid autoantibodies—Tg Ab and TPO Ab—are usually present in both Graves' disease and Hashimoto's thyroiditis, but TSH-R Ab [stim] is specific for Graves' disease. This may be a useful diagnostic test in the "apathetic" hyperthyroid patient or in the patient who presents with unilateral exophthalmos without obvious signs or laboratory manifestations of Graves' disease. The ^{123}I or technetium scan is useful to evaluate the size of the gland or the presence of "hot" or "cold" nodules. Since the ultrasensitive TSH test will detect TSH sup-

pression, TRH tests (see above) are rarely indicated. CT and MRI scans of the orbit have revealed muscle enlargement in most patients with Graves' disease even when there is no clinical evidence of ophthalmopathy. In patients with ophthalmopathy, orbital muscle enlargement may be striking (Figure 7–45).

Differential Diagnosis

Graves' disease occasionally presents in an unusual or atypical fashion, in which case the diagnosis may not be obvious. Marked muscle atrophy may suggest severe myopathy that must be differentiated from primary neurologic disorder. **Thyrotoxic periodic paralysis** usually occurs in Asian males and presents with a sudden attack of flaccid paralysis and hypokalemia. The paralysis usually subsides spontaneously and can be prevented by K^+ supplementation and beta-adrenergic blockade. The illness is cured by appropriate treatment of the thyrotoxicosis (see Chapter 24). Patients with **thyrocardiac disease** present primarily with symptoms of heart involvement—especially refractory atrial fibrillation insensitive to digoxin—or with high-output heart failure. About 50% of these patients have no evidence of underlying heart disease, and the cardiac problems are cured by treatment of the thyrotoxicosis. Some older patients will present with weight loss, small goiter, slow atrial fibrillation, and severe depression, with none of the clinical features of increased catecholamine reactivity. These placid patients have **"apathetic hyperthyroidism."** Finally, some young women may present with amenorrhea or infertility as the primary symptom.

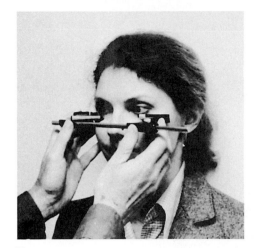

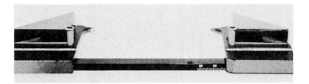

A   **B**

Figure 7–44. *A:* Hertel exophthalmometer. *B:* Proper use of the exophthalmometer. The edges of the instrument are placed on the lateral orbital ridges, and the distance from the orbital bone to the anterior cornea is read on the scale contained within the prisms.

In all of these instances, the diagnosis of hyperthyroidism can usually be made on the basis of the clinical and laboratory studies described above.

In the syndrome called **"familial dysalbuminemic hyperthyroxinemia,"** an abnormal albumin-like protein is present in serum that preferentially binds T_4 but not T_3. This results in elevation of serum T_4 and FT_4I, but free T_4, T_3, and TSH are normal. It is important to differentiate this euthyroid state from hyperthyroidism. In addition to the absence of clinical features of hyperthyroidism, a normal serum T_3 and a normal TSH level will rule out hyperthyroidism.

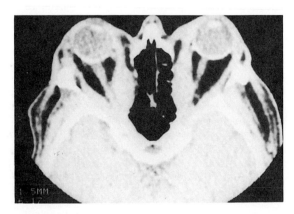

Figure 7–45. Orbital CT scan in a patient with severe ophthalmopathy and visual failure. Note the marked enlargement of extraocular muscles posteriorly, with compression of the optic nerve at the apex of the orbital cone.

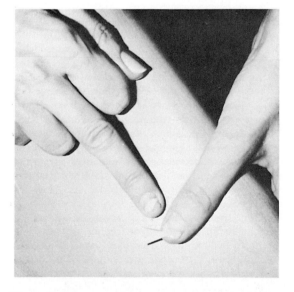

Figure 7–46. Onycholysis (separation of the nail from its bed) in Graves' disease usually resolves spontaneously as the patient improves.

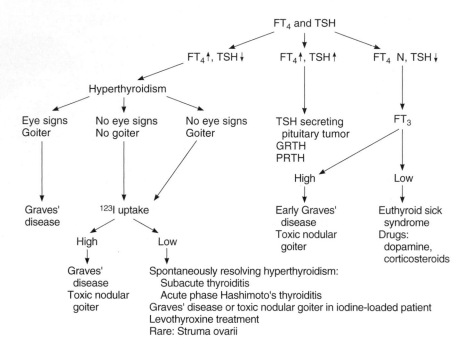

Figure 7–47. Laboratory tests useful in the differential diagnosis of hyperthyroidism. (See text for details.)

Complications

Thyrotoxic crisis ("thyroid storm") is the acute exacerbation of all of the symptoms of thyrotoxicosis, often presenting as a syndrome that may be of life-threatening severity. (See Chapter 24.) Occasionally, thyroid storm may be mild and present simply as an unexplained febrile reaction after thyroid surgery in a patient who has been inadequately prepared. More commonly, it occurs in a more severe form after surgery, radioactive iodine therapy, or parturition in a patient with inadequately controlled thyrotoxicosis—or during a severe, stressful illness or disorder such as uncontrolled diabetes, trauma, acute infection, severe drug reaction, or myocardial infarction. The clinical manifestations of thyroid storm are marked hypermetabolism and excessive adrenergic response. Fever ranges from 38 to 41 °C and is associated with flushing and sweating. There is marked tachycardia, often with atrial fibrillation and high pulse pressure and occasionally with heart failure. Central nervous system symptoms include marked agitation, restlessness, delirium, and coma. Gastrointestinal symptoms include nausea, vomiting, diarrhea, and jaundice. A fatal outcome will be associated with heart failure and shock.

At one time it was thought that thyroid storm was due to sudden release or "dumping" of stored thyroxine and triiodothyronine from the thyrotoxic gland. Care-ful studies have revealed, however, that the serum levels of T_4 and T_3 in patients with thyroid storm are not higher than in thyrotoxic patients without this condition. There is no evidence that thyroid storm is due to excessive production of triiodothyronine. There is evidence that in thyrotoxicosis the number of binding sites for catecholamines increases, so that heart and nerve tissues have increased sensitivity to circulating catecholamines. In addition, there is decreased binding to TBG, with elevation of free T_3 and T_4. The present theory is that in this setting, with increased binding sites available for catecholamines, an acute illness, infection, or surgical stress triggers an outpouring of catecholamines which, in association with high levels of free T_4 and T_3, precipitates the acute problem.

The most striking clinical diagnostic feature of thyrotoxic crisis is hyperpyrexia out of proportion to other findings. Laboratory findings include elevated serum T_4, FT_4, and T_3 as well as a suppressed TSH (see Chapter 24).

Treatment of Graves' Disease

Although autoimmune mechanisms are responsible for the syndrome of Graves' disease, management has been largely directed toward controlling the hyperthyroidism. Three good methods are available: (1) antithyroid drug therapy, (2) surgery, and (3) radioactive iodine therapy.

A. Antithyroid Drug Therapy

In general, antithyroid drug therapy is most useful in young patients with small glands and mild disease. The drugs (propylthiouracil or methimazole) are given until the disease undergoes spontaneous remission. This occurs in 20–40% of patients treated for 6 months to 15 years. Although this is the only therapy that leaves an intact thyroid gland, it does require a long period of observation, and the incidence of relapse is high, perhaps 50–60% even in selected patients. There may be a genetic predisposition to the failure to respond to antithyroid drug therapy. Antithyroid drug therapy is generally started with large divided doses; when the patient becomes clinically euthyroid, maintenance therapy may be achieved with a lower single morning dose. A common regimen consists of giving propylthiouracil, 100 mg every 6 hours initially, and then in 4–8 weeks reducing the dose to 50–200 mg once or twice daily. Propylthiouracil has one advantage over methimazole in that it partially inhibits the conversion of T_4 to T_3, so that it is effective in bringing down the levels of activated thyroid hormone more quickly. However, methimazole has a longer duration of action and is more useful if a single daily dose is desirable. A typical program would start with a 40-mg dose of methimazole each morning for 1–2 months; this dose would then be reduced to 5–20 mg each morning for maintenance therapy. The laboratory tests of most value in monitoring the course of therapy are serum FT_4 and TSH.

An alternative method of therapy utilizes the concept of a total block of thyroid activity. The patient is treated with methimazole until euthyroid (about 3–6 months), but instead of continuing to taper the dose of methimazole, at this point levothyroxine is added in a dose of about 0.1 mg/d. The patient then continues to receive the combination of methimazole 10 mg/d and levothyroxine 0.1 mg/d for another 12–24 months. At the end of this time, or when the size of the gland has returned to normal, methimazole is discontinued. This combined therapy will prevent the development of hypothyroidism due to excessive doses of methimazole, but the incidence of relapse is about the same as after treatment with methimazole alone.

1. Duration of therapy—The duration of therapy with antithyroid drugs in Graves' disease is quite variable and can range from 6 months to 20 years or more. A sustained remission may be predicted in about 80% of treated patients in the following circumstances: (1) if the thyroid gland returns to normal size; (2) if the disease can be controlled with a relatively small dose of antithyroid drugs; (3) if TSH-R Ab [stim] is no longer detectable in the serum; and (4) if the thyroid gland becomes normally suppressible following the administration of liothyronine.

2. Reactions to antithyroid drugs—Allergic reactions to antithyroid drugs involve either a rash (about 5% of patients) or agranulocytosis (about 0.5% of patients). The rash can be managed by simply administering antihistamines, and unless it is severe it is not an indication for discontinuing the medication. Agranulocytosis requires immediate cessation of all antithyroid drug therapy, institution of appropriate antibiotic therapy, and shifting to an alternative therapy, usually radioactive iodine. Agranulocytosis is usually heralded by sore throat and fever. Thus, all patients receiving antithyroid drugs are instructed that if sore throat or fever develops, they should stop the drug, obtain a white blood cell and differential count, and see their physician. If the white blood cell count is normal, the antithyroid drug can be resumed. Cholestatic jaundice, angioneurotic edema, hepatocellular toxicity, and acute arthralgia are serious but rare side effects that also require cessation of drug therapy.

B. Surgical Treatment

Subtotal thyroidectomy is the treatment of choice for patients with very large glands or multinodular goiters. The patient is prepared with antithyroid drugs until euthyroid (about 6 weeks). In addition, starting 2 weeks before the day of operation, the patient is given saturated solution of potassium iodide, 5 drops twice daily. This regimen has been shown empirically to diminish the vascularity of the gland and to simplify surgery.

There is disagreement about how much thyroid tissue should be removed. Total thyroidectomy is usually not necessary unless the patient has severe progressive ophthalmopathy (see below). However, if too much thyroid tissue is left behind, the disease will relapse. Most surgeons leave 2–3 g of thyroid tissue on either side of the neck. Many patients, however, require thyroid supplementation following thyroidectomy for Graves' disease.

Hypoparathyroidism and recurrent laryngeal nerve injury occur as complications of surgery in about 1% of cases.

C. Radioactive Iodine Therapy

In the USA, sodium iodide ^{131}I is the preferred treatment for most patients over age 21. In many patients without underlying heart disease, radioactive iodine may be given immediately in a dosage of 80–150 μCi/g of thyroid weight estimated on the basis of physical examination and sodium ^{123}I rectilinear scan. The dosage is corrected for iodine uptake according to the following formula:

$$^{131}\text{I}(\mu\text{Ci}/\text{g}) \times \begin{matrix} \text{Estimated} \\ \text{thyroid} \\ \text{weight (g)} \end{matrix} \times \cfrac{100}{\begin{matrix} 24-\text{hour} \\ \text{RAI uptake} \end{matrix}} = \begin{matrix} \text{Therapeutic} \\ \text{dose} - \text{of} \ ^{131}\text{I} \\ \text{in} \ \mu\text{Ci} \end{matrix}$$

Following the administration of radioactive iodine, the gland will shrink and the patient will become euthyroid over a period of 6–12 weeks.

In elderly patients and in those with underlying heart disease or other medical problems, severe thyrotoxicosis, or large glands (> 100 g), it is desirable to achieve a euthyroid state prior to ^{131}I therapy. For this purpose, pretreatment with methimazole rather than propylthiouracil is preferable because propylthiouracil may inhibit radioiodine uptake for weeks or months after discontinuation, whereas the inhibitory effect of methimazole on radioiodine uptake may dissipate in 24 hours. Patients usually are treated with methimazole until they are euthyroid; medication is then stopped for 5–7 days; and a dose of 100–150 mCi ^{131}I per gram of estimated thyroid weight (corrected for uptake) is calculated as described above. Because it is usually desirable to destroy most of the gland in patients with underlying medical problems, the dose of ^{131}I may be slightly larger than is ordinarily given.

The major complication of radioactive iodine therapy is hypothyroidism, which ultimately develops in 80% or more of patients who are adequately treated. However, this complication may indeed be the best assurance that the patient will not have a recurrence of hyperthyroidism. Serum FT_4 and TSH levels should be followed, and when hypothyroidism develops, prompt replacement therapy with levothyroxine, 0.05–0.2 mg daily, is instituted.

Hypothyroidism may occur after any type of therapy for Graves' disease—even after antithyroid drug therapy; in some patients, "burned-out" Graves' disease may be an end result of autoimmune thyroid disease. Accordingly, all patients with Graves' disease require lifetime follow-up to be certain that they remain euthyroid.

D. OTHER MEDICAL MEASURES

During the acute phase of thyrotoxicosis, beta-adrenergic blocking agents are extremely helpful. Propranolol, 10–40 mg every 6 hours, will control tachycardia, hypertension, and atrial fibrillation. This drug is gradually withdrawn as serum thyroxine levels return to normal. Adequate nutrition, including multivitamin supplements, is essential. Barbiturates accelerate T_4 metabolism, and phenobarbital may be helpful both for its sedative effect and to lower T_4 levels. Ipodate sodium or iopanoic acid has been shown to inhibit both thyroid hormone synthesis and release as well as peripheral conversion of T_4 to T_3. Thus, in a dosage of 1 g daily, this drug may help to rapidly restore the euthyroid state. It leaves the gland saturated with iodide, so it should not be used before ^{131}I therapy or antithyroid drug therapy with propylthiouracil or methimazole. Cholestyramine, 4 g orally three times daily, will lower serum T_4 by binding it in the gut. In a patient with a large toxic goiter and a severe allergic reaction to antithyroid drugs, ipodate sodium and beta blockade can be used effectively as preparation for surgery.

Choice of Therapy

Choice of therapy will vary with the nature and severity of the illness and prevailing customs. For example, in the USA, radioiodine therapy has been the preferred treatment for the average patient, whereas in Europe and Asia, antithyroid drug therapy is preferred. In the opinion of this author, most patients should be treated with antithyroid drugs until euthyroid. If there is a prompt response and the gland begins to shrink, the option of long-term antithyroid drug therapy with or without simultaneous levothyroxine therapy should be considered. If large doses of antithyroid drugs are required for control and the gland does not shrink in response to therapy, radioiodine would be the treatment of choice. If the gland is very large (> 150 g) or multinodular—or if the patient wishes to become pregnant very soon—thyroidectomy is a reasonable option. A serious allergic reaction to an antithyroid drug is an indication for radioiodine therapy.

Treatment of Complications

A. THYROTOXIC CRISIS

Thyrotoxic crisis (thyroid storm) requires vigorous management. Propranolol, 1–2 mg slowly intravenously or 40–80 mg every 6 hours orally, is helpful in controlling arrhythmias. In the presence of severe heart failure or asthma and arrhythmia, cautious intravenous administration of verapamil in a dose of 5–10 mg may be effective. Hormone synthesis is blocked by the administration of propylthiouracil, 250 mg every 6 hours. If the patient is unable to take medication by mouth, methimazole in a dose of 60 mg every 24 hours or propylthiouracil, 400 mg every 6 hours, can be given by rectal suppository or enema.* After admin-

---

*__Preparation of rectal methimazole:__ Dissolve 1200 mg methimazole in 12 mL of water to which has been added a mixture of 2 drops of Span 80 in 52 mL of cocoa butter warmed to 37 °C. Stir the mixture to form a water-oil emulsion, pour into 2.6 mL suppository molds, and cool. Each suppository will supply approximately 60 mg methimazole absorbed dose (Nabil et al, 1982).
__Preparation of rectal propylthiouracil:__ Dissolve 400 mg propylthiouracil in 60 mL of Fleet Mineral Oil for the first dose and then dissolve 400 mg propylthiouracil in 60 mL of Fleet Phospho-Soda for subsequent enemas.

istration of an antithyroid drug, hormone release is retarded by the administration of sodium iodide, 1 g intravenously over a 24-hour period, or saturated solution of potassium iodide, 10 drops twice daily. Ipodate sodium, 1 g daily given orally, or iohexol given intravenously may be used instead of sodium iodide, but this will block the definitive use of radioiodine therapy for 3–6 months. The conversion of T_4 to T_3 is blocked by the administration of ipodate sodium or iohexol and also by the combination of propranolol and propylthiouracil. The administration of hydrocortisone hemisuccinate, 50 mg intravenously every 6 hours, is additive. Supportive therapy includes a cooling blanket and acetaminophen to help control fever. Aspirin is probably contraindicated because of its tendency to bind to TBG and displace thyroxine, rendering more thyroxine available in the free state. Fluids, electrolytes, and nutrition are important. For sedation, phenobarbital is probably best because it accelerates the peripheral metabolism and inactivation of thyroxine and triiodothyronine, ultimately bringing these levels down. Oxygen, diuretics, and digitalis are indicated for heart failure. Finally, it is essential to treat the underlying disease process that may have precipitated the acute exacerbation. Thus, antibiotics, anti-allergy drugs, and postoperative care are indicated for management of these problems. As an extreme measure (rarely needed) to control thyrotoxic crisis, plasmapheresis or peritoneal dialysis may be used to remove high levels of circulating thyronines. (See Chapter 24.)

B. OPHTHALMOPATHY

Management of ophthalmopathy due to Graves' disease involves close cooperation between the endocrinologist and the ophthalmologist. The thyroid disease may be managed as outlined above, but in the opinion of this author, total surgical excision of the thyroid gland or total ablation of the thyroid gland with radioactive iodine is indicated. Although there is controversy over the need for total ablation, removal or destruction of the thyroid gland certainly prevents exacerbations and relapses of thyrotoxicosis, which may reactivate residual ophthalmopathy. Prednisone begun 24 hours after radioiodine in a dose of 40 mg/d, tapering the dose 10 mg every 2 weeks, will protect against exacerbation of ophthalmopathy following ^{131}I therapy. Keeping the patient's head elevated at night will diminish periorbital edema. For the severe acute inflammatory reaction, a short course of corticosteroid therapy is frequently effective, eg, prednisone, 100 mg daily orally in divided doses for 7–14 days, then every other day in gradually diminishing dosage for 6–12 weeks. If corticosteroid therapy is not effective, external x-ray therapy to the retrobulbar area may be helpful. The dose is usually 2000 cGy in ten fractions given over a period of 2 weeks. The lens and anterior chamber structures must be shielded.

In very severe cases where vision is threatened, orbital decompression can be used. One type of orbital decompression involves a transantral approach through the maxillary sinus, removing the floor and the lateral walls of the orbit. In the alternative anterior approach, the orbit is entered under the globe, and portions of the floor and the walls of the orbit are removed. Both approaches have been extremely effective, and exophthalmos can be reduced by 5–7 mm in each eye by these techniques. After the acute process has subsided, the patient is frequently left with double vision or lid abnormalities owing to muscle fibrosis and contracture. These can be corrected by cosmetic lid surgery or eye muscle surgery.

C. THYROTOXICOSIS AND PREGNANCY

Thyrotoxicosis during pregnancy presents a special problem. Radioactive iodine is contraindicated because it crosses the placenta freely and may injure the fetal thyroid. Two good alternatives are available. If the disease is detected during the first trimester, the patient can be prepared with propylthiouracil, and subtotal thyroidectomy can be performed safely during the mid trimester. It is essential to provide thyroid supplementation during the balance of the pregnancy. Alternatively, the patient can be treated with antithyroid drugs throughout the pregnancy, postponing the decision regarding long-term management until after delivery. The dosage of antithyroid drugs must be kept to the minimum necessary to control symptoms, because these drugs cross the placenta and may affect the function of the fetal thyroid gland. If the disease can be controlled by initial doses of propylthiouracil of 250 mg/d (in divided doses) or less and maintenance doses of 25–100 mg/d, the likelihood of fetal hypothyroidism is extremely small. The FT_4I or FT_4 should be maintained in the upper range of normal by appropriately reducing the propylthiouracil dosage. Supplemental thyroxine is not necessary. Breast feeding is not contraindicated, because propylthiouracil is not concentrated in the milk.

Graves' disease may occur in the newborn infant (**neonatal Graves' disease**). There seem to be two forms of the disease. In both types, the mother has a current or recent history of Graves' disease. In the first type, the child is born small, with weak muscles, tachycardia, fever, and frequently respiratory distress or neonatal jaundice. Examination reveals an enlarged thyroid gland and occasionally prominent, puffy eyes. The heart rate is rapid, temperature is elevated, and heart failure may ensue. Laboratory studies reveal an elevated FT_4I or FT_4, a markedly elevated T_3, and usually a low TSH—in contrast to normal infants, who have elevated

TSH at birth. Bone age may be accelerated. TSH-R Ab [stim] is usually found in the serum of both the infant and the mother. The pathogenesis of this syndrome is thought to involve transplacental transfer of TSH-R Ab [stim] from mother to fetus, with subsequent development of thyrotoxicosis. The disease is self-limited and subsides over a period of 4–12 weeks, coinciding with the fall in the child's TSH-R Ab [stim]. Therapy for the infant includes propylthiouracil in a dose of 5–10 mg/kg/d (in divided doses at 8-hour intervals); strong iodine (Lugol's) solution, 1 drop (8 mg potassium iodide) every 8 hours; and propranolol, 2 mg/kg/d in divided doses. In addition, adequate nutrition, antibiotics for infection if present, sedatives if necessary, and supportive therapy are indicated. If the child is very toxic, corticosteroid therapy (prednisone, 2 mg/kg/d) will partially block conversion of T_4 to T_3 and may be helpful in the acute phase. The above medications are gradually reduced as the child improves and can usually be discontinued by 6–12 weeks.

A second form of neonatal Graves' disease occurs in children from families with a high incidence of that disorder. Symptoms develop more slowly and may not be noted until the child is 3–6 months old. This syndrome is thought to be a true genetic inheritance of defective lymphocyte immunoregulation. It is much more severe, with a 20% mortality rate and evidence of persistent brain dysfunction even after successful treatment. The hyperthyroidism may persist for months or years and requires prolonged therapy.

Maternal sera may contain TSH-R blocking antibodies that can cross the placenta and produce transient hypothyroidism in the infant. This condition may need to be treated with T_4 supplementation for a short time.

Course & Prognosis

In general, the course of Graves' disease is one of remissions and exacerbations over a protracted period of time unless the gland is destroyed by surgery or radioactive iodine. Although some patients may remain euthyroid for long periods after treatment, many eventually develop hypothyroidism. Lifetime follow-up is therefore indicated for all patients with Graves' disease.

2. Other Forms of Thyrotoxicosis

Toxic Adenoma

(Plummer's Disease)

A functioning adenoma hypersecreting T_3 and T_4 will cause hyperthyroidism. These lesions start out as a "hot nodule" on the thyroid scan, slowly increase in size, and gradually suppress the other lobe of the gland (Figure

7–48). The typical patient is an older individual (usually over 40) who has noted recent growth of a long-standing thyroid nodule. Symptoms of weight loss, weakness, shortness of breath, palpitation, tachycardia, and heat intolerance are noted. Infiltrative ophthalmopathy is never present. Physical examination reveals a definite nodule on one side, with very little thyroid tissue on the other side. Laboratory studies usually reveal suppressed TSH and marked elevation in serum T_3 levels, often with only borderline elevation of thyroxine levels. The scan reveals that the nodule is "hot." Toxic adenomas are almost always follicular adenomas and almost never malignant. They are easily managed by administration of antithyroid drugs such as propylthiouracil, 100 mg every 6 hours, or methimazole, 10 mg every 6 hours, followed by treatment with radioactive iodine or unilateral lobectomy. Sodium ^{131}I in doses of 20–30 mCi is usually required to destroy the benign neoplasm. Radioactive iodine is preferable for smaller toxic nodules, but larger ones are best managed surgically.

Toxic Multinodular Goiter

This disorder usually occurs in older patients with longstanding multinodular goiter. Ophthalmopathy is extremely rare. Clinically, the patient presents with tachy-

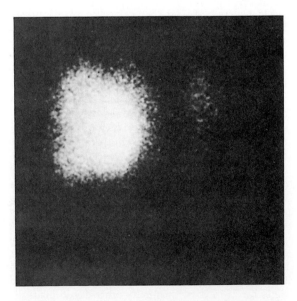

Figure 7–48. Solitary toxic nodule as it appears on ^{99m}Tc pertechnetate scan. Note suppression of contralateral lobe (left) by toxic nodule (right).

cardia, heart failure, or arrhythmia and sometimes weight loss, nervousness, weakness, tremors, and sweats. Physical examination reveals a multinodular goiter that may be small or quite large and may even extend substernally. Laboratory studies reveal a suppressed TSH and striking elevation in serum T_3 levels, with less striking elevation of serum T_4. Radioiodine scan reveals multiple functioning nodules in the gland or occasionally an irregular, patchy distribution of radioactive iodine (Figure 7–49).

Hyperthyroidism in patients with multinodular goiters can often be precipitated by the administration of iodides (often called "jodbasedow phenomenon," or iodide-induced hyperthyroidism). Some thyroid adenomas do not develop the Wolff-Chaikoff effect (see above) and cannot adapt to an iodide load. Thus, they are driven to excess hormone production by a high level of circulating iodide. This is one mechanism for the development of hyperthyroidism after administration of the antiarrhythmic drug amiodarone (see below).

The management of toxic nodular goiter is difficult. Control of the hyperthyroid state with antithyroid drugs followed by subtotal thyroidectomy would seem to be the therapy of choice, but often these patients are elderly and have other illnesses that make them poor candidates for surgery. The toxic nodules can be destroyed with ^{131}I, but the multinodular goiter will re-

main, and other nodules may become toxic, requiring repeated doses of [131]I.

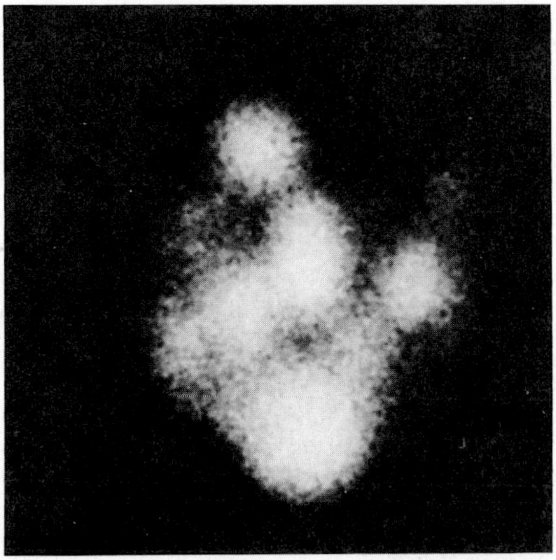

Amiodarone is an antiarrhythmic drug that contains 37.3% iodine. In the body, it is stored in fat, myocardium, liver, and lung and has a half-life of about 50 days. About 2% of patients treated with amiodarone develop amiodarone-induced thyrotoxicosis. In some patients, the thyrotoxicosis is due to the excess iodine; in others, it is due to an amiodarone-induced thyroiditis with dumping of stored hormone. Thyroid ultrasound with doppler examination of the thyroid circulation may be helpful in differentiating the two syndromes: The circulation is increased in iodide-induced hyperthyroidism and diminished in the chemically induced thyroiditis. Treatment is difficult. Iodide-induced thyrotoxicosis can be controlled with methimazole, 40–60 mg/d, and beta-adrenergic blockade. In addition, potassium perchlorate in a dose of 250 mg every 6 hours may be added to block further iodide uptake. However, long-term potassium chloride has been associated with aplastic anemia and requires monitoring. The chemical thyroiditis responds to prednisone therapy, which may be continued for several months. Total thyroidectomy is curative but is feasible only if the patient can withstand the stress of surgery. (See Chapter 24.)

Subacute or Chronic Thyroiditis

These entities will be discussed in a separate section, but it should be mentioned here that thyroiditis, either subacute or chronic, may present with an acute release of T_4 and T_3, producing symptoms of mild to severe thyrotoxicosis. These illnesses can be differentiated from other forms of thyrotoxicosis in that the radioiodine uptake is markedly suppressed, and the symptoms usually subside spontaneously over a period of weeks or months.

Thyrotoxicosis Factitia

This is a psychoneurotic disturbance in which the patient ingests excessive amounts of thyroxine or thyroid hormone, usually for purposes of weight control. The individual is often someone connected with the field of medicine who can easily obtain thyroid medication. Features of thyrotoxicosis, including weight loss, nervousness, palpitation, tachycardia, and tremor, may be present, but no goiter or eye signs. Characteristically, TSH is suppressed, serum T_4 and T_3 levels are elevated, serum thyroglobulin is low, and radioactive iodine uptake is nil. Management requires careful discussion of the hazards of long-term thyroxine therapy, particularly cardiovascular damage, muscle wasting, and osteoporosis. Formal psychotherapy may be necessary.

Figure 7–49. Toxic multinodular goiter as it appears on ^{99m}Tc pertechnetate scan. Note multiple functioning thyroid nodules. (Courtesy of JM Lowenstein.)

Rare Forms of Thyrotoxicosis

A. STRUMA OVARII

In this syndrome, a teratoma of the ovary contains thyroid tissue that becomes hyperactive. Mild features of thyrotoxicosis result, such as weight loss and tachycardia, but there is no evidence of goiter or eye signs. Serum FT_4 and T_3 are mildly elevated, serum TSH is suppressed, and radioiodine uptake in the neck is nil. Body scan reveals uptake of radioiodine in the pelvis. The disease is curable by removal of the teratoma.

B. THYROID CARCINOMA

Carcinoma of the thyroid, particularly follicular carcinoma, may concentrate radioactive iodine, but only rarely does it retain the ability to convert this iodide into active hormone. Only a few cases of metastatic thyroid cancer have presented with hyperthyroidism. The clinical picture consists of weakness, weight loss, palpitation, and a thyroid nodule but no ophthalmopathy. Body scan with ^{131}I reveals areas of uptake usually distant from the thyroid, eg, bone or lung. Treatment with large doses of radioactive iodine may destroy the metastatic deposits.

C. HYDATIDIFORM MOLE

Hydatidiform moles produce chorionic gonadotropin, which has intrinsic TSH-like activity. This may induce thyroid hyperplasia, increased iodine turnover, suppressed TSH, and mild elevation of serum T_4 and T_3 levels. It is rarely associated with overt thyrotoxicosis and is totally curable by removal of the mole.

D. "HAMBURGER THYROTOXICOSIS"

An epidemic of thyrotoxicosis in the midwestern United States was traced to hamburger made from "neck trim," the strap muscles from the necks of slaughtered cattle that contained beef thyroid tissue. The United States Department of Agriculture has now prohibited the use of this material for human consumption.

E. SYNDROME OF INAPPROPRIATE TSH SECRETION

A group of patients have been reported with elevated serum free thyroxine concentrations in association with elevated serum immunoreactive TSH. This has been called the "syndrome of inappropriate TSH secretion." Two types of problems are found: (1) TSH-secreting pituitary adenoma and (2) nonneoplastic pituitary hypersecretion of TSH.

Patients with **TSH-secreting pituitary adenomas** usually present with mild thyrotoxicosis and goiter, often with evidence of gonadotropic hormone deficiency such as amenorrhea or impotence. There are no eye signs of Graves' disease. Study reveals elevated total and free serum T_4 and T_3. Serum TSH, usually undetectable in Graves' disease, is within the normal range or even elevated. The TSH α subunit secretion from these tumors is markedly elevated; a molar ratio of α subunit:TSH greater than 5.7 is usually diagnostic of the presence of a TSH-secreting pituitary adenoma.* In addition, there is no hormonal response to TRH, and the increased radioactive iodine uptake is not suppressible with exogenous thyroid hormone. Visual field examination may reveal temporal defects, and CT or MRI of the sella usually reveals a pituitary tumor. Management usually involves control of the thyrotoxicosis with antithyroid drugs and removal of the pituitary tumor via transsphenoidal hypophysectomy. These tumors are often quite aggressive and may extend widely out of the sella. If the tumor cannot be completely removed, it may be necessary to treat residual tumor with radiation therapy and to control thyrotoxicosis with radioactive iodine. Long-acting somatostatin (octreotide) will suppress TSH secretion in many of these patients and may even inhibit tumor growth in some.

Nonneoplastic pituitary hypersecretion of TSH is essentially a form of pituitary (and occasionally peripheral) resistance to T_3 and T_4. This is discussed below.

THYROID HORMONE RESISTANCE SYNDROMES

Several forms of resistance to thyroid hormones have been reported: (1) generalized resistance to thyroid hormones (GRTH), (2) selective pituitary resistance to thyroid hormones (PRTH), and possibly (3) a selective peripheral resistance to thyroid hormones (perRTH).

Generalized resistance to thyroid hormones was first described in 1967 by Refetoff and coworkers as a familial syndrome of deaf mutism, stippled epiphyses, goiter, and abnormally high thyroid hormone levels with normal TSH. The clinical presentation in the more than 500 cases that have been reported has been variable; while most patients are euthyroid, many present with goiter, stunted growth, delayed maturation, attention deficits, hyperactivity disorders, and resting tachycardia. Seventy-five percent of reported cases are familial. Inheritance is autosomal dominant. Laboratory tests reveal elevated T_4, FT_4, T_3, and normal or elevated TSH. Dynamic tests to distinguish generalized resistance to thyroid hormones from TSH-secreting adenomas usually reveal an increase in TSH after administration of TRH, a fall in TSH with T_3 suppression, and a molar

---

*The α subunit:TSH molar ratio is calculated as follows: α subunit in $\mu g/L$ divided by TSH in $\mu U/L \times 10$. Normal range (for a patient with normal TSH and gonadotrophins) is < 5.7.

ratio of α subunit:TSH of less than 1. In addition, in patients with GRTH, pituitary MRI fails to demonstrate a microadenoma. Molecular studies have revealed point mutations in the carboxyl terminal ligand-binding portion of the human thyroid receptor beta gene (*TRβ*), which produces a defective thyroid hormone receptor (TR) that fails to bind T_3 but retains the ability to bind to DNA. In addition, the mutant TR occupies the TRE as an inactive dimer or heterodimer, perhaps inducing sustained gene repression (Figures 7–25 and 7–26). Different point mutations in different families may account in part for the differences in clinical expression of the syndrome. Furthermore, identification of the mutation in affected individuals may allow the use of molecular screening methods for the diagnosis of the syndrome in some families.

In most patients with generalized resistance to thyroid hormones, the increased levels of T_3 and T_4 will compensate in part for the receptor defect, and treatment is not necessary. In some children, administration of thyroid hormone may be necessary to correct defects in growth or mental development.

Selective pituitary resistance to thyroid hormones is less common and usually presents with symptoms of mild hyperthyroidism, goiter, elevated serum T_4 and T_3, and normal or elevated serum TSH. In this syndrome, T_3 receptors in peripheral tissues are normal, but there is a failure of T_3 to inhibit pituitary TSH secretion, resulting in inappropriate TSH secretion and TSH-induced hyperthyroidism. Differentiation from TSH-secreting pituitary adenoma can be made using the dynamic tests and MRI of the pituitary as outlined above.

This syndrome may be due in part to some abnormality in the pituitary type 2 5′-deiodinase with failure to convert intrapituitary T_4 to T_3, leading to PTHR. Ablation of the thyroid gland with ^{131}I or treatment with antithyroid drugs may lead to pituitary hyperplasia. However, administration of triiodothyroacetic acid (TRIAC) has been reported to suppress TSH, reduce the size of the goiter, lower serum T_4, and correct the hyperthyroidism.

Only one case of suspected selective peripheral resistance to T_3 has been reported, and it is not yet clear that this is a distinct entity.

TSH Receptor Gene Mutations

Mutations in the TSH receptor gene can produce a variety of clinical syndromes. Somatic mutations in the seven-transmembrane loop of the TSH-R may activate the receptor, producing solitary or multiple hyperfunctioning adenomas, whereas germline mutations may result in congenital hyperthyroidism in the newborn. Mutations in the extracellular amino terminal of the TSH-R produce resistance to TSH with uncompen-

sated or compensated hypothyroidism. The patient reported by Refetoff had normal FT_4 and FT_3 and normal growth and development but persistently elevated serum TSH. The patients reported by Medeiros-Neto were severely hypothyroid (cretinoid), with low FT_4 levels, elevated TSH, and no response to exogenous TSH. In this group, the defect may be in the coupling of TSH-R and the G_s protein necessary for activation of adenylyl cyclase.

NONTOXIC GOITER

Etiology

Nontoxic goiter usually represents enlargement of the thyroid gland from TSH stimulation, which in turn results from inadequate thyroid hormone synthesis. Table 7–11 lists some of the causes of nontoxic goiter.

Iodine deficiency was the most common cause of nontoxic goiter or "endemic goiter"; with the widespread use of iodized salt and the introduction of iodides into fertilizers, animal feeds, and food preservatives, iodide deficiency in developed countries has become relatively rare. It does not exist in the United States. However, there are large areas such as central Africa, the mountainous areas of central Asia, the Andes of central South America, and Indonesia (particularly New Guinea), where iodine intake is still markedly deficient. Optimal iodine requirements for adults are in the range of 150–300 µg/d. In endemic goiter areas, the daily intake (and urinary excretion) of iodine falls below 50 µg/d; in areas where iodine is extremely scarce, excretion falls below 20 µg/d. It is in these areas that 90% of the population will have goiters, and 5–15% of infants will be born with myxedematous or neurologic changes of cretinism. The variability in the extent of goiter in these areas may be related to the presence of other, unidentified goitrogens.

Dietary goitrogens are a rare cause of goiter, and of these the most common is iodide itself. Large amounts of iodide, as in amiodarone or kelp tablets, may in susceptible individuals produce goiter and hypothyroidism

Table 7–11. Etiology of nontoxic goiter.

1. Iodine deficiency
2. Goitrogen in the diet
3. Hashimoto's thyroiditis
4. Subacute thyroiditis
5. Inadequate hormone synthesis due to inherited defect in thyroidal enzymes necessary for T_4 and T_3 biosynthesis
6. Generalized resistance to thyroid hormone (rare)
7. Neoplasm, benign or malignant

(see above). Withdrawal of iodide reverses the process. Other goitrogens include lithium carbonate and some vegetable foodstuffs such as goitrin, found in certain roots and seeds; and cyanogenic glycosides, found in cassava and cabbage, that release thiocyanates which may cause goiter, particularly in the presence of iodide deficiency. In addition, compounds such as phenols, phthalates, pyridines, and polyaromatic hydrocarbons found in industrial waste water are weakly goitrogenic. The role of these vegetable and pollutant goitrogens in the production of goiter is not clearly established.

The most common cause of thyroid enlargement in developed countries is chronic thyroiditis (Hashimoto's thyroiditis; see below). Subacute thyroiditis causes thyroid enlargement with exquisite tenderness (see below).

Nontoxic goiter may be due to impaired hormone synthesis resulting from genetic deficiencies in enzymes necessary for hormone biosynthesis (thyroid dyshormonogenesis, or familial goiter). These effects may be complete, resulting in a syndrome of cretinism with goiter; or partial, resulting in nontoxic goiter with mild hypothyroidism. At least five separate biosynthetic abnormalities have been reported: (1) impaired transport of iodine; (2) deficient peroxidase with impaired oxidation of iodide to iodine and failure to incorporate iodine into thyroglobulin; (3) impaired coupling of iodinated tyrosines to triiodothyronine or tetraiodothyronine; (4) absence or deficiency of iodotyrosine deiodinase, so that iodine is not conserved within the gland; and (5) excessive production of metabolically inactive iodoprotein by the thyroid gland (Figure 7–9). The latter may involve impaired or abnormal thyroglobulin synthesis. In all of these syndromes, impaired production of thyroid hormones presumably results in TSH release and goiter formation.

Finally, thyroid enlargement can be due to a benign lesion, such as adenoma, or to a malignant one such as carcinoma.

Pathogenesis

The development of nontoxic goiter in patients with dyshormonogenesis or severe iodine deficiency involves impaired hormone synthesis and, secondarily, an increase in TSH secretion. TSH induces diffuse thyroid hyperplasia, followed by focal hyperplasia with necrosis and hemorrhage, and finally the development of new areas of focal hyperplasia. Focal or nodular hyperplasia usually involves a clone of cells that may or may not be able to pick up iodine or synthesize thyroglobulin. Thus, the nodules will vary from "hot" nodules that can concentrate iodine to "cold" ones that cannot, and from colloid nodules that can synthesize thyroglobulin to microfollicular ones that cannot. Initially, the hyperplasia is TSH-dependent, but later the nodules become TSH-independent, or autonomous. Thus, a diffuse nontoxic TSH-dependent goiter progresses over a period of time to a multinodular toxic or nontoxic TSH-independent goiter.

The mechanism for the development of autonomous growth and function of thyroid nodules may involve mutations that occur with TSH-induced cell division in an oncogene that activates the G_s protein in the cell membrane. Mutations of this oncogene, called the *gsp* oncogene, have been found in a high proportion of nodules from patients with multinodular goiter. Chronic activation of the G_s protein would result in thyroid cell proliferation and hyperfunction even when TSH is suppressed.

Clinical Features

A. SYMPTOMS AND SIGNS

Patients with nontoxic goiter usually present with thyroid enlargement, which, as noted above, may be diffuse or multinodular. The gland may be relatively firm but is often extremely soft. Over a period of time, the gland becomes progressively larger, so that in long-standing multinodular goiter, huge goiters may develop and extend inferiorly to present as substernal goiter. Facial flushing and dilation of cervical veins on lifting the arms over the head is a positive **Pemberton sign** and indicates obstruction. The patient may complain of pressure symptoms in the neck, particularly on moving the head upward or downward, and of difficulty in swallowing. Vocal cord paralysis due to recurrent laryngeal nerve involvement is rare. There may be symptoms of mild hypothyroidism, but most of these patients are euthyroid. Thyroid enlargement probably represents compensated hypothyroidism.

B. LABORATORY FINDINGS

Laboratory studies will reveal a low or normal free thyroxine and, usually, normal levels of TSH. The increased mass of thyroid tissue compensates for inefficient synthesis of hormone. In patients with dyshormonogenesis due to abnormal iodoprotein synthesis, PBI and serum thyroglobulin may be elevated out of proportion to serum T_4, because of secretion of nonhormonal organic iodide compounds. Radioiodine uptake may be high, normal, or low, depending upon the iodide pool and the TSH drive.

C. IMAGING STUDIES

Isotope scanning usually reveals a patchy uptake, frequently with focal areas of increased uptake corresponding to "hot" nodules and areas of decreased uptake corresponding to "cold" nodules. Radioactive iodine uptake of the "hot" nodules may not be suppressible on administration of thyroid hormones such as liothyronine. Thyroid ultrasound is a simple way to follow the growth of the goiter and in addition may reveal cystic changes in one or more of the nodules, representing previous hemorrhage and necrosis.

Differential Diagnosis

The major problem in differential diagnosis is to rule out cancer. This will be discussed in the section on thyroid carcinoma.

Treatment

With the exception of those due to neoplasm, the current management of nontoxic goiters consists simply of giving thyroid hormone until TSH is suppressed to 0.1–0.4 µU/L (normal range is 0.5–5 µU/L). This requires levothyroxine in doses of 0.1–0.2 mg (approximately 2.2 µg/kg, or 1 µg/lb) daily. This will correct hypothyroidism and often result in slow regression of the goiter. Long-standing goiters may have areas of necrosis, hemorrhage, and scarring as well as autonomously functioning nodules that will not regress on thyroxine therapy. However, the lesions will usually grow more slowly while the patient is taking thyroxine. In older patients with multinodular goiters, administration of levothyroxine must be done very cautiously since the "hot" nodules are autonomous and the combination of endogenous and exogenous hormone will rapidly produce toxic symptoms.

Surgery is indicated for goiters that continue to grow despite TSH suppression with T_4 or those that produce obstructive symptoms. Substernal extension of a goiter is usually an indication for surgical removal. The gross appearance of a multinodular goiter at the time of surgery is presented in Figure 7–50. Note that the left lobe of the gland extends downward from the middle of the thyroid cartilage to just above the clavicle. The pressure of this enlargement has caused deviation of the trachea to the right. The surface of the gland is irregular, with many large and small nodules. Although these multinodular goiters are rarely malignant, the size of the mass with resulting pressure symptoms requires subtotal thyroidectomy.

If the patient is not a suitable candidate for surgery, radioiodine ablation of functioning thyroid tissue may provide palliative relief of obstructive symptoms. An adequate dose of radioiodine will reduce the size of the goiter about 30%, but the residual tissue may regrow, with recurrence of symptoms.

Course & Prognosis

Patients with nontoxic goiter must usually take levothyroxine for life. They should avoid iodides, which may induce either hyperthyroidism or, in the absence of thy-

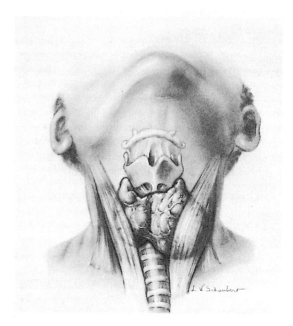

Figure 7–50. Multinodular goiter at the time of surgery. The asymmetric enlargement and the nodularity are apparent, as is the rightward deviation of the trachea resulting from marked enlargement of the lobe.

roxine therapy, hypothyroidism. Occasionally, single adenomas or several adenomas will become hyperfunctional, producing a toxic nodular goiter (discussed above). Nontoxic goiter is often familial, and other members of the family should be examined and observed for the possible development of goiter.

THYROIDITIS

1. Subacute Thyroiditis

Subacute thyroiditis (De Quervain's thyroiditis, or granulomatous thyroiditis) is an acute inflammatory disorder of the thyroid gland most likely due to viral infection. A number of viruses, including mumps virus, coxsackievirus, and adenoviruses, have been implicated, either by finding the virus in biopsy specimens taken from the gland or by demonstration of rising titers of viral antibodies in the blood during the course of the infection. Pathologic examination reveals moderate thyroid enlargement and a mild inflammatory reaction involving the capsule. Histologic features include destruction of thyroid parenchyma and the presence of many large phagocytic cells, including giant cells.

Clinical Features

A. SYMPTOMS AND SIGNS

Subacute thyroiditis usually presents with fever, malaise, and soreness in the neck, which may extend up to the angle of the jaw or toward the ear lobes on one or both sides of the neck. Initially, the patient may have symptoms of hyperthyroidism, with palpitations, agitation, and sweats. There is no ophthalmopathy. On physical examination, the gland is exquisitely tender, so that the patient will object to pressure upon it. There are no signs of local redness or heat suggestive of abscess formation. Clinical signs of toxicity, including tachycardia, tremor, and hyperreflexia, may be present.

B. LABORATORY FINDINGS

Laboratory studies will vary with the course of the disease (Figure 7–51). Initially, T_4 and T_3 are elevated, whereas serum TSH and thyroid radioactive iodine uptake are extremely low. The erythrocyte sedimentation rate is markedly elevated, sometimes as high as 100 mm/h by the Westergren scale. Thyroid autoantibodies are usually not detectable in serum. As the disease progresses, T_4 and T_3 will drop, TSH will rise, and symptoms of hypothyroidism are noted. Later, radioactive iodine uptake will rise, reflecting recovery of the gland from the acute insult.

Differential Diagnosis

Subacute thyroiditis can be differentiated from other viral illnesses by the involvement of the thyroid gland. It is differentiated from Graves' disease by the presence of low thyroid radioiodine uptake associated with elevated serum T_3 and T_4 and suppressed serum TSH and by the absence of thyroid antibodies.

Treatment

In most cases, only symptomatic treatment is necessary, eg, acetaminophen, 0.5 g four times daily. If pain, fever, and malaise are disabling, a short course of a nonsteroidal anti-inflammatory drug or a glucocorticoid such as prednisone, 20 mg three times daily for 7–10 days, may be necessary to reduce the inflammation. Levothyroxine, 0.1–0.15 mg once daily, is indicated during the hypothyroid phase of the illness in order to prevent reexacerbation of the disease induced by the rising TSH levels. In about 10% of patients, permanent hypothyroidism ensues and long-term levothyroxine therapy is necessary.

Course & Prognosis

Subacute thyroiditis usually resolves completely and spontaneously over weeks or months. Occasionally, the disease may begin to resolve and then suddenly get worse, sometimes involving first one lobe of the thyroid gland and then the other (migrating thyroiditis). Exacerbations often occur when the T_4 levels have fallen, the TSH level has risen, and the gland is starting to recover function. Rarely, the course may extend over several years, with repeated bouts of inflammatory disease.

2. Chronic Thyroiditis

Chronic thyroiditis (Hashimoto's thyroiditis, lymphocytic thyroiditis) is probably the most common cause of hypothyroidism and goiter in the United States. It is certainly the major cause of goiter in children and young adults and is probably the major cause of "idiopathic myxedema," which represents an end stage of Hashimoto's thyroiditis, with total destruction of the gland. **Riedel's struma** is probably a variant of Hashimoto's thyroiditis, with extensive fibrosis extending outside the gland and involving overlying muscle and surrounding tissues. Riedel's struma presents as a stony-hard mass that must be differentiated from thyroid cancer.

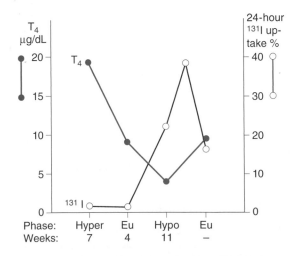

Figure 7–51. Changes in serum T_4 and radioactive iodine uptake in patients with subacute thyroiditis. In the initial phase, serum T_4 is elevated and the patient may have symptoms of thyrotoxicosis, but radioactive iodine uptake is markedly suppressed. The illness may pass through phases of euthyroidism and hypothyroidism before remission. (Data adapted, with permission, from Woolf PD, Daly R: Thyrotoxicosis with painless thyroiditis. Am J Med 1976;60:73.)

Etiology & Pathogenesis

Hashimoto's thyroiditis is thought to be an immunologic disorder in which lymphocytes become sensitized to thyroidal antigens and autoantibodies are formed that react with these antigens (see thyroid autoimmunity, above). In Hashimoto's thyroiditis, the three most important thyroid autoantibodies are thyroglobulin antibody (Tg Ab), thyroperoxidase antibody (TPO Ab), and TSH receptor blocking antibody (TSH-R Ab [block]). During the early phases of Hashimoto's thyroiditis, Tg Ab is markedly elevated and TPO Ab is slightly elevated. Later, Tg Ab may disappear, but TPO Ab will be present for many years. TSH-R Ab [block] is found in patients with **atrophic thyroiditis** and myxedema and in mothers giving birth to infants with no detectable thyroid tissue **(athyreotic cretins).** The pathology of Hashimoto's thyroiditis involves a heavy infiltration of lymphocytes totally destroying normal thyroidal architecture. Lymphoid follicles and germinal centers may be formed. The follicular epithelial cells are frequently enlarged and contain a basophilic cytoplasm (Hurthle cells). Destruction of the gland results in a fall in serum T_3 and T_4 and a rise in TSH. Initially, TSH may maintain adequate hormonal synthesis by the development of thyroid enlargement or goiter, but often the gland fails, and hypothyroidism with or without goiter ensues.

Hashimoto's thyroiditis is part of a spectrum of thyroid diseases that includes Graves' disease at one end and idiopathic myxedema at the other (Figure 7–52). It is familial and may be associated with other autoimmune diseases such as pernicious anemia, adrenocortical insufficiency, idiopathic hypoparathyroidism, myasthenia gravis, and vitiligo. **Schmidt's syndrome** consists of Hashimoto's thyroiditis, idiopathic adrenal insufficiency, hypoparathyroidism, diabetes mellitus, and ovarian insufficiency. Schmidt's syndrome represents destruction of multiple endocrine glands on an autoimmune basis (Chapter 4).

Clinical Features

A. SYMPTOMS AND SIGNS

Hashimoto's thyroiditis usually presents with goiter in a patient who is euthyroid or has mild hypothyroidism. The sex distribution is about four females to one male. The process is painless, and the patient may be unaware of the goiter unless it becomes very large. Older patients may present with severe hypothyroidism with only a small, firm atrophic thyroid gland (idiopathic myxedema).

B. LABORATORY FINDINGS

There are multiple defects in iodine metabolism. Peroxidase activity is decreased, so that organification of iodine is impaired. This can be demonstrated by a positive perchlorate discharge test (Figure 7–11). In addition, iodination of metabolically inactive protein material occurs, so that there will be a disproportionately high serum PBI and serum globulin compared with serum T_4. Radioiodine uptake may be high, normal, or low. Circulating thyroid hormone levels are usually normal or low, and if low, TSH will be elevated.

The most striking laboratory finding is the high titer of autoantibodies to thyroidal antigens in the serum. Serum tests for either Tg Ab or TPO Ab are positive in most patients with Hashimoto's thyroiditis. Another diagnostic test that may be helpful is the fine-needle aspiration biopsy, which reveals a large infiltration of lymphocytes as well as the presence of Hurthle cells.

Differential Diagnosis

Hashimoto's thyroiditis can be differentiated from other causes of nontoxic goiter by serum antibody studies and, if necessary, by fine-needle aspiration biopsy.

Idiopathic myxedema	Hashimoto's thyroiditis	"Euthyroid Graves' disease"	Graves' disease
Hypothyroid without goiter	Hypothyroid or euthyroid with goiter	Euthyroid with or without goiter	Hyperthyroid with goiter

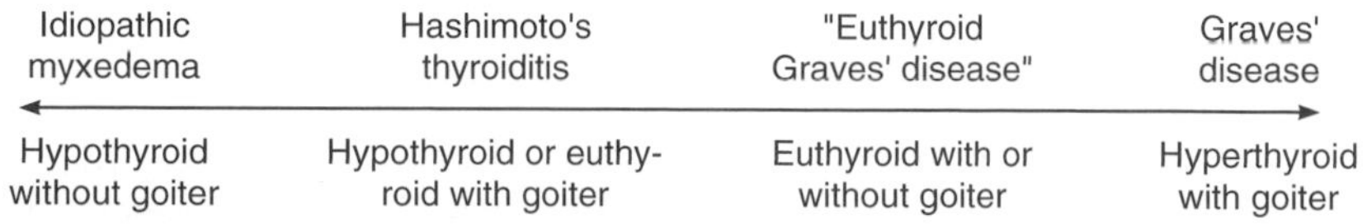

Figure 7–52. Spectrum of autoimmune disease of the thyroid gland. The clinical manifestations of autoimmune disease of the thyroid gland range from idiopathic myxedema, through nontoxic goiter, to diffuse toxic goiter, or Graves' disease. Progression of autoimmune disease from one form to another in the same patient can occasionally occur.

Complications & Sequelae

The major complication of Hashimoto's thyroiditis is progressive hypothyroidism. Although only 10–15% of young patients presenting with goiter and hypothyroidism seem to progress to permanent hypothyroidism, the high incidence of permanent hypothyroidism in older patients with positive antibody tests and elevated TSH levels suggests that long-term treatment is desirable. Rarely, a patient with Hashimoto's thyroiditis may develop lymphoma of the thyroid gland, but whether the two conditions are causally related is not clear. Thyroid lymphoma is characterized by rapid growth of the gland despite continued thyroid hormone therapy; the diagnosis of lymphoma must be made by surgical biopsy (see below).

There is no evidence that adenocarcinoma of the thyroid gland occurs more frequently in patients with Hashimoto's thyroiditis, but the two diseases—chronic thyroiditis and carcinoma—can coexist in the same gland. Cancer must be suspected when a solitary nodule or thyroid mass grows or fails to regress while the patient is receiving maximal tolerated doses of thyroxine. Fine-needle aspiration biopsy is helpful in this differential diagnosis.

Treatment

The indications for treatment of Hashimoto's thyroiditis are goiter or hypothyroidism; a positive thyroid antibody test does not require therapy. Sufficient levothyroxine is given to suppress TSH and allow regression of the goiter. Surgery is rarely indicated.

Course & Prognosis

Without treatment, Hashimoto's thyroiditis will usually progress from goiter and hypothyroidism to myxedema. The goiter and the myxedema are totally corrected by adequate thyroxine therapy. Hashimoto's thyroiditis may go through periods of activity when large amounts of T_4 and T_3 are released or "dumped," resulting in transient symptoms of thyrotoxicosis. This syndrome, which has been called **spontaneously resolving hyperthyroidism,** is characterized by low radioiodine uptake. However, it can be differentiated from subacute thyroiditis in that the gland is not tender, the erythrocyte sedimentation rate is not elevated, autoantibodies to thyroidal antigens are strongly positive, and fine-needle aspiration biopsy reveals lymphocytes and Hurthle cells. Therapy is symptomatic, usually requiring only propranolol, until symptoms subside; T_4 supplementation may then be necessary.

Because Hashimoto's thyroiditis may be part of a syndrome of multiple autoimmune diseases (Chapter 4), the patient should be monitored for other autoimmune diseases such as pernicious anemia, adrenal insufficiency, hypothyroidism, or diabetes mellitus. Patients with Hashimoto's thyroiditis may also develop true Graves' disease, occasionally with severe ophthalmopathy or dermopathy (Figure 7–52). The chronic thyroiditis may blunt the severity of the thyrotoxicosis, so that the patient may present with eye or skin complications of Graves' disease without marked thyrotoxicosis, a syndrome often called **euthyroid Graves' disease.** The thyroid gland will invariably be nonsuppressible, and this, plus the presence of thyroid autoantibodies, will help to make the diagnosis. The ophthalmopathy and dermopathy are treated as if thyrotoxic Graves' disease were present.

3. Other Forms of Thyroiditis

The thyroid gland may be subject to acute abscess formation in patients with septicemia or acute infective endocarditis. Abscesses cause symptoms of pyogenic infection, with local pain and tenderness, swelling, and warmth and redness of the overlying skin. Needle aspiration will confirm the diagnosis and identify the organism. Treatment includes antibiotic therapy and occasionally incision and drainage. A thyroglossal duct cyst may become infected and present as acute suppurative thyroiditis. This too will respond to antibiotic therapy and occasionally incision and drainage.

EFFECTS OF IONIZING RADIATION ON THE THYROID GLAND

Ionizing radiation can induce both acute and chronic thyroiditis. Thyroiditis may occur acutely in patients treated with large doses of radioiodine and may be associated with release of thyroid hormones and an acute thyrotoxic crisis. Such an occurrence is extremely rare, however, and pretreatment with antithyroid drugs to bring the patient to a euthyroid state prior to ^{131}I therapy will completely prevent this type of radiation thyroiditis.

External radiation was used many years ago for the treatment of respiratory problems in the newborn, thought to be due to thymic hyperplasia, and for the treatment of benign conditions such as severe acne and chronic tonsillitis or adenoiditis. This treatment was often associated with the later development of nodular goiter, hypothyroidism, or thyroid cancer. Another source of radiation exposure is fallout from atomic bomb testing or a nuclear reactor accident.

The incidence of thyroid lesions after irradiation is summarized in Table 7–12. As little as 6.5 cGy (1 cGy = 1 rad) to the thyroid gland received during the radia-

Table 7–12. Thyroid lesions after irradiation.

Areas Treated	Estimated Dose to Thyroid (cGy)	Incidence (%)		Source
		Nodular Goiter	Cancer	
Scalp	6.5	...	0.11	Modan et al (1974)
Thymus				
Total group	119	1.8	0.8	Hemplemann et al (1975)
Subgroup	399	7.6	5.0	
Neck, chest	807	27.2	5.7	Favus et al (1975)
	180–1500	26.2	6.8	Refetoff et al (1975)
Radiation fallout	< 50	...	0.4	Parker et al (1974)
	> 50	...	6.7	Sampson et al (1969)
	175 (γ) and 700–1400 (β)	39.6	5.7	Conrad et al (1970)
^{131}I therapy	≈10,000	0.17	0.08	Dobyns et al (1974)

tion treatment of tinea capitis has been reported to cause cancer in 0.11% of exposed children; the incidence of thyroid cancer in sibling controls was 0.02%. Radiation therapy to the thymus delivered to the thyroid dosages of 100–400 cGy, and the incidence of thyroid cancer attributed to this source ranged from 0.5% to 5%. X-ray therapy to the neck and chest given to children or adolescents for acne or chronic upper respiratory infections delivered thyroid doses ranging from 200 cGy to 1500 cGy, resulting in the development of nodular goiter in about 27% and thyroid cancer in 5–7% of the patients so treated. These tumors developed 10–40 years after radiation was administered, with a peak incidence at 20–30 years. Radiation fallout with a thyroid dose of 700–1400 cGy has produced nodular goiter in approximately 40% of exposed victims and thyroid cancer in about 6%. However, radioiodine therapy, which exposes the thyroid to a dosage of around 10,000 cGy, was rarely associated with the development of thyroid cancer, presumably because the thyroid gland is largely destroyed by these doses of radioiodine, so that—although the incidence of postradiation hypothyroidism is high—the incidence of thyroid cancer is extremely low. Ninety percent of patients with radiation-induced thyroid cancer develop papillary carcinoma; the remainder develop follicular carcinoma. Medullary carcinoma and anaplastic carcinomas have been rare following radiation exposure. Although the overall incidence of thyroid carcinoma in irradiated patients is low, data from several large series suggest that the incidence of cancer in a patient who presents with a solitary cold nodule of the thyroid gland and a history of therapeutic radiation of the head, neck, or chest is around 50%.

The most recent episode of radiation-induced thyroid neoplasia was the Chernobyl disaster in April 1986, at which time huge amounts of radioactive material, especially radioiodine, were released. As early as 4 years later, a striking increase in the incidence of thyroid nodules and thyroid cancer was noted in children in Gomel, an area in the Republic of Belarus, close to Chernobyl and heavily contaminated. A high proportion of the cancers arose in young children and developed after a very short latency period. The sex distribution was equal. Most of the cancers were papillary carcinomas and were very aggressive, with intraglandular, capsular, local, and lymph node invasion.

Patients who have been exposed to ionizing radiation should be followed carefully for life. Annual studies should include physical examination of the neck for goiter or nodules, and FT_4 or TSH determinations to rule out hypothyroidism. Periodic thyroid ultrasound may detect nodules that are not palpable. If a nodule is found, it should be scanned with ^{123}I, and if cold, fine-needle aspiration biopsy should be done. If the nodule is malignant, the patient should have total thyroidectomy; if benign, the patient should be treated with levothyroxine in a dose sufficient to suppress TSH. If the nodule persists or grows while T_4 therapy is being given, the thyroid gland should be surgically removed.

THYROID NODULES & THYROID CANCER

In 95% of cases, thyroid cancer presents as a nodule or lump in the thyroid. In occasional instances, particularly in children, enlarged cervical lymph nodes are the first sign of the disease, though on careful examination a small primary focus in the form of a thyroid nodule can often be felt. Rarely, distant metastasis in lung or bone is the first sign of thyroid cancer. Thyroid nodules are extremely common, particularly among women. The prevalence of thyroid nodules in the USA has been estimated to be about 4% of the adult population, with a female:male ratio of 4:1. In young children, the prevalence is less than 1%; in persons aged 11–18 years, about 1.5%; and in persons over age 60, about 5%.

In contrast to thyroid nodules, thyroid cancer is a rare condition, with a prevalence of 0.004% per year according to the Third National Cancer Survey. Thus, most thyroid nodules are benign, and it is important to identify those that are likely to be malignant.

1. Benign Thyroid Nodules

Etiology

Benign conditions that can produce nodularity in the thyroid gland are listed in Table 7–13. They include focal areas of chronic thyroiditis, a dominant portion of a multinodular goiter, a cyst involving thyroid tissue, parathyroid tissue, or thyroglossal duct remnants, and agenesis of one lobe of the thyroid, with hypertrophy of the other lobe presenting as a mass in the neck. It is usually the left lobe of the thyroid that fails to develop, and the hypertrophy occurs in the right lobe. Scarring in the gland following surgery—or regrowth of the gland after surgery or radioiodine therapy—can present with nodularity. Finally, benign neoplasms in the thyroid include follicular adenomas such as colloid or macrofollicular adenomas, fetal adenomas, embryonal adenomas, and Hurthle cell or oxyphil adenomas. Rare types of benign lesions include teratomas, lipomas, and hemangiomas. Except for thyroid hyperplasia of the right lobe of the gland in the presence of agenesis of the left lobe—and

Table 7–13. Etiology of benign thyroid nodules.

1. Focal thyroiditis
2. Dominant portion of multinodular goiter
3. Thyroid, parathyroid, or thyroglossal cysts
4. Agenesis of a thyroid lobe
5. Postsurgical remnant hyperplasia or scarring
6. Postradioiodine remnant hyperplasia
7. Benign adenomas:
   a. Follicular:
      Colloid or macrofollicular
      Fetal
      Embryonal
      Hürthle cell
   b. Rare: Teratoma, lipoma, hemangioma

some follicular adenomas—all of the above lesions present as "cold" nodules on isotope scanning.

Differentiation of Benign & Malignant Lesions

Risk factors that predispose to benign or malignant disease are set forth in Table 7–14 and discussed below.

A. History

A family history of goiter suggests benign disease, as does residence in an area of endemic goiter. However, a family history of medullary carcinoma or a history of recent thyroid growth, hoarseness, dysphagia, or obstruction strongly suggests cancer. The significance of exposure to ionizing radiation is discussed above.

B. Physical Characteristics

Physical characteristics associated with a low risk for thyroid cancer include older age, female sex, soft thyroid nodules, and the presence of a multinodular goiter. Individuals at higher risk for thyroid cancer include children, young adults, and males. A solitary firm or dominant nodule that is clearly different from the rest of the gland signifies an increased risk of malignancy. Vocal cord paralysis, enlarged lymph nodes, and suspected metastases are strongly suggestive of malignancy.

C. Serum Factors

A high titer of thyroid autoantibodies in serum suggests chronic thyroiditis as the cause of thyroid enlargement but does not rule out an associated malignancy. However, an elevated serum calcitonin, particularly in patients with a family history of medullary carcinoma, strongly suggests the presence of thyroid cancer. Elevated serum thyroglobulin following total thyroidectomy for papillary or follicular thyroid cancer usually indicates metastatic disease, but serum thyroglobulin is not usually helpful in determining the nature of a thyroid nodule.

D. Imaging Studies

Scanning procedures can be used to identify "hot" or "cold" nodules, ie, those that take up more or less radioactive iodine than surrounding tissue. Hot nodules are almost never malignant, whereas cold ones may be. Scintillation camera photographs with ^{99m}Tc pertechnetate give the best resolution (Figure 7–53). Thyroid ultrasound can distinguish cystic from solid lesions. A pure cyst is almost never malignant. Cystic lesions that have internal septa or solid lesions on ultrasound may be benign or malignant. CT scanning or MRI may be

Table 7–14. Risk factors useful in distinguishing benign from malignant thyroid lesions.

	More Likely Benign	More Likely Malignant
History	Family history of benign goiter Residence in endemic goiter area	Family history of medullary cancer of thyroid Previous therapeutic irradiation of head or neck Recent growth of nodule Hoarseness, dysphagia, or obstruction
Physical characteristics	Older woman Soft nodule Multinodular goiter	Child, young adult, male Solitary, firm nodule clearly different from rest of gland ("dominant nodule") Vocal cord paralysis, firm lymph nodes, distant metastases
Serum factors	High titer of thyroid autoantibodies	Elevated serum calcitonin
Scanning techniques ^{123}I or ^{99m}TcO$_4$	"Hot nodule"	"Cold nodule"
Echo scan	Cyst (pure)	Solid or semicystic
Biopsy (needle)	Benign appearance on cytologic examination	Malignant or suggestion of malignancy
Levothyroxine therapy (TSH suppression for 3–6 months)	Regression	No regression

helpful in defining substernal extension or deep thyroid nodules in the neck.

E. NEEDLE BIOPSY

The major advance in management of the thyroid nodule in recent years has been the fine-needle aspiration biopsy (see above). Large-needle core aspiration biopsies of thyroid nodules have been available since about 1930, but they are limited to large nodules and are relatively traumatic. Söderström in 1952 introduced the technique of fine-needle aspiration biopsy, which is simple, safe, reliable, and well-tolerated (Figure 7–54).

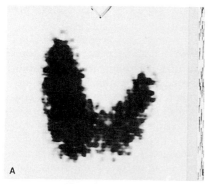 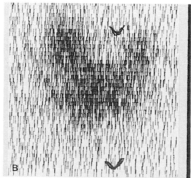 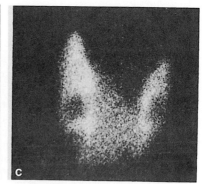

Figure 7–53. Demonstration of resolution obtained utilizing different scanning techniques: **A:** ^{123}I scintiscan with rectilinear scanner. **B:** Fluorescent scan with rectilinear scanner. **C:** ^{99m}Tc pertechnetate scan with the pinhole collimated gamma camera. Note the presence of two "cold" nodules, one in each lobe of the thyroid, easily detected in **C** but not clearly delineated in the other two scans. The lesion in the right lobe was palpable, about 1 cm in diameter, and was shown to be follicular carcinoma on needle biopsy. The lesion in the left lobe was either a metastatic tumor or a second primary follicular carcinoma. (Courtesy of MD Okerlund.)

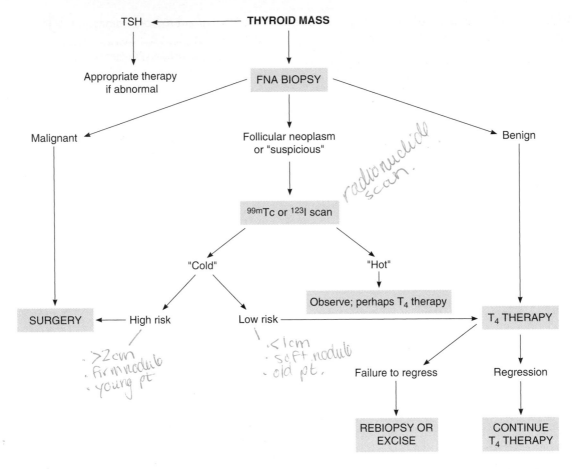

Figure 7–54. Decision matrix for workup of a thyroid nodule. See text for details. (FNA, fine-needle aspiration.)

Fine-needle aspiration biopsy separates thyroid nodules into three groups: (1) Malignant thyroid nodules: The technique is diagnostic in about 95% of all types of thyroid malignancies. (2) Follicular neoplasms: About 15% of these lesions are malignant and about 85% are benign, but these two groups cannot be distinguished by cytology. Thus, a diagnosis of follicular neoplasm is always suspicious for malignancy. On isotope scan, a "hot" follicular neoplasm is benign, and a "cold" follicular neoplasm may be benign or malignant. (3) Benign thyroid nodules. About 5% of fine-needle aspiration readings are false-positives and about 5% false-negatives. Thus, results are accurate in about 90% of cases, as demonstrated by subsequent surgery or long-term follow-up of patients with lesions originally reported to be benign. The results of the biopsy study must be interpreted by the clinician but are extremely useful for the diagnosis of malignancy in thyroid nodules.

F. SUPPRESSIVE THERAPY

Benign lesions may undergo spontaneous involution and regression, and some may be sufficiently TSH-dependent to shrink in response to thyroxine therapy. Some studies have shown no regression of solitary nodules following T_4 therapy, while others have shown a 20–30% reduction in size, particularly in multinodular goiters. However, malignant lesions are unlikely to regress either spontaneously or in response to T_4 therapy.

Management of Thyroid Nodules

A decision matrix for management of a thyroid nodule is presented in Figure 7–54. A patient with a thyroid nodule should have a serum TSH and fine-needle aspiration biopsy as the initial screening tests. If TSH is abnormal, appropriate therapy should be instituted. The biopsy will be reported as malignant, follicular neoplasm, benign, or unsatisfactory. If unsatisfactory, it should be repeated. If the nodule is malignant, the patient is referred directly to the surgeon. If the cytologic report shows that the nodule is benign, the patient is given thyroxine, and if the lesion regresses the patient is maintained on thyroxine indefinitely at a dose sufficient to suppress serum TSH. If there is no regression, the lesion is biopsied again—or, if it grows or changes in consistency, it may be excised. In patients who are reported to have follicular neoplasms, radionuclide scan is obtained. If the scan reveals the nodule to be hot, the patient is simply observed, with or without thyroxine therapy. If the lesion is cold and there is an increased chance of malignancy (large lesion over 2 cm in diameter, firm nodule, young patient), the patient might be referred directly to the surgeon. If the risk is low (small lesion 1 cm or less in diameter, soft nodule, older patient), the patient is given thyroxine. If thyroxine does not induce regression in the latter case, the lesion should probably be excised.

There are two groups that represent special problems: patients with thyroid cysts and patients who have received radiation therapy. Although thyroid cysts are almost always benign, cancer is occasionally found in the wall of the cyst. For this reason, recurrent cysts should be studied with ultrasonography, and if there is evidence of a septate lesion or growth in the wall of the lesion, surgical removal is indicated. In patients who have received radiation therapy, there may be multiple lesions, some benign and some malignant. Therefore, the presence of a cold nodule in a patient who has had radiation exposure is an indication for surgical removal.

If this protocol is followed, there will be a marked reduction in surgery for benign thyroid nodules, and the incidence of malignancy at the time of surgery will be about 40%. The cost savings is enormous, since unnecessary surgery is eliminated and the cost of the thyroid nodule workup is cut in half. In addition, there is no delay in making the diagnosis and referring the patient with thyroid cancer for appropriate therapy.

2. Thyroid Cancer

Pathology

The types and approximate frequency of malignant thyroid tumors are listed in Table 7–15.

A. PAPILLARY CARCINOMA

Papillary carcinoma of the thyroid gland usually presents as a nodule that is firm, solitary, "cold" on isotope scan, solid on thyroid ultrasound, and clearly different from the rest of the gland. In multinodular goiter, the cancer will usually be a "dominant nodule"—larger, firmer, and

Table 7–15. Approximate frequency of malignant thyroid tumors.

Papillary carcinoma (including mixed papillary and follicular)	75%
Follicular carcinoma	16%
Medullary carcinoma	5%
Undifferentiated carcinomas	3%
Miscellaneous (including lymphoma, fibrosarcoma, squamous cell carcinoma, malignant hemangioendothelioma, teratomas, and metastatic carcinomas)	1%

(again) clearly different from the rest of the gland. About 10% of papillary carcinomas, especially in children, present with enlarged cervical nodes, but careful examination will often reveal a "cold" nodule in the thyroid. Rarely, there will be hemorrhage, necrosis, and cyst formation in the malignant nodule, but on thyroid ultrasound of these lesions, clearly defined internal echoes will differentiate the semicystic malignant lesion from the nonmalignant "pure cyst." Finally, papillary carcinoma may be found incidentally as a microscopic focus of cancer in the middle of a gland removed for other reasons such as Graves' disease or multinodular goiter.

Microscopically, the tumor consists of single layers of thyroid cells arranged in vascular stalks, with papillary projections extending into microscopic cyst-like spaces. The nuclei of the cells are large and pale and frequently contain clear, glassy intranuclear inclusion bodies. About 40% of papillary carcinomas form laminated calcified spheres—often at the tip of a papillary projection—called "psammoma bodies," which are usually diagnostic of papillary carcinoma. These cancers usually extend by intraglandular metastasis and by local lymph node invasion. They grow very slowly and remain confined to the thyroid gland and local lymph nodes for many years. In older patients, they may become more aggressive and invade locally into muscles and trachea. In later stages, they can spread to the lung. Death is usually due to local disease, with invasion of deep tissues in the neck; less commonly, death may be due to extensive pulmonary metastases. In some older patients, a long-standing, slowly growing papillary carcinoma will begin to grow rapidly and convert to undifferentiated or anaplastic carcinoma. This "late anaplastic shift" is another cause of death from papillary carcinoma. Many papillary carcinomas secrete thyroglobulin, which can be used as a marker for recurrence or metastasis of the cancer.

B. FOLLICULAR CARCINOMA

Follicular carcinoma is characterized by the presence of small follicles, though colloid formation is poor. Indeed, follicular carcinoma may be indistinguishable from follicular adenoma except by capsular or vascular invasion. The tumor is somewhat more aggressive than papillary carcinoma and can spread either by local invasion of lymph nodes or by blood vessel invasion with distant metastases to bone or lung. Microscopically, the cells are cuboidal, with large nuclei, arranged around follicles that frequently contain dense colloid. These tumors often retain the ability to concentrate radioactive iodine, to form thyroglobulin, and, rarely, to synthesize T_3 and T_4. Thus, the rare "functioning thyroid cancer" is almost always a follicular carcinoma. This characteristic makes these tumors more likely to respond to radioactive iodine therapy. In untreated patients, death is due to local extension or to distant bloodstream metastasis with extensive involvement of bone, lungs, and viscera.

A variant of follicular carcinoma is the "Hürthle cell" carcinoma, characterized by large individual cells with pink-staining cytoplasm filled with mitochondria. They behave like follicular cancer except that they rarely take up radioiodine. Mixed papillary and follicular carcinomas behave more like papillary carcinoma. Thyroglobulin secretion by follicular carcinomas can be used to follow the course of disease.

C. Medullary Carcinoma

Medullary cancer is a disease of the C cells (parafollicular cells) derived from the ultimobranchial body and capable of secreting calcitonin, histaminase, prostaglandins, serotonin, and other peptides. Microscopically, the tumor consists of sheets of cells separated by a pink-staining substance that has characteristics of amyloid. This material stains with Congo red. Amyloid consists of chains of calcitonin laid down in a fibrillary pattern—in contrast to other forms of amyloid, which may have immunoglobulin light chains or other proteins deposited in a fibrillary pattern.

Medullary carcinoma is somewhat more aggressive than papillary or follicular carcinoma but not as aggressive as undifferentiated thyroid cancer. It extends locally into lymph nodes and into surrounding muscle and trachea. It may invade lymphatics and blood vessels and metastasize to lungs and viscera. Calcitonin and carcinoembryonic antigen (CEA) secreted by the tumor are clinically useful markers for diagnosis and follow-up.

About 80% of medullary carcinomas are sporadic, and the remainder are familial. There are three familial patterns: (1) familial medullary carcinoma without associated endocrine disease (FMTC); (2) MEN 2A, consisting of medullary carcinoma, pheochromocytoma, and hyperparathyroidism; and (3) MEN 2B, consisting of medullary carcinoma, pheochromocytoma, and multiple mucosal neuromas. There is also a variant of MEN 2A with cutaneous lichen amyloidosis, a pruritic skin lesion located on the upper back. The genes responsible for the familial syndromes have been mapped to the centromeric region of chromosome 10, which is the location of the *ret* proto-oncogene (a receptor-linked protein kinase gene), and mutations in exon 10, 11, or 16 of this proto-oncogene have been found in these syndromes (see below and Chapter 22).

If medullary carcinoma is diagnosed by fine-needle aspiration biopsy or at surgery, it is essential that the patient be screened for the other endocrine abnormalities found in MEN 2 and that family members be screened for medullary carcinoma and MEN 2 as well. Screening involves measurement of serum calcitonin after calcium infusion in patients who have demonstrated mutations in the *ret* proto-oncogene on DNA analysis (see below). Calcium gluconate is administered intravenously in a dose of 2 mg/kg given over 1 minute, and blood for calcitonin determination is obtained at 1, 2, 3, and 5 minutes after the infusion. Peak values occur 1–2 minutes after injection. Peak values of > 100 pg/mL in females and > 300 pg/mL in males are considered abnormal.

D. Undifferentiated (Anaplastic) Carcinoma

Undifferentiated thyroid gland tumors include small cell, giant cell, and spindle cell carcinomas. They usually occur in older patients with a long history of goiter in whom the gland suddenly—over weeks or months—begins to enlarge and produce pressure symptoms, dysphagia, or vocal cord paralysis. Death from massive local extension usually occurs within 6–36 months. These tumors are very resistant to therapy.

E. Miscellaneous Types

1. Lymphoma—The only type of rapidly growing thyroid cancer that is responsive to therapy is the lymphoma, which may develop as part of a generalized lymphoma or may be primary in the thyroid gland. Thyroid lymphoma occasionally develops in a patient with long-standing Hashimoto's thyroiditis and may be difficult to distinguish from chronic thyroiditis. It is characterized by lymphocyte invasion of thyroid follicles and blood vessel walls, which helps to differentiate thyroid lymphoma from chronic thyroiditis. If there is no systemic involvement, the tumor may respond dramatically to radiation therapy.

2. Cancer metastatic to the thyroid—Systemic cancers that may metastasize to the thyroid gland include cancers of the breast and kidney, bronchogenic carcinoma, and malignant melanoma. The primary site of involvement is usually obvious. Occasionally, the diagnosis is made by needle biopsy or open biopsy of a rapidly enlarging cold thyroid nodule. The prognosis is that of the primary tumor.

3. Molecular biology of thyroid neoplasms—Extensive studies have revealed evidence of gene mutations in both benign and malignant thyroid neoplasms (Figure 7–55). Activating mutations in the *gsp* oncogene or TSH-R in the thyroid follicular cell have been associated with increased growth and function in the "hot" or "toxic" thyroid nodule. Aberrant DNA methylation, activation of the *ras* oncogene and mutation of the *MEN1* gene located at 11q13 are associated with benign follicular adenomas. Loss of the *3P* suppressor gene may then result in the development of follicular carcinoma, and further loss of suppressor gene *P53* may allow progression to an anaplastic carcinoma. Mutations in the *ret* and *trk* oncogenes are associated with the development of papillary carcinomas—and again, loss of *P53* suppressor gene may allow progression to anaplastic carcinoma. This hypothesis suggests a progression from benign to malignant lesions and from differentiated to undifferentiated carcinoma. Indeed, in pathology specimens from older patients with long-standing goiters and recent rapid enlargement, we may see a transition from papillary or follicular thyroid carcinoma to anaplastic carcinoma, a phenomenon termed "late anaplastic shift."

As noted above, activating mutations of the *ret* proto-oncogene on chromosome 10 have been shown to be associated with MEN 2A, MEN 2B, and familial medullary thyroid carcinoma (FMTC). The *ret* oncogene encodes a receptor-linked tyrosine kinase. About 85–90% of the mutations found in MEN 2A and FMTC occur in exons 10 and 11, whereas about 95% of the mutations associated with MEN 2B are found in

exon 16 of the *ret* oncogene. These mutations can be demonstrated in DNA from peripheral white blood cells utilizing the polymerase chain reaction (PCR) and restriction fragment length polymorphism (RFLP). In patients with MEN 2 or FMTC who do not demonstrate a mutation in the *ret* oncogene, family unit linkage analysis may be used to identify gene carriers. Thus, families can be screened for the carrier state, and early diagnosis and treatment can be instituted (Figure 7–56). Somatic mutations in the *ret* oncogene occur in about 30% of sporadic MTC tumor cells, but this does not occur in white blood cells and does not represent a germline mutation. (See also Chapter 22.)

Management of Thyroid Cancer (Figure 7–57)

A. PAPILLARY AND FOLLICULAR CARCINOMA

These patients may be classified into low-risk and high-risk groups. The low-risk group includes patients under age 45 with primary lesions under 2 cm and no evidence of intra- or extraglandular spread. For these patients, lobectomy is adequate therapy. All other patients should be considered high-risk, and for these total thyroidectomy and—if there is evidence of lymphatic spread—a modified neck dissection are indicated. In the absence of evidence of lymphatic spread, prophylactic neck dissection is not necessary. However, for the high-risk group, postoperative radioiodine ablation of residual thyroid remnant is essential. After recovery from surgery, the patient receives liothyronine, 50–100 μg daily in divided doses for 4 weeks; the medication is then stopped for 2 weeks, and the patient is placed on a low-iodine diet. At the end of the 2-week period, the serum thyroglobulin level is determined and the patient is scanned at 24 and 72 hours after a dose of 2–4 mCi of ^{131}I. Liothyronine is used for replacement therapy because it is cleared from the blood rapidly; after 2 weeks off therapy, serum TSH is usually over 50 mU/L, which is necessary for good scanning studies. If there is evidence of residual radioactive iodine uptake in the neck or elsewhere or if there is a rise in serum thyroglobulin greater than 4 ng/mL, radioactive iodine (^{131}I) is effective treatment. (Therapeutic doses of ^{131}I range from 30 mCi to 200 mCi.) The scan is repeated at intervals of 12 months until serum thyroglobulin levels remain under 4 ng/mL and no further uptake is observed; the patient is then maintained on maximum replacement therapy with levothyroxine, 0.15–0.3 mg daily, to suppress serum TSH to undetectable levels. Once a negative scan has been achieved, recombinant human TSH (rhTSH) can be used instead of thyroxine withdrawal for follow-up evaluation. The patient continues to take the appropriate dose of levothyroxine but follows a low-iodine diet for at least 1

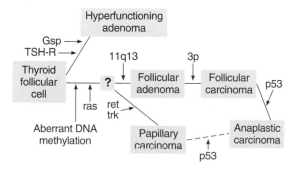

Figure 7–55. Molecular defects associated with development and progression of human thyroid neoplasms. The hypothetical role of specific mutational events in thyroid tumorigenesis is inferred from their prevalence in the various thyroid tumor phenotypes. (Reproduced, with permission, from Fagin JA: Genetic basis of endocrine disease 3: Molecular defects in thyroid gland neoplasia. J Clin Endocrinol Metab 75:1398, 1992.)

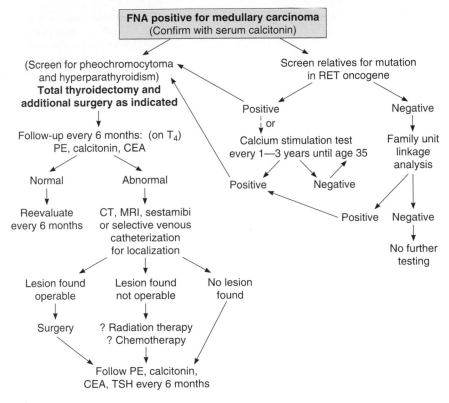

Figure 7–56. Decision matrix for the management of medullary thyroid carcinoma. See text for details. FNA, fine-needle aspiration biopsy; PE, physical examination.

week prior to the study. Then on day 1, blood is drawn for thyroglobulin (Tg) determination, and 0.9 mg of rhTSH is administered intramuscularly. On day 2, the patient receives rhTSH, 0.9 mg intramuscularly; on day 3, 4 mCi ^{131}I is given orally; and on day 5, blood is drawn for Tg determination and a neck scan and whole body scan are obtained. If serum Tg is < 2 ng/mL and the scans are negative, the study is negative for recurrence. If serum Tg rises above 4 ng/mL or if the scan is positive, the patient has persistent disease and should be treated with ^{131}I following the schedule of levothyroxine withdrawal as set forth above. If Tg is > 4 ng/mL and the scan is negative, thyroid ultrasound, CT, or MRI examination may reveal recurrent tumor that may be approached surgically.

Follow-up at intervals of 6–12 months should include careful examination of the neck for recurrent masses. If a lump is noted, needle biopsy is indicated to confirm or rule out cancer. Serum TSH should be checked to be certain it is adequately suppressed, and serum Tg should be < 2 ng/mL (2 μg/L). A rise in

serum Tg to > 4 ng/mL (10 μg/L) while TSH is suppressed suggests recurrence of the malignancy, which may be treated with ^{131}I as above.

Thyroglobulin antibodies in the patient's serum interfere with the thyroglobulin assay and may negate the value of the serum thyroglobulin determination. These patients may have to be followed with periodic visualization studies such as thyroid ultrasound or MRI. The patient with a rising thyroglobulin and a negative ^{131}I scan presents a difficult problem. Administration of a large dose of ^{131}I after appropriate preparation has been tried, but there is little evidence of long-term benefit. For patients with bone or brain metastases, combined external radiation and ^{131}I therapy may be effective. Chemotherapeutic programs are being studied, but no clearly effective protocol has yet been developed.

B. MEDULLARY CARCINOMA

Patients with medullary carcinoma should be followed in a similar way, except that the marker for recurrent medullary cancer is serum calcitonin or carcinoembry-

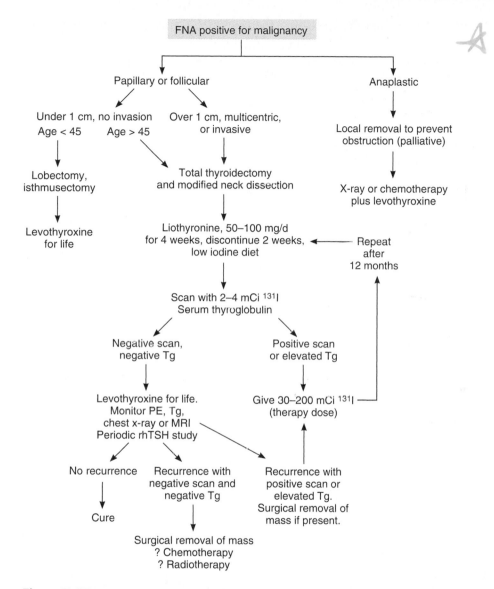

Figure 7–57. Decision matrix for the management of papillary, follicular, or anaplastic thyroid carcinoma. See text for details. FNA, fine-needle aspiration biopsy; PE, physical examination.

onic antigen (CEA). Family members of patients with a genetic *ret* oncogene mutation should be screened for the mutation as noted above (Figure 7–56). Histaminase and other peptides are also secreted by these tumors, but assays for these substances are not generally available. If a patient has a persistently elevated serum calcitonin concentration after total thyroidectomy and regional node dissection, MRI of the neck and chest or selective venous catheterization and sampling for serum

calcitonin may reveal the location of the metastases. Metastatic medullary carcinoma foci may be revealed by PET scan, indium-labeled somatostatin (octreotide), or sestamibi scan. If this fails to localize the lesion (as is often the case), the patient must be followed until the metastatic lesion shows itself as a palpable mass or a shadow on chest x-ray or MRI. Metastatic medullary carcinoma cannot be treated with ^{131}I; therefore, initial thorough surgical excision and postoperative levothyrox-

Table 7–16. Tumor (T), lymph node (N), and distant metastasis (M) classification and staging of thyroid cancer.[1]

DEFINITION of TNM

Primary Tumor (T)

Note: All categories may be subdivided: (a) solitary tumor, (b) multifocal tumor (the largest determines the classification).

TX	Primary tumor cannot be assessed
T0	No evidence of primary tumor
T1	Tumor 2 cm or less in greatest dimension limited to the thyroid
T2	Tumor more than 2 cm but not more than 4 cm in greatest dimension limited to the thyroid
T3	Tumor more than 4 cm in greatest dimension limited to the thyroid or any tumor with minimal extrathyroid extension (eg, extension to sternothyroid muscle or perithyroid soft tissues)
T4a	Tumor of any size extending beyond the thyroid capsule to invade subcutaneous soft tissues, larynx, trachea, esophagus, or recurrent laryngeal nerve
T4b	Tumor invades prevertebral fascia or encases carotid artery or mediastinal vessels

Anaplastic Carcinomas

T4a	Intrathyroidal anaplastic carcinoma—surgically resectable
T4b	Extrathyroidal anaplastic carcinoma—surgically unresectable

Regional Lymph Nodes (N)

Regional lymph nodes are the central compartment, lateral cervical, and upper mediastinal lymph nodes

NX	Regional lymph nodes cannot be assessed
N0	No regional lymph node metastasis
N1	Regional lymph node metastasis
N1a	Metastasis to Level VI (pretracheal, paratracheal, and prelaryngeal/Delphian lymph nodes)
N1b	Metastasis to unilateral, bilateral, or contralateral cervical or superior mediastinal lymph nodes

Distant Metastasis (M)

MX	Distant metastasis cannot be assessed
M0	No distant metastasis
M1	Distant metastasis

STAGE GROUPING

Separate stage groupings are recommended for papillary or follicular, medullary, and anaplastic (undifferentiated) carcinoma.

Papillary or follicular
Under 45 Years

Stage I	Any T	Any N	M0
Stage II	Any T	Any N	M1

Papillary or Follicular
45 Years and Older

Stage I	T1	N0	M0
Stage II	T2	N0	M0
Stage III	T3	N0	M0
	T1	N1a	M0
	T2	N1a	M0
	T3	N1a	M0
Stage IVA	T4a	N0	M0
	T4a	N1a	M0
	T1	N1b	M0
	T2	N1b	M0
	T3	N1b	M0
	T4a	N1b	M0
Stage IVB	T4b	Any N	M0
Stage IVC	Any T	Any N	M1

Medullary Carcinoma

Stage I	T1	N0	M0
Stage II	T2	N0	M0
Stage III	T3	N0	M0
	T1	N1a	M0
	T2	N1a	M0
	T3	N1a	M0
Stage IVA	T4a	N0	M0
	T4a	N1a	M0
	T1	N1b	M0
	T2	N1b	M0
	T3	N1b	M0
	T4a	N1b	M0
Stage IVB	T4b	Any N	M0
Stage IVC	Any T	Any N	M1

Anaplastic Carcinoma

All anaplastic carcinomas are considered Stage IV

Stage IVA	T4a	Any N	M0
Stage IVB	T4b	Any N	M0
Stage IVC	Any T	Any N	M1

[1]Reproduced with permission from: Greene FL et al (editors): *AJCC Cancer Staging Manual,* 6th ed., Springer, 2002.

ine therapy are essential. Chemotherapy for medullary carcinoma has not been effective.

C. ANAPLASTIC CARCINOMA

Anaplastic carcinoma of the thyroid has a very poor prognosis. Treatment consists of isthmusectomy (to confirm the diagnosis and to prevent tracheal compression) and palliative x-ray therapy (Figure 7–57). Thyroid lymphomas are quite responsive to x-ray therapy; giant cell, squamous cell, spindle cell, and anaplastic carcinomas are unresponsive. Chemotherapy is not very effective for anaplastic carcinomas. Doxorubicin, 75 mg/m^2 as a single injection or divided into three consecutive daily injections repeated at 3-week intervals, has been useful in some patients with disseminated thyroid cancer unresponsive to surgery, TSH suppression, or radiation therapy. This drug is quite toxic; side effects include cardiotoxicity, myelosuppression, alopecia, and gastrointestinal symptoms.

D. X-RAY THERAPY

Local x-ray therapy has been useful in the treatment of solitary metastatic lesions, particularly follicular or papillary tumors, that do not concentrate radioactive iodine. It is particularly effective in isolated nonfunctional bone metastases.

Course & Prognosis

The staging of cancer has been a useful method for prediction of the outcome of therapy. The International Union Against Cancer (UICC) and the American Joint Committee on Cancer (AJCC) have proposed the TNM (tumor, nodes, metastases) system for staging thyroid cancer (Table 7–16).

In this system, papillary and follicular thyroid carcinomas are grouped together and the staging is directly related to the age of the patient at the time of diagnosis. The cause-specific 5-year mortality rates in a group of 1500 patients studied by Hay were as follows: stage 1, 0%; stage 2, 0.6%; stage 3, 5.3%; and stage 4, 77%. Similarly, DeGroot and coworkers demonstrated 80–90% survival for stage 1 and stage 2 patients followed for up to 38 years; about 50% survival for stage 3 patients followed for 20 years; and 0% survival for stage 4 patients followed for 10 years. The TNM system may

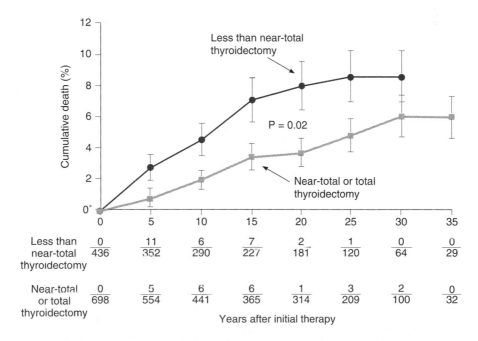

Figure 7–58. Improved survival in patients with papillary or follicular thyroid carcinoma following total or near-total thyroidectomy compared to less than near total thyroidectomy. (Reproduced, with permission, from Mazzaferri EL, Jhiang SM: Long term impact of initial surgical and medical therapy on papillary and follicular thyroid cancer. Am J Med 1994;97:418.)

underestimate the risk of recurrence and death in younger patients with aggressive disease. This is particularly true for patients under age 7 with local invasion or distant metastases, who should probably be grouped in stage 3 or stage 4. However, the system recognizes that for most younger patients, papillary and follicular thyroid carcinomas are relatively indolent and thus can be classified as stage 1 or stage 2.

Outcome is also dependent upon adequate therapy. There has been controversy over the extent of initial surgery for papillary and follicular thyroid cancer. As noted above, lesions under 1 cm with no evidence of local or distant metastases (T1, N0, M0) can probably be treated with lobectomy alone. However, in all other groups, total thyroidectomy and modified regional neck dissection (if gross evidence of spread is noted at the time of surgery) is indicated for two reasons: (1) it removes all local disease, and (2) it sets the stage for ^{131}I therapy and follow-up utilizing serum thyroglobulin measurements. Total or near-total thyroidectomy must be performed by an experienced thyroid surgeon to minimize the complications of surgery. The improvement in outcome following total thyroidectomy is presented in Figure 7–58.

A second factor in survival is the use of radioiodine for ablation of residual thyroid tissue after thyroidectomy and the treatment of residual or recurrent disease. Low doses of 30–50 mCi ^{131}I are used to ablate residual thyroid tissue, but larger doses of 100–200 mCi are necessary for the treatment of metastatic disease. Acute adverse effects of the larger doses include radiation sickness, sialitis, gastritis, and transient oligospermia. Cumulative doses of ^{131}I above 500 mCi may be associated with infertility in the female and azoospermia in the male, pancytopenia in about 4%, and leukemia in about 0.3% of patients. Radiation pneumonitis may occur in patients with diffuse pulmonary metastases, but this is minimized by utilization of high-dose treat-

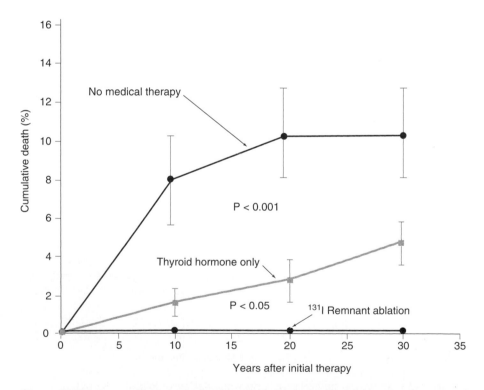

Figure 7–59. Cancer death rates after thyroid remnant ablation, thyroid hormone therapy alone, or no postoperative medical therapy. (Modified and reproduced, with permission, from Mazzaferri EL: Thyroid remnant ^{131}I ablation for papillary and follicular thyroid carcinoma. Thyroid 1997;7:265.)

ment no more than once a year. The effectiveness of ^{131}I therapy in reducing cancer mortality is presented in Figure 7–59.

A third factor in survival is the adequate use of TSH suppression therapy. T_4 in a dose of 2.2 µg/kg/d (1 µg/lb/d) will usually suppress TSH to 0.1 mU/L or less, which removes a major growth factor for papillary or follicular thyroid cancer (Figure 7–59). However, high-dose T_4 therapy is not without risk: angina, tachycardia, or heart failure in older patients or tachycardia and nervousness in younger patients. In addition, there is an increased risk of osteoporosis in postmenopausal women. Estrogen or bisphosphonate therapy may prevent bone loss in these patients, but the treatment program must be individualized.

Medullary carcinoma is more aggressive. It is most aggressive in patients with MEN 2B, less in the sporadic type, and least virulent in MEN 2A and FMTC. Early and adequate initial surgery is the best therapy; once the disease has started to metastasize, it is very difficult to control, though the more favorable types often progress very slowly. Anaplastic thyroid carcinomas have a very poor prognosis, with death anticipated to occur within 1 year.

REFERENCES

Anatomy

Gillam MP, Kopp P: Genetic regulation of thyroid development. Curr Opin Pediatr 2001;13:358. [PMID: 11717563]

Hegedus L: Thyroid ultrasound. Endocrinol Metab Clin North Am 2001;30:339. [PMID: 11444166]

Lindner HH: The thyroid gland. In: *Clinical Anatomy*. Appleton & Lange, 1989.

Monfared A et al: Microsurgical anatomy of the laryngeal nerves as related to thyroid surgery. Laryngoscope 2002;112:386. [PMID: 11889402]

Weber AL et al: The thyroid and parathyroid glands. CT and MRI imaging and correlation with pathology and clinical findings. Radiol Clin North Am 2000;38:1105. [PMID: 11054972]

Physiology

Baxter JD et al: Selective modulation of thyroid hormone receptor action. J Steroid Biochem Mol Biol 2001;76:31. [PMID: 11384861]

Bianco AC et al: Biochemistry, cellular and molecular biology, and physiological roles of the iodothyronine selenodeiodinases. Endocr Rev 2002;23:38. [PMID: 11844744]

Collu R: Genetic aspects of central hypothyroidism. J Endocrinol Invest 2000;23:125. [PMID: 10800768]

Delange F: Iodine deficiency in the world: where do we stand at the turn of the century? Thyroid 2001;11:437. [PMID: 11396702]

Dunn JT, Dunn AD: Update on intrathyroidal iodine metabolism. Thyroid 2001;11:407. [PMID: 11396699]

Gershengorn MC, Osman R: Minireview: Insights into G protein-coupled receptor function. Endocrinology 2001;142:2. [PMID: 11145559]

Glinoer D: Pregnancy and iodine. Thyroid 2001;11:471. [PMID: 11396705]

Koenig RJ: Thyroid hormone receptor coactivators and corepressors. Thyroid 1998;8:703. [PMID: 9737367]

Kohn LD et al: Effects of thyroglobulin and pendrin on iodide flux through the thyrocyte. Trends Endocrinol Metab 2001;12:10. [PMID: 11137035]

Kohrle J: Local activation and inactivation of thyroid hormones: the deiodinase family. Mol Cell Endocrinol 1999;151:103. [PMID: 10411325]

Kopp P: The TSH receptor and its role in thyroid disease. Cell Mol Life Sci 2001;58:1301. [PMID: 11577986]

Marino M, McCluskey RT: Role of thyroglobulin endocytic pathways in the control of thyroid hormone release. Am J Physiol Cell Physiol 2000;279:C1295. [PMID: 11029276]

Persani L: Hypothalamic thyrotropin-releasing hormone and thyrotropin biological activity. Thyroid 1998;8:941. [PMID: 9827663]

Rose SR: Disorders of thyrotropin synthesis, secretion, and function. Curr Opin Pediatr 2000;12:375. [PMID: 10943820]

Schussler GC: The thyroxine-binding proteins. Thyroid 2000;10:141. [PMID: 10718550]

Shen DH et al: Sodium iodide symporter in health and disease. Thyroid 2001;11:415. [PMID: 11396700]

St Germain DL, Galton VA: The deiodinase family of selenoproteins. Thyroid 1997;7:655. [PMID: 9292958]

Szkudlinski MW et al: Thyroid-stimulating hormone and thyroid-stimulating hormone receptor structure-function relationships. Physiol Rev 2002;82:473. [PMID: 11917095]

Weintraub BD, Szkudlinski MW: Development and in vitro characterization of human recombinant thyrotropin. Thyroid 1999;9:447. [PMID: 10365675]

Wilber JF, Xu AH: The thyrotropin-releasing hormone gene 1998: cloning, characterization, and transcriptional regulation in the central nervous system, heart, and testis. Thyroid 1998;8:897. [PMID: 9827656]

Winter WE, Signorino MR: Review: molecular thyroidology. Ann Clin Lab Sci 2001;31:221. [PMID: 11508826]

Wolffe AP et al: Thyroid hormone receptor, v-ErbA, and chromatin. Vitam Horm 2000;58:449. [PMID: 10668407]

Wonerow P et al: Thyrotropin receptor mutations as a tool to understand thyrotropin receptor action. J Mol Med 2001;79:707. [PMID: 11862314]

Wrutniak-Cabello C et al: Thyroid hormone action in mitochondria. J Mol Endocrinol 2001;26:67. [PMID: 11174855]

Wu Y, Koenig RJ: Gene regulation by thyroid hormone. Trends Endocrinol Metab 2000;11:207. [PMID: 10878749]

Yen PM: Physiological and molecular basis of thyroid hormone action. Physiol Rev 2001;81:1097. [PMID: 11427693]

Zhang J, Lazar MA: The mechanism of action of thyroid hormones. Annu Rev Physiol 2000;62:439. [PMID: 10845098]

Tests of Thyroid Function

Camacho PM, Dwarkanathan AA: Sick euthyroid syndrome. What to do when thyroid function tests are abnormal in critically ill patients. Postgrad Med 1999;105:215. [PMID: 10223098]

Dayan CM: Interpretation of thyroid function tests. Lancet 2001; 357:619. [PMID: 11558500]

Despres N, Grant AM: Antibody interference in thyroid assays: a potential for clinical misinformation. Clin Chem 1998; 44:440. [PMID: 9510847]

Fantz CR et al: Thyroid function during pregnancy. Clin Chem 1999;45:2250. [PMID: 10585360]

Fisher DA: Thyroid function in premature infants. The hypothyroxinemia of prematurity. Clin Perinatol 1998;25:999. [PMID: 9891626]

Klein I: Clinical, metabolic, and organ-specific indices of thyroid function. Endocrinol Metab Clin North Am 2001;30:415. [PMID: 11444169]

Nayar R, Frost AR: Thyroid aspiration cytology: a "cell pattern" approach to interpretation. Semin Diagn Pathol 2001;18:81. [PMID: 11403258]

Ross DS: Serum thyroid-stimulating hormone measurement for assessment of thyroid function and disease. Endocrinol Metab Clin North Am 2001;30:24. [PMID: 11444162]

Hypothyroidism

Cooper DS: Clinical practice. Subclinical hypothyroidism. N Engl J Med 2001;345:260. [PMID: 11474665]

Glinoer D: Potential consequences of maternal hypothyroidism on the offspring: evidence and implications. Horm Res 2001;55:109. [PMID: 11549871]

Greenspan SL, Greenspan FS: The effect of thyroid hormone on skeletal integrity. Ann Intern Med 1999;130:750. [PMID: 10357695]

Haddow JE et al: Maternal thyroid deficiency during pregnancy and subsequent neuropsychological development of the child. N Engl J Med 1999;341:549. [PMID: 1041459]

LaFranchi S: Congenital hypothyroidism: etiologies, diagnosis and management. Thyroid 1999;9:735. [PMID: 10447022]

Kopp P: Pendred's syndrome and genetic defects in thyroid hormone synthesis. Rev Endocr Metab Disord 2000;1:109. [PMID: 11704986]

Singer PA et al: Treatment guidelines for patients with hyperthyroidism and hypothyroidism. JAMA 1995;273:808. [PMID: 7532241]

Wiersinga WM: Thyroid hormone replacement therapy. Horm Res 2001;56(Suppl 1):74. [PMID: 11786691]

Hyperthyroidism

Alsanea O, Clark OH: Treatment of Graves' disease: the advantages of surgery. Endocrinol Metab Clin North Am 2000; 29:321. [PMID:10874532]

Bahn RS: Understanding the immunology of Graves' ophthalmopathy. Is it an autoimmune disease? Endocrinol Metab Clin North Am 2000;29:287. [PMID: 10874530]

Bartalena L et al: Management of Graves' ophthalmopathy: reality and perspectives. Endocr Rev 2000;21:168. [PMID: 10782363]

Fadel BM et al: Hyperthyroid heart disease. Clin Cardiol 2000;23:402. [PMID: 10875028]

Fontanilla JC et al: The use of oral radiographic contrast agents in the management of hyperthyroidism. Thyroid 2001;11:561. [PMID: 11442003]

Gough SC: The genetics of Graves' disease. Endocrinol Metab Clin North Am 2000;29:255. [PMID: 10874528]

Heufelder AE: Pathogenesis of ophthalmopathy in autoimmune thyroid disease. Rev Endocr Metab Disord 2000;1:87. [PMID: 11704996]

Koh LD et al: Graves' disease: a host defense mechanism gone awry. Int Rev Immunol 2000;19:633. [PMID: 11129119]

Kraiem Z, Newfield RS: Graves' disease in childhood. J Pediatr Endocrinol Metab 2001;229:43. [PMID: 11308041]

Manoukian MA et al: Clinical and metabolic features of thyrotoxic periodic paralysis in 24 episodes. Arch Intern Med 1999; 159:601. [PMID: 10090117]

Marcocci C et al: Graves' ophthalmopathy and ^{131}I therapy. Q J Nucl Med 1999;43:307. [PMID: 10731781]

Meurisse M et al: Iatrogenic thyrotoxicosis: causal circumstances, pathophysiology, and principles of treatment—review of the literature. World J Surg 2000;24:1377. [PMID: 11038210]

Murakami M et al: Gs alpha mutations in hyperfunctioning thyroid adenomas. Arch Med Res 1999;30:514. [PMID: 10714366]

Nabil N et al: Methimazole: an alternative route of administration. J Clin Endocrinol Metab 1982;54:180. [PMID: 7054215]

Pauwels EK et al: Health effects of therapeutic use of ^{131}I in hyperthyroidism. Q J Nucl Med 2000;44:333. [PMID: 11302261]

Smitt MC, Donaldson SS: Radiation therapy for benign disease of the orbit. Semin Radiat Oncol 1999;9:179. [PMID: 10092710]

Stanbury JB et al: Iodine-induced hyperthyroidism: occurrence and epidemiology. Thyroid 1998;8:83. [PMID: 9492158]

Volpe R: The immunomodulatory effects of anti-thyroid drugs are mediated via actions on thyroid cells, affecting thyrocyte-immunocyte signalling: a review. Curr Pharm Des 2001;7:451. [PMID: 11281852]

Woeber KA: Update on the management of hyperthyroidism and hypothyroidism. Arch Intern Med 2000;160:1067. [PMID: 10789598]

Thyroid Hormone Resistance

Chatterjee VK: Resistance to thyroid hormone, and peroxisome-proliferator-activated receptor gamma resistance. Biochem Soc Trans 2001;29:227. [PMID: 11356159]

Kopp P et al: Syndrome of resistance to thyroid hormone: insights into thyroid hormone action. Proc Soc Exp Biol Med 1996; 211:49. [PMID: 8594618]

Refetoff S: Resistance to thyroid hormone. Clin Lab Med 1993; 13:563. [PMID: 8222575]

Syndrome of Inappropriate TSH Secretion

Kourides IA: Inappropriate secretion of thyroid stimulating hormone. Curr Ther Endocrinol Metab 1997;6:187. [PMID: 9174701]

Losa M et al: Criteria of cure and follow-up of central hyperthyroidism due to thyrotropin-secreting pituitary adenomas. J Clin Endocrinol Metab 1996;81:3084. [PMID: 8768879]

Sanno N et al: Thyrotropin-secreting pituitary adenomas. Clinical and biological heterogeneity and current treatment. J Neurooncol 2001;54:179. [PMID: 11761434]

Multinodular Goiter

Bononi M et al: Surgical treatment of multinodular goiter: incidence of lesions of the recurrent nerves after total thyroidectomy. Int Surg 2000;85:190. [PMID: 11324993]

Derwahl M, Studer H: Nodular goiter and goiter nodules: Where iodine deficiency falls short of explaining the facts. Exp Clin Endocrinol Diabetes 2001;109:250. [PMID: 11507648]

Freitas JE: Therapeutic options in the management of toxic and nontoxic nodular goiter. Semin Nucl Med 2000;30:88. [PMID: 10787189]

Hurley DL, Gharib H: Evaluation and management of multinodular goiter. Otolaryngol Clin North Am 1996;29:527. [PMID: 8844728]

Maurer AH, Charkes ND: Radioiodine treatment for nontoxic multinodular goiter. J Nucl Med 1999;40:1313. [PMID: 10450683]

Nakhjavani M, Gharib H: Diffuse nontoxic and multinodular goiter. Curr Ther Endocrinol Metab 1997;6:109. [PMID: 9174716]

Siegel RD, Lee SL: Toxic nodular goiter. Toxic adenoma and toxic multinodular goiter. Endocrinol Metab Clin North Am 1998;27:151. [PMID: 9534034]

Singh B et al: Substernal goiter: a clinical review. Am J Otolaryngol 1994;15:409. [PMID: 7872476]

Thyroiditis

Barbesino G, Chiovato L: The genetics of Hashimoto's disease. Endocrinol Metab Clin North Am 2000;29:357. [PMID: 10874534]

Borgerson KL et al: The role of Fas-mediated apoptosis in thyroid autoimmune disease. Autoimmunity 1999;30:251. [PMID: 10524501]

McLachlan SM, Rapoport B: Autoimmune response to the thyroid in humans: thyroid peroxidase—the common autoantigenic denominator. Int Rev Immunol 2000;19:587. [PMID: 11129117]

Muller AF et al: Postpartum thyroiditis and autoimmune thyroiditis in women of childbearing age: recent insights and consequences for antenatal and postnatal care. Endocr Rev 2001; 22:605. [PMID: 11588143]

Ross DS: Syndromes of thyrotoxicosis with low radioactive iodine uptake. Endocrinol Metab Clin North Am 1998;27:169. [PMID: 9534035]

Schumm-Draeger PM et al: Prophylactic levothyroxine therapy in patients with Hashimoto's thyroiditis. Exp Clin Endocrinol Diabetes 1999;107 Suppl 3:S84. [PMID: 10522812]

Stafford EA, Rose NR: Newer insights into the pathogenesis of experimental autoimmune thyroiditis. Int Rev Immunol 2000; 19:501. [PMID: 11129113]

Vinuesa CG, Cook MC: The molecular basis of lymphoid architecture and B cell responses: implications for immunodeficiency and immunopathology. Curr Mol Med 2001;1:689. [PMID: 11899257]

Walfish PG: Thyroiditis. Curr Ther Endocrinol Metab 1997; 6:117. [PMID: 9174718]

Radiation Exposure

Gilbert ES et al: Health effects from fallout. Health Phys 2002; 82:726. [PMID: 12003021]

Inskip PD: Thyroid cancer after radiotherapy for childhood cancer. Med Pediatr Oncol 2001;36:568. [PMID: 11340614]

Rubino C et al: Thyroid cancer after radiation exposure. Eur J Cancer 2002;38:645. [PMID: 11916545]

Thyroid Nodules and Thyroid Cancer

Alsanea O, Clark OH: Familial thyroid cancer. Curr Opin Oncol 2001;13:44. [PMID: 11148685]

Basaria M et al: The use of recombinant thyrotropin in the follow-up of patients with differentiated thyroid cancer. Am J Med 2002;112:721. [PMID: 12079713]

Brandi ML et al: Guidelines for diagnosis and therapy of MEN type 1 and type 2. J Clin Endocrinol Metab 2001;86:5658. [PMID: 11739416]

Csako G et al: Assessing the effects of thyroid suppression on benign solitary thyroid nodules. A model for using quantitative research synthesis. Medicine (Baltimore) 2000;79:9. [PMID: 10670406]

Giuffrida D, Gharib H: Anaplastic thyroid carcinoma: current diagnosis and treatment. Ann Oncol 2000;11:1083. [PMID: 11061600]

Krohn K, Paschke R: Somatic mutations in thyroid nodular disease. Mol Genet Metab 2002;75:202. [PMID: 11914031]

Leenhardt L, Aurengo A: Post-Chernobyl thyroid carcinoma in children. Baillieres Best Pract Res Clin Endocrinol Metab 2000;14:667. [PMID: 11289741]

Lind P et al: The role of F-18FDG PET in thyroid cancer. Acta Med Austriaca 2000;27:38. [PMID: 10812462]

Mazzaferri EL: An overview of the management of papillary and follicular thyroid carcinoma. Thyroid 1999;9:421. [PMID: 10365671]

Meier CA: Thyroid nodules: pathogenesis, diagnosis and treatment. Baillieres Best Pract Res Clin Endocrinol Metab 2000; 14:559. [PMID: 11289735]

Modigliani E et al: Diagnosis and treatment of medullary thyroid cancer. Baillieres Best Pract Res Clin Endocrinol Metab 2000;14:631. [PMID: 11289739]

Moretti F et al: Molecular pathogenesis of thyroid nodules and cancer. Baillieres Best Pract Res Clin Endocrinol Metab 2000; 14:517. [PMID: 11289733]

Pacini F, Pinchera A: Serum and tissue thyroglobulin measurement: clinical applications in thyroid disease. Biochimie 1999;81:463. [PMID: 10403176]

Ringel MD: Molecular diagnostic tests in the diagnosis and management of thyroid carcinoma. Rev Endocr Metab Disord 2000;1:173. [PMID: 11705003]

Ruben Harach H: Familial nonmedullary thyroid neoplasia. Endocr Pathol 2001;12:97. [PMID: 11579685]

Sherman SI: The management of metastatic differentiated thyroid carcinoma. Rev Endocr Metab Disord 2000;1:165. [PMID: 11705002]

Singer PA et al: Treatment guidelines for patients with thyroid nodules and well-differentiated thyroid cancer. American Thyroid Association. Arch Intern Med 1996;156:2165. [PMID: 8885814]

Weiss RE, Lado-Abeal J: Thyroid nodules: diagnosis and therapy. Curr Opin Oncol 2002;14:46. [PMID: 11790980]

Wiersinga WM: Thyroid cancer in children and adolescents–consequences in later life. J Pediatr Endocrinol Metab 2001; 14(Suppl 5):1289. [PMID: 11964025]

Wong CK, Wheeler MH: Thyroid nodules: rational management. World J Surg 2000;24:934. [PMID: 10865037]

Metabolic Bone Disease

8

Dolores Shoback, MD, Robert Marcus, MD, & Daniel Bikle, MD, PhD

ADHR	Autosomal dominant hypophosphatemic rickets	**MEN**	Multiple endocrine neoplasia
AIRE	Autoimmune regulator	**ODF**	Osteoclast differentiation factor
BMD	Bone mineral density	**OPG**	Osteoprotegerin
BMU	Basic multicellular unit	**PHP**	Pseudohypoparathyroidism
CGRP	Calcitonin gene-related peptide	**PIP$_2$**	Phosphatidylinositol 4,5-biphosphate
DBP	Vitamin D-binding protein	**PPHP**	Pseudopseudohypoparathyroidism
DXA	Dual-energy x-ray absorptiometry	**PTH**	Parathyroid hormone
FBHH	Familial benign hypocalciuric hypercalcemia	**PTHrP**	Parathyroid hormone-related protein
		RANKL	Receptor activator of NF-κβ ligand
ICMA	Immunochemiluminescent assay	**SERMS**	Selective estrogen response modulators
IP$_3$	Inositol 1,4,5-triphosphate	**VDR**	Vitamin D receptor
IRMA	Immunoradiometric assay	**VDRE**	Vitamin D response element

CELLULAR & EXTRACELLULAR CALCIUM METABOLISM

The calcium ion plays a critical role in intracellular and extracellular events in human physiology. **Extracellular** calcium levels in humans are tightly regulated within a narrow physiologic range to provide for proper functioning of many tissues: excitation-contraction coupling in the heart and other muscles, synaptic transmission and other functions of the nervous system, platelet aggregation, coagulation, and secretion of hormones and other regulators by exocytosis. The level of **intracellular** calcium is also tightly controlled, at levels about 10,000-fold lower than extracellular calcium, in order for calcium to serve as an intracellular second messenger in the regulation of cell division, muscle contractility, cell motility, membrane trafficking, and secretion.

It is the concentration of ionized calcium ($[Ca^{2+}]$) that is regulated in the extracellular fluid. The ionized calcium concentration averages 1.25 ± 0.07 mmol/L (Table 8–1). However, only about 50% of the total calcium in serum and other extracellular fluids is present in the ionized form. The remainder is bound to albumin (about 40%) or complexed with anions such as phosphate and citrate (about 10%). The protein-bound and complexed fractions of serum calcium are metabolically inert and are not regulated by hormones; only the $[Ca^{2+}]$ serves a regulatory role, and only this fraction is itself regulated by the calciotropic hormones parathyroid hormone (PTH) and vitamin D. However, large increases in the serum concentrations of phosphate or citrate can, by mass action, markedly increase the complexed fraction of calcium. For example, massive transfusions of blood, in which citrate is used as an anticoagulant, can reduce the $[Ca^{2+}]$ enough to produce tetany. In addition, because calcium and phosphate circulate at concentrations close to saturation, a substantial rise in the serum concentration of either calcium or phosphate can lead to the precipitation of calcium phosphate salts in tissues, and this is a source of major clinical problems in patients with severe hypercalcemia (eg, malignant tumors) and in those with severe hyperphosphatemia (eg, in renal failure or rhabdomyolysis).

Table 8–1. Calcium concentrations in body fluids.

Total serum calcium	8.5–10.5 mg/dL (2.1–2.6 mmol/L)
Ionized calcium	4.4–5.2 mg/dL (1.1–1.3 mmol/L)
Protein-bound calcium	4.0–4.6 mg/dL (0.9–1.1 mmol/L)
Complexed calcium	0.7 mg/dL (0.18 mmol/L)
Intracellular free calcium	0.00018 mmol/L (180 nmol/L)

What is remarkable about calcium metabolism is that the extracellular fluid $[Ca^{2+}]$, which represents a tiny fraction of the total body calcium, can be so tightly regulated in the face of the rapid fluxes of calcium through it that take place during the course of calcium metabolism (Figure 8–1). The total calcium in extracellular fluid amounts to about 1% of total body calcium, with most of the remainder sequestered in bone. Yet from the extracellular fluid compartment, which contains about 900 mg of calcium, 10,000 mg/d is filtered at the glomerulus and 500 mg/d is added to a labile pool in bone; and to the extracellular fluid compartment are added about 200 mg absorbed from the diet, 9800 mg reabsorbed by the renal tubule, and 500 mg from bone.

The challenge of the calcium homeostatic system, then, is to maintain a constant level of $[Ca^{2+}]$ in the extracellular fluid, simultaneously providing adequate amounts of calcium to cells, to bone, and for renal excretion—and all the while compensating, on an hourly basis, for changes in daily intake of calcium, bone metabolism, and renal function. It is scarcely surprising that this homeostatic task requires two hormones, PTH and vitamin D, or that the secretion of each hormone is exquisitely sensitive to small changes in the serum calcium, or that each hormone is able to regulate calcium exchange across all three interfaces of the extracellular fluid: the gut, the bone, and the renal tubule. We will reexamine the integrated roles of PTH and vitamin D in calcium homeostasis after their actions and secretory control have been described.

The challenge of the cellular calcium economy is to maintain a cytosolic $[Ca^{2+}]$, or $[Ca^{2+}]_i$, of about 0.1 μmol/L, about 10,000-fold less than what is present outside cells, providing for rapid fluxes through the intracellular compartment as required for regulation while maintaining a large gradient across the cell membrane. The calcium gradient across the cell membrane is maintained by ATP-dependent calcium pumps and by a Na^+-Ca^{2+} exchanger. Calcium can enter cells through several types of calcium channels, some of which are voltage-operated or receptor-operated, to provide for rapid influx in response to depolarization or receptor stimulation. The cell also maintains large stores of calcium in microsomal and mitochondrial pools. Calcium can be released from microsomal stores rapidly by cellular signals such as 1,4,5-inositol trisphosphate (IP_3). Reuptake mechanisms are also present, so that cytosolic calcium transients can be rapidly terminated by returning calcium to storage pools or pumping it across the plasma membrane.

PARATHYROID HORMONE

Anatomy & Embryology of the Parathyroid Glands

Parathyroid hormone is secreted from four glands located adjacent to the thyroid gland in the neck. The glands weigh an average of 40 mg each. The two superior glands are usually found near the posterior aspect of the thyroid capsule; the inferior glands are most often located near the inferior thyroid margin. However, the exact location of the glands is variable, and 12–15% of normal persons have a fifth parathyroid gland. The parathyroid glands arise from the third and fourth branchial pouches. The inferior glands are actually those derived from the third branchial pouches. Beginning cephalad to the other pair, they migrate further caudad, and one of them sometimes follows the thymus gland into the superior mediastinum. The small size of the parathyroids and the vagaries of their location and number make parathyroid surgery a challenging enterprise for all but the expert surgeon.

The parathyroid glands are composed of epithelial cells and stromal fat. The predominant epithelial cell is the chief cell. The chief cell is distinguished by its clear cytoplasm from the oxyphil cell, which is slightly larger

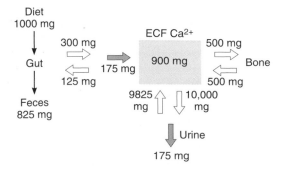

Figure 8–1. Calcium fluxes in a normal individual in a state of zero external mineral balance. The open arrows denote unidirectional calcium fluxes; the solid arrows denote net fluxes. (Reproduced, with permission, from Felig P et al [editors]: *Endocrinology and Metabolism,* 2nd ed. McGraw-Hill, 1987.)

and has eosinophilic granular cytoplasm. Both cell types contain PTH, and it is not known whether their secretory regulation differs.

Secretion of Parathyroid Hormone

In order to carry out its function to regulate the extracellular calcium concentration, PTH must be under exquisite control by the serum calcium concentration. Thus, the negative feedback relationship of PTH with serum $[Ca^{2+}]$ is steeply sigmoidal, with the steep portion of the curve corresponding exactly to the normal range of serum calcium—precisely the relationship to create a high "gain" controller and assure maintenance of the normal serum calcium concentration by PTH (Figure 8–2).

To sense the concentration of extracellular $[Ca^{2+}]$ and thereby regulate the secretion of PTH, the parathyroid cell relies on a sensor of extracellular calcium. This calcium sensor is a 120-kDa G protein-coupled receptor, with the canonical structure of the seven-transmembrane-domain receptors of this class (Figure 3–2.) The calcium receptor has sequence homologies to the metabotropic glutamate receptors of the central nervous system, the γ-aminobutyric acid receptor-B, and a large family of pheromone receptors. The large extracellular domain of the calcium receptor is thought to be involved in ion recognition, and it is likely that calcium binds directly to sites in this domain. Like other G protein-coupled receptors, the calcium receptor has seven serpentine membrane-spanning domains. The intracellular loops that connect these domains are directly involved in coupling the receptor to G proteins, probably those with alpha q and alpha i subunits.

Shortly after identification of the calcium receptor, it was shown that mutations in this receptor were responsible for familial benign hypocalciuric hypercalcemia, a disorder of calcium sensing by the parathyroid and kidney. The calcium receptor is not unique to the parathyroid. Calcium receptors are widely distributed in the brain, skin, growth plate, intestine, stomach, C cells, and other tissues. This receptor regulates the responses to calcium in thyroid C cells, which secrete calcitonin in response to high extracellular calcium, and in the distal nephron of the kidney, where the receptor regulates calcium excretion. The function of calcium receptors in many other sites is beginning to be addressed.

The primary cellular signal by which increased extracellular calcium inhibits the secretion of PTH is an increase in $[Ca^{2+}]_i$. The calcium receptor is directly coupled by G_q to the enzyme phospholipase C, which hydrolyzes the phospholipid phosphatidylinositol 4,5-bisphosphate (PIP_2) to liberate the intracellular messengers IP_3 and diacylglycerol (see Figure 3–5). IP_3 binds to a receptor in endoplasmic reticulum that releases calcium from membrane stores. The release of stored calcium raises the $[Ca^{2+}]_i$ rapidly and is followed by a sustained influx of extracellular calcium, through channels to produce a rise and a sustained plateau in $[Ca^{2+}]_i$. Increased intracellular calcium may be sufficient for inhibition of PTH release, but it is unclear whether calcium release from intracellular stores or sustained calcium influx from the cell exterior is most important. The other product of phospholipase C action is the lipid diacylglycerol, an activator of the calcium- and phospholipid-sensitive protein kinase, protein kinase C. The effects of protein kinase C on the release of PTH from the gland are complex. Calcium receptors also couple to the inhibition of cAMP generation, which also may play a role in setting the response of parathyroid cells to ambient calcium levels.

The initial effect of high extracellular calcium is to inhibit the secretion of preformed PTH from storage granules in the gland by blocking the fusion of storage granules with the cell membrane and release of their contents. In most cells, stimulation of exocytosis ("stimulus-secretion coupling") is a calcium-requiring

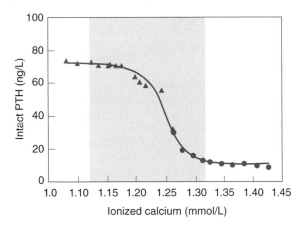

Figure 8–2. The relations between the serum ionized calcium level and the simultaneous serum concentration of intact PTH in normal humans. The serum calcium concentration was altered by the infusion of calcium (closed circles) or citrate (closed triangles). Parathyroid sensitivity to changes in serum calcium is maximal within the normal range (the shaded area). Low concentrations of PTH persist in the face of hypercalcemia. (Modified from Conlin PR et al: Hysteresis in the relationship between serum ionized calcium and intact parathyroid hormone during recovery from induced hyper- and hypocalcemia in normal humans. J Clin Endocrinol Metab 1989;69:593. By permission of the Journal of Clinical Endocrinology and Metabolism.)

process, which is inhibited by depletion of calcium. The parathyroid cell is necessarily an exception to this rule, because this cell must increase secretion of PTH when the calcium level is low. In the parathyroids, intracellular magnesium appears to serve the role in stimulus-secretion coupling that calcium does in other cells. As discussed below in the section on hypoparathyroidism, depletion of magnesium stores can paralyze the secretion of PTH, leading to reversible hypoparathyroidism.

Besides calcium, there are several regulators of PTH secretion. Hypermagnesemia inhibits PTH, and during the treatment of premature labor with infusions of magnesium sulfate a reduction in the PTH level and occasionally hypocalcemia are observed. Conversely, moderate hypomagnesemia can stimulate PTH secretion, even though prolonged depletion of magnesium will paralyze it. On a molar basis, magnesium is less potent in controlling the secretion than calcium. Catecholamines, acting through β-adrenergic receptors and cAMP, stimulate the secretion of PTH. This effect does not appear to be clinically significant. The hypercalcemia sometimes observed in patients with pheochromocytoma usually has another basis—secretion of parathyroid hormone-related protein (PTHrP) by the tumor.

Not only do changes in serum calcium regulate the secretion of PTH—they also regulate the synthesis of PTH at the level of stabilizing preproPTH mRNA levels and possibly enhancing gene transcription. It is estimated that glandular stores of PTH are sufficient to maintain maximal rates of secretion for no more than 1.5 hours, so increased synthesis is required to meet sustained hypocalcemic challenges.

Transcription of the PTH gene is also regulated by vitamin D: high levels of 1,25-dihydroxyvitamin D inhibit PTH gene transcription. This is one of many ways that the calciotropic hormones cooperatively regulate calcium homeostasis, and it has therapeutic implications. Vitamin D analogs are used to treat secondary hyperparathyroidism in dialysis patients with renal osteodystrophy.

Synthesis and Processing of Parathyroid Hormone

PTH is an 84-amino-acid peptide with a molecular weight of 9300. Its gene is located on chromosome 11. The gene encodes a precursor called preproPTH with a 29-amino-acid extension added at the amino terminal of the mature PTH peptide (Figure 8–3). This extension includes a 23-amino-acid signal sequence (the "pre" sequence) and a six-residue prohormone sequence. The signal sequence in preproPTH functions precisely as it does in most other secreted protein molecules, to allow recognition of the peptide by a signal recognition particle, which binds to nascent peptide chains as they emerge from the ribosome and guides them to the endoplasmic reticulum, where they are inserted through the membrane into the lumen (Figure 8–4). The process is discussed in detail in Chapter 2.

In the lumen of the endoplasmic reticulum, a signal peptidase cleaves the signal sequence from preproPTH to leave proPTH, which exits the endoplasmic reticulum and travels to the Golgi apparatus, where the "pro" sequence is cleaved from PTH by an enzyme called furin (Chapter 2). While preproPTH is evanescent, proPTH has a life span of about 15 minutes. The processing of proPTH is quite efficient, and proPTH, unlike other prohormones (eg, proinsulin), is not secreted. As it leaves the Golgi apparatus, PTH is repackaged into dense neuroendocrine-type secretory granules, where it is stored to await secretion.

Clearance & Metabolism of PTH

PTH secreted by the gland has a circulating half-life of 2–4 minutes. Intact PTH(1–84) is predominantly cleared in the liver and kidney. There, PTH is cleaved at the 33–34 and 36–37 positions to produce an amino terminal fragment and a carboxyl terminal fragment. Amino terminal fragments of PTH do circulate but not to the extent of carboxyl terminal fragments. The latter are cleared from blood by renal filtration, and they accumulate in chronic renal failure. Although the classic activities of PTH are encoded in the amino terminal portion of the molecule, mid region and carboxyl terminal fragments of the hormone may not be metabolically inert. Recent evidence suggests that they have their own receptors and may have their own biologic actions.

Assay of PTH

Modern assays of intact PTH(1–84) employ two-site immunoradiometric assay (IRMA) or immunochemiluminescent assay (ICMA) techniques, in which the normal range for PTH is 10–60 pg/mL (1–6 pmol/L). By utilizing antibodies to two determinants, one near the amino terminal of PTH and the other near the carboxyl terminal, these assays are designed to measure the intact, biologically active hormone specifically (Figure 8–5). In practice, such assays have sufficient sensitivity and specificity not only to detect increased levels of PTH in hyperparathyroid disorders but also to detect suppressed levels of PTH in patients with nonparathyroid hypercalcemia. The ability to detect suppression of

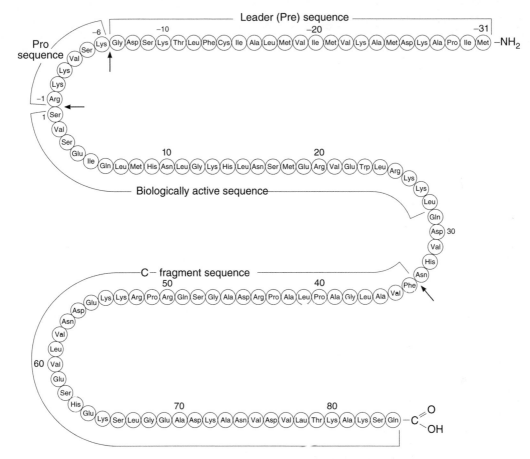

Figure 8–3. Primary structure of human preparathyroid hormone. The arrows indicate sites of specific cleavages which occur in the sequence of biosynthesis and peripheral metabolism of the hormone. The biologically active sequence is enclosed in the center of the molecule. (Reproduced, with permission, from Felig P, Baxter JD, Frohman LA [editors]: *Endocrinology and Metabolism,* 3rd ed. McGraw-Hill, 1995.)

PTH makes these assays powerful tools for the differential diagnosis of hypercalcemia: If hypercalcemia results from some form of hyperparathyroidism, then the serum PTH level will be high; if hypercalcemia has a nonparathyroid basis, then PTH will be suppressed. Recently, intact PTH assays have been refined so that the amino terminal antibody requires more than just the immediate amino terminal of the PTH molecule for its interaction. This improvement was made as a result of the recognition that antibodies used in first-generation intact PTH assays could recognize small amino terminal PTH fragments which are generated in vivo and may circulate to a significant extent in chronic renal failure. Two-site assays of intact PTH have essentially replaced earlier techniques, many of which also detected inert carboxyl terminal fragments as well as intact PTH. These assays could not detect suppression of PTH in nonparathyroid disorders and gave very high levels of immunoreactive PTH in chronic renal failure.

Biologic Effects of PTH

The function of PTH is to regulate serum calcium levels by concerted effects on three principal target organs: bone, intestinal mucosa, and kidney. The effect of PTH on intestinal calcium absorption is indirect, resulting from increased renal production of the intestinally active vitamin D metabolite 1,25-dihydroxyvitamin D. By its integrated effects on the kidney, gut, and bone, PTH acts to increase the inflow of calcium into

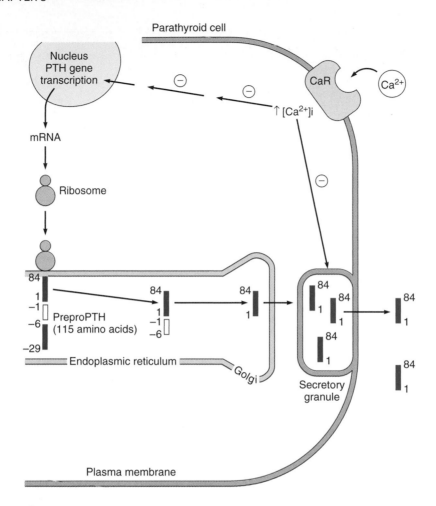

Figure 8–4. Biosynthetic events in the production of PTH within the parathyroid cell. PreproPTH gene is transcribed to its mRNA, which is translated on the ribosomes to preproPTH (amino acids −29 to +84). The pre- sequence is removed within the endoplasmic reticulum, yielding proPTH (−6 to +84). Mature PTH(1–84) released from the Golgi is packaged in secretory granules and released into the circulation in the presence of hypocalcemia. The calcium receptor senses changes in extracellular calcium that affect both the release of PTH and the transcription of the preproPTH gene. (Reproduced, with permission, from McPhee SJ et al [editors]: *Pathophysiology of Disease: An Introduction to Clinical Medicine.* Originally published by Appleton & Lange. Copyright © 1995 by The McGraw-Hill Companies, Inc.)

the extracellular fluid and thus defend against hypocalcemia. Removal of the parathyroid glands results in profound hypocalcemia and ultimately in tetany and death.

In the kidney, PTH has direct effects on the tubular reabsorption of calcium, phosphate, and bicarbonate. Although the bulk of calcium is resorbed from tubule fluid together with sodium in the proximal convoluted tubule, the fine tuning of calcium excretion occurs in the distal nephron. There, PTH markedly increases the reabsorption of calcium, predominantly in the distal convoluted tubule. Although calcium is actively transported against an electrochemical gradient, the precise nature of the calcium transport process that is regulated

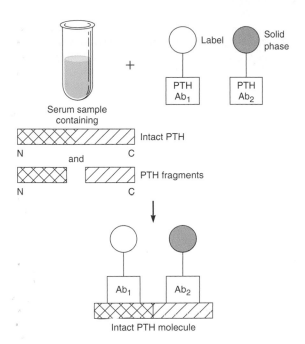

Figure 8–5. Schematic representation of the principle of the two-site assay for intact PTH. The label may be a luminescent probe or ^{125}I in the immunochemiluminescent or immunoradiometric assay, respectively. Two different region-specific antibodies are used (Ab1 and Ab$_2$). Only the hormone species containing both immunodeterminants is counted in the assay. (Reproduced, with permission, from McPhee SJ et al [editors]: *Pathophysiology of Disease: An Introduction to Clinical Medicine.* Originally published by Appleton & Lange. Copyright © 1995 by The McGraw-Hill Companies, Inc.)

by PTH is controversial. However, from a physiologic standpoint, the ability to limit renal losses of calcium is one important means by which PTH protects the serum calcium level.

PTH inhibits the reabsorption of phosphate in the renal proximal tubule. In this nephron segment, phosphate is transported across the apical membrane of the tubule cell by a specific sodium-phosphate cotransporter, with phosphate influx driven by the energy of the sodium gradient. The transport protein has been identified by molecular cloning. It is suspected that PTH may inhibit sodium-phosphate reabsorption by reducing the rate of insertion of transporters from a sequestered cytoplasmic pool into the apical membrane. In any case, the phosphaturic effect of PTH is profound. It is best quantified by calculating the tubule reabsorption of phosphate (TRP) from the clearances of phosphate and creatinine (TRP = $1 - C_p/C_{creat}$, normal range 80–97%), or by calculating the renal phosphate threshold (TmP/GFR) from a standard nomogram. Because it is primarily the renal phosphate threshold that sets the level of serum phosphorus, the phosphaturic effect of PTH is mirrored in the serum phosphorus level, eg, hypophosphatemia in hyperparathyroidism. Hyperparathyroid states may also be characterized by impaired bicarbonate reabsorption and a mild hyperchloremic metabolic acidosis, because of inhibition of Na^+-H^+ antiporter activity by PTH.

Though the hypocalciuric effect of PTH is readily understood as part of the concerted actions of the hormone to protect the serum calcium level, the utility of the phosphaturic effect of PTH is less obvious. One consideration is that the phosphaturic effect tends to prevent an increase in serum phosphate, which would otherwise result from the obligatory release of phosphate with calcium during bone resorption and would tend to dampen the homeostatic increase in serum calcium by complexing calcium in blood. An example is renal osteodystrophy. When phosphate clearance is impaired by renal failure, the hypocalcemic effect of phosphate released during bone remodeling is an important contributor to progressive secondary hyperparathyroidism as part of a positive feedback loop—the more that bone resorption is stimulated and phosphate released, the more hyperparathyroidism is induced.

Mechanism of Action of Parathyroid Hormone

There are two mammalian receptors for PTH. The first receptor to be identified recognizes PTH and PTH-related protein (PTHrP) and is designated the PTH and PTHrP receptor, or the PTH-1 receptor. The PTH-2 receptor is activated by PTH only. These receptors also differ in their tissue distribution. The PTH receptor-1 in kidney and bone is an 80,000-MW glycoprotein member of the G protein receptor superfamily. It has the canonical architecture of such receptors, with a large first extracellular domain, seven consecutive membrane-spanning domains, and a cytoplasmic tail (see Figure 3–2). PTH binds to sites in the large extracellular domain of the receptor. The hormone-bound form of the receptor then activates associated G proteins via several determinants in the intracellular loops. PTH receptors are only remotely related in sequence to most other G protein coupled receptors, but they are more closely related to a small subfamily of peptide hormone receptors, which includes those for secretin, VIP, ACTH, and calcitonin.

PTH itself has a close structural resemblance to a sister protein, PTHrP, and also resembles the peptides secretin, VIP, calcitonin, and ACTH. As noted above, the receptors for these related ligands are themselves members of a special family. These peptide hormones are characterized by an amino terminal α-helical domain, thought to be directly involved in receptor activation, and an adjacent α-helical domain which seems to be the primary receptor-binding domain. In the case of PTH, residues 1–6 are required for activation of the receptor; truncated analogs without these residues (eg, PTH[7–34]) can bind the receptor but cannot efficiently activate it and thus serve as competitive antagonists of PTH action. The primary receptor-binding domain consists of PTH(18–34). Although the intact form of PTH is an 84-amino-acid peptide, PTH (35–84) does not seem to have any important role in binding to the bone-kidney receptor. However, a separate PTH(35–84) receptor may exist; the carboxyl terminal PTH receptor could mediate an entirely new set of actions of PTH.

The PTH-1 receptor binds PTH and its sister hormone PTHrP with equivalent affinity. Inheritance of a constitutively active form of this receptor produces lifelong hypercalcemia as part of a rare heritable form of short-limbed dwarfism disorder called Jansen-type metaphysial chondrodysplasia. Homozygous inactivating mutations of the PTH-1 receptor gene are responsible for congenital Blomstrand's chondrodysplasia, a lethal developmental syndrome.

Physiologic activation of the receptor by binding of either PTH or PTHrP induces the active, GTP-bound state of two receptor-associated G proteins. G_s couples the receptor to the effector adenylyl cyclase and thereby to the generation of cAMP as a cellular second messenger. G_q couples the receptor to a separate effector system, phospholipase C, and thereby to an increase in $[Ca^{2+}]_i$ and to activation of protein kinase C (Figure 3–5). Although it is not clear which of the cellular messengers, cAMP or intracellular calcium, is responsible for each of the various cellular effects of PTH, there is evidence from an experiment of nature that cAMP is the intracellular second messenger for calcium homeostasis and renal phosphate excretion. The experiment is pseudohypoparathyroidism, in which null mutations in one allele of the stimulatory G protein subunit $G_s\alpha$ cause hypocalcemia and unresponsiveness of renal phosphate excretion to PTH.

PTHrP

When secreted in abundance by malignant tumors, PTHrP produces severe hypercalcemia by activating the PTH/PTHrP-1 receptor. However, the physiologic role of PTHrP is quite different from that of PTH. PTHrP is produced in many fetal and adult tissues. Based on gene knockout experiments and overexpression of PTHrP in individual tissues, we now know that PTHrP

is required for normal development as a regulator of the proliferation and mineralization of chondrocytes and as a regulator of placental calcium transport. In postnatal life, PTHrP appears to regulate the epithelial-mesenchymal interactions that are critical for development of the mammary gland, skin, and hair follicle. In most physiologic circumstances, PTHrP carries out local rather than systemic actions. PTHrP is discussed more fully in Chapter 21.

CALCITONIN

Calcitonin is a 32-amino-acid peptide whose principal function is to inhibit osteoclast-mediated bone resorption. Calcitonin is secreted by parafollicular C cells of the thyroid. These are neuroendocrine cells derived from the ultimobranchial body, which fuses with the posterior lobes of the thyroid to become C cells. C cells make up only about 0.1% of the mass of the thyroid.

The secretion of calcitonin is under the control of the serum $[Ca^{2+}]$. The C cell uses the same calcium receptor as the parathyroid cell to sense changes in the ambient calcium concentration, but the C cell increases secretion of calcitonin in response to hypercalcemia and shuts off hormone secretion during hypocalcemia.

The calcitonin gene is composed of six exons, and, through alternative exon splicing, it encodes two entirely different peptide products (Figure 8–6). In the thyroid C cell, the predominant splicing choice generates mature calcitonin (Figure 8–7), which is incorporated within a 141-amino-acid precursor. In other tissues, especially neurons of the central nervous system, a peptide called calcitonin gene-related peptide (CGRP) is produced from a 128-amino-acid precursor. CGRP is a 37-amino-acid peptide with considerable homology to calcitonin. The amino terminals of both peptides incorporates a seven-member disulfide-bonded ring (Figure 8–7). Acting through its own receptor, CGRP is among the most potent vasodilator substances known. There are two distinct genes encoding calcitonin and CGRP (CALC1 and CALC2). CALC1 can produce calcitonin and CGRP I, while CALC2 encodes CGRP II. This peptide differs from CGRP I by only three amino acids.

When administered intravenously, calcitonin produces a rapid and dramatic decline in levels of serum calcium and phosphorus, primarily through actions on bone. The major effect of the hormone is to inhibit osteoclastic bone resorption. After exposure to calcitonin, the morphology of the osteoclast changes rapidly. Within minutes, the cell withdraws its processes, shrinks in size, and retracts the ruffled border, the organelle of bone resorption, from the bone surface. Osteoclasts and cells of the proximal renal tubule express a

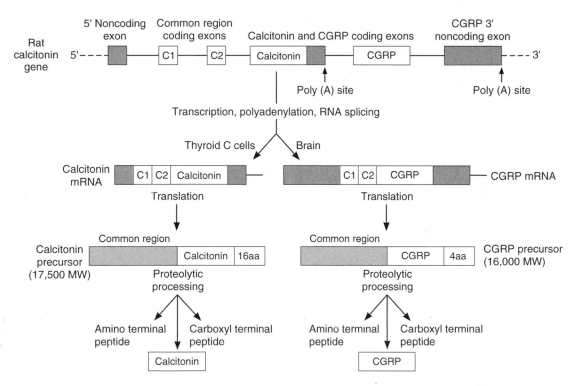

Figure 8–6. Alternative processing of the human calcitonin gene. Calcitonin is produced by thyroid C cells; CGRP is produced in the brain. (Modified and reproduced, with permission, from Rosenfeld MG et al: Production of a novel neuropeptide encoded by the calcitonin gene via tissue-specific RNA processing. Nature 1983;304:129.)

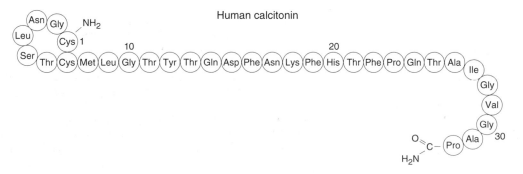

Figure 8–7. Amino acid sequence of human calcitonin, demonstrating its biochemical features, including an amino terminal disulfide bridge and carboxyl terminal prolinamide. (Reproduced, with permission, from McPhee SJ et al [editors]: *Pathophysiology of Disease: An Introduction to Clinical Medicine.* Originally published by Appleton & Lange. Copyright © 1995 by The McGraw-Hill Companies, Inc.)

calcitonin receptor. Like the PTH receptor, this is a serpentine G protein-coupled receptor with seven membrane-spanning regions which is coupled by G_s to adenylyl cyclase and thereby to the generation of cAMP in target cells. Calcitonin also has renal effects. At the kidney, calcitonin inhibits the reabsorption of phosphate, thus promoting renal phosphate excretion. Calcitonin also induces a mild natriuresis and increases the renal excretion of calcium. The renal effects of calcitonin are not essential for its acute effect on serum calcium levels, which results from blockade of bone resorption.

Although its secretory control by calcium and its antiresorptive actions enable calcitonin to counter PTH in the control of calcium homeostasis, thus engendering bihormonal regulation, it is actually unlikely that calcitonin plays an essential physiologic role in humans and other terrestrial animals. This surprising conclusion is supported by two lines of evidence. First, removal of the thyroid gland—the only known source of calcitonin in mammals—has no perceptible impact on calcium handling or bone metabolism. Second, secretion of extremely high calcitonin levels by medullary thyroid carcinoma, a malignancy of the C cell, likewise has no apparent effect on mineral homeostasis. Thus, in humans, calcitonin is a hormone in search of a function. It plays a much more obvious homeostatic role in salt-water fish, in which the major challenge is maintenance of blood calcium levels in the sea, where the ambient calcium concentration of sea water is very high.

Calcitonin is of clinical interest for two reasons. First, calcitonin is important as a tumor marker in medullary thyroid carcinoma. Second, calcitonin has found several therapeutic uses as an inhibitor of osteoclastic bone resorption. Calcitonin can be administered either parenterally or as a nasal spray and is used in the treatment of Paget's disease of bone, hypercalcemia, and osteoporosis.

VITAMIN D

Nomenclature

The term vitamin D (calciferol) refers to two secosteroids: vitamin D_2 (ergocalciferol) and vitamin D_3 (cholecalciferol) (Figure 8–8). Both are produced by photolysis from naturally occurring sterol precursors. Vitamin D_2 is the principal form of vitamin D available for pharmaceutical purposes other than as dietary supplements (Table 8–2). Vitamin D_3 is produced from 7-dehydrocholesterol, a precursor of cholesterol found in high concentration in the skin. Vitamins D_2 and D_3 are nearly equipotent in humans, so the term vitamin D, unless otherwise qualified, will be understood here to denote both. Vitamins D_2 and D_3 differ in their side chains: vitamin D_2 has a methyl group at C24 and a double bond at C22 to C23. These features alter the metabolism of vitamin D_2 compared with vitamin D_3; however, both are converted to 25-hydroxyvitamin D and 1,25-dihydroxyvitamin D_3.

In the process of forming vitamins D_2 and D_3, the B ring of the sterol precursor is cleaved, and the A ring is rotated around the C5 to C6 double bond so that the 3β-hydroxyl group is positioned below the plane of the A-ring. By convention, this hydroxyl group retains its designation as 3β, and the 1-position above the plane of the A-ring is designated 1α. Hydroxylations in the side-chain can lead to stereoisomers designated R and S. The natural position for the C24 hydroxyl group is R. Both the R and the S positions can be hydroxylated at C25 in the formation of $25,26(OH)_2D$.

Since vitamin D can be formed in vivo (in the epidermis) in the presence of adequate amounts of ultraviolet light, it is more properly considered a hormone (or prohormone) than a vitamin. To be biologically active, vitamin D must be metabolized further. The liver metabolizes vitamin D to its principal circulating form, $25(OH)D$. The kidney and other tissues metabolize $25(OH)D$ to a variety of other metabolites, the most important of which are $1,25(OH)_2D_3$ and, perhaps, $24,25(OH)_2D$. A large number of other metabolites have been identified, but their physiologic roles are unclear. They may only represent products destined for elimination. Normal circulating levels of the principal metabolites are listed in Table 8–3. The recommended daily allowance for vitamin D is 400 units. One unit equals 0.025 μg vitamin D.

Cutaneous Synthesis of Vitamin D

Vitamin D_3 is formed in the skin from 7-dehydrocholesterol, which is distributed throughout the epidermis and dermis but has its highest concentration in the lower layers of the epidermis, the stratum spinosum and stratum basale. These epidermal layers also account for the highest production of vitamin D. The cleavage of the B ring of 7-dehydrocholesterol to form previtamin D_3 (Figure 8–8) requires ultraviolet light. Following cleavage of the B ring, the previtamin D_3 undergoes thermal isomerization to vitamin D_3 but also to the biologically inactive compounds lumisterol and tachysterol. Formation of pre-D_3 is rapid and reaches a maximum within hours during exposure to solar or ultraviolet irradiation. The degree of epidermal pigmentation, the age of the skin, and the intensity of exposure all affect the time required to reach the maximum pre-D_3 concentration but do not alter that maximum. Continued ultraviolet light exposure then results in continued formation of the inactive compounds from pre-D_3. The formation of lumisterol is re-

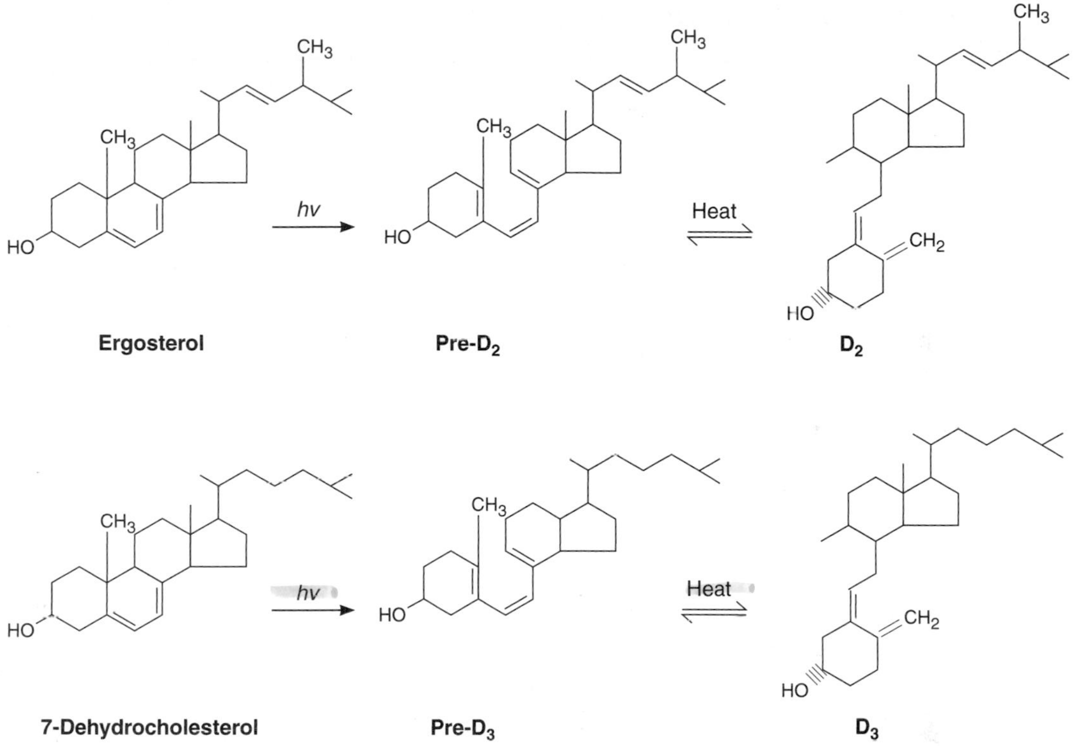

Figure 8–8. The photolysis of ergosterol and 7-dehydrocholesterol to vitamin D_2 (ergocalciferol) and vitamin D_3 (cholecalciferol), respectively. An intermediate is formed after photolysis, which undergoes a thermal-activated isomerization to the final form of vitamin D. The rotation of the A-ring puts the 3β-hydroxyl group into a different orientation with respect to the plane of the A-ring during production of vitamin D.

Table 8–2. Commonly used vitamin D metabolites and analogs.

	Cholecalciferol, Ergocalciferol	Dihydrotachysterol	Calcifediol	Calcitriol
Abbreviation	D_3, D_2	DHT	$25(OH)D_3$	$1,25(OH)_2D$
Physiologic dose	2.5–10 µg (1 µg = 40 units)	25–100 µg	1–5 µg	0.25–0.5 µg
Pharmacologic dose	0.625–5 mg	0.2–1 mg	20–200 µg	1–3 µg
Duration of action	1–3 months	1–4 weeks	2–6 weeks	2–5 days
Clinical applications	Vitamin D deficiency Vitamin D malabsorption Hypoparathyroidism Anticonvulsant therapy in institutionalized patients	Chronic renal failure Hypoparathyroidism	Vitamin D malabsorption Chronic renal failure	Chronic renal failure Hypoparathyroidism Hypophosphatemic rickets Acute hypocalcemia Vitamin D-dependent rickets types I and II

Table 8–3. Vitamin D and its metabolites.[1]

Name	Abbreviation	Generic Name	Serum Concentration[2]
Vitamin D	D	Calciferol	1.6 ± 0.4 ng/mL
Vitamin D_3	D_3	Cholecalciferol	
Vitamin D_2	D_2	Ergocalciferol	
25-Hydroxyvitamin D	25(OH)D	Calcifediol	26.5 ± 5.3 ng/mL
1,25-Dihydroxyvitamin D	1,25(OH)$_2$D	Calcitriol	34.1 ± 0.4 pg/mL
24,25-Dihydroxyvitamin D	24,25(OH)$_2$D		1.3 ± 0.4 ng/mL
25,26-Dihydroxyvitamin D	25,26(OH)$_2$D		0.5 ± 0.1 ng/mL

[1]Data from Lambert PW et al. In: Bikle D (editor): *Assay of Calcium Regulating Hormones.* Springer, 1983.
[2]Values differ somewhat from laboratory to laboratory depending on the methodology used and the sunlight exposure and dietary intake of vitamin D in the population study. Children tend to have higher 1,25(OH)$_2$D levels than do adults.

versible, so lumisterol can be converted back to pre-D_3 as pre-D_3 levels fall. Short exposure to sunlight causes prolonged release of vitamin D_3 from the exposed skin because of the slow conversion of pre-D_3 to vitamin D_3 and the conversion of lumisterol to pre-D_3. Prolonged exposure to sunlight does not produce toxic quantities of vitamin D_3 because of the photoconversion of pre-D_3 to lumisterol and tachysterol.

Vitamin D_3 transport from the skin into the circulation has not been thoroughly studied. Vitamin D_3 is carried in the bloodstream primarily bound to vitamin D-binding protein (DBP), an α-globulin produced in the liver. DBP has a lower affinity for vitamin D_3 than other vitamin D metabolites such as 25(OH)D and 24,25(OH)$_2$D. 7-Dehydrocholesterol, pre-D_3, lumisterol, and tachysterol bind to DBP even less well. Therefore, vitamin D_3 could be selectively removed from skin by the gradient established by selective binding to DBP. Since the deepest levels of the epidermis make the most vitamin D_3 when the skin is irradiated, the distance over which vitamin D_3 must diffuse to reach the circulation is short. However, simple diffusion is an unlikely means for so hydrophobic a molecule to enter the bloodstream. Epidermal lipoproteins may play a role in transport, but this remains to be established.

Dietary Sources & Intestinal Absorption

Dietary sources of vitamin D are clinically important because exposure to ultraviolet light may not be sufficient to maintain adequate production of vitamin D in the skin. The farther away from the equator one lives, the shorter the period of the year during which the in-

tensity of sunlight is sufficient to produce vitamin D_3. Most dairy products in the United States are supplemented with vitamin D. Unfortified dairy products contain little or no vitamin D. Although plants contain ergosterol, their content of vitamin D_2 is limited unless they are irradiated with ultraviolet light during processing. Vitamin D is found in high concentrations in fish oils, fish liver, and eggs. Vitamin D is absorbed from the diet in the small intestine with the help of bile salts. Drugs that bind bile salts such as colestipol will reduce vitamin D absorption. Most of the vitamin D passes into the lymph in chylomicrons, but a significant amount is absorbed directly into the portal system. The presence of fat in the lumen decreases vitamin D absorption. 25(OH)D is preferentially absorbed into the portal system and is less influenced by the amount of fat in the lumen. Biliary conjugates of the vitamin D metabolites have been identified, and an enterohepatic circulation of these metabolites has been established. Vitamin D is taken up rapidly by the liver and is metabolized to 25(OH)D. 25(OH)D is also transported in the blood bound to DBP. Little vitamin D is stored in the liver. Excess vitamin D is stored in adipose tissue and muscle.

Binding Proteins for Vitamin D Metabolites

As noted above, vitamin D metabolites are transported in the blood bound principally to DBP (85%) and albumin (15%). DBP binds 25(OH)D and 24,25 (OH)$_2$D with approximately 30 times greater affinity than it binds 1,25(OH)$_2$D$_3$ and vitamin D. DBP circulates at a concentration (5×10^{-6} mol/L) approximately

50 times greater than the total concentrations of the vitamin D metabolites. DBP levels are reduced in liver disease and in the nephrotic syndrome and increased during pregnancy and with estrogen administration but are not altered by states of vitamin D deficiency or excess. The high affinity of DBP for the vitamin D metabolites and the large excess binding capacity maintain the free and presumed biologically active concentrations of the vitamin D metabolites at very low levels—approximately 0.03% and 0.4% of the total 25(OH)D and 1,25(OH)$_2$D$_3$ levels, respectively. Liver disease reduces the total level of the vitamin D metabolites commensurate with the reduction in DBP and albumin levels, but the free concentrations of the vitamin D metabolites remain normal in most subjects. This fact must be borne in mind when evaluating a patient with liver disease and determining whether or not such a patient is truly vitamin D-deficient. Pregnancy, on the other hand, increases both the free and total concentrations by increasing DBP levels, altering the binding of the metabolites to DBP, and increasing the production of 1,25(OH)$_2$D$_3$. The binding of the vitamin D metabolites to DBP appears to occur at the same site, and saturation of this site by one metabolite can displace the other metabolites. This is an important consideration in vitamin D toxicity because the very high levels of 25(OH)D that mark this condition displace the often normal levels of 1,25(OH)$_2$D$_3$, leading to elevated free and biologically active concentrations of 1,25(OH)$_2$D$_3$. This phenomenon at least partially explains the hypercalcemia and hypercalciuria that mark vitamin D intoxication even in patients with normal total 1,25(OH)$_2$D$_3$ levels. At present, it is not clear whether DBP functions just to maintain a circulating reservoir of vitamin D metabolites or whether DBP participates in transporting the vitamin D metabolites to and within their target tissues. There is little evidence for a DBP receptor on cells. Independently of vitamin D, DBP binds to actin and appears to activate macrophages, suggesting that DBP has functions other than vitamin D metabolite transport.

Metabolism

The conversion of vitamin D to 25(OH)D occurs principally in the liver (Figure 8–9). Both mitochondria and microsomes have the capacity to produce 25(OH)D, but with different kinetics and probably with different enzymes. The mitochondrial enzyme has been identified as the 5β-cholestane-3α,7α,12α-triol-27(26)-hydroxylase (CYP27), a cytochrome P450 mixed-function oxidase, and its cDNA has been isolated. Regulation of 25(OH)D production is difficult to demonstrate. Drugs such as phenytoin and phenobarbital reduce serum 25(OH)D levels primarily by increased catabolism of 25(OH)D and vitamin D. Liver disease leads to reduced serum 25(OH)D levels, primarily because of reduced DBP synthesis and not reduced synthesis of 25(OH)D. Vitamin D deficiency is marked by low blood levels of 25(OH)D primarily because of lack of substrate for the 25-hydroxylase. Vitamin D intoxication, on the other hand, leads to increased levels of 25(OH)D because of the lack of feedback-inhibition.

Control of vitamin D metabolism is exerted principally in the kidney (Figure 8–9). 1,25(OH)$_2$D$_3$ and 24,25(OH)$_2$D are produced by cytochrome mixed-function oxidases in mitochondria of the proximal tubules. cDNAs encoding these enzymes have both been identified and show substantial homology to each other and to the 25-hydroxylase (CYP27). Their homology to other mitochondrial steroid hydroxylases is considerable, but not as high. Although the 24-hydroxylase is widely distributed, the 1-hydroxylase is more limited, being found only in the epidermis, placenta, bone, macrophages, and prostate in addition to kidney.

The kidney remains the principal source for circulating 1,25(OH)$_2$D$_3$. Production of 1,25(OH)$_2$D$_3$ in the kidney is stimulated by PTH and is inhibited by high blood levels of calcium and phosphate. Calcium and phosphate have both direct and indirect effects on 1,25(OH)$_2$D$_3$ production. In addition to direct actions on the 1-hydroxylase, calcium alters PTH secretion, and phosphate alters factors (possibly growth hormone) from the pituitary gland which regulate 1,25(OH)$_2$D$_3$ production as well. 1,25(OH)$_2$D$_3$ inhibits its own production and stimulates the production of 24,25(OH)$_2$D. Other hormones such as prolactin, growth hormone, and calcitonin may regulate 1,25(OH)$_2$D$_3$ production, but their roles under normal physiologic conditions in humans have not been demonstrated clearly.

Extrarenal production of 1,25(OH)$_2$D$_3$ is regulated differently in a cell-specific fashion. Cytokines such as γ-interferon and tumor necrosis factor-α stimulate 1,25(OH)$_2$D$_3$ production in macrophages and keratinocytes. 1,25(OH)$_2$D$_3$ and calcium are less inhibitory of 1,25(OH)$_2$D$_3$ production in macrophages. This is important in understanding the pathophysiology of hypercalcemia and the increased 1,25(OH)$_2$D$_3$ levels in patients with sarcoidosis, lymphomas, and other granulomatous diseases.

Mechanisms of Action

The main function of vitamin D metabolites is the regulation of calcium and phosphate homeostasis, which occurs in conjunction with PTH. The gut, kidney, and bone are the principal target tissues for this regulation. The major pathologic complication of vitamin D defi-

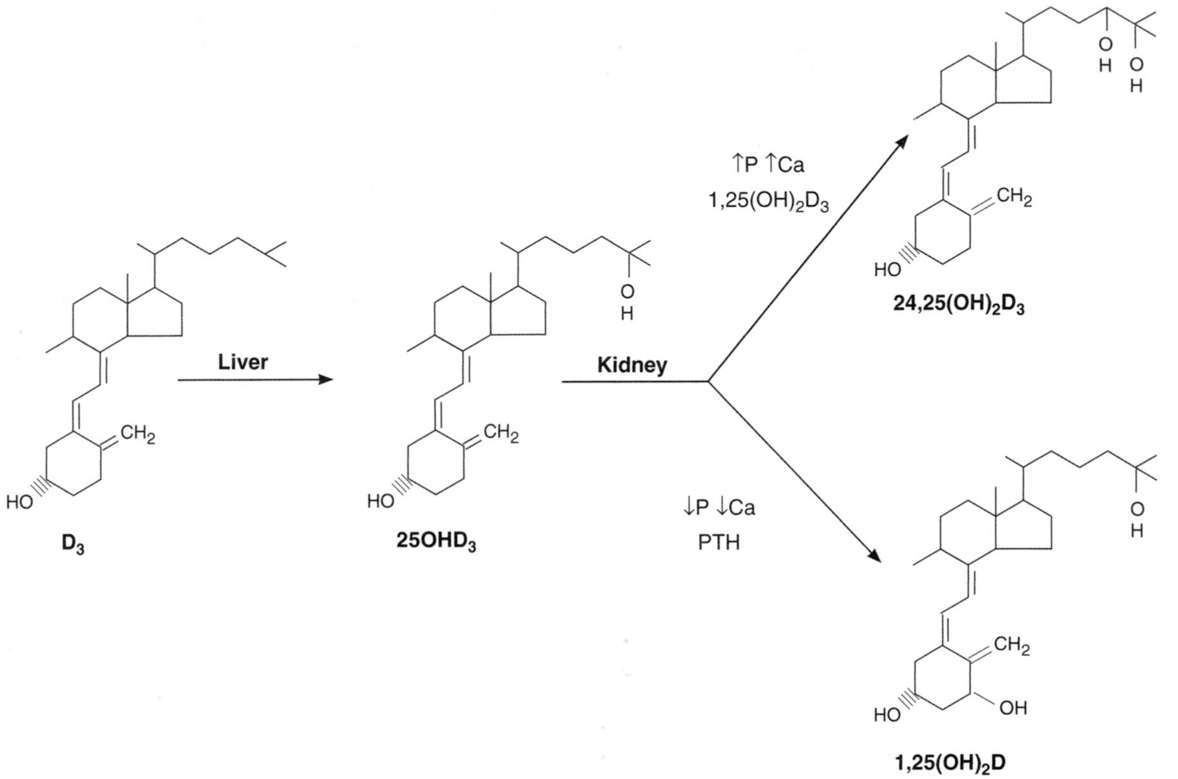

Figure 8–9. The metabolism of vitamin D. The liver converts vitamin D to 25(OH)D. The kidney converts 25(OH)D to 1,25(OH)$_2$D$_3$ and 24,25(OH)$_2$D. Control of metabolism is exerted primarily at the level of the kidney, where low serum phosphorus, low serum calcium, and high parathyroid hormone (PTH) levels favor production of 1,25(OH)$_2$D$_3$.

ciency is rickets (in children with open epiphyses) or osteomalacia (in adults), which in part results from a deficiency in calcium and phosphate required for bone mineralization. 1,25(OH)$_2$D$_3$ is the most biologically active if not the only vitamin D metabolite involved in maintaining calcium and phosphate homeostasis.

Most of the cellular processes regulated by 1,25(OH)$_2$D$_3$ involve the nuclear vitamin D receptor (VDR), a 50-kDa protein related by structural and functional homology to a large class of nuclear hormone receptors including the steroid hormone receptors, thyroid hormone receptors (TRs), retinoic acid and retinoid X receptors (RARs, RXRs), and endogenous metabolite receptors, including peroxisome proliferation activator receptors (PPARs), liver X receptors (LXRs), and farnesoid X receptors (FXRs). These receptors are transcription factors. The VDR, as is the case with TRs, RARs, PPARs, LXRs, and FXRs, generally acts by forming heterodimers with RXRs. The VDR-RXR complex then binds to specific regions within the regulatory portions of the genes whose expression is controlled by 1,25(OH)$_2$D$_3$ (Figure 8–10). The regulatory regions are called vitamin D response elements (VDREs) and are generally composed of two stretches of six nucleotides (each called a half-site) with a specific and nearly identical sequence separated by three nucleotides with a less specific sequence (a direct repeat with three base-pair separation; DR3). Exceptions to this rule can be found such as a VDR-RAR complex binding to a DR6 (direct repeat with six base-pair separation). Other nuclear hormone receptors bind to similar elements but with different spacing or orientation of the half-sites. The binding of the VDR-RXR complex to the VDRE then attracts a number of other proteins called coactivators which are thought to bridge the gap between the VDRE and the initiation complex (TATA box proteins) to signal the beginning of transcription. Many of these coactivators have histone acetyltransferase activity, which leads to an unraveling of the histone-chromatin complex encompassing the gene, thus

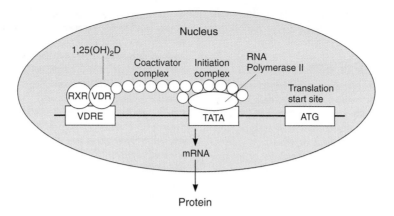

Figure 8–10. 1,25(OH)$_2$D$_3$-initiated gene transcription. 1,25(OH)$_2$D$_3$ enters the target cell and binds to its receptor, VDR. The VDR then heterodimerizes with the retinoid X receptor, RXR. This increases the affinity of the VDR/RXR complex for the vitamin D response element (VDRE), a specific sequence of nucleotides in the promoter region of the vitamin D responsive gene. Binding of the VDR/RXR complex to the VDRE attracts a complex of proteins termed coactivators to the VDR/RXR complex which span the gap between the VDRE and RNA polymerase II and other proteins in the initiation complex centered at or around the TATA box (or other transcription regulatory elements). Transcription of the gene is initiated to produce the corresponding mRNA, which leaves the nucleus to be translated to the corresponding protein.

allowing it to be activated. Not all actions of 1,25(OH)$_2$D$_3$ can be explained by changes in gene expression. An area of active investigation involves efforts to identify a membrane receptor for 1,25(OH)$_2$D$_3$ that may mediate the rapid effects of 1,25(OH)$_2$D$_3$ on calcium influx and protein kinase C activity observed in a number of tissues.

A. Intestinal Calcium Transport

Intestinal calcium transport is the best-understood target tissue response of 1,25(OH)$_2$D$_3$. Calcium transport through the intestinal epithelium proceeds by at least three distinct steps: (1) entrance into the cell from the lumen across the brush border membrane down a steep electrochemical gradient; (2) passage through the cytosol, probably within subcellular organelles such as mitochondria and dense bodies; and (3) removal from the cell against a steep electrochemical gradient at the basolateral membrane. Each of these steps is regulated by 1,25(OH)$_2$D$_3$. At the brush border, 1,25(OH)$_2$D$_3$ induces a change in the binding of calmodulin to brush border myosin 1, a unique form of myosin found only in the intestine, where it resides primarily in the microvillus bound to actin and to the plasma membrane.

The calmodulin-myosin 1 complex may provide the mechanism for removing calcium from the brush border after it crosses the membrane into the cell. Changes in the phospholipid composition of the brush border may explain the increased flux of calcium across this membrane after calcitriol administration. None of these changes require new protein synthesis. However, recent evidence indicates that a newly described calcium channel (CaT1) in the brush border membrane may be induced by 1,25(OH)$_2$D. This channel may be the major mechanism by which calcium enters the intestinal epithelial cell. The transport of calcium through the cytosol requires a vitamin D-inducible protein called calbindin. Calbindin exists either in a 28-kDa or 9-kDa form, depending on the species. Calbindin has a high affinity for calcium. If its synthesis is blocked, the calcium content of the cytosol and mitochondria increases, and efficiency of transport is reduced. At the basolateral membrane, calcium is removed from the cell by an ATP-driven pump, the Ca^{2+}-ATPase, a protein also induced by 1,25(OH)$_2$D$_3$. In mice in which the VDR is rendered nonfunctional (VDR "knockout"), intestinal calcium transport is markedly impaired, indicating the importance of VDR function—presumably regulation of gene expression— in governing intestinal calcium transport. The requirement for a functional VDR is less clear for other target tissues.

B. Actions of Vitamin D in Bone

The critical role of $1,25(OH)_2D_3$ in regulating bone formation and resorption is evidenced by the development of rickets in children who lack the ability to produce $1,25(OH)_2D_3$ (vitamin D-dependent rickets type 1 or pseudovitamin D-deficient rickets) or who lack a functioning VDR (vitamin D-dependent rickets type 2 or hereditary $1,25(OH)_2D_3$-resistant rickets). The appearance of bone in these conditions is quite similar to that in patients with vitamin D deficiency. The former have inactivating mutations in the 1-hydroxylase gene and can be treated successfully with calcitriol (but not with vitamin D), whereas the latter are resistant to calcitriol as well as to vitamin D. These experiments of nature, however, do not exclude the possibility that other vitamin D metabolites, in combination with $1,25(OH)_2D_3$, are essential for normal bone metabolism.

In vitamin D deficiency, all vitamin D metabolites are reduced, but $25(OH)D$ and $24,25(OH)_2D$ tend to be reduced out of proportion to $1,25(OH)_2D_3$, which may be maintained in the low normal range despite clear abnormalities in bone mineralization. Thus, it is reasonable to ask whether $1,25(OH)_2D_3$ is the only vitamin D metabolite of consequence for the regulation of skeletal homeostasis. In fact, a number of studies point to unique actions of $24,25(OH)_2D$ that cannot be replicated by $1,25(OH)_2D_3$, especially in cartilage, although this remains controversial. Studies in mice in which the 24-hydroxylase gene has been inactivated ("knocked out") support the concept that $24,25(OH)_2D$ has a role in bone formation that is not replaced by $1,25(OH)_2D_3$. This is an important concept in the treatment of vitamin D deficiency, which is best done with vitamin D or $25(OH)D$ rather than calcitriol alone, as the former serve as precursors for both $1,25(OH)_2D_3$ and $24,25(OH)_2D$.

The mechanisms by which $1,25(OH)_2D_3$ regulates skeletal homeostasis remain uncertain. Provision of adequate calcium and phosphate for mineralization is clearly important. The rickets of patients with defective VDRs (vitamin D-dependent rickets type 2) can be cured with calcium and phosphate infusions. Similarly, in mice in which the VDR is rendered nonfunctional ("knocked out"), rickets could be prevented with diets high in calcium and phosphate. Thus, even though the osteoblast, the cell responsible for forming new bone, contains a VDR and the transcription of a number of proteins in bone is transcriptionally regulated by $1,25(OH)_2D_3$, it is not clear how essential the direct actions of $1,25(OH)_2D_3$ on bone are for bone formation and mineralization.

In organ cultures of bone, the best established action of $1,25(OH)_2D_3$ is bone resorption. This is accompanied by an increase in osteoclast number and activity and decreased collagen synthesis. The increase in osteoclast activity is now known to be mediated by the production in osteoblasts of a membrane-bound protein called receptor activator of NF-κB ligand (RANKL), which acts on its receptor in osteoclasts and their precursors to stimulate osteoclast differentiation and activity. $1,25(OH)_2D_3$ is one of several hormones (PTH and selected cytokines are others) that stimulate RANKL production. Although vitamin D deficiency is not marked by decreased bone resorption (probably due to the elevated PTH levels, which could compensate for the lack of $1,25(OH)_2D_3$ at the level of RANKL production), the clinical evidence that the bones of patients with vitamin D deficiency are partially resistant to the actions of PTH may be explained by this mechanism.

$1,25(OH)_2D_3$ also promotes the differentiation of osteoblasts. This action is less well delineated than the promotion of osteoclast differentiation. Osteoblasts pass through a well-defined sequence of biochemical processes as they differentiate from proliferating osteoprogenitor cells to cells capable of producing and mineralizing matrix. The effect of $1,25(OH)_2D_3$ on the osteoblast depends on the stage of differentiation at which the $1,25(OH)_2D_3$ is administered. Early in the differentiation process (or in bone cells characterized as immature osteoblast-like cells), $1,25(OH)_2D_3$ stimulates collagen production and alkaline phosphatase activity. These functions are inhibited in more mature osteoblasts. On the other hand, osteocalcin production is stimulated by $1,25(OH)_2D_3$ only in mature osteoblasts. Experiments in vivo demonstrating that excessive $1,25(OH)_2D_3$ can inhibit normal bone mineralization—leading to the paradoxical appearance of osteomalacia—can be understood in the context of these differential effects of $1,25(OH)_2D_3$ on the osteoblast as it differentiates. Too much $1,25(OH)_2D_3$ can disrupt the differentiation pathway.

C. Actions of Vitamin D in Kidney

The kidney expresses VDR, and $1,25(OH)_2D_3$ stimulates calbindin and Ca^{2+}-ATPase in the distal tubule as well as $24,25(OH)_2D$ production in the proximal tubule. However, the role of $1,25(OH)_2D_3$ in regulating calcium and phosphate transport across the renal epithelium remains controversial. $25(OH)D$ may be more important than $1,25(OH)_2D_3$ in acutely stimulating calcium and phosphate reabsorption by the kidney tubules. In vivo studies are complicated by the effect of $1,25(OH)_2D_3$ on other hormones, particularly PTH, which appears to be more important than the vitamin D metabolites in regulating calcium and phosphate handling by the kidney.

D. Actions of Vitamin D in Other Tissues

An exciting recent discovery has been that VDRs are found in a large number of tissues beyond the classic target tissues—gut, bone, and kidney—and these tissues respond to $1,25(OH)_2D_3$. These tissues include elements of the hematopoietic and immune systems; cardiac, skeletal, and smooth muscle; brain, liver, breast, endothelium, skin (keratinocytes, melanocytes, and fibroblasts), and endocrine glands (pituitary, parathyroid, pancreatic islets [B cells], adrenal cortex and medulla, thyroid, ovary, and testis). Furthermore, malignancies developing in these tissues often contain VDRs and respond to the antiproliferative actions of $1,25(OH)_2D_3$.

The responses of these tissues to $1,25(OH)_2D_3$ are as varied as the tissues themselves. $1,25(OH)_2D_3$ regulates hormone production and secretion, including insulin from the pancreas, prolactin from the pituitary, and PTH from the parathyroid gland, just as it regulates cytokine production and secretion of interleukin-2 from lymphocytes and tumor necrosis factor from monocytes. Myocardial contractility and vascular tone are modulated by $1,25(OH)_2D_3$, as is liver regeneration. $1,25(OH)_2D_3$ reduces the rate of proliferation of many cell lines, including normal keratinocytes, fibroblasts, lymphocytes, and thymocytes as well as abnormal cells of mammary, skeletal, intestinal, lymphatic, and myeloid origin. Differentiation of numerous normal cell types, including keratinocytes, lymphocytes, hematopoietic cells, intestinal epithelial cells, osteoblasts, and osteoclasts as well as abnormal cells of the same lineage is enhanced by $1,25(OH)_2D_3$. Thus, the potential for manipulating a vast array of physiologic and pathologic processes with calcitriol and its analogs is enormous. This promise is starting to be realized in that vitamin D analogs are being used to treat psoriasis, uremic hyperparathyroidism, and osteoporosis. Trials of vitamin D analogs in the treatment of a variety of cancers are also being conducted. Thus, although regulation of bone mineral homeostasis remains the major physiologic function of vitamin D, clinical applications for these compounds are being found outside the classic target tissues.

INTEGRATED CONTROL OF MINERAL HOMEOSTASIS

Consider a person who switches from a high normal to a low normal intake of calcium and phosphate—from 1200 per day to 300 mg per day of calcium (the equivalent of leaving three glasses of milk out of the daily diet). The net absorption of calcium falls sharply, causing a transient decrease in the serum calcium level. The homeostatic response to this transient hypocalcemia is led by an increase in PTH, which stimulates the release of calcium and phosphate from bone and the retention of calcium by the kidney. The phosphaturic effect of PTH allows elimination of phosphate, which is resorbed from bone together with calcium. In addition, the increase in PTH, along with the fall in serum calcium and serum phosphorus, activates renal $1,25(OH)_2D_3$ synthesis. In its turn, $1,25(OH)_2D_3$ increases the fractional absorption of calcium and further increases bone resorption. External calcium balance is thus restored by increased fractional absorption of calcium and increased bone resorption at the expense of increased steady state levels of PTH and $1,25(OH)_2D_3$.

■ MEDULLARY THYROID CARCINOMA

Medullary carcinoma, a neoplasm of thyroidal C cells, accounts for 5–10% of all thyroid malignancies. Approximately 75% of medullary carcinomas are sporadic. The remainder are familial and associated with one of three heritable syndromes: familial isolated medullary carcinoma; multiple endocrine neoplasia 2A (MEN 2A), consisting of medullary carcinoma, pheochromocytoma, and primary hyperparathyroidism; or multiple endocrine neoplasia 2B (MEN 2B), consisting of medullary carcinoma, pheochromocytoma, multiple mucosal neuromas, and, rarely, primary hyperparathyroidism (Table 8–4). The MEN syndromes are more extensively discussed in Chapter 22.

Understanding of the pathogenesis of medullary carcinoma has been greatly enhanced by the identification of causative mutations in the *RET* proto-oncogene located on chromosome 10q11.2. The *RET* gene encodes a membrane tyrosine kinase receptor for whose ligands are in the glial cell line-derived neurotrophic factor (GDNF) family. This receptor is expressed developmentally in migrating neural crest cells that will give rise to hormone-secreting neuroendocrine cells (eg, C cells and adrenal medullary cells) and to the parasympathetic and sympathetic ganglia of the peripheral nervous system. Remarkably, different mutations in *RET* can produce five distinct diseases. Inheritance of certain activating mutations is responsible for MEN 2A and familial medullary thyroid carcinoma. Inheritance of a different set of activating mutations causes MEN 2B. In over half of sporadic medullary thyroid carcinomas, the tumor has a clonal somatic mutation (present in the tumor but not in genomic DNA), which is identical to one of the mutations that is responsible for the familial forms of medullary carcinoma. Almost certainly, such somatic mutations cause sporadic medullary carcinoma.

Table 8–4. Clinical features of multiple endocrine neoplasia syndromes.

MEN 1
  Parathyroid hyperplasia (very common)
  Pancreatic tumors (benign or malignant)
    Gastrinoma
    Insulinoma
    Glucagonoma, VIPoma (both rare)
  Pituitary tumor
    Growth hormone-secreting
    Prolactin-secreting
    ACTH-secreting
  Other tumors: lipomas, carcinoids, adrenal and thyroid
    adenomas
MEN 2A
  Medullary carcinoma of the thyroid
  Pheochromocytoma (benign or malignant)
  Parathyroid hyperplasia
MEN 2B
  Medullary carcinoma of the thyroid
  Pheochromocytoma
  Mucosal neuromas, ganglioneuromas
  Marfanoid habitus
  Hyperparathyroidism (very rare)

In addition to its role in medullary carcinoma, where the *RET* gene product is activated by point mutations, the *RET* gene is often rearranged in papillary carcinoma of the thyroid, giving rise to *RET* chimeric genes. Transgenic experiments indicate that the rearranged *RET* gene is sufficient to cause papillary thyroid carcinoma in mice. Finally, mutations that inactivate the *RET* gene produce Hirschsprung's disease, a congenital absence of the enteric parasympathetic ganglia, in which intestinal motility is disturbed, resulting in megacolon.

Medullary carcinoma is usually located in the middle or upper portions of the thyroid lobes. It is typically unilateral in sporadic cases but often multicentric and bilateral in familial forms of medullary carcinoma. Pathologically, medullary thyroid carcinoma was originally distinguished from other thyroid cancers by the presence of amyloid, eosinophilic material which stains with Congo red. Molecular studies have shown that amyloid consists of dense fibrillar deposits of protein in a β-pleated sheet structure. In the case of medullary carcinoma, the protein deposited as amyloid is procalcitonin or calcitonin itself. Thus, the pathologic diagnosis of medullary carcinoma can now be made by immunohistochemical staining for calcitonin.

The natural history of medullary carcinoma is variable. Sporadic tumors may be quite aggressive or very indolent; the mean five-year survival rate is about 50%.

The behavior of familial forms varies among syndromes. MEN 2B has the most aggressive form of medullary carcinoma, with a 2-year survival of about 50%; MEN 2A has a course similar to that of sporadic medullary carcinoma, and familial medullary carcinoma has the most indolent course of all. The tumor may spread to regional lymph nodes or undergo hematogenous spread to the lungs and other viscera. When metastatic, medullary thyroid carcinoma is sometimes associated with a chronic diarrhea syndrome. The pathogenesis of the diarrhea is unclear. In addition to calcitonin, these tumors secrete a variety of other bioactive products, including prostaglandins, serotonin, histaminase, and peptide hormones (ACTH, somatostatin, CRH). In some cases the associated diarrhea responds dramatically to treatment with long-acting somatostatin analogs such as octreotide, which block secretion of these bioactive products.

Calcitonin is a tumor marker for medullary thyroid carcinoma. It is most sensitive for this purpose when secretion is stimulated with provocative agents. The standard provocative tests used pentagastrin (0.5 μg/kg intravenously over 5 seconds) or a rapid infusion of calcium gluconate (2 mg calcium/kg over 1 minute). Blood samples are obtained at baseline and 1, 2, and 5 minutes after the stimulus. For maximal sensitivity both tests are usually combined, with the calcium infusion immediately followed by administration of pentagastrin. Although basal calcitonin levels are often normal in early tumors, calcitonin levels may be many times higher than normal in patients with disseminated medullary carcinoma. Despite this, the patients are uniformly normocalcemic. Although tumors secrete larger-MW forms of calcitonin with decreased biologic activity, monomeric calcitonin levels are often high as well. *RET* oncogene analysis has replaced provocative testing in most cases, though basal calcitonin levels can still be used to follow disease activity.

Members of families that carry *RET* mutations must be individually screened for medullary thyroid carcinoma and for the associated tumors which occur in MEN 2A and MEN 2B (Chapter 22). In the case of medullary thyroid carcinoma, the presence of the *RET* mutation in an individual will lead generally to the recommendation of a total thyroidectomy prior to the development of frank malignancy or abnormal calcitonin levels. It is now recommended in a kindred with a known *RET* mutation that children be screened at birth using genomic DNA. Early thyroidectomy can be performed in carriers of the trait, and further testing can be discontinued in genetically normal family members. The timing of prophylactic thyroidectomy in asymptomatic carriers of *RET* mutations, however, remains uncertain. Most experts favor surgery in early childhood. Because a limited number of mutations in *RET* cause over 95% of hereditary medullary thyroid carcinomas and up to 25% of sporadic disease, it is possible to screen many patients through commercial reference laboratories.

Apparently sporadic medullary thyroid carcinoma also calls for family studies, since up to 25% of new cases may actually be probands of families who harbor one of the familial syndromes. As in known familial cases, screening can be accomplished by provocative testing of the calcitonin response in first-degree relatives or by testing tumor and genomic DNA from the patient for *RET* mutations. Identification of a mutation that is present only in tumor tissue would establish the mutation as somatic and the tumor as a sporadic one. Identification of the same *RET* mutation in tumor and genomic DNA would make the diagnosis of a familial form of the disorder and would mandate careful screening of the family.

■ HYPERCALCEMIA

Clinical Features

A number of symptoms and signs accompany the hypercalcemic state: central nervous system effects such as lethargy, depression, psychosis, ataxia, stupor, and coma; neuromuscular effects such as weakness, proximal myopathy, and hypertonia; cardiovascular effects such as hypertension, bradycardia (and eventually asystole), and a shortened QT interval; renal effects such as stones, decreased glomerular filtration, polyuria, hyperchloremic acidosis, and nephrocalcinosis; gastrointestinal effects such as nausea, vomiting, constipation, and anorexia; eye findings such as band keratopathy; and systemic metastatic calcification. This constellation of clinical findings has led to the mnemonic for recalling the signs and symptoms of hypercalcemia: "stones, bones, abdominal groans, and psychic moans" (Figure 8–11).

Mechanisms

Although many disorders are associated with hypercalcemia (Table 8–5), they can produce hypercalcemia through only a limited number of mechanisms: (1) increased bone resorption, (2) increased gastrointestinal absorption of calcium, or (3) decreased renal excretion of calcium. While any of these mechanisms can be involved in a given patient, the common feature of virtually all hypercalcemic disorders is accelerated bone resorption. The only recognized hypercalcemic disorder in which bone resorption does not play a part is the milk-alkali syndrome.

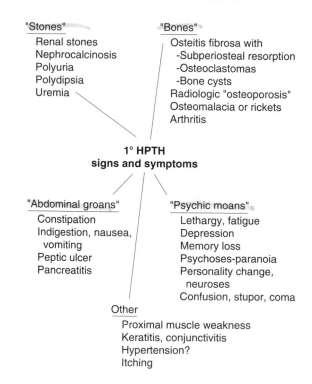

Figure 8–11. Signs and symptoms of primary hyperparathyroidism.

The central feature of the defense against hypercalcemia is suppression of PTH secretion. This reduces bone resorption, reduces renal production of $1,25(OH)_2D_3$ and thereby inhibits calcium absorption, and increases urinary calcium losses. The kidney plays a key role in the adaptive response to hypercalcemia as the only route of net calcium elimination, and the level of renal calcium excretion is markedly increased by the combined effects of an increased filtered load of calcium and the suppression of PTH. However, the patient who relies on the kidneys to excrete an increased calcium load is in precarious balance: Glomerular filtration is impaired by hypercalcemia; the urinary concentrating ability is diminished, predisposing to dehydration; poor mentation may interfere with access to fluids; and nausea and vomiting may further predispose to dehydration and renal azotemia. Renal insufficiency in turn compromises calcium clearance, leading to a downward spiral (Figure 8–12). Thus, once established, many hypercalcemic states are self-perpetuating or aggravated through the "vicious cycle of hypercalcemia." The only alternative to the renal route for elimination of calcium from the extracellular fluid is deposition as calcium phosphate and other salts in bone and soft tissues. Soft tissue calcification is observed with massive

Table 8–5. Causes of hypercalcemia.

Primary hyperparathyroidism
  Sporadic
  Associated with MEN 1 or MEN 2A
  Familial
  After renal transplantation

Variant forms of hyperparathyroidism
  Familial benign hypocalciuric hypercalcemia
  Lithium therapy
  Tertiary hyperparathyroidism in chronic renal failure

Malignancies
  Humoral hypercalcemia of malignancy
    Caused by PTHrP (solid tumors, adult T cell leukemia
      syndrome)
    Caused by 1,25(OH)$_2$D (lymphomas)
    Caused by ectopic secretion of PTH (rare)
  Local osteolytic hypercalcemia (multiple myeloma, leuke-
    mia, lymphoma)

Sarcoidosis or other granulomatous diseases

Endocrinopathies
  Thyrotoxicosis
  Adrenal insufficiency
  Pheochromocytoma
  VIPoma

Drug-induced
  Vitamin A intoxication
  Vitamin D intoxication
  Thiazide diuretics
  Lithium
  Milk-alkali syndrome
  Estrogens, androgens, tamoxifen (in breast carcinoma)

Immobilization

Acute renal failure

Idiopathic hypercalcemia of infancy

ICU hypercalcemia

Serum protein disorders

calcium loads, with massive phosphate loads (as in crush injuries and compartment syndromes), and when renal function is markedly impaired.

Differential Diagnosis

The differential diagnosis is set forth in Table 8–5. As a practical matter, the categories can be divided into primary hyperparathyroidism and everything else. Hyperparathyroidism is by far the commonest cause of hypercalcemia and has distinctive pathophysiologic features. Thus, the first step in the differential diagnosis is determination of PTH, using an assay for intact PTH (Figure

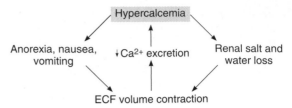

Figure 8–12. Once established, hypercalcemia can be maintained or aggravated as depicted. (Reproduced, with permission, from Felig P, Baxter JD, Frohman LA [editors]: *Endocrinology and Metabolism,* 3rd ed. McGraw-Hill, 1995.)

8–13). If the PTH level is high and thus inappropriate for hypercalcemia, little further workup is required except to consider the variant forms of hyperparathyroidism which are discussed below. If the PTH level is suppressed, then a search for other entities must be conducted. Most other entities in Table 8–5 are readily diagnosed by their distinctive features, as discussed below.

DISORDERS CAUSING HYPERCALCEMIA

1. Primary Hyperparathyroidism

Primary hyperparathyroidism is a hypercalcemic disorder that results from excessive secretion of PTH. With the advent of multiphasic screening of serum chemistries, we have come to recognize that primary hyperparathyroidism is a common and usually asymptomatic disorder. Its incidence is approximately 42 per 100,000, and its prevalence is up to 4 per 1000 in women over age 60. Primary hyperparathyroidism is approximately two to three times as common in women as in men.

Etiology & Pathogenesis

Primary hyperparathyroidism is caused by a single parathyroid adenoma in about 80% of cases and by primary hyperplasia of the parathyroids in about 15%. Parathyroid carcinoma is a rare cause of hyperparathyroidism, accounting for 1–2% of cases. Parathyroid carcinoma is often recognizable preoperatively because it presents with severe hypercalcemia or a palpable neck mass. Primary hyperparathyroidism can occur as part of at least three different familial endocrinopathies. All of them are autosomal dominant traits causing four-gland parathyroid hyperplasia. They include MEN 1, MEN 2A, and isolated familial hyperparathyroidism.

Thyroid adenomas have a clonal origin, indicating that they can be traced back to an oncogenic mutation in a single progenitor cell. A few of these mutations are identified or can tentatively be assigned a genomic locus. About 25% of sporadic parathyroid adenomas

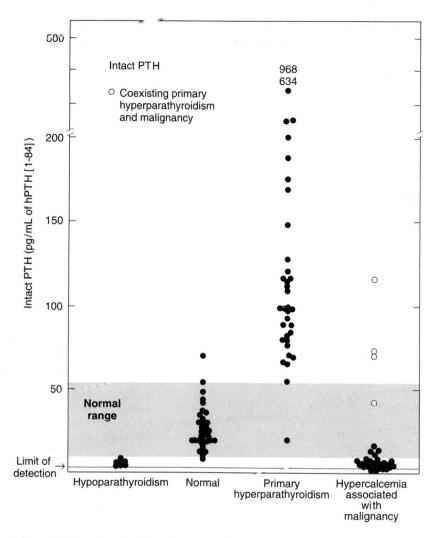

Figure 8–13. Clinical utility of immunoradiometric assay for intact PTH. (Reproduced, with permission, from Endres DB et al: Measurement of parathyroid hormone. Endocrinol Metab Clin North Am 1989;18:611.)

have chromosomal deletions involving chromosome 11q12–13 that are thought to eliminate the putative tumor suppressor gene *MENIN*. As reviewed below and in Chapter 22, loss of the functioning menin protein, a tumor suppressor gene, at this locus is the cause of parathyroid, pituitary, and pancreatic tumors in the MEN 1 syndrome. An additional 40% of parathyroid adenomas display allelic loss on chromosome 1p (1p32pter).

Another important locus on chromosome 11 that has been implicated in approximately 4% of sporadic parathyroid adenomas involves the *PRAD1* oncogene. In the initial elucidation of this pathogenetic mecha-

nism, a chromosomal rearrangement was found. Inversion of a piece of chromosome 11 brings the *PRAD1* cell cycle regulatory gene under the control of the PTH gene promoter. This rearrangement results in marked overexpression of *PRAD1* in the parathyroid. The *PRAD1* gene encodes a cell cycle regulatory protein, cyclin D, which is normally expressed at high levels in the G_1 phase of the cell cycle and permits entry of cells into the mitotic phase of the cycle. Thus, a parathyroid-specific disorder of cell cycle regulation leads to abnormal cell proliferation and ultimately excessive PTH production.

Parathyroid hyperplasia occurs spontaneously, accounting for 12–15% of cases of primary hyperparathyroidism and as part of three forms of familial hyperparathyroidism: MEN 1, MEN 2A, and isolated familial hyperparathyroidism. Parathyroid hyperplasia was traditionally viewed as an example of true hyperplasia, a polyclonal expansion of cell number. This occurs in other endocrine tissues when a trophic hormone is present in excess, eg, ACTH excess produces bilateral adrenal hyperplasia. Molecular analysis, however, has revised this view. MEN 1 is due to the inherited absence of one allele of the menin gene, which is a tumor suppressor gene. Somatic mutations in the *MENIN* gene that result in loss of the other allele's function produce tumors in endocrine tissues where the gene is expressed. In this view, multicentric somatic mutations would account for the occurrence of four-gland hyperparathyroidism. In MEN 2, the occurrence of parathyroid hyperplasia is presumably a consequence of expression of activating mutations of the *RET* gene in the four glands. Surprisingly, it has recently been shown that the majority of glands in spontaneous parathyroid hyperplasia are monoclonal, implying that they arose from a single progenitor cell, presumably as the result of a somatic mutation. Perhaps there is a parathyroid trophic hormone, eg, the *RET* receptor ligand, in some cases of parathyroid hyperplasia, and the increased mitotic rate in hyperplastic glands predisposes to clonal oncogenic mutations.

Parathyroid carcinomas frequently display loss of the retinoblastoma tumor-suppressor gene *RB*, another cell cycle regulator. Certain parathyroid carcinomas show loss of another tumor-suppressor, the *P53* gene. The *P53* and *RB* mutations do not commonly occur in parathyroid adenomas, whereas loss of one or both of these tumor suppressors is prevalent in many other kinds of carcinoma. It is thus likely that these abnormalities in parathyroid carcinoma account for its aggressiveness.

Several candidate parathyroid oncogenes have been eliminated by molecular analysis. Familial benign hypocalciuric hypocalcemia is caused typically by a germline inactivating mutation of one allele of the parathyroid calcium sensor. Somatic mutations of the parathyroid calcium sensor could theoretically produce isolated primary hyperparathyroidism, but such mutations appear to be very infrequent in sporadic hyperparathyroidism. Similarly, mutations in *RET* that cause MEN 2A are quite uncommon in sporadic parathyroid tumors.

Clinical Features

A. SYMPTOMS AND SIGNS

The typical clinical presentation of primary hyperparathyroidism has evolved considerably over the past two decades. As the disease is detected increasingly by multiphasic screening that includes determination of serum calcium levels, there has been a marked reduction in the frequency of the classic signs and symptoms of primary hyperparathyroidism, renal disease—renal stones, decreased renal function, and occasionally nephrocalcinosis—and the classic hyperparathyroid bone disease osteitis fibrosa cystica. In fact, about 85% of patients presenting today have neither bony nor renal manifestations of hyperparathyroidism and are regarded as asymptomatic or minimally symptomatic. At the same time, we have begun to recognize more subtle manifestations of hyperparathyroidism in some patients. This has presented a number of questions about the role of parathyroid surgery in primary hyperparathyroidism, which are discussed below (see Treatment).

1. Hyperparathyroid bone disease—The classic bone disease of hyperparathyroidism is osteitis fibrosa cystica. Formerly common, this disorder now occurs in less than 10% of patients. Clinically, osteitis fibrosa cystica causes bone pain and sometimes pathologic fractures. The most common laboratory finding is an elevation of the alkaline phosphatase level, reflecting high bone turnover. Histologically, there is an increase in the number of bone-resorbing osteoclasts, marrow fibrosis, and cystic lesions that may contain fibrous tissue (brown tumors) or cyst fluid. The most sensitive and specific radiologic finding of osteitis fibrosa cystica is subperiosteal resorption of cortical bone, best seen in high-resolution films of the phalanges (Figure 8–14A). A similar process in the skull leads to a salt-and-pepper appearance (Figure 8–14B). Bone cysts or brown tumors may be evident as osteolytic lesions. Dental films may disclose loss of the lamina dura of the teeth, but this is a nonspecific finding also seen in periodontal disease.

The other important consequence of hyperparathyroidism is osteoporosis. Unlike other osteoporotic disorders, hyperparathyroidism typically results in predominant loss of cortical bone (Figure 8–15). In general, both the mass and the mechanical strength of trabecular bone are relatively well maintained. Patients who are followed medically for mild primary hyperparathyroidism often do not experience progressive bone loss even when they are osteoporotic at diagnosis. This may be due to the fact that PTH under certain circumstances has anabolic effects on the skeleton to increase bone mass. Although osteoporosis is generally considered to be an indication for surgical treatment of primary hyperparathyroidism, its impact on morbidity is hard to assess (see Treatment of Hypercalcemia).

2. Hyperparathyroid kidney disease—Once common in primary hyperparathyroidism, kidney stones now occur in less than 15% of cases. These are usually

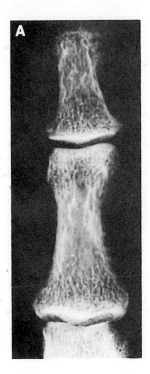
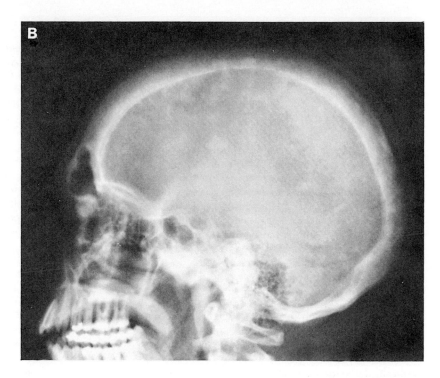

Figure 8–14. ***A:*** Magnified x-ray of index finger on fine-grain industrial film showing classic subperiosteal resorption in a patient with severe primary hyperparathyroidism. Note the left (radial) surface of the distal phalanx, where the cortex is almost completely resorbed, leaving only fine wisps of cortical bone. ***B:*** Skull x-ray from a patient with severe secondary hyperparathyroidism due to end-stage renal disease. Extensive areas of demineralization alternate with areas of increased bone density, resulting in the "salt and pepper" skull x-ray. (Both films courtesy of H Genant.)

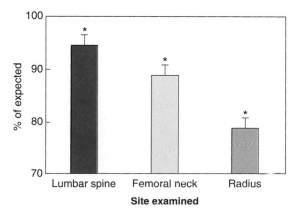

Figure 8–15. Bone density at several sites in primary hyperparathyroidism. (Reproduced, with permission, from Silverberg SJ, Shane E, Jacobs TP et al: Nephrolithiasis and bone involvement in primary hyperparathyroidism. Am J Med 1990;89:327.)

calcium oxalate stones. From the perspective of a stone clinic, only about 7% of calcium stone formers will prove to have primary hyperparathyroidism. They are difficult to manage medically, and stones constitute one of the agreed indications for parathyroidectomy. Clinically evident nephrocalcinosis rarely occurs, but a gradual loss of renal function is not uncommon. Renal function is stabilized after a successful parathyroidectomy, and otherwise unexplained renal insufficiency in the setting of primary hyperparathyroidism is also considered to be an indication for surgery because of the risk of progression. Chronic hypercalcemia can also compromise the renal concentrating ability, giving rise to polydipsia and polyuria.

3. Nonspecific features of primary hyperparathyroidism—Although stupor and coma occur in severe hypercalcemia, the degree to which milder impairments of central nervous system function affect the typical patient with primary hyperparathyroidism is unclear. Lethargy, fatigue, depression, difficulty in concentrating, and personality changes occur and in some patients appear to benefit from parathyroidectomy. Frank psychosis will also respond to surgery on occasion. Muscle weakness with characteristic electromyographic changes is also seen, and there is good evidence from controlled clinical trials that surgery can improve muscle strength. It was formerly thought that the incidence of hypertension was increased in primary hyperparathyroidism, but more recent evidence suggests that the appreciable incidence in this patient group is probably no greater than in age-matched controls, and parathyroidectomy appears to be of no benefit. Dyspepsia, nausea, and constipation all occur, probably as a consequence of hypercalcemia, but there is probably no increase in the incidence of peptic ulcer disease. The articular manifestations of primary hyperparathyroidism are several. Chondrocalcinosis occurs in up to 5% of patients, but acute attacks of pseudogout are less frequent.

B. LABORATORY FINDINGS

Hypercalcemia is virtually universal in primary hyperparathyroidism, though the serum calcium sometimes fluctuates into the upper normal range. In patients with subtle hyperparathyroidism, repeated serum calcium measurements over a period of time may be required to establish the pattern of intermittent hypercalcemia. Both total and ionized calcium are elevated, and in most clinical instances there is no advantage to measuring the ionized calcium level. Patients with normocalcemic primary hyperparathyroidism, in whom the possibility of subtle forms of vitamin D deficiency has been eliminated, are being recognized more frequently. In patients with primary hyperparathyroidism, the serum phosphorus level is low-normal (< 3.5 mg/dL) or low (< 2.5 mg/dL) because of the phosphaturic effect of PTH. A mild hyperchloremic metabolic acidosis may be manifest as hyperchloremia.

The diagnosis of primary hyperparathyroidism in a hypercalcemic patient can be made by determining the intact PTH level with a two-site assay. As shown in Figure 8–13, an elevated or even upper-normal level of PTH is clearly inappropriate in a hypercalcemic patient and establishes the diagnosis of hyperparathyroidism (or one of its variants—familial benign hypercalciuric hypercalcemia or lithium-induced hypercalcemia). The reliability of the two-site intact PTH assay allows the diagnosis of primary hyperparathyroidism to be definitive. In a patient with a high PTH level, there is no need to screen for metastatic malignancy, sarcoidosis, etc. Determinations of renal function and a plain abdominal radiograph for renal stones are often obtained for prognostic reasons. A determination of urinary calcium concentration and urinary creatinine excretion should be obtained to exclude familial benign hypocalciuric hypercalcemia.

Treatment

The definitive treatment of primary hyperparathyroidism is parathyroidectomy. The surgical strategy depends on the ability of localizing studies such as sestamibi scanning to identify one clearly abnormal gland and the availability of intraoperative PTH determinations to verify that the disease-producing lesion has been removed during surgery. If multiple enlarged glands are suspected, the likely diagnosis is parathyroid hyperplasia or double adenoma. In patients with hyperplasia, the preferred operation is a 3½-gland parathyroidectomy, leaving a remnant sufficient to prevent hypocalcemia. Double parathyroid adenomas are both removed in affected patients. The pathologist is of little help in distinguishing among normal tissue, parathyroid adenoma, and parathyroid hyperplasia: these in essence are surgical diagnoses, based on the size and appearance of the glands. The recurrence rate of hypercalcemia is high in patients who have parathyroid hyperplasia—particularly in those with one of the MEN syndromes, because of the inherited propensity for tumor growth. In such cases, the parathyroid remnant can be removed from the neck and implanted in pieces in forearm muscles to allow for easy subsequent removal of some additional parathyroid tissue if hypercalcemia recurs.

In competent hands, the cure rate of parathyroid adenoma is over 95%. The success rate in primary parathyroid hyperplasia is somewhat lower, because of missed glands and recurrent hyperparathyroidism in patients with MEN syndromes. There is a 20% incidence of persistent or recurrent hypercalcemia. However, parathyroidectomy is difficult surgery: the normal parathyroid gland weighs only about 40 mg and may be located throughout the neck or upper mediastinum. It is mandatory not only to locate a parathyroid adenoma but also to find the other gland or glands and determine whether they are normal. Complications of surgery include damage to the recurrent laryngeal nerve, which passes close to the posterior thyroid capsule, and inadvertent removal or devitalization of all parathyroid tissue, producing permanent hypoparathyroidism. In skilled hands, the incidence of these complications is less than 1%. It is critical that parathyroid surgery be performed by someone with specialized skill and experience. (See Chapter 26.)

Localization studies of the parathyroid glands in patients with primary hyperparathyroidism and intraoperative PTH testing are critical components of the contemporary management of patients presenting for initial surgical procedures. If these studies clearly indicate a single abnormal gland and if intraoperative PTH testing is available, surgical management now typically consists of unilateral exploration and limited parathyroidectomy. Localization studies continue to be essential in the management of patients with recurrent or persistent hyperparathyroidism. The most successful procedures are ^{99m}Tc-sestamibi scanning, computed tomography, MRI, and ultrasound. Individually, each has a sensitivity of 60–80% in experienced hands. Used in combination, they are successful in at least 80% of reoperated cases. Invasive studies, such as angiography and venous sampling, are rarely performed.

There is no definitive medical therapy for hyperparathyroidism. In postmenopausal women, estrogen replacement therapy in high doses (1.25 mg of conjugated estrogens or 30–50 μg of ethinyl estradiol) will produce an average decrease of 0.5–1 mg/dL in the serum calcium and an increase in bone mineral density. The effect of estrogen treatment is on the bone response to PTH. PTH levels do not fall. Limited data are available on bisphosphonates and selective estrogen response modulators. Calcimimetic agents that activate the parathyroid calcium-sensing receptor, currently in clinical trials, may offer an alternative to surgery in the future.

The relatively asymptomatic state of most patients today presents a dilemma: Which of them should be subjected to surgery? To answer this question definitively, it would be necessary to know more than we presently do about the natural history of untreated primary hyperparathyroidism. However, in observational studies over as many as 10 years, it is clear that most patients are stable with regard to serum calcium, stone disease, and renal function. Recent data also indicate that osteoporosis, when present, is usually nonprogressive (Figure 8–16). On the other hand, surgery is usually curative. In experienced hands, surgery has a low morbidity rate. Although parathyroid surgery has a substantial initial cost, over the long term the cost-benefit

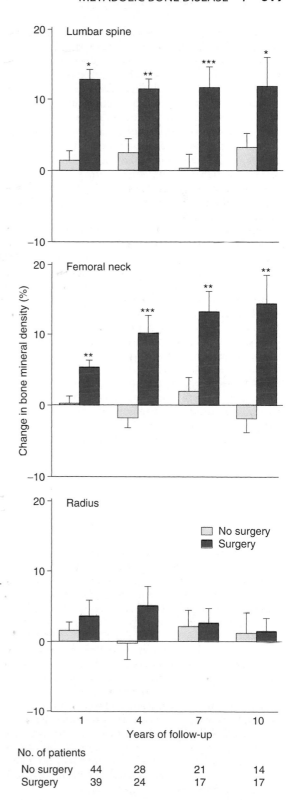

Figure 8–16. Mean changes in bone mineral density (BMD) measurements in patients who underwent parathyroidectomy (■) compared with medical follow-up (▨) during a 15-year observational study. BMD changes are reported compared with baseline and were statistically different from baseline as shown. (* p < .05, ** p < .01, *** p < .001.) The number of patients whose measurements are included are shown underneath each time-point. Radius BMD measurements did not change. (Reproduced and modified, with permission, from Silverberg SJ et al: A 10-year prospective study of primary hyperparathyroidism with or without parathyroid surgery. N Engl J Med 1999;341:1249. Copyright © 1999 by The Massachusetts Medical Society. All rights reserved.)

No. of patients				
No surgery	44	28	21	14
Surgery	39	24	17	17

ratio may be favorable when compared with a lifetime of medical follow-up. Moreover, there is a marked improvement in bone density after surgery (Figure 8–16), with sustained increases over at least 5 years postoperatively. These changes remain stable over years. Some surgeons also argue that the nonspecific symptoms often present may improve with surgery, but no controlled trial has excluded the placebo effect of surgery as a possible explanation for these results.

A 1990 NIH Consensus Development Conference considered the issue of surgery in primary hyperparathyroidism and arrived at the following recommendations: Surgery should be recommended (1) if the serum calcium is markedly elevated (above 11.4–12 mg/dL [2.8–3 mmol/L]); (2) if there has been a previous episode of life-threatening hypercalcemia; (3) if the creatinine clearance is reduced below 70% of normal; (4) if a kidney stone is present; (5) if the urinary calcium is markedly elevated (> 400 mg/24 h); (6) if bone mass is substantially reduced (less than 2 SD below normal for age, sex, and race, ie, two Z-scores below normal); or (7) if the patient is young (under 50 years of age, particularly premenopausal women). In addition, medical surveillance is not considered suitable for patients who request surgery, patients who are unlikely to comply with long-term follow-up schedules, or patients with a coexisting illness complicating their management. These recommendations remain provisional and are currently being revised in consideration of minimally invasive parathyroid surgery and the beneficial skeletal effects of parathyroidectomy in patients with mild disease.

Variants of Primary Hyperparathyroidism

A. FAMILIAL BENIGN HYPOCALCIURIC HYPERCALEMIA (FBHH)

Inherited as an autosomal dominant trait, this disorder is responsible for lifelong asymptomatic hypercalcemia, first detectable in cord blood. Hypercalcemia is usually mild (10.5–12 mg/dL [2.7–3 mmol/L]) and is often accompanied by mild hypophosphatemia and hypermagnesemia. The PTH level is normal or slightly elevated, indicating that this is a PTH-dependent form of hypercalcemia. The parathyroid glands are normal in size or slightly enlarged. The most notable laboratory feature of the disorder is hypocalciuria. The urinary calcium level is usually less than 50 mg/24 h, and the calcium/creatinine clearance ratio is less than 0.01 and calculated as follows:

$$\frac{Urine_{calcium} \times Serum_{creatinine}}{Serum_{calcium} \times Urine_{creatinine}}$$

Hypocalciuria is an intrinsic renal trait, as it persists even in patients who have undergone total parathyroidectomy.

Since familial benign hypocalciuric hypercalcemia is an asymptomatic trait, the most important role of diagnosis is to distinguish it from primary hyperparathyroidism and avoid an unnecessary parathyroidectomy. If subtotal parathyroidectomy is performed, the serum calcium invariably returns shortly to preoperative levels; these persons resist attempts to lower the serum calcium. Unfortunate patients with this variant who have undergone total parathyroidectomy are rendered hypoparathyroid and are dependent on calcium and vitamin D.

The diagnosis must be considered in patients with asymptomatic mild hypercalcemia who are relatively hypocalciuric. However, an unequivocal diagnosis cannot be made biochemically because the serum and urinary calcium and PTH levels all overlap with typical primary hyperparathyroidism. Family studies are necessary to make the diagnosis. The penetrance of the phenotype is 100%, and affected family members are hypercalcemic throughout life, so if the proband has the disorder, each first-degree relative who is screened will have a 50% chance of being hypercalcemic.

Most cases of familial benign hypocalciuric hypercalcemia are caused by loss-of-function mutations in the parathyroid calcium receptor. Loss of one functional receptor allele shifts the set-point for inhibition of PTH release to the right, producing hypercalcemia. The same receptor is expressed in the kidney, where it regulates renal calcium excretion. A variety of point mutations in several exons of the calcium receptor produce the familial benign hypocalciuric hypercalcemia phenotype. Thus, simple molecular genetic testing is impractical for diagnosis at present.

Children of two parents with the disorder may inherit a mutant allele from each parent, producing neonatal severe hypercalcemia, a life-threatening disorder in which failure to sense extracellular calcium causes severe hyperparathyroidism, requiring total parathyroidectomy soon after birth.

B. MEN SYNDROMES

As noted above, primary hyperparathyroidism is a feature of both MEN 1 and MEN 2A. The penetrance of primary hyperparathyroidism in MEN 1 is over 90% by age 40. Patients with the MEN 1 syndrome are thought to inherit a loss-of-function germline mutation of the tumor suppressor gene *MENIN* on chromosome 11q12–13. Menin is a nuclear protein which appears to interact with JunD, a member of the AP1 family of transcription factors. A gene deletion during mitosis of a parathyroid cell that resulted in loss of the remaining allele in that cell would abrogate the cell's growth control mechanism and permit clonal expansion of its progeny to generate the parathyroid tumor. A similar mechanism appears also to operate in a small fraction of sporadic parathyroid adenomas with 11q12–13 deletions.

The penetrance of primary hyperparathyroidism in MEN 2A is about 30%. As discussed in the section on medullary thyroid carcinoma, the disorder is caused by activating mutations in the *RET* gene, a tyrosine kinase growth factor receptor. Evidently, the *RET* gene product is less important for growth of the parathyroids than for thyroid C cells, since the penetrance of primary hyperparathyroidism is fairly low and since in MEN 2B a separate class of activating *RET* mutations produces medullary carcinoma and pheochromocytoma and very rarely primary hyperparathyroidism. The treatment for parathyroid hyperplasia in MEN 1 or MEN 2 is subtotal parathyroidectomy. The recurrence rate is higher than in sporadic parathyroid hyperplasia and may approach 50% in MEN 1.

C. LITHIUM THERAPY

Both in patients and in isolated parathyroid cells, exposure to extracellular lithium shifts the set-point for inhibition of PTH secretion to the right. Clinically, this results in hypercalcemia and a detectable or elevated level of PTH. Lithium treatment also produces hypocalciuria and is thus a virtual phenocopy of familial benign hypocalciuric hypercalcemia. Most patients with therapeutic lithium levels for bipolar affective disorder will have a slight increase in the serum calcium level, and up to 10% become mildly hypercalcemic, with PTH levels that are high normal or slightly elevated. Lithium treatment can also unmask underlying primary hyperparathyroidism. It is difficult to diagnose primary hyperparathyroidism in a lithium-treated patient, particularly when temporary cessation of lithium therapy is deemed dangerous. However, the likelihood of underlying primary hyperparathyroidism is high when the serum calcium is greater than 11.5 mg/dL, and the decision to undertake surgery must be based on such clinical criteria. Unfortunately, surgical cure of hyperparathyroidism rarely ameliorates the underlying psychiatric condition.

2. Malignancy-Associated Hypercalcemia

Malignancy-associated hypercalcemia is the second most common form of hypercalcemia, with an incidence of 15 cases per 100,000 per year—about one-half the incidence of primary hyperparathyroidism. It is, however, much less prevalent than primary hyperparathyroidism, because most patients have a very limited survival. Nonetheless, malignancy-associated hy-

percalcemia is the commonest cause of hypercalcemia in hospitalized patients. The clinical features and pathogenesis of malignancy-associated hypercalcemia are presented in Chapter 23. The treatment of nonparathyroid hypercalcemia is presented below.

3. Sarcoidosis & Other Granulomatous Disorders

Hypercalcemia is seen in up to 10% of subjects with sarcoidosis. A higher percentage have hypercalciuria. This is due to inappropriately elevated $1,25(OH)_2D_3$ levels. Provocative testing with vitamin D or 25(OH)D increases serum or urine calcium into the abnormal range in an even larger percentage of subjects, demonstrating that most patients with sarcoidosis have abnormal vitamin D metabolism. Lymphoid tissue and pulmonary macrophages from affected individuals contain 25(OH)D 1-hydroxylase activity which is not seen in normal individuals. 1-Hydroxylase activity in these cells is not readily inhibited by calcium or $1,25(OH)_2D_3$, indicating a lack of feedback-inhibition. This makes these subjects vulnerable to hypercalcemia or hypercalciuria during periods of increased vitamin D production (eg, summertime with increased sunlight exposure). In contrast, gamma interferon stimulates 1-hydroxylase activity in these cells, which makes such subjects more vulnerable to altered calcium homeostasis when their disease is active. Glucocorticoids, on the other hand, suppress the 1-hydroxylase activity, and this provides effective treatment for both the disease and this complication of it. The 1-hydroxylase enzyme, responsible for the overproduction of $1,25(OH)_2D_3$ in sarcoidosis, is thought to be the same as that in the kidney. Thus, it is unclear what the basis is for differences in regulation of its activity in sarcoid tissue compared with kidney.

Other granulomatous diseases are associated with abnormal vitamin D metabolism resulting in hypercalcemia and or hypercalciuria. These disorders include tuberculosis, berylliosis, disseminated coccidioidomycosis, histoplasmosis, leprosy, and pulmonary eosinophilic granulomatosis. Furthermore, a substantial number of subjects with Hodgkin's or non-Hodgkin's lymphomas develop hypercalcemia associated with inappropriately elevated $1,25(OH)_2D_3$ levels. Although most such patients are normocalcemic on presentation, they may be hypercalciuric, and this should be evaluated as part of the workup. Furthermore, hypercalcemia and hypercalciuria may not become apparent until situations such as increased sunlight exposure or vitamin D and calcium ingestion are experienced. Thus, one should remain alert to this complication even when the initial evaluation of serum calcium is within normal limits.

4. Endocrinopathies

Thyrotoxicosis

Mild hypercalcemia is found in about 10% of patients with thyrotoxicosis. The PTH is suppressed and the serum phosphorus is in the upper normal range. The serum alkaline phosphatase and urinary hydroxyproline may be mildly increased. Significant hypercalcemia is seen only in patients with severe thyrotoxicosis, particularly if they are temporarily immobilized. Thyroid hormone has direct bone-resorbing properties causing a high-turnover state, which often eventually progresses to mild osteoporosis.

Adrenal Insufficiency

Hypercalcemia can be a feature of acute adrenal crisis and responds rapidly to glucocorticoid therapy. Animal studies suggest that hemoconcentration is a critical factor. In experimental adrenal insufficiency, [Ca^{2+}] is normal.

5. Endocrine Tumors

Hypercalcemia in patients with pheochromocytoma is most often a manifestation of the MEN 2A syndrome, but hypercalcemia is found occasionally in uncomplicated pheochromocytoma, where it appears to result from secretion of PTHrP by the tumor. About 40% of tumors secreting vasoactive intestinal peptide (VIPomas) are associated with hypercalcemia. The cause is unknown. It is known, however, that at high levels VIP may activate the PTH/PTHrP receptor.

6. Thiazide Diuretics

The administration of thiazides and related diuretics such as chlorthalidone, metolazone, and indapamide can produce an increase in the serum calcium which is not fully accounted for by hemoconcentration. Hypercalcemia is mild and usually transient, lasting for days or weeks, but occasionally it persists. Thiazide administration can also exacerbate the effects of underlying primary hyperparathyroidism; in fact, thiazide administration was formerly used as a provocative test for hyperparathyroidism in patients with borderline hypercalcemia. Most patients with persistent hypercalcemia while receiving thiazides will prove to have primary hyperparathyroidism.

7. Vitamin D & Vitamin A

Hypervitaminosis D

Hypercalcemia may occur in individuals ingesting large doses of vitamin D either therapeutically or accidentally (eg, irregularities in milk product supplementation with vitamin D have been reported). The initial signs and symptoms of vitamin D intoxication include weakness, lethargy, headaches, nausea, and polyuria and are attributable to the hypercalcemia and hypercalciuria. Ectopic calcification may occur, particularly in the kidneys, resulting in nephrolithiasis or nephrocalcinosis; other sites include blood vessels, heart, lungs, and skin. Infants appear to be quite susceptible to vitamin D intoxication and may develop disseminated atherosclerosis, supravalvular aortic stenosis, and renal acidosis.

Hypervitaminosis D is readily diagnosed by the very high serum levels of 25(OH)D, because the conversion of vitamin D to 25(OH)D is not tightly regulated. In contrast, $1,25(OH)_2D_3$ levels are often normal, but not suppressed. This reflects the expected feedback regulation of $1,25(OH)_2D_3$ production by the elevated calcium and reduced PTH levels. Levels of free $1,25(OH)_2D_3$ when measured have been found to be increased. This is in part caused by the high levels of 25(OH)D that displace $1,25(OH)_2D_3$ from DBP, raising the ratio of free:total $1,25(OH)_2D_3$. The elevated free concentration of $1,25(OH)_2D_3$, plus the intrinsic biologic effects of the elevated 25(OH)D concentration, combine to increase intestinal calcium absorption and bone resorption. The hypercalciuria, which is invariably seen, may lead to dehydration and coma as a result of hyposthenuria, prerenal azotemia, and worsening hypercalcemia.

The dose of vitamin D required to induce toxicity varies among patients, reflecting differences in absorption, storage, and subsequent metabolism of the vitamin as well as in target tissue response to the active metabolites. For example, an elderly patient is likely to have reduced intestinal calcium transport and renal production of $1,25(OH)_2D_3$. Such an individual may be able to tolerate 50,000–100,000 units of vitamin D daily. However, patients with unsuspected hyperparathyroidism receiving such doses for the treatment of osteoporosis are more likely to experience hypercalcemia. Treatment consists of withdrawing the vitamin D, rehydration, reducing calcium intake, and administration of glucocorticoids, which antagonize the ability of $1,25(OH)_2D_3$ to stimulate intestinal calcium absorption. Excess vitamin D is slowly cleared from the body (weeks to months), so treatment is prolonged.

Hypervitaminosis A

Excessive ingestion of vitamin A, usually from self-medication with vitamin A preparations, causes a number of abnormalities, including gingivitis, cheilitis, erythema, desquamation, and hair loss. Bone resorption is increased, leading to osteoporosis and fractures, hypercalcemia, and hyperostosis. Excess vitamin A causes hepatosplenomegaly with hypertrophy of fat storage cells, fibrosis, and sclerosis of central veins. Many of these effects can be attributed to the effects of vitamin A on cellular membranes. Under normal circumstances, such effects are prevented because vitamin A is bound to retinal-binding protein (RBP), and its release from the liver is regulated. In vitamin A toxicity, however, these protective mechanisms are overcome, and retinol and its retinyl esters appear in blood unbound to RBP. The mechanism by which vitamin A stimulates bone resorption is not clear.

8. Milk-Alkali Syndrome

The ingestion of large quantities of calcium together with an absorbable alkali can produce hypercalcemia with alkalosis, renal impairment, and often nephrocalcinosis. The syndrome was more common when absorbable antacids were the standard treatment for peptic ulcer disease, but it is still seen occasionally. This is the only recognized example of pure absorptive hypercalcemia. The details of its pathogenesis are poorly understood.

9. Miscellaneous Conditions

Immobilization

In immobilized patients there is a marked increase in bone resorption, which often produces hypercalciuria and occasionally hypercalcemia, mainly in individuals with a preexisting high bone turnover state, such as adolescents and patients with thyrotoxicosis or Paget's disease. Intact PTH and PTHrP levels are suppressed. The disorder remits with the restoration of activity. If acute treatment is required, bisphosphonates appear to be the treatment of choice.

Acute Renal Failure

Hypercalcemia is often seen when renal failure is precipitated by rhabdomyolysis and usually occurs during the early recovery stage, presumably as calcium deposits are mobilized from damaged muscle tissue. It typically resolves over a few weeks.

TREATMENT OF HYPERCALCEMIA

Initial management of hypercalcemia consists of assessing the hydration state of the patient and rehydrating as necessary with saline. The first goal is to restore renal function, which is often impaired in hypercalcemia because of reduced glomerular filtration and dehydration. Hypercalcemia impairs the urinary concentrating ability, leading to polyuria, and at the same time impairs the sensorium, diminishing the sense of thirst. Once renal function is restored, renal excretion of calcium

can be further enhanced by inducing a saline diuresis. Because most of the filtered calcium is reabsorbed by bulk flow in the proximal tubule along with sodium chloride, a saline diuresis will markedly increase calcium excretion. However, a vigorous saline diuresis will also induce substantial urinary losses of potassium and magnesium, and these must be monitored and replaced as necessary.

After these initial steps, attention should be given to finding a suitable chronic therapy. It is important to start chronic therapy soon after hospitalization, as several of the most useful agents take up to 5 days to have their full effect. Intravenous bisphosphonates (pamidronate or zoledronic acid) are the first choice for most patients. Bisphosphonates act by inhibiting osteoclastic bone resorption. The initial dose of pamidronate is 60–90 mg by intravenous infusion over 4 hours, and the dose of zoledronic acid is 4 mg infused over 15 minutes. In two large trials, 88% and 70% of patients with malignancy-associated hypercalcemia normalized their serum calcium values after infusions of zoledronic acid (4 mg) and pamidronate (90 mg), respectively. Zoledronic acid produced a longer duration of response—32 days versus 18 days for pamidronate. The nadir of serum calcium does not occur until 4–5 days after administration of either agent. Re-treatment with either agent can be conducted after recurrence of hypercalcemia. Transient fever and myalgia occur in 20% of patients who undergo intravenous bisphosphonate therapy. Increased serum creatinine (≥ 0.5 mg/dL) occurs in about 15% of patients. Intravenous bisphosphonates should be used cautiously and at reduced doses when the baseline serum creatinine exceeds 2.5 mg/dL.

In patients with severe hypercalcemia and those with renal insufficiency that is refractory to rehydration, it may be necessary to use a second antiresorptive agent for a few days while awaiting the full therapeutic effect of bisphosphonates. For this purpose, synthetic salmon calcitonin may be administered at a dose of 4–8 IU/kg subcutaneously every 12 hours. This is a useful adjunct acutely, but most patients become totally refractory to calcitonin within a few days, so it is not suitable for chronic use.

The use of an antiresorptive agent together with saline diuresis provides for a two-pronged approach to hypercalcemia. Other agents besides bisphosphonates may be considered (eg, plicamycin or gallium nitrate), but their toxicity and lack of superior efficacy tend to discourage their use. Both agents act to inhibit osteoclastic bone resorption.

Glucocorticoid administration is first-line treatment for hypercalcemia in patients with multiple myeloma, lymphoma, sarcoidosis, or intoxication with vitamin D or vitamin A. Glucocorticoids are also beneficial in some patients with breast carcinoma. However, they are of little use in most other patients with solid tumors and hypercalcemia.

■ HYPOCALCEMIA

Classification

Both PTH and $1,25(OH)_2D_3$ function to maintain a normal serum calcium and are thus central to the defense against hypocalcemia. Hypocalcemic disorders are best understood as failures of the adaptive response. Thus, chronic hypocalcemia can result from a failure to secrete PTH, a failure to respond to PTH, a deficiency of vitamin D, or a failure to respond to vitamin D. Acute hypocalcemia is most often the consequence of an overwhelming challenge to the adaptive response such as rhabdomyolysis, in which a flood of phosphate from injured skeletal muscle inundates the extracellular fluid (Table 8–6).

Clinical Features

Most of the symptoms and signs of hypocalcemia occur because of increased neuromuscular excitability (tetany, paresthesias, seizures, organic brain syndrome) or because of deposition of calcium in soft tissues (cataract, calcification of basal ganglia).

A. NEUROMUSCULAR MANIFESTATIONS

Clinically, the hallmark of severe hypocalcemia is tetany. Tetany is a state of spontaneous tonic muscular contraction. Overt tetany is often heralded by tingling paresthesias in the fingers and about the mouth, but the classic muscular component of tetany is carpopedal spasm. This begins with adduction of the thumb, followed by flexion of the metacarpophalangeal joints, extension of the interphalangeal joints, and flexion of the wrists to produce the *main d'accoucheur* posture (Figure 8–17). These involuntary muscle contractions are painful. Although the hands are most typically involved, tetany can involve other muscle groups, including life-threatening spasm of laryngeal muscles. Electromyographically, tetany is typified by repetitive motor neuron action potentials, usually grouped as doublets. Tetany is not specific for hypocalcemia. It also occurs with hypomagnesemia and metabolic alkalosis, and the most common cause of tetany is respiratory alkalosis from hyperventilation.

Lesser degrees of neuromuscular excitability (eg, serum calcium 7–9 mg/dL) produce latent tetany, which can be elicited by testing for Chvostek's and

Table 8–6. Causes of hypocalcemia.

Hypoparathyroidism
Surgical
Idiopathic
Neonatal
Familial
Deposition of metals (iron, copper, aluminum)
Postradiation
Infiltrative
Functional (in hypomagnesemia)
Resistance to PTH action
Pseudohypoparathyroidism
Renal insufficiency
Medications that block osteoclastic bone resorption
Plicamycin
Calcitonin
Bisphosphonates
Failure to produce $1,25(OH)_2D$ normally
Vitamin D deficiency
Hereditary vitamin D-dependent rickets, type 1 (renal 25-OH-vitamin D 1α-hydroxylase deficiency)
Resistance to $1,25(OH)_2D$ action
Hereditary vitamin D-dependent rickets, type 2 (defective VDR)
Acute complexation or deposition of calcium
Acute hyperphosphatemia
Crush injury with myonecrosis
Rapid tumor lysis
Parenteral phosphate administration
Excessive enteral phosphate
Oral (phosphate-containing antacids)
Phosphate-containing enemas
Acute pancreatitis
Citrated blood transfusion
Rapid, excessive skeletal mineralization
Hungry bones syndrome
Osteoblastic metastasis
Vitamin D therapy for vitamin D deficiency

Trousseau's signs. Chvostek's sign is elicited by tapping the facial nerve about 2 cm anterior to the earlobe, just below the zygoma. The response is a contraction of facial muscles ranging from twitching of the angle of the mouth to hemifacial contractions. The specificity of the test is low; about 25% of normal individuals have a mild Chvostek sign. Trousseau's sign is elicited by inflating a blood pressure cuff to about 20 mm Hg above systolic pressure for 3 minutes. A positive response is carpal spasm. Trousseau's sign is more specific than Chvostek's, but 1–4% of normals have positive Trousseau signs.

Hypocalcemia predisposes to focal or generalized seizures. Other central nervous system effects of hypo-

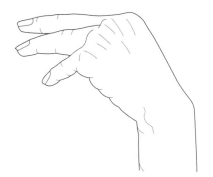

Figure 8–17. Position of fingers in carpal spasm due to hypocalcemic tetany. (Reproduced, with permission, from Ganong WF: *Review of Medical Physiology,* 16th ed. Originally published by Appleton & Lange. Copyright © 1993 by The McGraw-Hill Companies, Inc.)

calcemia include pseudotumor cerebri, papilledema, confusion, lassitude, and organic brain syndrome. Twenty percent of children with chronic hypocalcemia develop mental retardation. The basal ganglia are often calcified in patients with long-standing hypoparathyroidism or pseudohypoparathyroidism. This is usually asymptomatic but can produce a variety of movement disorders.

B. OTHER MANIFESTATIONS OF HYPOCALCEMIA

1. Cardiac effects—Repolarization is delayed, with prolongation of the QT interval. Excitation-contraction coupling may be impaired, and refractory congestive heart failure is sometimes observed, particularly in patients with underlying cardiac disease.

2. Ophthalmologic effects—Subcapsular cataract is common in chronic hypocalcemia, and its severity is correlated with the duration and level of hypocalcemia.

3. Dermatologic effects—The skin is often dry and flaky and the nails brittle. A dermatitis known as impetigo herpetiformis or pustular psoriasis is peculiar to hypocalcemia.

CAUSES OF HYPOCALCEMIA

1. Hypoparathyroidism

Hypoparathyroidism may be surgical, autoimmune, familial, or idiopathic. The signs and symptoms are those of chronic hypocalcemia. Biochemically, the hallmarks of hypoparathyroidism are hypocalcemia, hyperphosphatemia (because the phosphaturic effect of PTH is lost), and an inappropriately low or undetectable PTH level.

Surgical Hypoparathyroidism

The most common cause of hypoparathyroidism is surgery on the neck, with removal or destruction of the parathyroid glands. The operations most often associated with hypoparathyroidism are cancer surgery, total thyroidectomy, and parathyroidectomy, but the skill and experience of the surgeon are more important predictors than the nature of the operation. Tetany ensues 1 or 2 days postoperatively, but about half of patients with postoperative tetany will recover sufficiently not to require long-term replacement therapy. In these cases, a devitalized parathyroid remnant has recovered its blood supply and resumes secretion of PTH. In some patients, hypocalcemia may not become evident until years after the procedure. Surgical hypoparathyroidism is the presumptive diagnosis for hypocalcemia in any patient with a surgical scar on the neck.

In patients with severe hyperparathyroid bone disease preoperatively, a syndrome of postoperative hypocalcemia can follow successful parathyroidectomy. This is the "hungry bones syndrome," which results from such avid uptake of calcium and phosphate by the bones that the parathyroids, though intact, cannot compensate. The syndrome is usually seen in patients with an elevated preoperative serum alkaline phosphatase. It can usually be distinguished from surgical hypoparathyroidism by the serum phosphorus, which is low in the hungry bones syndrome because of skeletal avidity for phosphate, and high in hypoparathyroidism, and by the serum PTH, which will become appropriately elevated in the hungry bones syndrome.

Idiopathic Hypoparathyroidism

Acquired hypoparathyroidism is sometimes seen in the setting of polyglandular endocrinopathies. Most commonly, it is associated with primary adrenal insufficiency and mucocutaneous candidiasis in the syndrome of pluriglandular autoimmune endocrinopathy, or type I polyglandular autoimmune syndrome (Chapter 4). The typical age at onset of hypoparathyroidism is 5–9 years. A similar form of hypoparathyroidism can occur as an isolated finding. The age at onset of idiopathic hypoparathyroidism is 2–10 years, and there is a preponderance of female cases. Circulating parathyroid antibodies are common in both the polyglandular syndrome and in isolated hypoparathyroidism. Up to one-third of patients with the latter syndrome have antibodies that recognize the parathyroid calcium sensor, though the pathogenetic role of these autoantibodies is not yet clarified. Mutations have been uncovered in a protein termed AIRE (autoimmune regulator) that appears to be a transcription factor involved in endocrine and immune function.

Familial Hypoparathyroidism

Hypoparathyroidism can rarely present in a familial form, which may be transmitted as an autosomal dominant or an autosomal recessive trait. Two families with PTH gene mutations that interfere with the normal processing of PTH have been reported. Several families have also been shown to have point mutations in the parathyroid calcium-sensing receptor gene, which renders the protein constitutively active. This property enables the receptor to mediate suppression of PTH secretion at normal and subnormal serum calcium levels. Affected individuals have mild hypoparathyroidism which may require replacement therapy. The set-point for calcium-induced suppression of PTH secretion in these patients is shifted to the left. Thus, this syndrome is the mirror image of familial benign hypocalciuric hypercalcemia.

Other Causes of Hypoparathyroidism

Neonatal hypoparathyroidism can be part of the **Di-George syndrome** (dysmorphia, cardiac defects, immune deficiency, and hypoparathyroidism) due to a microdeletion on chromosome 22q11.2; the HDR syndrome (hypoparathyroidism, sensorineural deafness, and renal anomalies) due to the loss of a copy of the GATA3 transcription factor; and other rare conditions. Transfusion-dependent individuals with thalassemia or red cell aplasia who survive into the third decade of life are susceptible to hypoparathyroidism as the result of **iron deposition** in the glands. **Copper deposition** can cause hypoparathyroidism in Wilson's disease. **Aluminum deposition** in dialysis patients blunts the parathyroid reserve. Infiltration with metastatic carcinoma is a rare cause of hypoparathyroidism.

Severe **magnesium depletion** temporarily paralyzes the parathyroid glands, preventing secretion of PTH. Magnesium depletion also blunts the actions of PTH to counteract the hypocalcemia. This is seen with magnesium losses due to gastrointestinal and renal disorders and alcoholism. The syndrome responds immediately to infusion of magnesium. As discussed above in the section on regulation of parathyroid hormone secretion, magnesium is probably required for stimulus-secretion coupling in the parathyroids.

2. Pseudohypoparathyroidism

Pseudohypoparathyroidism is a heritable disorder of target-organ unresponsiveness to parathyroid hormone. Biochemically, it mimics hormone-deficient forms of hypoparathyroidism, with hypocalcemia and hyperphosphatemia, but the PTH level is elevated and there is a markedly blunted response to the administration of PTH (see Diagnosis, below).

Clinical Features

Two distinct forms of pseudohypoparathyroidism are recognized. Pseudohypoparathyroidism type 1B is a disorder of isolated resistance to PTH, which presents with the biochemical features of hypocalcemia, hyperphosphatemia and secondary hyperparathyroidism. Pseudohypoparathyroidism type 1A has, in addition to these biochemical features, a characteristic somatic phenotype known as Albright's hereditary osteodystrophy. This consists of short stature, a round face, short neck, brachydactyly (short digits), and subcutaneous ossifications. Because of shortening of the metacarpal bones—most often the fourth and fifth metacarpals—affected digits have a dimple, instead of a knuckle, when a fist is made (Figure 8–18). In addition, primary hypothyroidism occurs commonly, and many patients have abnormalities of reproductive function—oligomenorrhea in females and infertility in males. Interestingly, certain individuals in families with pseudohypoparathyroidism inherit the somatic phenotype of Albright's hereditary osteodystrophy without any disorder of calcium metabolism; this state, which mimics pseudohypoparathyroidism, is called **pseudopseudohypoparathyroidism.**

Pathophysiology

Pseudohypoparathyroidism type 1A is caused by loss of one functional allele of the gene encoding the G protein subunit $G_s\alpha$. This is predicted to produce a 50% deficiency of the alpha subunits of the heterotrimeric G_s, which couples the PTH receptor to adenylyl cyclase. Patients with pseudohypoparathyroidism type 1A have a markedly blunted response of urinary cAMP to administration of PTH. Since G_s also couples many other receptors to adenylyl cyclase, the expected result of this mutation would be a generalized disorder of hormonal unresponsiveness. The high prevalence of primary hypothyroidism and primary hypogonadism indicates that in fact resistance to TSH, LH, and FSH are commonly present, but the response to other hormones (eg, ACTH, glucagon) is fairly normal. Thus, a 50% loss of the α_s protein produces resistance to some hormones but not others. $G_s\alpha$ is also deficient in individuals with pseudopseudohypoparathyroidism, who have Albright's hereditary osteodystrophy but normal responsiveness to PTH. Thus, the mutation in the $G_s\alpha$ gene invariably produces Albright's hereditary osteodystrophy but only sometimes produces resistance to PTH, suggesting that the occurrence of resistance may be determined by other factors (Table 8–7).

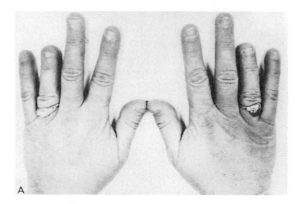

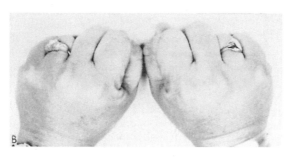

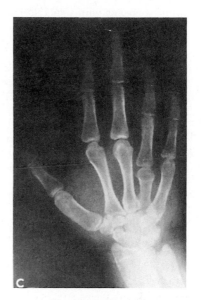

Figure 8–18. Hands of a patient with pseudohypoparathyroidism. **A:** Note the short fourth finger. **B:** Note the "absent" fourth knuckle. **C:** Film shows the short fourth metacarpal. (Reproduced, with permission, from Potts JT: Pseudohypoparathyroidism: Clinical features; signs and symptoms; diagnosis and differential diagnosis. In: *The Metabolic Basis of Inherited Disease,* 4th ed. Stanbury JB, Wyngaarden JB, Fredrickson DS [editors]. McGraw-Hill, 1978.)

In pseudohypoparathyroidism type 1B, where there is resistance to PTH but no somatic phenotype, levels of $G_s\alpha$ protein in red blood cell or fibroblast membranes are normal. The disorder, however, has also been linked to the GNAS1 locus, but it does not involve mutations in the coding region of $G_s\alpha$. It is likely that abnormal methylation of GNAS1 regulatory sequences is involved in the pathogenesis of PHP1b.

Genetics

Pseudohypoparathyroidism type 1A is inherited as an autosomal dominant trait. Few cases of male-to-male transmission are recognized, but this is probably because of male infertility in affected individuals. Individuals who have acquired the trait from their fathers almost always present with pseudopseudohypoparathyroidism and lack hormone resistance. When inheritance is from the mother, pseudohypoparathyroidism with hormone resistance is almost always present. These fea-

Table 8–7. Features of pseudohypoparathyroidism (PHP).

	PHP 1A	PPHP[1]	PHP 1B
Hypocalcemia	Yes	No	Yes
Response to PTH	No	Yes	No
Albright's hereditary osteodystrophy	Yes	Yes	No
$G_s\alpha$ mutation	Yes	Yes	No
Generalized unresponsiveness	Yes	No	No

[1]Pseudopseudohypoparathyroidism.

tures suggest genomic imprinting, where the maternal allele is preferentially expressed in the kidney.

Diagnosis

Several disorders present with hypocalcemia and secondary hyperparathyroidism (eg, vitamin D deficiency), but when these features occur together with hyperphosphatemia or Albright's hereditary osteodystrophy, this suggests the diagnosis of pseudohypoparathyroidism. To confirm that resistance to PTH is present, the patient is challenged with PTH (the Ellsworth-Howard test). For this purpose, synthetic human PTH(1–34) (teriparatide acetate, 3 IU/kg body weight) is infused intravenously over 10 minutes during a water diuresis, and urine is collected during the hour preceding the infusion, during the half-hour following the infusion, 30–60 minutes after the infusion, and 1–2 hours after the infusion and assayed for cAMP and creatinine. Data are expressed as nanomoles of cAMP per liter of glomerular filtrate, based on creatinine measurements. Normally, there is an increase in urinary cAMP of > 300 nmol/L glomerular filtrate after administration of PTH. The use of the urinary phosphate response as a gauge of PTH responsiveness is much less reliable.

3. Vitamin D Deficiency

Pathogenesis

Vitamin D deficiency results from one or a combination of three causes: inadequate sunlight exposure, inadequate nutrition, and malabsorption. In addition, drugs that activate the catabolism of vitamin D and its metabolites, such as phenytoin and phenobarbital, can precipitate vitamin D deficiency in subjects with marginal vitamin D status. Although the human skin is capable of producing sufficient amounts of vitamin D if exposed to sunlight of adequate intensity, institutionalized patients frequently do not get adequate exposure. Furthermore, the fear of skin cancer has led many to avoid sunlight exposure or to apply protective agents that block the UV portion of sunlight from reaching the lower reaches of the epidermis where most of the vitamin D is produced. Heavily pigmented and elderly individuals have less efficient production of vitamin D for a given exposure to UV irradiation. The intensity of sunlight is an important factor that limits effective vitamin D production as a function of season (summer greater than winter) and latitude (less intense the higher the latitude). The supplementation of dairy products has reduced the incidence of vitamin D deficiency in the United States, but a number of countries do not follow this practice. Even in the United States, vitamin D deficiency may occur in children of vegetarian mothers who avoid milk products (and presumably have reduced vitamin D stores) and in children who are not weaned to vitamin D-supplemented milk by age 2. Breast milk contains little vitamin D. Elderly people who avoid dairy products as well as sunlight are likewise at risk. Individuals with a variety of small bowel diseases, partial gastrectomy, pancreatic diseases, and biliary tract diseases have reduced capacity to absorb the vitamin D in the diet.

Clinical Features

The clinical features of individuals with vitamin D deficiency will be discussed more thoroughly in the section on osteomalacia and rickets. Vitamin D deficiency should be suspected in individuals complaining of lethargy, proximal muscle weakness, and bone pain who on routine biochemical evaluation have low or low normal serum calcium and phosphate and low urine calcium. A low serum 25(OH)D level is diagnostic in this setting. $1,25(OH)_2D_3$ levels are often normal and reflect the increased 1-hydroxylase activity in these subjects which is responding appropriately to the increased PTH levels as well as the low serum calcium and phosphate levels.

Treatment

The goal in treating vitamin D deficiency is to normalize the clinical, biochemical, and radiologic abnormalities without producing hypercalcemia, hyperphosphatemia, hypercalciuria, nephrolithiasis, or ectopic calcification. To realize this goal, patients must be followed carefully. As the bone lesions heal or the underlying disease improves, the dosage of vitamin D, calcium, or phosphate needs to be adjusted to avoid such complications. Simple nutritional vitamin D deficiency responds to oral doses of 2000–4000 units of vitamin D per day taken for several months and then followed by replacement doses of up to 800 units/d. Patients with malabsorption may respond to larger amounts of vitamin D (25,000–100,000 units/d or one to three times per week). 25(OH)D (50–100 μg/d) is better-absorbed than vitamin D and may be used if malabsorption of vitamin D is a limiting factor. Calcitriol is not appropriate therapy for patients with vitamin D deficiency because of the likely requirement for vitamin D metabolites other than $1,25(OH)_2D_3$ in the healing of rachitic bone. Vitamin D therapy should be supplemented with 1–3 g of elemental calcium per day. Care must be taken in managing patients with vitamin D deficiency who also have elevated PTH levels as long-standing vitamin D deficiency may produce a degree of autonomy in the parathyroid glands such that rapid replacement with calcium and vitamin D could result in hypercalcemia or hypercalciuria. A listing of available vitamin D metabolites and analogs with their main indications for clinical use is set forth in Table 8–2.

4. Vitamin D-Dependent Rickets Type I

Vitamin D-dependent rickets type I, also known as pseudovitamin D deficiency, is a rare autosomal recessive disease in which there is a low level of $1,25(OH)_2D_3$ but normal levels of $25(OH)D$ and rickets. The disease is due to mutation in the $25(OH)D$ 1-hydroxylase gene which renders it nonfunctional. Both alleles need to be defective in order for the disease to be manifest. Although affected patients do not respond to doses of vitamin D that are effective in subjects with vitamin D deficiency, they can respond to pharmacologic doses of vitamin D and to physiologic doses of calcitriol, which is the preferred treatment.

5. Vitamin D-Dependent Rickets Type II

Vitamin D-dependent rickets type II, also known as hereditary $1,25(OH)_2D_3$-resistant rickets, is a rare autosomal recessive disease that presents in childhood with rickets similar to that seen in patients with vitamin D deficiency. Many of these patients also have alopecia, which is not characteristic of vitamin D deficiency. The biochemical changes are similar to those reported in subjects with vitamin D deficiency except that the $1,25(OH)_2D_3$ levels are generally very high. The disease is caused by inactivating mutations in the VDR gene. The location of the mutation can affect the severity of the disease. These patients are treated with large doses of calcitriol and dietary calcium, and may show partial or complete remission as they grow older. An animal model of this disease (inactivation of the VDR by homologous recombination or "knockout") demonstrates that the bone disease can be corrected with high dietary intake of calcium and phosphate, although the alopecia is not altered. This disease points to a role for the VDR in epidermis and hair development that is independent of its activity in bone.

6. Other Hypocalcemic Disorders

Hypoalbuminemia produces a low total serum calcium concentration because of a reduction in the bound fraction of calcium, but the ionized calcium is normal. The ionized calcium level can be determined directly, or the effect of hypoalbuminemia can be roughly corrected using the following formula:

$$\text{Corrected serum calcium} = \text{Measured serum calcium} + (0.8)(4 - \text{Measured serum albumin})$$

Thus, in a patient with a serum calcium of 7.8 mg/dL and a serum albumin of 2 mg/dL, the corrected serum calcium is $7.8 + (0.8)(4 - 2) = 9.4$ mg/dL.

Several disorders produce acute hypocalcemia despite intact homeostasis, simply because they overwhelm the adaptive mechanisms. Acute hyperphosphatemia that results from rhabdomyolysis or tumor lysis, often in the setting of renal insufficiency, may produce severe symptomatic hypocalcemia. Transfusion of citrated blood causes acute hypocalcemia by complexation of calcium as calcium citrate. In this instance, total calcium may be normal but the ionized fraction is reduced. In acute pancreatitis, hypocalcemia is an ominous prognostic sign. The mechanism of hypocalcemia is sequestration of calcium by saponification with fatty acids, which are produced in the retroperitoneum by the action of pancreatic lipases. Skeletal mineralization, when very rapid, can cause hypocalcemia. This is seen in the "hungry bones syndrome," which was discussed above in the section on surgical hypoparathyroidism, and occasionally with widespread osteoblastic metastases from prostatic carcinoma.

TREATMENT OF HYPOCALCEMIA

Acute Hypocalcemia

Patients with tetany should receive intravenous calcium as calcium chloride (272 mg calcium per 10 mL), calcium gluconate (90 mg calcium per 10 mL), or calcium gluceptate (90 mg calcium per 10 mL). Approximately 200 mg of elemental calcium can be given over several minutes. The patient must be observed for stridor and the airway secured if necessary. Oral calcium and a rapidly acting preparation of vitamin D should be started. If necessary, calcium can be infused in doses of 400–1000 mg/24 h until oral therapy has taken effect. Intravenous calcium is irritating to the veins. Caution must be exercised in patients taking digitalis, since they are predisposed to toxicity by infusion of calcium.

Chronic Hypocalcemia

The objective of chronic therapy is to keep the patient free of symptoms and to maintain a serum calcium of approximately 8.5–9.2 mg/dL. With lower serum calcium levels, the patient may not only experience symptoms but may be predisposed over time to cataracts. With serum calcium concentrations in the upper normal range, there may be marked hypercalciuria, which occurs because the hypocalciuric effect of PTH has been lost. This may predispose to nephrolithiasis, nephrocalcinosis, and chronic renal insufficiency. In addition, the patient with a borderline elevated calcium is at increased risk of overshooting the therapeutic goal, with symptomatic hypercalcemia.

The mainstays of treatment are calcium and vitamin D. Oral calcium can be given in a dose of 1.5–3 g of elemental calcium per day. These large doses of calcium reduce the necessary dose of vitamin D and allow for rapid normalization of calcium if vitamin D intoxication subsequently occurs. Numerous preparations of calcium are available. A short-acting preparation of vitamin D (calcitriol) and the very long-acting preparations such as vitamin D_2 (ergocalciferol) are available (Table 8–2). By far the most inexpensive regimens are those that use ergocalciferol. In addition to economy, they have the advantage of rather easy maintenance in most patients. The disadvantage is that ergocalciferol can slowly accumulate and produce delayed and prolonged vitamin D intoxication. Caution must be exercised in the introduction of other drugs that influence calcium metabolism. For example, thiazide diuretics have a hypocalciuric effect. By reducing urinary calcium excretion in treated patients, whose other adaptive mechanisms, PTH and $1,25(OH)_2D_3$, are nonoperative and who are thus absolutely dependent on renal excretion of calcium to maintain the serum calcium level, thiazides may produce severe hypercalcemia. In a similar way, intercurrent illnesses that compromise renal function may produce dangerous hypercalcemia in the patient who is maintained on large doses of vitamin D. Short-acting preparations are less prone to some of these effects but may require more frequent titration and are much more expensive than vitamin D_2.

■ BONE ANATOMY & REMODELING

FUNCTIONS OF BONE

Bone has three major functions. (1) It provides rigid support to extremities and body cavities containing vital organs. In disease situations in which bone is weak or defective, erect posture may be impossible, and vital organ function may be compromised. An example is the cardiopulmonary dysfunction that occurs in patients with severe kyphosis due to vertebral collapse. (2) Bones are crucial to locomotion in that they provide efficient levers and sites of attachment for muscles. With bony deformity, these levers become defective, and severe abnormalities of gait develop. (3) Bone provides a large reservoir of ions, such as calcium, phosphorus, magnesium, and sodium, that are critical for life and can be mobilized when the external environment fails to provide them.

STRUCTURE OF BONE

Bone is not only rigid and resists forces that would ordinarily break brittle materials but is also light enough to be moved by muscle contractions. Cortical bone, composed of densely packed layers of mineralized collagen, provides rigidity and is the major component of tubular bones (Figure 8–19). Trabecular (cancellous) bone is spongy in appearance, provides strength and elasticity, and constitutes the major portion of the axial skeleton. Disorders in which cortical bone is defective or scanty lead to fractures of the long bones, whereas disorders in which trabecular bone is defective or scanty lead preferentially to vertebral fractures. Fractures of long bones may also occur because normal trabecular bone reinforcement is lost.

Two-thirds of the weight of bone is due to mineral; the remainder is due to water and type I collagen. Minor organic components such as proteoglycans, lipids, acidic proteins containing γ-carboxyglutamic acid, osteonectin, osteopontin, and growth factors are probably important, but their functions are poorly understood.

Bone Mineral

The mineral of bone is present in two forms. The major form consists of hydroxyapatite in crystals of varying maturity. The remainder is amorphous calcium phosphate, which lacks a coherent x-ray diffraction pattern, has a lower calcium-to-phosphate ratio than pure hydroxyapatite, occurs in regions of active bone formation, and is present in larger quantities in young bone.

Bone Cells

Bone is composed of three types of cells: the osteoblast, the osteocyte, and the osteoclast.

A. OSTEOBLAST:

The osteoblast is the principal bone-forming cell. It arises from a pool of mesenchymal precursor cells in the bone marrow which, as they differentiate, acquire a set of characteristics including PTH and vitamin D receptors; surface expression of alkaline phosphatase; and expression of bone matrix protein genes—type I collagen, osteocalcin, etc. Differentiated osteoblasts are directed to the bone surface, where they line regions of new bone formation, laying down bone matrix (osteoid) in orderly lamellae and inducing its mineralization (Figure 8–20). In the mineralization process, hydroxyapatite crystals are deposited on the collagen layers to produce lamellar bone. Mineralization requires an adequate supply of extracellular calcium and phosphate as well as the enzyme

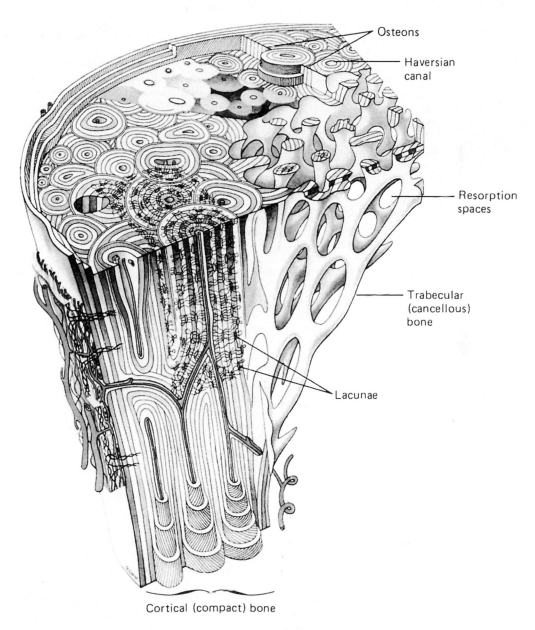

Osteons

Haversian canal

Resorption spaces

Trabecular (cancellous) bone

Lacunae

Cortical (compact) bone

Figure 8–19. Diagram of some of the measures of the microstructure of mature bone seen in both transverse (top) and longitudinal section. Areas of cortical (compact) and trabecular (cancellous) bone are included. (Reproduced, with permission, from *Gray's Anatomy,* 35th ed. Warwick R, Williams PL [editors]. Longman, 1973.)

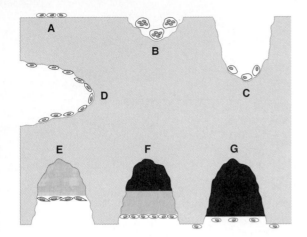

Figure 8–20. The remodeling cycle. **A:** Resting trabecular surface. **B:** Multinucleated osteoclasts dig a cavity of approximately 20 microns. **C:** Completion of resorption to 60 microns by mononuclear phagocytes. **D:** Recruitment of osteoblast precursors to the base of the resorption cavity. **E:** Secretion of new matrix (gray shading) by osteoblasts. **F:** Continued secretion of matrix, with initiation of calcification (black areas). **G:** Completion of mineralization of new matrix. Bone has returned to quiescent state, but a small deficit in bone mass persists.

alkaline phosphatase, which is secreted in large amounts by active osteoblasts. The fate of senescent osteoblasts is not well defined. Some probably become flattened, inactive lining cells on trabecular bone surfaces, and some are buried in cortical bone as osteocytes.

B. OSTEOCYTE:

Osteoblasts that are trapped in cortical bone during the remodeling process become osteocytes. Protein synthetic activity decreases markedly, and the cells develop multiple processes that reach out through lacunae in bone tissue to communicate with nutrient capillaries, with processes of other osteocytes within a unit of bone (osteon) and also with the cell processes of surface osteoblasts (Figure 8–19). The physiologic importance of osteocytes is controversial, but they are believed to act as a cellular syncytium that permits translocation of mineral in and out of regions of bone removed from surfaces.

C. OSTEOCLAST:

The osteoclast is a multinucleated giant cell that is specialized for resorption of bone. Osteoclasts are terminally differentiated cells that arise continuously from hematopoietic precursors in the monocyte lineage and

do not divide. In a process that requires hematopoietic growth factors such as macrophage colony-stimulating factor (M-CSF, also called CSF-1) and is accelerated by cytokines such as interleukin-6 and by the systemic calciotropic hormones PTH and vitamin D, osteoclast precursors gradually mature, acquire the capacity to produce osteoclast-specific enzymes, and finally fuse to produce the mature multinucleate cell (Figure 8–21).

To resorb bone, the motile osteoclast alights on a bone surface and seals off an area by forming an adhesive ring. Having isolated an area of bone surface, the osteoclast develops above the surface an elaborately invaginated plasma membrane structure called the **ruffled border** (Figure 8–22). The ruffled border is a distinctive organelle, but it acts essentially as a huge lysosome that dissolves bone mineral by secreting acid onto the isolated bone surface and simultaneously breaks down bone matrix by secretion of catheptic proteases. The resulting collagen peptides have pyridinoline structures that can be assayed in urine as a measure of bone resorption rates. Bone resorption can be controlled in two ways: by regulating the formation of osteoclasts to change their number or by regulating the activity of the mature osteoclast. The mature osteoclast has receptors for calcitonin but does not appear to have PTH or vitamin D receptors.

BONE REMODELING

Bone remodeling is a continuous process of breakdown and renewal that occurs throughout life. During childhood and adolescence, remodeling proceeds at a vigorous rate but is quantitatively overwhelmed by the concomitant occurrence of bone modeling and linear growth. Once peak bone mass has been established, remodeling supervenes as the common mechanism by which bone mass is modified for the remainder of a person's life. Each remodeling event is carried out by individual "bone remodeling units" (BMUs) on bone surfaces throughout the skeleton (Figure 8–20). Normally, about 90% of these surfaces lie dormant, covered by a thin layer of lining cells. Following physical or biochemical signals, precursor cells from the bone marrow migrate to specific loci on the bone surface, where they fuse into multinucleated bone-resorbing cells—osteoclasts—that dig a cavity into the bone.

Cortical bone is remodeled from within by cutting cones, groups of osteoclasts that cut tunnels through the compact bone (Figure 8–23). They are followed by trailing osteoblasts that line the tunnels with a cylinder of new bone which progressively narrows the tunnels until all that remains are the tiny haversian canals by which the cells left behind as resident osteocytes are fed. The packet of new bone formed by a single cutting cone is called an osteon (Figure 8–19).

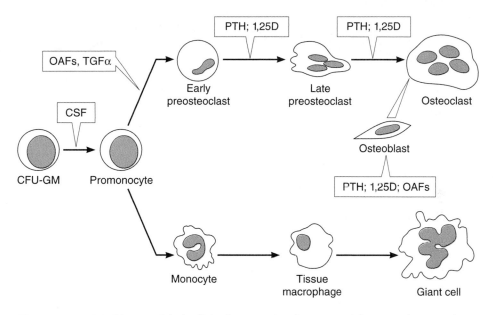

Figure 8–21. Working model of cells in the osteoclast lineage and the sites of action of various growth and differentiation factors. (Reproduced, with permission, from Favus MJ [editor]: *Primer on the Metabolic Bone Diseases and Disorders of Mineral Metabolism,* 2nd ed. Raven Press, 1993.)

By contrast, trabecular resorption creates scalloped areas of the bone surface called Howship's lacunae. Two to 3 months after initiation, the resorption phase reaches completion, having created a cavity about 60 μm deep. This is accompanied by ingress from marrow stroma into the base of the resorption cavity of precursors for bone-forming osteoblasts. These cells develop an osteoblastic phenotype, expressing characteristic bone-specific proteins such as alkaline phosphatase, osteopontin, and osteocalcin, and begin to replace the resorbed bone by elaborating new bone matrix. Once the newly formed osteoid reaches a thickness of about 20 μm, mineralization begins. Completion of a full remodeling cycle normally lasts about 6 months (Figure 8–20).

How do osteoclasts and osteoblasts communicate to achieve the coupling that ensures bone balance? It appears that the important signals are local, not systemic. Although complete understanding of this process has not been achieved, evidence suggests that two proteins derived from osteoblasts comprise an effective bone turnover regulatory system: The first component of this system is an osteoclast differentiation factor called RANK ligand (RANKL) that binds to its receptor, RANK receptor, which activates NF-κB on the surface of osteoclast precursors to directly stimulate osteoclast production. The second component, osteoprotegerin (OPG), is a soluble protein that binds to RANKL and

thereby inhibits its ability to interact with RANK. According to current views of this system, when peripheral signals instruct the osteoblast to increase bone remodeling, RANKL is secreted and binds to RANK, its natural receptor, thereby initiating the proliferation of new osteoclasts. When circumstances favor decreasing the rate of remodeling, RANKL production abates and increased OPG binds to residual RANKL, thereby minimizing the binding of RANKL to RANK and downregulating osteoclast production.

Bone remodeling does not absolutely require systemic hormones except to maintain intestinal absorption of minerals and thus ensure an adequate supply of calcium and phosphorus. For example, bone is normal, aside from low turnover, in patients with hypoparathyroidism. However, systemic hormones use the bone pool as a source of minerals for regulation of extracellular calcium homeostasis. When they do, the coupling mechanism ensures that bone is replenished. For example, when bone resorption is activated by PTH to provide calcium to correct hypocalcemia, bone formation will also increase, tending to replenish lost bone. One probable mechanism of coupling has to do with the apparent absence of PTH receptors and VDRs on osteoclasts. This means that other bone cells that have receptors for these hormones, such as osteoblasts, must receive the hormonal signal and pass it along to the os-

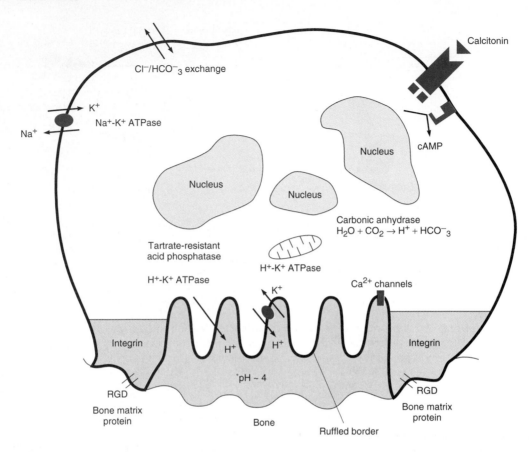

Figure 8–22. Osteoclast-mediated bone resorption. The osteoclast attaches to the bone surface via integrin-mediated binding to bone matrix bone proteins. When enough integrin binding has occurred, the osteoclast is anchored and a sealed space is formed. The repeatedly folded plasma membrane creates a "ruffled" border. Secreted into the sealed space are acid and enzymes forming an extracellular "lysosome." (Reproduced, with permission, from Felig P, Baxter JD, Frohman LA [editors]: *Endocrinology and Metabolism,* 3rd ed. McGraw-Hill, 1995.)

teoclast. This would allow for bone formation to be activated along with bone resorption.

If the replacement of resorbed bone matched the amount that was removed, remodeling would lead to no net change in bone mass. However, small bone deficits persist on completion of each cycle, reflecting inefficiency in remodeling dynamics. Consequently, lifelong accumulation of remodeling deficits underlies the well-documented phenomenon of age-related bone loss, a process that begins shortly after growth stops. Alterations in remodeling activity represent the final pathway through which diverse stimuli, such as dietary insufficiency, hormones, and drugs affect bone balance. A change in whole body remodeling rate can be brought about through distinct perturbations in remodeling dynamics. Changes in hormonal milieu often increase the activation of remodeling units. Examples include hyperthyroidism, hyperparathyroidism, and hypervitaminosis D. Other factors may impair osteoblastic functional adequacy, such as high doses of glucocorticoids or ethanol. Yet other perturbations, such as estrogen deficiency, may augment osteoclastic resorptive capacity. At any given time, a transient deficit in bone exists called the remodeling space, representing sites of bone resorption that have not yet filled in. In response to any stimulus that alters the birth rate of new remodeling units, the remodeling space will either increase or decrease accordingly until a new steady state is established, and this adjustment will be seen as an increase or decrease in bone mass.

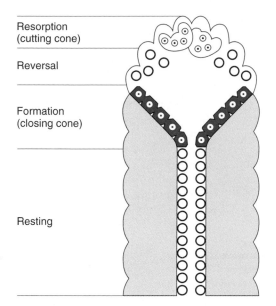

Resorption
(cutting cone)

Reversal

Formation
(closing cone)

Resting

Figure 8–23. Schematic representation of the four principal stages involved in the formation of a new basic structural unit in cortical bone. (Reproduced, with permission, from Felig P, Baxter JD, Frohman LA [editors]: *Endocrinology and Metabolism,* 3rd ed. McGraw-Hill, 1995.)

■ OSTEOPOROSIS

Osteoporosis is a condition of low bone mass and microarchitectural disruption that results in fractures with minimal trauma. Osteoporotic fractures are a major public health problem for older women and men in Western society, and billions of dollars are spent annually for acute hospital care of hip fracture alone. The consequences of vertebral deformity are less readily measured, but chronic pain, inability to conduct daily activities, and psychologic depression may be devastating.

The term "primary osteoporosis" denotes reduced bone mass and fractures in postmenopausal women (postmenopausal osteoporosis) or in older men and women ("senile" osteoporosis). "Secondary osteoporosis" is bone loss resulting from specific clinical disorders, such as thyrotoxicosis or hyperadrenocorticism (Table 8–8). States of estrogen-dependent bone loss, such as exercise-related amenorrhea or prolactin-secreting tumors, are conventionally treated as special cases of primary osteoporosis.

Fractures constitute the only clinically relevant consequence to having a fragile skeleton. At any age,

Table 8–8. Representative examples of "secondary" osteoporosis.

Chronic glucocorticoid exposure
Thyroid hormone excess
Immobilization
Chronic heparin therapy
Anticonvulsants
Hypervitaminosis A
Mastocytosis

women experience twice as many osteoporosis-related fractures as men do, reflecting gender-related differences in skeletal properties as well as the almost universal loss of bone at menopause. Currently increasing in prevalence, osteoporotic fractures in older men should not be considered of trivial importance (Figure 8–24). Fractures attributed to bone fragility are those due to trauma equal to or less than a fall from a standing position. Common sites of fragility-related fractures include vertebral bodies, the distal forearm, and the proximal femur, but since the skeletons of patients with osteoporosis are diffusely fragile, other sites, such as ribs and long bones, also fracture with high frequency. Vertebral compression fractures are the most common fragility-related fractures. Pain sufficient to require medical attention occurs in approximately one-third of vertebral fractures, the majority being detected only as height loss or spinal deformity (kyphosis) occurs. Both skeletal and extraskeletal factors determine fracture risk (Table 8–9).

Gain, Maintenance, & Loss of Bone

The amount of bone mineral present at any time in adult life represents that which has been gained at skeletal maturity (peak bone mass) minus that which has been subsequently lost. Bone acquisition is almost complete by 17 years in girls and by 20 years in boys. Heredity accounts for most of the variance in bone acquisition. Specific genes implicated in bone acquisition include those affecting body size, hormone responsiveness, and bone-specific proteins (Table 8–10). Other factors include circulating gonadal steroids, physical activity, and nutrient intake.

Bone gained during adolescence accounts for about 60% of final adult bone mass. Assuming adequate exposure to key nutrients, physical activity, and reproductive hormones, adolescent growth supports acquisition of the maximum bone mass permitted by genetic endowment. Estradiol plays a decisive role in the initiation of adolescent growth and bone acquisition. Rare examples have been reported of young men bearing

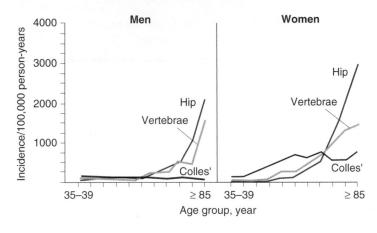

Figure 8–24. Incidence rates for the three common osteoporotic fractures (Colles', hip, and vertebral) in men and women, plotted as a function of age at the time of the fracture. (Reproduced, with permission, from Cooper C, Melton LJ III: Epidemiology of osteoporosis. Trends Endocrinol Metab 1992;314:224.)

mutations in the estradiol receptor or in aromatase, the enzyme that converts androgen to estrogen. Although these men had normal or increased circulating concentrations of testosterone, estradiol was either absent or totally ineffective. In all cases, severe deficits in bone density were observed and the patients had not undergone the anticipated acceleration in linear growth at the time of puberty. In the patients with aromatase deficiency, substantial gains in bone were observed shortly after initiating estrogen therapy.

Adolescent bone acquisition falters in the face of inadequacies in diet, physical activity, or reproductive function, resulting in a lower peak bone mass (acquisitional osteopenia) and less reserve to accommodate future losses. Recent trends in habitual physical activity and calcium intake for North American teenagers, particularly girls, offer little encouragement in this regard. A list of representative states of acquisitional osteopenia is presented in Table 8–11.

Once peak bone mass is achieved, bone mass remains fairly stable until about age 50 (Figure 8–25). Successful bone maintenance requires continued attention to the same "hygienic" factors that influenced

bone acquisition: diet, physical activity, and reproductive status. Maintenance of bone requires sufficiency in all areas, and deficiency in one is not compensated by the others. For example, amenorrheic athletes lose bone despite frequent high-intensity physical activity and supplemental calcium intake. Successful bone maintenance is also jeopardized by known toxic exposures such as smoking, alcohol excess, and immobility as well as by systemic illnesses and many medications. Based on the above considerations, a rational osteoporosis prevention strategy can be formulated (Table 8-12).

Bone Loss Associated with Estrogen Deficiency

Estrogen deprivation promotes bone remodeling by releasing constraints on osteoblastic production of skeletally active cytokines which, in turn, stimulate the proliferation of osteoclast precursors. The primary cytokine involved in this process appears to be interleukin-6. Estradiol suppresses IL-6 secretion by marrow stromal osteoblastic cells, and treatment of mice with neutralizing IL-6 antibodies suppresses osteoclast production after oophorectomy. Estradiol directly suppresses IL-6 production in human osteoblasts, and IL-6 gene knock-

Table 8–9. Factors affecting fracture risk.

Skeletal factors
  Bone age
  Bone size
  Bone mineral density and quality
  Bone turnover rate
Extrinsic factors (susceptibility to falls)
  Vision
  Muscle strength
  Neuropathy
  General frailty
  Small animals underfoot in household

Table 8–10. Genetic polymorphisms implicated in the acquisition of bone and regulation of bone mass in humans.

Somatotrophic axis (IGF-1 gene polymorphism)
Vitamin D receptor
Estradiol receptor
Type I collagen
Transforming growth factor-β

Table 8–11. Examples of disorders associated wtih acquisitional osteopenia.

Anorexia nervosa
Ankylosing spondylitis
Childhood immobilization ("therapeutic rest")
Cystic fibrosis
Delayed puberty
Exercise-associated amenorrhea
Galactosemia
Intestinal or renal disease
Marfan's syndrome
Osteogenesis imperfecta

Table 8–12. A strategy to prevent osteoporosis at all ages.

Regular physical activity of reasonable intensity
Adequate nutrient intake
Sensible intake of calories and all macronutrients
Meet age-appropriate dietary guidelines for calcium intake
Treatment of hypogonadism with timely, sustained hormone replacement (or effective surrogate medication)

---

out prevents bone loss in oophorectomized mice. Thus, a strong case implicates IL-6 as a critical molecule by which osteoblasts signal increased bone remodeling and suggests that this link is a major site for estrogen action in bone. Subsidiary roles for IL-1 and IL-11 have also been described. As discussed above, the RANK-RANKL-OPG system acts as a bone regulatory system through which osteoblast signals stimulate the produc-

tion of osteoclasts. With estrogen deficiency, OPG secretion is low, permitting a robust response of osteoclast precursors to RANKL. With estrogen sufficiency, increased local concentrations of OPG bind to RANKL, reduce osteoclast production, and thereby decrease bone turnover.

With accelerated bone turnover, delivery of calcium from bone to the circulation increases, and the resultant subtle increase in plasma calcium concentration suppresses the secretion of PTH, thereby enhancing calciuria, suppressing renal production of 1,25 dihydroxyvitamin D, and reducing intestinal calcium absorption

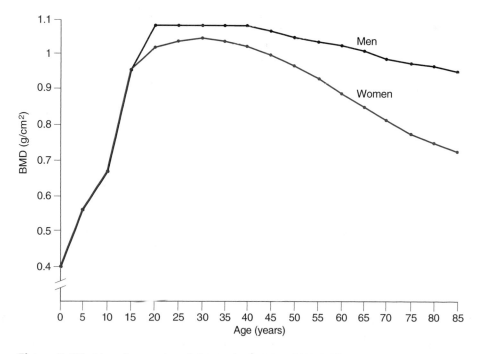

Figure 8–25. Mean bone mineral density by DXA in white males (upper curve) and females (lower curve) aged 5–85 years. (The data are from Southard RN et al: Bone mass in healthy children: Measurement with quantitative DXA. Radiology 1991;179:735; and from Kelly TL: Bone mineral reference databases for American men and women. J Bone Miner Res 1990;5[Suppl 2]:702. Courtesy of Hologic, Inc.)

efficiency. At menopause, loss of endogenous estrogen promotes an increase in daily calcium loss from 20 mg to about 60 mg, reflecting a relative increase in bone resorption over formation activity. Although small, this magnitude of change in mineral balance would account after a decade for about 13% of an original whole body calcium mass of 1000 g, equivalent to a standard deviation in bone mineral density (BMD), and would lead to a two- to threefold increase in the risk for fracture (Figure 8–25). In contrast, women who receive estrogen replacement as they enter menopause show calcium balance and rates of mineral turnover similar to those of premenopausal women. To accommodate menopausal changes in calcium economy by dietary means alone, a rise in daily calcium intake from 1000 mg to about 1500 mg would be necessary.

Bone Loss in Later Life

Progressive deficits in renal and intestinal function impair whole body calcium economy during normal human aging. These deficits include progressive inefficiency of vitamin D production by the skin as well as declining ability to convert 25-hydroxyvitamin D to 1,25-dihydroxyvitamin D in the kidney. Consequently, intestinal calcium absorption becomes less efficient, leading to modest reductions in plasma ionized calcium activity and compensatory hypersecretion of PTH. PTH maintains blood calcium concentrations by activating new bone remodeling units, though as a result of its inherent inefficiency, increased bone remodeling leads to accelerated bone loss. Little can be done to counteract remodeling inefficiency, but the impact of these physiologic deficits can be minimized by suppressing the stimulus for PTH secretion by consuming adequate amounts of dietary calcium (about 1500 mg/d) and vitamin D (about 400–800 units/d).

Diagnosis of Osteoporosis

Diagnosis may be obvious in patients who have sustained fragility fractures (Figure 8–26), but noninvasive methods to estimate bone mineral density may be required to identify high-risk patients who have not yet sustained a fracture. Several techniques have been developed for this purpose, but dual-energy x-ray absorptiometry (DXA) currently offers the most precise measurements at multiple skeletal sites for the least amount of radiation exposure.

Bone mineral density (BMD) is a highly significant predictor of fracture risk. Each standard deviation below age-predicted mean values confers a two- to threefold increased risk for fracture over time (Figure 8–27). A World Health Organization panel offered an absolute BMD standard to make the diagnosis of osteoporosis. By this criterion, a person whose BMD value falls more than 2.5 SD below the average value for a 25-year-old Caucasian woman is stated to have osteoporosis, and individuals whose BMDs fall between −1.0 and −2.5 SD below the standard are said to have **osteopenia.** Although useful, this concept still presents difficulties, particularly with respect to its validity for men and to non-Caucasian populations. Absolute reliance on a BMD standard for diagnosis fails to account for the fact that BMD predicts fracture risk along a continuous, progressive relationship and ignores contributions of other factors to bone fragility. The latter include bone size and geometry as well as qualitative abnormalities of the matrix and mineral of osteoporotic bone (Table 8–13). Thus, the primary diagnostic value of densitometry is not to confer a specific diagnosis of osteoporosis but to predict an individual's long-term fracture risk.

TREATMENT OF OSTEOPOROSIS

Drugs used for prevention and treatment of osteoporosis act either by decreasing the rate of bone resorption, thereby slowing the rate of bone loss, or by increasing bone formation. All drugs currently approved in the United States for this indication inhibit resorption (Table 8–14). Because of the coupled nature of bone resorption and formation, these agents ultimately decrease the rate of bone formation. Thus, increases in BMD, representing a reduction of the remodeling space to a new steady-state level, are commonly observed during the first year or two of therapy, after which BMD values reach a plateau.

Specific Antiresorptive Agents

A. CALCIUM

In childhood and adolescence, adequate substrate is required for bone accretion. Clinical trials indicate that supplemental calcium promotes adolescent bone acquisition, but its impact on peak bone mass is not known. In the seventh decade and beyond, supplemental calcium suppresses bone turnover, increases bone mass, and has been shown in clinical trials to decrease fracture incidence. Studies confirming the clinical efficacy of various pharmacologic agents to increase BMD or decrease fracture have been done in the setting of calcium sufficiency. Thus, adequate intake of calcium should be considered a basic approach for prevention and treatment of osteoporosis in all patients (Table 8–15).

Patients who are unable or unwilling to increase dietary calcium by diet alone may choose from many

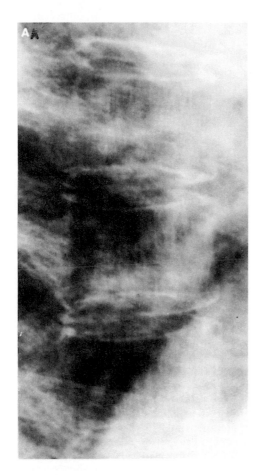
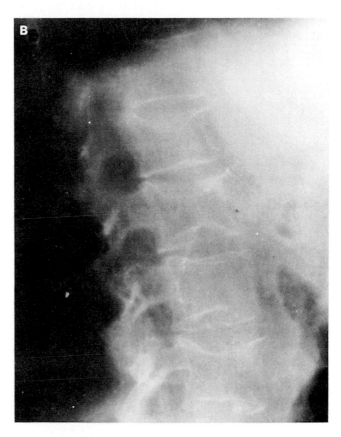

Figure 8–26. ***A:*** Magnified x-rays of thoracic vertebrae from a woman with osteoporosis. Note the relative prominence of vertical trabeculae and the absence of horizontal trabeculae. ***B:*** Lateral x-ray of the lumbar spine of a woman with postmenopausal osteoporosis. Note the increased density of the superior and inferior cortical margins of vertebrae, the marked demineralization of vertebral bodies, and the central compression of articular surfaces of vertebral bodies by intervertebral disks. (Courtesy of G Gordan.)

palatable, low-cost calcium preparations, the most frequently prescribed being the carbonate salt (Table 8–16). Others include the lactate, gluconate, and citrate salts and hydroxyapatite. Absorption of most commonly prescribed calcium products is reasonable. For many patients, cost and palatability outweigh modest differences in efficacy. The usual dose of calcium is about 1000 mg/d—approximately the amount contained in a quart of vitamin D-supplemented milk. Added to the 500–600 mg of dietary calcium present in the typical diet of elderly men and women, this provides a total daily intake of about 1500 mg. Calcium carbonate requires an acid environment for optimal absorption. For older individuals who may have hypo- or achlorhydria, taking calcium carbonate tablets with

meals generally provides adequate acidity for this requirement.

B. Vitamin D and Calcitriol

In recent years, it has become necessary to reassess our concepts of vitamin D sufficiency. Although circulating 25(OH)D concentrations above 8 ng/mL appear adequate for preventing osteomalacia, a strong case can now be made that values below 25–30 ng/mL are associated with hypersecretion of PTH and increased bone turnover. In some regions, healthy adults show average 25(OH)D concentrations of 30 ng/mL or above, but in others, such as New England or in states farther north than Missouri, the ultraviolet component of sunlight fails to contain sufficient amounts at the critical region

A

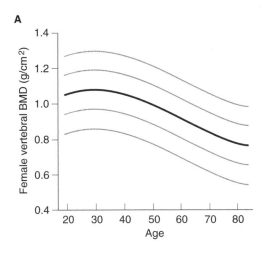

B

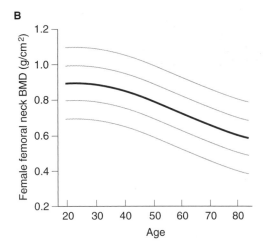

Figure 8–27. Bone density of **(A)** the lumbar spine (L2–4) and **(B)** femoral neck. The bold line represents the mean of 650 women with no overt bone disease; the thinner lines represent 1 SD and 2 SD above and below the mean. (Courtesy of Hologic, Inc.)

of approximately 270–310 nm to support cutaneous vitamin D synthesis. In those areas, vitamin D insufficiency is very common, particularly in frail or hospitalized patients. Vitamin D supplementation (400–800 IU/d) improves intestinal calcium absorption, suppresses PTH and bone remodeling, and increases bone mass in individuals with marginal or deficient vitamin D status.

The use of potent vitamin D analogs or metabolites—such as calcitriol—to treat osteoporosis is distinct from ensuring vitamin D nutritional adequacy. In the treatment of osteoporosis, the rationale is to exploit the ability of these compounds to interact with the vitamin D receptor in parathyroid cells to suppress PTH secretion directly and reduce bone turnover. Clinical experience with calcitriol remains mixed. Higher doses impose an added risk of hypercalciuria and hypercalcemia but appear more likely to improve bone mass. Potent vitamin D metabolites and analogs are still considered experimental and should be preferably used in the context of a clinical trial.

Table 8–13. Qualitative abnormalities in osteoporotic bone.

Heterogeneity of matrix mineralization
Trabecular disruption
Cortical porosity
Cement line accumulation
Unremodeled fatigue damage

C. ESTROGEN

Clinical trials clearly establish that timely replacement of estrogen conserves bone mass. Although such conservation is likely to confer protection against fracture, estimates of the antifracture efficacy of estrogen are based largely on observational data rather than on clinical trials. The minimum daily estrogen dose for skeletal protection of women within 10 years of menopause appears to be 0.625 mg/d of conjugated equine estrogens or its equivalent. This dose, given for 3 years, can be expected to increase BMD about 5% at the lumbar spine and 2.5% at the proximal femur. Long-term treatment at this dosage prevents bone loss in about 95% of women who adhere to therapy. In older women who

Table 8–14. Pharmacologic approaches to osteoporosis.

Antiresorptive agents
Calcium
Vitamin D and calcitriol
Estrogen
SERMs
Calcitonin
Bisphosphonates
Bone-forming agents[1]
Fluoride
Androgens
Parathyroid hormone

[1]Not yet approved in the United States.

Table 8–15. Calcium nutrition and osteoporosis.

Optimal daily calcium intakes	
(NIH Consensus Statement, 1994)	
Children	
1–5 years	800 mg
6–10 years	800–1200 mg
Adolescents	1200–1500 mg
Adults 25–50 years	1000 mg
Women	
Pregnant or lactating	1200 mg
Postmenopausal, on estrogen	1000 mg
Postmenopausal, not on estrogen	1500 mg
Elderly (age > 65)	1500 mg
Actual daily calcium intake (average in	550 mg
women aged 65)	
Calcium sources	
Dairy product-free diet	400 mg
Cow's milk (8 oz)	300 mg
Calcium carbonate (500 mg)	200 mg

also receive adequate calcium supplementation, 0.3 mg of conjugated estrogens has been shown to be effective. Both oral and transdermal estrogen offer skeletal protection. Estrogen cessation leads rapidly to bone loss, and protection against fracture dissipates within a few years of stopping even after prolonged treatment. Thus, for persistent skeletal benefit, estrogen must be considered lifelong therapy. Standard practice recommends cyclic or continuous administration of progestational drugs to women with an intact uterus, and the skeletal response to estrogen appears not to be affected by progestin use. For women without a uterus, estrogen therapy is continuous and does not require adding a progestin. The optimal time to institute estrogen replacement is early menopause, when bone turnover accelerates. However, beneficial skeletal effects of estro-

Table 8–16. Calcium preparations in common use.

Trade Name	Form of Salt	Elemental Calcium per Tablet (mg)
Os-Cal[1]	Carbonate	250
Os-Cal 500	Carbonate	500
Generic oyster shell calcium	Carbonate	500
Tums	Carbonate	200
Posture	Phosphate	600
Citracal	Citrate	200
PhosLo	Acetate	169

[1]Contains 125 IU cholecalciferol.

gen are observed when estrogen is started even after age 65. Many older women will not accept cyclic bleeding or other anticipated side effects of estrogen, so the decision to initiate estrogen in elderly women must be individualized. Some women find the decision easy; for others, a careful weighing of risks and benefits may be required. Bone densitometry is of use in advising undecided women (Figure 8–28). Since women whose BMD is in the lower range of normal have a substantially increased risk of future fractures, they can be encouraged to consider replacement therapy. Conversely, women whose BMD is in the upper normal range can be encouraged to make their decision based on other issues, such as their experience of hot flushes and the risk for cardiovascular disease and breast cancer.

D. Selective Estrogen Response Modulators (SERMs)

The past decade has witnessed the design and development of several molecules that act as estrogens on some tissues but as antiestrogens on others. The first of these to reach clinical practice was tamoxifen, which is a full estrogen agonist on bone, liver, and uterus but an antiestrogen at the breast and brain. More recently, raloxifene has been introduced for skeletal protection. This compound is an estrogen agonist at bone and liver, resulting in conservation of BMD and lowering of LDL cholesterol concentrations, but it is inert at the endometrium and a potent antiestrogen at the breast. Raloxifene has been shown to decrease the vertebral fracture incidence in older osteoporotic women and has received FDA approval for both prevention and treatment of osteoporosis in postmenopausal women.

E. Calcitonin

An inhibitor of osteoclastic bone resorption, calcitonin increases spine BMD in osteoporotic patients by 10–15%. Although this maximal calcitonin effect is accomplished with injectable salmon calcitonin, this agent has been largely supplanted by a more convenient nasal spray that has been approved for osteoporosis treatment and which, although it produces only modest changes in BMD, has been shown to reduce vertebral fracture incidence. In menopausal women who cannot or will not accept estrogen replacement or raloxifene, calcitonin affords reasonable conservation of bone mass.

F. Bisphosphonates

Alendronate, a potent antiresorptive drug, has been shown to increase BMD, reduce by 50% the incidence of vertebral and cortical bone fractures—including hip fracture—and diminish height loss in postmenopausal women with established osteoporosis. For older women

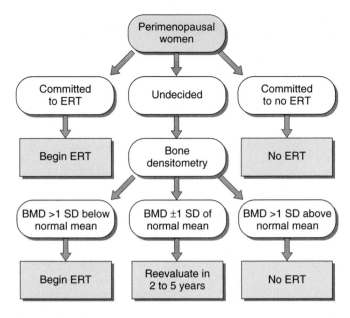

Figure 8–28. Algorithm for making decisions about the use of estrogen replacement therapy to prevent osteoporosis in post-menopausal women. (Reproduced, with permission, from Riggs BL, Melton LJ III: The prevention and treatment of osteoporosis. N Engl J Med 1992;327:620.)

with low bone mass who have not sustained fractures, alendronate also decreases the incidence of vertebral fractures. Alendronate and a related bisphosphonate, risedronate, are both approved for prevention and treatment of osteoporosis, including that associated with glucocorticoid use. These drugs are generally well tolerated, though they have been associated with esophagitis in some patients. For adequate absorption, they must be taken only with water after an overnight fast and at least 30 minutes before consuming other food, liquids, or medications. The patient should remain upright after swallowing the tablet to minimize the chance of esophageal distress.

Bone-Forming Agents

A. FLUORIDE

Although fluoride salts definitely increase BMD, particularly at the spine, considerable doubt remains about their ability to reduce fracture. A recent trial of sustained-release fluoride, which is associated with lower blood fluoride levels, showed a dramatic reduction in new vertebral fractures, but a European trial of monofluorophosphate showed no benefit. The status of slow-release fluoride remains under FDA review.

B. ANDROGEN

Testosterone increases bone mass of hypogonadal men. Androgens also improve bone mass in osteoporotic women, but therapy is frequently limited by virilizing side effects. Nandrolone decanoate, 50 mg intramuscularly every 3 weeks, and the androgenic progestin norethisterone acetate increased BMD in osteoporotic women without bothersome side effects. Fracture data do not yet permit a conclusion about the clinical utility of these agents.

C. PARATHYROID HORMONE

Fractures, skeletal deformity, and bone pain are well-described manifestations of bone disease associated with severe primary hyperparathyroidism. It may seem counterintuitive, therefore, to suggest that administration of PTH to individuals with low bone mass may not only improve BMD but also reduce the risk for fractures—yet that is what experience over the past 2 decades suggests. The decisive element that determines the effects of PTH to be destructive or therapeutic is whether PTH concentrations in blood are elevated constantly or only intermittently. In severe hyperparathyroidism, PTH concentrations remain high, varying little throughout the day. In most cases of mild hyperparathyroidism seen today, PTH concentrations are lower, sometimes within the normal range. In such patients, normal and even increased lumbar spine BMD are commonly observed. Administration of PTH as daily pulse injections has been shown to increase BMD in both animals and humans. Abundant evidence now indicates that PTH is truly an osteotropic agent, and several laboratories have shown increases in axial bone mineral density of patients with osteoporosis. In a large clinical trial conducted in postmenopausal women with osteoporosis, recombinant human PTH (1–34), given for approximately 1½ years, reduced the incidence of vertebral fractures by over 50% and of nonvertebral fractures by 53%. During the course of this trial, a long-term carcinogenicity study showed that rats given near-lifetime daily injections of rhPTH (1–34) showed a dose-related incidence of osteosarcoma. Clinical studies with this agent were immediately suspended pending a thorough review of all relevant information by an independent group of cancer biologists, who concluded that the rat osteosarcoma finding was not likely to predict a relationship to osteosarcoma in humans. Consequently, human trials with rhPTH (1–34) were resumed. As of this writing, rhPTH (1–34) is awaiting FDA approval for treatment of patients with osteoporosis at high risk for fracture.

NONPHARMACOLOGIC ASPECTS OF OSTEOPOROSIS MANAGEMENT

Much of the day-to-day management of osteoporotic patients involves issues that are not specific for bone. These include depression, pain control, maintaining nutritional status, exercise, and assisting the patient to organize activities of daily living.

Minimal attention has been devoted to the role of exercise for patients with established osteoporosis. Patients and physicians often show reluctance to participate in exercise because of concerns for additional injury. However, activity avoidance aggravates bone loss and places the skeleton in even greater jeopardy, whereas improving muscle strength, particularly of the back extensor groups, constitutes a powerful means for reducing pain and increasing functional capacity.

Although exercise may improve bone density in patients with osteoporosis, gains have been small, and one may ask what the real benefits could be from such limited improvement. Many older individuals have such little proximal femur strength that even large increases in BMD would not permit a direct fall onto the trochanter without fracture. Since the great majority of hip fractures are the immediate result of a fall, strategies aimed at reduction of falls may be more effective in reducing the incidence of hip fracture than those aimed

specifically at increasing bone mass. Muscle weakness is an important predictor of falls risk, and decreased muscle mass and strength are consequences of normal human aging. Resistance exercise, ie, weight training, promotes muscle strength even in very old men and women, and evidence suggests that increased lower extremity strength may reduce falls risk by improving postural stability. Thus, a widely disseminated program of leg-strengthening exercise could lower the risk of falling and reduce hip fracture incidence even if no changes in bone mineral were achieved.

Several additional measures may lower the risk of fracture for osteoporotic patients. Proper footwear and installation of safety features around the home may minimize the risk of falling. Such features include bathroom safety rails and night-lights, rails and lighting for stairways, and elimination of floor clutter. Assorted canes and walking aids can be recommended to patients with unsteady gait. Physicians may need to overcome substantial patient resistance, but these aids can be life-saving. Corsets and other support garments stabilize posture and relieve strain on paraspinous muscles. Metal braces may be indicated at times, but they are expensive, poorly accepted by most patients, and frequently end up unused. Patients should be encouraged to schedule daily rest periods. An hour or so of comfortable repose can restore sufficient energy to allow patients to participate in evening activities. Many patients are severely incapacitated by pain and depression, so that successful management requires timely and effective use of appropriate analgesic and antidepressant medications.

GLUCOCORTICOID-INDUCED OSTEOPOROSIS

Few skeletal disorders prove as vexing to treat as glucocorticoid-induced osteoporosis. Recent years have witnessed important progress in understanding this condition as well as in achieving partial reversal of established disease. In children, chronic exposure to glucocorticoid impairs skeletal growth. Glucocorticoid-induced deficits in childhood bone mass reflect failure of normal skeletal acquisition occasionally compounded by bone loss. In adults, glucocorticoid-induced skeletal deficits exclusively reflect bone loss due to uncoupling of the normal relationship between the resorption and formation phases of bone remodeling. When adults are administered high doses of glucocorticoid for more than several days, rapid bone loss ensues, leading to BMD deficits within a few months. Bone loss in the axial (central) skeleton exceeds that in appendicular (peripheral) bone, reflecting greater investment of trabecular bone in axial regions. The magnitude of axial bone loss typically approaches 40% of initial values, which translates into a high incidence of vertebral compression fractures. Peripheral bone loss is more likely to be about 20%. Skeletal fragility is not the only risk factor for fracture in steroid-treated patients, since glucocorticoids (and the illnesses for which they are prescribed) are also associated with muscle weakness, which may be profound and which itself creates instability and increases the risk for falling.

Glucocorticoid-induced bone loss generally follows sustained administration of systemic doses greater than 5 mg/d of prednisone or its equivalent. Skeletal consequences depend on the condition being treated. A week-long course at high dosage for treatment of poison oak dermatitis is not an important risk, but even low-dose steroids may place frail elders with rheumatic conditions in considerable jeopardy. Used according to manufacturer recommendations, most steroid inhalers available in the United States are of little concern since systemic absorption of glucocorticoids is insubstantial. However, excessive use of standard preparations may achieve systemic concentrations adequate to suppress the hypothalamic-pituitary axis and predictably lead to loss of bone. Patients receiving maintenance hydrocortisone dosages (eg, 20 mg/d) for adrenocortical insufficiency do not generally have an increased skeletal risk. However, based on accurate measurements of steroid production rates in normal humans, maintenance doses of hydrocortisone are now estimated to be lower (ie, 15 mg/d) than have traditionally been recommended (about 30 mg/d). Patients who continue to be treated according to older recommendations may be at risk for excessive bone loss.

Pathophysiology

Glucocorticoids affect human mineral balance through functional alterations in the kidney, intestine, and skeleton.

A. RENAL CALCIUM LOSSES

Within a few days after initiating therapy, direct inhibition of renal tubular calcium reabsorption leads to hypercalciuria, which is magnified by excessive dietary sodium and attenuated by thiazide diuretics.

B. INTESTINAL CALCIUM LOSSES

Glucocorticoids given in high doses for several weeks directly inhibit intestinal calcium absorption, lowering plasma ionized calcium activity. This is thought to stimulate compensatory hypersecretion of PTH, which restores ionized calcium activity by increasing the efficiency of renal calcium reabsorption and by activating bone turnover to increase delivery of calcium to the circulation from bone. Thus, the dominant model for conceptualizing steroid-induced changes in bone homeostasis requires an increase in activity of the parathyroid axis. The operative term in this model is "activity," because it has been very difficult to show with consistency that plasma PTH concentrations are actually elevated in steroid-treated patients. Evidence suggests that expression of PTH action in bone and kidney may be enhanced by glucocorticoids, so the described model does not require increased PTH concentrations for validity. Consistent effects of glucocorticoids on the production, clearance, and circulating concentrations of vitamin D metabolites have not been demonstrable, so it appears that the intestinal actions of glucocorticoids are independent of the vitamin D system.

C. SKELETAL LOSSES

Glucocorticoids interact with the skeleton at multiple sites. In mice, they directly promote osteoclastic bone resorption, an effect that seems not to occur in humans. Glucocorticoids inhibit osteoblastic maturation and activity, and recent information indicates that glucocorticoids shift multipotent stem cell maturation away from osteoblastic lineage toward other cell lines, particularly adipocytes. Glucocorticoids also promote apoptosis in osteoblasts. In composite, the most coherent basis for glucocorticoid-associated bone loss is suppression of bone formation activity.

High-dose glucocorticoid administration suppresses gonadotropin secretion and creates a hypogonadal state in both men and women. Thus, a component of the bone loss in some steroid-treated patients is likely to be related to loss of gonadal function.

Prevention & Treatment of Glucocorticoid-Related Osteoporosis

A. REDUCTION OF STEROID DOSE

Given the poor response of established glucocorticoid-related osteoporosis to available therapies, prevention remains the approach most likely to give a favorable outcome. The most important aspect of a sound preventive strategy is to limit exposure to glucocorticoids and to find alternative treatments if possible. Opportunities should be sought for initiating dose reduction or switching to nonsystemic forms of steroids. Unfortunately, the use of alternate-day steroids, which is known to protect growth in steroid-treated children, appears not to offer skeletal protection to steroid-treated adults. The possibility that a bone-sparing glucocorticoid might be developed has been under consideration for many years but no such agent has yet been approved in the United States. In patients who require immunosuppression following organ transplantation, widespread use of cyclosporine and tacrolimus has permitted reductions in glucocorticoid use. However, these newer drugs also promote bone loss, so their net effect on bone status may be just as worrisome.

B. CALCIUM AND VITAMIN D

Providing supplemental calcium and vitamin D to glucocorticoid-treated patients will normalize plasma ionized calcium activity, suppress PTH secretion, and reduce bone remodeling, thereby reducing the number of remodeling units in action at a given time. So long as the patient continues to take glucocorticoids, however, suppression of osteoblast function is not reversed. Patients should receive 1500 mg/d of supplemental calcium. Vitamin D has been given at dosages of 400 IU/d to 50,000 IU three times per week. Periodic surveillance of glucocorticoid-treated patients for urinary calcium excretion is warranted, since they would be at higher risk for developing kidney stones as a consequence of hypercalciuria.

C. PHYSICAL ACTIVITY

Skeletal immobilization precipitates bone loss, so, inactivity must be avoided in steroid-treated patients. Some conditions such as polymyalgia rheumatica respond exuberantly to steroid therapy, giving patients a rapid and complete recovery of function. These patients may have little difficulty maintaining a vigorous schedule of weight-bearing activities during treatment. Patients with other conditions may not regain full mobility and may have residual functional disabilities. It is particularly important for such patients to receive physical therapy or other appropriate assistance for maintaining and restoring functional capacity.

D. HORMONE REPLACEMENT THERAPY

In some rheumatologic conditions (eg, systemic lupus erythematosus), estrogens have been traditionally avoided. If there are no contraindications to estrogen administration, replacement therapy will counteract the negative skeletal consequences of pituitary-gonadal suppression.

Pharmacologic Therapy of Glucocorticoid-Related Osteoporosis

Given that the primary skeletal abnormality induced by glucocorticoids is inhibition of bone formation, the potential benefits of antiresorptive therapy are not immediately obvious. Evidence from clinical trials of glucocorticoid-treated patients indicates clinical utility for calcitriol, with calcitonin being of only marginal value. However, enthusiasm for calcitriol is tempered by its significant risk for producing unacceptable degrees of hypercalciuria, if calcium intake is not restricted. Recent interest has centered around the use of bisphosphonates. Well-conducted trials have shown unequivocal benefit in terms of conserving and even increasing bone density. In a study of patients who had been treated with glucocorticoids for variable periods of time, 48 weeks of daily alendronate (5 mg/d or 10 mg/d) significantly increased BMD of the spine and hip compared with a control group, leading ultimately to a substantial reduction in the incidence of vertebral fracture. Similar results have been observed with risedronate, and both drugs are approved for prevention and treatment of glucocorticoid-induced osteoporosis.

Promoters of Bone Formation

It is reasonable to assume that an agent which directly promotes osteoblast function would be ideal for counteracting the effects of glucocorticoids. Several compounds have generated interest. There is strong evidence that PTH may exert a true bone anabolic effect. In a recent study, hPTH (1–34), an active fragment of human PTH, was given to estrogen-replaced postmenopausal women who were taking glucocorticoids, primarily for rheumatoid arthritis. Over 1 year of follow-up, lumbar spine BMD in the group receiving the PTH analog increased by 35% (measured by computed tomography) and by 11% (measured by DXA). By contrast, patients receiving hormone replacement therapy alone showed BMD changes of less than 2%. The differential response between CT and DXA reflects the fact that CT specifically measures trabecular bone, which appears to have been the primary responding tissue, whereas DXA measures both trabecular bone and the surrounding cortex. These results suggest that PTH may have great clinical utility in glucocorticoid-treated patients and emphasize the need for a longer-term controlled clinical trial of this agent.

■ OSTEOMALACIA & RICKETS

Osteomalacia and rickets are caused by the abnormal mineralization of bone and cartilage. Osteomalacia is a bone defect in which the epiphysial plates have closed (ie, in adults). Rickets occurs in growing bone (ie, in children). Abnormal mineralization in growing bone affects the transformation of cartilage into bone at the zone of provisional calcification. As a result, an enormous profusion of disorganized, nonmineralized, degenerating cartilage appears in this region, leading to widening of the epiphysial plate (observed radiologically as a widened radiolucent zone) with flaring or cupping and irregularity of the epiphysial-metaphysial junctions. This latter problem gives rise to the clinically obvious beaded swellings along the costochondral junctions known as the "rachitic rosary" and the swelling at the ends of the long bones. Growth is retarded by the failure to make new bone. Once bone growth has ceased (ie, after closure of the epiphysial plates), the clinical evidence for defective mineralization becomes more subtle, and special diagnostic procedures may be required for its detection.

Pathogenesis

The best-known cause of abnormal bone mineralization is vitamin D deficiency (see above). Vitamin D, through its biologically active metabolites, ensures that the calcium and phosphate concentrations in the extracellular milieu are adequate for mineralization. Vitamin D may also permit osteoblasts to produce a bone matrix that can be mineralized and then allows them to mineralize that matrix in a normal fashion. Phosphate deficiency can also cause defective mineralization, as in diseases in which phosphate is lost in the urine or poorly absorbed in the intestine. Phosphate deficiency may act independently or in conjunction with other predisposing abnormalities since most hypophosphatemic disorders associated with osteomalacia or rickets also affect the vitamin D endocrine system. Dietary calcium deficiency has been shown to lead to rickets in children in the absence of vitamin D deficiency and may contribute to the osteomalacia of elderly adults who are also susceptible to vitamin D deficiency.

Osteomalacia or rickets may develop despite adequate levels of calcium, phosphate, and vitamin D if the bone matrix cannot undergo normal mineralization as a result of enzyme deficiencies such as decreased alkaline phosphatase in patients with hypophosphatasia or in the presence of inhibitors of mineralization such as aluminum, fluoride, and etidronate. Table 8–17 lists diseases associated with osteomalacia or rickets according to their presumed mechanism. Several diseases appear under several headings indicating that they contribute to the bone disease by several mechanisms.

Diagnosis

The following discussion refers primarily to vitamin D deficiency. In children, the presentation of rickets is generally obvious from a combination of clinical and radiologic evidence. The diagnostic challenge is to determine the cause. In adults, the clinical, radiologic, and biochemical evidence for osteomalacia is often subtle. In situations in which osteomalacia should be suspected (malnutrition, malabsorption, unexpected osteopenia), the clinician must decide whether to obtain a bone biopsy for histomorphometric examination. This decision must rest on the availability of resources to take and examine the biopsy specimen, the index of suspicion coupled with the lack of certainty from other diagnostic procedures, and the degree to which the therapeutic approach will be altered by the additional information. In many cases, a clinical trial will suffice to establish the diagnosis without the need for bone biopsy.

Table 8–17. Causes of osteomalacia.

Disorders in the vitamin D endocrine system
  Decreased bioavailability
    Insufficient sunlight exposure
    Nutritional vitamin D deficiency
    Nephrotic syndrome (urinary loss)
    Malabsorption (fecal loss)
      Billroth type II gastrectomy
      Sprue
      Regional enteritis
      Jejunoileal bypass
      Pancreatic insufficiency
      Cholestatic disorders
      Cholestyramine
  Abnormal metabolism
    Liver disease
    Chronic renal failure
    Vitamin D-dependent rickets type I
    Tumoral hypophosphatemic osteomalacia
    X-linked hypophosphatemia
    Chronic acidosis
    Anticonvulsants
  Abnormal target tissue response
    Vitamin D-dependent rickets type II
    Gastrointestinal disorders

Disorders of phosphate homeostasis
  Decreased intestinal absorption
    Malnutrition
    Malabsorption
    Antacids containing aluminum hydroxide
  Increased renal loss
    X-linked hypophosphatemic rickets
    Tumoral hypophosphatemic osteomalacia
    De Toni-Debré-Fanconi

Calcium deficiency

Primary disorders of bone matrix
  Hypophosphatasia
  Fibrogenesis imperfecta ossium
  Axial osteomalacia

Inhibitors of mineralization
  Aluminum
    Chronic renal failure
    Total parenteral nutrition
  Etidronate
  Fluoride

Clinical Features

A. Symptoms and Signs

The clinical presentation of rickets depends on the age of the patient and, to some extent, the cause of the syndrome (Figure 8–29). The affected infant or young child may be apathetic, listless, weak, hypotonic, and

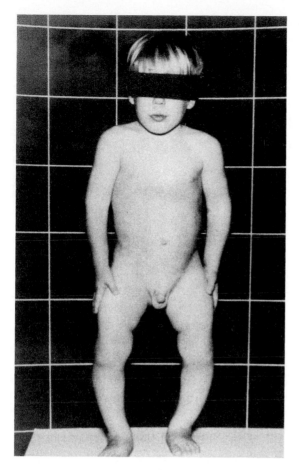

Figure 8–29. The clinical appearance of a young child with rickets. The most striking abnormalities are the bowing of the legs and protuberant abdomen. Flaring of the ends of the long bones can also be appreciated. (Photograph courtesy of S Arnaud.)

growing poorly. A soft, somewhat misshapen head with widened sutures and frontal bossing may be observed. Eruption of teeth may be delayed, and teeth that do appear may be pitted and poorly mineralized. The enlargement and cupping of the costochondral junctions produce the "rachitic rosary" on the thorax. The tug of the diaphragm against the softened lower ribs may produce an indentation at the point of insertion of the diaphragm (Harrison's groove). Muscle hypotonia can result in a pronounced "potbelly" and a waddling gait. The limbs may become bowed, and joints may swell because of flaring at the ends of the long bones (including phalanges and metacarpals). Pathologic fractures may occur in patients with florid rickets. After the epiphyses have closed, the clinical signs of rickets or osteo-

malacia are subtle and cannot be relied upon to make the diagnosis. Patients with severe osteomalacia complain of bone pain and proximal muscle weakness. Difficulty climbing stairs or rising from chairs may be reported and should be looked for. Such individuals may have a history of fractures and be diagnosed as having osteoporosis. Distinguishing osteoporosis from osteomalacia on clinical grounds alone is at times quite difficult.

B. LABORATORY FINDINGS

1. Biochemistry—Vitamin D deficiency results in decreased intestinal absorption of calcium and phosphate. In conjunction with the resulting secondary hyperparathyroidism, vitamin D deficiency leads to an increase in bone resorption, increased excretion of urinary phosphate, and increased renal tubular reabsorption of calcium. The net result tends to be a low-normal serum calcium level, low serum phosphorus level, elevated serum alkaline phosphatase level, increased PTH level, decreased urinary calcium level, and increased urinary phosphate level. Finding a low 25(OH)D level, in combination with these other biochemical alterations, strengthens the diagnosis of vitamin D deficiency. The $1,25(OH)_2D_3$ level may be normal, making this determination less useful for the diagnosis of osteomalacia. Both 25(OH)D and $1,25(OH)_2D_3$ levels may be reduced in patients with liver disease or nephrotic syndrome because the binding proteins for the vitamin D metabolites are low secondary to decreased production (liver disease) or increased renal losses (nephrotic syndrome; see below). Such individuals may have normal free concentrations of these metabolites and so are not vitamin D-deficient. Other factors, such as age and diet, must be considered. For example, serum phosphorus values are normally lower in adults than in children. Dietary history is important, since urinary phosphate excretion and, to a lesser extent, urinary calcium excretion reflect dietary phosphate and calcium content. Since phosphate excretion depends on the filtered load (the product of the glomerular filtration rate and plasma phosphate concentration), urinary phosphate levels may be reduced despite the presence of hyperparathyroidism, when serum phosphate levels are particularly low. Expressions of renal phosphate clearance that account for these variables (eg, renal threshold for phosphate, or T_mP/GFR) are a better indicator of renal phosphate handling than is total phosphate excretion. The T_mP/GFR can be calculated from a nomogram using measurements of a fasting serum and urine phosphorus concentration.

2. Histologic examination—Transcortical bone biopsy is the definitive means of making the diagnosis of osteomalacia. A rib or the iliac crest is the site at which biopsy is usually performed. To assess osteoid content and mineral appositional rate, the bone biopsy specimen is processed without decalcification. This requires special equipment. In osteomalacia, bone is mineralized poorly and slowly, resulting in wide osteoid seams (>12 μm) and a large fraction of bone covered by unmineralized osteoid. States of high bone turnover (increased bone formation and resorption), such as hyperparathyroidism, can also cause wide osteoid seams and an increased osteoid surface, producing a superficial resemblance to osteomalacia. Therefore, the rate of bone turnover should be determined by labeling bone with tetracycline, which provides a fluorescent marker of the calcification front. When two doses of tetracycline are given at different times, the distance between the two labels divided by the time interval between the two doses equals the mineral appositional rate. The normal appositional rate is approximately 0.74 μm/d. Mineralization lag time—the time required for newly formed osteoid to be mineralized—can be calculated by dividing osteoid seam width by the appositional rate corrected by the linear extent of mineralization of the calcification front (a measure of the bone surface that is undergoing active mineralization as measured by tetracycline incorporation). Mineralization lag time is normally about 20–25 days. Bone formation rate is calculated as the product of the appositional rate times the linear extent of mineralization of the calcification front. Depressed appositional rate, increased mineralization lag time, and reduced bone formation rate clearly distinguish osteomalacia from high-turnover states such as hyperparathyroidism. Low-turnover states, as can be seen in various forms of osteoporosis, also have low appositional and bone formation rates, but these conditions are distinguished from osteomalacia by normal or reduced osteoid surface and volume.

C. Imaging Studies

The radiologic features of rickets can be quite striking, especially in the young child. In growing bone, the radiolucent epiphyses are wide and flared, with irregular epiphysial-metaphysial junctions. Long bones may be bowed. The cortices of the long bones are often indistinct. Occasionally, evidence of secondary hyperparathyroidism—subperiosteal resorption in the phalanges and metacarpals and erosion of the distal ends of the clavicles—is observed. Pseudofractures (also known as Looser's zones or Milkman's fractures) are an uncommon but nearly pathognomonic feature of rickets and osteomalacia (Figure 8–30). These radiolucent lines are most often found along the concave side of the femoral neck, pubic rami, ribs, clavicles, and lateral aspects of the scapulae. Pseudofractures may result from unhealed microfractures at points of stress or at the entry point of blood vessels into bone. They may

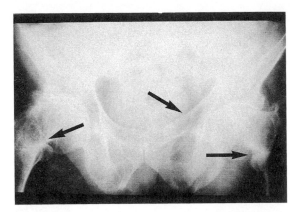

Figure 8–30. X-ray of the pelvis of an elderly woman with osteomalacia. Note marked bowing of both femoral necks, with pseudofractures of the medial aspect of the femoral necks and the superior aspect of the left pubic ramus (arrows). (Photograph courtesy of H Genant.)

progress to complete fractures that go unrecognized and thus lead to substantial deformity and disability. Bone density is not a reliable indicator of osteomalacia, since bone density can be decreased in patients with vitamin D deficiency or increased in patients with chronic renal failure. In adults with normal renal function, radiologic evidence of a mineralization defect is often subtle and not readily distinguished from osteoporosis, with which it often coexists.

Treatment

The treatment of vitamin D deficiency is covered under that heading. The treatment of other diseases causing rickets/osteomalacia is found below under the specific diseases.

NEPHROTIC SYNDROME

Nephrotic syndrome may lead to osteomalacia because of losses of vitamin D metabolites in the urine. Vitamin D metabolites are tightly bound to DBP, an α-globulin, and less tightly bound to albumin as described above. Patients with the nephrotic syndrome may lose large amounts of DBP and albumin in their urine and so deplete their vitamin D stores. Such patients can have very low levels of vitamin D metabolites in their serum, though the free concentrations are less affected. Thus, the measurement of total 25(OH)D or 1,25(OH)$_2$D$_3$ may be misleading with respect to the severity of the vitamin D deficiency. Although bone disease has been recognized as a complication of the nephrotic syndrome, the prevalence of osteomalacia in this population is unknown. If vitamin D deficiency is suspected, treatment with vitamin D is indicated with the proviso that normal total levels of 25(OH)D and $1,25(OH)_2D_3$ are not the goal. Blood levels of calcium, phosphorus, and PTH are a more reliable guide to treatment.

HEPATIC OSTEODYSTROPHY

Hepatic osteodystrophy is the bone disease associated with liver failure. In the United States, patients with liver failure generally have osteoporosis, not osteomalacia. Both osteomalacia and osteoporosis are found in patients with liver disease in Great Britain, where vitamin D deficiency is more common. Although the liver is the site of the first step in the bioactivation of vitamin D—the conversion of vitamin D to 25(OH)D—this process is not tightly controlled, and until the liver disease is severe it is not rate-limiting. Neither cholestatic nor parenchymal liver disease has much effect on 25(OH)D production until the late stages of liver failure. The low levels of 25(OH)D and $1,25(OH)_2D_3$ associated with liver disease can usually be attributed to the reduced production of DBP and albumin, poor nutrition, or malabsorption rather than a deficiency in the vitamin D 25-hydroxylase. As in patients with the nephrotic syndrome, the low total levels of the vitamin D metabolites may be misleading, as they reflect a reduction in DBP and albumin rather than a reduction in the free concentrations of these metabolites.

DRUG-INDUCED OSTEOMALACIA

Phenytoin and phenobarbital are anticonvulsants that induce drug-metabolizing enzymes in the liver which alter the hepatic metabolism of vitamin D and its metabolites. This action is not limited to anticonvulsants as the antituberculosis drug rifampin has been reported to do likewise. This effect may account for the lower circulating levels of 25(OH)D found in patients treated with such drugs. Levels of $1,25(OH)_2D_3$ are less affected. Chronic anticonvulsant or antituberculosis therapy does not appear to lead to clinically significant bone disease except in subjects with other predisposing factors such as inadequate sunlight exposure (institutionalized patients) and poor nutrition. Children may be more vulnerable than adults. In animal studies, phenytoin has been noted to exert a direct inhibitory effect on bone mineralization, but the relevance of this observation to the human use of this drug is uncertain. The decrease in 25(OH)D levels in patients taking these drugs can be readily reversed with supplemental vitamin D administration.

HYPOPHOSPHATEMIC DISORDERS

Phosphate Deficiency

Chronic hypophosphatemia may lead to rickets or osteomalacia independently of other predisposing abnormalities. The principal diseases in which hypophosphatemia is associated with osteomalacia or rickets, however, also include other abnormalities that can interfere with bone mineralization. Chronic phosphate depletion is caused by dietary deficiency (as in strict vegetarians), decreased intestinal absorption, or increased renal clearance (renal wasting). Acute hypophosphatemia can result from movement of phosphate into cells (eg, after infusion of insulin and glucose), but this condition is transient and does not result in bone disease.

Seventy to 90 percent of dietary phosphate is absorbed under normal conditions in the jejunum. This process is not tightly regulated, though $1,25(OH)_2D_3$ stimulates phosphate absorption, a factor that needs to be considered when calcitriol is being used to treat other conditions. Meat and dairy products are the principal dietary sources of phosphate. The incidence of osteomalacia in vegetarians who avoid all meat and dairy products is unknown, but its occurrence has been reported. Intrinsic small bowel disease and small bowel surgery interfere with phosphate absorption and, if coupled with diarrhea or steatorrhea, can result in phosphate depletion. A number of widely used antacids (eg, Mylanta, Maalox, Basaljel, and Amphojel) contain aluminum hydroxide, which binds phosphate and prevents its absorption. Patients who ingest large amounts of these antacids may become phosphate-depleted. When this occurs in the setting of renal failure—in which these antacids are used to control serum phosphate—overzealous reduction in serum phosphate plus the added insult of aluminum intoxication in these individuals, who also have reduced $1,25(OH)_2D_3$ production, can produce profound osteomalacia. Eighty-five to 90 percent of the phosphate filtered by the glomerulus is reabsorbed, primarily in the proximal tubule. This process is regulated by PTH, which reduces renal tubular phosphate reabsorption, and probably also by various vitamin D metabolites that appear to increase renal tubular phosphate reabsorption. Many diseases that affect renal handling of phosphate are associated with osteomalacia—especially those also associated with abnormalities in vitamin D metabolism, as discussed below.

Treatment of phosphate deficiency is generally geared to correction of the primary problem. Oral preparations of phosphate (and the amounts required to provide 1 g of elemental phosphorus) include Fleet Phospho-soda (6.12 mL) and Neutra-Phos (300 mL). These preparations are usually given in amounts that provide 1–3 g of phosphorus daily in divided doses, though diarrhea may limit the dose. Careful attention to both serum calcium and serum phosphorus concentrations is required to avoid hypocalcemia or ectopic calcification.

X-Linked & Autosomal Dominant Hypophosphatemia

X-linked hypophosphatemia (formerly called vitamin D-resistant rickets) is characterized by renal phosphate wasting, hypophosphatemia, and decreased $1,25(OH)_2D_3$ production relative to the degree of hypophosphatemia. Clinical presentation is variable, but children often present with florid rickets. This dominant disorder affects males more severely than females. A similar but genetically distinct syndrome, autosomal dominant hypophosphatemic rickets, is less common, affects females to the same extent as males, and may present later in life (second to fourth decades). Animal studies have indicated that the cause of the renal phosphate wasting in X-linked hypophosphatemia is humoral rather than a structural defect in the phosphate transporter itself. Recent evidence strongly suggests that this humoral factor is FGF23. It is presumed to be responsible for both the reduction in phosphate reabsorption in the renal proximal tubule as well as the inadequate response of the proximal tubule to the ensuing hypophosphatemia with respect to $1,25(OH)_2D_3$ production. The gene responsible for X-linked hypophosphatemia has recently been identified and is called *PHEX* (originally called *PEX*) for phosphate-regulating gene with homologies to endopeptidases located on the X chromosome. As is implicit in this ambiguous name, the role of *PHEX* in renal phosphate transport is not clear. The prevailing hypothesis is that *PHEX* cleaves and so inactivates FGF23, thus relieving the inhibition of phosphate reabsorption and $1,25(OH)_2$ production. Autosomal dominant hypophosphatemic rickets appears to be due to a mutation in FGF23 that renders it resistant to cleavage by *PHEX*. Recent evidence suggests that the defects in X-linked hypophosphatemia and autosomal dominant hypophosphatemia may not be restricted to the proximal renal tubule but may affect osteoblast function as well, a cell in which *PHEX* is expressed. With the recent cloning of *PHEX* and FGF23, our understanding of this disease should rapidly increase. Treatment of X-linked hypophosphatemia generally requires a combination of phosphate (1–4 g/d in divided doses) combined with calcitriol (1–3 μg/d) as tolerated. Vitamin D is less effective than calcitriol and should no longer be used for this condition. Appropriate therapy heals the rachitic lesions and increases growth velocity. A frequent complication of this treatment, however, is the development of hyperparathyroidism, which may become autonomous and require parathyroidectomy.

Treatment with phosphate and calcitriol may also lead to ectopic calcification, including nephrocalcinosis. Thus, these patients need to be followed closely.

Tumor-Induced Osteomalacia

The association of osteomalacia and hypophosphatemia with tumors primarily of mesenchymal origin has been recognized for half a century. The cause of this syndrome has until recently remained obscure. Removal of the tumors, which are often small and hard to find, cures the disease. Although most implicated tumors are mesenchymal, including fibromas and osteoblastomas, other tumors, including breast, prostate, and lung carcinomas, multiple myeloma, and chronic lymphocytic leukemia, have been associated with this syndrome. The patient generally presents with bone pain, muscle weakness, and osteomalacia. Symptoms may occur for years before the diagnosis is made. Renal phosphate wasting, hypophosphatemia, and normal serum calcium and 25(OH)D levels but inappropriately low $1,25(OH)_2D_3$ levels characterize the disease. Thus, it resembles X-linked hypophosphatemia or autosomal dominant hypophosphatemic rickets. Tumor extracts contain material—as yet not fully characterized—which inhibits renal phosphate transport and $1,25(OH)_2D_3$ production, suggesting that a phosphatonin-like substance is involved. Thus, it was of great interest to observe that these tumors overproduce FGF23. Recent evidence strongly indicates that production by the tumor of one species of fibroblast growth factor, FGF-23, underlies all of the metabolic abnormalities associated with hypophosphatemic syndrome.

The best treatment is removal of the tumor, but this is not always possible. Phosphate and calcitriol have been the mainstays of treatment but with limited success, and patients should be dosed to tolerance as in X-linked hypophosphatemia. Recently, the demonstration of somatostatin receptors on one such tumor led to successful correction of hypophosphatemia by use of the somatostatin analog octreotide.

De Toni-Debré-Fanconi Syndrome & Hereditary Hypophosphatemic Rickets with Hypercalciuria

The De Toni-Debré-Fanconi syndrome includes a heterogeneous group of disorders affecting the proximal tubule and leading to phosphaturia and hypophosphatemia, aminoaciduria, glycosuria, bicarbonaturia, and proximal renal tubular acidosis. Not all features must be present to make the diagnosis. Damage to the renal proximal tubule secondary to genetic or environmental causes is the underlying cause. This syndrome may be divided into two types depending on whether vitamin D metabolism is also abnormal. In the more common type I, $1,25(OH)_2D_3$ production is reduced relative to the degree of hypophosphatemia. In type II disease, $1,25(OH)_2D_3$ production is appropriately elevated in response to the hypophosphatemia, and this leads to hypercalciuria.

The type II Fanconi's syndrome shares the principal features of hereditary hypophosphatemic rickets with hypercalciuria. It is a rare disorder of uncertain genetic mode of transmission that is heterogeneous in clinical presentation but in severely affected individuals begins in childhood with bone pain and skeletal deformities. The syndrome is characterized by renal phosphate wasting and hypophosphatemia, hypercalciuria and normal serum calcium, and elevated $1,25(OH)_2D_3$ levels. The osteomalacia associated with these renal phosphate-wasting syndromes is probably the result of the hypophosphatemia, with contributions from the acidosis and decreased $1,25(OH)_2D_3$ levels in the type I syndrome.

The ideal treatment is correction of the underlying defect, which may or may not be identified and reversible. Otherwise, treatment includes phosphate supplementation in all cases, correction of the acidosis, and $1,25(OH)_2D_3$ replacement in the type I syndrome.

CALCIUM DEFICIENCY

Calcium deficiency may contribute to the mineralization defect that complicates gastrointestinal disease and proximal tubular disorders, but it is less well established as a cause of osteomalacia than is vitamin D or phosphate deficiency. In carefully performed studies of children who ingested a low-calcium diet in Africa, there was clinical, biochemical, and histologic evidence of osteomalacia. The serum phosphorus and 25(OH)D and $1,25(OH)_2D_3$ levels were normal; serum alkaline phosphatase level was elevated; and serum and urine calcium levels were low. Since intestinal absorption of calcium decreases with age, the daily requirement for calcium increases from approximately 800 mg in young adults to 1400 mg in the elderly. Calcium deficiency can result not only from inadequate dietary intake but also from excessive fecal and urinary losses. Except in cases in which a renal leak of calcium plays an important role in the etiology of calcium deficiency (certain forms of idiopathic hypercalciuria or following glucocorticoid therapy for inflammatory diseases), urinary calcium excretion provides a useful means to determine the appropriate level of oral calcium replacement. Because of its low cost and high percentage of elemental calcium, calcium carbonate is the treatment of choice.

PRIMARY DISORDERS OF THE BONE MATRIX

Several diseases lead to abnormalities in bone mineralization because of intrinsic defects in the matrix or in the osteoblast producing that matrix. With the exception of osteogenesis imperfecta, these tend to be rare. Examples are listed below.

Osteogenesis Imperfecta

Osteogenesis imperfecta is a hereditable disorder of connective tissue due to a qualitative or quantitative abnormality in type I collagen, the most abundant collagen in bone. The disease is typically transmitted in an autosomal dominant mode, though autosomal recessive inheritance has also been described. Clinical expression is highly variable, depending on the location and type of mutation observed. Although skeletal deformity and fracture are the hallmarks of this disease, other tissues are often affected, including the teeth, skin, ligaments, and scleras. Routine biochemical studies of bone and mineral metabolism are generally normal, though elevated serum alkaline phosphatase and increased urine excretion of hydroxyproline and calcium are often found. Bone histology shows abundant disorganized, poorly mineralized matrix but with a high rate of bone turnover as reflected by increased tetracycline labeling.

Treatment is supportive and includes orthopedic, rehabilitative, and dental intervention as appropriate. Bisphosphonates have recently been shown to be of use.

Hypophosphatasia

Hypophosphatasia, transmitted in an autosomal recessive or dominant pattern, has considerable variability in clinical expression ranging from a severe form of rickets in children to a predisposition to fractures in adults. The biochemical hallmarks are low serum and tissue levels of alkaline phosphatase (liver-bone-kidney but not intestine-placenta) and increased urinary levels of phosphoethanolamine. Serum calcium and phosphorus levels may be high, and many patients have hypercalciuria. Levels of vitamin D metabolites and PTH are generally normal. In some families, a mutation in the alkaline phosphatase gene has been identified. Radiologic examination shows osteopenia, with the frequent occurrence of stress fractures and chondrocalcinosis. Bone biopsy specimens show osteomalacia. It is not clear why these patients develop osteomalacia or rickets. Skeletal alkaline phosphatase cleaves pyrophosphate, an inhibitor of bone mineralization. Thus, patients deficient in alkaline phosphatase may be unable to hydrolyze this inhibitor and so develop a mineralization defect.

There is no established medical therapy. Use of vitamin D or its metabolites may further increase the already elevated serum calcium and phosphorus and should not be used.

Fibrogenesis Imperfecta Ossium

Fibrogenesis imperfecta ossium is a rare, painful disorder that affects middle-aged subjects in what appears to be a sporadic fashion. Serum alkaline phosphatase activity is increased. The bones have a dense, amorphous mottled appearance radiologically and a disorganized arrangement of collagen with decreased birefringence histologically when viewed with polarized light microscopy. Presumably, the disorganized collagen matrix retards normal bone mineralization.

There is no specific therapy.

Axial Osteomalacia

This rare disease involves only the axial skeleton and affects mostly middle aged or elderly males. Most cases are sporadic. It is not particularly painful. Alkaline phosphatase activity may be increased, but calcium, phosphorus, and vitamin D metabolite levels are normal. Histologically, the bone shows increased osteoid and reduced tetracycline incorporation. The reason for the mineralization disorder is uncertain.

No effective medical therapy has been established.

INHIBITORS OF MINERALIZATION

Several drugs are known to cause osteomalacia or rickets by inhibiting mineralization. However, the mechanisms by which this occurs are not fully understood.

Aluminum

Aluminum-induced bone disease is found primarily in patients with renal failure on chronic hemodialysis and in patients being treated with total parenteral nutrition (TPN). With the recognition of this complication and the switch to deionized water for dialysis, decreased use of aluminum-containing antacids, and the use of purified amino acids rather than casein hydrolysates (which contained large amounts of aluminum) for TPN, the incidence and prevalence of this complication has been markedly reduced. The problem, however, still exists. As described under renal osteodystrophy, the bone disease is osteomalacia and can be severe and painful. Aluminum deposits in the mineralization front and appears to inhibit the mineralization process.

Removal of the aluminum with deferoxamine chelation therapy is the treatment of choice.

Etidronate

This first-generation bisphosphonate possesses an unwelcome side effect: the ability to inhibit bone mineralization at doses greater than 5–10 mg/kg/d. This side effect is not found at clinically effective doses of newer bisphosphonates.

Fluoride

Fluoride is a potent stimulator of bone formation. If administered at high doses with inadequate calcium supplementation, the bone formed as a result is poorly mineralized. The mechanisms underlying the effects of fluoride on osteoblast function and bone mineralization remain unclear.

■ PAGET'S DISEASE OF BONE (OSTEITIS DEFORMANS)

Paget's disease is a focal disorder of bone remodeling that leads to greatly accelerated rates of bone turnover, disruption of the normal architecture of bone, and sometimes to gross deformities of bone. As a focal disorder it is not, strictly speaking, a metabolic bone disease. Paget's disease is highly prevalent in northern Europe, particularly in England and Germany, where up to 4% of people over age 40 are affected. It is also common in the United States but is unusual in Africa and Asia.

Etiology

It has long been thought that Paget's disease, with its late onset and spotty involvement of the skeleton, might be due to a chronic slow virus infection of bone. Inclusion bodies that resemble paramyxovirus inclusions have been identified in pagetic osteoclasts, and the presence of measles virus transcripts has recently been detected by molecular biologic techniques. However, considerably more work would be required to prove the infectious etiology of Paget's disease. There are also familial clusters of the disease, with up to 20% of patients in some studies having afflicted first-degree relatives.

Pathology

At the microscopic level, the disorder is characterized by highly vascular and cellular bone, consistent with its high metabolic activity. The osteoclasts are sometimes huge and bizarre, with up to 100 nuclei per cell. Because pagetic osteoclasts initiate the bone remodeling cycle in a chaotic fashion, the end result of remodeling is a mosaic pattern of lamellar bone. Paget's disease (and other high turnover states) can also produce woven bone—bone that is laid down rapidly and in a disorganized fashion, without the normal lamellar architecture.

Pathogenesis

Abnormal osteoclastic bone resorption is the probable initiating event in Paget's disease. Not only are the osteoclasts very abnormal histologically and prone to unruly behavior, but some forms of the disease are marked by an early resorptive phase in which pure osteolysis occurs without an osteoblastic response. Additionally, Paget's disease responds dramatically to inhibitors of osteoclastic bone resorption.

The rate of bone resorption is often increased by as much as 10- to 20-fold, and this is reflected in biochemical indices of bone resorption, including urinary excretion of collagen metabolites like hydroxyproline and pyridinoline cross-linked peptides of collagen. Over the skeleton as a whole, osteoblastic new bone formation responds appropriately to this challenge. Even though local disparities in remodeling may result in areas with the radiographic appearance of osteolysis or dense new bone, there is a linear relationship between biochemical markers of bone resorption (eg, urinary hydroxyproline) and biochemical markers of bone formation (eg, alkaline phosphatase). Because this tight coupling is maintained in Paget's disease in the face of enormously increased skeletal turnover rates, systemic mineral homeostasis is usually unperturbed.

Clinical Features

A. SYMPTOMS AND SIGNS

Paget's disease may affect any of the bones, but the most common sites are the sacrum and spine (50% of patients), the femur (46%), the skull (28%), and the pelvis (22%). The clinical features of Paget's disease are pain, fractures, deformity, and manifestations of the neurologic, rheumatologic, or metabolic complications of the disease. However, at least two-thirds of patients are asymptomatic. Thus, Paget's disease is often discovered as an incidental radiologic finding or during the investigation of an elevated alkaline phosphatase level. On physical examination, enlargement of the skull, frontal bossing, or deafness may be evident. Involvement of the weight-bearing long bones of the lower extremity often results in bowing. The femur and tibia bow anteriorly and laterally, but the fibula is almost never affected by Paget's disease. Cutaneous erythema and warmth, as well as bone tenderness, may be evident over affected areas of the skeleton, reflecting greatly increased blood flow through pagetic bone. The findings

of pain, warmth, and erythema led to the appellation osteitis deformans, though Paget's disease is not truly an inflammatory disorder. The most common fractures in Paget's disease are vertebral crush fractures and incomplete "fissure" fractures through the cortex, usually on the convex surface of the tibia or femur. Affected bones may fracture completely; when they do, healing is usually rapid and complete—the increased metabolic activity of pagetic bone seems to favor fracture healing.

B. LABORATORY FINDINGS

The serum alkaline phosphatase activity and urinary hydroxyproline excretion are usually increased, sometimes to a very high degree. Levels of the newer biochemical markers of bone turnover are also high, but it is not clear that their determination offers any special benefit. The serum osteocalcin concentration is usually increased to a lesser extent than the alkaline phosphatase activity. The serum calcium and phosphorus concentrations and the urinary calcium excretion are normal, though if a patient sustains a fracture and becomes immobilized, hypercalciuria and hypercalcemia may occur.

C. IMAGING STUDIES

The early stages of Paget's disease are often osteolytic. Examples are erosion of the temporal bone of the skull, osteoporosis circumscripta, and pagetic lesions in the extremities, which begin in the metaphysis and migrate down the shaft as a V-shaped resorptive front (Figure 8–31). Over years or even decades, the typical mixed picture of late Paget's disease evolves. Trabeculae are thickened and coarse. The bone may be enlarged or bowed. In the pelvis, the iliopectineal line or pelvic brim is often thickened (Figure 8–32). In the spine, osteoblastic lesions of the vertebral bodies may present a "picture-frame" appearance or a homogeneously increased density, the "ivory vertebra." Associated osteoarthritis may present with narrowing of the joint space (Figure 8–32). Osteosarcoma may present with cortical destruction or a soft tissue mass (Figure 8–32). Radionuclide bone scanning with technetium-labeled bisphosphonates or other bone-seeking agents is uniformly positive in active Paget's disease and is useful for surveying the skeleton when a focus of Paget's disease has been found radiographically (Figure 8–33).

Complications

Complications of Paget's disease may be neurologic, rheumatologic, neoplastic, or cardiac (Table 8–18).

A. NEUROLOGIC

The brain, spinal cord, and peripheral nerves are all at risk. Sensorineural deafness occurs in up to 50% of pa-

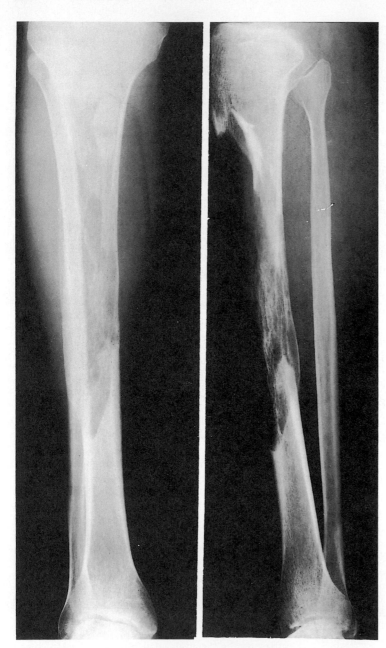

Figure 8–31. Lytic Paget's disease in the tibia before (left) and after (right) immobilization in a cast. The lytic area has a flame- or V-shaped leading edge (**left**). (Reproduced, with permission, from Strewler GJ: Paget's disease of bone. West J Med 1984;140:763.)

tients in whom the skull is involved, and compression of the other cranial nerves can also occur. At the base of the skull, Paget's disease can produce platybasia and basilar impression of the brain stem, with symptoms of brain stem compression, obstructive hydrocephalus, or vertebrobasilar insufficiency. Spinal stenosis is common in vertebral Paget's disease, in part because the pagetic vertebra can be enlarged, and may spread posteriorly

when collapse occurs, but spinal stenosis responds well to medical treatment of the disease. Peripheral nerve entrapment syndromes include carpal and tarsal tunnel syndromes.

B. RHEUMATOLOGIC

Osteoarthritis is common in Paget's disease. It may be an unrelated finding in elderly patients with the disor-

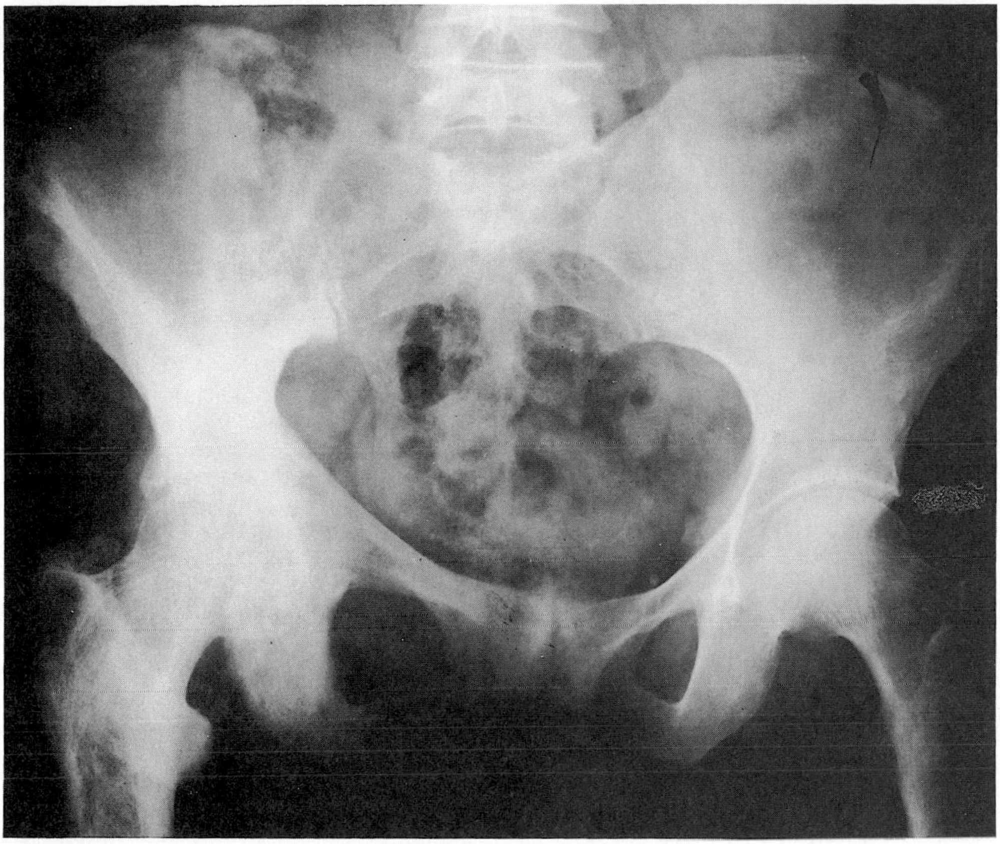

Figure 8–32. Paget's disease of the right femur and pelvis. The right femur displays cortical thickening and coarse trabeculation. The right ischium is enlarged, with sclerosis of ischial and pubic rami and the right ilium. Two complications of Paget's disease are present. There is concentric bilateral narrowing of the hip joint space, signifying osteoarthritis. The destructive lesion interrupting the cortex of the right ilium is an osteosarcoma. (Reproduced, with permission, from Strewler GJ: Paget's disease of bone. West J Med 1984;140:763.)

der, or it may result directly from pagetic deformities and their effects on wear and tear in the joints. Arthritis presents a conundrum to the clinician attempting to relieve pain, as it may be difficult to determine whether the pain originates in pagetic bone or in the nearby joint. An association of osteitis deformans and gout was first noted by James Paget himself, and asymptomatic hyperuricemia is also common.

C. Neoplastic

The most terrible complication of Paget's disease is development of bone sarcoma. The tumor arises in pagetic bone, typically in individuals with polyostotic involvement, and may present with soft tissue swelling, increased pain, or a rapidly increasing alkaline phosphatase. Osteosarcoma, chondrosarcoma, and giant cell tumors all occur in Paget's disease, with a combined incidence of about 1%. Because osteosarcoma is otherwise uncommon in the elderly, fully 30% of elderly patients with osteosarcoma have underlying Paget's disease.

D. Cardiac

High-output congestive heart failure occurs rarely and is due to markedly increased blood flow to bone, usually in patients with more than 50% involvement of the skeleton.

Treatment

In a patient known to have Paget's disease, bone pain that is unresponsive to nonsteroidal anti-inflammatory

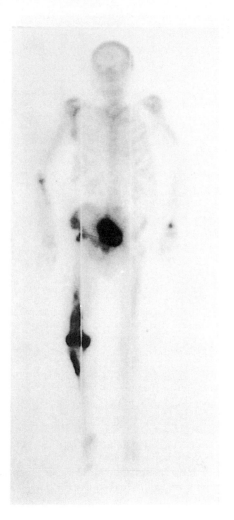

Figure 8–33. Bone scan of a patient with Paget's disease of the skull, spine, pelvis, right femur, and acetabulum. Note localization of bone-seeking isotope (^{99m}Tc-labeled bisphosphonate) in these areas.

Table 8–18. Complications of Paget's disease.

Rheumatologic
  Osteoarthritis
  Gout
  Calcific periarthritis
  Rheumatoid arthritis
Neurologic
  Basilar impression
  Cranial nerve dysfunction (especially deafness)
  Spinal cord and root compression
  Peripheral nerve entrapment (carpal and tarsal tunnel syndromes)
Metabolic
  Immobilization hypercalciuria-hypercalcemia
  Urolithiasis
Neoplastic
  Bone sarcoma
  Giant cell tumor

sometimes treated in the hope of arresting the progress of deformities (eg, bowing of the extremities and resultant osteoarthritis), but it is not certain whether medical treatment can achieve this aim or whether it will arrest the progression of deafness in patients with skull involvement.

Three classes of agents are used in the treatment of Paget's disease: the calcitonins, the bisphosphonates, and plicamycin. All are inhibitors of osteoclastic bone resorption.

A. CALCITONIN-SALMON

Calcitonin-salmon is administered initially at a dosage of 50–100 IU daily until symptoms are improved; thereafter, many patients can be maintained on 50 units three times a week. Improvement in pain is usually evident within 2–6 weeks. On average, the alkaline phosphatase and urinary hydroxyproline will fall by 50% within 3–6 months, with the alkaline phosphatase lagging slightly behind the hydroxyproline. Many patients will have a sustained response to treatment extending over years, and the biochemical parameters are often suppressed for 6 months to 1 year after treatment is discontinued. Up to 20% of patients receiving chronic calcitonin treatment will develop late resistance to calcitonin, which may be antibody-mediated. Human calcitonin therapy has been uniformly effective in these patients. A nasal spray preparation is now available, but data on its efficacy in Paget's disease are limited.

B. BISPHOSPHONATES

The bisphosphonate etidronate disodium has long been available for treatment of Paget's disease and was shown

agents deserves a trial of specific therapy. As noted above, it may not be easy to differentiate pagetic bone pain from that due to osteoarthritis. The other indications for treatment of Paget's disease are controversial. Treatment has been advocated for neurologic compression syndromes, as preparation for surgery, and to prevent deformities. Neurologic deficits often respond to medical treatment, and a trial of treatment is often warranted. Pretreatment for 2–3 months before orthopedic surgery will prevent excessive bleeding and postoperative hypercalcemia, but satisfactory bone healing usually occurs without medical treatment. Paget's disease is to be beneficial in controlled clinical trials. It is administered in a dose of 5 mg/kg/d for 6 months, and about 60% of patients will show a biochemical response. However, some patients will experience worsening of bone pain or lytic bone lesions, and etidronate can impair bone mineralization, particularly at higher doses.

Three newer oral bisphosphonates are available for treatment of Paget's disease and appear to offer advantages over etidronate, both in terms of drug potency and in a decreased risk for impaired bone mineralization. Alendronate is administered at a dose of 40 mg daily for 6 months. On average, alkaline phosphatase activity is suppressed by about 80% on such treatment. Biochemical remissions are often prolonged for more than 1 year after the drug is stopped. The main side effect is significant gastrointestinal upset, requiring discontinuation of therapy in about 6% of patients. Two additional oral bisphosphonates have shown treatment efficacy and are approved for treatment of Paget's disease: tiludronate, given at a dosage of 400 mg/d for 6–12 months; and risedronate, given at a dosage of 30 mg/d for 2 months. For some patients, particularly those with gastrointestinal intolerance to oral bisphosphonates, it may be more convenient or more timely to administer an equivalent dose of bisphosphonate intravenously. Pamidronate, an amino-bisphosphonate closely related to alendronate, has been used for this purpose. In the United States, pamidronate is approved only for treatment of hypercalcemia. Intravenous infusions of pamidronate (60 or 90 mg) produce a high remission rate and a durable response. The principal side-effect observed with intravenous administration is an acute phase response, including fever and myalgia, that occurs in about 20% of patients and may last for several days after a dose.

C. PLICAMYCIN

Plicamycin is a cytotoxic antibiotic that has been used as a "last resort" in Paget's disease unresponsive to less toxic agents. With the advent of the newer bisphosphonates, there are few indications for treatment with plicamycin.

■ RENAL OSTEODYSTROPHY

Pathogenesis

Metabolism of $25(OH)D$ to $1,25(OH)_2D_3$ and $24,25(OH)_2D$ in the kidney is tightly regulated. Renal disease results in reduced circulating levels of both of these metabolites. With the reduction in $1,25(OH)_2D_3$ levels, intestinal calcium absorption falls, and bone resorp-

tion appears to become less sensitive to PTH—a result that leads to hypocalcemia. Phosphate excretion by the diseased kidney is decreased, resulting in hyperphosphatemia, which amplifies the fall in serum calcium. The fall in serum calcium combined with the low levels of $1,25(OH)_2D_3$ (which is an inhibitor of PTH secretion) results in hyperparathyroidism. The net effect of deficient $1,25(OH)_2D_3$ and $24,25(OH)_2D$ and excess PTH on bone is complex (Figure 8–34). Patients may have osteitis fibrosa (reflecting excessive PTH), osteomalacia (in part reflecting decreased vitamin D metabolites), or a combination of the two. One particularly debilitating form of renal osteodystrophy is found in a small percentage of patients on hemodialysis in whom only osteomalacia occurs. Some of these patients have increased aluminum content in their bones, particularly in the region where mineralization is occurring (calcification front), and this appears to inhibit mineralization. Other patients do not have aluminum excess but have low bone turnover. These patients are particularly prone to develop symptoms of bone pain, fractures, and muscle weakness.

Clinical Features

Most patients with renal osteodystrophy have osteitis fibrosa alone or in combination with osteomalacia. If not well controlled, these patients will have a low serum level of calcium and high serum levels of phosphorus, alkaline phosphatase, and PTH. A few patients develop severe secondary hyperparathyroidism in which the PTH level increases dramatically and stays elevated even with restoration of the serum calcium to normal. Such patients are prone to developing hypercalcemia with the usual replacement doses of calcium (some-

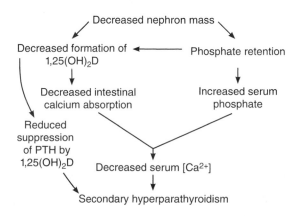

Figure 8–34. Schema for the pathogenesis of renal osteodystrophy.

times referred to as tertiary hyperparathyroidism). Another subset of patients with renal osteodystrophy present with relatively normal levels of PTH and alkaline phosphatase. Their serum calcium levels are often elevated after treatment with small doses of calcitriol. These patients have pure osteomalacia on bone biopsy and generally suffer from aluminum intoxication (see above).

Treatment

Patients with renal osteodystrophy generally respond to calcitriol (0.5–1 μg/d) or dihydrotachysterol (0.25–0.5 mg/d), calcium supplementation (1–3 g/d), and phosphate restriction. Because of the concern about aluminum intoxication, calcium carbonate is generally used as a first agent to block intestinal phosphate absorption, reserving aluminum hydroxide for situations in which calcium carbonate is not effective in maintaining normal serum phosphorus levels. The goal is to achieve and maintain normal serum levels of calcium, phosphorus, PTH, and alkaline phosphatase. This regimen treats osteitis fibrosa more effectively than osteomalacia. Patients with aluminum intoxication are very sensitive to and respond poorly to calcitriol and calcium, with rapid onset of hypercalcemia and little improvement in their bone disease. These patients may respond to chelation therapy with deferoxamine, a drug also used for iron chelation. Severe secondary hyperparathyroidism also creates management problems, as these patients also are prone to the development of hypercalcemia with calcium supplementation. Intravenous doses of calcitriol following hemodialysis may preferentially inhibit PTH secretion with less effect on raising serum calcium. Several analogs of calcitriol, which have less effect on raising serum calcium than calcitriol itself, are currently approved or in clinical trials for the management of such patients, as is a calcimimetic compound that inhibits PTH secretion by activating the calcium receptor of the parathyroid gland.

REFERENCES

Calcium Metabolism

Bushinsky DA, Monk RD: Electrolyte quintet: Calcium. Lancet 1998;352:306. [PMID: 9690425]

Parathyroid Hormone

Goltzman D: Interactions of PTH and PTHrP with the PTH/PTHrP receptor and with downstream signaling pathways: exceptions that provide the rules. J Bone Min Res 1999;14:173. [PMID: 9933469]

John MR et al: A novel immunoradiometric assay detects full-length human PTH but not amino-terminally truncated frag-

ments: implications for PTH measurements in renal failure. J Clin Endocrinol Metab 1999;84:4287. [PMID: 10566687]

Kronenberg HM et al: Functional analysis of the PTH/PTHrP network of ligands and receptors. Rec Prog Horm Res 1998; 53:283. [PMID: 9769712]

Schipani E et al: A novel parathyroid hormone (PTH)/PTH-related peptide receptor mutation in Jansen's metaphyseal chondrodysplasia. J Clin Endocrinol Metab 1999;84:3052. [PMID: 10487664]

Strewler GJ: The physiology of parathyroid hormone-related protein. N Engl J Med 2000;342:177. [PMID: 10639544]

Zhang P et al: A homozygous inactivating mutation in the parathyroid hormone/parathyroid hormone-related peptide receptor causing Blomstrand chondrodysplasia. J Clin Endocrinol Metab 1998;83:3365. [PMID: 9745456]

Calcitonin

Martin TJ: Calcitonin, an update. Bone 1999;24(5 Suppl):63S. [PMID: 10321932]

Vitamin D

Fu GK et al: Cloning of human 25-hydroxyvitamin D-1 alpha-hydroxylase and mutations causing vitamin D-dependent rickets type 1. Mol Endocrinol 1997;11:1961. [PMID: 9415400]

Haussler MR et al: The nuclear vitamin D receptor: biological and molecular regulatory properties revealed. J Bone Min Res 1998;13:325. [PMID: 9525333]

Li YC et al: Normalization of mineral ion homeostasis by dietary means prevents hyperparathyroidism, rickets, and osteomalacia, but not alopecia in vitamin D receptor-ablated mice. Endocrinology 1998;139:4391. [PMID: 9751523]

Okuda K et al: Recent progress in enzymology and molecular biology of enzymes involved in vitamin D metabolism. J Lipid Res 1995;36:1641. [PMID: 7595086]

Pettifor JM et al: Serum levels of free 1,25-dihydroxyvitamin D in vitamin D toxicity. Ann Intern Med 1995;122:511. [PMID: 7872586]

Rachez C et al: The DRIP complex and SRC-1/p160 coactivators share similar nuclear receptor binding determinants but constitute functionally distinct complexes. Mol Cell Biol 2000;20:2718. [PMID: 10733574]

Medullary Thyroid Carcinoma

Eng C: RET proto-oncogene in the development of human cancer. J Clin Oncol 1999;17:380. [PMID: 10458257]

Hansford JR, Mulligan LM: Multiple endocrine neoplasia type 2 and RET: from neoplasia to neurogenesis. J Med Genet 2000;37:817. [PMID: 11073534]

Lee NC, Norton JA: Multiple endocrine neoplasia type 2B—genetic basis and clinical expression. Surg Oncol 2000;9:111. [PMID: 11356339]

Ponder BA: The phenotypes associated with ret mutations in the multiple endocrine neoplasia type 2 syndrome. Cancer Res 1999;59(7 Suppl):1736S. [PMID: 10197589]

Wells SA Jr, Franz C: Medullary carcinoma of the thyroid gland. World J Surg 2000;24:952. [PMID: 10865039]

Hypercalcemic Disorders

Agarwal SK et al: Menin interacts with the AP1 transcription factor JunD and represses JunD-activated transcription. Cell 1999; 96:143. [PMID: 9989505]

Brandi ML et al: Guidelines for diagnosis and therapy of MEN type 1 and type 2. J Clin Endocrinol Metab 2001;86:5658. [PMID: 11739416]

Brown EM: Familial hypocalciuric hypercalcemia and other disorders with resistance to extracellular calcium. Endocrinol Metab Clin North Am 2000;29:503. [PMID: 11033758]

Carling T et al: Familial hypercalcemia and hypercalciuria caused by a novel mutation in the cytoplasmic tail of the calcium receptor. J Clin Endocrinol Metab 2000;85:2042. [PMID: 10843194]

Conron M, Young C, Beynon HL: Calcium metabolism in sarcoidosis and its clinical implications. Rheumatology (Oxford) 2000;39:707. [PMID: 10908687]

Dackiw AP et al: Relative contributions of technetium Tc 99m sestamibi scintigraphy, intraoperative gamma probe detection, and the rapid parathyroid hormone assay to the surgical management of hyperparathyroidism. Arch Surg 2000;135:550. [PMID: 10807279]

Dempster DW et al: On the mechanism of cancellous bone preservation in postmenopausal women with mild primary hyperparathyroidism. J Clin Endocrinol Metab 1999;84:1562. [PMID: 10323380]

Guo SS, Sawicki MP: Molecular and genetic mechanisms of tumorigenesis in multiple endocrine neoplasia type-1. Mol Endocrinol 2001;15:1653. [PMID: 11579199]

Hendy GN: Molecular mechanisms of primary hyperparathyroidism. Rev Endocr Metab Disord 2000;1:297. [PMID: 11706744]

Hoff AO, Cote GJ, Gagel RF: Multiple endocrine neoplasias. Annu Rev Physiol 2000;62:377. [PMID: 10845096]

Howe JR: Minimally invasive parathyroid surgery. Surg Clin North Am 2000;80:1399. [PMID: 11059711]

Kinder BK, Stewart AF: Hypercalcemia. Curr Probl Surg 2002;39:349. [PMID: 11976629]

Major P et al: Zoledronic acid is superior to pamidronate in the treatment of hypercalcemia of malignancy: a pooled analysis of two randomized, controlled clinical trials. J Clin Oncol 2001;19:558. [PMID: 11208851]

Mak TW et al: Effects of lithium therapy on bone mineral metabolism: a two-year prospective longitudinal study. J Clin Endocrinol Metab 1998;83:3857. [PMID: 9814458]

Mallya SM, Arnold A: Cyclin D1 in parathyroid disease. Front Biosci 2000;5:D367. [PMID: 10704427]

Marx SJ: Hyperparathyroid and hypoparathyroid disorders. N Engl J Med 2000;343:1863. [PMID: 11117980]

NIH Consensus Development Conference: Diagnosis and management of asymptomatic primary hyperparathyroidism. Ann Intern Med 1991;114:593.

Schussheim DH et al: Multiple endocrine neoplasia type 1: new clinical and basic findings. Trends Endocrinol Metab 2001; 12:173. [PMID: 11295574]

Shane E: Clinical review 122: Parathyroid carcinoma. J Clin Endocrinol Metab 2001;86:485. [PMID: 11157996]

Silverberg SJ et al: A 10-year prospective study of primary hyperparathyroidism with or without parathyroid surgery. N Engl J Med 1999;341:1249. [PMID: 10528034]

Silverberg SJ et al: Therapeutic controversies in primary hyperparathyroidism. J Clin Endocrinol Metab 1999;84:2275. [PMID: 10404790]

Simonds WF et al: Familial isolated hyperparathyroidism: clinical and genetic characteristics of 36 kindreds. Medicine (Baltimore) 2002;81:1. [PMID: 11807402]

Thakker RV: Multiple endocrine neoplasia. Horm Res 2001;56 (Suppl 1):67. [PMID: 11786689]

Vieth R: Vitamin D supplementation, 25-hydroxyvitamin D concentrations, and safety. Am J Clin Nutr 1999;69:842. [PMID: 10232622]

Weigel RJ: Nonoperative management of hyperparathyroidism: present and future. Curr Opin Oncol 2001;12:33. [PMID: 11148683]

Hypocalcemic Disorders

Bastepe M et al: Positional dissociation between the genetic mutation responsible for pseudohypoparathyroidism type Ib and the associated methylation defect at exon A/B: evidence for a long-range regulatory element within the imprinted GNAS1 locus. Hum Mol Genet 2001;10:1231. [PMID: 11406605]

Bastepe M, Juppner H: Pseudohypoparathyroidism. New insights into an old disease. Endocrinol Metab Clin North Am 2000; 29:569. [PMID: 11033761]

Betterle C, Greggio NA, Volpato M: Clinical review 93: Autoimmune polyglandular syndrome type 1. J Clin Endocrinol Metab 1998;83:1049. [PMID: 9543115]

Brasier AR, Nussbaum SR: Hungry bone syndrome: Clinical and biochemical predictors of its occurrence after parathyroid surgery. Am J Med 1988;84:654.

Cuneo BF: 22q11.2 deletion syndrome: DiGeorge, velocardiofacial, and conotruncal anomaly face syndromes. Curr Opin Pediatr 2001;13:465. [PMID: 11801894]

Garfield N, Karaplis AC: Genetics and animal models of hypoparathyroidism. Trends Endocrinol Metab 2001;12:288. [PMID: 11504667] (The underlying basis for hypoparathyroid disorders is provided using recent evidence from animal models.)

Levine MA: Clinical spectrum and pathogenesis of pseudohypoparathyroidism. Rev Endocr Metab Disord 2000;1:265. [PMID: 11706740]

Mancilla EE, De Luca F, Baron J: Activating mutations of the Ca^{2+}-sensing receptor. Molec Genet Metab 1998;64:198. [PMID: 9719629]

Obermayer-Straub P, Manns MP: Autoimmune polyglandular syndromes. Baillieres Clin Gastroenterol 1998;12:293. [PMID: 9890074]

Pattou F et al: Hypocalcemia following thyroid surgery: incidence and prediction of outcome. World J Surg 1998;22:718. [PMID: 9606288]

Tengan CH et al: Mitochondrial encephalomyopathy and hypoparathyroidism associated with a duplication and a deletion of mitochondrial deoxyribonucleic acid. J Clin Endocrinol Metab 1998;83:125. [PMID: 9435428]

Umpaichitra V, Bastian W, Castells S: Hypocalcemia in children: pathogenesis and management. Clin Pediatr (Phila) 2001; 40:305. [PMID: 11824172]

Van Esch H, Devriendt K: Transcription factor GATA3 and the human HDR syndrome. Cell Mol Life Sci 2001;58:1296. [PMID: 11577985]

Bone Anatomy & Remodeling

Aubin JE et al: Osteoblast and chondroblast differentiation. Bone 1995;17:77S. [PMID: 8619383]

Einhorn TA: The bone organ system: form and function. In: *Osteoporosis*. Marcus R, Feldman D, Kelsey J (editors). Academic Press, 1996.

Marcus R: Normal and abnormal bone remodeling in man. Ann Rev Med 1987;117:129. [PMID: 3555287]

Miller PD et al: Practical clinical application of biochemical markers of bone turnover: Consensus of an Expert Panel. J Clin Densitom 1999;2:323. [PMID: 10548827]

Suda T et al: Modulation of osteoclast differentiation by local factors. Bone 1995;17:87S. [PMID: 8579904]

Osteoporosis

Bikle DD et al: Bone disease in alcohol abuse. Ann Intern Med 1985;103:42. [PMID: 2988390]

Black D et al: Randomization of alendronate or risk of fracture in women with existing vertebral fractures.The Fracture Intervention Trial Research Group. Lancet 1996;348:1535. [PMID: 8950879]

Chapuy MC et al: Vitamin D_3 and calcium to prevent hip fractures in elderly women. N Engl J Med 1992;327:1637. [PMID: 1331788]

Civitelli R: Calcitonin. In: *Osteoporosis*. Marcus R, Feldman D, Kelsey J (editors). Academic Press, 1996.

Cummings SR et al: Bone density at various sites for prediction of hip fractures. Lancet 1993;341:72. [PMID: 8093403]

Cummings SR et al: Risk factors for hip fracture in white women. Study of Osteoporotic Fractures Research Group. N Engl J Med 1995;332:767. [PMID: 7862179]

Cummings SR, Black D: Bone mass measurements and risk of fracture in Caucasian women: A review of findings from prospective studies. Am J Med 1995;98:24S. [PMID: 7709929]

Effects of hormone therapy on bone mineral density. Results from the Postmenopausal Estrogen/Progestin Interventions (PEPI) Trial. The Writing Group for the PEPI Trial. JAMA 1996; 276:1389. [PMID: 8892713]

Grady D et al: Hormone therapy to prevent disease and prolong life in postmenopausal women. Ann Intern Med 1992; 117:1016. [PMID: 1443971]

Johnston CC et al: Calcium supplementation and increases in bone mineral density in children. N Engl J Med 1992;327:82. [PMID: 1603140]

Kanis JA et al: The diagnosis of osteoporosis. J Bone Min Res 1994;9:1137. [PMID: 7976495]

Lane NE et al: Parathyroid hormone treatment can reverse corticosteroid-induced osteoporosis: results of a randomized controlled clinical trial. J Clin Invest 1998;102:1627. [PMID: 9788977]

Lindsay R, Cosman F: Estrogen and osteoporosis. In: *Osteoporosis*, 2nd ed. Marcus R et al (editors). Academic Press, 2001.

Lindsay R et al: Randomised controlled study of effect of parathyroid hormone on vertebral-bone mass and fracture incidence among postmenopausal women on oestrogen with osteoporosis. Lancet 1997;350:550. [PMID: 9284777]

Marcus R: The nature of osteoporosis. In: *Osteoporosis*. Marcus R, Feldman D, Kelsey J (editors). Academic Press, 1996.

Neer RM et al: Effect of parathyroid hormone (1–34) on fractures and bone mineral density in postmenopausal women with osteoporosis. N Engl J Med 2001;344:1434.

Pak CYC et al: Treatment of postmenopausal osteoporosis with slow-release sodium fluoride. Final report of a randomized controlled trial. Ann Intern Med 1995;123:401. [PMID: 7639438]

Recker RR et al: Correcting calcium nutritional deficiency prevents spine fractures in elderly women. J Bone Min Res 1996;11: 1961. [PMID: 8970899]

Riggs BL, Melton LJ 3d: The prevention and treatment of osteoporosis. N Engl J Med 1992;327:620. [PMID: 1640955]

Wahner HW: Use of densitometry in management of osteoporosis. In: *Osteoporosis*. Marcus R, Feldman D, Kelsey J (editors). Academic Press, 1996.

Osteomalacia

The ADHR Consortium: Autosomal dominant hypophosphataemic rickets is associated with mutations in FGF23. Nat Genet 2000;26:345. [PMID: 11062477]

Francis RM, Selby PL: Osteomalacia. Baillieres Clin Endocrinol Metab 1997;11:145. [PMID: 9222490]

Hutchison FN, Bell NH: Osteomalacia and rickets. Semin Nephrol 1992;12:127. [PMID: 1561493]

Lips P: Vitamin D deficiency and secondary hyperparathyroidism in the elderly: consequences for bone loss and fractures and therapeutic implications. Endocr Rev 2001;22:477. [PMID: 11493580]

Thomas MK et al: Hypovitaminosis D in medical inpatients. N Engl J Med 1998;338:777. [PMID: 9504937]

Tovey FI et al: A review of postgastrectomy bone disease. J Gastroenterol Hepatol 1992;7:639. [PMID: 1486191]

White KE et al: The autosomal dominant hypophosphatemic rickets (ADHR) gene is a secreted polypeptide overexpressed by tumors that cause phosphate wasting. J Clin Endocrinol Metab 2001;86:497. [PMID: 11157998]

Paget's Disease

Grauer A et al: Discussion: Newer bisphosphonates in the treatment of Paget's disease of bone: where we are and where we want to go. J Bone Miner Res 1999;14(Suppl 2):74. [PMID: 10510218]

Lyles KW et al: A clinical approach to diagnosis and management of Paget's disease of bone. J Bone Miner Res 2001;16:1379. [PMID: 11499860]

Noor M, Shoback D: Paget's disease of bone: diagnosis and treatment update. Curr Rheumatol Rep 2000;2:67. [PMID: 11123042]

Reddy SV et al: Paget's disease of bone: a disease of the osteoclast. Rev Endocr Metab Disord 2001;2:195. [PMID: 11705325]

Singer FR et al: Risedronate, a highly effective oral agent in the treatment of patients with severe Paget's disease. J Clin Endocrinol Metab 1998;83:1906. [PMID: 9626117]

Siris E et al: Comparative study of alendronate versus etidronate for the treatment of Paget's disease of bone. J Clin Endocrinol Metab 1996;81:961. [PMID: 8772558]

Siris ES et al: Risedronate in the treatment of Paget's disease of bone: an open label, multicenter study. J Bone Min Res 1998;13:1032. [PMID: 9626635]

Renal Osteodystrophy

Coburn JW, Elangovan L: Prevention of metabolic bone disease in the pre-end-stage renal disease setting. J Am Soc Nephrol 1998;9(12 Suppl):S71. [PMID: 11443772]

Goodman WG: Calcimimetic agents for the treatment of hyperparathyroidism. Curr Opin Nephrol Hypertens 2001;10:575. [PMID: 11496049]

Hruska K: New concepts in renal osteodystrophy. Nephrol Dial Transplant 1998;13:2755. [PMID: 9829475]

Martin KJ, Gonzalez EA: Strategies to minimize bone disease in renal failure. Am J Kidney Dis 2001;38:1430. [PMID: 11728986]

Mucsi I, Hercz G: Relative hypoparathyroidism and adynamic bone disease. Am J Med Sci 1999;317:405. [PMID: 10372841]

Sakhaee K, Gonzalez GB: Update on renal osteodystrophy: pathogenesis and clinical management. Am J Med Sci 1999;317:251. [PMID: 10210362]

Glucocorticoids & Adrenal Androgens

David C. Aron, MD, MS, James W. Findling, MD, & J. Blake Tyrrell, MD

ACTH	Adrenocorticotropic hormone	**LH**	Luteinizing hormone
ADH	Antidiuretic hormone (vasopressin)	**LPH**	Lipotropin
APCED	Autoimmune polyendocrinopathy-candidiasis-ectodermal dystrophy syndrome (autoimmune polyglandular syndrome type 1)	**PEPCK**	Phosphoenolpyruvate carboxykinase
		PLA	Phospholipase A
		PMN	Polymorphonuclear neutrophil
		PNMT	Phenylethanolamine-N-methyltransferase
AVP	Arginine vasopressin		
cAMP	Cyclic adenosine monophosphate	**PRA**	Plasma rennin activity
CBG	Corticosteroid-binding globulin	**PRL**	Prolactin
CRH	Corticotropin-releasing hormone	**PTH**	Parathyroid hormone
DHEA	Dehydroepiandrosterone acetate	**REM**	Rapid eye movement
DOC	Deoxycorticosterone	**SHBG**	Sex hormone-binding globulin
GH	Growth hormone	**StAR**	Steroidogenic acute regulatory protein
GIP	Gastrointestinal inhibitory polypeptide	**TBG**	Thyroxine-binding globulin
GnRH	Gonadotropin-releasing hormone	**TRH**	Thyrotropin-releasing hormone
HLA	Human leukocyte antigen	**TSH**	Thyroid-stimulating hormone (thyrotropin)
HPLC	High-performance liquid chromatography		
IPSS	Inferior petrosal sinus sampling	**VLCFA**	Very long chain fatty acid
IRMA	Immunoradiometric assay		

The adrenal cortex produces many steroid hormones of which the most important are cortisol, aldosterone, and the adrenal androgens. Disorders of the adrenal glands lead to classic endocrinopathies such as Cushing's syndrome, Addison's disease, hyperaldosteronism, and the syndromes of congenital adrenal hyperplasia. This chapter describes the physiology and disorders of the glucocorticoids and the adrenal androgens. Disorders of aldosterone secretion are discussed in Chapter 10 and congenital defects in adrenal hormone biosynthesis in Chapters 10 and 14. Hirsutism and virilization (which reflect excess androgen action) are discussed in Chapter 13.

Advances in diagnostic procedures have simplified the evaluation of adrenocortical disorders; in particular, the assay of plasma glucocorticoids, androgens, and ACTH has allowed more rapid and precise diagnosis. In addition, advances in surgical and medical treatment have improved the outlook for patients with these disorders.

EMBRYOLOGY & ANATOMY

Embryology

The adrenal cortex is of mesodermal origin and derives from a single cell lineage characterized by expression of certain transcription factors such as steroidogenic factor 1. At 2 months' gestation, the cortex, already identifiable as a separate organ, is composed of a **fetal zone** and a **definitive zone** similar to the adult adrenal cortex. The adrenal cortex then increases rapidly in size; at mid gestation, it is considerably larger than the kidney and much larger than the adult gland in relation to total body mass. The fetal zone makes up the bulk of the weight of the adrenal cortex at this time. Factors shown to be important in adrenal development, especially early on, include steroidogenic factor 1 and DAX1, the product of the dosage-sensitive sex reversal-adrenal hypoplasia gene, among others; mutations of the *DAX1* gene are associated with congenital adrenal hypoplasia.

The fetal adrenal is under the control of ACTH by mid pregnancy, but the fetal zone is deficient in the activity of 3β-hydroxysteroid dehydrogenase (see section on biosynthesis of cortisol and adrenal androgens, below) and thus produces mainly dehydroepiandrosterone (DHEA) and DHEA sulfate, which serve as precursors of maternal-placental estrogen production after conversion in the liver to 16α-hydroxylated derivatives. The definitive zone synthesizes a number of steroids and is the major site of fetal cortisol synthesis. Mutations of the ACTH- or melanocortin-2 receptor gene are associated with familial glucocorticoid deficiency.

Anatomy

The anatomic relationship of the fetal and definitive zones is maintained until birth, at which time the fetal zone gradually disappears, with a consequent decrease in adrenocortical weight in the 3 months following delivery. During the next 3 years, the adult adrenal cortex develops from cells of the outer layer of the cortex and differentiates into the three adult zones: glomerulosa, fasciculata, and reticularis–adrenal zonation.

The adult adrenal glands, with a combined weight of 8–10 g, lie in the retroperitoneum above or medial to the upper poles of the kidneys (Figure 9–1). A fibrous capsule surrounds the gland; the cortex comprises 90% of the adrenal weight, the inner medulla about 10%.

The adrenal cortex is richly vascularized and receives its main arterial supply from branches of the inferior phrenic artery, the renal arteries, and the aorta. These small arteries form an arterial plexus beneath the capsule and then enter a sinusoidal system that penetrates

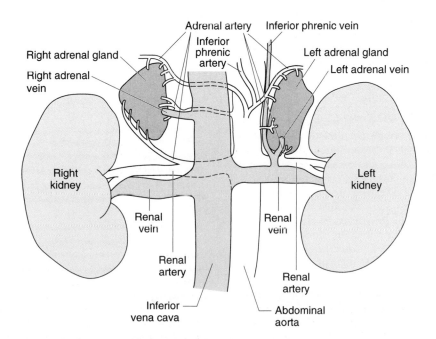

Figure 9–1. Location and blood supply of the adrenal glands (schematic). (Reproduced, with permission, from Miller WL, Tyrrell JB: The adrenal cortex. In: *Endocrinology and Metabolism*, 4th ed. Felig P et al [editors]. McGraw-Hill, 2002.)

the cortex and medulla, draining into a single central vein in each gland. The right adrenal vein drains directly into the posterior aspect of the vena cava; the left adrenal vein enters the left renal vein. These anatomic features account for the fact that it is relatively easier to catheterize the left adrenal vein than it is to catheterize the right adrenal vein.

Microscopic Anatomy

Histologically, the adult cortex is composed of three zones: an outer zona glomerulosa, a zona fasciculata, and an inner zona reticularis (Figure 9–2). However, the inner two zones appear to function as a unit (see below). The **zona glomerulosa,** which produces aldosterone and constitutes about 15% of adult cortical volume, is deficient in 17α-hydroxylase activity and thus cannot produce cortisol or androgens (see below and Chapter 10). The zona glomerulosa lacks a well-defined structure, and the small lipid-poor cells are scattered beneath the adrenal capsule. The **zona fasciculata** is the thickest layer of the adrenal cortex, making up about 75% of the cortex, and produces cortisol and androgens. The cells of the zona fasciculata are larger and contain more lipid and thus are termed "clear cells." These cells extend in columns from the narrow zona reticularis to either the zona glomerulosa or to the capsule. The inner **zona reticularis** surrounds the medulla and also produces cortisol and androgens. The "compact" cells of this narrow zone lack significant lipid content but do contain lipofuscin granules. The zonae fasciculata and reticularis are regulated by ACTH; excess or deficiency of this hormone alters their structure and function. Thus, both zones atrophy when ACTH is deficient; when ACTH is present in excess, hyperplasia and hypertrophy of these zones occur. In addition, chronic stimulation with ACTH leads to a gradual depletion of the lipid from the clear cells of the zona fasciculata at the junction of the two zones; these cells thus attain the characteristic appearance of the compact reticularis cells. With chronic excessive stimulation, the compact reticularis cells extend outward and may reach the outer capsule. It is postulated that the zona fasciculata cells can respond acutely to ACTH stimulation with increased cortisol production, whereas the reticularis cells maintain basal glucocorticoid secretion and that induced by prolonged ACTH stimulation.

BIOSYNTHESIS OF CORTISOL & ADRENAL ANDROGENS

Steroidogenesis

The major hormones secreted by the adrenal cortex are cortisol, the androgens, and aldosterone. The carbon atoms in the steroid molecule are numbered as shown in Figure 9–3, and the major biosynthetic pathways and hormonal intermediates are illustrated in Figures 9–4 and 9–5.

The scheme of adrenal steroidogenic synthesis has been clarified by analysis of the steroidogenic enzymes. Most of these enzymes belong to the family of cytochrome P450 oxygenases (see Table 9–1 for current and historical nomenclature conventions). In mitochondria, the *CYP11A* gene, located on chromosome 15, encodes P450scc, the enzyme responsible for cholesterol side chain cleavage. *CYP11B1,* a gene located on chromosome 8, encodes P450c11, another mitochondrial enzyme, which mediates 11β-hydroxylation in the zona reticularis and zona fasciculata. This reaction converts 11-deoxycortisol to cortisol and 11-deoxycorticosterone to corticosterone. In the zona glomerulosa, *CYP11B2,* also located on chromosome 8, encodes the enzyme P450aldo, also known as aldosterone synthase. P450aldo mediates 11β-hydroxylation, 18-hydroxylation, and 18-oxidation to convert 11-deoxycorticosterone → corticosterone → 18-hydroxycorticosterone → aldosterone. In the endoplasmic reticulum, gene *CYP17,* located on chromosome 10, encodes a single enzyme, P450c17, which mediates both 17α-hydroxylase activity and 17,20-lyase activity, and the gene *CYP21A2* encodes the enzyme P450c21, which mediates 21-hydroxylation of both progesterone and 21-hydroxyprogesterone. The 3β-hydroxysteroid dehydrogenase:$\Delta^{5,4}$-isomerase activities are mediated by a single non-P450 microsomal enzyme (Figure 9–4).

A. ZONES AND STEROIDOGENESIS

Because of enzymatic differences between the zona glomerulosa and the inner two zones, the adrenal cortex functions as two separate units, with differing regulation and secretory products. Thus, the zona glomerulosa, which produces aldosterone, lacks 17α-hydroxylase activity and cannot synthesize 17α-hydroxypregnenolone and 17α-hydroxyprogesterone, which are the precursors of cortisol and the adrenal androgens. The synthesis of aldosterone by this zone is primarily regulated by the renin-angiotensin system and by potassium (see Chapter 10).

The zona fasciculata and zona reticularis (Figure 9–4) produce cortisol, androgens, and small amounts of estrogens. These zones, primarily regulated by ACTH, do not express the gene *CYP11B2* (encoding P450aldo) and therefore cannot convert 11-deoxycorticosterone to aldosterone. (See Chapter 10.)

B. CHOLESTEROL UPTAKE AND SYNTHESIS

Synthesis of cortisol and the androgens by the zonae fasciculata and reticularis begins with cholesterol, as does the synthesis of all steroid hormones. Plasma lipoproteins are the major source of adrenal choles-

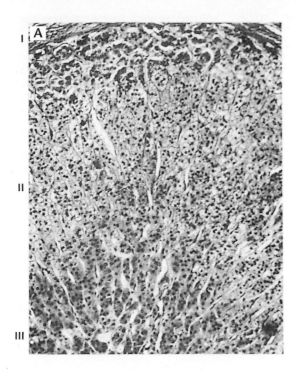

Figure 9–2. Photomicrograph of the adrenal cortex (H&E stain). **A:** A low-power general view. I, the glomerulosa; II, the fasciculata; III, the reticularis. (Reproduced, with permission, from Junqueira LC, Carneiro J: *Basic Histology,* 7th ed. McGraw-Hill, 1992.) **B.** Electron micrograph of a normal adrenocortical steroid-producing cell. M, large mitochondria with tubular cristae; SER, smooth endoplasmic reticulum; L, lipid vacuole. (Courtesy of Dr. Medhat O. Hasan, Pathology Department, Louis Stokes Cleveland Department of Veterans Affairs Medical Center.)

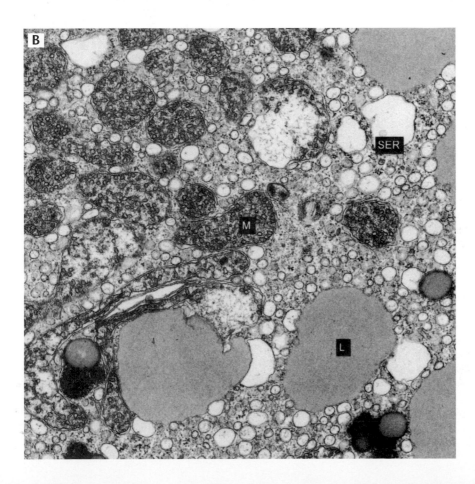

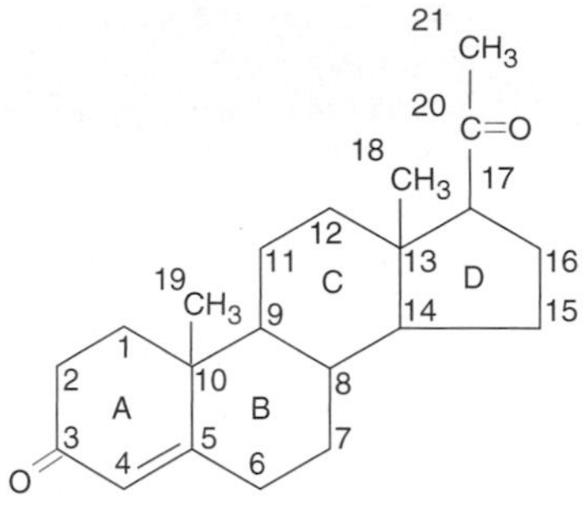

Figure 9–3. Structure of adrenocortical steroids. The letters in the formula for progesterone identify the A, B, C, and D rings; the numbers show the positions in the basic C-21 steroid structure. The angular methyl groups (positions 18 and 19) are usually indicated simply by straight lines, as in the lower formula. Dehydroepiandrosterone is a "17-ketosteroid" formed by cleavage of the side chain of the C-21 steroid 17-hydroxypregnenolone and its replacement by an O atom. (Reproduced, with permission, from Ganong WF: *Review of Medical Physiology*, 14th ed. McGraw-Hill, 1989.)

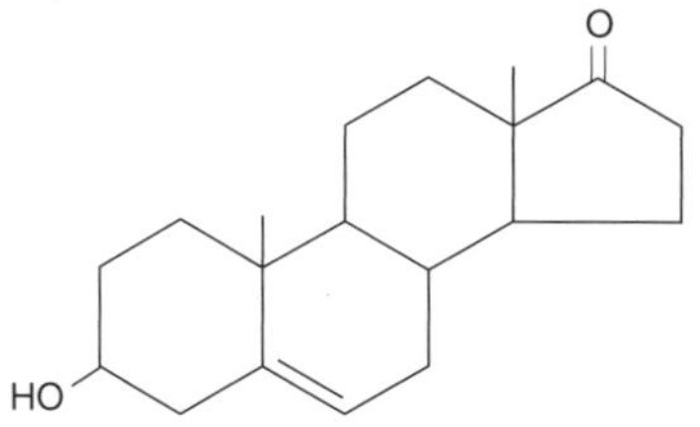

terol, though synthesis within the gland from acetate also occurs. Low-density lipoprotein (LDL) accounts for about 80% of cholesterol delivered to the adrenal gland. A small pool of free cholesterol within the adrenal is available for rapid synthesis of steroids when the adrenal is stimulated. When stimulation occurs, there is also increased hydrolysis of stored cholesteryl esters to free cholesterol, increased uptake from plasma lipoproteins, and increased cholesterol synthesis within the gland. The acute response to a steroidogenic stimulus is mediated by the steroidogenic acute regulatory protein (StAR). This mitochondrial phosphoprotein enhances cholesterol transport from the outer to the inner mitochondrial membrane. Mutations in the StAR gene result in congenital lipoid adrenal hyperplasia with severe cortisol and aldosterone deficiencies at birth.

C. Cholesterol Metabolism

The conversion of cholesterol to pregnenolone is the rate-limiting step in adrenal steroidogenesis and the major site of ACTH action on the adrenal. This step occurs in the mitochondria and involves two hydroxylations and then the side-chain cleavage of cholesterol. A single enzyme, CYP11A, mediates this process; each step requires molecular oxygen and a pair of electrons. The latter are donated by NADPH to adrenodoxin reductase, a flavoprotein, and then to adrenodoxin, an iron-sulfur protein, and finally to CYP11A. Both adrenodoxin reductase and adrenodoxin are also involved in the action of CYP11B1 (see above). Electron transport to microsomal cytochrome P450 involves P450 reductase, a flavoprotein distinct from adrenodoxin reductase. Pregnenolone is then transported outside the mitochondria before further steroid synthesis occurs.

D. Synthesis of Cortisol

Cortisol synthesis proceeds by 17α-hydroxylation of pregnenolone by CYP17 within the smooth endoplasmic reticulum to form 17α-hydroxypregnenolone. This steroid is then converted to 17α-hydroxyprogesterone after conversion of its 5,6 double bond to a 4,5 double bond by the 3β-hydroxysteroid dehydrogenase:$\Delta^{5,4}$-oxosteroid isomerase enzyme complex, which is also located within the smooth endoplasmic reticulum. An alternative but apparently less important pathway in the zonae fasciculata and reticularis is from pregnenolone $\rightarrow$ progesterone $\rightarrow$ 17α-hydroxyprogesterone (Figure 9–4).

The next step, which is again microsomal, involves the 21-hydroxylation by CYP21A2 of 17α-hydroxyprogesterone to form 11-deoxycortisol; this compound is further hydroxylated within mitochondria by 11β-hydroxylation (CYP11B1) to form cortisol. The zona fasciculata and zona reticularis also produce 11-deoxycorticosterone (DOC), 18-hydroxydeoxycorticosterone, and corticosterone. However, as noted above, the absence of the mitochondrial enzyme CYP11B2 prevents production of aldosterone by these zones of the adrenal cortex (Figure 9–5). Cortisol secretion under basal (ie, nonstressed) conditions ranges from 8 to 25 mg/d (22–69 µmol/d), with a mean of about 9.2 mg/d (25 µmol/d)—rates lower than most previous calculations.

E. Synthesis of Androgens

The production of adrenal androgens from pregnenolone and progesterone requires prior 17α-hydroxylation (CYP17) and thus does not occur in the zona glomerulosa. The major quantitative production of an-

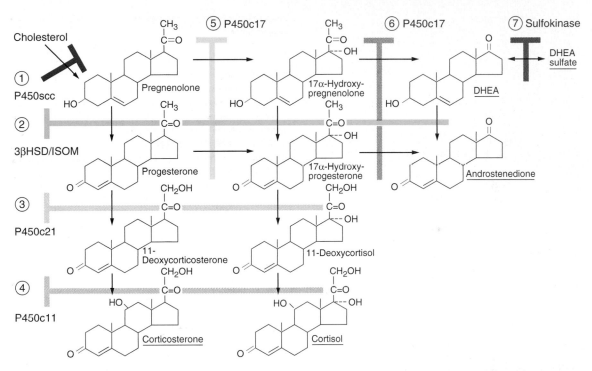

Figure 9–4. Steroid biosynthesis in the zona fasciculata and zona reticularis of the adrenal cortex. The major secretory products are underlined. The enzymes for the reactions are numbered on the left and at the top of the chart, with the steps catalyzed shown by the shaded bars. ① P450scc, cholesterol 20,22-hydroxylase:20,22 desmolase activity; ② 3βHSD/ISOM, 3-hydroxysteroid dehydrogenase:δ^5-oxosteroid isomerase activity; ③ P450c21, 21α-hydroxylase activity; ④ P450c11 = 11β-hydroxylase activity; ⑤ P450c17, 17α-hydroxylase activity; ⑥ P450c17, 17,20-lyase/desmolase activity; ⑦ sulfokinase. (See also Figures 7–1, 9–2, 10–4, and 11–13.) (Modified and reproduced, with permission, from Ganong WF: *Review of Medical Physiology,* 16th ed. McGraw-Hill, 1993.)

drogens is by conversion of 17α-hydroxypregnenolone to the 19-carbon compounds (C-19 steroids) DHEA and its sulfate conjugate DHEA sulfate. Thus, 17α-hydroxypregnenolone undergoes removal of its two-carbon side chain at the C$_{17}$ position by microsomal 17,20-desmolase (CYP17), yielding DHEA with a keto group at C$_{17}$. DHEA is then converted to DHEA sulfate by a reversible adrenal sulfokinase. The other major adrenal androgen, androstenedione, is produced mostly from DHEA, mediated by CYP17, and possibly from 17α-hydroxyprogesterone, also by CYP17. Androstenedione can be converted to testosterone, though adrenal secretion of this hormone is minimal. The adrenal androgens, DHEA, DHEA sulfate, and androstenedione, have minimal intrinsic androgenic activity, and they contribute to androgenicity by their peripheral conversion to the more potent androgens testosterone and dihydrotestosterone. Although DHEA and DHEA sulfate are secreted in greater quan-

tities, androstenedione is qualitatively more important, since it is more readily converted peripherally to testosterone (see Chapter 12).

Regulation of Secretion

A. SECRETION OF CRH AND ACTH

ACTH is the trophic hormone of the zonae fasciculata and reticularis and the major regulator of cortisol and adrenal androgen production, although other factors produced within the adrenal including neurotransmitters, neuropeptides, and nitric oxide also play a role. ACTH in turn is regulated by the hypothalamus and central nervous system via neurotransmitters and corticotropin-releasing hormone (CRH) and arginine vasopressin (AVP). The neuroendocrine control of CRH and ACTH secretion involves three mechanisms (see below and Chapter 5).

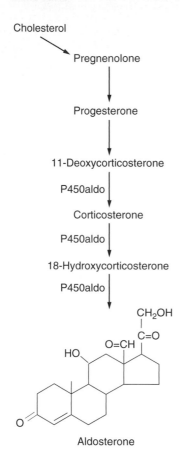

Figure 9–5. Steroid biosynthesis in the zona glomerulosa. The steps from cholesterol to 11-deoxycorticosterone are the same as in the zona fasciculata and zona reticularis. However, the zona glomerulosa lacks 17α-hydroxylase activity and thus cannot produce cortisol. Only the zona glomerulosa can convert corticosterone to 18-hydroxycorticosterone and aldosterone. The single enzyme P450aldo catalyzes the conversion of 11-deoxycorticosterone → corticosterone → 18-hydroxycorticosterone → aldosterone. (See also Figures 7–1, 9–2, and 10–4.) (Modified and reproduced, with permission, from Ganong WF: *Review of Medical Physiology,* 16th ed. McGraw-Hill, 1993.)

B. ACTH EFFECTS ON THE ADRENAL CORTEX

ACTH administration leads to the rapid synthesis and secretion of steroids; plasma levels of these hormones rise within minutes. ACTH increases RNA, DNA, and protein synthesis. Chronic stimulation leads to adrenocortical hyperplasia and hypertrophy; conversely, ACTH deficiency results in decreased steroidogenesis and is accompanied by adrenocortical atrophy, decreased gland weight, and decreased protein and nucleic acid content.

C. ACTH AND STEROIDOGENESIS

ACTH binds to high-affinity plasma membrane receptors, thereby activating adenylyl cyclase and increasing cAMP, which in turn activates intracellular phosphoprotein kinases (Figure 9–6), including steroidogenic acute regulatory protein (StAR). ACTH action results in increased free cholesterol formation as a consequence of increased cholesterol esterase activity and decreased cholesteryl ester synthetase as well as increased lipoprotein uptake by the adrenal cortex. This process stimulates the rate-limiting step—cholesterol delivery to the side-chain cleavage enzyme (P450scc or CYP11A1) for conversion to Δ^5-pregnenolone, thereby initiating steroidogenesis.

D. NEUROENDOCRINE CONTROL

Cortisol secretion is closely regulated by ACTH, and plasma cortisol levels parallel those of ACTH (Figure 9–7). There are three mechanisms of neuroendocrine control: (1) episodic secretion and the circadian rhythm of ACTH, (2) stress responsiveness of the hypothalamic-pituitary adrenal axis, and (3) feedback inhibition by cortisol of ACTH secretion.

1. Circadian rhythm—Circadian rhythm is superimposed on episodic secretion; it is the result of central nervous system events that regulate both the number and magnitude of CRH and ACTH secretory episodes. Cortisol secretion is low in the late evening and continues to decline in the first several hours of sleep, at which time plasma cortisol levels may be undetectable. During the third and fifth hours of sleep there is an increase in secretion; but the major secretory episodes begin in the sixth to eighth hours of sleep (Figure 9–7) and then begin to decline as wakefulness occurs. About half of the total daily cortisol output is secreted during this period. Cortisol secretion then gradually declines during the day, with fewer secretory episodes of decreased magnitude; however, there is increased cortisol secretion in response to eating and exercise.

Although this general pattern is consistent, there is considerable intra- and interindividual variability, and the circadian rhythm may be altered by changes in sleep pattern, light-dark exposure, and feeding times. The rhythm is also changed by (1) physical stresses such as major illness, surgery, trauma, or starvation; (2) psychologic stress, including severe anxiety, endogenous depression, and the manic phase of manic-depressive psychosis; (3) central nervous system and pituitary disorders; (4) Cushing's syndrome; (5) liver disease and other conditions that affect cortisol metabolism; (6) chronic renal failure; and (7) alcoholism. Cyproheptadine inhibits the circadian rhythm, possibly by its an-

Table 9–1. The main components of the steroidogenic pathway.[1]

Enzyme	Gene	Chromosomal Location	Enzyme Activity (or Activities)	Subcellular Localization	Characteristic Features of Normal Tissue-Specific Expression
Steroidogenic acute regulatory protein (StAR)	StAR	8p11.2	Activation of peripheral type benzodiazepine receptor	Outer mitochondrial membrane	All steroid hormone-producing cells except the placenta, Schwann cells, and the brain
Peripheral type benzodiazepine receptor	PDA	22q13.31	Regulated cholesterol channel	Forms channel at the contact sites between the outer and inner mitochondrial membranes	All steroid hormone-producing cells
P450scc	CYP11A	15q23–24	Cholesterol-20,22-desmolase	Matrix side of inner mitochondrial membrane	All steroid hormone-producing cells
3β-Hydroxysteroid dehydrogenase (HSD) isomerase	3β-Hydroxysteroid dehydrogenase type I	1p13, the HSD3B1 and HSD3B2 loci are located 1–2 cM from the centromeric marker D1Z5	3β-Hydroxysteroid dehydrogenase, $\Delta^{5,4}$-oxosteroid	Smooth endoplasmic reticulum	Expressed in syncytiotrophoblast cells, sebaceous glands
	3β-Hydroxysteroid dehydrogenase type II				Expressed in the definitive adrenal cortex and the gonads. Absent from the fetal zone of the adrenal cortex.
P450c21	CYP21B	6p21.3 (close to HLA locus)	21-Hydroxylase	Smooth endoplasmic reticulum	Only in adrenal cortex (all zones); low levels in fetal zone
	CYP21A	6p21.3 (close to HLA locus)	Pseudogene	N/A	N/A
P450c11	CYP11B1	8q21–22	11β-Hydroxylase	Matrix side of inner mitochondrial membrane	Only expressed in zona fasciculata and zona reticularis of the adrenal cortex; low levels in fetal zone
P450aldo	CYP11B2	8q24.3	Aldosterone synthase: 11β-hydroxylase, 18-hydroxylase, 18-oxidase	Matrix side of inner mitochondrial membrane	Only expressed in the zona glomerulosa of the adrenal cortex; low levels in fetal zone
P450c17	CYP17	10q24–25	17α-Hydroxylase, 17,20-lyase	Smooth endoplasmic reticulum	Absent from the zona glomerulosa in adults, the placenta, and the definitive zone of fetal adrenal cortex until the third trimester
P450arom	CYP19	15q	Aromatase	Smooth endoplasmic reticulum	

[1]Modified from Kacsoh B. *Endocrine Physiology*. McGraw-Hill, 2000.

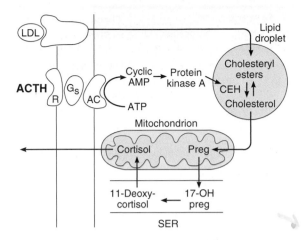

Figure 9–6. Mechanism of action of ACTH on cortisol-secreting cells in the inner two zones of the adrenal cortex. When ACTH binds to its receptor (R), adenylyl cyclase (AC) is activated via G$_s$. The resulting increase in cAMP activates protein kinase A, and the kinase phosphorylates cholesteryl ester hydrolase (CEH), increasing its activity. Consequently, more free cholesterol is formed and converted to pregnenolone in the mitochondria. Note that in the subsequent steps in steroid biosynthesis, products are shuttled between the mitochondria and the smooth endoplasmic reticulum (SER). (Reproduced, with permission, from Ganong WF: *Review of Medical Physiology*, 16th ed. McGraw-Hill, 1993.)

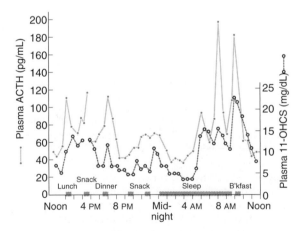

Figure 9–7. Fluctuations in plasma ACTH and glucocorticoids (11-OHCS) throughout the day. Note the greater ACTH and glucocorticoid rises in the morning before awakening. (Reproduced, with permission, from Krieger DT et al: Characterization of the normal temporal pattern of corticosteroid levels. J Clin Endocrinol Metab 1971;32:266.)

tiserotonergic effects, whereas other drugs usually have no effect.

2. Stress responsiveness—Plasma ACTH and cortisol secretion are also characteristically responsive to physical stress. Thus, plasma ACTH and cortisol are secreted within minutes following the onset of stresses such as surgery and hypoglycemia, and these responses abolish circadian periodicity if the stress is prolonged. Stress responses originate in the central nervous system and increase hypothalamic CRH and thus pituitary ACTH secretion. Stress responsiveness of plasma ACTH and cortisol is abolished by prior high-dose glucocorticoid administration and in spontaneous Cushing's syndrome; conversely, the responsiveness of ACTH secretion is enhanced following adrenalectomy. Regulation of the hypothalamic-pituitary-adrenal axis is linked to that of the immune system. For example, interleukin-1 (IL-1) stimulates ACTH secretion, and cortisol inhibits IL-1 synthesis.

3. Feedback inhibition—The third major regulator of ACTH and cortisol secretion is that of feedback inhibition by glucocorticoids of CRH, ACTH, and cortisol secretion. Glucocorticoid feedback inhibition occurs at both the pituitary and hypothalamus and involves two distinct mechanisms—fast and delayed feedback inhibition.

Fast feedback inhibition of ACTH secretion is rate-dependent—ie, it depends on the rate of increase of the glucocorticoid but not the dose administered. This phase is rapid (within minutes) and transient (lasting < 10 minutes), suggesting mediation by a noncytosolic glucocorticoid receptor mechanism. **Delayed feedback inhibition** is both time- and dose-dependent. With continued glucocorticoid administration, ACTH levels continue to decrease and become unresponsive to stimulation, ultimately resulting in suppression of CRH and ACTH release and atrophy of the zonae fasciculata and reticularis. The suppressed hypothalamic-pituitary-adrenal axis fails to respond to stress and stimulation. Delayed feedback appears to act via the classic glucocorticoid receptor mechanism (see below).

E. ACTH EFFECTS ON REGULATION OF ANDROGEN PRODUCTION

Adrenal androgen production in adults is also regulated by ACTH; both DHEA and androstenedione exhibit circadian periodicity in concert with ACTH and cortisol. In addition, plasma concentrations of DHEA and androstenedione increase rapidly with ACTH administration and are suppressed by glucocorticoid administration. DHEA sulfate, because of its slow metabolic clearance rate, does not exhibit a diurnal rhythm. The existence of a separate anterior pituitary hormone that regulates adrenal androgen secretion has been postulated but not yet proved.

CIRCULATION OF CORTISOL & ADRENAL ANDROGENS

Cortisol and the adrenal androgens circulate bound to plasma proteins. The plasma half-life of cortisol (60–90 minutes) is determined by the extent of plasma binding and by the rate of metabolic inactivation.

Plasma Binding Proteins

Cortisol and adrenal androgens are secreted in an unbound state; however, these hormones bind to plasma proteins upon entering the circulation. Cortisol binds mainly to corticosteroid-binding globulin (CBG, transcortin) and to a lesser extent to albumin, whereas the androgens bind chiefly to albumin. Bound steroids are biologically inactive; the unbound or free fraction is active. The plasma proteins may provide a pool of circulating cortisol by delaying metabolic clearance, thus preventing more marked fluctuations of plasma free cortisol levels during episodic secretion by the gland. Because there are no binding proteins in saliva, salivary cortisol reflects free cortisol.

Free & Bound Cortisol

Under basal conditions, about 10% of the circulating cortisol is free, about 75% is bound to CBG, and the remainder is bound to albumin. The plasma free cortisol level is approximately 1 µg/dL, and it is this biologically active cortisol which is regulated by ACTH.

A. CORTICOSTEROID-BINDING GLOBULIN (CBG)

CBG has a molecular weight of about 50,000, is produced by the liver, and binds cortisol with high affinity. The CBG in plasma has a cortisol-binding capacity of about 25 µg/dL. When total plasma cortisol concentrations rise above this level, the free concentration rapidly increases and exceeds its usual fraction of 10% of the total cortisol. Other endogenous steroids usually do not appreciably affect cortisol binding to CBG; an exception is in late pregnancy, when progesterone may occupy about 25% of the binding sites on CBG. Synthetic steroids do not bind significantly to CBG—with the exception of prednisolone. CBG levels are increased in high-estrogen states (pregnancy; estrogen or oral contraceptive use), hyperthyroidism, diabetes, certain hematologic disorders, and on a genetic basis. CBG concentrations are decreased in familial CBG deficiency, hypothyroidism, and protein deficiency states such as severe liver disease or nephrotic syndrome.

B. ALBUMIN

Albumin has a much greater capacity for cortisol binding but a lower affinity. It normally binds about 15% of the circulating cortisol, and this proportion increases when the total cortisol concentration exceeds the CBG binding capacity. Synthetic glucocorticoids are extensively bound to albumin; eg, about 75% of dexamethasone in plasma is bound to albumin.

C. ANDROGEN BINDING

Androstenedione, DHEA, and DHEA sulfate circulate weakly bound to albumin. However, testosterone is bound extensively to a specific globulin, sex hormone-binding globulin (SHBG). (See Chapters 12 and 13.)

METABOLISM OF CORTISOL & ADRENAL ANDROGENS

The metabolism of the steroids renders them inactive and increases their water solubility, as does their subsequent conjugation with glucuronide or sulfate groups. These inactive conjugated metabolites are more readily excreted by the kidney. The liver is the major site of steroid catabolism and conjugation, and 90% of these metabolized steroids are excreted by the kidney.

Conversion & Excretion of Cortisol

Cortisol is modified extensively before excretion in urine; less than 1% of secreted cortisol appears in the urine unchanged.

A. HEPATIC CONVERSION

Hepatic metabolism of cortisol involves a number of metabolic conversions of which the most important (quantitatively) is the irreversible inactivation of the steroid by Δ^4-reductases, which reduce the 4,5 double bond of the A ring. Dihydrocortisol, the product of this reaction, is then converted to tetrahydrocortisol by a 3-hydroxysteroid dehydrogenase. Cortisol is also converted extensively by 11β-hydroxysteroid dehydrogenase to the biologically inactive cortisone, which is then metabolized by the enzymes described above to yield tetrahydrocortisone. Tetrahydrocortisol and tetrahydrocortisone can be further altered to form the cortoic acids. These conversions result in the excretion of approximately equal amounts of cortisol and cortisone metabolites. Cortisol and cortisone are also metabolized to the cortols and cortolones and to a lesser extent by other pathways, eg, to 6β-hydroxycortisol.

B. HEPATIC CONJUGATION

Over 95% of cortisol and cortisone metabolites are conjugated by the liver and then reenter the circulation to be excreted in the urine. Conjugation is mainly with glucuronic acid at the 3α-hydroxyl position.

C. Variations in Clearance and Metabolism

The metabolism of cortisol is altered by a number of circumstances. It is decreased in infants and in the elderly. It is impaired in chronic liver disease, leading to decreased renal excretion of cortisol metabolites; however, the plasma cortisol level remains normal. Hypothyroidism decreases both metabolism and excretion; conversely, hyperthyroidism accelerates these processes. Cortisol clearance may be reduced in starvation and anorexia nervosa and is also decreased in pregnancy because of the elevated CBG levels. The metabolism of cortisol to 6β-hydroxycortisol is increased in the neonate, in pregnancy, with estrogen therapy, and in patients with liver disease or severe chronic illness. Cortisol metabolism by this pathway is also increased by drugs that induce hepatic microsomal enzymes, including barbiturates, phenytoin, mitotane, aminoglutethimide, and rifampin. These alterations generally are of minor physiologic importance, since secretion, plasma levels, and cortisol half-life are normal. However, they result in decreased excretion of the urinary metabolites of cortisol measured as 17-hydroxycorticosteroids. These conditions and drugs have a greater influence on the metabolism of synthetic glucocorticoids and may result in inadequate plasma levels of the administered glucocorticoid because of rapid clearance and metabolism.

D. Cortisol-Cortisone Shunt

Aldosterone is the principal mineralocorticoid controlling sodium and potassium exchange in the distal nephron. Mineralocorticoid receptors in the kidney are responsible for this effect, and the sensitivities of both the glucocorticoid receptor and the mineralocorticoid receptor for cortisol in vitro are similar. Small changes in aldosterone affect sodium and potassium exchange in the kidney while free and biologically active cortisol does not, yet cortisol circulates in much higher concentration. This apparent paradox is explained by an intracellular enzyme—11β-hydroxysteroid dehydrogenase type 2 (11β-HSD2)—that metabolizes cortisol to the inactive cortisone and protects the mineralocorticoid receptor from cortisol binding (Figure 9–8). However, when circulating cortisol is extremely high (as in severe Cushing's syndrome), this prereceptor metabolism of cortisol is overwhelmed and the mineralocorticoid receptor is activated by cortisol, resulting in volume expansion, hypertension, and hypokalemia. The active ingredient of licorice (glycyrrhizic acid) actually inhibits 11β-HSD2 and gives cortisol free access to the unprotected mineralocorticoid receptor in the kidney, causing hypokalemia and hypertension. In addition, some tissues can actually convert the inactive cortisone to cortisol with the isoform called 11β-hydroxysteroid dehydrogenase type 1 (11β-HSD1). The skin expresses this enzyme, explaining why cortisone cream can be effective. More importantly, the liver expresses 11β-HSD1 and can activate cortisone to cortisol, thereby completing the "cortisol-cortisone shunt" such that the kidney inactivates cortisol to cortisone and the liver can reactivate cortisone to cortisol. The expression of 11β-HSD1 in adipose tissue may contribute to abdominal obesity seen in syndrome X without biochemical hypercortisolism.

Conversion & Excretion of Adrenal Androgens

Adrenal androgen metabolism results either in degradation and inactivation or the peripheral conversion of these weak androgens to their more potent derivatives testosterone and dihydrotestosterone. DHEA is readily converted within the adrenal to DHEA sulfate, the adrenal androgen secreted in greatest amount. DHEA secreted by the gland is also converted to DHEA sulfate by the liver and kidney, or it may be converted to Δ⁴-androstenedione. DHEA sulfate may be excreted without further metabolism; however, both it and DHEA are also metabolized to 7α- and 16α-hydroxylated derivatives and by 17β reduction to Δ⁵-androstenediol and its sulfate. Androstenedione is converted either to testosterone or by reduction of its 4,5 double bond to etiocholanolone or androsterone, which may be further converted by 17α reduction to etiocholanediol and androstanediol, respectively. Testosterone is converted to dihydrotestosterone in androgen-sensitive tissues by 5β reduction, and it in turn is mainly metabolized by 3α reduction to androstanediol. The metabolites of these androgens are conjugated either as glucuronides or sulfates and excreted in the urine. (See Figure 12–2.)

■ BIOLOGIC EFFECTS OF ADRENAL STEROIDS

GLUCOCORTICOIDS

Although glucocorticoids were originally so called because of their influence on glucose metabolism, they are currently defined as steroids that exert their effects by binding to specific cytosolic receptors which mediate the actions of these hormones. These glucocorticoid receptors are present in virtually all tissues, and glucocorticoid-receptor interaction is responsible for most of the

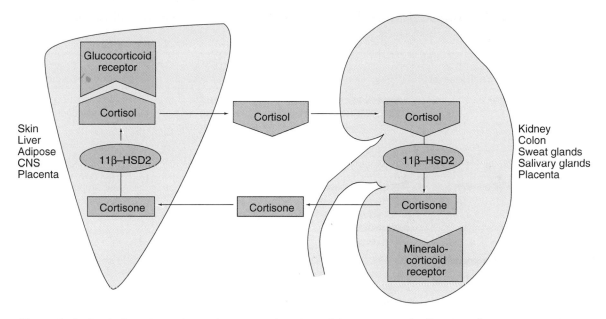

Figure 9–8. Cortisol-cortisone shunt. Contrasting functions of the isozymes of 11β-HSD. 11β-HSD2 is an exclusive 11β-dehydrogenase that acts in classical aldosterone target tissues to exclude cortisol from otherwise nonselective mineralocorticoid receptors. Inactivation of cortisol also occurs in placenta. 11β-HSD1 is a predominant 11β-reductase in vivo that acts in many tissues to increase local intracellular glucocorticoid concentrations and thereby maintain adequate exposure of relatively low affinity glucocorticoid receptors to their ligand. (Modified from Seckl JR, Walker BR: Minireview: 11beta-hydroxysteroid dehydrogenase type 1—a tissue-specific amplifier of glucocorticoid action. Endocrinology 2001;142:1371.)

known effects of these steroids. Alterations in the structure of the glucocorticoids have led to the development of synthetic compounds with greater glucocorticoid activity. The increased activity of these compounds is due to increased affinity for the glucocorticoid receptors and delayed plasma clearance, which increases tissue exposure. In addition, many of these synthetic glucocorticoids have negligible mineralocorticoid effects and thus do not result in sodium retention, hypertension, and hypokalemia. This section describes the molecular mechanisms of glucocorticoid action and the effects on individual metabolic functions and tissues (Table 9–2).

Molecular Mechanisms

Glucocorticoid action is initiated by entry of the steroid into the cell and binding to the cytosolic **glucocorticoid receptor proteins.** (See Figures 3–11, 3–12, and 3–13.) The most abundant cytoplasmic glucocorticoid receptor complex includes two subunits of the 90-kDa heat shock protein hsp90. After binding, the hsp90 subunits dissociate and activated hormone-receptor complexes enter the nucleus and interact with nuclear chromatin acceptor sites. The DNA binding domain of the receptor is a cysteine-rich region which, when it chelates zinc, assumes a conformation called a "zinc finger." The receptor-glucocorticoid complex acts via two mechanisms: (1) binding to specific sites in nuclear DNA, the glucocorticoid regulatory elements; and (2) interactions with other transcription factors such as nuclear factor κB, an important regulator of cytokine genes. These result in altered expression of specific genes and the transcription of specific mRNAs. The resulting proteins elicit the glucocorticoid response, which may be inhibitory or stimulatory depending on the specific gene and tissue affected. Although glucocorticoid receptors are similar in many tissues, the proteins synthesized in response to glucocorticoids vary widely and are the result of expression of specific genes in different cell types. The mechanisms underlying this specific regulation are unknown. Analyses of cloned complementary DNAs for human glucocorticoid receptors have revealed marked structural and amino acid sequence homology between glucocorticoid receptors and receptors for other steroid hormones (eg, mineralocorticoids, estrogen, progesterone) as well as for thyroid

Table 9–2. The main targets and actions of glucocorticoids and the consequences of Cushing's disease and Addison's disease.[1]

Target System	Specific Target	Physiologic Function	Cushing's Disease	Addison's Disease
Intermediary metabolism	Liver	Increased expression of gluconeogenic enzymes, phosphoenolpyruvate kinase, glucose-6-phosphatase, and fructose-2,6-bisphosphatase	Increased hepatic glucose output; together with insulin, increased hepatic glycogen stores	Diminished hepatic glucose output and glycogen stores
	Adipose tissue	Permissive for lipolytic signals (catecholamines, GH) leading to elevated plasma FFA to fuel gluconeogenesis	Overall effect (together with insulin): central obesity (truncal obesity, moon facies, and buffalo hump)	Decreased adiposity and decreased lipolysis
	Skeletal muscle	Degradation of fibrillar muscle proteins by activating the ubiquitin pathway, thereby providing substrate for gluconeogenesis	Muscle weakness and wasting mainly in proximal muscles; increased urinary nitrogen excretion (urea from amino acids)	Muscle weakness, decreased muscle glycogen stores; decreased urinary nitrogen excretion
	Plasma glucose	Maintains plasma glucose during fasting (antihypoglycemic action); increases plasma glucose during stress (hyperglycemic action)	Impaired glucose tolerance, insulin-resistant diabetes mellitus; increased plasma glucose is mainly due to decreased peripheral glucose utilization	Hypoglycemia, increased insulin sensitivity
Calcium homeostasis	Kidney	Decreased reabsorption of calcium	Hypercalciuria without hypercalcemia leading to secondary hyperparathyroidism; retardation of bone growth and bone age by direct action and by decreasing GH; osteoporosis in adults	Retardation of bone growth mainly through decreased GH; hypercalcemia possible
	Bone, cartilage	Inhibition of collagen synthesis and bone deposition		
	Gastrointestinal tract	Inhibition of calcium, magnesium, and phosphate absorption by antagonizing calcitriol		
Other endocrine systems	Hypothalamus, pituitary	Decreases endogenous opioid production; depresses gonadotroph responsiveness to GnRH; stimulates GH gene expression by the pituitary; inhibits GH secretion via the hypothalamus	Scanty menses due to suppressed gonadotroph sensitivity to GnRH; suppressed GH secretion by hypothalamic action; minimal suppression of the TRH-TSH axis	Scanty menses by upregulated CRH-endogenous opioid pathway-mediated suppression of GnRH; suppressed GH secretion; hypothyroidism (if present) is due to direct autoimmune action

(continued)

Table 9–2. The main targets and actions of glucocorticoids and the consequences of Cushing's disease and Addison's disease.[1] (continued)

Target System	Specific Target	Physiologic Function	Cushing's Disease	Addison's Disease
	Pancreas	Inhibits insulin secretion by decreasing the efficacy of cytoplasmic Ca^{2+} on the exocytotic process	Absolute hyperinsulinemia with relative hypoinsulinemia (lower plasma insulin than expected for the degree of hyperglycemia)	Absolute hypoinsulinemia with relative hyperinsulinemia
	Adrenal medulla	Increases PNMT expression and activity (epinephrine synthesis)	Increased responses to sympathoadrenal activation	Decreased responses to sympathoadrenal activation
	Carrier proteins (CBG, SHBG, TBG)	Decreases all major hormone-binding proteins	Decreased in total T_4, free T_4 remains normal	
Immune system	Thymus, lymphocytes	Causes age-related involution of the thymus. Induces thymic atrophy.	Immunocompromised state; lymphocytopenia	Relative lymphocytosis in peripheral blood
	Monocytes	Inhibits monocyte proliferation and antigen presentation; decreased production of Il-1, Il-6, and TNFα	Monocytopenia in peripheral blood	Monocytosis in peripheral blood
	Granulocytes	Demargination of neutrophils by suppressing the expression of adhesion molecules	Peripheal blood: granulocytosis, eosinopenia	Peripheal blood: granulocytopenia, eosinophilia
	Inflammatory response	Inhibition of inflammation by inhibiting PLA_2, thereby inhibiting production of leukotrienes and prostaglandin; suppresses COX-2 expression		
	Erythrocytes	No significant effect	Increased hemoglobin and hematocrit are due to ACTH-mediated overproduction of androgens	Anemia is more pronounced in women and is due to loss of adrenal androgens: Anemia may be related to direct autoimmune targeting of gastric parietal cells
Skin and connective tissue		Antiproliferative for fibroblasts and keratinocytes	Easy bruisability due to dermal atrophy; striae or sites of increased tension, especially sites of adipose tissue accumulation; poor wound healing; hirsutism and acne are due to ACTH-mediated increase of adrenal androgens; hyperpigmentation is a direct effect of ACTH on melanocortin 1 receptors	The darkening of the skin is due to ACTH-mediated stimulation of epidermal melanocortin 1 receptors; vitiligo may occur due to direct autoimmune destruction of melanocytes in circumscribed areas

(continued)

Table 9–2. The main targets and actions of glucocorticoids and the consequences of Cushing's disease and Addison's disease.[1] (continued)

Target System	Specific Target	Physiologic Function	Cushing's Disease	Addison's Disease
Breast	Mammary epithelium	Mandatory requirement for location	Cushing's disease may be associated with galactorrhea	Addison's disease is not associated with galactorrhea
Lung	Type II alveolar cell	Stimulation of surfactant production		
Cardiovascular system	Heart	Increased contractility	Hypertension	Lower peripheral resistance; hypertension with further postural decrease in blood pressure (orthostatic hypotension); low-voltage ECG
	Vasculature	Increased vascular reactivity to vasoconstrictors (catecholamines, angiotensin II)		
Na⁺, K⁺, and ECF volume	Kidney	Increased GFR and non-physiologic actions on mineralocorticoid receptors	Hypokalemic alkalosis, increased ECF volume due to mineralocorticoid activity (increased DOC, saturation of type 11β-hydroxysteroid dehydrogenase by high levels of cortisol).	Hyponatremia, hyperkalemic acidosis, and decreased ECF volume are mainly due to loss of mineralocorticoid activity.
	Posterior pituitary		Hypophosphatemia due to SIADH	SIADH mainly via hypovolemia-related baroreceptor mechanism
Psychiatric parameters of CNS function	Mood	Eucortisolemia maintains emotional balance	Initially, euphoria; long-term, depression	Depression
	Appetite	Increases appetite	Hyperphagia	Decreased appetite in spite of improved taste and smell
	Sleep	Suppression of REM sleep	Sleep disturbances	
	Memory	Sensitizes hippocampal glutamate receptors, induces atrophy of dendrites	Impaired memory, bilateral hippocampal atrophy	
	Eye	Increasing intraocular pressure	Cataract formation; increased intraocular pressure	Decreased intraocular pressure

[1]Modified from Kacsoh B: *Endocrine Physiology.* McGraw-Hill, 2000.

hormone and the oncogene v-*erb* A. Although the steroid-binding domain of the glucocorticoid receptor confers specificity for glucocorticoid binding, glucocorticoids such as cortisol and corticosterone bind to the mineralocorticoid receptor with an affinity equal to that of aldosterone. Mineralocorticoid receptor speci-

ficity is maintained by the expression of 11β-hydroxysteroid dehydrogenase in classic mineralocorticoid-sensitive tissues—the cortisol-cortisone shunt.

Although glucocorticoid-receptor complexes and their subsequent regulation of gene expression are responsible for most glucocorticoid effects, other effects may occur through different mechanisms such as plasma membrane alteration.

Glucocorticoid Agonists & Antagonists

The study of glucocorticoid receptors has led to the definition of glucocorticoid agonists and antagonists. These studies have also identified a number of steroids with mixed effects termed partial agonists, partial antagonists, or partial agonist–partial antagonists.

A. AGONISTS

In humans, cortisol, synthetic glucocorticoids (eg, prednisolone, dexamethasone), corticosterone, and aldosterone are glucocorticoid agonists. The synthetic glucocorticoids have substantially higher affinity for the glucocorticoid receptor, and these have greater glucocorticoid activity than cortisol when present in equimolar concentrations. Corticosterone and aldosterone have substantial affinity for the glucocorticoid receptor; however, their plasma concentrations are normally much lower than that of cortisol, and thus these steroids do not have significant physiologic glucocorticoid effects.

B. ANTAGONISTS

Glucocorticoid antagonists bind to the glucocorticoid receptors but do not elicit the nuclear events required to cause a glucocorticoid response. These steroids compete with agonist steroids such as cortisol for the receptors and thus inhibit agonist responses. Other steroids have partial agonist activity when present alone; ie, they elicit a partial glucocorticoid response. However, in sufficient concentration, they compete with agonist steroids for the receptors and thus competitively inhibit agonist responses; ie, these partial agonists may function as partial antagonists in the presence of more active glucocorticoids. Steroids such as progesterone, 11-deoxycortisol, DOC, testosterone, and 17β-estradiol have antagonist or partial agonist-partial antagonist effects; however, the physiologic role of these hormones in glucocorticoid action is probably negligible, because they circulate in low concentrations. The antiprogestational agent RU 486 (mifepristone) has substantial glucocorticoid antagonist properties and has been used to block glucocorticoid action in patients with Cushing's syndrome.

Intermediary Metabolism (Table 9–2)

Glucocorticoids in general inhibit DNA synthesis. In addition, in most tissues they inhibit RNA and protein synthesis and accelerate protein catabolism. These actions provide substrate for intermediary metabolism; however, accelerated catabolism also accounts for the deleterious effects of glucocorticoids on muscle, bone, connective tissue, and lymphatic tissues. In contrast, RNA and protein synthesis in liver is stimulated.

A. HEPATIC GLUCOSE METABOLISM

Glucocorticoids increase hepatic gluconeogenesis by stimulating the gluconeogenetic enzymes phosphoenolpyruvate carboxykinase and glucose 6-phosphatase. They have a permissive effect in that they increase hepatic responsiveness to the gluconeogenetic hormone glucagon, and they also increase the release of substrates for gluconeogenesis from peripheral tissues, particularly muscle. This latter effect may be enhanced by the glucocorticoid-induced reduction in peripheral amino acid uptake and protein synthesis. Glucocorticoids also increase glycerol and free fatty acid release by lipolysis and increase muscle lactate release. They enhance hepatic glycogen synthesis and storage by stimulating glycogen synthetase activity and to a lesser extent by inhibiting glycogen breakdown. These effects are insulin-dependent.

B. PERIPHERAL GLUCOSE METABOLISM

Glucocorticoids also alter carbohydrate metabolism by inhibiting peripheral glucose uptake in muscle and adipose tissue. This effect and the others described above may result in increased insulin secretion in states of chronic glucocorticoid excess.

C. EFFECTS ON ADIPOSE TISSUE

In adipose tissue, the predominant effect is increased lipolysis with release of glycerol and free fatty acids. This is partially due to direct stimulation of lipolysis by glucocorticoids, but it is also contributed to by decreased glucose uptake and enhancement by glucocorticoids of the effects of lipolytic hormones. Although glucocorticoids are lipolytic, increased fat deposition is a classic manifestation of glucocorticoid excess. This paradox may be explained by the increased appetite caused by high levels of these steroids and by the lipogenic effects of the hyperinsulinemia that occurs in this state. The reason for abnormal fat deposition and distribution in states of cortisol excess is unknown. In these instances, fat is classically deposited centrally in the face, cervical area, trunk, and abdomen; the extremities are usually spared.

D. SUMMARY

The effects of the glucocorticoids on intermediary metabolism can be summarized as follows: (1) Effects are minimal in the fed state. However, during fasting, glucocorticoids contribute to the maintenance of plasma glucose levels by increasing gluconeogenesis, glycogen deposition, and the peripheral release of substrate. (2) Hepatic glucose production is enhanced, as is hepatic RNA and protein synthesis. (3) The effects on muscle are catabolic, ie, decreased glucose uptake and metabolism, decreased protein synthesis, and increased release of amino acids. (4) In adipose tissue, lipolysis is stimulated. (5) In glucocorticoid deficiency, hypoglycemia may result, whereas in states of glucocorticoid excess there may be hyperglycemia, hyperinsulinemia, muscle wasting, and weight gain with abnormal fat distribution.

Effects on Other Tissues & Functions (Table 9–2)

A. CONNECTIVE TISSUE

Glucocorticoids in excess inhibit fibroblasts, lead to loss of collagen and connective tissue, and thus result in thinning of the skin, easy bruising, stria formation, and poor wound healing.

B. BONE

The physiologic role of glucocorticoids in bone metabolism and calcium homeostasis is unknown; however, in excess, they have major deleterious effects. Glucocorticoids directly inhibit bone formation by decreasing cell proliferation and the synthesis of RNA, protein, collagen, and hyaluronate. Glucocorticoids also directly stimulate bone-resorbing cells, leading to osteolysis and increased urinary hydroxyproline excretion. In addition, they potentiate the actions of PTH and 1,25-dihydroxycholecalciferol (1,25[OH]$_2$D$_3$) on bone, and this may further contribute to net bone resorption.

C. CALCIUM METABOLISM

Glucocorticoids also have other major effects on mineral homeostasis. They markedly reduce intestinal calcium absorption, which tends to lower serum calcium. This results in a secondary increase in PTH secretion, which maintains serum calcium within the normal range by stimulating bone resorption. In addition, glucocorticoids may directly stimulate PTH release. The mechanism of decreased intestinal calcium absorption is unknown, though it is not due to decreased synthesis or decreased serum levels of the active vitamin D metabolites; in fact, 1,25(OH)$_2$D$_3$ levels are normal or even increased in the presence of glucocorticoid excess. Increased 1,25(OH)$_2$D$_3$ synthesis in this setting may result from decreased serum phosphorus levels (see below), increased PTH levels, and direct stimulation by glucocorticoids of renal 1α-hydroxylase. Glucocorticoids also increase urinary calcium excretion, and hypercalciuria is a consistent feature of cortisol excess. They also reduce the tubular reabsorption of phosphate, leading to phosphaturia and decreased serum phosphorus concentrations.

Thus, glucocorticoids in excess result in negative calcium balance, with decreased calcium absorption and increased urinary calcium excretion. Serum calcium levels are maintained, but at the expense of net bone resorption. Decreased bone formation and increased resorption ultimately result in the disabling osteoporosis that is often a major complication of spontaneous and iatrogenic glucocorticoid excess (see Chapter 8).

D. GROWTH AND DEVELOPMENT

Glucocorticoids accelerate the development of a number of systems and organs in fetal and differentiating tissues, although the mechanisms are unclear. As discussed above, glucocorticoids are generally inhibitory, and these stimulatory effects may be due to glucocorticoid interactions with other growth factors. Examples of these development-promoting effects are increased surfactant production in the fetal lung and the accelerated development of hepatic and gastrointestinal enzyme systems.

Glucocorticoids in excess inhibit growth in children, and this adverse effect is a major complication of therapy. This may be a direct effect on bone cells, although decreased growth hormone (GH) secretion and somatomedin generation also contribute (see Chapter 6).

E. BLOOD CELLS AND IMMUNOLOGIC FUNCTION

1. Erythrocytes—Glucocorticoids have little effect on erythropoiesis and hemoglobin concentration. Although mild polycythemia and anemia may be seen in Cushing's syndrome and Addison's disease, respectively, these alterations are more likely to be secondary to altered androgen metabolism.

2. Leukocytes—Glucocorticoids influence both leukocyte movement and function. Thus, glucocorticoid administration increases the number of intravascular polymorphonuclear leukocytes (PMNs) by increasing PMN release from bone marrow, by increasing the circulating half-life of PMNs, and by decreasing PMN movement out of the vascular compartment. Glucocorticoid administration reduces the number of circulating lymphocytes, monocytes, and eosinophils, mainly by increasing their movement out of the circulation. The converse—ie, neutropenia, lymphocytosis, monocytosis, and eosinophilia—is seen in adrenal insufficiency. Glucocorticoids also decrease the migration of inflammatory cells (PMNs, monocytes, and lymphocytes) to sites of injury, and this is probably a major mechanism of the anti-inflammatory actions and increased susceptibility to infection that occur following chronic administration. Glucocorticoids also decrease lymphocyte production and the mediator and effector functions of these cells.

3. Immunologic effects—Glucocorticoids influence multiple aspects of immunologic and inflammatory responsiveness, including the mobilization and function of leukocytes, as discussed above. They inhibit phospholipase A_2, a key enzyme in the synthesis of prostaglandins. This inhibition is mediated by a class of peptides called lipocortins or annexins. They also impair release of effector substances such as the lymphokine interleukin-1, antigen processing, antibody production and clearance, and other specific bone marrow-derived and thymus-derived lymphocyte functions. The immune system, in turn, affects the hypothalamic-pituitary-adrenal axis; interleukin-1 stimulates the secretion of CRH and ACTH.

F. CARDIOVASCULAR FUNCTION

Glucocorticoids may increase cardiac output, and they also increase peripheral vascular tone, possibly by augmenting the effects of other vasoconstrictors, eg, the catecholamines. Glucocorticoids also regulate expression of adrenergic receptors. Thus, refractory shock may occur when the glucocorticoid-deficient individual is subjected to stress. Glucocorticoids in excess may cause hypertension independently of their mineralocorticoid effects. Although the incidence and the precise cause of this problem are unclear, it is likely that the mechanism involves the renin-angiotensin system; glucocorticoids regulate renin substrate, the precursor of angiotensin I.

G. RENAL FUNCTION

These steroids affect water and electrolyte balance by actions mediated either by mineralocorticoid receptors (sodium retention, hypokalemia, and hypertension) or via glucocorticoid receptors (increased glomerular filtration rate due to increased cardiac output or due to direct renal effects on salt and water retention). Thus, corticosteroids such as betamethasone or dexamethasone that have little mineralocorticoid activity increase sodium and water excretion. Glucocorticoid-deficient subjects have decreased glomerular filtration rates and are unable to excrete a water load. This may be further aggravated by increased ADH secretion, which may occur in glucocorticoid deficiency.

H. CENTRAL NERVOUS SYSTEM FUNCTION

Glucocorticoids readily enter the brain, and although their physiologic role in central nervous system function is unknown, their excess or deficiency may profoundly alter behavior and cognitive function.

1. **Excessive glucocorticoids**—In excess, the glucocorticoids initially cause euphoria; however, with prolonged exposure, a variety of psychologic abnormalities occur, including irritability, emotional lability, and depression. Hyperkinetic or manic behavior is less common; overt psychoses occur in a small number of patients. Many patients also note impairment in cognitive functions, most commonly memory and concentration. Other central effects include increased appetite, decreased libido, and insomnia, with decreased REM sleep and increased stage II sleep.

2. **Decreased glucocorticoids**—Patients with Addison's disease are apathetic and depressed and tend to be irritable, negativistic, and reclusive. They have decreased appetite but increased sensitivity of taste and smell mechanisms.

I. EFFECTS ON OTHER HORMONES

1. **Thyroid function**—Glucocorticoids in excess affect thyroid function. Although basal TSH levels are usually normal, TSH synthesis and release are inhibited by glucocorticoids, and TSH responsiveness to thyrotropin-releasing hormone (TRH) is frequently subnormal. Serum total thyroxine (T_4) concentrations are usually low normal because of a decrease in thyroxine-binding globulin, but free T_4 levels are normal. Total and free T_3 (triiodothyronine) concentrations may be low, since glucocorticoid excess decreases the conversion of T_4 to T_3 and increases conversion to reverse T_3. Despite these alterations, manifestations of hypothyroidism are not apparent.

2. **Gonadal function**—Glucocorticoids also affect gonadotropin and gonadal function. In males, they inhibit gonadotropin secretion, as evidenced by decreased responsiveness to administered gonadotropin-releasing hormone (GnRH) and subnormal plasma testosterone concentrations. In females, glucocorticoids also suppress LH responsiveness to GnRH, resulting in suppression of estrogens and progestins with inhibition of ovulation and amenorrhea.

J. MISCELLANEOUS EFFECTS

1. **Peptic ulcer**—The role of steroid excess in the production or reactivation of peptic ulcer disease is controversial. However, there appears to be a modest independent effect of glucocorticoids to promote peptic ulcer disease (relative risk about 1.4), and when this effect is combined with that of nonsteroidal anti-inflammatory drugs there is a synergistic interaction that considerably increases the risk.

2. **Ophthalmologic effects**—Intraocular pressure varies with the level of circulating glucocorticoids and parallels the circadian variation of plasma cortisol levels. In addition, glucocorticoids in excess increase intraocular pressure in patients with open-angle glaucoma. Glucocorticoid therapy may also cause cataract formation. Central serous chorioretinopathy, an accumulation of subretinal detachment, may also complicate endogenous or exogenous glucocorticoid excess.

ADRENAL ANDROGENS

The direct biologic activity of the adrenal androgens (androstenedione, DHEA, and DHEA sulfate) is minimal, and they function primarily as precursors for peripheral conversion to the active androgenic hormones testosterone and dihydrotestosterone. Thus, DHEA sulfate secreted by the adrenal undergoes limited conversion to DHEA; this peripherally converted DHEA and that secreted by the adrenal cortex can be further converted in peripheral tissues to androstenedione, the immediate precursor of the active androgens.

The actions of testosterone and dihydrotestosterone are described in Chapter 12. This section will deal only with the adrenal contribution to androgenicity.

Effects in Males

In males with normal gonadal function, the conversion of adrenal androstenedione to testosterone accounts for less than 5% of the production rate of this hormone, and thus the physiologic effect is negligible. In adult males, excessive adrenal androgen secretion has no clinical consequences; however, in boys, it causes premature penile enlargement and early development of secondary sexual characteristics.

Effects in Females

In females, the adrenal substantially contributes to total androgen production by the peripheral conversion of androstenedione to testosterone. In the follicular phase of the menstrual cycle, adrenal precursors account for two-thirds of testosterone production and one-half of dihydrotestosterone production. During midcycle, the ovarian contribution increases, and the adrenal precursors account for only 40% of testosterone production.

In females, abnormal adrenal function as seen in Cushing's syndrome, adrenal carcinoma, and congenital adrenal hyperplasia results in excessive secretion of adrenal androgens, and their peripheral conversion to testosterone results in androgen excess, manifested by acne, hirsutism, and virilization.

LABORATORY EVALUATION

Cortisol and the adrenal androgens are measured by specific plasma assays. Certain urinary assays, particularly measurement of 24-hour urine free cortisol, are also useful. In addition, plasma concentrations of ACTH can be determined. The plasma steroid methods commonly used measure the total hormone concentration and are therefore influenced by alterations in plasma binding proteins. Furthermore, since ACTH and the plasma concentrations of the adrenal hormones fluctuate markedly (Figure 9–7), single plasma measurements are frequently unreliable. Thus, plasma levels must be interpreted cautiously, and more specific diagnostic information is usually obtained by performing appropriate dynamic tests (stimulation and suppression) or other tests that reflect cortisol secretory rate.

Plasma ACTH

A. METHODS OF MEASUREMENT

Plasma ACTH measurements are extremely useful in the diagnosis of pituitary-adrenal dysfunction. The normal range for plasma ACTH, using a sensitive immunometric assay (IMA), is 9–52 pg/mL (2–11.1 pmol/L).

B. INTERPRETATION

Plasma ACTH levels are most useful in differentiating pituitary causes from adrenal causes of adrenal dysfunction: (1) In **adrenal insufficiency** due to primary adrenal disease, plasma ACTH levels are elevated. Conversely, in pituitary ACTH deficiency and secondary hypoadrenalism, plasma ACTH levels are "normal" or less than 10 pg/mL (2.2 pmol/L). (2) In **Cushing's syndrome** due to primary glucocorticoid-secreting adrenal tumors, plasma ACTH is suppressed, and a level less than 5 pg/mL (1.1 pmol/L) is diagnostic. In patients with Cushing's disease (pituitary ACTH hypersecretion), plasma ACTH levels are normal or elevated. Plasma ACTH levels are usually markedly elevated in the ectopic ACTH syndrome, but there is a considerable amount of overlap with levels seen in Cushing's disease. In addition, values lower than expected may be observed rarely in ectopic ACTH syndrome when the two-site immunoradiometric assay is used; this assay does not detect high-molecular-weight precursors of ACTH. (3) Plasma ACTH levels are also markedly elevated in patients with the common forms of **congenital adrenal hyperplasia** and are useful in the diagnosis and management of these disorders (see Chapters 10 and 14).

Plasma Cortisol

A. METHODS OF MEASUREMENT

The most common methods of measurement of plasma cortisol are radioimmunoassay and high-performance liquid chromatography. These methods measure total cortisol (both bound and free) in plasma. Since cortisol is present in saliva in its unbound or free state, salivary cortisol measurements provide a simple and accurate assessment of free cortisol concentration.

Radioimmunoassays of plasma cortisol depend on inhibition of binding of radiolabeled cortisol to an antibody by the cortisol present in a plasma sample. Current assays are very sensitive, so that small plasma volumes can be used. In addition, cross-reactivity of current antisera with other endogenous steroids is minimal, and radioimmunoassay thus gives a reliable measurement of total plasma cortisol levels. Cross-reactivity with some synthetic glucocorticoids, eg, prednisone, is variable. Other commonly used drugs and medications do not interfere with this assay.

B. INTERPRETATION

The diagnostic utility of single plasma cortisol concentrations is limited by the episodic nature of cortisol secretion and its appropriate elevations during stress. As explained below, more information is obtained by dynamic testing of the hypothalamic-pituitary-adrenal axis.

1. Normal values—Normal plasma cortisol levels vary with the method used. With radioimmunoassay levels at 8 AM range from 3 to 20 μg/dL (80–550 nmol/L) and average 10–12 μg/dL (275.9–331.1 nmol/L). Values obtained later in the day are lower and at 4 PM are approximately half of morning values. At 10 PM to 2 AM, the plasma cortisol concentrations by these methods are usually under 3 μg/dL (80 nmol/L). The normal salivary cortisol level at midnight is < 0.15 μg/dL (4 nmol/L).

2. Levels during stress—Cortisol secretion increases in patients who are acutely ill, during surgery, and following trauma. Plasma concentrations may reach 40–60 μg/dL (1100–1655 nmol/L).

3. High-estrogen states—The total plasma cortisol concentration is also elevated with increased CBG binding capacity, which occurs most commonly when circulating estrogen levels are high, eg, during pregnancy and when exogenous estrogens or oral contraceptives are being used. In these situations, plasma cortisol may reach levels two to three times normal.

4. Other conditions—CBG levels may be increased or decreased in other situations, as discussed above in the sections on circulation and metabolism. Total plasma cortisol concentrations may also be increased in severe anxiety, endogenous depression, starvation, anorexia nervosa, alcoholism, and chronic renal failure.

Late-Night Salivary Cortisol

Most patients with Cushing's syndrome have an abnormal circadian rhythm characterized by failure to decrease cortisol secretion during the normal nadir in the late evening, usually between 11:00 PM and midnight. This may account for the disrupted sleep cycles and some of the psychologic problems seen in these patients. Several studies have demonstrated that an elevated midnight serum cortisol level (with a blood sample obtained during sleeping) is highly accurate in differentiating patients with Cushing's syndrome from

normal subjects and from patients with pseudo-Cushing conditions such as depression or alcoholism. In one study, a midnight serum cortisol of > 5.2 μg/dL (140 nmol/L) yielded a sensitivity of 100% and a specificity of 77% for the diagnosis of Cushing's syndrome. Since obtaining such cortisol measurements is impractical on an ambulatory basis, many clinicians are now using late-night salivary cortisol measurements as a means of establishing the presence or absence of Cushing's syndrome. Cortisol in the saliva is in equilibrium with the free and biologically active cortisol in the blood. The concentration of cortisol is not affected by salivary flow or composition and is stable at room temperature for many days. Saliva can easily be sampled at home by the patient using a variety of techniques, including the use of a commercially available sampling device. Recent studies have demonstrated that late-night salivary cortisol measurements provide a sensitivity and specificity for the diagnosis of Cushing's syndrome of > 90%, and this procedure is emerging as possibly the simplest and most effective screening tool for patients in whom the diagnosis of hypercortisolism is suspected. Reference ranges for late-night salivary cortisol concentrations are dependent on the assays employed.

Urinary Corticosteroids

A. FREE CORTISOL

1. Methods of measurement—The assay of unbound cortisol excreted in the urine is an excellent method for the diagnosis of Cushing's syndrome. Normally, less than 1% of the secreted cortisol is excreted unchanged in the urine. However, in states of excess secretion, the binding capacity of CBG is exceeded, and plasma free cortisol therefore increases, as does its urinary excretion. Urine free cortisol is measured in a 24-hour urine collection by high-performance liquid chromatography (HPLC), radioimmunoassay, and most recently by gas chromatography-mass spectroscopy.

2. Normal values—HPLC provides the most specific measurement of cortisol and is the current procedure of choice. The normal range for urine free cortisol assayed by HPLC is 5–50 μg/24 h (14–135 nmol/24 h). The normal range for urine free cortisol is 20–90 μg/24 h (50–250 nmol/24 h) when radioimmunoassay techniques are used.

3. Diagnostic utility—This method is particularly useful in differentiating simple obesity from Cushing's syndrome, since urine free cortisol levels are not elevated in obesity, as are the urinary 17-hydroxycorticosteroids (see below). The levels may be elevated in the same conditions that increase plasma cortisol (see above), including a slight elevation during pregnancy.

This test is not useful in adrenal insufficiency, because of the lack of sensitivity of the method at low levels and because low cortisol excretion is often found in normal persons.

B. 17-HYDROXYCORTICOSTEROIDS

These urinary steroids should not be measured at present because of the greater utility of plasma cortisol and urine free cortisol measurements.

Dexamethasone Suppression Tests

A. LOW-DOSE TEST

This procedure is used to establish the presence of Cushing's syndrome regardless of its cause. Dexamethasone, a potent glucocorticoid, normally suppresses pituitary ACTH release with a resulting fall in plasma and urine corticosteroids, thus assessing feedback inhibition of the hypothalamic-pituitary-adrenal axis. In Cushing's syndrome, this mechanism is abnormal, and steroid secretion fails to be suppressed in the normal way. Dexamethasone in the doses used does not interfere with the measurement of plasma and urinary cortisol.

The overnight 1 mg dexamethasone suppression test is a suitable screening test for Cushing's syndrome. Dexamethasone, 1 mg orally, is given as a single dose at 11:00 PM, and the following morning a plasma sample is obtained for cortisol determination. Cushing's syndrome is probably excluded if the serum or plasma cortisol level is less than 1.8 µg/dL (50 nmol/L). If the level is greater than 10 µg/dL (276 nmol/L)—in the absence of conditions causing false-positive responses—Cushing's syndrome is the probable cause, and the diagnosis should be confirmed with other procedures.

Eighty to 99 percent of patients with Cushing's syndrome have abnormal responses. False-negative results are more common in mild hypercortisolism and may also occur in patients in whom dexamethasone metabolism is abnormally slow, since plasma levels of dexamethasone in these patients are higher than normally achieved and result in apparently normal suppression of cortisol. Simultaneous measurement of plasma dexamethasone and cortisol levels will identify these patients.

False-positive results occur in hospitalized and chronically ill patients. Acute illness, depression, anxiety, alcoholism, high-estrogen states, and uremia may also cause false-positive results. Patients taking phenytoin, barbiturates, and other inducers of hepatic microsomal enzymes may have accelerated metabolism of dexamethasone and thus fail to achieve adequate plasma levels to suppress ACTH.

B. HIGH-DOSE TESTS

High dose dexamethasone suppression testing has historically been used to differentiate Cushing's disease (pituitary ACTH hypersecretion) from ectopic ACTH and adrenal tumors. This rationale has been based on the fact that in some patients with Cushing's disease, the hypothalamic-pituitary-adrenal axis is suppressible with supraphysiologic doses of glucocorticoids, whereas cortisol secretion is autonomous in patients with adrenal tumors and in most patients with the ectopic ACTH syndrome. Unfortunately, exceptions to these rules are so common that high-dose dexamethasone suppression testing must be interpreted with extreme caution.

1. Overnight high-dose dexamethasone suppression test—This simple test is preferable to the 2-day high-dose dexamethasone suppression test described below. After a baseline morning cortisol specimen is obtained, a single dose of dexamethasone, 8 mg orally, is administered at 11:00 PM and plasma cortisol is measured at 8:00 AM the following morning. Generally, patients with Cushing's disease will suppress plasma cortisol level to less than 50% of baseline values—in contrast to patients with the ectopic ACTH syndrome, who fail to suppress to this level. Patients with cortisol-producing adrenal tumors will also fail to suppress: their cortisol secretion is autonomous, and ACTH secretion is already suppressed by the high endogenous levels of cortisol.

2. Two-day high-dose dexamethasone suppression test—This test is performed by administering dexamethasone, 2 mg orally every 6 hours for 2 days. Twenty-four-hour urine samples are collected before and on the second day of dexamethasone administration. Patients with Cushing's disease have a reduction of urine cortisol excretion to less than 50% of baseline values, whereas those with adrenal tumors or the ectopic ACTH syndrome usually have little or no reduction in urinary cortisol excretion. However, some patients with an ectopic ACTH-secreting neoplasm suppress steroid secretion with high doses of dexamethasone, and some patients with pituitary ACTH-dependent Cushing's syndrome fail to suppress to these levels. The diagnostic sensitivity, specificity, and accuracy of the high-dose dexamethasone suppression test are only about 80%. An analysis of the standard low- and high-dose dexamethasone suppression tests has shown better specificity and accuracy by utilizing new criteria. The decrease in urine free cortisol of more than 90% in the high-dose test had 100% diagnostic specificity for Cushing's disease and excluded ectopic ACTH syndrome in one series. However, several exceptions to these new criteria have been observed; and it has become increasingly clear that high-dose dexamethasone suppression testing, regardless of the criteria employed, cannot distinguish pituitary from nonpituitary ACTH hypersecretion with certainty.

Pituitary-Adrenal Reserve

Determinations of pituitary-adrenal reserve are used to evaluate the patient's adrenal and pituitary reserve and to assess the ability of the hypothalamic-pituitary-adrenal axis to respond to stress. ACTH administration directly stimulates adrenal secretion; metyrapone inhibits cortisol synthesis, thereby stimulating pituitary ACTH secretion; and insulin-induced hypoglycemia stimulates ACTH release by increasing CRH secretion. More recently, CRH has been utilized to directly stimulate pituitary corticotrophs to release ACTH. The relative utility of these procedures is discussed below in the section on adrenocortical insufficiency and also in Chapter 5.

A. ACTH STIMULATION TESTING

1. Procedure and normal values—The rapid ACTH stimulation test measures the acute adrenal response to ACTH and is used to diagnose both primary and secondary adrenal insufficiency. A synthetic human α^{1-24}-ACTH called tetracosactrin or cosyntropin is used. Fasting is not required, and the test may be performed at any time of the day. A baseline cortisol sample is obtained; cosyntropin is administered in a dose of 0.25 mg intramuscularly or intravenously; and additional samples for plasma cortisol are obtained at 30 or 60 minutes following the injection. Because the peak concentration of ACTH with this test achieves a pharmacologic level exceeding 10,000 pg/mL, this study assesses maximal adrenocortical capacity. The peak cortisol response, 30–60 minutes later, should exceed 18–20 μg/dL (> 497–552 nmol/L). The 30-minute peak cortisol response to ACTH is constant and is unrelated to the basal cortisol level. In fact, there is no difference in the peak cortisol level at 30 minutes regardless of whether 250 μg, 5 μg, or even 1 μg of ACTH is administered. Use of a 1 μg dose of ACTH provides a more sensitive indication of adrenocortical function and has been better able to differentiate a subgroup of patients on long-term corticosteroid therapy who responded normally to the regular 250 μg test but who have a reduced response to 1 μg. The low-dose (1 μg) ACTH stimulation test is gaining greater acceptance and may emerge as the diagnostic procedure of choice in suspected adrenal insufficiency, though it is still controversial.

2. Subnormal responses—If the cortisol response to the rapid ACTH stimulation test is inadequate, adrenal insufficiency is present. In primary adrenal insufficiency, destruction of cortical cells reduces cortisol secretion and increases pituitary ACTH secretion. Therefore, the adrenal is already maximally stimulated, and there is no further increase in cortisol secretion when exogenous ACTH is given; ie, there is decreased adrenal reserve. In secondary adrenal insufficiency due to ACTH deficiency, there is atrophy of the zonae fasciculata and reticularis, and the adrenal thus is either hyporesponsive or unresponsive to acute stimulation with exogenous ACTH. In either primary or secondary types, a subnormal response to the rapid ACTH stimulation test accurately predicts deficient responsiveness of the axis to insulin hypoglycemia, metyrapone, and surgical stress.

3. Normal responses—A normal response to the rapid ACTH stimulation test excludes both primary adrenal insufficiency (by directly assessing adrenal reserve) and overt secondary adrenal insufficiency with adrenal atrophy. However, a normal response does not rule out partial ACTH deficiency (decreased pituitary reserve) in patients whose basal ACTH secretion is sufficient to prevent adrenocortical atrophy. These patients may be unable to further increase ACTH secretion and thus may have subnormal pituitary ACTH responsiveness to stress or hypoglycemia. In such patients, further testing with metyrapone, hypoglycemia, or CRH may be indicated. For further discussion, see the section on diagnosis of adrenocortical insufficiency.

B. METYRAPONE TESTING

Metyrapone testing has been used to diagnose adrenal insufficiency and to assess pituitary-adrenal reserve. The test procedures are detailed in Chapter 5. Metyrapone blocks cortisol synthesis by inhibiting the 11β-hydroxylase enzyme that converts 11-deoxycortisol to cortisol. This stimulates ACTH secretion, which in turn increases the secretion and plasma levels of 11-deoxycortisol. The overnight metyrapone test is most commonly used and is best suited to patients with suspected pituitary ACTH deficiency; patients with suspected primary adrenal failure are usually evaluated with the rapid ACTH stimulation test as described above and discussed in the section on diagnosis of adrenocortical insufficiency. The normal response to the overnight metyrapone test is a plasma 11-deoxycortisol level greater than 7 ng/dL (0.2 nmol/L) and a plasma ACTH level greater than 100 pg/mL (22 pmol/L) and indicates both normal ACTH secretion and adrenal function. A subnormal response establishes adrenocortical insufficiency. A normal response to metyrapone accurately predicts normal stress responsiveness of the hypothalamic-pituitary axis and correlates well with responsiveness to insulin-induced hypoglycemia. Metyrapone is not routinely available except directly from the manufacturer, Novartis Pharmaceuticals, at 1-800-988-7768.

C. Insulin-Induced Hypoglycemia Testing

The details of this procedure are described in Chapter 5. Hypoglycemia induces a central nervous system stress response, increases CRH release, and in this way increases ACTH and cortisol secretion. It therefore measures the integrity of the axis and its ability to respond to stress. The normal plasma cortisol response is an increment greater than 8 μg/dL (220 nmol/L) and a peak level greater than 18–20 μg/dL (497–552 nmol/L). The plasma ACTH response to hypoglycemia is usually greater than 100 pg/mL (22 pmol/L). A normal plasma cortisol response to hypoglycemia excludes adrenal insufficiency and decreased pituitary reserve. Thus, patients with normal responses do not require cortisol therapy during illness or surgery.

D. CRH Testing

The procedure for CRH testing is described in Chapter 5. ACTH responses are exaggerated in patients with primary adrenal failure and absent in patients with hypopituitarism. Delayed responses may occur in patients with hypothalamic disorders. CRH testing has also been used to differentiate among the causes of Cushing's syndrome (see below).

Androgens

Androgen excess is usually evaluated by the measurement of basal levels of these hormones, since suppression and stimulation tests are not as useful as in disorders affecting the glucocorticoids.

A. Plasma Levels

Assays are available for total plasma levels of DHEA, DHEA sulfate, androstenedione, testosterone, and dihydrotestosterone. Traditional measurement of urinary androgen metabolites measured as urinary 17-ketosteroids should no longer be used.

Because it is present in greater quantities, DHEA sulfate can be measured directly in unextracted plasma. However, because of their similar structures and lower plasma concentrations, the other androgens require extraction and purification steps prior to assay. This is accomplished by solvent extraction followed by chromatography, and the purified steroids are then measured by radioimmunoassay or competitive protein-binding radioassay. These methods allow measurement of multiple steroids in small volumes of plasma.

B. Free Testosterone

Plasma free testosterone (ie, testosterone not bound to SHBG) can be measured and is a more direct measure of circulating biologically active testosterone than the total plasma level. These methods require separation of the bound and free hormone prior to assay and are technically difficult. The plasma free testosterone concentration in normal women averages 5 pg/mL (17 pmol/L), representing approximately 1% of the total testosterone concentration. In hirsute women, average levels are 16 pg/mL (55 pmol/L), with a wide range (see Chapter 13).

■ DISORDERS OF ADRENOCORTICAL INSUFFICIENCY

Deficient adrenal production of glucocorticoids or mineralocorticoids results in adrenocortical insufficiency, which is either the consequence of destruction or dysfunction of the cortex (primary adrenocortical insufficiency, or Addison's disease) or secondary to deficient pituitary ACTH secretion (secondary adrenocortical insufficiency). Glucocorticoid therapy is the most common cause of secondary adrenocortical insufficiency.

PRIMARY ADRENOCORTICAL INSUFFICIENCY (Addison's Disease)

Etiology & Pathology (Figure 9–9)

The etiology of primary adrenocortical insufficiency has changed over time. Prior to 1920, tuberculosis was the major cause of adrenocortical insufficiency. Since 1950, autoimmune adrenalitis with adrenal atrophy has accounted for about 80% of cases. It is associated with a high incidence of other immunologic and autoimmune endocrine disorders (see below). Causes of primary adrenal insufficiency are listed in Table 9–3. Primary adrenocortical insufficiency, or Addison's disease, is rare, with a reported prevalence of 110 per million population in the United Kingdom and 60 per million in Denmark. It is more common in females, with a female:male ratio of 2.6:1. Addison's disease is usually diagnosed in the third to fifth decades. As patients with malignant disease and with AIDS live longer, more cases of adrenal insufficiency will be seen.

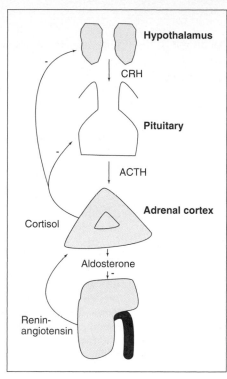

Normal state

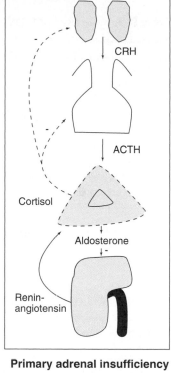

Primary adrenal insufficiency

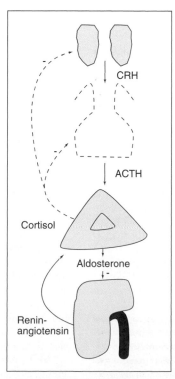

Secondary adrenal insufficiency (ACTH deficiency)

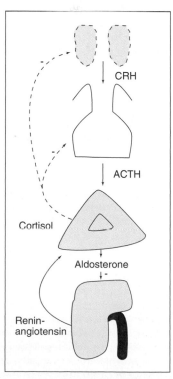

Tertiary adrenal insufficiency (CRH deficiency)

Figure 9–9. Hypothalamic-pituitary axis in adrenal insufficiency of different causes. These panels illustrate hormone secretion in the normal state (upper left), primary adrenal insufficiency (upper right), secondary adrenal insufficiency–ACTH deficiency (lower left), and tertiary adrenal insufficiency–CRH deficiency (lower right). Renin-angiotensin system is also illustrated. In contrast to normal secretion and hormone levels, decreased hormonal secretion is indicated by a dotted line and increased secretion by a dark solid line.

Table 9–3. Causes of primary adrenocortical insufficiency.

Autoimmune
Metastatic malignancy or lymphoma
Adrenal hemorrhage
Infectious
    Tuberculosis, CMV, fungi (histoplasmosis, coccidioidomy-
      cosis), HIV
Adrenoleukodystrophy
Infiltrative disorders
    Amyloidosis, hemochromatosis
Congenital adrenal hyperplasia
Familial glucocorticoid deficiency and hypoplasia
Drugs
    Ketoconazole, metyrapone, aminoglutethimide, trilostane,
      mitotane, etomidate

A. Autoimmune Adrenocortical Insufficiency

The adrenals are small and atrophic, and the capsule is thickened. The adrenal medulla is preserved, though cortical cells are largely absent, show degenerative changes, and are surrounded by a fibrous stroma and the characteristic lymphocytic infiltrates.

Autoimmune Addison's disease is frequently accompanied by other immune disorders. There are two different syndromes in which autoimmune adrenal insufficiency may occur. The best-characterized one is known as autoimmune polyendocrinopathy-candidiasis-ectodermal dystrophy syndrome (APCED), or autoimmune polyglandular disease type I. This is an autosomal recessive disorder that usually presents in childhood and is accompanied by hypoparathyroidism, adrenal failure, and mucocutaneous candidiasis. APCED results from a mutation of the autoimmune regulator gene *(AIRE),* which is located on chromosome 21q22.3. These patients have a defect in T cell-mediated immunity, especially toward the candida antigen. This disorder has no relationship to HLA and is often associated with hepatitis, dystrophy of dental enamel and nails, alopecia, vitiligo, and keratopathy and may be accompanied by hypofunction of the gonads, thyroid, pancreatic B cell, and gastric parietal cells. Autoantibodies against the cholesterol side-chain cleavage enzyme (P450scc, CYP11A1) and others have been described in patients with this disorder.

The more common presentation of autoimmune adrenocortical insufficiency is associated with HLA-related disorders including type I diabetes mellitus, autoimmune thyroid disease, alopecia areata, vitiligo, and celiac sprue. This disorder is often referred to as polyglandular autoimmune syndrome type II (or Schmidt's syndrome). The genetic susceptibility to this disorder is linked to HLA-DR3 or DR4 (or both). These patients have antiadrenal cytoplasmic antibodies that may be important in the pathogenesis of this disorder, and autoantibodies directed against 21α-hydroxylase (P450c21, CYP21A2) have recently been identified. (See Chapter 4.)

B. Adrenal Hemorrhage

Bilateral adrenal hemorrhage is now a relatively common cause of adrenal insufficiency in the United States. The diagnosis is usually made in critically ill patients in whom a CT scan of the abdomen is done. Bilateral adrenal enlargement is found, leading to an assessment of adrenocortical function. Anatomic factors predispose the adrenal glands to hemorrhage. The adrenal glands have a rich arterial blood supply, but they are drained by a single vein. Adrenal vein thrombosis may occur during periods of stasis or turbulence, thereby increasing adrenal vein pressure and resulting in a "vascular dam." This causes hemorrhage into the gland and is followed by adrenocortical insufficiency.

Most patients with adrenal hemorrhage have been taking anticoagulant therapy for an underlying coagulopathy or are predisposed to thrombosis. Heparin-induced thrombocytopenia syndrome may be accompanied by adrenal vein thrombosis and hemorrhage. The primary antiphospholipid antibody syndrome (lupus anticoagulant) has emerged as one of the more common causes of adrenal hemorrhage.

C. Infections

Although tuberculosis may represent a common cause of primary adrenal insufficiency in the rest of the world, it is a rare cause of this problem in the United States. Clinically significant adrenal insufficiency appears to occur in only about 5% of patients with disseminated tuberculosis. With the use of antituberculous chemotherapy, it may even be reversible if detected in early stages. It is important to recognize that rifampin may accelerate the metabolic clearance of cortisol, thereby increasing the replacement dose needed in these patients.

Most if not all systemic fungal infections can involve and destroy the adrenal cortex. Histoplasmosis is the most common fungal infection causing adrenal hypofunction in the United States. Of note, the antifungal agent ketoconazole inhibits adrenal cytochrome P450 steroidogenic enzymes which are essential for cortisol biosynthesis. Thus, ketoconazole treatment in patients with marginal adrenocortical reserve due to fungal disease may precipitate adrenal crisis.

AIDS has been associated with pathologic involvement of the adrenal gland. Although adrenal necrosis is commonly seen in postmortem examination of patients with AIDS, primary adrenal insufficiency appears to complicate only approximately 5% of patients with this disorder. Primary adrenal insufficiency in AIDS is usually caused by opportunistic infections such as cytomegalovirus and tuberculosis. Adrenocortical insufficiency usually occurs as a late manifestation in AIDS patients with very low CD4 counts. (See Chapter 25.)

D. ADRENOLEUKODYSTROPHY

X-linked adrenoleukodystrophy is an important cause of adrenal insufficiency in men. This disorder represents two distinct entities that may cause malfunction of the adrenal cortex and demyelination in the central nervous system. These disorders are characterized by abnormally high levels of very long chain fatty acids (VLCFAs) due to their defective beta oxidation within peroxisomes. The abnormal accumulation of VLCFAs in the brain, adrenal cortex, testes, and liver result in the clinical manifestations of this disorder.

Adrenoleukodystrophy has an incidence of approximately one in 25,000 and is an X-linked disorder (chromosome Xq28) with incomplete penetrance. Molecular analysis is available clinically and can be used both in family screening and in prenatal evaluation. Two clinical phenotypes have been described. Cerebral adrenoleukodystrophy usually presents in childhood, and its neurologic symptoms include cognitive dysfunction, behavioral problems, emotional lability, and visual and gate disturbances. It may progress to dementia. Because 30% of these patients develop adrenal insufficiency before the onset of neurologic symptoms, a young man with primary adrenal insufficiency should always be screened for adrenoleukodystrophy. A clinically milder phenotype, adrenomyeloneuropathy, usually presents in the second to fourth decades of life. Spinal cord and peripheral nerve demyelination occur over years and may result in loss of ambulation, cognitive dysfunction, urinary retention, and impotence. Once again, adrenal insufficiency may occur before the onset of neurologic symptoms.

The diagnosis of adrenoleukodystrophy can be confirmed by demonstration of the defect in fatty acid metabolism with the abnormal accumulation of saturated VLCFAs, especially C26:0 fatty acid.

E. METASTATIC ADRENAL DISEASE

There is a common misconception that metastatic cancer to the adrenal glands rarely causes adrenal insufficiency. Prospective studies show that approximately 20% of patients with adrenal metastasis have a subnormal cortisol response to ACTH. The adrenal glands are common sites of metastasis for lung, gastrointestinal, breast, and renal neoplasia. In addition, non-Hodgkin's and Hodgkin's lymphoma may present with involvement of the adrenal glands, primary adrenal insufficiency, and bilateral adrenal enlargement.

F. FAMILIAL GLUCOCORTICOID DEFICIENCY

Familial glucocorticoid deficiency is a rare disorder in which there is hereditary adrenocortical unresponsiveness to ACTH. This leads to adrenal insufficiency with subnormal glucocorticoid and adrenal androgen secretion as well as elevated plasma ACTH levels. As a rule, aldosterone secretion is preserved. At least two distinct types of this disorder have been described. One type is associated with mutations in the ACTH receptor on the cells of the adrenal cortex. Another type is often associated with achalasia and alacrima (Allgrove's syndrome; triple A syndrome) and progressive neurologic impairment, but no mutations in the ACTH receptor have been seen in these patients. The responsible gene is on chromosome 12 (12q13) and encodes a protein belonging to the WD repeat proteins. Its function remains unknown.

G. CORTISOL RESISTANCE

Primary cortisol resistance is an unusual disorder representing target cell resistance to cortisol due to either qualitative or quantitative abnormalities of glucocorticoid receptor. This disorder is characterized by hypercortisolism without clinical manifestations of glucocorticoid excess. Pituitary resistance to cortisol results in hypersecretion of ACTH, which stimulates the adrenal gland to produce excessive amounts of cortisol, mineralocorticoids and adrenal androgens. The increased production of these nonglucocorticoid adrenal steroids may cause hypertension, hypokalemia, virilization, and sexual precocity. Because cortisol is essential for life, this disorder actually represents partial rather than complete resistance.

H. OTHER CAUSES OF ADRENAL INSUFFICIENCY

Drugs associated with primary adrenal insufficiency include the antifungal agent ketoconazole and the antiparasitic agent suramin as well as the steroid synthesis inhibitors aminoglutethimide and metyrapone. Critically ill patients with severe inflammatory disorders (eg, septic shock) may have relatively low cortisol levels. Neither the pathogenesis nor the clinical significance of the finding is clear.

Pathophysiology

Loss of more than 90% of both adrenal cortices results in the clinical manifestations of adrenocortical insufficiency. Gradual destruction such as occurs in the idiopathic and invasive forms of the disease leads to chronic adrenocortical insufficiency. However, more rapid destruction occurs in many cases; about 25% of patients are in crisis or impending crisis at the time of diagnosis. With gradual adrenocortical destruction, the initial phase is that of decreased adrenal reserve; ie, basal steroid secretion is normal, but secretion does not increase in response to stress. Thus, acute adrenal crisis can be precipitated by the stresses of surgery, trauma, or infection, which require increased corticosteroid secretion. With further loss of cortical tissue, even basal secretion of mineralocorticoids and glucocorticoids becomes deficient, leading to the manifestations of chronic adrenocortical insufficiency. Destruction of the adrenals by hemorrhage results in sudden loss of both glucocorticoid and mineralocorticoid secretion, accompanied by acute adrenal crisis.

With decreasing cortisol secretion, plasma levels of ACTH are increased because of decreased negative feedback inhibition of their secretion. In fact, an elevation of plasma ACTH is the earliest and most sensitive indication of suboptimal adrenocortical reserve.

Clinical Features

A. SYMPTOMS AND SIGNS

Cortisol deficiency causes weakness, fatigue, anorexia, nausea and vomiting, hypotension, hyponatremia, and hypoglycemia. Mineralocorticoid deficiency produces renal sodium wasting and potassium retention and can lead to severe dehydration, hypotension, hyponatremia, hyperkalemia, and acidosis.

1. Chronic primary adrenocortical insufficiency— The chief symptoms (Table 9–4) are hyperpigmentation, weakness and fatigue, weight loss, anorexia, and gastrointestinal disturbances.

Hyperpigmentation is the classic physical finding, and its presence in association with the above manifestations should suggest primary adrenocortical insufficiency. Generalized hyperpigmentation of the skin and mucous membranes is one of the earliest manifestation of Addison's disease. It is increased in sun-exposed areas and accentuated over pressure areas such as the knuckles, toes, elbows, and knees. It is accompanied by increased numbers of black or dark-brown freckles. The classic hyperpigmentation of the buccal mucosa and gums is preceded by generalized hyperpigmentation of the skin; adrenal insufficiency should also be suspected when there is increased pigmentation of the palmar creases, nail beds, nipples, areolae, and perivaginal and perianal mucosa. Scars that have formed after the onset of ACTH excess become hyperpigmented, whereas older ones do not.

General weakness, fatigue and malaise, anorexia, and weight loss are invariable features of the disorder. Weight loss may reach 15 kg with progressive adrenal failure. Gastrointestinal disturbances, especially nausea and vomiting, occur in most patients; diarrhea is less frequent. An increase in gastrointestinal symptoms during an acute adrenal crisis may confuse the diagnosis by suggesting a primary intra-abdominal process.

Hypotension is present in about 90% of patients and is accompanied by orthostatic symptoms and occasionally syncope. In more severe chronic cases and in acute crises, recumbent hypotension or shock is almost invariably present. Vitiligo occurs in 4–17% of patients with autoimmune Addison's disease but is rare in Addison's disease due to other causes. Salt craving occurs in about 20% of patients.

Severe hypoglycemia may occur in children. This finding is unusual in adults but may be provoked by fasting, fever, infection, or nausea and vomiting, especially in acute adrenal crisis. Hypoglycemia occurs more commonly in secondary adrenal insufficiency.

Amenorrhea is common in Addison's disease. It may be due to weight loss and chronic illness or to primary ovarian failure. Loss of axillary and pubic hair may occur in women as a result of decreased secretion of adrenal androgens.

2. Acute adrenal crisis—Acute adrenal crisis represents a state of acute adrenocortical insufficiency and occurs in patients with Addison's disease who are exposed to the stress of infection, trauma, surgery, or dehydration due to salt deprivation, vomiting, or diarrhea.

The symptoms are listed in Table 9–5. Anorexia and nausea and vomiting increase and worsen the volume depletion and dehydration. Hypovolemic shock frequently occurs, and adrenal insufficiency should be considered in any patient with unexplained vascular collapse. Abdominal pain may occur and mimic an acute abdominal emergency. Weakness, apathy, and confusion are usual. Fever is usual and may be due to infection or to hypoadrenalism per se. Hyperpigmentation is present unless the onset of adrenal insufficiency is rapid and should suggest the diagnosis.

Table 9–4. Clinical features of primary adrenocortical insufficiency.[1]

	Percent
Weakness, fatigue, anorexia, weight loss	100
Hyperpigmentation	92
Hypotension	88
Gastrointestinal disturbances	56
Salt craving	19
Postural symptoms	12

[1]Reproduced, with permission, from Baxter JD, Tyrrell JB, in: *Endocrinology and Metabolism.* Felig P, Baxter JD, Frohman LA (editors). 3rd ed. McGraw-Hill, 1995.

Table 9–5. Clinical features of adrenal hemorrhage.[1]

	Percent
General features	
Hypotension and shock	74
Fever	59
Nausea and vomiting	46
Confusion, disorientation	41
Tachycardia	28
Cyanosis or lividity	28
Local features	
Abdominal, flank, or back pain	77
Abdominal or flank tenderness	38
Abdominal distention	28
Abdominal rigidity	20
Chest pain	13
Rebound tenderness	5

[1]Reproduced, with permission, from Baxter JD, Tyrrell JB, in: *Endocrinology and Metabolism.* Felig P, Baxter JD, Frohman LA (editors). 3rd ed. McGraw-Hill, 1995.

Additional findings that suggest the diagnosis are hyponatremia, hyperkalemia, lymphocytosis, eosinophilia, and hypoglycemia.

Shock and coma may rapidly lead to death in untreated patients. (See Chapter 24.)

3. Acute adrenal hemorrhage—(See Table 9–6.) Bilateral adrenal hemorrhage and acute adrenal destruction in an already compromised patient with major medical illness follow a progressively deteriorating course. The usual manifestations are abdominal, flank, or back pain and abdominal tenderness. Abdominal distention, rigidity, and rebound tenderness are less frequent. Hypotension, shock, fever, nausea and vomiting, confusion, and disorientation are common; tachycardia and cyanosis are less frequent.

With progression, severe hypotension, volume depletion, dehydration, hyperpyrexia, cyanosis, coma, and death ensue.

Table 9–6. Clinical features of acute adrenal crisis.

Hypotension and shock
Fever
Dehydration, volume depletion
Nausea, vomiting, anorexia
Weakness, apathy, depressed mentation
Hypoglycemia

The diagnosis of acute adrenal hemorrhage should be considered in the deteriorating patient with unexplained abdominal or flank pain, vascular collapse, hyperpyrexia, or hypoglycemia.

B. LABORATORY AND ELECTROCARDIOGRAPHIC FINDINGS AND IMAGING STUDIES

1. Gradual adrenal destruction—Hyponatremia and hyperkalemia are classic manifestations of the glucocorticoid and mineralocorticoid deficiency of primary adrenal insufficiency and should suggest the diagnosis. Hematologic manifestations include normocytic, normochromic anemia, neutropenia, eosinophilia, and a relative lymphocytosis. Azotemia with increased concentrations of blood urea nitrogen and serum creatinine is due to volume depletion and dehydration. Mild acidosis is frequently present. Hypercalcemia of mild to moderate degree occurs in about 6% of patients.

Abdominal radiographs reveal adrenal calcification in half the patients with tuberculous Addison's disease and in some patients with other invasive or hemorrhagic causes of adrenal insufficiency. Computed tomography (CT scan) is a more sensitive detector of adrenal calcification and adrenal enlargement. Bilateral adrenal enlargement in association with adrenal insufficiency may be seen with tuberculosis, fungal infections, cytomegalovirus, malignant and nonmalignant infiltrative diseases, and adrenal hemorrhage.

Electrocardiographic features are low voltage, a vertical QRS axis, and nonspecific ST–T wave abnormalities secondary to abnormal electrolytes.

2. Acute adrenal hemorrhage—Hyponatremia and hyperkalemia occur in only a small number of cases, but azotemia is a usual finding. Increased circulating eosinophils may suggest the diagnosis. The diagnosis is frequently established only when imaging studies reveal bilateral adrenal enlargement.

SECONDARY ADRENOCORTICAL INSUFFICIENCY

Etiology

Secondary adrenocortical insufficiency due to ACTH deficiency is most commonly a result of exogenous glucocorticoid therapy. Pituitary or hypothalamic tumors are the most common causes of naturally occurring pituitary ACTH hyposecretion. These and other less common causes are reviewed in Chapter 5.

Pathophysiology

ACTH deficiency is the primary event and leads to decreased cortisol and adrenal androgen secretion. Aldosterone secretion remains normal except in a few cases.

In the early stages, basal ACTH and cortisol levels may be normal; however, ACTH reserve is impaired, and ACTH and cortisol responses to stress are therefore subnormal. With further loss of basal ACTH secretion, there is atrophy of the zonae fasciculata and reticularis of the adrenal cortex; and, therefore, basal cortisol secretion is decreased. At this stage, the entire pituitary adrenal axis is impaired; ie, there is not only decreased ACTH responsiveness to stress but also decreased adrenal responsiveness to acute stimulation with exogenous ACTH.

The manifestations of glucocorticoid deficiency are similar to those described for primary adrenocortical insufficiency. However, since aldosterone secretion by the zona glomerulosa is usually preserved, the manifestations of mineralocorticoid deficiency are absent.

Clinical Features

A. SYMPTOMS AND SIGNS

Secondary adrenal insufficiency is usually chronic, and the manifestations may be nonspecific. However, acute crisis can occur in undiagnosed patients or in corticosteroid-treated patients who do not receive increased steroid dosage during periods of stress.

The clinical features of secondary adrenal insufficiency differ from those of primary adrenocortical insufficiency in that pituitary secretion of ACTH is deficient and hyperpigmentation is therefore not present. In addition, mineralocorticoid secretion is usually normal. Thus, the clinical features of ACTH and glucocorticoid deficiency are nonspecific.

Volume depletion, dehydration, and hyperkalemia are usually absent. Hypotension is usually not present except in acute presentations. Hyponatremia may occur as a result of water retention and inability to excrete a water load but is not accompanied by hyperkalemia. Prominent features are weakness, lethargy, easy fatigability, anorexia, nausea, and occasionally vomiting. Arthralgias and myalgias also occur. Hypoglycemia is occasionally the presenting feature. Acute decompensation with severe hypotension or shock unresponsive to vasopressors may occur.

B. ASSOCIATED FEATURES

Patients with secondary adrenal insufficiency commonly have additional features that suggest the diagnosis. A history of glucocorticoid therapy or, if this is not available, the presence of cushingoid features suggests prior glucocorticoid use. Hypothalamic or pituitary tumors leading to ACTH deficiency usually cause loss of other pituitary hormones (hypogonadism and hypothyroidism). Hypersecretion of GH or prolactin (PRL) from a pituitary adenoma may be present.

C. LABORATORY FINDINGS

Findings on routine laboratory examination consist of normochromic, normocytic anemia, neutropenia, lymphocytosis, and eosinophilia. Hyponatremia is not uncommon and may be the presenting laboratory abnormality. Hyponatremia is due to the lack of glucocorticoid negative feedback on AVP as well as the reduction in glomerular filtration associated with hypocortisolism. Serum potassium, creatinine, and bicarbonate and blood urea nitrogen are usually normal; plasma glucose may be low, though severe hypoglycemia is unusual.

DIAGNOSIS OF ADRENOCORTICAL INSUFFICIENCY

Although the diagnosis of adrenal insufficiency should be confirmed by assessment of the pituitary adrenal axis, therapy should not be delayed nor should the patient be subjected to procedures that may increase volume loss and dehydration and further contribute to hypotension. If the patient is acutely ill, therapy should be instituted and the diagnosis established when the patient is stable.

Diagnostic Tests

Since basal levels of adrenocortical steroids in either urine or plasma may be normal in partial adrenal insufficiency, tests of adrenocortical reserve are necessary to establish the diagnosis (Figure 9–10). These tests are described in the section on laboratory evaluation and in Chapter 5.

Rapid ACTH Stimulation Test

The rapid ACTH stimulation test assesses adrenal reserve and is the initial procedure in the assessment of possible adrenal insufficiency, either primary or secondary. As previously discussed, the low-dose ACTH (1 μg cosyntropin) stimulation test has been shown to represent a more physiologic stimulus to the adrenal cortex and may emerge as a more sensitive indicator of suboptimal adrenal function.

Subnormal responses to exogenous ACTH administration are an indication of decreased adrenal reserve and establish the diagnosis of adrenocortical insufficiency. Further diagnostic procedures are not required, since subnormal responses to the rapid ACTH stimulation test indicate lack of responsiveness to metyrapone, insulin-induced hypoglycemia, or stress. However, this test does not permit differentiation of primary and secondary causes. This is best accomplished by measurement of basal plasma ACTH levels, as discussed below.

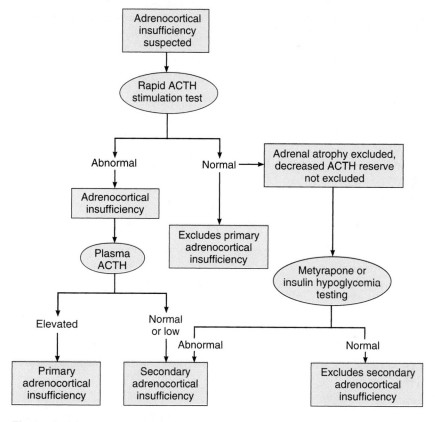

Figure 9–10. Evaluation of suspected primary or secondary adrenocortical insufficiency. Boxes enclose clinical decisions, and circles enclose diagnostic tests. (Redrawn and reproduced, with permission, from Miller WL, Tyrrell JB: The adrenal cortex. In: *Endocrinology and Metabolism.* Felig P et al [editors]. McGraw-Hill, 1995.)

A normal response to the rapid ACTH stimulation test excludes primary adrenal failure, since a normal cortisol response indicates normal cortical function. However, normal responsiveness does not exclude partial secondary adrenocortical insufficiency in those few patients with decreased pituitary reserve and decreased stress responsiveness of the hypothalamic-pituitary-adrenal axis who maintain sufficient basal ACTH secretion to prevent adrenocortical atrophy. If this situation is suspected clinically, pituitary ACTH responsiveness may be tested directly with metyrapone or insulin-induced hypoglycemia. (See section on laboratory evaluation and below.)

Plasma ACTH Levels

If adrenal insufficiency is present, plasma ACTH levels are used to differentiate primary and secondary forms. In patients with primary adrenal insufficiency, plasma ACTH levels exceed the upper limit of the normal range (> 52 pg/mL [11 pmol/L]) and usually exceed 200 pg/mL (44 pmol/L). Plasma ACTH concentration is "normal" or less than 10 pg/mL (2.2 pmol/L) in patients with secondary adrenal insufficiency (Figure 9–11). However, the basal ACTH level must always be interpreted in light of the clinical situation, especially because of the episodic nature of ACTH secretion and its short plasma half-life. For example, ACTH levels will frequently exceed the normal range during the recovery of the hypothalamic-pituitary-adrenal (HPA) axis from secondary adrenal insufficiency and may be confused with levels seen in primary adrenal insufficiency. Patients with primary adrenal insufficiency consistently have elevated ACTH levels. In fact, the ACTH concentration will be elevated early in the course of adrenal insufficiency even before a significant reduction in the basal cortisol level or its response to exogenous ACTH occurs. Therefore, plasma ACTH measure-

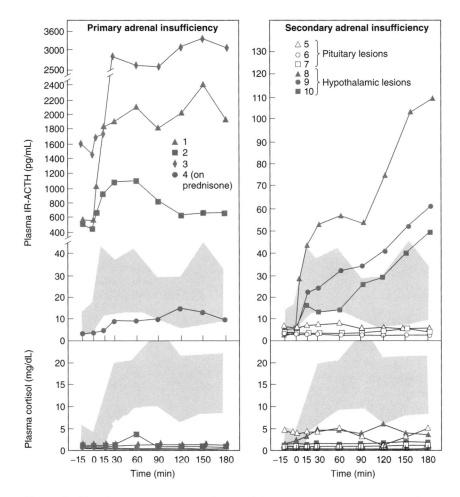

Figure 9–11. Plasma ACTH (top) and cortisol (bottom) responses to CRH in subjects with primary adrenal insufficiency (left) or secondary adrenal insufficiency (right). Patients with hypothalamic lesions had clearly distinct ACTH responses to CRH, different from those in three patients with pituitary adrenal insufficiency. **Shaded area:** Absolute range from 15 normal subjects. (IR-ACTH, ACTH by IRMA.) (Reproduced, with permission, from Schulte HM et al: The corticotropin-releasing hormone stimulation test: A possible aid in the evaluation of patients with adrenal insufficiency. J Clin Endocrinol Metab 1984;58:1064.)

ments serve as a valuable screening study for primary adrenal insufficiency.

Partial ACTH Deficiency

When partial ACTH deficiency and decreased pituitary reserve are suspected despite normal responsiveness to the rapid ACTH stimulation test, the following procedures may be used for more direct assessment of hypothalamic-pituitary function:

A. METHODS OF TESTING

The overnight metyrapone test is used in patients with suspected hypothalamic or pituitary disorders when hypoglycemia is contraindicated and in those with prior glucocorticoid therapy. Insulin-induced hypoglycemia is used in patients with suspected hypothalamic or pituitary tumors, since both ACTH and GH responsiveness can be assessed (see Chapter 5).

B. INTERPRETATION

A normal response to either metyrapone or hypoglycemia excludes secondary adrenocortical insufficiency. (See section on laboratory evaluation.) Subnormal responses, in the presence of a normal response to ACTH administration, establish the diagnosis of secondary adrenal insufficiency.

TREATMENT OF ADRENOCORTICAL INSUFFICIENCY

The aim of treatment of adrenocortical insufficiency is to produce levels of glucocorticoids and mineralocorticoids equivalent to those achieved in an individual with normal hypothalamic-pituitary-adrenal function under similar circumstances.

Acute Addisonian Crisis (Table 9–7)

Treatment for acute addisonian crisis should be instituted as soon as the diagnosis is suspected. Therapy includes administration of glucocorticoids; correction of dehydration, hypovolemia, and electrolyte abnormalities; general supportive measures; and treatment of coexisting or precipitating disorders.

A. CORTISOL (HYDROCORTISONE)

Parenteral cortisol in soluble form (hydrocortisone hemisuccinate or phosphate) is the glucocorticoid preparation most commonly used. When administered in supraphysiologic doses, hydrocortisone has sufficient sodium-retaining potency so that additional mineralocorticoid therapy is not required in patients with primary adrenocortical insufficiency.

Table 9–7. Treatment of acute adrenal crisis.

Glucocorticoid replacement
 (1) Administer hydrocortisone sodium phosphate or sodium succinate, 100 mg intravenously every 6 hours for 24 hours.
 (2) When the patient is stable, reduce the dosage to 50 mg every 6 hours.
 (3) Taper to maintenance therapy by day 4 or 5 and add mineralocorticoid therapy as required.
 (4) Maintain or increase the dose to 200–400 mg/d if complications persist or occur.
General and supportive measures
 (1) Correct volume depletion, dehydration, and hypoglycemia with intravenous saline and glucose.
 (2) Evaluate and correct infection and other precipitating factors.

Cortisol in doses of 100 mg intravenously is given every 6 hours for the first 24 hours. The response to therapy is usually rapid, with improvement occurring within 12 hours or less. If improvement occurs and the patient is stable, 50 mg every 6 hours is given on the second day, and in most patients the dosage may then be gradually reduced to approximately 10 mg three times daily by the fourth or fifth day. (See section on maintenance therapy, below.)

1. In severely ill patients, especially in those with additional major complications (eg, sepsis), higher cortisol doses (100 mg intravenously every 6–8 hours) are maintained until the patient is stable.

2. In primary Addison's disease, mineralocorticoid replacement, in the form of fludrocortisone (see below), is added when the total cortisol dosage has been reduced to 50–60 mg/d.

3. In secondary adrenocortical insufficiency with acute crisis, the primary requirement is glucocorticoid replacement and is satisfactorily supplied by the administration of cortisol, as outlined above. If the possibility of excessive fluid and sodium retention in such patients is of concern, equivalent parenteral doses of synthetic steroids such as prednisolone or dexamethasone may be substituted.

4. Intramuscular cortisone acetate is contraindicated in acute adrenal failure for the following reasons: (1) absorption is slow; (2) it requires conversion to cortisol in the liver; (3) adequate plasma levels of cortisol are not obtained; and (4) there is inadequate suppression of plasma ACTH levels, indicating insufficient glucocorticoid activity.

B. INTRAVENOUS FLUIDS

Intravenous glucose and saline are administered to correct volume depletion, hypotension, and hypoglycemia. Volume deficits may be severe in Addison's disease, and hypotension and shock may not respond to vasopressors unless glucocorticoids are administered. Hyperkalemia and acidosis are usually corrected with cortisol and volume replacement; however, an occasional patient may require specific therapy for these abnormalities. (See also Chapter 24.)

Maintenance Therapy (Table 9–8)

Patients with Addison's disease require life-long glucocorticoid and mineralocorticoid therapy. Cortisol (hydrocortisone) is the glucocorticoid preparation of first choice. The basal production rate of cortisol is approximately $8–12$ $mg/m^2/d$. The maintenance dose of hydrocortisone is usually 15–30 mg daily in adults. The oral dose is usually divided into 10–20 mg in the morning on arising and 5–10 mg later in the day. Cortisol in

Table 9–8. Regimen for maintenance therapy of primary adrenocortical insufficiency.[1]

---

(1) Hydrocortisone, 15–20 mg in AM and 10 mg orally at 4–5 PM.
(2) Fludrocortisone, 0.05–0.1 mg orally in AM.
(3) Clinical follow-up: Maintenance of normal weight, blood pressure, and electrolytes with regression of clinical features.
(4) Patient education plus identification card or bracelet.
(5) Increased hydrocortisone dosage during "stress."

---

[1]Reproduced, with permission, from Miller WL, Tyrrell JB, in: *Endocrinology and Metabolism,* 3rd ed. Felig P, Baxter JD, Frohman LA (editors). McGraw-Hill, 1995.

twice-daily doses gives satisfactory responses in most patients; however, some patients may require only a single morning dose, and others may require three doses daily to maintain well-being and normal energy levels. Insomnia is a side effect of glucocorticoid administration and can usually be prevented by administering the last dose at 4:00–5:00 PM.

Fludrocortisone (9α-fluorocortisol) is used for mineralocorticoid therapy; the usual doses are 0.05–0.2 mg/d orally in the morning. Because of the long half-life of this agent, divided doses are not required. About 10% of addisonian patients can be managed with cortisol and adequate dietary sodium intake alone and do not require fludrocortisone.

Secondary adrenocortical insufficiency is treated with the cortisol dosages described above for the primary form. Fludrocortisone is rarely required. The recovery of normal function of the hypothalamic-pituitary-adrenal axis following suppression by exogenous glucocorticoids may take weeks to years, and its duration is not readily predictable. Consequently, prolonged replacement therapy may be required. Recent studies have pointed to the potential benefits of DHEA in doses of 50 mg/d in terms of improvement in well-being.

Response to Therapy

General clinical signs, such as good appetite and sense of well-being, are the guides to the adequacy of replacement. Obviously, signs of Cushing's syndrome indicate overtreatment. It is generally expected that the daily dose of hydrocortisone should be doubled during periods of minor stress, and the dose needs to be increased to as much as 200–300 mg/d during periods of major stress, such as a surgical procedure. Patients receiving excessive doses of glucocorticoids are also at risk for increased bone loss and clinically significant osteoporosis. Therefore, the replacement dose of glucocorticoid

should be maintained at the lowest amount needed to provide the patient with a proper sense of well-being. Traditionally, assessment of the adequacy of glucocorticoid replacement has involved clinical, but not biochemical measures. Two major factors have prompted a reassessment of this issue. First, there is a greater appreciation of the potential risks of overtreatment or undertreatment. Recent evidence suggests that subclinical Cushing's syndrome associated with adrenal incidentalomas contributes to poor control of blood sugar and blood pressure in diabetic patients, decreased bone density, and increased serum lipid levels. The levels of cortisol secretion by many incidentalomas are similar to those observed in patients with adrenal insufficiency receiving mild cortisol overreplacement. In addition, studies in patients receiving glucocorticoid replacement therapy demonstrate an inverse relationship between dose and bone mineral density and a positive correlation between dose and markers of bone resorption. Second, there is recognition that there is considerable variation among individuals in terms of the plasma levels of cortisol achieved with orally administered hydrocortisone or cortisol.

The measurement of urine free cortisol does not provide a reliable index for appropriate glucocorticoid replacement. Similarly, ACTH measurements are not a good indication of the adequacy of glucocorticoid replacement; marked elevations of plasma ACTH in patients with chronic adrenal insufficiency are often not suppressed into the normal range despite adequate hydrocortisone replacement. Plasma cortisol day curves—multiple samples for plasma cortisol concentration—have been proposed but not yet widely adopted.

Adequate treatment results in the disappearance of weakness, malaise, and fatigue. Anorexia and other gastrointestinal symptoms resolve, and weight returns to normal. The hyperpigmentation invariably improves but may not entirely disappear. Inadequate cortisol administration leads to persistence of these symptoms of adrenal insufficiency, and excessive pigmentation will remain.

Adequate mineralocorticoid replacement may be determined by assessment of blood pressure and electrolyte composition. With adequate treatment, the blood pressure is normal without orthostatic change, and serum sodium and potassium remain within the normal range. Some endocrinologists monitor plasma renin activity (PRA) as an objective measure of fludrocortisone replacement. Upright PRA levels are usually < 5 ng/mL/h in adequately replaced patients. Hypertension and hypokalemia result if the fludrocortisone dose is excessive. Conversely, undertreatment may lead to fatigue and malaise, orthostatic symptoms, and subnormal supine or upright blood pressure, with hyperkalemia and hyponatremia.

Prevention of Adrenal Crisis

The development of acute adrenal insufficiency in previously diagnosed and treated patients is almost entirely preventable in cooperative individuals. The essential elements are patient education and increased glucocorticoid dosages during illness.

The patient should be informed about the necessity for lifelong therapy, the possible consequences of acute illness, and the necessity for increased therapy and medical assistance during acute illness. An identification card or bracelet should be carried or worn at all times.

The cortisol dose should be increased by the patient to 60–80 mg/d with the development of minor illnesses; the usual maintenance dosage may be resumed in 24–48 hours if improvement occurs. Increased mineralocorticoid therapy is not required.

If symptoms persist or become worse, the patient should continue increased cortisol doses and call the physician.

Vomiting may result in inability to ingest or absorb oral cortisol, and diarrhea in addisonian patients may precipitate a crisis because of rapid fluid and electrolyte losses. Patients must understand that if these symptoms occur, they should seek immediate medical assistance so that parenteral glucocorticoid therapy can be given.

Steroid Coverage for Surgery (Table 9–9)

The normal physiologic response to surgical stress involves an increase in cortisol secretion. The increased glucocorticoid activity may serve primarily to modulate the immunologic response to stress. Thus, patients with primary or secondary adrenocortical insufficiency scheduled for elective surgery require increased gluco-

Table 9–9. Steroid coverage for surgery.[1]

(1) Correct electrolytes, blood pressure, and hydration if necessary.
(2) Give hydrocortisone sodium phosphate or sodium succinate, 100 mg intramuscularly, on call to operating room.
(3) Give 50 mg intramuscularly or intravenously in the recovery room and then every 6 hours for the first 24 hours.
(4) If progress is satisfactory, reduce dosage to 25 mg every 6 hours for 24 hours and then taper to maintenance dosage over 3–5 days. Resume previous fludrocortisone dose when the patient is taking oral medications.
(5) Maintain or increase hydrocortisone dosage to 200–400 mg/d if fever, hypotension, or other complications occur.

[1]Reproduced, with permission, from Miller WL, Tyrrell JB, in: *Endocrinology and Metabolism*, 3rd ed. Felig P, Baxter JD, Frohman LA (editors). McGraw-Hill, 1995.

corticoid coverage. This problem is most frequently encountered in patients with pituitary-adrenal suppression due to exogenous glucocorticoid therapy. The principles of management are outlined in Table 9–9. **Note:** Intramuscular cortisone acetate should not be used, for the reasons discussed above in the section on treatment of acute addisonian crisis.

PROGNOSIS OF ADRENOCORTICAL INSUFFICIENCY

Before glucocorticoid and mineralocorticoid therapy became available, primary adrenocortical insufficiency was invariably fatal, with death usually occurring within 2 years after onset. Survival now depends upon the underlying cause of the adrenal insufficiency. In patients with autoimmune Addison's disease, survival approaches that of the normal population, and most patients lead normal lives. In general, death from adrenal insufficiency now occurs only in patients with rapid onset of disease who may die before the diagnosis is established and appropriate therapy started.

Secondary adrenal insufficiency has an excellent prognosis with glucocorticoid therapy.

Adrenal insufficiency due to bilateral adrenal hemorrhage is still often fatal, with most cases being recognized only at autopsy.

◼ CUSHING'S SYNDROME

Chronic glucocorticoid excess, whatever its cause, leads to the constellation of symptoms and physical features known as Cushing's syndrome. It is most commonly iatrogenic, resulting from chronic glucocorticoid therapy. "Spontaneous" Cushing's syndrome is caused by abnormalities of the pituitary or adrenal or may occur as a consequence of ACTH or CRH secretion by nonpituitary tumors (**ectopic ACTH syndrome; ectopic CRH syndrome**). Cushing's *disease* is defined as the specific type of Cushing's syndrome due to excessive pituitary ACTH secretion from a pituitary tumor. This section will review the various types of spontaneous Cushing's syndrome and discuss their diagnosis and therapy. (See also Chapter 5.)

Classification & Incidence

Cushing's syndrome is conveniently classified as either ACTH-dependent or ACTH-independent (Table 9–10).

The ACTH-dependent types of Cushing's syndrome—ectopic ACTH syndrome and Cushing's dis-

Table 9–10. Cushing's syndrome: differential diagnosis.

ACTH-dependent
   Pituitary adenoma (Cushing's disease)
   Nonpituitary neoplasm (ectopic ACTH)
ACTH-independent
   Iatrogenic (glucocorticoid, megestrol acetate)
   Adrenal neoplasm (adenoma, carcinoma)
   Nodular adrenal hyperplasia
      Primary pigmented nodular adrenal disease
      Massive macronodular adrenonodular hyperplasia
      Food-dependent (GIP-mediated)
   Factitious

---

ease—are characterized by chronic ACTH hypersecretion, which results in hyperplasia of the adrenal zonae fasciculata and reticularis and therefore increased adrenocortical secretion of cortisol, androgens, and DOC.

ACTH-independent Cushing's syndrome may be caused by a primary adrenal neoplasm (adenoma or carcinoma) or nodular adrenal hyperplasia. In these cases, the cortisol excess suppresses pituitary ACTH secretion.

A. CUSHING'S DISEASE

This is the most frequent type of Cushing's syndrome and is responsible for about 70% of reported cases. Cushing's disease is much more common in women than in men (female:male ratio of about 8:1) and the age at diagnosis is usually 20–40 years but may range from childhood to 70 years.

B. ECTOPIC ACTH HYPERSECRETION

This disorder accounts for approximately 15–20% of patients with ACTH-dependent Cushing's syndrome. The production of ACTH from a tumor of nonpituitary origin may result in severe hypercortisolism, but many of these patients lack the classic features of glucocorticoid excess. This presumably reflects the acuteness of the clinical course in the ectopic ACTH syndrome. The clinical presentation of ectopic ACTH secretion is most frequently seen in patients with small cell carcinoma of the lung; this tumor is responsible for about 50% of cases of this syndrome, though ectopic ACTH hypersecretion is estimated to occur in only 0.5–2% of patients with small cell carcinoma. The prognosis in these patients is very poor, with a short mean survival. The ectopic ACTH syndrome may also present in a fashion identical to classic Cushing's disease and pose a challenging diagnostic dilemma. The majority of these tumors are also located in the lung (bronchial carcinoids) and may be radiologically inapparent at the time of the presentation. The ectopic ACTH syndrome is more common in men, and the peak age incidence is 40–60 years.

C. PRIMARY ADRENAL TUMORS

Primary adrenal tumors cause approximately 10% of cases of Cushing's syndrome. Most of these patients have benign adrenocortical adenomas. Adrenocortical carcinomas are uncommon, with an incidence of approximately 2 per million per year. Both adrenocortical adenomas and carcinomas are more common in women.

D. CHILDHOOD CUSHING'S SYNDROME

Cushing's syndrome in childhood and adolescence is distinctly unusual. However, in contrast to the incidence in adults, adrenal carcinoma is the most frequent cause (51%), and adrenal adenomas are present in 14%. These tumors are more common in girls than in boys, and most occur between the ages of 1 and 8 years. Cushing's disease is more common in the adolescent population and accounts for 35% of cases; most of these patients are over 10 years of age at diagnosis, and the sex incidence is equal.

Pathology

A. ANTERIOR PITUITARY GLAND

1. Pituitary adenomas—Pituitary adenomas are present in over 90% of patients with Cushing's disease. These tumors are typically smaller than those secreting GH or PRL; 80–90% are less than 10 mm in diameter. A small group of patients have larger tumors (> 10 mm); these macroadenomas are frequently invasive, leading to extension outside the sella turcica. Malignant pituitary tumors occur rarely.

Microadenomas are located within the anterior pituitary; they are not encapsulated but surrounded by a rim of compressed normal anterior pituitary cells. With routine histologic stains, these tumors are composed of compact sheets of well-granulated basophilic cells in a sinusoidal arrangement. ACTH, β-LPH, and β-endorphin have been demonstrated in these tumor cells by immunocytochemical methods. Larger tumors may appear chromophobic on routine histologic study; however, they also contain ACTH and its related peptides. These ACTH-secreting adenomas typically show Crooke's changes (a zone of perinuclear hyalinization that is the result of chronic exposure of corticotroph cells to hypercortisolism). Electron microscopy demonstrates secretory granules that vary in size from 200 to 700 nm. The number of granules varies in individual cells; they may be dispersed throughout the cytoplasm or concentrated along the cell membrane. A typical feature of these adenomas is the presence of bundles of perinuclear microfilaments (average 7 nm in diameter) surrounding the nucleus; these are responsible for Crooke's hyaline changes visible on light microscopy.

2. Hyperplasia—Diffuse hyperplasia of corticotroph cells has been reported rarely in patients with Cushing's disease.

3. Other conditions—In patients with adrenal tumors or ectopic ACTH syndrome, the pituitary corticotrophs show prominent Crooke hyaline changes and perinuclear microfilaments. The ACTH content of corticotroph cells is reduced consistent with their suppression by excessive cortisol secretion present in these conditions.

B. ADRENOCORTICAL HYPERPLASIA

Bilateral hyperplasia of the adrenal cortex occurs with chronic ACTH hypersecretion. Two types have been described: simple and bilateral nodular hyperplasia.

1. Simple adrenocortical hyperplasia—This condition is usually due to Cushing's disease. Combined adrenal weight (normal, 8–10 g) is modestly increased, ranging from 12 g to 24 g. On histologic study, there is equal hyperplasia of the compact cells of the zona reticularis and the clear cells of the zona fasciculata; consequently, the width of the cortex is increased. Electron microscopy reveals normal ultrastructural features. When ACTH levels are very high as in the **ectopic ACTH syndrome**, the adrenals are frequently larger, with combined weights up to or more than 50 g. The characteristic microscopic feature is marked hyperplasia of the zona reticularis; columns of compact reticularis cells expand throughout the zona fasciculata and into the zona glomerulosa. The zona fasciculata clear cells are markedly reduced.

2. Bilateral nodular hyperplasia—Bilateral nodular hyperplasia with Cushing's syndrome has been identified as a morphologic consequence of several unique pathophysiologic disorders. Long-standing ACTH hypersecretion—either pituitary or nonpituitary—may result in nodular enlargement of the adrenal gland. These focal nodules are often mistaken for adrenal neoplasms and have led to unnecessary as well as unsuccessful unilateral adrenal surgery. In occasional cases these nodules may, over a period of time, even become autonomous or semiautonomous. Removal of the ACTH-secreting neoplasm will result in regression of the adrenal nodules as well as resolution of hypercortisolism unless the nodules have already developed significant autonomy.

Several types of ACTH-independent nodular adrenal hyperplasia have been described. Bilateral macronodular adrenal hyperplasia (and occasionally a unilateral adrenocortical tumor) may be under the control of abnormal or ectopic hormone receptors. Aberrant regulation of cortisol production and adrenal growth have been shown in some of these patients to be mediated by the abnormal adrenal expression of receptors for a variety of hormones. The best-characterized appears to be the expression of glucose-dependent insulinotropic polypeptide (GIP), whose adrenal expression has resulted in the modulation of cortisol production after physiologic postprandial fluctuation of endogenous levels of GIP, causing a state of "food-dependent Cushing's syndrome." Other abnormal hormone receptors that have been described in association with endogenous hypercortisolism with this phenomenon include vasopressin, beta-adrenergic agonists, hCG-LH, and serotonin. The identification of an abnormal adrenal receptor raises the possibility of new pharmacologic approaches to control of hypercortisolism by suppressing the endogenous ligands or by blocking the abnormal receptor with specific antagonists.

Another unusual adrenal-dependent cause of Cushing's syndrome associated with bilateral adrenal nodular hyperplasia has been referred to as primary pigmented nodular adrenocortical disease. This is a familial disorder with an autosomal dominant inheritance pattern usually presenting in adolescence or young adulthood. The disorder is associated with unusual conditions such as myxomas (cardiac, cutaneous, and mammary), spotty skin pigmentation, endocrine overactivity, sexual precocity, acromegaly, and schwannomas—the Carney complex. Activating mutations in protein kinase A have recently been shown to be present in many of these patients. Interestingly, the adrenal glands in this syndrome are often small or normal in size and have multiple black and brown nodules with intranodular cortical atrophy.

Finally, in McCune-Albright syndrome, activating mutations of $G_s\alpha$ leads to constitutive steroidogenesis in adrenal nodules carrying the mutation.

C. ADRENAL TUMORS

Adrenal tumors causing Cushing's syndrome are independent of ACTH secretion and are either adenomas or carcinomas.

1. Glucocorticoid-secreting adrenal adenomas—These adenomas are encapsulated, weigh 10–70 g, and range in size from 1 cm to 6 cm. Microscopically, clear cells of the zona fasciculata type predominate, although cells typical of the zona reticularis are also seen.

2. Adrenal carcinomas—Adrenal carcinomas are usually > 4 cm when diagnosed and often weigh over 100 g, occasionally exceeding 1 kg. They may be palpable as abdominal masses. Grossly, they are encapsulated and highly vascular; necrosis, hemorrhage, and cystic degeneration are common, and areas of calcification may be present. The histologic appearance of these carcinomas varies considerably; they may appear to be benign or may exhibit considerable pleomorphism. Vascular or capsular invasion is predictive of malignant behavior, as is local extension. These carcinomas invade local structures (kidney, liver, and retroperitoneum) and metastasize hematogenously to liver and lung.

3. Uninvolved adrenal cortex—The cortex contiguous to the tumor and that of the contralateral gland are atrophic in the presence of functioning adrenal adenomas and carcinomas. The cortex is markedly thinned, whereas the capsule is thickened. Histologically, the zona reticularis is virtually absent; the remaining cortex is composed of clear fasciculata cells. The architecture of the zona glomerulosa is normal.

Etiology & Pathogenesis

A. CUSHING'S DISEASE

The causes and natural history of Cushing's disease are reviewed in Chapter 5. Current evidence is consistent with the view that spontaneously arising corticotroph-cell pituitary adenomas are the primary cause and that the consequent ACTH hypersecretion and hypercortisolism lead to the characteristic endocrine abnormalities and hypothalamic dysfunction. This is supported by evidence showing that selective removal of these adenomas by pituitary microsurgery reverses the abnormalities and is followed by return of the hypothalamic-pituitary-adrenal axis to normal. In addition, molecular studies have shown that nearly all corticotroph adenomas are monoclonal.

Although these primary pituitary adenomas are responsible for the great majority of cases, a few patients have been described in whom pituitary disease has been limited to corticotroph-cell hyperplasia; these may be secondary to excessive CRH secretion by rare, benign hypothalamic gangliocytoma.

B. ECTOPIC ACTH SYNDROME AND ECTOPIC CRH SYNDROME

Ectopic ACTH syndrome arises when nonpituitary tumors synthesize and hypersecrete biologically active ACTH. The related peptides β-LPH and β-endorphin are also synthesized and secreted, as are inactive ACTH fragments. Production of CRH has also been demonstrated in ectopic tumors secreting ACTH, but whether CRH plays a role in pathogenesis is unclear. A few cases in which nonpituitary tumors produced only CRH have been reported.

Ectopic ACTH syndrome occurs predominantly in only a few tumor types (Table 9–11); small cell carcinoma of the lung causes half of cases. Other tumors causing the syndrome are carcinoid tumors of lung, thymus, gut, pancreas, or ovary; pancreatic islet cell tumors; medullary thyroid carcinoma; and pheochromocytoma and related tumors. Other rare miscellaneous tumor types have also been reported (see Chapter 21).

Table 9–11. Tumors causing the ectopic ACTH syndrome.[1]

Small cell carcinoma of the lung (50% of cases)
Pancreatic islet cell tumors
Carcinoid tumors (lung, thymus, gut, pancreas, ovary)
Medullary carcinoma of the thyroid
Pheochromocytoma and related tumors

[1]Modified and reproduced, with permission, from Miller WL, Tyrrell JB, in: *Endocrinology and Metabolism,* 3rd ed. Felig P, Baxter JD, Frohman LA (editors). McGraw-Hill, 1995.

C. ADRENAL TUMORS

Glucocorticoid-producing adrenal adenomas and carcinomas arise spontaneously. They are not under hypothalamic-pituitary control and autonomously secrete adrenocortical steroids. Rarely, adrenal carcinomas develop in the setting of chronic ACTH hypersecretion in patients with either Cushing's disease and nodular adrenal hyperplasia or congenital adrenal hyperplasia.

Pathophysiology (Table 9–11, Figure 9–12)

A. CUSHING'S DISEASE

In Cushing's disease, ACTH hypersecretion is random and episodic and causes cortisol hypersecretion with absence of the normal circadian rhythm. Feedback inhibition of ACTH (secreted from the pituitary adenoma) by physiologic levels of glucocorticoids is suppressed; thus, ACTH hypersecretion persists despite elevated cortisol secretion and results in chronic glucocorticoid excess. The episodic secretion of ACTH and cortisol results in variable plasma levels that may at times be within the normal range. However, elevation of urine free cortisol or demonstration of elevated late-night serum or salivary cortisol levels because of the absence of diurnal variability confirms cortisol hypersecretion (see sections on laboratory evaluation and diagnosis of Cushing's syndrome). The overall increase in glucocorticoid secretion causes the clinical manifestations of Cushing's syndrome; however, ACTH and β-LPH secretion are not usually elevated sufficiently to cause hyperpigmentation.

1. Abnormalities of ACTH secretion—Despite ACTH hypersecretion, stress responsiveness is absent; stimuli such as hypoglycemia or surgery fail to further elevate ACTH and cortisol secretion. This is probably due to suppression of hypothalamic function and CRH secretion by hypercortisolism, resulting in loss of hypothalamic control of ACTH secretion (see Chapter 5).

2. Effect of cortisol excess—Cortisol excess not only inhibits normal pituitary and hypothalamic function,

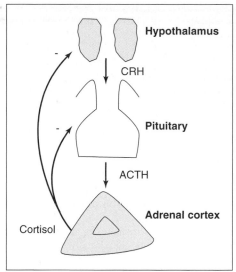

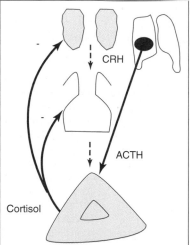

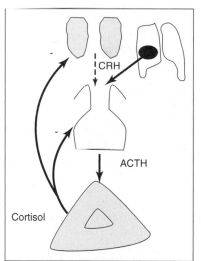

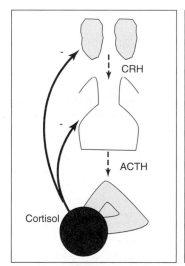

Figure 9–12. Hypothalamic-pituitary axis in Cushing's syndrome of different causes. These panels illustrate hormone secretion in the normal state (upper left), and four types of cortisol excess: Pituitary ACTH-dependent {with an ACTH-secreting pituitary tumor} (upper right), adrenal tumor (lower left), ectopic ACTH syndrome due to an ACTH-secreting lung cancer (lower middle), and ectopic CRH syndrome due to a CRH-secreting lung tumor. In contrast to normal secretion and hormone levels, decreased hormonal secretion is indicated by a dotted line and increased secretion by a dark solid line.

affecting ACTH, thyrotropin, GH, and gonadotropin release, but also results in all the systemic effects of glucocorticoid excess described in previous sections and in the section on clinical features below.

3. Androgen excess—Secretion of adrenal androgens is also increased in Cushing's disease, and the degree of androgen excess parallels that of ACTH and cortisol. Thus, plasma levels of DHEA, DHEA sulfate, and androstenedione may be moderately elevated in Cushing's disease; the peripheral conversion of these hormones to testosterone and dihydrotestosterone leads to androgen excess. In women, this causes hirsutism, acne, and amenorrhea. In men with Cushing's disease, cortisol suppression of LH secretion decreases testosterone secretion by the testis, resulting in decreased libido and impotence. The increased adrenal androgen secretion is insufficient to compensate for the decreased gonadal testosterone production.

B. ECTOPIC ACTH SYNDROME

Hypersecretion of ACTH and cortisol is usually greater in patients with ectopic ACTH syndrome than in those with Cushing's disease. ACTH and cortisol hypersecretion is randomly episodic, and the levels are often greatly elevated. Usually, ACTH secretion by ectopic tumors is not subject to negative-feedback control; ie, secretion of ACTH and cortisol is nonsuppressible with pharmacologic doses of glucocorticoids (see section on diagnosis).

Plasma levels, secretion rates, and urinary excretion of cortisol, the adrenal androgens, and DOC are often markedly elevated; despite this, the typical features of Cushing's syndrome are usually absent, presumably because of rapid onset of hypercortisolism, anorexia, and other manifestations of the associated malignant disease. Features of mineralocorticoid excess (hypertension and hypokalemia) are frequently present and have been attributed to increased secretion of DOC and the mineralocorticoid effects of cortisol. With ectopic CRH secretion, pituitary ACTH cell hyperplasia and ACTH hypersecretion are observed along with resistance to negative feedback by cortisol.

C. ADRENAL TUMORS

1. Autonomous secretion—Primary adrenal tumors, both adenomas and carcinomas, autonomously hypersecrete cortisol. Circulating plasma ACTH levels are suppressed, resulting in cortical atrophy of the uninvolved adrenal. Secretion is randomly episodic, and these tumors are typically unresponsive to manipulation of the hypothalamic-pituitary axis with pharmacologic agents such as dexamethasone and metyrapone.

2. Adrenal adenomas—Adrenal adenomas causing Cushing's syndrome typically present solely with clinical manifestations of glucocorticoid excess, since they usually secrete only cortisol. Thus, the presence of androgen or mineralocorticoid excess should suggest that the tumor is an adrenocortical carcinoma.

3. Adrenal carcinomas—Adrenal carcinomas frequently hypersecrete multiple adrenocortical steroids and their precursors. Cortisol and androgens are the steroids most frequently secreted in excess; 11-deoxycortisol is often elevated, and there may be increased secretion of DOC, aldosterone, or estrogens. Plasma cortisol and urine free cortisol are often markedly increased; androgen excess is usually even greater than that of cortisol. Thus, high levels of plasma DHEA, DHEA sulfate, and of testosterone typically accompany the cortisol excess. Clinical manifestations of hypercortisolism are usually severe and rapidly progressive in these patients. In women, features of androgen excess are prominent; virilism may occasionally occur. Hypertension and hypokalemia are frequent and most commonly result from the mineralocorticoid effects of cortisol; less frequently, DOC and aldosterone hypersecretion also contribute.

Clinical Features (Table 9–12)

A. SYMPTOMS AND SIGNS

1. Obesity—Obesity is the most common manifestation, and weight gain is usually the initial symptom. It is classically central, affecting mainly the face, neck, trunk, and abdomen, with relative sparing of the extremities. Generalized obesity with central accentuation is equally common, particularly in children.

Accumulation of fat in the face leads to the typical "moon facies," which is present in 75% of cases and is accompanied by facial plethora in most patients. Fat accumulation around the neck is prominent in the supraclavicular and dorsocervical fat pads; the latter is responsible for the "buffalo hump."

Obesity is absent in a handful of patients who do not gain weight; however, they usually have central redistribution of fat and a typical facial appearance.

2. Skin changes—Skin changes are frequent, and their presence should arouse a suspicion of cortisol excess. Atrophy of the epidermis and its underlying connective tissue leads to thinning (a transparent appearance of the skin) and facial plethora. Easy bruisability following minimal trauma is present in about 40%. Striae occur in 50% but are very unusual in patients over 40 years of age; these are typically red to purple, depressed below the skin surface secondary to loss of underlying connective tissue, and wider (not infrequently 0.5–2 cm) than the pinkish white striae that may occur with pregnancy or rapid weight gain. These striae are most commonly

Table 9–12. Clinical features of Cushing's syndrome (% prevalence).

General
  Obesity 90%
  Hypertension 85%
Skin
  Plethora 70%
  Hirsutism 75%
  Striae 50%
  Acne 35%
  Bruising 35%
Musculoskeletal
  Osteopenia 80%
  Weakness 65%
Neuropsychiatric 85%
  Emotional lability
  Euphoria
  Depression
  Psychosis
Gonadal dysfunction
  Menstrual disorders 70%
  Impotence, decreased libido 85%
Metabolic
  Glucose intolerance 75%
  Diabetes 20%
  Hyperlipidemia 70%
  Polyuria 30%
  Kidney stones 15%

abdominal but may also occur over the breasts, hips, buttocks, thighs, and axillae.

Acne may result from hyperandrogenism presenting as pustular lesions or as papular lesions from the glucocorticoid excess.

Minor wounds and abrasions may heal slowly, and surgical incisions sometimes undergo dehiscence.

Mucocutaneous fungal infections are frequent, including tinea versicolor, involvement of the nails (onychomycosis), and oral candidiasis.

Hyperpigmentation of the skin is rare in Cushing's disease or adrenal tumors but is common in ectopic ACTH syndrome.

3. Hirsutism—Hirsutism is present in about 80% of female patients owing to hypersecretion of adrenal androgens. Facial hirsutism is most common, but increased hair growth may also occur over the abdomen, breasts, chest, and upper thighs. Acne and seborrhea usually accompany hirsutism. Virilism is unusual except in cases of adrenal carcinoma, in which it occurs in about 20%.

4. Hypertension—Hypertension is a classic feature of spontaneous Cushing's syndrome; it is present in about

75% of cases, and the diastolic blood pressure is greater than 100 mm Hg in over 50%. Hypertension and its complications contribute greatly to the morbidity and mortality rates in spontaneous Cushing's syndrome.

5. Gonadal dysfunction—This is very common as a result of elevated androgens (in females) and cortisol (in males and to a lesser extent in females). Amenorrhea occurs in 75% of premenopausal women and is usually accompanied by infertility. Decreased libido is frequent in males, and some have decreased body hair and soft testes.

6. Central nervous system and psychologic disturbances—Psychologic disturbances occur in the majority of patients. Mild symptoms consist of emotional lability and increased irritability. Anxiety, depression, poor concentration, and poor memory may also be present. Euphoria is frequent, and occasional patients manifest overtly manic behavior. Sleep disorders are present in most patients, with either insomnia or early morning awakening.

Severe psychologic disorders occur in a few patients and include severe depression, psychosis with delusions or hallucinations, and paranoia. Some patients have committed suicide. Loss of brain volume that is at least partially reversible following correction of hypercortisolism has been observed.

7. Muscle weakness—This occurs in about 60% of cases; it is more often proximal and is usually most prominent in the lower extremities. Hypercortisolism is associated with both low fat-free muscle mass and low total body protein.

8. Osteoporosis—Owing to the profound effects of glucocorticoids on the skeleton, patients with Cushing's syndrome frequently have evidence of significant osteopenia and osteoporosis. Patients may present with frequent unexplained fractures, typically of the feet, ribs, or vertebrae. Back pain may be the initial complaint. Compression fractures of the spine are demonstrated radiographically in 15–20% of patients. In fact, unexplained osteopenia in any young or middle-aged adult should always prompt an evaluation for Cushing's syndrome even in the absence of any other signs or symptoms of cortisol excess. Although avascular necrosis of bone has been associated with exogenous glucocorticoid administration, the problem is rarely observed in patients with endogenous hypercortisolism, suggesting a role for the underlying disorders in patients for whom glucocorticoids are prescribed.

9. Renal calculi—Calculi secondary to glucocorticoid-induced hypercalciuria occur in approximately 15% of patients, and renal colic may occasionally be a presenting complaint.

10. Thirst and polyuria—Polyuria is rarely due to overt hyperglycemia. Polyuria is usually due to glucocorticoid inhibition of vasopressin (antidiuretic hormone) secretion and the direct enhancement of renal free water clearance by cortisol.

B. LABORATORY FINDINGS

Routine laboratory examinations are described here. Specific diagnostic tests to establish the diagnosis of Cushing's syndrome are discussed in the section on diagnosis.

High normal hemoglobin, hematocrit, and red cell counts are usual; polycythemia is rare. The total white count is usually normal; however, both the percentage of lymphocytes and the total lymphocyte count may be subnormal. Eosinophils are also depressed, and a total eosinophil count less than 100/μL is present in most patients. Serum electrolytes, with rare exceptions, are normal in Cushing's disease; however, hypokalemic alkalosis occurs when there is marked steroid hypersecretion with the ectopic ACTH syndrome or adrenocortical carcinoma.

Fasting hyperglycemia or clinical diabetes occurs in only 10–15% of patients; postprandial hyperglycemia is more common. Glycosuria is present in patients with fasting or postprandial hyperglycemia. Most patients have secondary hyperinsulinemia and abnormal glucose tolerance tests.

Serum calcium is normal; serum phosphorus is low normal or slightly depressed. Hypercalciuria is present in 40% of cases.

C. IMAGING STUDIES

Routine radiographs may reveal cardiomegaly due to hypertensive or atherosclerotic heart disease or mediastinal widening due to central fat accumulation. Vertebral compression fractures, rib fractures, and renal calculi may be present.

D. ELECTROCARDIOGRAPHIC FINDINGS

Hypertensive, ischemic, and electrolyte-induced changes may be present on the ECG.

Features Suggesting a Specific Cause

A. CUSHING'S DISEASE

Cushing's disease typifies the classic clinical picture: female predominance, onset generally between ages 20 and 40, and a slow progression over several years. Hyperpigmentation and hypokalemic alkalosis are rare; androgenic manifestations are limited to acne and hirsutism. Secretion of cortisol and adrenal androgens is only moderately increased.

B. ECTOPIC ACTH SYNDROME (CARCINOMA)

In contrast, this syndrome occurs predominantly in males, with the highest incidence between ages 40 and 60. The clinical manifestations of hypercortisolism are frequently limited to weakness, hypertension, and glucose intolerance; the primary tumor is usually apparent. Hyperpigmentation, hypokalemia, and alkalosis are common, as are weight loss and anemia. The hypercortisolism is of rapid onset, and steroid hypersecretion is frequently severe, with equally elevated levels of glucocorticoids, androgens, and DOC.

C. ECTOPIC ACTH SYNDROME (BENIGN TUMOR)

A minority of patients with ectopic ACTH syndrome due to more "benign" tumors, especially bronchial carcinoids, present a more slowly progressive course, with typical features of Cushing's syndrome. These patients may be clinically identical with those having pituitary-dependent Cushing's disease, and the responsible tumor may not be apparent. Hyperpigmentation, hypokalemic alkalosis, and anemia are variably present. Further confusion may arise, since a number of these patients with occult ectopic tumors may have ACTH and steroid dynamics typical of Cushing's disease (see below).

D. ADRENAL ADENOMAS

The clinical picture in patients with adrenal adenomas is usually that of glucocorticoid excess alone, and androgenic effects such as hirsutism are absent. Onset is gradual, and hypercortisolism is mild to moderate. Plasma androgens are usually in the low normal or subnormal range.

E. ADRENAL CARCINOMAS

In general, adrenal carcinomas have a rapid onset of the clinical features of excessive glucocorticoid, androgen, and mineralocorticoid secretion and are rapidly progressive. Marked elevations of both cortisol and androgens are usual; hypokalemia is common, as are abdominal pain, palpable masses, and hepatic and pulmonary metastases.

Diagnosis

The clinical suspicion of Cushing's syndrome must be confirmed with biochemical studies. Initially, a general assessment of the patient regarding the presence of other illnesses, drugs, alcohol, or psychiatric problems must be done since these factors may confound the evaluation. In the majority of cases, the biochemical differential diagnosis of Cushing's syndrome can be easily performed in the ambulatory setting (Figure 9–13).

A. DEXAMETHASONE SUPPRESSION TEST

The overnight 1 mg dexamethasone suppression test is a valuable screening test in patients with suspected hypercortisolism. This study employs the administration of 1 mg of dexamethasone at bedtime (11:00 PM), with

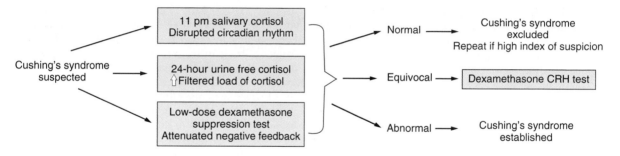

Figure 9–13. The diagnosis of Cushing's syndrome. (DST, dexamethasone suppression test; IRMA, immunoradiometric assay; IPSS, inferior petrosal sinus sampling; ISP:P, inferior petrosal sinus:peripheral ACTH ratio; CRH, corticotropin-releasing hormone.)

determination of a plasma cortisol early the following the morning. Normal subjects should suppress plasma cortisol to less than 1.8 μg/dL (50 nmol/L) following an overnight 1 mg test. Although a level of less than 5 μg/dL has been used in the past, several false negative studies have been discovered using this test criterion. False-negative results may occur in some patients with mild hypercortisolism and exquisite negative feedback sensitivity to glucocorticoids and in those with intermittent hypercortisolism. This test should only be employed as a screening tool for the consideration of Cushing's syndrome and biochemical confirmation must rely on urine free cortisol excretion. False positive results with the overnight 1 mg dexamethasone suppression test may be caused by patients receiving drugs that accelerate dexamethasone metabolism (phenytoin, phenobarbital, rifampin). False-positive results also occur in patients with renal failure, in patients suffering from endogenous depression, or in any patients undergoing a stressful event or serious illness.

The 2-day low-dose dexamethasone suppression test cannot be used to reliably exclude the diagnosis of Cushing's syndrome and its use is no longer recommended.

B. URINE FREE CORTISOL

The most useful clinical study in the confirmation of Cushing's syndrome is the determination of urine free cortisol measured by HPLC or gas chromatography-mass spectroscopy in a 24-hour urine collection. This method is highly accurate and specific. Commonly used drugs and medications do not interfere; however, carbamazepine causes falsely elevated results with HPLC since the drug elutes with cortisol. Urinary free cortisol is usually less than 50 μg/24 h (< 135 nmol/24 h) measured by HPLC. Urine free cortisol determinations usually provide clear discrimination between patients with hypercortisolism and obese non-Cushing

patients, though exceptions occur. Less than 5% of obese subjects will have mild elevations of urine free cortisol.

C. DIURNAL RHYTHM

The absence of diurnal rhythm has been considered a hallmark of the diagnosis of Cushing's syndrome. Normally, cortisol is secreted episodically with a diurnal rhythm paralleling the secretion of ACTH. Levels are usually highest early in the morning and decrease gradually throughout the day, reaching the nadir in the late evening. Because normal levels of plasma cortisol cover a broad range, the levels found in Cushing's syndrome may often be normal. Documenting the presence or absence of diurnal rhythm is difficult, since single determinations obtained in the morning or evening are usually uninterpretable because of the pulsatility of pathologic and physiologic ACTH and cortisol secretion. Nonetheless, serum cortisol levels exceeding 7 μg/dL (193 nmol/L) at midnight in nonstressed patients provide good specificity for the diagnosis of Cushing's syndrome. Since cortisol is secreted as free cortisol, the measurement of salivary cortisol may provide a simple and more convenient means of probing nighttime cortisol secretion in a practical fashion. Recent studies have shown that patients with Cushing's syndrome have midnight salivary cortisol levels that usually exceed 0.1 μg/dL (2.8 nmol/L).

Problems in Diagnosis

A major diagnostic problem is distinguishing patients with mild Cushing's syndrome from those with mild physiologic hypercortisolism due to conditions that are classified as "pseudo-Cushing's syndrome." These include the depressed phase of affective disorder, alcoholism, withdrawal from alcohol intoxication, or eating disorders such as anorexia and bulimia nervosa. These conditions may have biochemical features of Cushing's syndrome, including elevations of urine free cortisol, disruptions in the normal diurnal pattern of cortisol secretion, and lack of suppression of cortisol after the overnight 1 mg dexamethasone suppression test. Although the history and physical examination may provide specific clues to the appropriate diagnosis, definitive biochemical confirmation may be difficult and may require repeated testing. The most definitive study available for distinguishing mild Cushing's syndrome from pseudo-Cushing conditions is the use of dexamethasone suppression followed by corticotropin-releasing hormone (CRH) stimulation. This new test takes advantage of the overt sensitivity of patients with Cushing's syndrome to both dexamethasone and CRH by combining these tests in order to provide greater accuracy in the diagnosis. This study involves the administration of dexamethasone, 0.5 mg every 6 hours for eight doses, followed immediately by a CRH stimulation test, starting 2 hours after the completion of the low-dose dexamethasone suppression. A plasma cortisol concentration greater than 1.4 μg/dL (38.6 nmol/L) measured 15 minutes after administration of CRH correctly identifies the majority of patients with Cushing's syndrome.

Differential Diagnosis

The differential diagnosis of Cushing's syndrome is usually very difficult and should always be performed with consultation by an endocrinologist. The introduction of several technologic advances over the past 10–15 years, including a specific and sensitive immunoradiometric assay for ACTH, CRH stimulation test, inferior petrosal sinus sampling (IPSS), and CT and MRI of the pituitary and adrenal glands have all provided means for an accurate differential diagnosis (Figure 9–13).

A. PLASMA ACTH

Initially, the differential diagnosis for Cushing's syndrome must distinguish between ACTH-dependent Cushing's syndrome (pituitary or nonpituitary ACTH-secreting neoplasm) and ACTH-independent hypercortisolism. The best way to distinguish these forms of Cushing's syndrome is measurement of plasma ACTH by immunoradiometric assay (IRMA). The development of this sensitive and specific test has made it possible to reliably identify patients with ACTH-independent Cushing's syndrome. The ACTH level is less than 5 pg/mL (1.1 pmol/L) and exhibits a blunted response to CRH (peak response < 10 pg/mL [2.2 pmol/L]) in patients with cortisol-producing adrenal neoplasms, autonomous bilateral adrenal cortical hyperplasia, and factitious Cushing's syndrome (Figure 9–14). Patients

with ACTH-secreting neoplasms usually have plasma ACTH levels greater than 10 pg/mL (2.2 pmol/L) and frequently greater than 52 pg/mL (11.5 pmol/L). The major challenge in the differential diagnosis of ACTH-dependent Cushing's syndrome is identifying the source of the ACTH-secreting tumor. The vast majority of these patients (90%) have a pituitary tumor, while the others harbor a nonpituitary neoplasm. Diagnostic studies needed to differentiate these two entities must yield nearly perfect sensitivity, specificity, and accuracy. Although plasma ACTH levels are usually higher in patients with ectopic ACTH than those with pituitary ACTH-dependent Cushing's syndrome, there is considerable overlap between these two entities. Many of the ectopic ACTH-secreting tumors are radiologically occult at the time of presentation and may not become clinically apparent for many years after the initial diagnosis. However, an enhanced ACTH response for CRH administration is more frequently found in Cushing's syndrome compared with ectopic ACTH syndrome, but the CRH test is much less accurate than petrosal sinus sampling (see below).

B. PITUITARY MRI

When ACTH-dependent Cushing's syndrome is present, MRI of the pituitary gland with gadolinium enhancement should be performed and will identify an adenoma in 50–60% of the patients. If the patient has classic clinical laboratory findings of pituitary ACTH-dependent hypercortisolemia and an unequivocal pituitary lesion on MRI, the likelihood of Cushing's disease is 98–99%. However, it must be emphasized that approximately 10% of the population in the age group from 20 to 50 years will have incidental tumors of the pituitary demonstrable by MRI. Therefore, some patients with ectopic ACTH syndrome will have radiographic evidence of a pituitary lesion.

C. HIGH-DOSE DEXAMETHASONE SUPPRESSION

Traditionally, the high-dose dexamethasone suppression test has been utilized in the differential diagnosis of Cushing's syndrome. However, the diagnostic accuracy of this procedure is only 70–80% which is actually less than the pretest probability of Cushing's disease—on average about 90%. Thus, the authors no longer recommend this test.

D. INFERIOR PETROSAL SINUS SAMPLING (IPSS)

The most definitive means of accurately distinguishing pituitary from nonpituitary ACTH-dependent Cushing's syndrome is the use of bilateral simultaneous IPSS with CRH stimulation, and this procedure is the next step in the evaluation of patients with ACTH-dependent Cushing's syndrome when MRI does not reveal

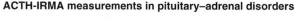

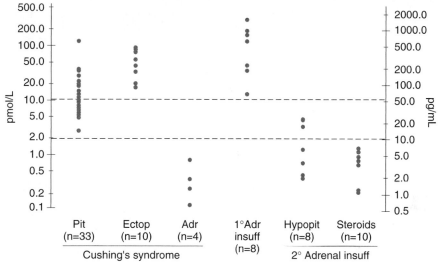

Figure 9–14. Plasma ACTH-IRMA (pmol/L or pg/mL) of patients with pituitary-adrenal disorders. Dashed horizontal lines indicate normal range. (Reproduced, with permission, from Findling JW: Clinical application of a new immunoradiometric assay for ACTH. Endocrinologist 1992;2:360.)

a definite adenoma. This study takes advantage of the means by which pituitary hormones reach the systemic circulation. Blood leaves the anterior lobe of the pituitary and drains into the cavernous sinuses, which then empty into the inferior petrosal sinuses and subsequently into the jugular bulb and vein. Simultaneous inferior petrosal sinus and peripheral ACTH measurement before and after CRH stimulation can reliably confirm the presence or absence of an ACTH-secreting pituitary tumor. An inferior petrosal sinus to peripheral (IPS:P) ratio greater than 2.0 after CRH is consistent with a pituitary ACTH-secreting tumor, and an IPS:P ratio less than 1.8 supports the diagnosis of ectopic ACTH. Interpetrosal sinus gradients have been utilized for preoperative localization of corticotroph adenomas, albeit with mixed results.

Bilateral IPSS with CRH stimulation does require a skilled interventional radiologist, but in experienced hands the procedure has yielded a diagnostic accuracy approaching 100% in identifying the source of ACTH-dependent Cushing's syndrome.

E. Occult Ectopic ACTH

If the IPSS study is consistent with a nonpituitary ACTH-secreting tumor, a search for an occult ectopic ACTH-secreting tumor is needed. Since the majority of these lesions are in the thorax, high-resolution CT of the chest may be useful; MRI of the chest appears to

have even better sensitivity in finding these lesions, which are usually small bronchial carcinoid tumors. Unfortunately, utilization of a radiolabeled somatostatin analog scan (octreotide acetate scintigraphy) has not been useful in localizing these tumors.

F. Adrenal Localizing Procedures

CT scan (Figure 9–15) and MRI are used to define adrenal lesions. Their primary use is to localize adrenal tumors in patients with ACTH-independent Cushing's syndrome. Most adenomas exceed 2 cm in diameter; carcinomas are usually much larger.

Treatment

A. Cushing's Disease

The aim of treatment of Cushing's syndrome is to remove or destroy the basic lesion and thus correct hypersecretion of adrenal hormones without inducing pituitary or adrenal damage, which requires permanent replacement therapy for hormone deficiencies.

Treatment of Cushing's disease is currently directed at the pituitary to control ACTH hypersecretion; available methods include microsurgery, various forms of radiation therapy, and pharmacologic inhibition of ACTH secretion. Treatment of hypercortisolism per se by surgical or medical adrenalectomy is less commonly used. These methods are discussed in Chapter 5.

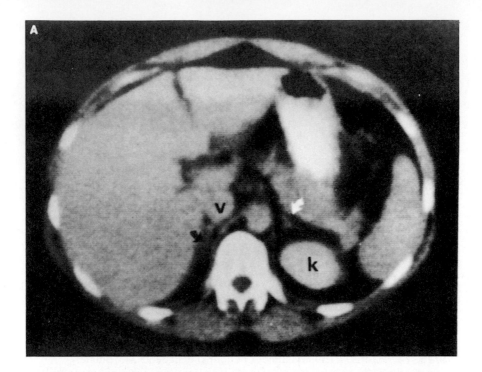

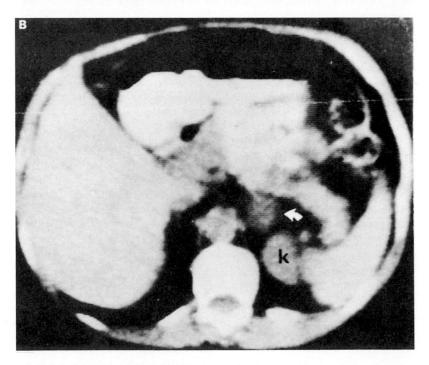

Figure 9–15. Adrenal CT scans in Cushing's syndrome. **A:** Patient with ACTH-dependent Cushing's syndrome. The adrenal glands are not detectably abnormal by this procedure. The curvilinear right adrenal (black arrow) is shown posterior to the inferior vena cava (V) between the right lobe of the liver and the right crus of the diaphragm. The left adrenal (white arrow) has an inverted Y appearance anteromedial to the left kidney (K). **B:** A 3-cm left adrenal adenoma (white arrow) is shown anteromedial to the left kidney (K). (Reproduced, with permission, from Korobkin M et al: Computed tomography in the diagnosis of adrenal disease. AJR Am J Roentgenol 1979;132:231.)

B. Ectopic ACTH Syndrome

Cure of ectopic ACTH syndrome is usually possible only in cases involving the more "benign" tumors such as bronchial or thymic carcinoids, or pheochromocytomas. Treatment is made difficult by the presence of metastatic malignant tumors and accompanying severe hypercortisolism. Therapy directed to the primary tumor is usually unsuccessful, and other means must be used to correct the steroid-excess state.

Severe hypokalemia may require potassium replacement in large doses and spironolactone to block mineralocorticoid effects.

Drugs that block steroid synthesis (ketoconazole, metyrapone, and aminoglutethimide) are useful, but they may produce hypoadrenalism, and steroid secretion must be monitored and replacement steroids given if necessary. The dosage of ketoconazole is 400–800 mg/d in divided doses and is usually well tolerated.

Because of its slow onset of action and its side effects, mitotane is less useful, and several weeks of therapy may be required to control cortisol secretion (see below and comment there about the availability of mitotane).

Bilateral adrenalectomy may be necessary if hypercortisolism cannot be controlled in other ways.

C. Adrenal Tumors

1. Adrenal adenomas—Patients with adrenal adenomas are successfully treated by unilateral adrenalectomy, and the outlook is excellent. Laparoscopic adrenal surgery has become widely used in patients with benign or small adrenal tumors and has significantly reduced the duration of the hospital stay. Since the hypothalamic-pituitary axis and the contralateral adrenal are suppressed by prolonged cortisol secretion, these patients have postoperative adrenal insufficiency and require glucocorticoid therapy both during and following surgery until the remaining adrenal recovers.

2. Adrenal carcinomas—Therapy in cases of adrenocortical carcinoma is less satisfactory, since the tumor has frequently already metastasized (usually to the retroperitoneum, liver, and lungs) by the time the diagnosis is made.

a. Operative treatment—Surgical cure is rare, but excision serves to reduce the tumor mass and the degree of steroid hypersecretion. Persisting nonsuppressible steroid secretion in the immediate postoperative period indicates residual or metastatic tumor.

b. Medical treatment—Mitotane is the drug of choice.[1] The dosage is 6–12 g/d orally in three or four divided doses. The dose must often be reduced because of side effects in 80% of patients (diarrhea, nausea and vomiting, depression, somnolence). About 70% of patients achieve a reduction of steroid secretion, but only 35% achieve a reduction in tumor size.

Ketoconazole, metyrapone, or aminoglutethimide (singly or in combination) are useful in controlling steroid hypersecretion in patients who do not respond to mitotane.

Radiotherapy and conventional chemotherapy have not been useful in this disease.

D. Nodular Adrenal Hyperplasia

When pituitary ACTH dependency can be demonstrated, macronodular hyperplasia may be treated like other cases of Cushing's disease. When ACTH dependency is not present, as in micronodular hyperplasia and in some cases of macronodular hyperplasia, bilateral adrenalectomy is appropriate.

Prognosis

A. Cushing's Syndrome

Untreated Cushing's syndrome is frequently fatal, and death may be due to the underlying tumor itself, as in the ectopic ACTH syndrome and adrenal carcinoma. However, in many cases, death is the consequence of sustained hypercortisolism and its complications, including hypertension, cardiovascular disease, stroke, thromboembolism, and susceptibility to infection. In older series, 50% of patients died within 5 years after onset.

B. Cushing's Disease

With current refinements in pituitary microsurgery and heavy particle irradiation, the great majority of patients with Cushing's disease can be treated successfully, and the operative mortality and morbidity rates that attended bilateral adrenalectomy are no longer a feature of the natural history of this disease. Survival in these patients is considerably longer than in older series. However, survival is still less than that of age-matched controls; the increased mortality rate is due to cardiovascular causes. Patients with Cushing's disease who have large pituitary tumors at the time of diagnosis have a much less satisfactory prognosis and may die as a consequence of tumor invasion or persisting hypercortisolism.

C. Adrenal Tumors

The prognosis in adrenal adenomas is excellent. In adrenal carcinoma, the prognosis is almost universally poor, and the median survival from the date of onset of symptoms is about 4 years.

---

[1]Mitotane has been withdrawn from the market in the USA but is available on a compassionate basis.

D. Ectopic ACTH Syndrome

Prognosis is also poor in patients with ectopic ACTH syndrome due to the nature of the malignancy producing the hormone, and in these patients with severe hypercortisolism, survival is frequently only days to weeks. Some patients respond to tumor resection or chemotherapy. The prognosis is better in patients with benign tumors producing the ectopic ACTH syndrome.

■ HIRSUTISM & VIRILISM

Excessive adrenal or ovarian secretion of androgens or excessive conversion of androgens in peripheral tissues leads to hirsutism and virilism (see Chapter 13). As previously discussed, the adrenal secretory products DHEA, DHEA sulfate, and androstenedione are weak androgens; however, the peripheral conversion to testosterone and dihydrotestosterone can result in a state of androgen excess.

Excessive androgen production is seen in both adrenal and ovarian disorders. Adrenal causes include Cushing's syndrome, adrenal carcinoma, and congenital adrenal hyperplasia (see previous sections and Chapter 14). Mild adult-onset cases of congenital adrenal enzyme deficiencies have been described; these appear to be relatively uncommon. Biochemical diagnosis of late-onset 21-hydroxylase deficiency is best achieved by measurement of the 17-hydroxyprogesterone response to ACTH. Ovarian causes are discussed in Chapter 13.

In children, androgen excess is usually due to premature adrenarche, congenital adrenal hyperplasia or adrenal carcinoma. In women, hirsutism accompanied by amenorrhea, infertility, ovarian enlargement, and elevated plasma LH levels is typical of the polycystic ovary syndrome, whereas in Cushing's syndrome hirsutism is accompanied by features of cortisol excess. Late-onset 21-hydroxylase deficiency is accompanied by elevated levels of plasma 17-hydroxyprogesterone, especially following ACTH administration. Virilism and severe androgen excess in adults are usually due to androgen-secreting adrenal or ovarian tumors; virilism is unusual in the polycystic ovary syndrome and rare in Cushing's disease. In the absence of these syndromes, hirsutism in women is usually idiopathic or due to milder forms of polycystic ovary syndrome. Exogenous androgen administration (eg, DHEA) should also be considered.

The diagnosis and therapy of hirsutism are discussed in Chapter 13.

■ INCIDENTAL ADRENAL MASS

The incidental adrenal mass has become a common diagnostic problem, since approximately 2% of patients undergoing CT studies of the abdomen are found to have focal enlargement of the adrenal gland. Adrenal masses in the adult may represent functional or nonfunctional cortical adenomas or carcinoma, pheochromocytomas, cysts, myelolipomas, or metastasis from other tumors. Congenital adrenal hyperplasia may also present as a focal enlargement of the adrenal gland, and adrenal hemorrhage will also cause enlargement, though usually bilateral.

The appropriate diagnostic approach to patients with an incidentally discovered adrenal mass is unresolved. The roentgenographic appearance taken in context with the clinical setting may provide some insight. The size of the lesion is important. Primary adrenocortical carcinoma is rare in adrenal masses smaller than 4 cm; however, the presence of unilateral bilateral adrenal masses (> 3 cm) in a patient with a known malignancy (particularly lung, gastrointestinal, renal, or breast) probably represents metastatic disease. Adrenal lesions smaller than 3 cm in patients with a known malignancy actually represent metastases in only 20–30% of cases.

Other CT findings may be informative. The presence of fat within the adrenal mass may suggest a myelolipoma which is usually a benign lesion. Adrenocortical adenomas are usually round masses with smooth margins, and adrenal cysts can also be identified with either CT or ultrasound examination. Lesions with low density (< 10 Hounsfield units) on unenhanced CT scans are usually benign. Adrenal hemorrhage usually has irregular borders with some lack of homogeneity. Primary adrenocortical carcinoma usually presents as a lesion greater than 5 cm with irregular borders. MRI of the adrenal gland is usually not necessary but may be helpful in selected patients. Typically, malignancies and pheochromocytomas tend to have bright signal intensity with T2-weighted images, in contrast to benign lesions of the adrenal gland; however, exceptions to this rule have been seen, limiting the clinical utility of this technique.

Malignancy

Primary adrenocortical carcinoma usually presents with a large lesion, and most authorities recommend removing all adrenal masses greater than 4–5 cm. One series of 45 adrenal masses greater than 5 cm showed 30 benign lesions (16 pheochromocytomas, six adenomas, four adrenal cysts, two myelolipomas, one hematoma, one ganglioneuroma) and 15 malignancies (seven adrenocortical carcinomas, five adrenal metastases, and three adrenal lymphomas. Lesions less than 4–5 cm in diameter are of concern only in patients with a known malignancy or in those in whom there is a high index of suspicion based on other clinical information. In patients with primary malignancies of the lung, gastrointestinal tract, kidney, or breast, an ultrasound or CT-guided needle biopsy may be helpful in establishing the presence or absence of metastatic disease. Metastatic disease can be identified with an accuracy of 75–85% in such patients; however, there are both false-negative and false-positive findings. Percutaneous adrenal biopsy really has no demonstrated efficacy in patients with adrenal masses and no history of a malignancy. Percutaneous adrenal biopsy should be reserved for patients in whom the presence or absence of adrenal metastases may alter the therapy or prognosis of the patient.

Endocrine Evaluation

The appropriate biochemical evaluation with an incidental adrenal mass is also controversial. An expert panel from the NIH found that the available evidence suggests that an overnight (1 mg) dexamethasone suppression test and determination of fractionated urinary or plasma metanephrines should be performed and that in patients with hypertension, serum potassium and a plasma aldosterone concentration/plasma renin activity ratio should be determined to evaluate for primary aldosteronism. However, good clinical judgment is essential, and repeat CT imagining in 6–12 months was also recommended to exclude neoplastic disease. Hormonal abnormalities may develop over time, and follow-up testing has been recommended by some depending upon the clinical context.

Cortisol-Producing Adenoma

The most common functioning lesion in patients with an incidentally discovered adrenal mass appears to be the autonomous secretion of cortisol. Approximately 5–15% of patients with adrenal incidentalomas ranging from 2–5 cm in diameter have pathologic cortisol secretion. These benign adrenal adenomas secrete small amounts of cortisol that are often not sufficient to elevate urine cortisol excretion but are able to cause some suppression of the hypothalamic-pituitary axis. These patients can be easily identified by their failure to suppress cortisol to less than 1.8 μg/dL (50 nmol/L) following an overnight 1 mg dexamethasone suppression test (using a dose of 3 mg or higher will reduce the number of false-positive results). In addition, the basal levels of ACTH in these patients are subnormal or frankly suppressed. The cortisol secretion by the tumor probably results in blunting of diurnal variation and eventually in lack of suppression by dexamethasone. The low plasma ACTH level exhibits a blunted response to CRH administration. Removal of these "silent" adrenocortical adenomas may be followed by clinically significant secondary adrenal insufficiency. Therefore, an overnight dexamethasone suppression test or measurement of plasma ACTH should be performed before surgical removal of any unknown adrenal neoplasm. These patients have been described as having "preclinical" or "subclinical" Cushing's syndrome. The natural history of this autonomous cortisol secretion is unknown. Many of these patients described with this problem have hypertension, obesity, or diabetes, and improvements in these clinical problems have been reported following resection of these cortisol-producing adenomas. Consequently, adrenalectomy is recommended in young patients with preclinical Cushing's syndrome and in patients with clinical problems, potentially aggravated by glucocorticoid excess.

Pheochromocytoma

Pheochromocytoma is a potentially life-threatening tumor that may present as an incidental adrenal mass. Surprisingly, pheochromocytoma may account for as many as 2–3% of incidental adrenal lesions. Many of these patients will have hypertension and symptoms associated with catecholamine excess such as headache, diaphoresis, palpitations, or nervousness (see Chapter 11).

Aldosterone-Producing Adenoma

Although aldosterone-producing adenomas are more common than either pheochromocytomas or cortisol-producing adenomas, they actually represent a very unusual cause of an incidentally discovered adrenal mass. This appears to be due to the fact that aldosterone-producing adenomas are usually small and frequently missed with CT imaging of the adrenal gland. Because most of these patients have hypertension, this diagnosis needs to be considered only in patients with hypertension. The presence of hypokalemia should arouse suspicion of this diagnosis. It is virtually always present in patients with aldosterone-producing adenomas greater than 3 cm. It can be conclusively excluded by a single measurement of aldosterone and PRA. If the aldosterone (ng/dL):PRA (ng/mL/h) ratio is less than 30 and plasma aldosterone is less than 20 ng/dL, an aldosterone-producing adenoma is excluded.

GLUCOCOCORTICOID THERAPY FOR NONENDOCRINE DISORDERS

Principles

Glucocorticoids have been used for their anti-inflammatory and immunosuppressive activity in treatment of a wide variety of disorders. These include rheumatologic disorders (eg, rheumatoid arthritis and systemic lupus erythematosus), pulmonary diseases (eg, asthma), renal disease (eg, glomerulonephritis), and many others. Because of their side effects, glucocorticoids should be used in the minimum effective dose and for the shortest possible duration of therapy.

Synthetic Glucocorticoids

Steroid compounds have been synthesized taking advantage of chemical alterations to the steroid nucleus that enhance glucocorticoid activity relative to mineralocorticoid activity. For example, prednisone has a double bond between positions 1 and 2 of cortisol and an 11-keto group instead of a hydroxyl group. It has three to five times more glucocorticoid activity than cortisol and relatively little mineralocorticoid activity. It must be converted to prednisolone by reduction of the 11-keto group to a hydroxyl group in order to be biologically active, a process that may be reduced in the presence of liver disease. Dexamethasone has the same additional double bond, a fluoro atom in the 9α position and a 16α-methyl group. This results in ten to twenty times the glucocorticoid activity of cortisol and negligible mineralocorticoid activity. Many other compounds have been synthesized. Although most synthetic glucocorticoids exhibit little binding to CBG, their plasma half-lives are longer than that of cortisol.

Modes of Administration

Glucocorticoids may be administered parenterally, orally, or topically. Absorption rates from intramuscular and intra-articular sites depend on the particular glucocorticoid and its formulation. Transdermal absorption also depends on the severity of the inflammatory disorder, the area of the body to which the drug is applied, the presence of vehicles that enhance absorption (eg, urea), and the use of an occlusive dressing. Inhaled glucocorticoids vary in their bioavailability; the technique of administration (eg, use of spacers) also affects the amount of drug delivered to the lungs.

Side Effects

In general, the severity of the side effects is a function of dose and duration of therapy, but there is marked individual variation.

A. Hypothalamic-Pituitary-Adrenal (HPA) Axis Suppression

Glucocorticoids suppress CRH and ACTH secretion (negative feedback). Suppression of the HPA axis may occur with doses of prednisone greater than 5 mg/d. It is difficult, however, to predict the development or degree of suppression in any given individual. In general, patients who develop clinical features of Cushing's syndrome or who have received glucocorticoids equivalent to 10–20 mg of prednisone per day for 3 weeks or more should be assumed to have clinically significant HPA axis suppression. Patients treated with alternate-day steroid regimens exhibit less suppression than those who receive steroids daily.

B. Cushing's Syndrome

Glucocorticoid administration will result in the development of cushingoid features. Of special concern is steroid-induced osteoporosis, particularly in patients for whom a long course of steroid therapy is anticipated. The severity of systemic effects of inhaled glucocorticoids varies among different preparations. However, they are associated with both local effects (dysphonia and oral candidiasis) and systemic effects, especially glaucoma, cataracts, osteoporosis, and growth retardation in children.

C. Steroid Withdrawal

Because of their adverse effects, glucocorticoids must be tapered downward as the clinical situation permits. Tapering regimens are essentially empirical. Factors that may limit the ability to taper the dose down to physiologic replacement levels include recrudescence of disease and steroid withdrawal syndrome. The latter appears in a variety of patterns. Patients may develop fatigue, arthralgias, and desquamation of the skin. Psychologic dependence has also been described. Even after the dose has been reduced to physiologic levels, HPA axis suppression (ie, secondary adrenal insufficiency) persists for an average of 9–10 months but may continue for as long as 1–2 years.

REFERENCES

General

Alesci S et al: Adrenal androgens regulation and adrenopause. Endocr Regul 2001;35:95. [PMID: 11563938]

Bornstein SR, Chrousos GP: Adrenocorticotropin (ACTH)- and non-ACTH-mediated regulation of the adrenal cortex: neural and immune inputs. J Clin Endocrinol Metab 1999;84:1729. [PMID: 10323408]

Bornstein SR, Vaudry H: Paracrine and neuroendocrine regulation of the adrenal gland—basic and clinical aspects. Horm Metab Res 1998;30:292. [PMID: 9694552]

Bottner A, Bornstein SR: Lessons learned from gene targeting and transgenesis for adrenal physiology and disease. Rev Endocr Metab Disord 2001;2:275. [PMID: 11705133]

Burchard K: A review of the adrenal cortex and severe inflammation: quest of the "eucorticoid" state. J Trauma 2001;51:800. [PMID: 11586182]

Christenson LK, Strauss JF 3rd: Steroidogenic acute regulatory protein: an update on its regulation and mechanism of action. Arch Med Res 2001;32:576. [PMID: 11750733]

Ehrhart-Bornstein M et al: Intraadrenal interactions in the regulation of adrenocortical steroidogenesis. Endocr Rev 1998;19: 101. [PMID: 9570034]

Jin Y, Penning TM: Steroid 5α-reductases and 3α-hydroxysteroid dehydrogenases: key enzymes in androgen metabolism. Best Prac Res Clin Endocrinol Metab 2001;15:79. [PMID: 11469812]

Kacsoh B: *Endocrine Physiology.* McGraw-Hill, 2000.

Kraan GP et al: The daily cortisol production reinvestigated in healthy men. The serum and urinary cortisol production rates are not significantly different. J Clin Endocrinol Metab 1998;83:1247. [PMID: 9543150]

McKenna TJ et al: A critical review of the origin and control of adrenal androgens. Baillieres Clin Obstet Gynaecol 1997; 1:229. [PMID: 9536209]

Miller DB, O'Callaghan JP: Neuroendocrine aspects of the response to stress. Metabolism 2002;51(6 Suppl 1):5. [PMID:12040534]

Miller WL, Tyrrell JB: The adrenal cortex. In: *Endocrinology and Metabolism,* 4th ed. Felig P, Baxter JD, Frohman LA (editors). McGraw-Hill, 2002.

Parker KL et al: Steroidogenic factor 1: an essential mediator of endocrine development. Recent Prog Horm Res 2002;57:19. [PMID: 12017543]

Parker KL, Schimmer BP. Genetics of the development and function of the adrenal cortex. Rev Endocr Metab Disord 2001;2:245. [PMID: 11705131]

Rainey WE et al: Dissecting human adrenal androgen production. Trends Endocrinol Metab 2002;13:234. [PMID: 12128283]

Rainey WE: Adrenal zonation: clues from 11β-hydroxylase and aldosterone synthase. Mol Cell Endocrinol 1999;151:151. [PMID: 10411330]

Sandeep TC, Walker BR: Pathophysiology of modulation of local glucocorticoid levels by 11β-hydroxysteroid dehydrogenases. Trends Endocrinol Metab 2001;12:446. [PMID: 11701343]

Seckl JR, Walker BR: Minireview: 11β-Hydroxysteroid dehydrogenase type 1—A tissue-specific amplifier of glucocorticoid action. Endocrinology 2001;142:1371. [PMID: 11250914]

Stewart PM, Tomlinson JW: Cortisol, 11β-hydroxysteroid dehydrogenase type 1 and central obesity. Trends Endocrinol Metab 2002;13:94. [PMID: 11893517]

Tomlinson JW, Stewart PM: Cortisol metabolism and the role of 11β-hydroxysteroid dehydrogenase. Best Prac Res Clin Endocrinol Metab 2001;15:61. [PMID: 11469811]

Turnbull AV, Rivier CL: Regulation of the hypothalamic-pituitary-adrenal axis by cytokines: actions and mechanisms of action. Physiol Rev 1999;79:1. [PMID: 9922367]

Van den Berghe G: Neuroendocrine pathobiology of chronic critical illness. Crit Care Clin 2002;18:509. [PMID: 12140911]

Walker BR: Steroid metabolism in metabolic syndrome X. Best Prac Res Clin Endocrinol Metab 2001;15:111. [PMID: 11469814]

Biologic Effects and Glucocorticoid Therapy

Andrews RC, Walker BR: Glucocorticoids and insulin resistance: old hormones, new targets. Clin Sci 1999;96:513. [PMID: 10209084]

Angeli A et al: Modulation by cytokines of glucocorticoid action. Ann N Y Acad Sci 1999;876:210. [PMID: 10415612]

Borski RJ: Nongenomic membrane actions of glucocorticoids in vertebrates. Trends Endocrinol Metab 2000;11:427.

Bourdeau I et al: Loss of brain volume in endogenous Cushing's syndrome and its reversibility after correction of hypercortisolism. J Clin Endocrinol Metab 2002;87:1949. [PMID: 11994323]

Cadepond F, Ulmann A, Baulieu EE: RU486 (mifepristone): mechanisms of action and clinical uses. Annu Rev Med 1997;48:129. [PMID: 9046951]

Chrousos GP et al: Hypothalamic-pituitary-adrenal axis suppression and inhaled corticosteroid therapy. 2. Review of the literature. Neuroimmunomodulation 1998;5:288. [PMID: 9762011]

Chrousos GP, Harris AG: Hypothalamic-pituitary-adrenal axis suppression and inhaled corticosteroid therapy. 1. General principles. Neuroimmunomodulation 1998;5:277. [PMID: 9762010]

Garbe E et al: Inhaled and nasal glucocorticoids and the risks of ocular hypertension or open-angle glaucoma. JAMA 1997;277: 722. [PMID: 9042844]

Garbe E, Suissa S: Inhaled corticosteroids and the risk of cataracts. N Engl J Med 1997;337:1555. [PMID: 9380124]

Gold PW et al: Divergent endocrine abnormalities in melancholic and atypical depression: clinical and pathophysiologic implications. Endocrinol Metab Clin North Am 2002;31:37. [PMID: 12055990]

Jenkins BD et al: Novel glucocorticoid receptor coactivator effector mechanisms. Trends Endocrinol Metab 2001;12;122. [PMID: 11306337]

Jones A et al: Inhaled corticosteroid effects on bone metabolism in asthma and mild chronic obstructive pulmonary disease. Cochrane Database Syst Rev 2002:CD003537. [PMID: 11869676]

Karin M, Chang L: AP-1—glucocorticoid receptor crosstalk taken to a higher level. J Endocrinol 2002;169:447. [PMID 11375114]

Kino T, Chrousos GP: Glucocorticoid and mineralocorticoid resistance/hypersensitivity syndromes. J Endocrinology 2001;169: 437. [PMID 11375113]

Patel L et al: Symptomatic adrenal insufficiency during inhaled corticosteroid treatment. Arch Dis Child 2001;85:330. [PMID: 11567945]

Pirlich M et al: Loss of body cell mass in Cushing's syndrome: effect of treatment. J Clin Endocrinol Metab 2002;87:1078. [PMID: 11889168]

Reichardt HM et al: New insights into glucocorticoid and mineralocorticoid signaling: lessons from gene targeting. Adv Pharmacol 2000;47:1. [PMID 10582083]

Reynolds RM et al: Skeletal muscle glucocorticoid receptor density and insulin resistance. JAMA 2002;287:2505. [PMID: 12020330]

Sartor O, Cutler GB Jr: Mifepristone: treatment of Cushing's syndrome. Clin Obstet Gynecol 1996;39:506. [PMID: 8734015]

Sizonenko PC: Effects of inhaled or nasal glucocorticosteroids on adrenal function and growth. J Pediatr Endocrinol Metab 2002;15:5. [PMID: 11822580]

Ullian ME: The role of corticosteroids in the regulation of vascular tone. Cardiovasc Res 1999;41:55. [PMID: 10325953]

Vgontzas AN, Chrousos GP: Sleep, the hypothalamic-pituitary-adrenal axis, and cytokines: multiple interactions and disturbances in sleep disorders. Endocrinol Metab Clin North Am 2002;31:15. [PMID: 12055986]

Laboratory Evaluation

Andrew R: Clinical measurement of steroid metabolism. Best Pract Res Clin Endocrinol Metab 2001;15:1. [PMID: 11469808]

Grinspoon SK, Biller BM: Laboratory assessment of adrenal insufficiency. J Clin Endocrinol Metab 1994;79:923. [PMID: 7962298]

Kane KF et al: Assessing the hypothalamo-pituitary-adrenal axis in patients on long-term glucocorticoid therapy: the short Synacthen versus the insulin tolerance test. Q J Med 1999;88:263. [PMID: 7796076]

Mayenknecht J et al: Comparison of low and high dose corticotropin stimulation tests in patients with pituitary disease. J Clin Endocrinol Metab 1998;83:1558. [PMID: 9589655]

Newell-Price J et al: Optimal response criteria for the human CRH test in the differential diagnosis of ACTH-dependent Cushing's syndrome. J Clin Endocrinol Metab 2002;87:1640. [PMID: 11932295]

Oelkers W: The role of high- and low-dose corticotropin tests in the diagnosis of secondary adrenal insufficiency. Eur J Endocrinol 1998;139:567. [PMID: 9916857]

Suliman AM et al: The low-dose ACTH test does not provide a useful assessment of the hypothalamic-pituitary-adrenal axis in secondary adrenal insufficiency. Clin Endocrinol (Oxf) 2002;56:533. [PMID: 11966747]

Adrenal Insufficiency

Beishuizen A, Thijs LG: Relative adrenal failure in intensive care: an identifiable problem requiring treatment? Best Pract Res Clin Endocrinol Metab 2001;15:513. [PMID: 11800521]

Betterle C et al: Autoimmune adrenal insufficiency and autoimmune polyendocrine syndromes: Autoantibodies, autoantigens, and their applicability in diagnosis and disease prediction. Endocr Rev 2002;23:327. [PMID: 12050123]

Brown CJ, Buie WD: Perioperative stress dose steroids: do they make a difference? J Am Coll Surg 2001;193:678. [PMID: 11768685]

Coursin DB, Wood KE: Corticosteroid supplementation for adrenal insufficiency. JAMA 2002;287:236. [PMID: 11779267]

Glowniak JV, Loriaux DL: A double-blind study of perioperative steroid requirements in secondary adrenal insufficiency. Surgery 1997;121:123. [PMID: 9037222]

Gurnell EM, Chatterjee VK: Dehydroepiandrosterone replacement therapy. Eur J Endocrinol 2001;145:1103. [PMID: 11454504]

Howlett TA: An assessment of optimal hydrocortisone replacement therapy. Clin Endocrinol (Oxf) 1997;46:263. [PMID: 9156032]

Hunt P et al: Improvement in mood and fatigue after dehydroepiandrosterone replacement in Addison's disease in a randomized, double blind trial. J Clin Endocrinol Metab 2000;85:4650. [PMID: 11134123]

Inder WJ, Hunt PJ: Glucocorticoid replacement in pituitary surgery: guidelines for perioperative assessment and management. J Clin Endocrinol Metab 2002;87:2745. [PMID: 12050244]

Jeffcoate W: Assessment of corticosteroid replacement therapy in adults with adrenal insufficiency. Ann Clin Biochem 1999;36:151. [PMID: 10370729]

Kumar PG, Laloraya M, She JX: Population genetics and functions of the autoimmune regulator (AIRE). Endocrinol Metab Clin North Am 2002;31:321. [PMID: 12092453]

Lamberts SW, Bruining HA, de Jong FH: Corticosteroid therapy in severe illness. N Engl J Med 1997;337:1285. [PMID: 9345079]

Lehmann SG, Lalli E, Sassone-Corsi P: X-linked adrenal hypoplasia congenita is caused by abnormal nuclear localization of the DAX-1 protein. Proc Natl Acad Sci U S A 2002;99:8225. [PMID: 12034880]

Lovas K, Husebye ES: High prevalence and increasing incidence of Addison's disease in western Norway. Clin Endocrinol (Oxf) 2002;56:787. [PMID: 12072049]

Mackenzie JS, Burrows L, Burchard KW: Transient hypoadrenalism during surgical critical illness. Arch Surg 1998;133:1998. [PMID: 9484735]

Mayo J et al: Adrenal function in the human immunodeficiency virus-infected patient. Arch Intern Med 2002;162:1095. [PMID: 12020177]

Norbiato G et al: Glucocorticoids and the immune function in the human immunodeficiency virus infection: a study in hypercortisolemic and cortisol-resistant patients. J Clin Endocrinol Metab 1997;82:3260. [PMID: 9329349]

Oelkers W: Adrenal insufficiency. N Engl J Med 1996;335:1206. [PMID: 8815944]

Perheentupa J: APS-I/APCED: The clinical disease and therapy. Endocrinol Metab Clin North Am 2002;31:295. [PMID: 12092452]

Robles DT et al: The genetics of autoimmune polyendocrine syndrome type II. Endocrinol Metab Clin North Am 2002;31:353. [PMID: 12092455]

Schatz DA, Winter WE: Autoimmune polyglandular syndrome II: Clinical syndrome and treatment. Endocrinol Clin North Am 2002;31:339. [PMID: 12092454]

Shenker Y, Skatrud JB. Adrenal insufficiency in critically ill patients. Am J Respir Crit Care Med 2001;163:1520. [PMID: 11401866]

Subramanian S et al: Clinical adrenal insufficiency in patients receiving megestrol therapy. Arch Intern Med 1997;157:1008. [PMID: 9140272]

Vermes I, Beishuizen A: The hypothalamic-pituitary-adrenal response to critical illness. Best Pract Res Clin Endocrinol Metab 2001;15:495. [PMID: 11800520]

Cushing's Syndrome

Aron DC, Tyrrell JB (editors): Cushing's syndrome. Endocrinol Metab Clin North Am 1994;23:451, 925.

Aron DC, Raff H, Findling JW: Effectiveness versus efficacy: the limited value in clinical practice of high dose dexamethasone suppression testing in the differential diagnosis of ACTH-dependent Cushing's syndrome. J Clin Endocrinol Metab 1997;82:1780. [PMID: 9177382]

Beuschlein F, Hammer GD: Ectopic pro-opiomelanocortin syndrome. Endocrinol Metab Clin North Am 2002;31:191. [PMID: 12055989]

Cavagnini F, Pecori Giraldi F: Epidemiology and follow-up of Cushing's disease. Ann Endocrinol (Paris) 2001;62:168. [PMID: 11353889]

Chee GH et al: Transsphenoidal pituitary surgery in Cushing's disease: can we predict outcome? Clin Endocrinol (Oxf) 2001;54:617. [PMID: 11380492]

Findling JW, Raff H: Diagnosis and differential diagnosis of Cushing's syndrome. Endocrinol Metab Clin North Am 2001; 30:729. [PMID: 11571938]

Lebrethon MC et al: Food-dependent Cushing's syndrome: characterization and functional role of gastric inhibitory polypeptide receptor in the adrenals of three patients. J Clin Endocrinol Metab 1998;83:4515. [PMID: 9851802]

Lindholm J et al: Incidence and late prognosis of Cushing's syndrome: a population-based study. J Clin Endocrinol Metab 2001;86:117. [PMID: 11231987]

Newell-Price J et al: Optimal response criteria for the human CRH test in the differential diagnosis of ACTH-dependent Cushing's syndrome. J Clin Endocrinol Metab 2002;87:1640. [PMID: 11932295]

Newell-Price J, Grossman A: Biochemical and imaging evaluation of Cushing's syndrome. Minerva Endocrinol 2002;27:95. [PMID: 11961502]

Newell-Price J: Transsphenoidal surgery for Cushing's disease: defining cure and following outcome. Clin Endocrinol (Oxf) 2002;56:19. [PMID: 11849241]

Quddisi S, Browne P, Hirsch IB: Cushing's syndrome due to surreptitious glucocorticoid administration. JAMA 1998;158: 294. [PMID: 9472211]

Raff H, Raff JL, Findling JW: Late-night salivary cortisol as a screening test for Cushing's syndrome. J Clin Endocrinol Metab 1998;83:2681. [PMID: 9709931]

Savage MO et al: Cushing's disease in childhood: presentation, investigation, treatment and long-term outcome. Horm Res 2001;55(Suppl 1):24. [PMID: 11408758]

Stratakis CA, Kirschner LS, Carney JA: Clinical and molecular features of the Carney complex: diagnostic criteria and recommendations for patient evaluation. J Clin Endocrinol Metab 2001;86:4041. [PMID: 11549623]

Swearingen B et al: Long-term mortality after transsphenoidal surgery for Cushing disease. Ann Intern Med 1999;130:821. [PMID: 10366371]

Hirsutism and Virilization

Azziz R, Carmina E, Sawaya ME: Idiopathic hirsutism. Endocr Rev 2000;21:347. [PMID: 10950156]

Cabrera MS et al: Long term outcome in adult males with classic congenital adrenal hyperplasia. J Clin Endocrinol Metab 2001;86:3070. [PMID: 11443169]

Miller WL: Congenital adrenal hyperplasia in the adult patient. Adv Intern Med 1999;44:155. [PMID: 9929708]

Moran C et al: 21-Hydroxylase-deficient nonclassic adrenal hyperplasia is a progressive disorder: a multicenter study. Am J Obstet Gynecol 2000;183:1468. [PMID: 11120512]

New MI: Diagnosis and management of congenital adrenal hyperplasia. Annu Rev Med 1998;49:311. [PMID: 9509266]

Rumsby G et al: Genotype-phenotype analysis in late onset 21-hydroxylase deficiency in comparison to the classical forms. Clin Endocrinol (Oxf) 1998;48:707. [PMID: 9713558]

Incidentally Discovered Adrenal Masses and Adrenal Cancer

Aron DC (editor): Incidentalomas. Endocrinol Metab Clin North Am 2000;29:1.

Boushey RP, Dackiw AP: Adrenal cortical carcinoma. Curr Treat Options Oncol 2001;2:355. [PMID: 12057116]

Caoili EM et al: Adrenal masses: characterization with combined unenhanced and delayed enhanced CT. Radiology 2002; 222:629.

Icard P et al: Adrenocortical carcinomas: surgical trends and results of a 253-patient series from the French Association of Endocrine Surgeons study group. World J Surg 2001;25:891. [PMID: 11572030]

Endocrine Hypertension

10

Burl R. Don, MD, Morris Schambelan, MD, & Joan C. Lo, MD

ACE	Angiotensin-converting enzyme	**DOC**	Deoxycorticosterone
ACTH	Adrenocorticotropic hormone	**EDRF**	Endothelium-derived relaxing factor
ANP	Atrial natriuretic peptide	**GFR**	Glomerular filtration rate
ARB	Angiotensin receptor blocker	**MRA**	Magnetic resonance angiography
BNP	Brain natriuretic peptide	**SGK**	Serum and glucocorticoid-regulated kinase
CBG	Corticosteroid-binding globulin		
CNP	C-type natriuretic peptide	**THE**	Tetrahydrocortisone
DHEA	Dehydroepiandrosterone	**THF**	Tetrahydrocortisol
DHEAS	Dehydroepiandrosterone sulfate	**WNK**	With no K (K lysine)

Arterial hypertension is a prominent component of a number of endocrine disorders, most prominently those involving the adrenal glands (pheochromocytoma, primary aldosteronism) and the pituitary (ACTH-producing tumors). Although the kidney is not an endocrine organ per se, its role as both the origin of and target tissue for the hormones that comprise the renin-angiotensin-aldosterone system makes hypertensive disorders of renal origin an appropriate subject for a chapter on endocrine hypertension. Hypertension may also be a prominent feature of other endocrine disorders such as acromegaly, thyrotoxicosis, hypothyroidism, and hyperparathyroidism, but these topics are considered elsewhere in this volume and will not be discussed in any detail here.

■ HYPERTENSION OF ADRENAL ORIGIN

SYNTHESIS, METABOLISM, & ACTION OF MINERALOCORTICOID HORMONES

The biosynthetic pathways of the mineralocorticoid hormones are shown in Figure 10–1. The major adrenal secretory products with mineralocorticoid activity are al-

dosterone and 11-deoxycorticosterone (DOC). Cortisol also has high intrinsic mineralocorticoid activity, but, as discussed in a subsequent section, its actions in the kidney are blunted by local degradation. Aldosterone is produced exclusively in the zona glomerulosa and is primarily controlled by the renin-angiotensin system. Other regulators include Na$^+$ and K$^+$ levels, ACTH, and dopamine. With the exception of 18-hydroxycorticosterone, the precursors of aldosterone that originate in the zona glomerulosa are normally present in very low concentrations in the peripheral blood. In the zona fasciculata, the two major biosynthetic pathways are under the control of ACTH. The major product formed by the 17-hydroxy pathway is cortisol. The principal steroid product of the 17-deoxy pathway with significant mineralocorticoid activity is DOC. Corticosterone and 18-hydroxydeoxycorticosterone are also produced in substantial amounts, but these steroids have relatively little mineralocorticoid activity in humans.

Aldosterone binds weakly to corticosteroid-binding globulin (CBG)—in contrast to steroids made in the zona fasciculata—and circulates mostly bound to albumin. Free aldosterone comprises 30–50% of its total plasma concentration, whereas the free fractions of the steroid products of the zona fasciculata comprise 5–10% of their total concentration. Consequently, aldosterone has a relatively short half-life, on the order of 15–20 minutes. Aldosterone is rapidly inactivated in the liver, with formation of tetrahydroaldosterone.

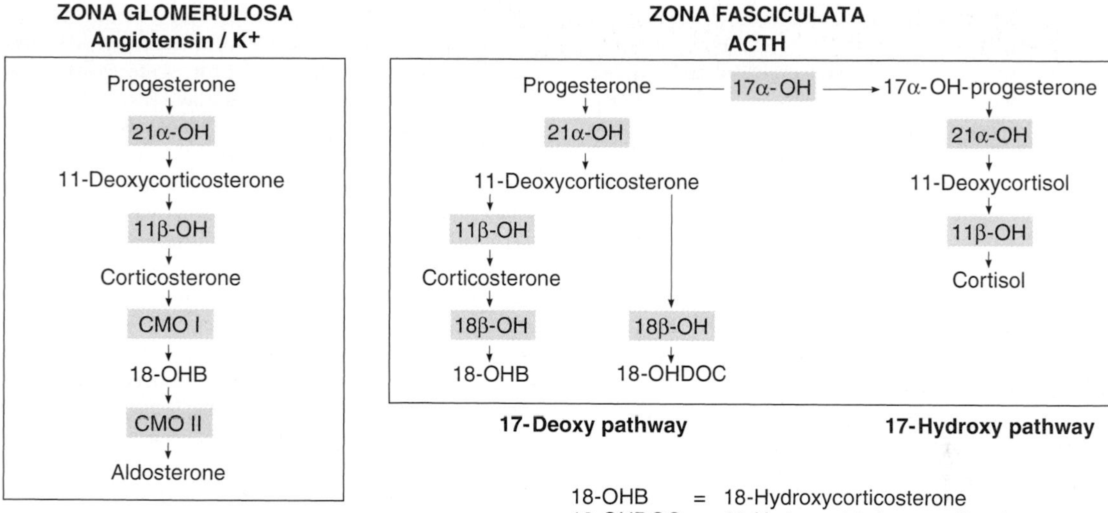

ZONA GLOMERULOSA
Angiotensin / K⁺

Progesterone
↓
21α-OH
↓
11-Deoxycorticosterone
↓
11β-OH
↓
Corticosterone
↓
CMO I
↓
18-OHB
↓
CMO II
↓
Aldosterone

ZONA FASCICULATA
ACTH

Progesterone ——— 17α-OH ——→ 17α-OH-progesterone
↓   ↓
21α-OH   21α-OH
↓   ↓
11-Deoxycorticosterone   11-Deoxycortisol
↓   ↓
11β-OH   11β-OH
↓   ↓
Corticosterone   Cortisol
↓   ↓
18β-OH   18β-OH
↓   ↓
18-OHB   18-OHDOC

17-Deoxy pathway   **17-Hydroxy pathway**

18-OHB	=	18-Hydroxycorticosterone
18-OHDOC	=	18-Hydroxy-11-deoxycorticosterone
CMO I	=	Corticosterone methyloxidase I (18β-hydroxylase) activity
CMO II	=	Corticosterone methyloxidase II (18β-hydrogenase) activity

(CMO I and CMO II are also called aldosterone synthase)

ACTH	=	Adrenocorticotropic hormone
17α-OH	=	P450c17 (17α-hydroxylase) activity
21α-OH	=	P450c21 (21α-hydroxylase) activity
11β-OH	=	P450c11 (11β-hydroxylase) activity
18β-OH	=	P450c11 (18β-hydroxylase) activity

Figure 10–1. Biosynthetic pathways of the mineralocorticoids. (See also Figures 2–6, 9–4, 9–5, and 14–13. And see Table 9–1 for current gene symbols for steroidogenic enzymes.)

Another metabolite, aldosterone-18-glucuronide, is formed by the kidney and usually represents 5–10% of the secreted aldosterone. A small amount of free aldosterone appears in the urine and can be easily quantitated. Aldosterone secretion rates vary from 50 to 250 µg/d on Na⁺ intakes in the range of 100–150 mmol/d.

DOC is secreted at approximately the same rate as aldosterone. However, like cortisol, DOC is almost totally bound to CBG, with less than 5% appearing in the free form. It is metabolized in the liver to tetrahydrodeoxycorticosterone, conjugated with glucuronic acid, and excreted in the urine. There is virtually no free DOC detectable in the urine.

Mineralocorticoid activity reflects the availability of free hormone and the affinity of the hormone for the receptor. Aldosterone and DOC have approximately equal and high affinities for the mineralocorticoid receptor and circulate at roughly similar concentrations, but aldosterone is quantitatively the most important because much more of it is free. Cortisol has an affinity for the receptor similar to that of aldosterone and its free levels in the circulation are about 100-fold higher than those of aldosterone. Because of this, cortisol is the major steroid that occupies the mineralocorticoid receptors in many tissues such as the pituitary and heart; however, at normal circulating levels, cortisol does not contribute much to mineralocorticoid action in typical target tissues (kidney, colon, salivary glands) because of local conversion (via 11β-hydroxysteroid dehydrogenase) to cortisone. Cortisol can lead to mineralocorticoid hypertension when this conversion is blunted by deficiency or inhibition of this enzyme (discussed subsequently).

Aldosterone and other mineralocorticoids influence certain ion-transporting epithelia with high Na⁺-K⁺ ATPase levels. The principal effects of the mineralocorticoids are on maintenance of normal Na⁺ and K⁺ concentrations and extracellular fluid volume. Mineralocorticoids cross the cell membrane and combine with a mineralocorticoid receptor in the cytosol (see Chapter 3 and Figure 3–12). The active steroid-receptor complex moves into the nucleus of the target cell, where it alters the rate of transcription of mineralocorticoid-responsive genes with subsequent changes in the levels of specific mRNAs and their protein products. The aldosterone-induced proteins include factors that regulate the luminal Na⁺ channel, facilitating movement of Na⁺ into cells, and components of the Na⁺-K⁺ ATPase pump. The principal early effect of aldosterone (beginning in less than 1 hour) is on the Na⁺ channel. Without altering overall channel abundance, aldosterone increases the apical membrane targeting, or the probability of open channels, already synthesized, in the collecting tubule and part of the distal convoluted tubule. Recently, a key mediator of the early response was identified as an aldosterone-regulated kinase (serum glucocorticoid-regulated kinase; SGK) that increases Na^+ channel activity. The later effects (occurring 6–24 hours after hormone administration) of aldosterone include activation of Na^+-K^+ ATPase and alterations in cell morphology and energy metabolism. Some or all of these may be due to the altered intracellular Na^+ concentrations that result from the primary effect on the Na^+ channel. In addition to directly enhancing Na^+ absorption, the major effect of these aldosterone-induced changes in ion transport is to increase the difference in electrical potential across the renal tubule. The increased luminal negativity augments tubular secretion of K^+ by the principal cell and H^+ by the intercalated cell (Figure 10–2). Tubular Na^+, via the Na^+ pump, enters the extracellular fluid and helps maintain its normal composition and volume. All of these events occur in other secretory systems as well and can be measured in saliva, sweat, and feces.

PATHOGENESIS OF MINERALOCORTICOID HYPERTENSION

Mineralocorticoid hormones produce hypertension by several mechanisms (Figure 10–3). The initiating events are the physiologic consequences of mineralocorticoid-induced expansion of plasma and extracellular fluid volume. Insights into these early mechanisms come from studies in normal subjects given high doses of mineralocorticoids and from sequential observations made following discontinuation of spironolactone therapy in patients with aldosterone-secreting adenomas. Initially, Na^+ and fluid retention occur, with an increase in body weight, extracellular fluid volume, and cardiac output. After gaining 1–2 L of additional extracellular fluid, the phenomenon of Na^+ "escape" follows, so that a new steady state is achieved. Renal K^+ wasting persists and arterial blood pressure continues to increase, however. Typically, the chronic stage of mineralocorticoid excess is characterized by an increase in total peripheral vascular resistance and normalization of stroke volume and cardiac output. The increase in peripheral vascular resistance is related in part to increased sensitivity to catecholamines even without a distinct increment in plasma epinephrine or norepinephrine levels. An additional mechanism may be a direct central action of aldosterone: Intracerebroventricular infusion of aldosterone to rats produced hypertension that could not be reversed or prevented by infusion, at the same site, of a competitive aldosterone antagonist.

Primary mineralocorticoid excess is manifested by hypertension, hypokalemia, and suppression of the renin-angiotensin system. Primary aldosteronism is the prototypic disorder and will be described in the greatest detail. Clinically similar syndromes can result from increased adrenal production of other steroids with mineralocorticoid activity (eg, DOC), failure to inactivate cortisol (eg, syndrome of apparent mineralocorticoid excess), or as a consequence of mineralocorticoid-independent augmentation of renal Na^+ reabsorption due to a constitutively activated epithelial Na^+ channel (eg, Liddle's syndrome). The presence of these latter disorders is often suggested by clinical findings of primary

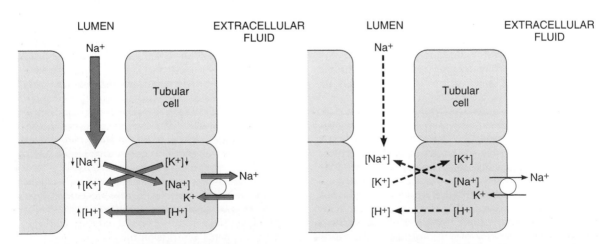

Figure 10–2. Mineralocorticoid action. On the left, rates of tubular sodium delivery together with increased mineralocorticoid action lead to K^+ and H^+ secretion and Na^+ movement into extracellular fluid. On the right, similar amounts of mineralocorticoid are ineffective when tubular sodium is reduced (eg, by dietary sodium restriction).

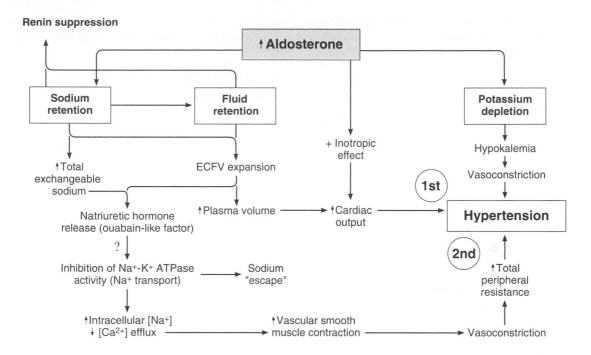

Figure 10–3. Mechanisms involved in mineralocorticoid hypertension. First, there is sodium retention, fluid retention, expansion of extracellular fluid volume and plasma volume, increased cardiac output, and hypertension. Second, there is vasoconstriction and increased total peripheral resistance and hypertension. (ECFV, extracellular fluid volume.) (See text for details.)

mineralocorticoid excess in a patient with subnormal aldosterone levels.

ALDOSTERONE & THE HEART

Over the last few years, there has been increasing interest in the effects of aldosterone on the myocardium—independent of changes attributable to chronic arterial hypertension. Aldosterone excess has been shown to result in cardiac fibrosis in animals, and studies in patients with primary aldosteronism suggest that aldosterone excess is associated with alterations in myocardial texture as assessed by echocardiography. Aldosterone also appears to be important in the pathophysiology of heart failure as demonstrated by the Randomized Aldactone Evaluation Study (RALES), in which treatment with spironolactone led to a substantial reduction in morbidity and mortality in patients with severe heart failure.

PRIMARY ALDOSTERONISM

Increased production of aldosterone by abnormal zona glomerulosa tissue (adenoma or hyperplasia) initiates the series of events, described in the preceding sections, that result in the typical clinical manifestations of the syndrome of primary aldosteronism. A benign aldosterone-producing adenoma, as originally described by Conn, accounts for 75% of cases of primary aldosteronism. Idiopathic hyperaldosteronism, a disorder with many similar clinical features, accounts for most of the remaining cases. In idiopathic hyperaldosteronism the adrenals are either normal in appearance or, more commonly, reveal bilateral (or, rarely, unilateral) micro- or macronodular adrenal hyperplasia.

Increased renal Na$^+$ retention results in expansion of the extracellular fluid volume and increased total body Na$^+$ content. Although the effects on the kidney are greatest quantitatively, other mineralocorticoid target tissues are also affected. Fecal excretion of Na$^+$, for example, can be decreased to almost nil, with a measurable effect on the rectal potential difference. Salivary electrolyte ratios can also reflect the influence of hyperaldosteronism on that target tissue. The expanded extracellular fluid and plasma volumes are sensed by stretch receptors at the juxtaglomerular apparatus and Na$^+$ flux at the macula densa, with resultant suppression of renin secretion, measured as suppressed plasma renin activity. Suppression of the renin-angiotensin system, while not of itself diagnostic of primary aldosteronism, is thus a major feature of this disorder.

In addition to Na^+ retention, K^+ depletion develops, decreasing the total body and plasma concentration of K^+. The extrusion of K^+ from its intracellular reservoir is followed by the intracellular movement of H^+ and, together with aldosterone-dependent increases in renal secretion of H^+, results in metabolic alkalosis. With moderate K^+ depletion, decreased carbohydrate tolerance (as evidenced by an abnormal glucose tolerance test) and resistance to vasopressin (as evidenced by impaired urinary concentrating ability) occur. Severe K^+ depletion blunts baroreceptor function, occasionally producing postural hypotension.

Primary aldosteronism is a disease of the zona glomerulosa. Other adrenal products formed in this zone such as DOC, corticosterone, and 18-hydroxycorticosterone may be present in increased amounts in the blood or urine of persons with an aldosterone-producing adenoma (Figure 10–1). Cells of this zone do not have the ability to make cortisol (owing to the absence of the CYP17, 17α-hydroxylase system). Thus, there are no abnormalities in either cortisol production or metabolism. Plasma and urine cortisol levels are normal.

Clinical Features

Patients typically come to medical attention because of symptoms of hypokalemia or detection of previously unsuspected hypertension during the course of a routine physical examination. The medical history reveals no characteristic symptoms other than nonspecific complaints of fatigue, loss of stamina, weakness, and lassitude—all of which are symptoms of K^+ depletion. If K^+ depletion is more severe, increased thirst, polyuria (especially nocturnal), and paresthesias may also be present. Headaches are frequent.

Excessive production of mineralocorticoids produces no characteristic physical findings. Blood pressure in patients with primary aldosteronism can range from borderline elevation to severely hypertensive levels. The mean blood pressure in the 136 patients reported by the Glasgow Hypertension Study unit was 205/123 mm Hg, with no significant difference between the groups with adenoma or hyperplasia. Accelerated or malignant hypertension is extremely rare. Retinopathy is mild, and hemorrhages are rarely present. Orthostatic decreases in blood pressure without reflex tachycardia are observed in the severely K^+-depleted patient because of blunting of the baroreceptors. A positive Trousseau or Chvostek sign may be suggestive of alkalosis accompanying severe K^+ depletion. The heart is usually only mildly enlarged, and electrocardiographic changes reflect modest left ventricular hypertrophy and K^+ depletion. Clinical edema is uncommon.

Initial Diagnosis

A. HYPOKALEMIA

Detection of spontaneous hypokalemia is often the initial clue that suggests a diagnosis of primary aldosteronism in a patient with hypertension. During the investigation, a high-K^+ diet or KCl supplements should be avoided, and all previous diuretic therapy must be discontinued for at least 3 weeks before a valid serum or plasma K^+ measurement can be obtained. The most common cause of hypokalemia in patients with hypertension is diuretic therapy.

In some series, up to 20% of patients with primary aldosteronism have had normal or low-normal serum K^+ concentrations. Serum K^+ concentration is closely related to and determined to a great extent by NaCl intake (Figure 10–2). A low Na^+ diet, by reducing delivery of Na^+ to aldosterone-sensitive sites in the distal nephron, can reduce renal K^+ secretion and thus correct hypokalemia. By the same token, increased distal delivery of Na^+ accompanying a high Na^+ diet can enhance K^+ loss, particularly when aldosterone is being secreted autonomously and is therefore not subject to normal suppression by the high Na^+ intake. These physiologic relationships serve to illustrate the importance of controlling the dietary Na^+ intake when evaluating patients suspected of having primary aldosteronism. In the presence of normal renal function and autonomous aldosterone production, salt loading will usually unmask hypokalemia. Normokalemic hyperaldosteronism under these conditions has been reported but is rare.

B. SALT INTAKE

In the USA, Japan, and many European countries, the average person consumes more than 120 mmol of Na^+ per day—enough to allow hypokalemia to become manifest. If a dietary history of high salt intake is obtained and K^+ concentrations are normal, a diagnosis of primary aldosteronism is unlikely. Patients who report a low Na^+ intake should be advised to take an unrestricted diet plus 1 g of NaCl with each meal for 4 days; blood samples for electrolyte determinations should be obtained in the fasting state on the following morning. This dietary regimen is also useful because it prepares the patient for optimal measurement of renin and aldosterone levels.

C. ASSESSMENT OF THE RENIN-ANGIOTENSIN-ALDOSTERONE SYSTEM

Assessment of the renin-angiotensin system can be accomplished by a random plasma renin activity measurement. If plasma renin activity is normal or high in a patient who has not been receiving diuretic therapy for at least 3 weeks, it is very unlikely that an aldosterone-producing adenoma is present. Some patients with idiopathic hyperaldosteronism may have low-normal levels of plasma renin activity, however. On the other hand, a subnormal plasma renin level is not alone sufficient to establish a diagnosis of primary aldosteronism, since a large subgroup of patients with essential hypertension have low plasma renin levels.

If hypokalemia and suppressed renin activity are detected, plasma and urinary aldosterone measurements should be obtained while the patient is taking an unrestricted salt diet with NaCl supplementation or if the dietary history reveals a high salt intake, as previously described. This is crucial, because with any significant diminution of salt intake, plasma aldosterone concentration and aldosterone production normally increase.

Assessment of aldosterone production can best be accomplished by measurement of urinary aldosterone excretion over a 24-hour period. Most laboratories measure excretion of the 18-glucuronide metabolite. The normal rates of urinary excretion of aldosterone-18-glucuronide range from 5 μg to 20 μg/24 h (14–56 nmol/24 h). In one large series, the mean values in patients with aldosterone-producing adenoma and idiopathic hyperaldosteronism were 45.2 ± 4 μg/24 h (125 ± 9 nmol/24 h) and 27.1 ± 2 μg/24 h (75 ± 5 nmol/24 h), respectively. Urinary measurements are superior to random measurements of plasma aldosterone for the detection of abnormal production of aldosterone but are not always able to discriminate between patients with adenoma and those with idiopathic hyperaldosteronism.

Samples for measurement of plasma aldosterone concentration should ideally be obtained at around 8:00 AM after at least 4 hours of recumbency and under the same dietary conditions as described above for measurement of urinary aldosterone. This measurement not only confirms the presence of hyperaldosteronism but also provides insight into the probable underlying pathology. When obtained under these conditions, a plasma aldosterone concentration greater than 25 ng/dL (695 pmol/L) usually indicates the presence of an aldosterone-producing adenoma (Figure 10–4).

Some investigators have advocated the use of the aldosterone:renin ratio as a means of screening for and perhaps establishing a diagnosis of primary aldosteronism. A ratio in excess of 30 (assuming that aldosterone levels are reported in nanograms per deciliter and renin levels in nanograms per milliliter per hour) is usually considered abnormal. However, since a low renin level (eg, 0.1 ng/mL/h) can result in an elevated ratio even when aldosterone levels are in the low normal range (eg, 3 ng/dL), use of the ratio in the absence of a con-

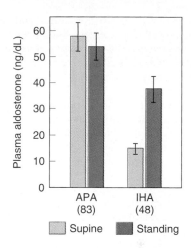

Figure 10–4. Response of plasma aldosterone to postural stimulation in primary aldosteronism. (APA, aldosterone-producing adenoma; IHA, idiopathic hyperaldosteronism.)

comitantly elevated aldosterone level should be discouraged.

Determining the plasma aldosterone level after 2–4 hours in the upright posture (which normally activates the renin system, with a resultant increase in the plasma aldosterone level), may be helpful in determining the cause of primary aldosteronism. Ninety percent of patients with adenoma will show no significant change or a frank decrease in plasma aldosterone levels, whereas aldosterone levels almost always increase in those with idiopathic hyperaldosteronism (Figure 10–4). The difference is due to (1) the profound suppression of the renin system by excessive aldosterone production in patients with an adenoma; (2) the influence of ACTH, to which the adenoma is still responsive and which normally decreases between 8 AM and 12 noon; and (3) decreased responsiveness of adenomas to angiotensin II. In contrast, in patients with idiopathic hyperaldosteronism, increased sensitivity of the gland to small increases in renin (and presumably of angiotensin II) levels that occur in the upright posture leads to an increased aldosterone level. Serum cortisol levels must be measured simultaneously. An increase in serum cortisol implies an ACTH discharge and invalidates the information obtained from the maneuver.

Measurement of other adrenal steroids may add to the precision of diagnosis. Plasma DOC, corticosterone, and, particularly, 18-hydroxycorticosterone levels are frequently increased in patients with adenoma, whereas they are rarely if ever increased in patients with idiopathic hyperaldosteronism. Increased urinary excretion of 18-hydroxycortisol and 18-oxocortisol, which is a characteristic finding in individuals with the dexamethasone-suppressible form of primary aldosteronism (described in a subsequent section), may also be present in some patients with aldosterone-producing adenomas.

The procedures just discussed can confirm a diagnosis of primary aldosteronism and differentiate adenoma from idiopathic hyperaldosteronism in most cases. Localization studies can also provide additional information. When uncertainty persists, the saline infusion test may also be useful.

D. SALINE INFUSION TEST

Saline loading establishes aldosterone unresponsiveness to volume expansion and thereby identifies autonomy in patients with aldosterone-producing adenomas. Two liters of isotonic NaCl are administered over 2–4 hours. Blood samples for aldosterone and cortisol measurements are obtained before and after the infusion. Expansion of the extracellular fluid volume reduces plasma aldosterone concentration promptly in patients with "essential" hypertension but fails to suppress plasma aldosterone concentration into the normal range in patients with adenoma or hyperplasia. Moreover, the saline infusion test typically distinguishes patients with primary aldosteronism from those with low-renin essential hypertension. The ratio of aldosterone to cortisol is typically greater than 3.0 following administration of saline in patients with an aldosterone-producing adenoma, reflecting the limited effect of volume expansion in the setting of marked suppression of the renin-angiotensin system.

Rare Forms of Primary Aldosteronism

A. DEXAMETHASONE (GLUCOCORTICOID)-REMEDIABLE ALDOSTERONISM

Dexamethasone-remediable aldosteronism is a rare form of genetic hypertension that has been recognized with increasing frequency since the molecular basis of this disorder was established. It is inherited in an autosomal dominant fashion. The primary defect is a gene duplication that results from an unequal crossing over event that fuses the regulatory region of the 11β-hydroxylase gene to the coding sequence of aldosterone synthase. This chimeric gene leads to ACTH-dependent expression of aldosterone synthase in the zona fasciculata, thereby resulting in the synthesis of aldosterone, 18-hydroxycortisol, and 18-oxocortisol (phenotypic markers of this disorder). Patients present with hypertension and biochemical features of mineralocorticoid excess (eg, suppressed plasma renin activity, increased aldosterone secretion) which are ameliorated with glucocorticoid administration. However, the response to dexamethasone suppression may dissipate over the long term in many patients, and additional antihypertensive therapy may thus be necessary. The presence of glucocorticoid-remediable aldosteronism should be considered in any family in which more than one individual is found to have primary aldosteronism. The diagnosis can easily be established by measurement of the marker steroids (18-oxocortisol or 18-hydroxycortisol) or by detection of the abnormal gene in DNA samples obtained from peripheral blood leukocytes.

B. ALDOSTERONE-PRODUCING ADRENOCORTICAL CARCINOMA

Malignant adrenocortical tumors producing aldosterone in the absence of hypercortisolism are rare, accounting for less than 3% of cases of primary aldosteronism. In general, the biochemical and hormonal features and the response to dynamic tests are similar to those typical in adenoma except that the magnitude of the abnormalities is usually greater. Hypercortisolism as well as hyperandrogenism or hyperestrogenism may occur during the progression of the disease.

Management of Aldosterone-Producing Adenomas

A. LOCATION OF ADENOMA

Once the biochemical diagnosis is secure, procedures that identify the likely site of an adenoma can aid in establishing the appropriate surgical approach. A number of techniques have been developed including adrenal venography, adrenal scintigraphy, adrenal vein catheterization with sampling for aldosterone measurements, and CT or MRI imaging. The diagnostic information provided by CT scanning or MRI in locating adenomas has proved to be both accurate and practical and is the initial procedure of choice. Adrenal venography was associated with a number of problems, such as extravasation of dye, hemorrhage, and adrenal infarction and is no longer utilized. Scanning using intravenously administered ^{131}I-iodocholesterol can identify the site of an adenoma in about 80% of patients, although the success rate decreases markedly if tumors are less than 1 cm in diameter. The procedure takes several visits to accomplish, however. The use of ^{131}I-labeled 6β-iodomethyl-19-norcholesterol reduces the interval between injection and scintiscanning to about 3–7 days.

Patients suspected of having an aldosterone-producing adenoma (younger age, more severe hypertension, more profound hypokalemia, and higher aldosterone secretion) who are found to have a unilateral adrenal nodule greater than 1 cm should proceed to unilateral laparoscopic adrenalectomy. Patients with less severe biochemical findings may have idiopathic hyperaldosteronism with an adrenal incidentaloma. For such patients and for those with equivocal CT findings (eg, adrenal nodules < 1 cm or bilateral adrenal abnormalities), adrenal vein sampling provides the most accurate means of differentiating a unilateral aldosterone-producing adrenal adenoma from idiopathic hyperaldosteronism.

Adrenal vein catheterization to obtain samples for measurement and comparison of aldosterone levels in the venous effluent of both adrenal glands continues to be useful in lateralizing tumors after other techniques fail and biochemical evidence still supports the diagnosis of adenoma. The success of this procedure is highly dependent on the skill and experience of the interventional radiologist. Cortisol levels should always be measured simultaneously to confirm the source of the sample and the extent of contamination with nonadrenal venous blood. Treatment with ACTH prior to and during the study (cosyntropin, 50 µg/h, given as a continuous infusion initiated 30 minutes prior to the study) is also recommended to magnify the differences between affected and unaffected sides and to avoid variable ACTH stimulation during the procedure. An adrenal vein to inferior vena cava cortisol gradient greater than 5:1 generally confirms successful adrenal vein catheterization. When comparing adrenal vein samples, the aldosterone level should be corrected for dilutional effects by dividing by the cortisol level. The finding of a ratio of the adrenal vein aldosterone levels so corrected that exceeds 4:1 is consistent with a unilateral aldosterone-producing adenoma.

B. Treatment Options

Treatment depends for the most part on the accuracy of diagnosis. In patients with an aldosterone-producing adenoma and no contraindication to surgery, unilateral adrenalectomy is recommended. The degree of reduction of blood pressure and correction of hypokalemia achieved with prior spironolactone therapy provides a good indication of the likely response to surgery; in fact, greater reduction often occurs postoperatively, presumably because of a greater reduction of extracellular fluid volume. The surgical cure rate of hypertension associated with adenoma is excellent—more than 70% have benefited in several large series—with reduction of hypertension in the remainder.

Subtotal adrenalectomy will correct hypokalemia in patients with idiopathic aldosteronism, but hypertension is rarely cured. Therefore, other antihypertensive measures (including spironolactone) should be used to control hypertension, and such patients should not be routinely sent to surgery. A subset of patients with primary aldosteronism but no identifiable adenoma may benefit from surgical reduction of adrenal mass, ie,

subtotal or total adrenalectomy. This group (referred to as primary adrenal hyperplasia) typically responds to stimulatory and suppressive maneuvers in a manner similar to patients with an aldosterone-producing adenoma. Pathologic examination of the adrenal tissue usually discloses micro- or macronodular hyperplasia. The autonomy of aldosterone production in this condition is difficult to explain, but the disease may be compared to the autonomy of cortisol production in nodular dysplasia associated with Cushing's syndrome.

C. Preoperative Preparation

Ideally, patients should be treated preoperatively with spironolactone until the blood pressure and serum K+ are normal. This drug is particularly beneficial because of its unique mechanism of action in blocking the mineralocorticoid receptor. Spironolactone reduces the volume of the expanded extracellular fluid toward normal, promotes K+ retention, and restores normal serum K+ concentration. It often has the additional desirable effect of activating (after 1–2 months) the suppressed renin-angiotensin system and, consequently, of aldosterone secretion by the contralateral adrenal gland. Postoperative hypoaldosteronism with hyperkalemia is unlikely with this treatment. Preoperative treatment will also permit reversal to some extent of some of the changes in target organs that were produced by the hypertensive and hypokalemic states. Spironolactone is usually well tolerated; the side effects of rashes, gynecomastia, impotence, and epigastric discomfort are rare over a short time interval. Once blood pressure and serum K+ levels are normal on an initial dose of 200–300 mg/d, the dose can be tapered to a maintenance dose of approximately 100 mg/d until the time of surgery. In patients who develop one or more of these side effects, the K+-sparing diuretic amiloride, in doses of 20–40 mg/d, can be used as an alternative. Other antihypertensive drugs may also be required and should be used to obtain optimal blood pressure control. Calcium channel blockers appear to be effective in this setting.

D. Surgical and Postoperative Medical Treatment

When the diagnosis and lateralization are certain, surgical removal of the adenoma is advised. Current preoperative lateralization techniques easily identify the site of tumor, which can be removed via a laparoscope in virtually all cases.

Over 70% of patients with primary aldosteronism who have undergone surgery have had unilateral adenoma. Bilateral tumors are rare. The characteristic adenoma is readily identified by its golden-yellow color. In addition, small satellite adenomas are often found, and distinction from micro- or macronodular hyperplasia is occasionally difficult. In patients with adenoma, the contiguous adrenal gland can show hyperplasia throughout the gland. Hyperplasia is also present in the contralateral adrenal gland but is not associated with aldosterone abnormalities after removal of the primary adenoma.

If the tumor is identified at surgery in a patient who had a unilateral lesion detected preoperatively, exploration of the contralateral adrenal is not indicated. If surgery is contraindicated or refused, prolonged treatment with spironolactone can be effective. The initial dose of 200–400 mg of spironolactone per day must be continued for 4–6 weeks before the full effect on blood pressure is realized. With prolonged treatment, aldosterone production does not increase even though K^+ replenishment and activation of the renin-angiotensin system occur. In addition, spironolactone directly inhibits aldosterone synthesis by adenomas. A chronic dose of 75–100 mg is usually sufficient to maintain a normal blood pressure.

Patients who have had unilateral adrenalectomy for removal of an aldosterone-producing tumor occasionally have a transient period of relative hypomineralocorticoidism with negative Na^+ balance, K^+ retention, and mild acidosis. Full recovery of the chronically unstimulated, contralateral zona glomerulosa usually takes place in 4–6 months following surgery but may take longer. Restitution of the suppressed renin-angiotensin system to normal is required for a completely normal adrenocortical response similar to the need for recovery of pituitary function after removal of a cortisol-producing adenoma (Cushing's syndrome). No specific treatment is usually necessary other than adequate Na^+ intake. A small percentage of patients (1%) do not have normal recovery of their renin-angiotensin-aldosterone system and require mineralocorticoid replacement (fludrocortisone) therapy for life. Preexisting renal disease that impairs renin secretion is usually evident in such individuals.

SYNDROMES DUE TO EXCESS DEOXYCORTICOSTERONE PRODUCTION

Deoxycorticosterone is the second most important naturally occurring mineralocorticoid hormone. Accordingly, excess DOC production should be suspected in any hypertensive patient with hypokalemia and suppression of renin and aldosterone production.

17α-Hydroxylase Deficiency

17α-Hydroxylase deficiency syndrome is usually recognized at the time of puberty in young adults by the presence of hypertension, hypokalemia, and primary amenorrhea (with sexual infantilism) in the female or pseudohermaphroditism in the male (Chapter 14). In contrast to the clinical manifestations in 21- and 11β-hydroxylation deficiencies, there is no virilization or restricted growth. Patients often present with eunuchoid proportions and appearance. The virtual absence of 17α-hydroxyprogesterone, pregnanetriol, and 17-ketosteroids is diagnostic of this type of hydroxylase deficiency.

The key location of the 17α-hydroxylating system (cytochrome P450c17α) in the steroid biosynthetic pathway prevents normal production of androgens and estrogens (Figure 9–4). There has been no instance in which the adrenal defect has appeared without a concomitant gonadal defect. The defect occurs in a single gene (in chromosome 10), which codes for the enzyme or the expression of the enzyme. The diminution of cortisol production induces increased production of ACTH. Initially, activity of the entire biosynthetic pathway of non-17-hydroxylated steroids is increased—namely, progesterone, DOC, corticosterone, 18-hydroxydeoxycorticosterone, 18-hydroxycorticosterone, and aldosterone. Subsequently, expansion of extracellular fluid and blood volumes, hypertension, and profound suppression of the renin-angiotensin system results, in most cases, in reduced aldosterone levels. Thus, the principal steroids present in excess are DOC, corticosterone, 18-hydroxycorticosterone, and 18-hydroxydeoxycorticosterone.

11β-Hydroxylase Deficiency

Congenital adrenal hyperplasia due to 11β-hydroxylase deficiency is usually recognized in newborns and infants because of virilization and the presence of both hypertension and hypokalemia. Plasma androgens, 11-deoxycortisol, 17α-hydroxyprogesterone, urinary 17-ketosteroids, and 17-hydroxycorticosteroids are increased. (See Chapter 14 and Figure 14–14.)

The defect in the gene (mapped to chromosome 8) is usually partial, so that some cortisol is produced, but it does not increase with further stimulation by ACTH. Blood levels and production rates of cortisol are usually within normal limits. A partial defect of 11β-hydroxylation results in increased production and blood levels of DOC, 11-deoxycortisol (Figure 10–1), and androgens. Hypertension results from excessive production of DOC by mechanisms similar to those previously described for aldosterone.

The blood levels and production rates of aldosterone are low-normal or reduced. Two mechanisms are proposed. Originally, a partial deficiency of the 11β-hydroxylation activity in the zona glomerulosa was postulated, with a block in aldosterone synthesis. This concept was supported by the observation that after normalization of DOC production and correction of the hypertension (by ACTH suppression), aldosterone production remained normal or reduced and a Na^+-losing state could be provoked. Currently, it is felt that there is no zona glomerulosa defect but that suppression of renin by the increased production of DOC reduces the production of aldosterone in the zona glomerulosa. Thus, after chronic salt restriction and ACTH suppression, both renin and aldosterone dynamics return to normal, implying an intact zona glomerulosa.

Treatment of 17α- & 11β-Hydroxylase Deficiency

Treatment of both of these disorders is similar to that of all non-Na^+-losing forms of congenital adrenal hyperplasia. Treatment with physiologic replacement doses of glucocorticoid, such as hydrocortisone or dexamethasone, restores blood pressure to normal levels, corrects K^+ depletion, reduces excessive DOC and corticosterone production in 17α-hydroxylase deficiency, and reduces DOC and 11-deoxycortisol production in 11β-hydroxylase deficiency. In 17α hydroxylase deficiency syndrome, restoration of normal levels of DOC results in a return of plasma renin activity and aldosterone to normal values. A delay in return of the suppressed renin-aldosterone system toward normal can result in hypovolemic crises with the initial natriuresis and diuresis. It may take several years before the aldosterone and renin systems become normal. The amount of glucocorticoid administered must be carefully determined because of apparently exquisite tissue sensitivity to glucocorticoid hormones. Addition of estrogen-progestin combined cyclic therapy may be necessary in the adult patient with 17α-hydroxylase deficiency (see Chapter 14).

Androgen- & Estrogen-Producing Adrenal Tumors

Most of the C-19 steroids produced by the adult adrenocortical zona reticularis have weak androgen activity, especially dehydroepiandrosterone (DHEA) and its sulfate (DHEAS) as well as androstenedione. Disturbances in both internal zona reticularis regulatory mechanisms (ie, enzyme activity) and its extra-adrenal regulators (ACTH and an androgen-stimulating peptide of possible hypothalamic-pituitary origin) may lead to excessive adrenal sex steroid production, resulting in syndromes of hirsutism and virilization in the female or feminization in men.

Although the zona reticularis has no intrinsic capacity to synthesize any effective glucocorticoid or mineralocorticoid, it has the potential, under conditions of chronic stimulation by ACTH, to transform some cellular function into the fasciculata cell type (by the induction of specific enzyme complexes) and produce cortisol and presumably other typical zona fasciculata steroids.

Some patients with malignancies originating in the zona reticularis (androgen- or estrogen-producing tumors, or both types) may have clinical features of mineralocorticoid excess, with hypertension, hypokalemia, and renin suppression. Aldosterone levels are generally not elevated and are often reduced. Urinary or plasma steroid profiling in some of these patients suggests that there may be inhibition of 11β-hydroxylase activity in association with the increased production of androgens or estrogens. Administration of methylandrostanediol to experimental animals and testosterone to humans suggests that exogenous androgen excess can block the conversion of 11-deoxycortisol and DOC to cortisol and corticosterone, respectively. Excessive secretion of DOC could then lead to a state of mineralocorticoid excess. Increased urinary excretion of DOC metabolites or plasma DOC concentrations have been found in several patients with androgen- or estrogen-producing adrenocortical carcinomas who have hypertension and hypokalemia.

The inhibition of 11β-hydroxylase in these carcinomas may be due to inactivation of the enzyme cytochrome CYP11B1 (formerly P450c11) by the high intra-adrenal concentration of androgens (androstenedione) that act as a pseudosubstrate for the reaction. This mechanism is similar to that occurring in Cushing's syndrome, in which cortisol appears to serve as the enzymatic inhibitor.

Syndrome of Primary Cortisol Resistance

Peripheral resistance to cortisol action is a very rare condition—reported only in a few families—in which hypertension, hypokalemia, and renin suppression are associated with elevated plasma and urinary levels of cortisol without causing clinical manifestations of Cushing's syndrome. The basic defect is at the level of the glucocorticoid receptor; both the number of receptors and the affinity of the receptors for cortisol are reduced in the target tissues. In this condition, plasma levels of ACTH are elevated as a result of block of cortisol feedback at the corticotroph. Cortisol production is thus increased, but it does not result in the typical clinical stigmas of hypercortisolism. However, chronic stimulation by excess ACTH of the 17-deoxy pathway of the zona fasciculata results in abnormal production of DOC and corticosterone, causing hypertension, hypokalemia, and suppression of renin and aldosterone production. Adrenal androgen production also increases under ACTH stimulation, and affected women may present with hirsutism, menstrual irregularities, and virilization. The clinical and biochemical abnormalities are partially relieved by treatment with high doses of dexamethasone.

CUSHING'S SYNDROME

Hypertension is a common finding of endogenous hypercortisolism (present in more than 80% of cases; see Chapter 9) but occurs in only 10–20% of patients receiving therapy with synthetic glucocorticoids. ACTH-dependent hypercortisolism (Cushing's disease and ectopic ACTH production) is frequently accompanied by increased levels of other ACTH-dependent steroids, especially DOC and corticosterone. Elevated DOC (Figure 10–5) and cortisol levels probably contribute to the mineralocorticoid excess state. Plasma renin activity varies but is typically normal as a consequence of concomitant increase in the production of angiotensinogen. Serum K^+ levels are also normal in most patients, implying the absence of a mineralocorticoid excess state. However, a small subset of patients have hypokalemia and suppressed plasma renin levels. Most of these patients have ectopic ACTH hypersecretion or adrenal tumors. Even when there is evidence for mineralocorticoid excess (suppressed plasma renin and hypokalemia), levels of aldosterone and 18-hydroxycorticosterone are consistently within or below the low normal range.

Hypertension in Cushing's syndrome is usually more frequent in patients with adrenocortical hyperplasia (due to ACTH excess) than in patients with cortical adenomas, which implies that, in addition to cortisol, other ACTH-dependent steroids (eg, DOC, corticosterone, or 18-hydroxydeoxycorticosterone) may contribute to the development or maintenance of hypertension. In addition, urinary excretion of the potent naturally occurring mineralocorticoid 19-nor-DOC, produced in the kidney by the conversion of an oxygenated form of DOC, is elevated in both the primary (adrenal) and secondary (pituitary) forms of Cushing's syndrome.

Since most patients with Cushing's syndrome do not have findings consistent with hypermineralocorticoidism (eg, hypokalemia and hyporeninemia), glucocorticoids appear to cause hypertension by mineralocorticoid-independent mechanisms (Figure 10–6). These include increased production of angiotensin II due to glucocorticoid-induced increases in the hepatic synthesis of angiotensinogen; enhanced glucocorticoid-mediated vascular reactivity to vasoconstrictors; inhibition of extraneuronal uptake and degradation of catecholamines; inhibition of vasodilatory systems such as kinins and prostaglandins; shift in Na^+ from the intracellular to the extracellular compartment, resulting in increased plasma volume; and an increase in cardiac output from the increased production of epinephrine

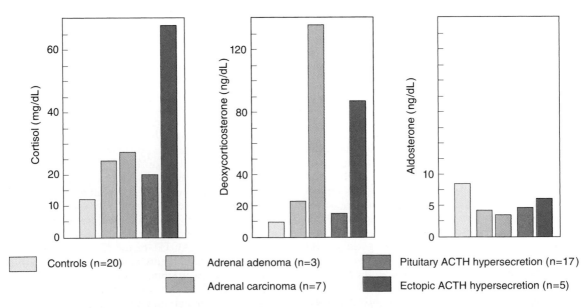

Figure 10–5. Basal cortisol, deoxycorticosterone, and aldosterone levels in patients with Cushing's syndrome according to etiology.

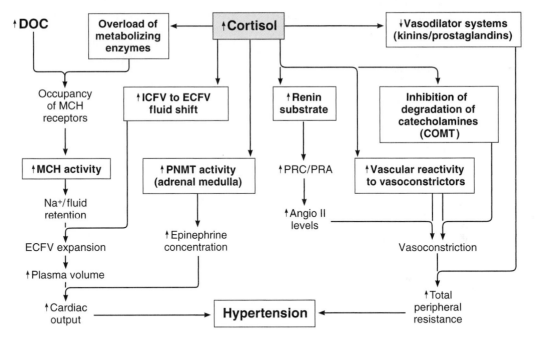

Figure 10–6. Mechanisms involved in glucocorticoid hypertension. (DOC, deoxycorticosterone; MCH, mineralocorticoid hormone; ECFV, extracellular fluid volume; ICFV, intracellular fluid volume; PRC, plasma renin concentration; PRA, plasma renin activity; COMT, catechol-*O*-methyltransferase; PNMT, phenylethanolamine-*N*-methyltransferase.)

due to enhanced phenylethanolamine-*N*-methyltransferase activity in the adrenal medulla.

PSEUDOHYPERALDOSTERONISM

The term pseudohyperaldosteronism comprises a heterogeneous group of disorders in which the clinical features are consistent with mineralocorticoid excess yet endogenous mineralocorticoid secretion is abnormally low owing to suppressed renin production. Renin secretion is suppressed by increased Na$^+$ retention and volume expansion, resulting either from the presence of endogenous or exogenous mineralocorticoids or mineralocorticoid-like substances or from a mineralocorticoid-independent increase in renal tubular sodium transport. Hypertension, hypokalemia, and metabolic alkalosis are the usual manifestations. In addition to the syndromes that result from excess production of DOC as described above, continuous use of fluorinated steroids with powerful mineralocorticoid-like activity contained in some topical preparations such as nasal sprays and dermatologic creams can be associated with hypertension, hypokalemia, and renin and aldosterone suppression. Withdrawal of these medications or adjustment of the dosage easily controls undesirable side

effects. Pseudohyperaldosteronism can also occur as a prominent feature of several rare syndromes, the pathophysiologic features of which have only recently been established. These are described in the following sections.

Syndrome of Apparent Mineralocorticoid Excess (11β-Hydroxysteroid Dehydrogenase Deficiency)

A rare disorder, initially designated as the syndrome of apparent mineralocorticoid excess, is characterized by findings suggestive of a hypermineralocorticoid state (hypertension, hypokalemia, suppressed renin levels, and amelioration by spironolactone) despite low levels of aldosterone and DOC. Most of the reported cases have been in children who have severe—often lethal—hypertension. Although the pathogenesis remained elusive for more than a decade, it is now evident that the primary abnormality in this disorder is reduced peripheral metabolism of cortisol due to a mutation in the gene encoding 11β-hydroxysteroid dehydrogenase type 2, the isoenzyme that is present in greatest abundance in the renal tubule. Impaired conversion of cortisol to cortisone (Figure 10–7) in the cells of the renal tubule

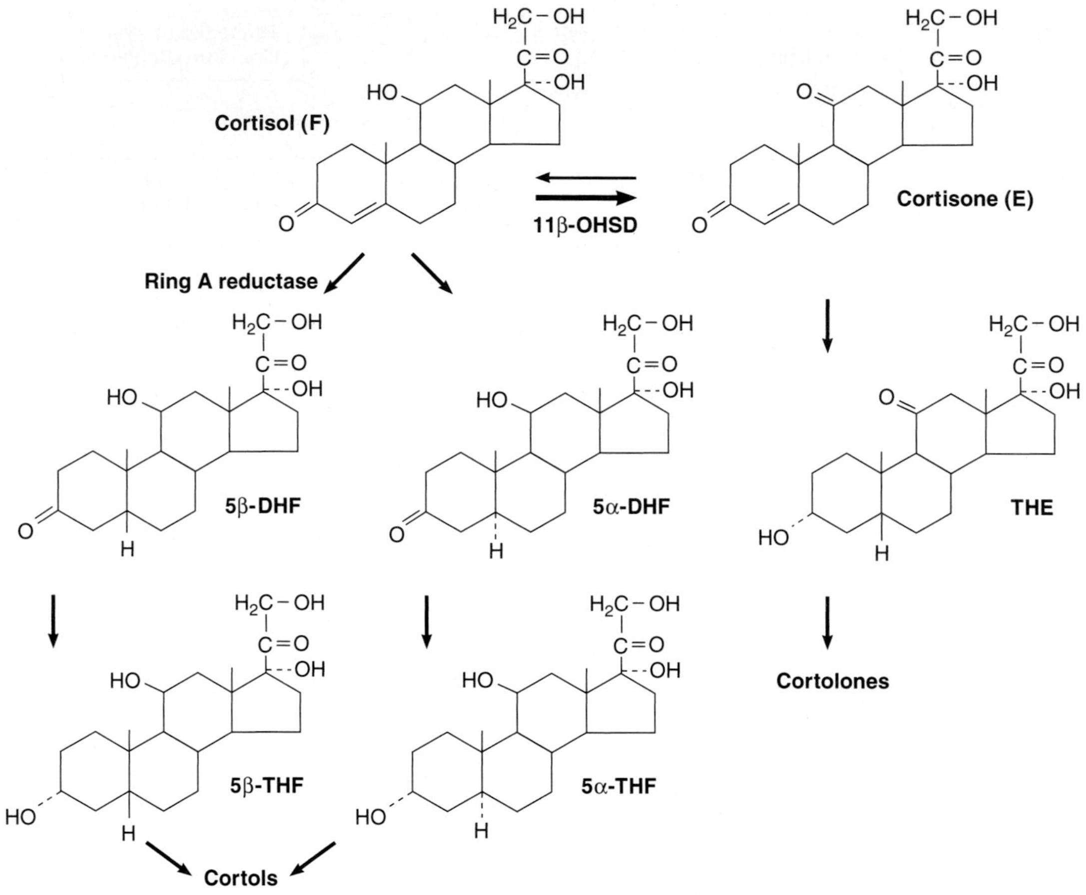

Figure 10–7. Principal pathways of cortisol metabolism. (11β-OHSD, 11β-hydroxysteroid dehydrogenase; DHF, dihydrocortisol; THF, tetrahydrocortisol; THE, tetrahydrocortisone.)

results in an accumulation of cortisol and subsequent occupancy of mineralocorticoid receptors. Despite normal plasma cortisol levels, urinary cortisol is increased, reflecting impairment of the kidney's ability to convert cortisol to cortisone. The increased urinary excretion of tetrahydrocortisol (THF) and reduced excretion of tetrahydrocortisone (THE) leads to a marked increase in the THF/THE ratio (Figure 10–8), a finding considered diagnostic of this disorder. Treatment consists of the administration of small doses of dexamethasone (0.75–1 mg/d) to suppress ACTH and to limit thereby the production of cortisol and its accumulation in mineralocorticoid target tissues in the kidney.

Chronic Ingestion of Licorice

Chronic ingestion of large amounts of substances containing "mineralocorticoid-like activity"—eg, certain candies, infusions, and some chewing tobaccos containing licorice—results in a syndrome of hypertension, hypokalemia, renal Na⁺ retention, volume expansion, suppressed plasma renin activity, and metabolic alkalosis. Aldosterone secretion and excretion are low or undetectable, however, as are other mineralocorticoid precursors in the aldosterone pathway. The responsible agent for this syndrome is the active principle of licorice, glycyrrhizic acid, and its metabolite glycyrrhetinic acid, that are present in certain commercially available products. Both of these alkaloids inhibit 11β-hydroxysteroid dehydrogenase in the kidney, which increases free cortisol locally to act as the mineralocorticoid in a manner similar to the syndrome of apparent mineralocorticoid excess. Pseudohyperaldosteronism can be induced by licorice and its derivatives such as carbenoxolone (an anti-gastric ulcer drug), the Na⁺ hemisuccinate of 18β-glycyrrhetinic acid. Electrolyte

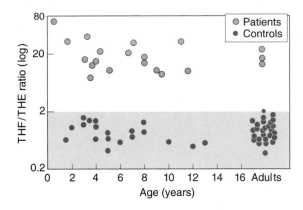

Figure 10–8. Ratio of the urinary metabolites of cortisol (THF, tetrahydrocortisol; 5α-THF, allotetrahydrocortisol) to cortisone (THE, tetrahydrocortisone) in the syndrome of apparent mineralocorticoid excess. (Modified from Shackleton CHL, Stewart PM: The hypertension of apparent mineralocorticoid excess syndrome. In: *Endocrine Hypertension.* Biglieri EG [editor]. Raven Press, 1990.)

abnormalities and hypertension disappear within a few weeks upon discontinuation of licorice ingestion or withdrawal of carbenoxolone treatment.

Liddle's Syndrome

In 1963, Liddle and colleagues reported the results of studies in a large family in which the affected members had clinical manifestations resembling those of classic primary aldosteronism: hypertension, hypokalemia with renal K⁺ wasting, metabolic alkalosis, and suppressed plasma renin activity. Aldosterone production, however, was negligible. The inheritance pattern in this large family was that of an autosomal dominant disorder, and the phenotype was soon identified in several additional families as well as in sporadic cases.

Although these findings suggested the possibility of excessive production of another mineralocorticoid to explain the clinical manifestations, in contrast to patients with excess DOC production or those with the syndrome of apparent mineralocorticoid excess, administration of the mineralocorticoid antagonist spironolactone did not correct either the hypertension or the hypokalemia. Furthermore, the adrenocortical synthesis-blocking agent metyrapone, which inhibits 11β- and 18-hydroxylation of aldosterone precursors, also had no effect. In contrast, administration of triamterene, a diuretic agent with K⁺-sparing activity independent of mineralocorticoid antagonism, was effective in correcting the abnormalities. The investigators proposed that a primary abnormality in the renal tubule that enhanced Na⁺ reabsorption was responsible.

Recent studies in the original kindred of Liddle as well as in individuals from several other kindreds similarly affected proved this hypothesis to be remarkably prescient. Using linkage analysis as well as electrophysiologic techniques, it has been established that patients with Liddle's syndrome have a defect in the cytoplasmic domain of either the β or γ subunit of the epithelial Na⁺ channel that results in constitutive activation of the channel. Since amiloride as well as triamterene are relatively specific inhibitors of this channel, treatment with these agents will correct the electrolyte abnormalities and ameliorate the hypertension as well.

TYPE II PSEUDOHYPOALDOSTERONISM (Arnold-Healy-Gordon Syndrome)

The term type II pseudohypoaldosteronism has been used to describe a rare autosomal dominant clinical syndrome in which hypertension is present in association with hyperkalemia, impairment of renal K⁺ excretion, hyperchloremic metabolic acidosis, and hyporeninemic hypoaldosteronism. The glomerular filtration rate (GFR) is usually normal. Mineralocorticoid resistance is apparent by persistence of hyperkalemia and a subnormal kaliuretic response to large doses of exogenously administered mineralocorticoid hormone. However, in contrast to patients with the classic form of mineralocorticoid resistance (type I pseudohypoaldosteronism), salt wasting is not present and both the antinatriuretic and antichloruretic responses to mineralocorticoid are intact.

An impairment in renal K⁺ secretion was initially proposed as the primary defect. However, whereas fractional renal K⁺ excretion was subnormal and increased only minimally when Na⁺ was delivered to distal nephron segments as NaCl, distal renal K⁺ secretion increased greatly when Na⁺ was delivered distally in the presence of non-Cl⁻ anions (sulfate and bicarbonate). These findings indicate that the renal K⁺ secretory mechanism is intact and suggest that the primary defect is related to increased Cl⁻ reabsorption in the distal nephron. This, in turn, would (1) limit the Na⁺ and mineralocorticoid-dependent driving force for K⁺ and H⁺ secretion, resulting in hyperkalemia and acidosis; and (2) augment distal NaCl reabsorption, resulting in hyperchloremia, volume expansion, and hypertension. Consistent with the presence of such a "chloride shunt," restriction of dietary NaCl or administration of a chloruretic diuretic (furosemide, thiazides) ameliorates hyperkalemia and acidosis in such patients. It is now known that two separate mutations in the WNK family of serine-threonine kinases (WNK 1 and WNK 4) are responsible for type II pseudohypoaldosteronism. Both kinases localize to distal nephron segments known to play a key role in the transport of ions that are altered in this syndrome.

■ HYPERTENSION OF RENAL ORIGIN

THE RENIN-ANGIOTENSIN SYSTEM

The term "renin" was first suggested by Tigerstedt and Bergman in 1898 to denote the pressor material in saline extracts of rabbit kidneys. Pioneer studies by Page and Helmer and Braun-Menendez in the 1930s demonstrated that renin enzymatically cleaves an α_2-globulin substrate (angiotensinogen) to form a decapeptide (angiotensin I) that is subsequently cleaved by angiotensin-converting enzyme (ACE) to form an octapeptide (angiotensin II) with potent vasoconstrictor effects. During this same period, Goldblatt noted that reducing the flow of blood to the kidney in experimental animals was followed by an increase in blood pressure. Subsequently, these two landmark observations were found to be related; reducing blood flow to the kidney stimulates the renin-angiotensin system, resulting in an increase in blood pressure. The integration of these concepts is a key paradigm in understanding blood pressure regulation and has served as one of the important models in evaluating mechanisms of hypertension.

Renin

As the afferent arteriole enters the glomerulus (Figure 10–9), the smooth muscle cells become modified to perform a secretory function. These juxtaglomerular cells produce and secrete renin, a proteolytic enzyme with a molecular weight of approximately 40,000. In close proximity to the juxtaglomerular cells are specialized tubular cells of the cortical thick ascending limb of the loop of Henle known as the macula densa. The juxtaglomerular cells of the afferent arteriole and the macula densa are referred to collectively as the juxtaglomerular apparatus and the interplay of these specialized cells has an important role in the regulation of renin secretion.

The synthesis of renin involves a series of steps beginning with the translation of renin mRNA into preprorenin. The 23-amino-acid amino terminal sequence of preprorenin directs trafficking of the protein into the

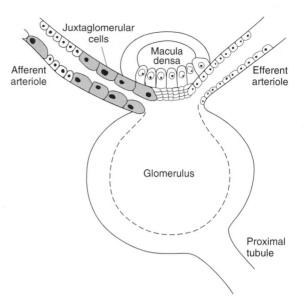

Figure 10–9. Diagram of a glomerulus, showing juxtaglomerular apparatus and macula densa.

endoplasmic reticulum, where it is subsequently cleaved, resulting in the formation of prorenin. Prorenin is glycosylated in the Golgi apparatus and is either secreted directly into the circulation by a nonregulated constitutive pathway or is processed in secretory granules to form active renin. Although prorenin constitutes 50–90% of the total circulating renin, it has no clear physiologic role. Prorenin can be converted into renin in vitro by a number of methods, but it is unlikely that significant extrarenal conversion of prorenin occurs in vivo. Plasma prorenin levels tend to be elevated in patients with type 1 diabetes mellitus in association with microvascular complications.

The release of renin from secretory granules into the circulation is controlled by three major effectors: (1) baroreceptors in the wall of the afferent arteriole that are stimulated by decreases in renal arteriolar perfusion pressure, perhaps mediated by local production of prostaglandins; (2) cardiac and systemic arterial receptors that activate the sympathetic nervous system, resulting in increased circulating catecholamines and increased direct neural stimulation of juxtaglomerular cells via β_1-adrenergic receptors; and (3) cells of the macula densa that appear to be stimulated by a reduction in Na^+ or Cl^- ion concentrations in the tubular fluid delivered to this site. The Cl^- ion may be the primary mediator of this effect.

Once secreted, renin initiates a series of steps beginning with the enzymatic cleavage of a decapeptide, angiotensin I from the amino terminal of angiotensinogen. Angiotensin I is then converted to the octapeptide angiotensin II (Figure 10–10) by angiotensin-converting enzyme (ACE). The concentration of ACE is greatest in the lung. It is also localized to the luminal membrane of vascular endothelial cells, the glomerulus, the brain, and other organs. The half-life of angiotensin II in plasma is less than 1 minute as a result of the action of multiple angiotensinases located in most tissues of the body.

Angiotensinogen

Angiotensinogen (renin substrate) is an α_2-globulin secreted by the liver. It has a molecular weight of approximately 60,000 and is usually present in human plasma at a concentration of 1 mmol/L. Although the rate of production of angiotensin II is normally determined by changes in plasma renin concentration, the concentration of angiotensinogen is below the V_{max} for the reaction. Thus, if angiotensinogen concentration increases, the amount of angiotensin produced at the same plasma renin concentration will increase. As will be discussed later, increased levels of angiotensinogen have been noted in patients with essential hypertension, and there appears to be linkage between a variant allele for the angiotensinogen gene and the presence of essential hypertension in selected populations. Hepatic production of angiotensinogen is increased by glucocorticoids and by estrogens. Stimulation of angiotensinogen production by estrogen-containing contraceptive pills may contribute to some of the hypertension encountered as a side effect of this treatment.

In situations such as Na^+ depletion, where there is a sustained high circulating level of renin, the rate of breakdown of angiotensinogen is greatly increased. Because the plasma concentration of angiotensinogen remains constant in these situations, hepatic production must increase to match the increased rate of breakdown. The mechanism of this increase is not clear, though angiotensin II itself is known to be a stimulus to angiotensinogen production.

Angiotensin-Converting Enzyme

Angiotensin-converting enzyme is a dipeptidyl carboxypeptidase, a glycoprotein of MW 130,000–160,000, that cleaves dipeptides from a number of substrates. In addition to angiotensin I, these include bradykinin, enkephalins, and substance P. Inhibitors of ACE are widely used to prevent the formation of angiotensin II in the circulation and thus block its biologic effects (Figure 10–10). Since ACE acts on a number of substrates, blockade of the enzyme may not always exert its effects solely via the renin-angiotensin system. In fact, the increased kinin levels caused by inhibitors of ACE may contribute to the hypotensive action of this class of drugs by releasing nitric oxide from vascular endothelial cells. Bradykinin antagonists can blunt the hypotensive effect of ACE inhibitors. In-

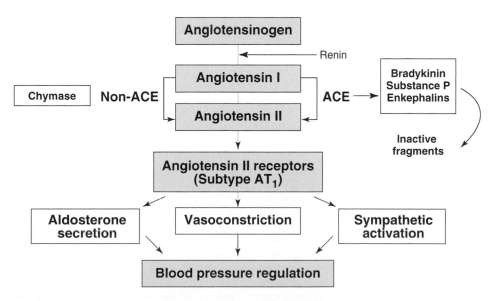

Figure 10–10. The renin-angiotensin-aldosterone axis. Angiotensin II is a critical hormone in the control of blood pressure.

creased kinins may contribute to another effect of ACE inhibitors—ie, the ability to improve insulin sensitivity—which can lower the blood glucose in patients with type 2 diabetes. In addition, the accumulation of kinins may account for two of the most significant side effects of ACE inhibitors: cough, angioedema, and anaphylaxis.

In addition to ACE, a serine protease known as chymase has been shown to convert angiotensin I to angiotensin II. This enzyme has been identified in various tissues, most notably the cardiac ventricles. Thus, there appears to be an ACE-independent pathway for the production of angiotensin II.

Angiotensin II

Similar to other peptide hormones, angiotensin II binds to receptors on the plasma membrane of target cells. Two major classes of angiotensin II receptors (AT1 and AT2) have been characterized and their respective mRNAs isolated and cloned. AT1 appears to mediate virtually all the known cardiovascular, renal, and adrenal-stimulatory effects of angiotensin II; AT2 may be involved in cell differentiation and growth. Both receptors have a seven-transmembrane-spanning motif. AT1 is linked to a G protein that activates phospholipase C, resulting in the hydrolysis of phosphoinositide to form inositol triphosphate and diacylglycerol. Generation of these second messengers results in a cascade of intracellular events including increases in calcium concentration, activation of protein kinases, and perhaps decreases in intracellular cAMP. The precise signaling mechanism associated with the AT2 receptor is still unknown.

Angiotensin II is a potent pressor agent, exerting its effects on peripheral arterioles to cause vasoconstriction and thus increasing total peripheral resistance. Vasoconstriction occurs in all tissue beds, including the kidney, and has been implicated in the phenomenon of renal autoregulation. Angiotensin may also increase the rate and strength of cardiac contraction. The possible role of increased circulating levels of angiotensin II in the pathogenesis of hypertension is discussed below.

Angiotensin II also acts directly on the adrenal cortex to stimulate aldosterone secretion and in most situations is the most important regulator of aldosterone secretion. Angiotensin thus plays a central role in regulating Na^+ balance. For example, during dietary Na^+ depletion, extracellular fluid volume is reduced. Subsequent stimulation of the renin-angiotensin system is important in two ways: Its vasoconstrictor actions help to maintain blood pressure in the face of reduced extracellular fluid volume, whereas its actions to stimulate aldosterone secretion and thus Na^+ retention allow volume to be conserved.

During chronic intravascular volume depletion, such as occurs during a low Na^+ intake, the persistent increases in angiotensin II levels results in AT1 receptor down-regulation in the vasculature. In this setting, there is less vasoconstriction for a given plasma level of angiotensin II. In contrast, intravascular volume depletion increases the number of AT1 receptors in the adrenal glomerulosa, resulting in augmented aldosterone secretion. It has been suggested that these opposite and apparently contradictory effects of chronic intravascular volume depletion on responsiveness of the vasculature and the adrenal glomerulosa to angiotensin II may be physiologically appropriate; in the setting of a low-Na^+ diet, the greater increase in aldosterone secretion allows Na^+ reabsorption to occur without a major rise in blood pressure. As will be discussed later, this so-called "Na^+ modulation" of adrenal and vascular responsiveness to angiotensin II may be modified in some patients with essential hypertension.

Angiotensin II modulates activity at sympathetic nerve endings in peripheral blood vessels and in the heart. It increases sympathetic activity partly by facilitating adrenergic transmitter release and partly by increasing the responsiveness of smooth muscle to norepinephrine. Angiotensin II also stimulates the release of catecholamines from the adrenal medulla.

A number of angiotensin receptor antagonists or blockers (ARBs) have been developed. The current clinically available ARBs only reduce AT1 activity—there is no change in AT2 receptor-mediated effects. In contrast, inhibition of angiotensin II formation with an ACE inhibitor will diminish the activity of both receptor subtypes. The ARBs do not directly affect bradykinin levels. Given that ACE inhibitors may reduce blood pressure in part by augmenting bradykinin levels and that angiotensin II formation can occur despite ACE inhibition, combination ACE inhibitor and ARB therapy may have an additive effect in lowering blood pressure. Clinical trials are currently investigating whether combination ACE inhibitor and ARB therapy confers additional benefit for lowering blood pressure and preventing end-organ damage.

Blockade of the formation or peripheral effects of angiotensin II is useful therapeutically. For example, in low-output congestive cardiac failure, plasma levels of angiotensin II are high. These high circulating levels promote salt and water retention and, by constricting arterioles, raise peripheral vascular resistance, thus increasing cardiac afterload. Treatment with ACE inhibitors or ARBs results in peripheral vasodilation, thereby improving tissue perfusion and cardiac performance as well as aiding renal elimination of salt and water. The use of ACE inhibitors as well as of AT1 receptor antagonists in the treatment of hypertension is discussed in a subsequent section.

Effects of Angiotensin II in the Brain

Angiotensin II is a polar peptide that does not cross the blood-brain barrier. Circulating angiotensin II, however, may affect the brain by acting through one or more of the circumventricular organs. These specialized regions within the brain lack a blood-brain barrier, so that receptive cells in these areas are sensitive to plasma composition. Of particular significance to the actions of angiotensin are the subfornical organ, the organum vasculosum of the lamina terminalis, and the area postrema. (See Chapter 5 and Figure 5–7.)

Angiotensin II is a potent dipsogen when injected directly into the brain or administered systemically. The major receptors for the dipsogenic action of circulating angiotensin II are located in the subfornical organ. Angiotensin II also stimulates vasopressin secretion, particularly in association with raised plasma osmolality. As such, the renin-angiotensin system may have an important part to play in the control of water balance, particularly during hypovolemia.

Production of angiotensin II in the brain has been implicated in several models of hypertension. Angiotensin also acts on the brain to increase blood pressure, though its effects at this site seem to be less potent than those exerted directly in the systemic circulation. In most animals, the receptors are located in the area postrema. Other central actions of angiotensin II include stimulation of ACTH secretion, suppression of plasma renin activity, and stimulation of Na^+ craving, particularly in association with raised mineralocorticoid levels. The full implications of these (and other) central actions of angiotensin remain to be elucidated.

Local Renin-Angiotensin Systems

In addition to the circulating renin-angiotensin system, there is an increasing appreciation that all of the components of the renin-angiotensin system may be present in various tissues and function thereby to promote local production of angiotensin II. Such tissues include the kidney, brain, heart, ovary, adrenal, testis, and peripheral blood vessels. In the kidney, for example, local generation of angiotensin II directly stimulates Na^+ reabsorption in the early proximal tubule, in part by activation of the Na^+-H^+ antiporter in the luminal membrane. Angiotensin II of either local or systemic origin is also of critical importance in the maintenance of GFR during hypovolemia and reduced renal arterial flow. Angiotensin II appears to induce a relatively greater increase in efferent arteriole vasoconstriction, resulting in an increase in hydraulic pressure in the glomerular capillary. This increased pressure protects against a fall in GFR during a reduction in renal perfusion.

THE RENIN-ANGIOTENSIN SYSTEM & HYPERTENSION

Essential Hypertension

Blood pressure is the product of cardiac output and peripheral vascular resistance. The hemodynamic abnormality that appears to underlie essential hypertension is an elevation in peripheral vascular resistance. The determinants of peripheral vascular resistance include a complex array of systemic and locally produced hormones and growth factors as well as neurogenic factors. However, the specific factor or factors that underlie the pathogenesis of essential hypertension remain to be determined. Since the original observation that impaired renal perfusion leads to secretion of renin and an increase in blood pressure, the renin-angiotensin system has been implicated in the etiology of essential hypertension.

In the early 1970s, Laragh and his colleagues suggested that plasma renin activity could be used to categorize the relative contributions of vasoconstriction and intravascular volume expansion in patients with essential hypertension. This so-called "renin profiling" divided patients with essential hypertensive into two subgroups: those with high renin levels, who were said to have a vasoconstrictor mechanism; and those with low renin levels, who were said to have a volume-expanded mechanism. While this bipolar model of hypertension is intellectually attractive, it has not generally been supported by hemodynamic measurements, and for that reason renin profiling of patients with essential hypertension is not generally advocated as part of routine practice.

As noted earlier, dietary Na^+ restriction enhances the adrenal but reduces the vascular response to angiotensin II; Na^+ loading produces the opposite effect. Thus, for normal subjects ingesting a high-Na^+ diet, the Na^+-induced modulation of adrenal and vascular activities increases renal blood flow while attenuating renal reabsorption of Na^+; both events facilitate excretion of the Na^+ load. It has been observed that about one-half of patients with essential hypertension with normal or high plasma renin levels may not modulate their adrenal and vascular responsiveness to a Na^+ load. These so-called "nonmodulators" do not increase their renal blood flow in response to a high-salt diet or increase aldosterone secretion in response to a low-salt diet. Thus, according to this model, these patients have an impaired ability to excrete a Na^+ load, leading to elevations in blood pressure. The proponents of this hypothesis suggest that there is an abnormality related either to local angiotensin II production or the angiotensin receptor such that target tissue responsiveness is not modified when Na^+ intake is altered. Adrenal and vascular responsiveness can be restored in these patients by reducing angiotensin II levels using ACE inhibitors.

Approximately 25% of patients with essential hypertension have low plasma renin levels. There is an increased frequency in blacks and the elderly, and it has been suggested that the increases in blood pressure in this population are more likely to be salt-sensitive and that the greatest antihypertensive response may be achieved with a diuretic or calcium channel blocker. Although it was initially suggested that ACE inhibitors would not be effective in this low-renin hypertensive population, recent studies suggest that plasma renin levels are not predictive of efficacy of this class of drugs. Conceivably, ACE inhibitors may be effective in this population by increasing levels of bradykinin or by reducing local angiotensin II generation in the kidney, brain, and vasculature. This notion is supported by recent experimental studies in transgenic rats harboring a mouse renin gene. These rats experience a severe and lethal form of hypertension that can be ameliorated by treatment with an ACE inhibitor or angiotensin II receptor antagonist. Although plasma renin activity, plasma angiotensin II levels and renal vein renin content are subnormal, adrenal renin content and plasma prorenin levels are increased in this model, and adrenalectomy attenuates the hypertension. This lends further support to the concept that measurements of systemic renin activity may not reflect the relative importance of local renin-angiotensin systems and their potential role in the pathogenesis of hypertension.

Recent studies using techniques of molecular genetics have further implicated the renin-angiotensin system in the pathogenesis of essential hypertension. A genetic linkage has been described between an allele of the angiotensinogen gene and essential hypertension in affected siblings. It is interesting to note that there is a correlation between plasma concentration of angiotensinogen and blood pressure and that increased levels of angiotensinogen are observed in patients with essential hypertension. Furthermore, normotensive offspring of hypertensive patients tend to have higher levels of angiotensinogen compared with normal control subjects.

Renovascular Hypertension

The most common cause of renin-dependent hypertension is renovascular hypertension. Various studies have reported it to be present in 1–4% of patients with hypertension, and it is the most common correctable cause of secondary hypertension. Both renovascular disease, defined as the presence of lesions in the renal artery, and renovascular hypertension, defined as renovascular disease that is causal of hypertension, are less common in African-Americans. Renovascular hypertension is usually due either to atherosclerosis or to fibromuscular hyperplasia of the renal arteries. These lesions result in decreased perfusion in the renal segment distal to the obstructed vessel, resulting in increased renin release and angiotensin II production. Blood pressure increase and high angiotensin II levels suppress renin release from the contralateral kidney. Consequently, total plasma renin activity may be only slightly elevated or even normal. Other anatomic lesions may cause hypertension as well: renal infarction, solitary cysts, hydronephrosis, and other parenchymal lesions.

Because of the relatively low incidence of the disorder, screening all hypertensives for renovascular hypertension is generally not recommended. Instead, most physicians look for indications that the hypertension may not be idiopathic before deciding to evaluate the patient for renovascular hypertension. The following clinical conditions are settings in which renovascular hypertension should be suspected: (1) severe hypertension (diastolic blood pressure greater than 120 mm Hg) with either progressive renal insufficiency or refractoriness to aggressive medical therapy; (2) accelerated or malignant hypertension with grade III or grade IV retinopathy; (3) moderate to severe hypertension in a patient with diffuse atherosclerosis or an incidentally detected asymmetry of kidney size; (4) an acute elevation in plasma creatinine concentration in a hypertensive patient that is either unexplained or follows therapy with an ACE inhibitor; (5) an acute rise in blood pressure over a previously stable baseline; (6) a systolic-diastolic abdominal bruit; (7) onset of hypertension below age 20 or above age 50; (8) moderate to severe hypertension in patients with recurrent acute pulmonary edema; (9) hypokalemia with normal or elevated plasma renin levels in the absence of diuretic therapy; and (10) a negative family history of hypertension. An acute deterioration in renal function following therapy with an ACE inhibitor or an ARB should suggest the possibility of bilateral renal artery stenosis. In that situation, both kidneys are dependent on angiotensin II to maintain intraglomerular pressure by its vasoconstrictor effect on the efferent arteriole; loss of this angiotensin II-mediated vasoconstriction will result in a decrease in intraglomerular pressure and GFR.

The standard test for diagnosing renal vascular disease is renal arteriography. Because of risks such as contrast-induced acute tubular necrosis, attempts have made to use newer noninvasive imaging tests and pharmacologic probes as screening tests for renovascular disease. Current noninvasive screening tests for renovascular disease include (1) captopril stimulation with measurement of plasma renin activity; (2) captopril renography; (3) Doppler ultrasound; (4) magnetic resonance angiography; and (5) spiral CT scan.

Basal plasma renin levels by themselves do not serve to diagnose renovascular hypertension inasmuch as levels are increased in only 50–80% of affected patients. The administration of the ACE inhibitor captopril normally induces a reactive hyperreninemia by preventing the negative feedback exerted by angiotensin II. This response is exaggerated in patients with renal artery stenosis such that renin levels measured 1 hour after the oral administration of captopril are much greater than those observed in patients with essential hypertension. The sensitivity and specificity of this test has been reported to range from 93% to 100% and from 80% to 95%, respectively. The test has less sensitivity in blacks, in the young, and in patients with reduced renal function as well as in the presence of concomitant antihypertensive therapy.

Normally, stenosis of a renal artery stimulates the renin-angiotensin system of the ipsilateral kidney such that angiotensin II-mediated vasoconstriction of the efferent arteriole helps maintain intraglomerular pressure and filtration. Administration of an ACE inhibitor (eg, captopril) will result in a reduction in angiotensin II production and thus lower intraglomerular pressure and GFR. Performance of a renal isotope scan prior to and after the administration of captopril scan can optimize detection of unilateral renal ischemia. If there is a relative decrease in isotope uptake in one kidney compared with the other or a delay in peak uptake of isotope, renovascular disease should be suspected. The sensitivity of an ACE inhibitor-augmented renal scan for significant renal artery stenosis is about 90% in high-risk patients. However, the sensitivity is reduced in patients with bilateral renal artery stenosis and in low-risk patients.

The combination of direct ultrasound imaging of the renal arteries (B-mode imaging) and measurement of renal arterial flow by Doppler technique has recently been become a popular screening test for renal artery stenosis. Studies suggest that the positive and negative predictive values for these procedures are in the upper 90% range. Having an experienced operator is important to achieve this level of performance. Visualization of the renal arteries can be impaired by the presence of a large amount of bowel gas, obesity, recent surgery, or the presence of an accessory renal artery.

Magnetic resonance angiography (MRA) has recently been advocated as a good screening test for renal artery stenosis. Initial sensitivities have been reported in the 92–97% range. A recent study suggests that spiral CT scan may be the most sensitive noninvasive imaging test to evaluate for renal artery stenosis, with sensitivity and specificity of 98% and 94%, respectively. These results are promising, and more studies are needed to clarify the utility of these imaging tests for renal vascular disease.

Given that there is no noninvasive imaging test that is sensitive enough to totally exclude renal artery stenosis, clinicians are frequently confronted with the dilemma of when and how a patient with hypertension should be evaluated for renovascular hypertension. Based on the index of clinical suspicion (Table 10–1), Mann and Pickering have developed a practical algorithm for the evaluation of renovascular hypertension and for the selection of patients for renal arteriography (Figure 10–11).

Table 10–1. Testing for renovascular hypertension: Clinical index of suspicion as a guide to workup.[1]

Low index (should not be tested)
Borderline, mild, or moderate hypertension in the absence of clinical clues

Moderate index (noninvasive tests recommended)
Severe hypertension (diastolic blood pressure > 120 mm Hg)
Hypertension refractory to standard therapy
Abrupt onset of sustained moderate to severe hypertension at age < 20 or > 50 years
Hypertension with a suggestive abdominal bruit (long, high-pitched, and localized to the region of the renal artery)
Moderate hypertension (diastolic blood pressure exceeding 105 mm Hg) in a smoker, a patient with evidence of occlusive vascular disease (cerebrovascular, coronary, peripheral vascular), or a patient with unexplained but stable elevation of serum creatinine
Normalization of blood pressure by an angiotensin-converting enzyme inhibitor in a patient with moderate or severe hypertension (particularly in a smoker or a patient with recent onset of hypertension)

High index (may consider proceeding directly to arteriography)
Severe hypertension (diastolic blood pressure > 120 mm Hg) with either progressive renal insufficiency or refractoriness to aggressive treatment (particularly in a patient who has been a smoker or has other evidence of occlusive arterial disease)
Accelerated or malignant hypertension (grade III or grade IV retinopathy)
Hypertension with recent elevation of serum creatinine, either unexplained or reversibly induced by an angiotensin-converting enzyme inhibitor
Moderate to severe hypertension with incidentally detected asymmetry of renal size

[1]Reprinted, with permission, from Mann SJ, Pickering TG: Detection of renovascular hypertension. State of the art: 1992. Ann Intern Med 1992;117:845.

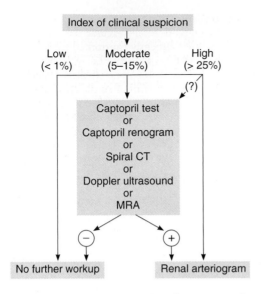

Figure 10–11. Suggested workup for renovascular hypertension. (Reproduced, with permission, from Mann SJ, Pickering TG: Detection of renovascular hypertension. State of the art: 1992. Ann Intern Med 1992;117:845.)

Anatomic correction is the preferred therapy for renovascular hypertension when it is possible and the patient is considered able to tolerate the procedure. The arteriographic finding of a greater than 75% stenosis in either or both renal arteries suggests that the patient may have physiologically significant renal artery stenosis. Prior to correction of a stenotic renal artery, it had been suggested that measurements of renal vein renins be performed to determine whether the stenosis is hemodynamically significant. In selective venous sampling, blood samples are obtained from the venous effluent of the affected portion of the kidney and from the contralateral kidney. The renin level is ordinarily significantly higher in the sample from the affected kidney than in that from the contralateral kidney. When the value for the affected kidney sample is divided by the value for the unaffected sample, a ratio greater than 1.5 generally indicates a functional abnormality, though a lower ratio does not exclude the diagnosis. Giving an ACE inhibitor prior to the renal vein sampling may increase the sensitivity of this test. Over 90% of patients with renal artery stenosis and lateralizing renal vein renins will have an improvement in blood pressure control following therapy. However, since many patients with renal vein renin ratios less than 1.5 (nonlateralizing) will have an amelioration of their hypertension after angioplasty or surgery, it is no longer routine to perform such studies in patients with a high-grade renal artery stenosis. Measurement of renal vein renin levels may be helpful in evaluating hypertensive patients with bilateral or segmental renal artery stenosis in order to determine which kidney or region of a kidney is the source of the augmented renin release. A recent study suggests that calculating the resistance index ([1 − end-diastolic velocity divided by maximal systolic velocity] × 100) using duplex Doppler ultrasonography may be helpful in predicting the success rates of revascularization procedures for the treatment of renovascular hypertension. Patients with resistance indices > 80 generally had a poor surgical outcome, with renal function decreasing in about 80% of the patients, and only one patient had a significant decline in blood pressure. In contrast, over 90% of patients with a resistance index < 80 had an improvement in blood pressure control after revascularization procedures. An elevated resistance index is probably indicative of intrarenal vascular disease and possible glomerulosclerosis, and revascularization of the main renal arteries thus may not improve blood pressure control and renal function.

Anatomic correction can be performed either with percutaneous angioplasty (with or without stent placement) or with surgical intervention. The best method of treating patients with renovascular hypertension remains a matter of speculation since there have been no truly randomized trials that have compared angioplasty with or without stent versus surgery versus medical therapy. Angioplasty is the procedure of choice for renovascular hypertension due to fibromuscular dysplasia, with cure rates between 50% and 85%, improvement in 30–35%, and failure rates less than 15%. For atherosclerotic renal artery stenosis, the optimal treatment regimen is much less clear. The technical success rates vary with the site of the lesion. In general, lesions within the main renal artery are most amenable to angioplasty, whereas ostial lesions do not respond as well to angioplasty and require stent placement. Using angioplasty alone for the treatment of atherosclerotic renal artery disease results in cure rates for hypertension between 8% and 20%, improvement in 50–60%, and failure rates between 20% and 30%. In addition, with angioplasty alone, there is an 8–30% restenosis rate at 2 years. Patients with bilateral renal artery disease or chronic hypertension have even less impressive improvement in hypertension with angioplasty alone. Recently, the placement of stents in the renal arteries has been used to improve the efficacy of angioplasty. Cure or improvement in hypertension has been reported in 65–88% of patients, with restenosis rates of only 11–14% in a number of uncontrolled studies. Another major issue in the treatment of renovascular disease is to determine which patients would benefit from procedures designed to preserve or improve renal function, especially if the patient has bilateral renal artery stenosis that results in reduced renal blood flow and glomerular filtration. A discussion of this interesting issue is beyond the scope of this chapter.

Surgical correction of renal artery stenosis usually involves endarterectomy or a bypass procedure. Although surgical correction is generally more effective than angioplasty in curing hypertension, operative mortality can be much greater, especially in older patients with concomitant cardiovascular and cerebrovascular disease. In most medical centers, the current revascularization procedure of choice is percutaneous angioplasty with stent implantation, especially in patients with ostial or proximal lesions. Surgical revascularization is considered if angioplasty fails or if the patient requires concomitant aortic surgery.

Renovascular hypertension can also be treated medically; this treatment is used when the patient is considered unable to tolerate a surgical procedure or the diagnosis is uncertain. In fact, recent randomized controlled trials in patients with renovascular hypertension have suggested that there may not be a clear benefit of revascularization over conservative medical therapy. The ACE inhibitors and selective AT1 antagonists are particularly effective, although they can lower intrarenal efferent arteriolar resistance and so decrease renal function in patients with bilateral renal artery stenosis. Renovascular hypertension may also respond to beta-adrenergic antagonists and calcium channel blockers.

Renin-Secreting Tumors

Renin-secreting tumors are extremely rare. The tumors are usually hemangiopericytomas containing elements of the juxtaglomerular cells. They can be located by CT scan and the presence confirmed by measurement of renin in the venous effluent. Other renin-secreting neoplasms (eg, Wilms' tumor) have been reported, including a pulmonary tumor that secreted excessive amounts of renin, producing hypertension and hypokalemia with secondary aldosteronism.

Accelerated Hypertension

Accelerated hypertension is characterized by marked elevations of diastolic blood pressure that can be abrupt in onset. This disorder is associated with progressive arteriosclerosis. The plasma levels of renin and aldosterone may be extremely high. It is believed that the intense vasospastic events that occur and the excessive renal cortical nephrosclerosis lead to hyperreninemia and accelerate the hypertensive process. Vigorous antihypertensive therapy usually will result in a reduction in the vasospastic process and an amelioration of hyperreninemia with time.

Estrogen Therapy

Aldosterone levels may be increased during treatment with replacement estrogen therapy or oral contraceptives. This is due to an increase in angiotensinogen production and presumed increase in angiotensin II levels. Aldosterone levels increase secondarily, but hypokalemia rarely occurs during estrogen administration.

■ OTHER HORMONE SYSTEMS & HYPERTENSION

INSULIN

Hyperinsulinemia and insulin resistance have been implicated as potential factors in the generation of hypertension, particularly in obese patients. It has been argued that insulin resistance is present in most obese patients with hypertension and in some nonobese hypertensive patients. In the setting of obesity, there is impaired insulin-mediated glucose uptake resulting in both type 2 diabetes mellitus and increased insulin secretion by the pancreas (hyperinsulinemia). The distribution of body fat may also be a key factor, inasmuch as hypertension and insulin resistance are seen more commonly in patients with abdominal obesity (upper body, male-type fat distribution). The association of hypertension, diabetes mellitus, abdominal obesity, and hyperlipidemia has been referred to as "syndrome X" or the syndrome of insulin resistance.

The hypertension observed in this clinical syndrome may be due in part to the hyperinsulinemia. Insulin accentuates the activity of the sympathetic nervous system, leading to greater vasoconstriction. In addition, insulin increases Na^+ reabsorption by the kidney, resulting in increased intravascular volume and blood pressure. Although insulin usually induces vasodilation to counterbalance these pressor forces, in the setting of obesity this action is attenuated. Thus, in these insulin-resistant states, it is postulated that the stimulation of both the sympathetic nervous system and renal Na^+ reabsorption by hyperinsulinemia combined with impaired vasodilation results in increased blood pressure. It is noteworthy that weight loss lowers both blood pressure, insulin levels, and insulin resistance in these patients.

Increased insulin levels alone are probably not sufficient to cause hypertension given the observations that experimental animals receiving high doses of insulin and patients with insulinomas do not develop hypertension. In addition, there are a substantial number of patients with obesity, insulin resistance, and type 2 diabetes mellitus who do not have hypertension (eg, Pima Indians). Thus, there is probably a critical interplay of genetic and hormonal factors in the pathogenesis of hypertension in patients with insulin resistance. (See Chapter 18.)

NATRIURETIC PEPTIDES

Extracts of atrial but not ventricular tissue cause marked natriuresis when injected into rats. The material is contained in densely staining granules in the atria of most mammalian species. Atrial natriuretic peptide (ANP) is a 28-amino-acid peptide derived from cleavage of the carboxyl terminal of a 126-amino-acid precursor located primarily in the storage vesicles of atrial cells. At least three other natriuretic peptides have subsequently been identified: a brain natriuretic peptide (BNP; 32-amino acids), C-type peptide (CNP; 22-amino acids), and a renal natriuretic peptide (urodilatin; 32-amino acids). Although originally described in the brain, the major source of BNP is the cardiac ventricle, and its action is similar to that of ANP. CNP is mainly produced in the brain, where it serves as a neurotransmitter and in endothelial cells, where it may regulate vasoconstriction. Urodilatin is produced in the kidney, where it acts locally to affect Na⁺ transport.

These natriuretic peptides bind to membrane receptors linked to guanylyl cyclase, resulting in production of the second messenger, cGMP. The major effects seen following the administration of ANP are vasodilation, hyperfiltration, and natriuresis. Although the peptide can cause relaxation of vascular smooth muscle, the fall in blood pressure is thought to be due largely to reduction of venous return and depression of cardiac output in intact animals. In the kidney, ANP increases GFR probably by inducing a relative afferent arteriolar dilation and efferent arteriolar vasoconstriction and an increase in glomerular permeability. The natriuresis is due both to the increase in GFR and to the direct inhibition by ANP of Na⁺ and water reabsorption by inner medullary and cortical collecting duct cells. ANP inhibits secretion of renin, aldosterone, vasopressin, and ACTH as well as the stimulation of heart rate mediated by the baroreceptors.

Maneuvers that expand plasma volume and increase atrial pressure are associated with increased levels of ANP in plasma. Thus, when blood volume increases, the associated increase in atrial pressure and atrial stretch may trigger secretion of the peptide and lead to natriuresis and blood pressure reduction. However, the precise role ANP plays in the control of Na⁺ balance, blood volume, and blood pressure regulation under normal physiologic conditions is not clear, and there are no known roles for impaired ANP secretion in the pathogenesis or maintenance of essential hypertension. Because of the pharmacologic effects of the natriuretic peptides to induce vasodilation, hyperfiltration, and natriuresis, studies are under way to determine if these peptides may have a therapeutic role in the treatment of hypertension, heart failure, and renal failure. Whether ANP will be a useful therapy for congestive heart failure is uncertain inasmuch as patients with chronically increased atrial pressures already have increased plasma levels of the peptide.

ENDOTHELIUM-DERIVED RELAXING FACTOR

The vascular endothelium produces a labile substance, endothelium-derived relaxing factor (EDRF), that mediates the vasorelaxant actions of various endogenous hormones including acetylcholine. EDRF has been identified as nitric oxide, which is synthesized from the guanidine nitrogen atom of the amino acid L-arginine by the enzyme nitric oxide synthase. Nitric oxide diffuses within the cell or to adjacent cells such as smooth muscle cells, where it stimulates soluble guanylyl cyclase. The resultant increase in cyclic guanosine monophosphate leads to a relaxation of vascular smooth muscle cells and therefore vasodilation (see Chapter 3). A number of recent studies in laboratory animals and human subjects have shown that nitric oxide synthesized by the vascular endothelium is an important determinant of resting peripheral vascular resistance and blood pressure. In anesthetized rabbits, inhibition of the activity of nitric oxide synthase using substituted arginine analogs (L-monomethyl arginine) acutely increased blood pressure. This hypertensive effect can be reversed by the infusion of arginine. In normal subjects, infusion of L-arginine decreases peripheral vascular resistance, causing hypotension and a reflex tachycardia. Because of this apparently important role of nitric oxide in maintaining basal blood pressure, it has been proposed that the nitric oxide pathway may be abnormal in patients with hypertension. This view has been supported by recent studies in humans. For example, patients with essential hypertension have a diminished vasoconstrictor response to an infusion of arginine analogs and a reduced arterial vasodilatory response to acetylcholine, suggesting that both the basal and stimulated release of nitric oxide is reduced in this disease. In contrast, the response to the endothelium-independent vasodilator nitroprusside was normal in patients with essential hypertension, suggesting that abnormality is a result of reduced nitric oxide production by the endothelium rather than impaired response in the vascular smooth muscle. The mechanisms responsible for this endothelial dysfunction are not known.

ENDOTHELIN

In addition to the production of the potent vasodilator, nitric oxide, the vascular endothelium produces a potent vasoconstrictor peptide, endothelin. At least three endothelin peptides have been identified: endothelin-1, endothelin-2, and endothelin-3. The predominant vascular vasoconstrictor, endothelin-1, is formed from proendothelin-1 by the action of a metalloprotease, endothelin-converting enzyme. Endothelin-1 binds to receptors in vascular smooth muscle which are linked to phospholipase C, resulting in the hydrolysis of phosphoinositide to inositol triphosphate.

Increased endothelin activity has been observed in disorders associated with vasoconstriction such as malignant hypertension, heart failure, pulmonary hypertension, contrast-induced acute tubular necrosis, and myocardial infarction. A rare tumor, hemangioendothelioma, can cause hypertension by the secretion of large quantities of endothelin. In addition, the hypertension associated with the use of cyclosporine may be due to increased endothelin production. However, a conclusive role for endothelin in the pathogenesis of essential hypertension has not been demonstrated.

KALLIKREIN-KININ SYSTEM

Kinins are potent vasodilators formed in blood vessels. They are cleaved from the precursor kininogen by the enzymatic action of kallikrein. Kallikrein activity has been noted to be reduced in patients with essential hypertension, suggesting lower vasodilatory kinin production. ACE is known to inactivate bradykinin, leading to the suggestion that the hypotensive effect of ACE inhibitors may be due, in part, to increased bradykinin levels. Moreover, the improved insulin sensitivity and glucose utilization observed in diabetic patients treated with ACE inhibitors may be the result of increased kinin levels rather than reduced angiotensin II production.

OTHER HORMONES & AUTACOIDS

Prostaglandins, vasopressin, calcitonin gene-related peptide, parathyroid hormone, and parathyroid hormone-related peptide are vasoactive hormones or autacoids that have been implicated in the regulation of blood pressure. Although vasopressin is both a potent vasoconstrictor and a prime factor in water reabsorption by the kidney, it does not appear to be a factor in the pathogenesis of essential hypertension. Calcitonin gene-related peptide is a potent vasodilator produced in the central nervous system and in autonomic nerves innervating blood vessels. It has been suggested that calcitonin gene-related peptide may mediate the hypotensive effect of calcium supplements given to hypertensive patients. Both infusions of parathyroid hormone and parathyroid hormone-related peptide can produce hypotension. Thus, the hypertension commonly seen in primary hyperparathyroidism is probably due to other factors.

SYMPATHETIC NERVOUS SYSTEM

Increased activity of the sympathetic nervous system has been implicated as a contributing factor in the pathogenesis of essential hypertension. This may be due to both genetic and environmental factors. Some patients with hypertension, particularly during the early stages, as well as normotensive offspring of hypertensive patients have enhanced sympathetic nervous system activity. It has been postulated that impaired baroreceptor function may prevent the normal inhibitory check on increases in sympathetic activity. In addition, the role of stress in the generation and maintenance of hypertension probably is mediated, in part, by activation of the sympathetic nervous system. The mechanisms by which increased sympathetic nervous system activity and catecholamines increase blood pressure is multifactorial, including augmented vasoconstriction, increased cardiac output, increased activity of the renin-angiotensin system, and enhanced Na^+ reabsorption by the kidney. Disorders of catecholamine metabolism are discussed in further detail in Chapter 11.

REFERENCES

Chen S-Y et al: Epithelial sodium channel regulated by aldosterone-induced protein sgk. Proc Natl Acad Sci USA 1999;96:2514. [PMID: 10051674]

Dluhy RG, Lifton RP: Glucocorticoid-remediable aldosteronism. Endocrinol Metab Clin North Am 1994;23:285. [PMID: 8070423]

Lifton RP et al: A chimaeric 11β-hydroxylase/aldosterone synthase gene causes glucocorticoid-remediable aldosteronism and human hypertension. Nature 1992;355:262. [PMID: 1731223]

Lifton RP, Gharavi AG, Geller DS: Molecular mechanisms of human hypertension. Cell 2001;104:545. [PMID:11239411]

Mann SJ, Pickering TG: Detection of renovascular hypertension. State of the art: 1992. Ann Intern Med 1992;117:845. [PMID: 1416561]

Pedersen EB: New tools in diagnosing renal artery stenosis. Kidney Int 2000;57:2657. [PMID:10844642]

Radermacher J, et al: Use of doppler ultrasonography to predict the outcome of therapy for renal-artery stenosis. N Engl J Med 2001;344:410. [PMID: 11172177]

Safian RD, Textor SC: Renal-artery stenosis. N Engl J Med 2001; 344:431. [PMID:11172181]

Schambelan M: Licorice ingestion and blood pressure regulating hormones. Steroids 1994;59:127. [PMID: 8191541]

Schiffrin EL: Endothelin: Potential role in hypertension and vascular hypertrophy. Hypertension 1995;25:1135. [PMID: 7768553]

Shen WT et al: Laparoscopic vs open adrenalectomy for the treatment of primary hyperaldosteronism. Arch Surg 1999;134:628. [PMID: 10367872]

Shimkets RA et al: Liddle's syndrome: Heritable human hypertension caused by mutations in the β subunit of the epithelial sodium channel. Cell 1994;79:407. [PMID: 7954808]

Stowasser M: New perspectives on the role of aldosterone excess in cardiovascular disease. Clin Exp Pharmacol Physiol 2001;28:783. [PMID:11553016]

White PC: Disorders of aldosterone biosynthesis and action. N Engl J Med 1994;331:250. [PMID: 8015573]

Wilson FH et al: Human hypertension caused by mutations in WNK kinases. Science 2001;293:1107. [PMID: 11498583]

Wilson RC et al: Several homozygous mutations in the gene for 11β-hydroxysteroid dehydrogenase type 2 in patients with apparent mineralocorticoid excess. J Clin Endocrinol Metab 1995;80:3145. [PMID: 7593417]

Young WF Jr et al: Primary aldosteronism: Adrenal venous sampling. Surgery 1996;120:913. [PMID: 8957473]

Adrenal Medulla

Paul A. Fitzgerald, MD, & Alan Goldfien, MD

ACTH	Adrenocorticotropic hormone	**IP$_3$**	Inositol trisphosphate
ATP	Adenosine triphosphate	**MAO**	Monoamine oxidase
cAMP	Cyclic adenosine monophosphate	**MEN**	Multiple endocrine neoplasia
CgA	Chromogramin A	**MIBG**	Metaiodobenzylguanidine
COMT	Catechol-O-methyltransferase	**PGE**	Prostaglandin E
CRH	Corticosteroid-releasing hormone	**PNMT**	Phenylethanolamine-N-methyl-transferase
DBH	Dopamine β-hydroxylase		
DHMA	Dihydroxymandelic acid	**VIP**	Vasoactive intestinal polypeptide
DHPG	Dihydroxphenylglycol	**VMA**	Vanillylmandelic acid (3-methoxy-4-hydroxymandelic acid)
HPLC	High-pressure liquid chromatography		

The adrenal medulla is a specialized part of the sympathetic nervous system that secretes catecholamines. The sympathetic nervous system typically secretes **norepinephrine** as a local neurotransmitter directly in target organs. In comparison, the adrenal medulla is important for its secretion of **epinephrine** and other substances into the general circulation for widespread distribution and effect. Although the adrenal medulla is not critically necessary for survival, its secretion of epinephrine and other compounds helps maintain the body's homeostasis during stress. Investigations of the adrenal medulla and the sympathetic nervous system have led to the discovery of different catecholamine receptors and the production of a wide variety of sympathetic agonists and antagonists with diverse clinical applications.

Pheochromocytomas are tumors that arise from the adrenal medulla whereas **paragangliomas** arise from extra-adrenal sympathetic ganglia. These tumors can secrete excessive amounts of norepinephrine and epinephrine, causing a dangerous exaggeration of the stress response.

HISTORY

The adrenal medulla was initially distinguished from the adrenal cortex in the early 19th century. Pheochromocytomas were first described by Fränkel in 1886

after the sudden death of an 18-year-old woman who had been experiencing episodes of palpitations, pounding heart, headaches, retinitis, pallor, and vomiting. Autopsy disclosed bilateral adrenal tumors, ventricular hypertrophy, and nephrosclerosis. In 1896, Manasse found that chromium salts turned such tumors dark brown, a reaction typical of adrenal medullary tissue. They were later termed "chromaffin" tumors.

In 1901, the substrate of the chromaffin reaction was chemically identified as 3,4-dihydroxyphenyl-2-methylaminoethanol by two independent researchers: J. Takamine named the substance "adrenaline" in the *Journal of Physiology* in London, while T.B. Aldrich called it "epinephrine" in the *American Journal of Physiology*. To this day, the substance is generally termed "adrenaline" in the United Kingdom and "epinephrine" in the United States. Norepinephrine was synthesized in 1904.

Alezais and Peyronin coined the term "paranglioma" in 1908 to denote chromaffin tumors arising from the paraganglia. In 1912, Pick coined the word "pheochromocytoma" from Greek *phaios* "dusky," *chroma* "color," and *kytos* "cell." The term refers to the color change that occurs in such tumor tissue when exposed to certain fixatives: Dichromate stain (eg, Zenker's, Helly's, or Orth's stain) produces a brownish-yellow coloration of cells with neurosecretory granules. Cells that contain epinephrine turn dark brown, whereas cells that contain norepinephrine turn pale yellow. Dilute Giemsa-Schmorl stain colors pheochromocytoma tissue green.

The first successful surgical resections of pheochromocytomas were performed in 1926 by C.H. Mayo at the Mayo Clinic and by Roux in Switzerland. In 1929, Rabin discovered that pheochromocytomas contain a pressor substance that could explain the clinical manifestations. However, it was not until 1939 that a patient with a pheochromocytoma was documented to have high blood levels of epinephrine. In 1946, von Euler found that the heart contains norepinephrine and that norepinephrine is the neurotransmitter for the sympathetic nervous system. In 1948, Alquist proposed the existence of two groups of adrenergic receptors that he designated α and β based on the relative potencies of a series of adrenergic agonists. In 1950, von Euler and Engel reported that urinary epinephrine and norepinephrine excretion was higher in patients with pheochromocytomas. Urinary collections for vanillylmandelic acid (VMA) were used to diagnose pheochromocytoma after Armstrong determined that VMA was a catecholamine metabolite. LaBrosse reported urinary normetanephrine excretion in 1958. Von Euler was awarded the Nobel Prize for Physiology in 1970.

ANATOMY

Embryology
(Figure 11–1)

The sympathetic nervous system arises in the fetus from the primitive cells of the neural crest (sympathogonia). At about the fifth week of gestation, these cells migrate from the primitive spinal ganglia in the thoracic region to form the sympathetic chain posterior to the dorsal aorta. They then begin to migrate anteriorly to form the remaining ganglia.

At 6 weeks of gestation, groups of these primitive cells migrate along the central vein and enter the fetal adrenal cortex to form the adrenal medulla, which is detectable by the eighth week. The adrenal medulla at this time is composed of sympathogonia and pheochromoblasts, which then mature into pheochromocytes. The cells appear in rosette-like structures, with the more primitive cells occupying a central position. Storage granules can be found in these cells by electron microscopy at 12 weeks. Pheochromoblasts and pheochromocytes also collect on both sides of the aorta to form the paraganglia. The principal collection of these cells is found at the level of the inferior mesenteric artery. They fuse anteriorly to form the organ of Zuckerkandl, which is quite prominent in fetal life. This organ is thought to be a major source of catecholamines during the first year of life, after which it begins to atrophy.

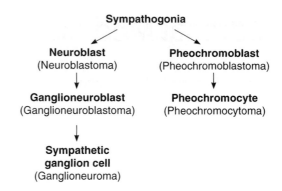

Figure 11–1. The embryonic development of adrenergic cells and tumors that develop from them (in parentheses). Sympathogonia are primitive cells derived from the neural crest. Neuroblasts are also called sympathoblasts; ganglion cells are the same as sympathocytes; and pheochromocytes are mature chromaffin cells.

The adrenal medullas are very small and amorphous at birth but develop into recognizable adult form by the sixth month of postnatal life. Pheochromocytes (chromaffin cells) also are found scattered throughout the abdominal sympathetic plexuses as well as in other parts of the sympathetic nervous system.

Gross Structure

The anatomic relationships between the adrenal medulla and the adrenal cortex differ in different species. These organs are completely separate structures in the shark. They remain separate but in close contact in amphibians, and there is some intermingling in birds. In mammals, the medulla is surrounded by the adrenal cortex. In humans, the adrenal medulla occupies a central position in the widest part of the gland, with only small portions extending into the narrower parts. It constitutes approximately one-tenth of the weight of the gland, although the proportions vary from individual to individual. There is no clear demarcation between cortex and medulla. The central vein is usually surrounded by a cuff of adrenal cortical cells, and there may be islands of cortex elsewhere in the medulla.

Microscopic Structure

The **chromaffin cells,** or **pheochromocytes,** of the adrenal medulla are large ovoid columnar cells arranged in clumps or cords around blood vessels. These cells have large nuclei and a well-developed Golgi apparatus. They contain large numbers of vesicles or granules containing catecholamines. Vesicles containing norepinephrine are darker than those containing epinephrine.

The pheochromocytes may be arranged in nests, alveoli, or cords and are surrounded by a rich network of capillaries and sinusoids. The adrenal medulla also contains some sympathetic ganglion cells, singly or in groups. Ganglion cells are also found in association with the viscera, the carotid body, the glomus jugulare, and the cervical and thoracic ganglia.

Nerve Supply

The cells of the adrenal medulla are innervated by preganglionic fibers of the sympathetic nervous system, which release acetylcholine and enkephalins at the synapses. Most of these fibers arise from a plexus in the capsule of the posterior surface of the gland and enter the adrenal glands in bundles of 30–50 fibers without synapsing. They follow the course of the blood vessels into the medulla without branching into the adrenal cortex. Some reach the wall of the central vein, where they synapse with small autonomic ganglia. However, most fibers end in relationship to the pheochromocytes.

Blood Supply

The human adrenal gland derives blood from the superior, middle, and inferior adrenal branches of the inferior phrenic artery, directly from the aorta and from the renal arteries. Upon reaching the adrenal gland, these arteries branch to form a plexus under the capsule supplying the adrenal cortex. A few of these vessels, however, penetrate the cortex, passing directly to the medulla. The medulla is also nourished by branches of the arteries supplying the central vein and cuff of cortical tissue around the central vein. Capillary loops passing from the subcapsular plexus of the cortex also supply blood as they drain into the central vein. It would appear, then, that most of the blood supply to the medullary cells is via a portal vascular system arising from the capillaries in the cortex. There is also a capillary network of lymphatics that drain into a plexus around the central vein.

In mammals, the enzyme that catalyzes the conversion of norepinephrine to epinephrine (phenylethanolamine-*N*-methyltransferase; PNMT) is induced by cortisol. The chromaffin cells containing epinephrine therefore receive most of their blood supply from the capillaries draining the cortical cells, whereas cells containing predominantly norepinephrine are supplied by the arteries that directly supply the medulla. (See Biosynthesis, below.)

On the right side, the central vein is short and drains directly into the vena cava, although some branches go to the surface of the gland and reach the azygos system. On the left, the vein is somewhat longer and drains into the renal vein.

■ HORMONES OF THE ADRENAL MEDULLA

CATECHOLAMINES

Biosynthesis & Metabolism (Figures 11–2 and 11–3)

Catecholamines are molecules that have a catechol nucleus consisting of benzene with two hydroxyl side groups plus a side-chain amine. Catecholamines include dopamine, norepinephrine, and epinephrine (Figure 11–2).

Catechol

Catecholamines are widely distributed in plants and animals. In mammals, **epinephrine** is synthesized mainly in the adrenal medulla, whereas **norepinephrine** is found not only in the adrenal medulla but also in the central nervous system and in the peripheral sympathetic nerves. **Dopamine,** the precursor of norepinephrine, is found in the adrenal medulla and in noradrenergic neurons. It is present in high concentrations in the brain, in specialized interneurons in the sympathetic ganglia, and in the carotid body, where it serves as a neurotransmitter. Dopamine is also found in specialized mast cells and in enterochromaffin cells.

Chromogranin A (CgA) is a peptide that is stored and released with catecholamines by exocytosis; catestatin is a fragment of the prohormone that inhibits further catecholamine release by acting as an antagonist at the neuronal cholinergic receptor. CgA levels tend to be somewhat higher in patients with hypertension than in matched normotensive individuals. However, interestingly, lower catestatin levels have been noted in the offspring of hypertensive individuals. In white individuals, those with lower catestatin levels tend to have greater

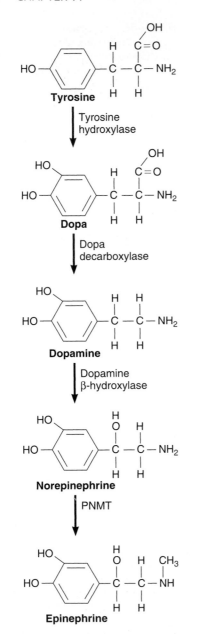

Figure 11–2. Biosynthesis of catecholamines. (PNMT, phenylethanolamine-*N*-methyltransferase.)

adrenergic pressor responses. Thus, relative deficiencies in catestatin may increase the risk for later development of essential hypertension.

The proportions of epinephrine and norepinephrine found in the adrenal medulla vary with the species (Table 11–1). In humans, the adrenal medulla contains 15–20% norepinephrine.

A. CONVERSION OF TYROSINE TO DOPA

The catecholamines are synthesized from **tyrosine,** which may be derived from ingested food or synthesized from phenylalanine in the liver. Tyrosine circulates at a concentration of 1–1.5 mg/dL of blood. It enters neurons and chromaffin cells by an active transport mechanism and is converted to L-dihydroxyphenylalanine (L-dopa). The reaction is catalyzed by **tyrosine hydroxylase,** which is transported via axonal flow to the nerve terminal. Tyrosine hydroxylase is the rate-limiting step in catecholamine synthesis. It is transcriptionally activated by acetylcholine through the nicotinic cholinergic receptor, which in turn activates protein kinase A via cAMP. Tyrosine hydroxylase activity may be inhibited by a variety of compounds. Alpha-methyltyrosine is effective and is sometimes used in the therapy of malignant pheochromocytomas.

B. CONVERSION OF DOPA TO DOPAMINE

Dopa is converted to dopamine by the enzyme aromatic L-amino acid decarboxylase (dopa decarboxylase). This enzyme is found in all tissues, with the highest concentrations in liver, kidney, brain, and vas deferens. The various enzymes have different substrate specificities depending upon the tissue source. Competitive inhibitors of dopa decarboxylase such as methyldopa are converted to substances (an example is α-methylnorepinephrine) that are then stored in granules in the nerve cell and released in place of norepinephrine. These products (false transmitters) were thought to mediate the antihypertensive action of drugs at peripheral sympathetic synapses but are now believed to stimulate the alpha receptors of the inhibitory corticobulbar system, reducing sympathetic discharge peripherally.

C. CONVERSION OF DOPAMINE TO NOREPINEPHRINE

Dopamine enters granulated storage vesicles where it is hydroxylated to norepinephrine by the enzyme dopamine-β-hydroxylase (DBH), which is found within the vesicle membrane. Norepinephrine is then stored in the vesicle. The granulated storage vesicle migrates to the cell surface and secretes its contents via exocytosis; both norepinephrine and DBH are released during exocytosis. After secretion, most norepinephrine is avidly recycled back into the nerve. Normally, most circulating norepinephrine originates from diffusion out of nonadrenal sympathetic nerve cells.

D. CONVERSION OF NOREPINEPHRINE TO EPINEPHRINE

Norepinephrine can diffuse into the cytoplasm from storage granules. In certain cells (particularly the adrenal medulla), norepinephrine is converted to epinephrine in the cytoplasm, catalyzed by 4-phenylethanolamine-*N*-methyltransferase (PNMT). Epinephrine can then return to the vesicle, diffuse from the cell, or undergo ca-

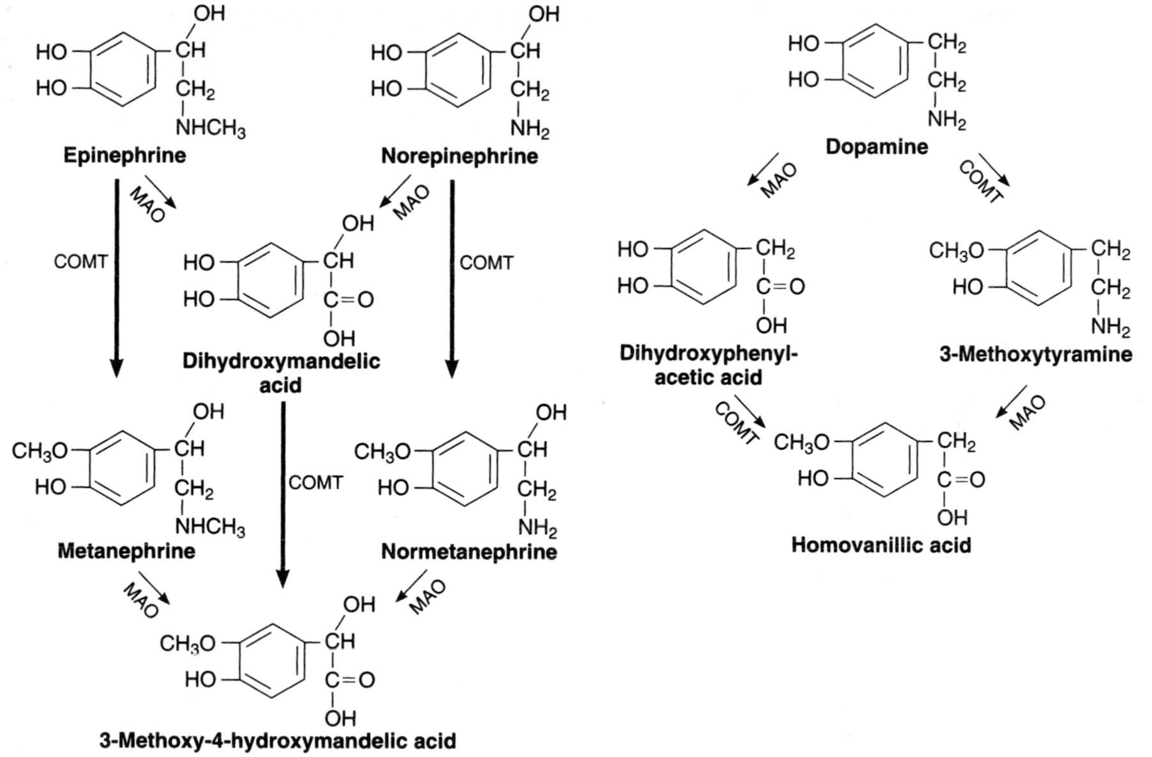

Figure 11–3. Metabolism of catecholamines by catechol-*O*-methyltransferase (COMT) and monoamine oxidase (MAO).

tabolism. High concentrations of cortisol enhance the expression of the gene encoding PNMT. Cortisol is present in high concentrations in most areas of the adrenal medulla due to venous blood flow from the adjacent adrenal cortex. This accounts for the fact that in the normal human adrenal medulla, about 80% of the

Table 11–1. Approximate percentages of total adrenal medullary catecholamines present as norepinephrine in various species.

Whale	70	Horse	25
Chicken	70	Squirrel	25
Lion	55	Cow	25
Frog	50	Human	20
Pig	45	Guinea pig	15
Cat	40	Rat	15
Gazelle	35	Zebra	13
Sheep	35	Rabbit	5
Goat	35	Baboon	0
Dog	30		

catecholamine content is epinephrine while only 20% is norepinephrine. Serum epinephrine levels fall precipitously after resection of both normal adrenals, while norepinephrine concentrations do not decline.

The enzyme PNMT is found in many tissues outside the adrenal medulla. PNMT that is identical to adrenal PNMT has been found in the lung, kidney, pancreas, and cancer cells. Therefore, nonadrenal tissue is capable of synthesizing epinephrine if norepinephrine is available as a substrate. However, nonadrenal production of epinephrine usually contributes minimally to circulating levels. PNMT is found in human lung; in vivo exposure of bronchial epithelial cell lines to dexamethasone increases the expression of PNMT. Thus, glucocorticoids could potentially increase local concentrations of epinephrine in the lung; this might be one potential mechanism for the effectiveness of systemic and inhaled glucocorticoids in asthma. PNMT activity is also found in red blood cells, where its activity is increased by hyperthyroidism and decreased by hypothyroidism. Renal PNMT activity is such that the kidney may synthesize up to one-half of the epinephrine found in the urine in normal individuals.

Catecholamine biosynthesis is coupled to secretion, so that the stores of norepinephrine at the nerve endings remain relatively unchanged even in the presence of marked nerve activity. In the adrenal medulla, it is possible to deplete stores with prolonged hypoglycemia. Biosynthesis appears to be increased during nerve stimulation by activation of tyrosine hydroxylase. Prolonged stimulation leads to the induction of increased amounts of this enzyme.

Storage

Catecholamines are found in the adrenal medulla and various sympathetically innervated organs, and their concentration reflects the density of sympathetic neurons. The adrenal medulla contains about 0.5 mg/g; the spleen, vas deferens, brain, spinal cord, and heart contain 1–5 μg/g; liver, gut, and skeletal muscle contain 0.1–0.5 μg/g. Catecholamines are stored in electron-dense granules approximately 1 μm in diameter that contain catecholamines and ATP in a 4:1 molar ratio, several neuropeptides, calcium, magnesium, and water-soluble proteins called **chromogranins** (see above). The interior surface of the membrane contains dopamine β-hydroxylase and ATPase. The Mg^{2+}-dependent ATPase facilitates the uptake and inhibits the release of catecholamines by the granules. Adrenal medullary granules appear to contain and release a number of active peptides including adrenomedullin, ACTH, vasoactive intestinal peptide (VIP), chromogranins, and enkephalins. The peptides derived from the chromogranins are physiologically active and may modulate catecholamine release.

Secretion (Table 11–2)

Adrenal medullary catecholamine secretion is increased by exercise, angina pectoris, myocardial infarction, hemorrhage, ether anesthesia, surgery, hypoglycemia, anoxia and asphyxia, and many other stressful stimuli. The rate of secretion of epinephrine increases more than that of norepinephrine in the presence of hypoglycemia and most other stimuli. However, anoxia and asphyxia produce a greater increase in adrenal medullary release of norepinephrine than is observed with other stimuli.

Secretion of the adrenal medullary hormones is mediated by the release of acetylcholine from the terminals of preganglionic fibers. The resulting depolarization of the axonal membrane triggers an influx of calcium ion. The contents of the storage vesicles, including the chromogranins and soluble dopamine β-hydroxylase, are released by exocytosis by the calcium ion increase. Membrane-bound dopamine β-hydroxylase is not released. **Tyramine,** however, releases norepinephrine primarily from the free store in the cytosol. Cocaine and monoamine oxidase inhibitors inhibit the effect of tyramine but do not affect the release of catecholamines by nervous stimulation. The rate of release in response to nerve stimulation is increased or decreased by a wide variety of neurotransmitters acting at specific receptors on the presynaptic neuron. Norepinephrine has an important role in modulating its own release by activating the α_2 receptors on the presynaptic membrane. Alpha$_2$ receptor antagonists inhibit this reaction. Conversely, presynaptic beta receptors enhance norepinephrine release, whereas beta receptor blockers decrease it. The accumulation of excess catecholamines that are not in the storage granules is prevented by the presence of intraneuronal monoamine oxidase.

Transport

When released into the circulation, catecholamines are bound to albumin or a closely associated protein with low affinity and high capacity.

Table 11–2. Range of plasma catecholamine levels observed in healthy subjects and patients.

	Norepinephrine	Epinephrine
Healthy subjects		
Basal	150–400 pg/mL (0.9–2.4 nmol/L)	25–100 pg/mL (0.1–0.6 nmol/L)
Ambulatory	200–800 pg/mL (1.2–4.8 nmol/L)	30–100 pg/mL (0.1–1 nmol/L)
Exercise	800–4000 pg/mL (4.8–24 nmol/L)	100–1000 pg/mL (0.5–5 nmol/L)
Symptomatic hypoglycemia	200–1000 pg/mL (1.2–6 nmol/L)	1000–5000 pg/mL (5–25 nmol/L)
Patients		
Hypertension	200–500 pg/mL (1.2–3 nmol/L)	20–100 pg/mL (0.1–0.6 nmol/L)
Surgery	500–2000 pg/mL (3–12 nmol/L)	199–500 pg/mL (0.5–3 nmol/L)
Myocardial infarction	1000–2000 pg/mL (6–12 nmol/L)	800–5000 pg/mL (4–25 nmol/L)

Metabolism & Inactivation of Catecholamines (Figures 11–3 and 11–4)

Catecholamines are quickly metabolized into inactive compounds, including metanephrines, VMA, and conjugated catecholamines.

Excess intracellular norepinephrine is inactivated primarily by deamination, catalyzed mainly by monoamine oxidase (MAO), at the outer mitochondrial membrane. (MAO regulates the catecholamine content of neurons; levels of MAO are increased by progesterone and decreased by estrogen.) The resultant aldehyde is then oxidized to 3,4-dihydroxymandelic acid (DHMA) or dihydroxyphenylglycol (DHPG); the latter are catalyzed by the enzyme catechol-*O*-methyltransferase (COMT) to VMA, which is then excreted. In pheochromocytomas, membrane-bound COMT metabolizes epinephrine into metanephrine; it converts norepinephrine into normetanephrine. These metanephrine metabolites are then secreted directly into the circulation. Thus, in patients with pheochromocytomas, about 93% of circulating normetanephrine comes from direct secretion from the tumor rather than from peripheral metabolism.

Catecholamines that are released at the synapse bind to their receptors with relatively low affinity and dissociate rapidly (Figure 11–4). About 15% of norepinephrine escapes from synapses into the systemic circulation. About 85% of synaptic catecholamines are reabsorbed by the nerves from which they were released or by the target cells, after which they may be stored for re-release or metabolized and released as described above. The catecholamine uptake mechanism is saturable, energy-requiring, stereoselective, and sodium-dependent. Synaptic catecholamine uptake is blocked by tricyclic antidepressants, phenothiazines, amphetamine derivatives, and cocaine.

Peripheral circulating norepinephrine is metabolized largely to normetanephrine by COMT, with the methyl donor being *S*-adenosylmethionine (SAM). COMT is an enzyme found in most tissues, especially blood cells, liver, kidney, and vascular smooth muscle. Epinephrine is similarly catabolized to metanephrine, some of which is then converted to VMA (Figure 11–3). Catecholamines may also be inactivated by conjugation of their phenolic hydroxyl group with sulfate or glucuronide; this reaction occurs mainly in the liver, gut, and red blood cells.

Catecholamines and metabolites are excreted in the urine. Normally, the proportions of urine catecholamines and metabolites are approximately 50% metanephrines, 35% VMA, 10% conjugated catecholamines and other metabolites, and < 5% free catecholamines.

Adrenergic Receptors

Adrenergic receptors were first classified by the relative potencies of a series of adrenergic agonists and antagonists. Each of the subtypes is now known to be coded for by one or more separate genes (Table 11–3). The physiologic effects mediated by them are summarized in Table 11–4.

The adrenergic receptors are transmembrane proteins with an extracellular amino terminus and an intracellular carboxyl terminus. Each of their seven hydrophobic regions spans the cell membrane (see Figure 3–2). Although these regions of the adrenergic receptor subtypes exhibit significant amino acid homology, differences in the fifth and sixth segments determine the specificity of agonist binding. Differences in the fifth and seventh segments determine which of the guanylyl nucleotide binding proteins (G proteins) is coupled to the receptor. The G proteins consist of α, β, and γ subunits. There are many G proteins that have different α subunits while the β and γ subunits are similar. When hormone binds to the receptor, the β and γ subunits dissociate from the α subunits, allowing GDP to be replaced by GTP on the α subunits and causing the β and γ subunits to dissociate from it. The GTP-bound α subunits activate the postreceptor pathways. (See Figure 11–5.)

A. ALPHA-ADRENERGIC RECEPTORS

The α_1 subtypes are postsynaptic receptors that typically mediate vascular and other smooth muscle contraction. When agonist binds to this receptor, the alpha subunit of the guanylyl nucleotide binding protein G_q is released and activates phospholipase C. This enzyme catalyzes the conversion of phosphatidylinositol phosphate to 1,4,5-inositol trisphosphate (IP_3) and diacylglycerol. IP_3 releases calcium ion from intracellular stores to stimulate physiologic responses. Diacylglycerol activates kinase C, which in turn phosphorylates a series of other proteins that initiate or sustain effects stimulated by the release of IP_3 and calcium ion (Figure 3–4). Epinephrine and norepinephrine are potent agonists for this receptor, while isoproterenol is weakly active.

Alpha$_2$ receptors were first identified at the presynaptic sympathetic nerve ending and, when activated, served to inhibit the release of norepinephrine. However, these receptors have been found in platelets and postsynaptically in the nervous system, adipose tissue, and smooth muscle.

Agonist binding to the α_2 receptor releases G_i alpha, which inhibits the enzyme adenylyl cyclase and reduces the formation of cAMP. Prazosin is a selective antagonist at the α_1 receptor and yohimbine is selective for the α_2, whereas phentolamine and phenoxybenzamine act at both (Table 11–3).

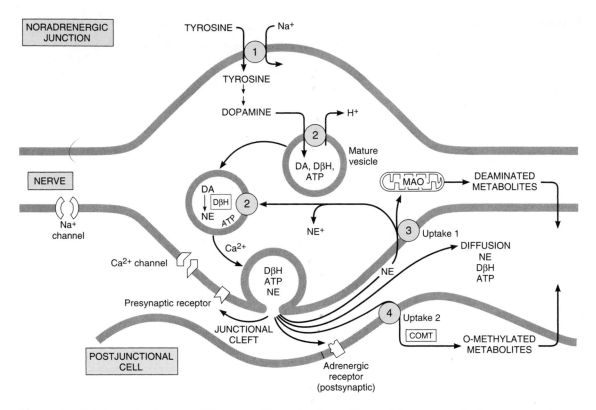

Figure 11–4. Schematic diagram of the neuroeffector junction of the peripheral sympathetic nervous system. The nerves terminate in complex networks with enlargements that form synaptic junctions with effector cells. The neurotransmitter at these junctions is norepinephrine, which is synthesized from tyrosine. Tyrosine uptake ① is linked to sodium uptake and transport into the varicosity where the secretory vesicles form. Tyrosine is hydroxylated by tyrosine hydroxylase to dopa, which is then decarboxylated by dopa decarboxylate to dopamine in the cytoplasm. Dopamine (DA) is transported into the vesicle by a carrier mechanism ② that can be blocked by reserpine. The same carrier transports norepinephrine (NE) and several other amines into these granules. Dopamine is converted to norepinephrine through the catalytic action of dopamine β-hydroxylase (DβH). ATP is also present in high concentration in the vesicle. Release of transmitter occurs when an action potential is conducted to the varicosity by the action of voltage-sensitive sodium channels. Depolarization of the synaptic membrane opens voltage-sensitive calcium channels and results in an increase in intracellular calcium. The elevated calcium facilitates exocytotic fusion of vesicles with the surface membrane and expulsion of norepinephrine, ATP, and some of the dopamine β-hydroxylase. Release is blocked by drugs such as guanethidine and bretylium. Norepinephrine reaching either pre- or postsynaptic receptors modifies the function of the corresponding cells. Norepinephrine also diffuses out of the cleft, or it may be transported into the cytoplasm of the varicosity (uptake 1, blocked by cocaine, tricyclic antidepressants) ③ or into the postjunctional cell (uptake 2) ④. (Reproduced, with permission, from Katzung BG [editor]: *Basic & Clinical Pharmacology,* 5th ed. McGraw-Hill, 1992.) (**Note:** In pheochromocytomas, membrane-bound COMT within tumor cells metabolizes epinephrine and norepinephrine directly into metanephrine and normetanephrine, respectively, which are then released.)

Table 11–3. Adrenoceptor types and subtypes.[1]

Receptor	Agonist	Antagonist	Effects	Gene on Chromosome
Alpha₁ type Alpha₁A	Phenylephrine, methoxamine	Prazosin, corynanthine WB4101	↑ IP_3, DAG common to all	C5
Alpha₁B		CEC (irreversible)		C8
Alpha₁D		WB4101		C20
Alpha₂ type Alpha₂A	Clonidine, BHT920 Oxymetazoline	Rauwolscine, yohimbine	↓ cAMP common to all ↑ K^+ channels; ↓ Ca^{2+} channels	C10
Alpha₂B		Prazosin	↓ cAMP; ↓ Ca^{2+} channels	C2
Alpha₂C		Prazosin	↓ cAMP	C4
Beta type Beta₁	Isoproterenol Dobutamine	Propranolol Betaxolol	↑ cAMP common to all ↑ cAMP	C10
Beta₂	Procaterol, terbutaline	Butoxamine	↑ cAMP	C5
Beta₃	BRL37344		↑ cAMP	C8
Dopamine type D₁	Dopamine Fenoldopam		↑ cAMP	C5
D₂	Bromocriptine		↓ cAMP; ↑ K^+ channels; ↓ Ca^{2+} channels	C11
D₃ (D₂-like)	Quinpirol	AJ76	↓ cAMP; ↑ K^+ channels; ↑ Ca^{2+} channels	C3
D₄ (D₂-like)		Clozapine	↓ cAMP	C11
D₅ (D₁-like)			↑ cAMP	C4

[1]Reproduced, with permission, from Katzung BJ (editor): *Basic and Clinical Pharmacology*, 8th ed. McGraw-Hill, 2001.
Key: BRL37344 = Sodium-4-{2-[2-hydroxy-(3-chlorophenyl)ethylamino]propyl}phenoxyacetate
BHT920 = 6-Allyl-2-amino-5,6,7,8-tetrahydro-4*H*-thiazolo-[4,5-*d*]azepine
CEC = Chloroethylclonidine
DAG = Diacylglycerol
IP₃ = Inositol trisphophate
WB4101 = *N*-[2-(2,6-dimethoxyphenoxy)ethyl]-2,3-dihydro-1,4-benzodioxan-2-methanamine

B. BETA-ADRENERGIC RECEPTORS

Agonist binding to the beta-adrenergic receptors activates adenylyl cyclase via the G_s alpha subunit to increase the production of cAMP, which in turn converts protein kinase A to its active form. Kinase A then phosphorylates a variety of proteins, including enzymes, ion channels, and receptors (see Figure 3–4). There are three major beta-receptor subtypes. The β₁ receptor, which mediates the direct cardiac effects, is more responsive to isoproterenol than to epinephrine or norepinephrine, whose potencies are similar. The β₂ receptor mediates vascular, bronchial, and uterine smooth muscle relaxation, probably by phos-phorylating myosin light chain kinase. Isoproterenol is also the most potent agonist at this receptor, but epinephrine is much more potent than norepinephrine. Beta₂ receptor polymorphisms are associated with differences in sensitivity to albuterol in asthmatics and with obesity in women. The β₃ receptors regulate energy expenditure and lipolysis. Homozygous mutations in the β₃ gene in Pima Indians are associated with earlier onset of type 2 diabetes. Resting autonomic nervous system activity is reduced in homozygous and heterozygous patients with Trp(64)-Arg polymorphism of the β₃ receptor. In the heart, β₃ stimulation causes decreased ventricular contraction by increasing nitric oxide.

Table 11–4. Adrenergic responses
of selected tissues.

Organ or Tissue	Receptor	Effect
Heart (myo-cardium)	β_1	Increased force of contraction Increased rate of contraction
Blood vessels	α	Vasoconstriction
	β_2	Vasodilation
Kidney	β	Increased renin release
Gut	α, β	Decreased motility and increased sphincter tone
Pancreas	α	Decreased insulin release Decreased glucagon release
	β	Increased insulin release Increased glucagon release
Liver	α, β	Increased glycogenolysis
Adipose tissue	β	Increased lipolysis
Most tissues	β	Increased calorigenesis
Skin (apocrine glands on hands, axillae, etc)	α	Increased sweating
Bronchioles	β_2	Dilation
Uterus	α	Contraction
	β_2	Relaxation

C. DOPAMINE RECEPTORS

Dopaminergic receptors are found in the central nervous system, presynaptic adrenergic nerve terminals, pituitary, heart, renal and mesenteric vascular beds, and other sites. Five subtypes of the dopaminergic receptor, D_1 to D_5, have been identified. The binding affinity of the D_1 receptor is greater for dopamine than for haloperidol; the reverse is true for the D_2 receptor. The effects of the D_1 receptor are mediated by stimulation of the adenylyl cyclase system and are found postsynaptically in the brain. Those in the pituitary are D_2 receptors that inhibit the formation of cAMP, open potassium channels, and decrease calcium influx.

Regulation of Activity

The major physiologic control of sympathoadrenal activity is exerted by alterations in the rate of secretion of the catecholamines. However, the receptors and postreceptor events serve as sites of fine regulation.

As noted above, presynaptically, norepinephrine released during nerve stimulation binds to alpha receptors and reduces the amount of norepinephrine released.

The number of receptors on the effector cell surface can be reduced by binding of agonist to receptor (antagonists do not have the same effect). This reduction is called "down-regulation." Thyroid hormone, however, has been shown to increase the number of beta receptors in the myocardium. Estrogen, which increases the number of alpha receptors in the myometrium, increases the affinity of some vascular alpha receptors for norepinephrine.

The mechanisms involved in some of these changes are known. For example phosphorylation of the beta-adrenergic receptor by beta-adrenergic receptor kinase results in their sequestration into membrane vesicles, internalization, and degradation. The phosphorylated receptor also has a greater affinity for β-arrestin, another regulatory protein, which prevents its interaction with $G_s\alpha$.

The finding that most cells in the body have adrenergic receptors has led to an appreciation of the important regulatory role of the peripheral sympathetic nervous system. In contrast, the effects of the adrenal medulla are mediated via the circulating catecholamines and, therefore, are much more generalized in nature. Furthermore, adrenal medullary secretion increases significantly only in the presence of stress or marked deviation from homeostatic or resting conditions.

Catecholamine Actions (Figure 11–4)

Dopamine is an important central neurotransmitter and a precursor to norepinephrine. Circulating dopamine is not normally a significant catecholamine; the presence of dopamine in the urine is mainly due to high renal concentrations of dopa decarboxylase. Higher serum concentrations of dopamine stimulate vascular D_1 receptors, causing vasodilation and increased renal blood flow. Extremely high serum levels of dopamine are required to activate vascular alpha receptors enough to cause vasoconstriction.

Norepinephrine is synthesized in the adrenal medulla, sympathetic paraganglia, brain, and spinal cord nerve cells. However, most norepinephrine is found in the synaptic vesicles of postganglionic autonomic nerves in organs that have rich sympathetic innervations: the heart, salivary glands, vascular smooth muscle, liver, spleen, kidneys, and muscles. A single sympathetic nerve cell may have up to 25,000 synaptic bulges along the length of its axon; each synapse synthesizes norepinephrine and stores it in adrenergic synaptic vesicles adjacent to target cells.

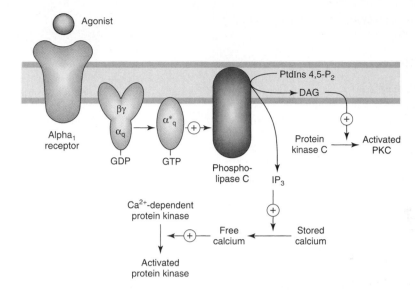

Figure 11–5. Activation of α_1 responses. Stimulation of α_1 receptors by catecholamines leads to the activation of a G_q coupling protein. The alpha subunit of this G protein activates the effector, phospholipase C, which leads to the release of IP_3 (inositol 1,4,5-trisphosphate) and DAG (diacylglycerol) from phosphatidylinositol 4,5-bisphosphate (PtdIns 4,5-P_2). IP_3 stimulates the release of sequestered stores of calcium, leading to an increased concentration of cytoplasmic Ca^{2+}. Ca^{2+} may then activate Ca^{2+}-dependent protein kinases, which in turn phosphorylate their substrates. DAG activates protein kinase C. See text for additional effects of α_1 receptor activation. (Reproduced, with permission, from Katzung BJ [editor]: *Basic & Clinical Pharmacology*, 8th ed. McGraw-Hill, 2001.)

Norepinephrine stimulates α_1-adrenergic receptors, which increases the influx of calcium into the target cell. Vascular α_1-adrenergic receptors are found in the heart, papillary dilator muscles, and smooth muscle. Activation of α_1-adrenergic receptors causes hypertension, increased cardiac contraction, and dilation of the pupils. α_1-Adrenergic activation stimulates sweating from nonthermoregulatory apocrine "stress" sweat glands, which are located variably on the palms, axillae, and forehead. Norepinephrine's activation of β-adrenergic receptors causes an influx of calcium into the target cell. Norepinephrine has great affinity for β_1-adrenergic receptors (increases cardiac contraction and rate); stimulation of the heart rate is opposed by simultaneous vagal stimulation. Norepinephrine has less affinity for β_2-adrenergic receptors (vasodilation, hepatic glycogenolysis). With higher norepinephrine levels, hypermetabolism and hyperglycemia are noted. Norepinephrine also activates β_3-adrenergic receptors on fat cells, causing lipolysis and an increase in serum levels of free fatty acids.

Epinephrine also stimulates α_1- and β_1-adrenergic receptors, with the same effects noted above for norepinephrine. However, epinephrine also activates β_2 receptors, causing vasodilation in skeletal muscles. Epinephrine thus has a variable effect on blood pressure ranging from hypertension to hypotension (rare). Hypoglycemia is a strong stimulus for the adrenal medulla to secrete epinephrine, which increases hepatic glycogenolysis. Epinephrine also stimulates lipolysis, resulting in increased serum levels of free fatty acids. Epinephrine also increases the basal metabolic rate. Epinephrine does not cross the blood-brain barrier well. However, high serum levels of epinephrine do stimulate the hypothalamus, resulting in unpleasant sensations ranging from nervousness to an "overwhelming sense of impending doom." These manifestations are distinct from those of noncatecholamine amphetamines, which enter the central nervous system more readily and have other stimulatory effects.

Physiologic Effects

A. Cardiovascular Effects

Catecholamines increase the rate and force of contraction and increase the irritability of the myocardium, primarily by activating β_1 receptors. The contractile effects of the catecholamines on vascular smooth muscle are regulated by α_1, α_2, and β_2 receptors. Contraction is mediated by the α_1 receptor, and although beta receptors are present and cause dilatation, other mechanisms of vascular dilatation are probably more important in vasoregulatory control. The release or injection of catecholamines can therefore be expected to increase heart rate and cardiac output and cause peripheral vasoconstriction—all leading to an increase in blood pressure. These events are modulated by reflex mechanisms, so that, as the blood pressure increases, reflex stimulation may slow the heart rate and tend to reduce cardiac output. Although norepinephrine in the usual doses will have these effects, the effect of epinephrine may vary depending on the smooth muscle tone of the vascular system at the time. For example, in an individual with increased vascular tone, the net effect of small amounts of epinephrine may be to reduce the mean blood pressure through vasodilation despite increasing the heart rate and cardiac output. In an individual with a reduction in vascular tone, the mean blood pressure would be expected to increase. In addition to the reflex mechanisms, vascular output is integrated by the central nervous system, so that, under appropriate circumstances, one vascular bed may be dilated while others remain unchanged. The central organization of the sympathetic nervous system is such that its ordinary regulatory effects are quite discrete—in contrast to periods of stress, when stimulation may be rather generalized and accompanied by release of catecholamines into the circulation. The infusion of catecholamines leads to a rapid reduction in plasma volume, presumably to accommodate the reduced volume of the arterial and venous beds (Figure 11–6).

B. Effects on Extravascular Smooth Muscle

The catecholamines also regulate the activity of smooth muscle in tissues other than blood vessels. These effects include relaxation and contraction of uterine myometrium, relaxation of intestinal and bladder smooth muscle, contraction of the smooth muscle in the bladder and intestinal sphincters, and relaxation of tracheal smooth muscle and pupillary dilatation.

C. Metabolic Effects

The catecholamines increase oxygen consumption and heat production. Although the effects appear to be me-

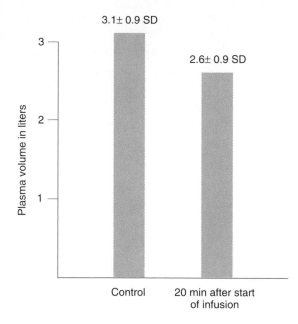

Figure 11–6. Changes in plasma volume produced by infusion of norepinephrine for 20 minutes in a dose sufficient to increase mean arterial pressure from 96 ± 10 mm Hg to 150 ± 16 mm Hg. (Data from Finnerty FA Jr, Buchholz JH, Guillaudeu RL: Blood volumes and plasma protein during arterenol-induced hypertension. J Clin Invest 1958;37:425.)

diated by the beta receptor, the mechanism is unknown. The catecholamines also regulate glucose and fat mobilization from storage depots. Glycogenolysis in heart muscle and in liver leads to an increase in available carbohydrate for utilization. Stimulation of adipose tissue leads to lipolysis and the release of free fatty acids and glycerol into the circulation for utilization at other sites. In humans, these effects are mediated by the beta receptor.

The plasma levels of catecholamines required to produce some cardiovascular and metabolic effects in humans are shown in Table 11–5.

The catecholamines have effects on water, sodium, potassium, calcium, and phosphate excretion in the kidney. However, the mechanisms and the significance of these changes are not clear.

The Regulatory Role of Catecholamines in Hormone Secretion

The sympathetic nervous system plays an important role in the regulation and integration of hormone secretion at two levels. Centrally, norepinephrine and dopamine

Table 11–5. Approximate circulating plasma levels of epinephrine and norepinephrine required to produce hemodynamic and metabolic changes during infusions of epinephrine and norepinephrine.[1]

	Norepinephrine	Epinephrine
Systolic blood pressure	↑ at 2500 pg/mL (15 nmol/L)	↑ at 500 pg/mL (3 nmol/L)
Diastolic blood pressure	↑ at 2500 pg/mL (15 nmol/L)	↓ at 500 pg/mL (3 nmol/L)
Pulse	↓ at 2500 pg/mL (15 nmol/dL)	↑ at 250 pg/mL (1.5 nmol/L)
Plasma glucose	↑ at 2500 pg/mL (15 nmol/L)	↑ at 250–500 pg/mL (1.5–3 nmol/L)

[1]Data from Silverberg AB et al: Am J Physiol 1978;234:E252; and from Clutter WE et al: J Clin Invest 1980;66:94.

play important roles in the regulation of secretion of the anterior pituitary hormones. Dopamine, for example, has been identified as the prolactin-inhibiting hormone, and the hypothalamic releasing hormones appear to be under sympathetic nervous system control. Peripherally, the secretion of renin by the juxtaglomerular cells of the kidney is regulated by the sympathetic nervous system via the renal nerves and circulating catecholamines. The catecholamines release renin via a beta receptor mechanism. The B cell of the pancreatic islets is stimulated by activation of the beta receptors in the presence of alpha-adrenergic blockade. However, the dominant effect of norepinephrine or epinephrine is inhibition of insulin secretion, which is mediated by the alpha receptor. Similar effects have been observed in the secretion of glucagon by pancreatic A cells. The catecholamines have also been found to increase the release of thyroxine, calcitonin, parathyroid hormone, and gastrin by a beta receptor-mediated mechanism.

OTHER HORMONES

In addition to the catecholamines, the chromaffin cells of the adrenal medulla and peripheral sympathetic neurons synthesize and secrete opiate-like peptides, including met- and leu-enkephalin (see Chapter 5). They are stored in the large, dense-cored vesicles with the catecholamines in the adrenal medulla and at sympathetic nerve endings. These peptides are also found in the terminals of the splanchnic fibers that innervate the adrenal medulla. The observation that naloxone increases plasma catecholamine levels suggests that these peptides may inhibit sympathetic activity.

Adrenomedullin, a peptide originally isolated from pheochromocytoma tissue, is produced in the adrenal medulla. It consists of 52 amino acids, has slight homology with calcitonin gene-related peptide, and exerts its effects by elevation of cAMP levels. It exhibits potent depressor and vasorelaxant activity. It has also been found in the heart, lung, kidney, and brain as well as vascular endothelium. Adrenomedullin is a vasodilatory and natriuretic peptide and is secreted by the heart in heart failure. Adrenomedullin circulates in blood, and plasma levels in patients with hypertension have been reported to be higher than those of normotensive controls. It is thought to play a role in blood pressure regulation. The amino terminal 20-amino-acid peptide of proadrenomedullin from which adrenomedullin is derived is also found in the same tissues. This peptide also exhibits hypotensive effects, but it appears to do so by inhibiting neural transmission at sympathetic nerve endings rather than directly relaxing vascular smooth muscle like adrenomedullin.

Vasopressin is produced by the adrenal medulla. Its receptors (V1a and V1b) are also present and are thought to regulate catecholamine secretion. Extracts of normal adrenals have also been found to contain corticotropin-releasing factor, growth hormone-releasing hormone, somatostatin, and peptide histidine methionine. Although these and other active peptides are secreted by tumors of the adrenal medulla and contribute to the symptomatology, little is known of their function in the normal gland.

■ DISORDERS OF ADRENAL MEDULLARY FUNCTION

ADRENAL MEDULLARY HYPOFUNCTION

Hypofunction of the adrenal medulla alone probably occurs only in individuals receiving adrenocortical steroid replacement therapy following adrenalectomy. Such individuals with otherwise intact sympathetic nervous systems suffer no clinically significant disability. Patients with autonomic insufficiency, which includes deficiency of adrenal medullary epinephrine secretion, can be demonstrated to have minor defects in recovery from insulin-induced hypoglycemia (Figure 11–7). It should be noted, however, that in patients with diabetes mellitus in whom the glucagon response is also deficient, the additional loss of adrenal medullary response leaves them more susceptible to severe bouts of hypoglycemia. This is the result of a decrease in the warning symptoms as well as an impaired response. (See Chapter 18.) Patients with generalized autonomic insufficiency usually have orthostatic hypotension. The causes of disorders associated with autonomic insufficiency are listed in Table 11–6.

Table 11–6. Disorders associated with autonomic insufficiency.

Familial dysautonomia
Shy-Drager syndrome
Parkinson's disease
Tabes dorsalis
Syringomyelia
Cerebrovascular disease
Autonomic neuropathy due to diabetes
Idiopathic orthostatic hypotension
Sympathectomy
Drugs: antihypertensives, antidepressants

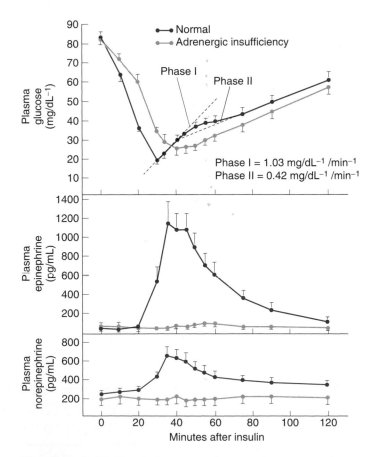

Phase I = 1.03 mg/dL^{-1} /min^{-1}
Phase II = 0.42 mg/dL^{-1} /min^{-1}

Figure 11–7. Plasma glucose, epinephrine, and norepinephrine levels after insulin administration in 14 normal subjects (•–•) and seven patients with idiopathic orthostatic hypotension (•–•) with low or absent epinephrine responses. Results are expressed as mean ± SEM. (Reproduced, with permission, from Polinsky RJ et al: The adrenal medullary response to hypoglycemia in patients with orthostatic hypotension. J Clin Endocrinol Metab 1980;51:1404.)

When a normal individual stands, a series of physiologic adjustments occur that maintain blood pressure and ensure adequate circulation to the brain. The initial lowering of the blood pressure stimulates the baroreceptors, which then activate central reflex mechanisms that cause arterial and venous constriction, increase cardiac output, and activate the release of renin and vasopressin. Interruption of afferent, central, or efferent components of this autonomic reflex results in autonomic insufficiency.

The treatment of symptomatic orthostatic hypotension is dependent upon maintenance of an adequate blood volume. If physical measures such as raising the foot of the bed at night and using support garments do not alleviate the condition, pharmacologic measures may be used. Although agents producing constriction of the vascular bed, including ephedrine, phenylephrine, metaraminol, monoamine oxidase inhibitors, levodopa, propranolol, and indomethacin, have been used, volume expansion with fludrocortisone is the most effective treatment. Octreotide alone or in combination with the adrenergic agonist midodrine have also been shown to be effective in many patients.

ADRENAL MEDULLARY HYPERFUNCTION

The adrenal medulla is not known to play a significant role in essential hypertension. However, the role of the sympathetic nervous system in the regulation of blood flow and blood pressure has led to extensive investigations of its role in various types of hypertension. Some of the abnormalities observed, such as a resetting of baroreceptor activity, are thought to be secondary to the change in blood pressure. Others, such as the increased cardiac output found in early essential hypertension, have been thought by some investigators to play a primary role.

Catecholamines can increase blood pressure by increasing cardiac output, by increasing peripheral resistance through their vasoconstrictive action on the arteriole, and by increasing renin release from the kidney, leading to increased circulating levels of angiotensin II. Although many studies show an increase in circulating free catecholamine levels, evidence of increased sympathetic activity has not been a uniform finding in patients with essential hypertension.

■ PHEOCHROMOCYTOMA

Pheochromocytomas are rare tumors. The National Cancer Registry in Sweden has reported that pheochromocytomas are discovered in about two patients per million people yearly. However, autopsy series suggest a higher incidence. The reported incidence in autopsy series has varied from about 250 cases per million to 1300 cases per million in a Mayo Clinic autopsy series. Retrospectively, 61% of pheochromocytomas at autopsy occurred in patients who were known to have had hypertension; about 91% had the typical but nonspecific symptoms associated with secretory pheochromocytomas. In one autopsy study, a large number of patients with pheochromocytoma had nonclassic symptoms such as abdominal pain, vomiting, dyspnea, heart failure, hypotension, or sudden death (Table 11–7). Considering these autopsy data, it is clear that the great majority of pheochromocytomas are not diagnosed during life. This is due to the protean manifestations of pheochromocytoma. Clearly, physicians must become more vigilant for pheochromocytoma and employ appropriate screening tests for all patients in whom pheochromocytoma enters into the differential diagnosis. Pheochromocytomas occur in both sexes and at any age but are most common in the fourth and fifth decades.

Hypertension, defined as either a systolic or diastolic blood pressure over 140/90 mm Hg, is an extremely common condition, affecting about 20% of all American adults and over 50% of adults over 60 years. The incidence of pheochromocytoma is estimated to be < 0.1% of the entire hypertensive population, but it is higher in certain subgroups whose hypertension is labile or severe. Screening for pheochromocytoma should be considered for such patients with severe hypertension and also for hypertensive patients with suspicious symptoms, eg, headaches, palpitations, sweating episodes, or unexplained bouts of abdominal or chest pains (Tables 11–8 and 11–9).

Pathology of Pheochromocytomas & Related Tumors

Pheochromocytomas are usually located in the adrenals (90% in adults, 70% in children), occurring more frequently on the right than on the left. In one series, right-sided pheochromocytomas were described as producing paroxysmal hypertension more often than sustained hypertension, whereas the opposite was true for

Table 11–7. Causes of death in patients with unsuspected pheochromocytomas.

Myocardial infarction
Cerebrovascular accident
Arrhythmias
Irreversible shock
Renal failure
Dissecting aortic aneurysm

Table 11–8. Patients to be screened for pheochromocytoma.

Young hypertensives
Hypertensive patients with–
    Symptoms listed in Table 11–9
    Weight loss
    Seizures
    Orthostatic hypotension
    Unexplained shock
    Family history of pheochromocytoma or medullary carcinoma of thyroid
    Neurofibromatosis and other neurocutaneous syndromes
    Mucosal neuromas
    Hyperglycemia
    Cardiomyopathy
Marked lability of blood pressure
Family history of pheochromocytoma
Shock or severe pressor responses with–
    Induction of anesthesia
    Parturition
    Surgery
    Invasive procedures
    Antihypertensive drugs
Radiologic evidence of adrenal mass

tumors arising from the left adrenal. Adrenal pheochromocytomas are bilateral in about 10% of adults and 35% of children. They may present at any age but appear more commonly in the fourth and fifth decades.

Most sporadic pheochromocytomas are encapsulated by either a true capsule or a pseudocapsule consisting of the adrenal capsule. Pheochromocytomas are

Table 11–9. Common symptoms in patients with hypertension due to pheochromocytoma.

Symptoms during or following paroxysms
    Headache
    Sweating
    Forceful heartbeat with or without tachycardia
    Anxiety or fear of impending death
    Tremor
    Fatigue or exhaustion
    Nausea and vomiting
    Abdominal or chest pain
    Visual disturbances

Symptoms between paroxysms
    Increased sweating
    Cold hands and feet
    Weight loss
    Constipation

firm in texture. Hemorrhages that occur within a pheochromocytoma can give the tumor a mottled or dark red appearance. Larger tumors frequently have large areas of hemorrhagic necrosis that have undergone cystic degeneration; viable tumor may be found in the cyst wall. Calcifications are often present. Pheochromocytomas can rarely invade adjacent organs; tumors may extend into the adrenal vein and the vena cava, resulting in pulmonary tumor emboli. Pheochromocytomas vary tremendously in size, ranging from microscopic to 3600 g. The "average" pheochromocytoma weighs about 100 g and is 4.5 cm in diameter.

Paragangliomas are extra-adrenal pheochromocytomas that arise from sympathetic ganglia (Figure 11–8). They account for about 10% of pheochromocytomas in adults and about 30% in children. About 85% are intra-abdominal, where they are typically found in the juxtarenal or para-aortic region, particularly in the perinephric, periaortic, and bladder regions. Retroperitoneal paragangliomas are more likely to be malignant (30–50%) and present with pain or a mass. They tend to metastasize to the lungs, lymph nodes,

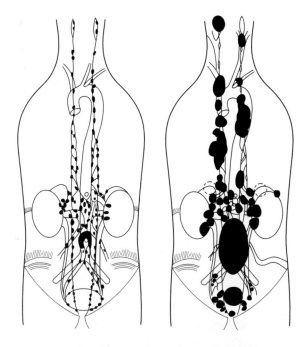

Figure 11–8. Left: Anatomic distribution of extra-adrenal chromaffin tissue in the newborn. **Right:** Locations of extra-adrenal pheochromocytomas reported before 1965. (Reproduced, with permission, from Coupland R: *The Natural History of the Chromaffin Cell.* Longmans, Green, 1965.)

and bones. Paragangliomas can be locally invasive and may destroy adjacent vertebrae and cause spinal cord compression. Pelvic paragangliomas may involve the bladder wall, obstruct the ureters, and metastasize to regional lymph nodes. About 36–60% of paragangliomas are functional, secreting norepinephrine and normetanephrine. Functional status is not known to affect survival. Nonfunctional paragangliomas can often concentrate MIBG or secrete chromogranin A. Paragangliomas of the bladder cause symptoms upon micturition. Large perinephric tumors can cause renal artery stenosis. Vaginal tumors can cause dysfunctional vaginal bleeding.

Paragangliomas may also arise in the anterior or posterior mediastinum or the heart. Central nervous system locations include the sella turcica, petrous ridge, and pineal region; cauda equina paraganglioma can cause increased intracranial pressure.

Nonchromaffin paragangliomas of neuroectodermal chemoreceptors are known as chemodectomas or glomus tumors; they are typically found in the head and neck, particularly near the carotid body, glomus jugulare, jugulotympanic region, or in the lung. Chemodectomas rarely secrete catecholamines.

Neuroblastomas, ganglioneuroblastomas, and **ganglioneuromas** are sympathetic nervous system tumors that are related to pheochromocytomas and likewise arise from primitive sympathogonia (Figure 11–1). These neuroblastic tumors account for 10% of childhood cancers. They develop from sympathetic tissue in the adrenal gland neck, posterior mediastinum, retroperitoneum, or pelvis. They differ in their degree of maturation and malignancy. Neuroblastoma tumors derive from immature neuroblasts, are generally aggressive, and tend to occur in very young children.

Ganglioneuroblastomas are composed of a mixture of neuroblasts and more mature gangliocytes; these develop in older children and tend to run a more benign course. Ganglioneuromas are the most benign of these tumors and are composed of gangliocytes and mature stromal cells. However, individual tumors can behave differently and some neuroblastomas are more indolent, depending upon the nature of their tumor oncogene mutations. Despite catecholamine secretion, children with neuroblastomas tend to be more symptomatic from their metastases than from catecholamine secretion. Tumors tend to concentrate radiolabeled metaiodobenzylguanidine (MIBG), making it a useful imaging and therapeutic agent. Treatment of malignant tumors consists of surgery, chemotherapy, external beam radiation to skeletal metastases, and high-dose ^{131}I-MIBG therapy for patients with MIBG-avid tumors. The mortality rate is high for children with neuroblastomas despite recent advances in treatment.

Genetic Conditions Associated with Pheochromocytomas

Most pheochromocytomas occur sporadically, though a substantial proportion of these tumors are found to have developed a somatic mutation similar to those seen in germline mutations that give rise to familial syndromes. Over 10% of pheochromocytomas are hereditary and occur as a feature of certain familial syndromes. Genetic testing is advisable for anyone with a family history of pheochromocytomas, paragangliomas, or bilateral pheochromocytomas. Genetic screening is also performed for patients with other manifestations of genetic syndromes noted below. Such screening can be done for MEN 2 *RET* oncogene mutations and *VHL* mutations. Mutations in the newly sequenced genes encoding succinate dehydrogenase subunit B (SDHB) and succinate dehydrogenase subunit D (SDHD) also predispose carriers to develop pheochromocytomas and glomus tumors.

A. MULTIPLE ENDOCRINE NEOPLASIA TYPE 2 (MEN 2)

MEN 2 is an autosomal dominant disorder caused by a mutation in the *ret* proto-oncogene (see Chapter 22). MEN 2 kindreds can be grouped into two distinct subtypes. In either subtype, pheochromocytomas usually develop in the adrenals; extra-adrenal paragangliomas are rare. Patients tend to have hypertension, usually paroxysmal. Each specific type of mutation in the *RET* codon determines each kindred's idiosyncrasies, such as the age at onset and the aggressiveness of medullary thyroid carcinoma. For example, patients with the 634-point mutation are more prone to develop pheochromocytoma and hyperparathyroidism. Plasma catecholamines may be normal; however, plasma concentrations of metanephrine are elevated early in most patients with pheochromocytomas associated with MEN 2, making this the screening test of choice for these patients.

1. MEN 2a (Sipple's syndrome)—Patients with this genetic condition may develop medullary thyroid carcinoma, hyperparathyroidism, pheochromocytoma, or adrenal medullary hyperplasia. Patients with MEN 2a also have a high incidence of lichen planus amyloidosis and Hirschsprung's disease. In patients with an MEN 2a genetic defect, the ultimate occurrence of medullary thyroid carcinoma is nearly 100%. However, the incidence of pheochromocytoma varies in different kindreds, ranging from 6% to 100% (average 40%), depending upon the kindred. Pheochromocytomas tend to present in middle age, often without hypertension. The incidence of hyperparathyroidism has also varied, averaging 35%. Anyone belonging to an MEN 2a kindred should have genetic testing for *ret* proto-oncogene mutations prior to 6 years of age to determine if they carry the genetic mutation that will require prophylactic thyroidectomy and close surveillance.

2. MEN 2b—Patients with this genetic condition are prone to develop aggressive medullary thyroid carcinoma, mucosal neuromas (visible in the eye and mouth), thick corneal nerves, intestinal ganglioneuromas, a marfanoid habitus, and pheochromocytoma or adrenal medullary hyperplasia. In patients with MEN 2b, medullary thyroid carcinoma tends to be aggressive and occurs at an earlier age than in patients with MEN 2a. Anyone belonging to a kindred with MEN 2b should have genetic testing immediately for RET proto-oncogene mutations. If an individual is found to carry the family's proto-oncogene mutation, early prophylactic thyroidectomy is advisable and long-term close surveillance is required.

B. VON HIPPEL-LINDAU DISEASE

In von Hippel-Lindau disease, a mutation of the *VHL* tumor suppressor gene causes an autosomal dominant predisposition to hemangioblastomas in the retina, cerebellum, and spinal cord. About 10–20% of patients with von Hippel-Lindau disease ultimately develop a pheochromocytoma; such patients are usually those having a *VHL* missense mutation rather than a deletion or frameshift mutation. Kidney cysts, renal cell carcinomas, and pancreatic cysts also occur.

In a French series of 36 patients with pheochromocytomas and von Hippel-Lindau disease, pheochromocytomas were the presenting tumor in 53%. Pheochromocytomas tended to develop at an early age and were bilateral in 42%; concurrent paragangliomas were present in 11%. Three of the 36 patients had a malignant pheochromocytoma. In 18% of these patients with von Hippel-Lindau disease, pheochromocytoma was the only known manifestation.

Plasma normetanephrine levels are usually elevated when patients with von Hippel-Lindau disease develop a pheochromocytoma. Therefore, it is advisable for patients with a *VHL* gene mutation to be screened regularly with plasma normetanephrine levels; patients with *VHL* missense mutations particularly require regular and frequent screening.

C. VON RECKLINGHAUSEN'S (TYPE 1) NEUROFIBROMATOSIS (NF-1)

Up to 5% of patients with von Recklinghausen's neurofibromatosis may ultimately develop pheochromocytomas. Such pheochromocytomas can grow to large size. Patients may develop hypertension, but some patients may be surprisingly asymptomatic despite increased catecholamine secretion. Patients with NF-1 are prone to develop vascular anomalies such as coarctation of the aorta and renal artery dysplasia, which can produce hypertension and mimic a pheochromocytoma.

Von Recklinghausen's disease is caused by a mutation in the NF-1 tumor suppressor gene mapped to chromosome 17q11.2; it is autosomal dominant, though about half of the cases seem sporadic. It is a common condition, with an incidence of 3000 cases per million population. Patients develop visible subcutaneous neurofibromas and schwannomas of cranial and vertebral nerve roots. Skeletal abnormalities are common. Hypothalamic hamartomas may occur and cause precocious puberty. Optic gliomas may affect vision. Patients may also have axillary freckles and multiple cutaneous pigmented café au lait spots that grow in size and number with age; most patients ultimately develop more than six spots measuring > 1.5 cm in diameter.

D. FAMILIAL PHEOCHROMOCYTOMAS

Pheochromocytomas may also occur as an isolated familial genetic syndrome. Pheochromocytomas are more likely to be bilateral, and adrenal medullary hyperplasia is common. Individuals with such genetic proclivity require frequent clinical and biochemical screening for pheochromocytoma.

E. FAMILIAL PARAGANGLIOMAS

Certain kindreds have a genetic proclivity to develop multicentric extra-adrenal paragangliomas. This syndrome has been attributed to mutations in three genes: *SDHB, SDHC,* and *SDHD.*

F. CARNEY'S TRIAD

Multicentric paragangliomas occur in patients with Carney's triad. It generally presents in women under age 40 and consists of paragangliomas, indolent gastric leiomyosarcomas, and pulmonary chondromas. (This condition is entirely different from Carney's complex.)

Physiology of Pheochromocytoma & Paraganglioma

Pheochromocytomas are tumors that arise from the adrenal medulla. Paraganglioma is a term used to describe extra-adrenal tumors that arise from nonadrenal chromaffin tissue. Although some pheochromocytomas do not secrete catecholamines, most synthesize catecholamines at increased rates that may be up to 27 times the synthetic rate of the normal adrenal medulla (Figure 11–9). This persistent hypersecretion of catecholamines by most pheochromocytomas is probably due to lack of feedback inhibition on tyrosine hydroxylase. Catecholamines are then produced in quantities that greatly exceed the vesicular storage capacity and accumulate in the cytoplasm. Catecholamines that are in the cytoplasm are subject to intracellular metabolism; the excess catecholamines and their metabolites diffuse out of the pheochromocytoma cell into the circulation.

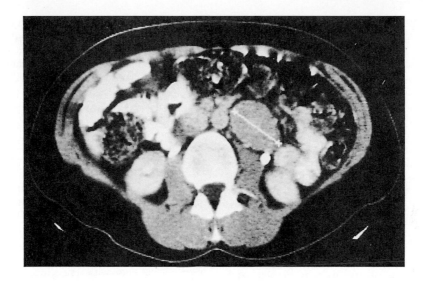

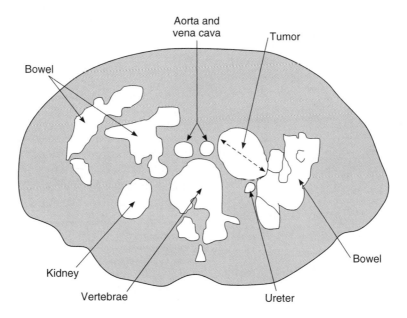

Figure 11–9. Left infrarenal paraganglioma shown by CT scanning. The lower diagram identifies many of the visible structures.

In contrast to the normal adrenal medulla, pheochromocytoma cells ordinarily contain more norepinephrine than epinephrine. In adults, approximately 90% of tumors arise from the adrenal medulla. Pheochromocytomas that secrete epinephrine are particularly likely to be found in the adrenal medulla. Extra-adrenal paragangliomas rarely secrete epinephrine—this is due to their lack of immediate proximity to the adrenal cortex, which ordinarily provides the high concentrations of cortisol needed for induction of the enzyme PNMT, which catalyzes the conversion of norepinephrine to epinephrine.

Surprisingly, the serum levels of catecholamine do not correlate well with tumor size. This appears to be due to the rapid production and secretion of catecholamines by small tumors and the slower secretion of catecholamines by larger tumors. Furthermore, much of the size of larger tumors is due to hemorrhagic necrosis and cystic formation.

Severe hypertensive episodes occur in most patients with pheochromocytomas. Exocytosis of catecholamines from the pheochromocytoma can play a role in such paroxysms, but most pheochromocytomas have minor sympathetic innervation. Instead, hypertensive crises are often caused by spontaneous hemorrhages within the tumor or by pressure on the tumor causing the release of blood from venous sinusoids that are rich in catecholamines. Thus, catecholamines can be released by physical stimuli such as bending or twisting or by micturition in patients with bladder paragangliomas. Of course, surgical manipulation of such tumors releases catecholamines and can cause life-threatening hypertensive crises.

Chronically high circulating levels of catecholamines may cause normal sympathetic axons to become saturated with catecholamines due to active catecholamine neuronal uptake. This may account for the paroxysms of hypertension that are triggered by pain, emotional upset, intubation, anesthesia, or surgical skin incisions. Adrenergic catecholamine saturation may also explain the elevations in serum and urine catecholamines that can occur for 10 days or longer after a successful surgical resection of a pheochromocytoma.

Many pheochromocytomas secrete significant amounts of neuropeptide Y (NPY). NPY is a 36-amino-acid peptide that is a very potent nonadrenergic vasoconstrictor and vascular growth factor.

Tyr-Pro-Ser-Lys-Pro-Asp-Asn-Pro-Gly-Glu-Asp-Ala-
Pro-Ala-Glu-Asp-Met-Ala-Arg-Tyr-Tyr-Ser-Ala-Leu-
Arg-His-Tyr-Ile-Asn-Leu-Ile-Thr-Arg-Gln-Arg-Tyr-NH$_2$

Neuropeptide Y

NPY is found in adrenergic neurosecretory granules and is secreted along with norepinephrine. Patients with essential hypertension have not been found to have elevated levels of NPY. However, in a series of eight patients with pheochromocytomas, NPY levels were elevated twofold to 465-fold above the normal reference range. In another series, 59% of adrenal pheochromocytomas were found to secrete NPY during surgical resection; high serum levels of NPY were observed to correlate with measures of vascular resistance, independent of norepinephrine. NPY appears to contribute to hypertension in most patients with pheochromocytoma. In contrast, few paragangliomas secrete NPY.

Neuron-specific enolase (NSE) is a neuroendocrine glycolytic enzyme. Serum levels of NSE have been reported to be normal in patients with benign pheochromocytoma but are elevated in about half of patients with malignant pheochromocytomas. Therefore, an elevated serum level of NSE indicates that a given pheochromocytoma is likely to be malignant.

Secretion of Other Peptides (Table 11–10)

Although pheochromocytomas secrete mainly catecholamines and their metabolites, they also secrete many other peptide hormones, many of which contribute to a patient's clinical symptoms. Secretion of parathyroid hormone-related peptide (PTHrP) can cause hypercalcemia. Ectopic ACTH production can cause Cushing's syndrome. Secretion of neuropeptide Y contributes to hypertension. Erythropoietin secretion can cause erythrocytosis. Leukocytosis is frequently seen in patients with pheochromocytoma, probably caused by cytokine release from the tumor. IL-6 secretion can cause fevers. Most pheochromocytomas secrete chromogranin A, and serum chromogranin A levels may be assayed as a tumor marker for pheochromocytoma. Pheochromocytomas may also secrete other peptides that are included in Table 11–10.

Table 11–10. Peptides that may be secreted by pheochromocytomas. Pheochromocytomas are variable in their secretion of different peptides. Not all peptides have been documented to produce clinical manifestations. See text.

Catecholamines	Galanin
Epinephrine	Gonadotropin-releasing hormone
Norepinephrine	(GnRH)
Metanephrines	Growth hormone (GH)
Metanephrine	Interleukin-6 (IL-6)
Normetanephrine	Motilin
Dopamine	Neuron-specific enolase
Adrenocorticotropic	Neuropeptide Y (NPY)
hormone (ACTH)	Neurotensin
Adrenomedullin	Parathyroid hormone-related
Atrial natriuretic factor	peptide (PTHrP)
Beta-endorphin	Peptide histidine-isoleucine
Calbindin	Renin
Calcitonin	Serotonin
Cholecystokinin	Somatostatin
Chromogranin A (CgA)	Substance P
Cytokines	Vasoactive intestinal polypeptide
Enkephalins	(VIP)
Erythropoietin	

Manifestations of Pheochromocytoma

A. SYMPTOMS OF PHEOCHROMOCYTOMA

Over one-third of pheochromocytomas cause death prior to diagnosis, death being caused by a fatal cardiac arrhythmia or stroke. Adult patients with a pheochromocytoma usually have paroxysmal symptoms, which may last minutes or hours; symptoms usually begin abruptly and subside slowly. Symptoms typically include episodes of headaches (80%), diaphoresis (70%), and palpitations (60%). Other symptoms may include anxiety (50%), a sense of dread, tremor (40%, particularly with epinephrine-secreting tumors), or paresthesias. Recurrent chest discomfort is a frequent complaint. Many patients experience visual changes during acute attacks (Tables 11–8 and 1–9).

Sweating (initially palms, axillae, head, and shoulders) usually occurs. Drenching sweats can occur, usually as a paroxysm subsides. Reflex thermoregulatory eccrine sweating occurs later in an attack, dissipating the heat that was acquired during the prolonged vasoconstriction that occurred during the paroxysm.

Gastrointestinal symptoms predominate in certain patients. Abdominal pain and vomiting are frequent symptoms. The abdominal pain may be due to ischemic enterocolitis. Pain may also be caused by the growth of a large intra-abdominal tumor. Constipation is common, and toxic megacolon may rarely occur.

These episodic paroxysms may not recur for months or may recur many times daily. Each patient tends to have a different pattern of symptoms, with the frequency or severity of episodes usually increasing over time. Attacks can occur spontaneously or may occur with bladder catheterization, anesthesia, and surgery. Some patients' attacks have been precipitated by nasal decongestants. Paroxysms can be induced by seemingly benign activities such as bending, rolling over in bed, exertion, abdominal palpation, or micturition (with bladder paragangliomas). There is an amazing interindividual variability in the manifestations of pheochromocytomas. Most patients have dramatic symptoms, but other patients with incidentally discovered secretory pheochromocytomas are completely asymptomatic. Patients who develop pheochromocytomas as part of MEN 2 or von Hippel-Lindau disease are especially prone to be normotensive and asymptomatic.

Children with pheochromocytomas or paragangliomas tend to present with a symptom complex that is different from that of adults. Children are more prone to diaphoresis, visual changes, and sustained (rather than episodic) hypertension. Children are more likely to have paroxysms of nausea, vomiting, and headache. They are also prone to weight loss, polydip-sia, polyuria, and convulsions. Edema and erythema of the hands occur quite frequently and are rather unique to children with pheochromocytoma. Children are more likely to have multiple tumors and paragangliomas. In one series, 39% of affected children had bilateral adrenal pheochromocytomas, an adrenal pheochromocytoma plus a paraganglioma, or multiple paragangliomas; a single paraganglioma occurred in an additional 14% of children.

B. SIGNS OF PHEOCHROMOCYTOMA

In adults, hypertension is considered to be present with blood pressures > 140 mm Hg systolic or > 90 mm Hg diastolic. In children, blood pressures increase with age, such that maximal normal ranges are age-dependent; blood pressures at the 95th percentile for age are as follows: < 6 months, 110/60 mm Hg; 3 years, 112/80 mm Hg; 5 years, 115/84 mm Hg; 10 years, 130/92 mm Hg; and 15 years, 138/95 mm Hg.

Hypertension is present in 90% of patients in whom a pheochromocytoma is diagnosed. Blood pressure patterns vary among patients with pheochromocytomas. Adults most commonly have sustained but variable hypertension, with severe hypertension during symptomatic episodes. Paroxysms of severe hypertension occur in about 50% of adults and in about 8% of children with pheochromocytoma. Other patients may be completely normotensive, may be normotensive between paroxysms, or may have stable sustained hypertension.

Hypertension can be mild or severe and resistant to treatment. Severe hypertension may be noted during induction of anesthesia for unrelated surgeries. Although hypertension usually accompanies paroxysmal symptoms and may be elicited by the above activities, this is not always the case.

Patients with sustained hypertension usually exhibit orthostatic changes in blood pressure. Blood pressure may drop, even to hypotensive levels, after the patient arises from a supine position and stands for 3 minutes; such orthostasis, especially when accompanied by a rise in heart rate, is typical of pheochromocytoma. Epinephrine secretion from a pheochromocytoma may cause episodic hypotension and even syncope. Therefore, the determination of orthostatic blood pressure and pulse rate should be a standard component in the evaluation and follow-up of patients with pheochromocytoma. Orthostasis is due to vasomotor adrenergic receptor desensitization; patients may have a diminished intravascular volume.

Left ventricular hypertrophy develops commonly in hypertensive patients with pheochromocytoma. High levels of catecholamines can also cause myocarditis and a dilated cardiomyopathy; full recovery from cardiomyopathy may occur after surgical resection of a pheochromocytoma. In some patients, myocardial scarring and fibrosis lead to irreversible cardiomyopathy and heart failure. Sudden arrhythmias often occur and may be fatal.

Palpitations are a frequent complaint, and cardiac arrhythmias are common. Sinus tachycardia is common, particularly in patients with epinephrine-secreting pheochromocytomas. The heart rate will often increase when standing. There can be an initial tachycardia during a paroxysm, followed by a reflex bradycardia. As a result of severe peripheral vasoconstriction, the radial pulse can become thready or even nonpalpable during a hypertensive crisis. Vasoconstriction is also responsible for the pallor and mottled cyanosis that can occur with paroxysms of hypertension. Reflex vasodilation usually follows an attack and can cause facial flushing. After an especially intense and prolonged attack of hypertension, shock may ultimately occur. This may be due to loss of vascular tone, low plasma volume, arrhythmias, or cardiac damage.

During pregnancy, a maternal pheochromocytoma can cause sustained hypertension or paroxysmal hypertension that is typically mistaken for eclampsia. Women may suffer from peripartum shock or postpartum fever that can mimic rupture or infection of the uterus.

Most patients lose some weight. More severe weight loss (> 10% of basal weight) occurs in about 15% of patients overall and in 41% of those with sustained and prolonged hypertension. Fevers are quite common and may be mild or severe, even as high as 41 °C; up to 70% of patients have unexplained low-grade elevations in temperature of 0.5 °C or more. Such fevers have been attributed to the secretion of IL-6. Distention of the neck veins is common during an attack, and the thyroid may increase in size transiently. Large pheochromocytomas or their metastases may be palpable. Some may grow so large that they impinge on the renal artery, causing renovascular hypertension. Other complications include cerebrovascular accident, malignant nephrosclerosis, and hypertensive retinopathy. Rarely, pheochromocytomas can secrete ACTH in amounts sufficient to stimulate the excessive production of cortisol, with resultant Cushing's syndrome.

About 15% of pheochromocytomas are malignant. Metastases are usually functional and can cause recurrent hypertension and symptoms many months or years after an operation that had been thought to be curative. Metastases can cause a variety of problems. Metastases to the skull are common and are frequently palpable. Therefore, the cranium should be palpated carefully in all patients with pheochromocytomas, particularly when metastases are suspected. Skull metastases can protrude from the cranium as soft masses with a consistency similar to that of sebaceous cysts. Metastases also have a predilection for the ribs, causing chest pain. Metastases to the spine cause back pain or neurologic

symptoms due to impingement on the spinal cord or nerve roots. Paragangliomas often arise adjacent to vertebrae and can directly invade them. Pulmonary and mediastinal metastases can cause dyspnea, hemoptysis, pleural effusion, or Horner's syndrome. Metastases involving the thoracic duct can cause chylothorax. Pheochromocytomas may recur within the abdomen as metastases in mesenteric nodes or as masses arising from peritoneal seeding originating from the original tumor. Metastases to the liver can cause hepatomegaly.

C. NORMOTENSION DESPITE HIGH PLASMA LEVELS OF NOREPINEPHRINE

Interestingly, many patients with pheochromocytomas and paragangliomas have no hypertension despite having chronically elevated serum levels of norepinephrine. This phenomenon has been variably called desensitization, tolerance, or tachyphylaxis.

Patients can be genetically prone to adrenergic desensitization. Some patients are homozygous for certain polymorphisms of β_2-adrenergic receptors that allow continued β_2-adrenergic-mediated vasodilation, thus counteracting the pressor effects of circulating epinephrine and norepinephrine caused by stimulation of vascular α_1-adrenergic receptors.

Adrenergic desensitization can also be caused by adrenergic receptors undergoing sequestration, downregulation, or phosphorylation. Desensitization does not account for all patients who are normotensive in the face of elevated serum levels of norepinephrine; some such patients can still have hypertensive responses to norepinephrine. Cosecretion of dopa may reduce blood pressure through a central nervous system action. Similarly, cosecretion of dopamine may directly dilate mesenteric and renal vessels and thus modulate the effects of norepinephrine. Adrenergic desensitization also appears to be one cause of the cardiovascular collapse that can occur abruptly following the removal of a pheochromocytoma in some patients.

Biochemical Testing

A. CATECHOLAMINES AND METANEPHRINES

The best methodology for assaying catecholamine and metanephrine levels (urine or plasma) has become high-pressure liquid chromatography (HPLC) with electrochemical detection (ECD). This methodology has proved superior to other assays because of its specificity and ease of use. However, misleadingly elevated levels of at least one catecholamine or metanephrine determination occur in up to 10% of patients with essential hypertension. These elevations are typically < 50% above the maximum normal and are usually normal upon retesting while avoiding medications, foods, and stresses that might cause misleadingly high catecholamine determinations. Patients with pheochromocytomas typically have elevations of catecholamines or metanephrines that are more than twice normal, particularly after a paroxysm.

Urine fractionated catecholamines and fractionated metanephrines are listed in Table 11–11. A single 24-hour urine specimen is collected for the above determinations, plus creatinine. The container is acidified with 10–25 mL of 6-N HCl for preservation of the catecholamines; the acid does not interfere with metanephrine and creatinine assays. The acid preservative may be omitted for children for safety reasons, in which case the specimen should be kept cold and processed immediately. The laboratory requisition form should request (1) assays for fractionated catecholamines, fractionated metanephrines, and creatinine performed on the same specimen; and (2) assay by an endocrine reference laboratory using high-pressure liquid chromatography (HPLC) followed by electrochemical detection.

A single-void urine specimen may be collected on first morning void or following a paroxysm. No acid preservative is used on single-void specimens, since it dilutes the specimen and is not required. For single-void collections, patients are instructed to void and discard the urine immediately at the onset of a paroxysm and then collect the next voided urine. The laboratory requisition should request "spot urine for total metanephrine (by HPLC and electrochemical detection) and creatinine concentrations." It is prudent to contact the laboratory technician and explain that the specimen is meant to be a single-void urine and not a 24-hour specimen or else the specimen may be rejected. Patients with pheochromocytomas generally excrete over 2.2 µg metanephrine/mg creatinine.

Urinary dopamine determination is not a sensitive test for pheochromocytomas. However, in patients with established pheochromocytomas, a normal urine dopamine is fairly predictive of benignity, whereas elevated urine dopamine excretion is seen in both benign and malignant pheochromocytomas.

Plasma catecholamine or metanephrine levels are not usually required. However, since catecholamines are metabolized within tumor cells, plasma levels of free metanephrines and normetanephrines are exceptionally sensitive and can be used as screening tests for pheochromocytoma, particularly when screening for pheochromocytoma in patients with established MEN 2 or von Hippel-Lindau disease. Plasma metanephrine is elevated in most patients with MEN 2, whereas plasma normetanephrine is usually elevated in patients with von Hippel-Lindau disease. Normal ranges for plasma metanephrines in children are different from those of adults and have been reported by Weise et al (see references). Plasma concentrations of norepinephrine do not correlate with blood pressure. Stimulation or suppression tests are not recommended.

There is no single test that is absolutely sensitive and specific for pheochromocytoma. Urinary metanephrines have a sensitivity of about 97%. Sensitivities of other tests are somewhat lower: urinary norepinephrine 93%, plasma norepinephrine 92%, urinary vanillylmandelic acid (VMA) 90%, plasma epinephrine 67%, urinary epinephrine 64%, plasma dopamine 63%.

B. Serum Chromogranin A

Chromogranin A may be determined by immunoradiometric (IRMA) assays. Chromogranins are acidic glycoproteins that are found in neurosecretory granules. They have been categorized into three classes: chromogranins A (CgA), B (secretogranin I), and C (secretogranin II).

Table 11–11. Maximal normal concentrations of the catecholamines and their metabolism in urine.[1] Substances interfering with their measurement are listed.

Compound	Excreted	Interfering Substances (See Table 11–12)
Epinephrine Norepinephrine Dopamine	24 µg/24 h (131 nmol/24 h) 100 µg/24 h (591 nmol/24 h) 480 µg/24 h (3139 nmol/24 h)	May be increased by highly fluorescent compounds such as tetracyclines and quinidine; by foods (eg, bananas contain significant amounts of norepinephrine) and drugs containing catecholamines; and by levodopa, methyldopa, and ethanol.
Metanephrine Normetanephrine	230 µg/24 h (1166 nmol/24 h) 540 µg/24 h (2738 nmol/24 h)	Increased by catecholamines, monoamine oxidase inhibitors, and other agents, depending on the method.
Vanillylmandelic acid Homovanillic acid	7 mg/24 h (35 µmol/24 h) 8.8 mg/24 h (48 µmol/24 h)	Increased by catecholamines, by foods containing vanillin, or by levodopa. Decreased by clofibrate, disulfiram, and monoamine oxidase inhibitors.

[1]Values may be higher under conditions of unusual stress, illness, or strenuous activity.

The serum CgA assay has become useful for the diagnosis of pheochromocytoma. However, CgA undergoes extensive tumor-specific cleavages so that only certain serum assays are useful for clinical diagnosis.

Serum CgA levels have a circadian rhythm in normal individuals, with lowest levels found at 8 AM and higher levels in the afternoon and at 11 PM. CgA levels are not elevated in essential hypertension. CgA is also secreted from extra-adrenal sympathetic nerves. Median morning CgA measurements have been reported to be 43 ng/mL in normals and 34 ng/mL in patients who have bilateral adrenalectomies.

Serum CgA levels are elevated in the great majority of patients with pheochromocytomas. The serum levels of CgA correlate with tumor mass, making CgA a useful tumor marker. However, smaller tumors may not be diagnosed. Serum CgA levels tend to be particularly elevated in patients with malignant pheochromocytoma. In one series, average serum CgA levels were 48 ng/mL in normals, 188 ng/mL in benign pheochromocytoma, and 2932 ng/mL in malignant pheochromocytoma.

Serum CgA can be elevated even in patients with "biochemically silent" tumors. In patients with normal renal function, serum CgA has a sensitivity of 83–90% and a specificity of 96% for diagnosis of these tumors. However, the usefulness of serum CgA levels is negated by any degree of renal failure because of its excretion by the kidneys; even mild azotemia causes serum levels to be elevated. However, in patients with normal renal function, a high serum level of CgA along with high urine or plasma catecholamines or metanephrines is virtually diagnostic of pheochromocytoma.

C. OTHER LABORATORY TESTS

Measurements of urinary vanillylmandelic acid (VMA) or dopamine have not increased the sensitivity or specificity of pheochromocytoma diagnosis. However, some centers have traditionally used a combination of urinary VMA and metanephrine determinations with good results. Clonidine suppression testing of plasma catecholamines is unnecessary and cumbersome. Glucagon stimulation testing is dangerous and no longer useful. Serum renin levels are not typically suppressed in patients with pheochromocytomas, since catecholamines stimulate renin release and some tumors may secrete renin ectopically.

Patients with pheochromocytoma are frequently found to have an increased white blood count with a high absolute neutrophil count. Counts as high as 23,600/μL have been reported. Hyperglycemia is noted in about 35% of patients with pheochromocytoma, but frank diabetes mellitus is uncommon. The erythrocyte sedimentation rate (ESR) is elevated in some patients. Hypercalcemia is common and may be caused by bone metastases or tumoral secretion of PTHrP. Erythrocytosis sometimes occurs, caused by ectopic secretion of erythropoietin.

Factors That May Cause Misleading Biochemical Testing for Pheochromocytoma

Several different methods may be employed for assay of urine and plasma catecholamines and metanephrines. Each assay uses different methods and internal standards. Most assays now employ high-pressure liquid chromatography (HPLC) with electrochemical detection (ECD). Such assays can be affected by interference from a diverse range of drugs and foods. These substances cause unusual shapes of the peaks on the HPL chromatogram. Not all of these assays are the same, and the potential for interference will depend upon the particular method employed. Therefore, it is best to check with the reference laboratory that runs the test or provides the test kit.

A. DRUGS (SEE TABLE 11–12)

Certain radiopaque contrast media can falsely lower urinary metanephrine determinations in some assays for up to 12 hours following administration. Such agents are those that contain meglumine acetrizoate or meglumine diatrizoate (eg, Renografin, Hypaque-M, Renovist, Cardiografin, Urografin, and Conray). However, diatrizoate sodium is an intravenous contrast agent that does not cause such interference and should be requested if a CT scan must be performed prior to testing for metanephrines. Many other drugs cause interference in the older fluorometric assays for VMA and metanephrines.

B. FOODS

Even using newer HPLC-ECD assay techniques, certain foods can cause misleading results in assays for catecholamines and metanephrines (Table 11–12). Coffee (even if decaffeinated) contains substances that can be converted into a catechol metabolite (dihydrocaffeic acid) that may cause confusing peaks on an HPL chromatogram. Caffeine inhibits the action of adenosine; one action of adenosine is to inhibit the release of catecholamines. Heavy caffeine consumption causes a persistent elevation in norepinephrine production and raises blood pressure an average of 4 mm Hg systolic. Bananas contain considerable amounts of tyrosine, which can be converted to dopamine by the central nervous system; dopamine is then converted to epinephrine and norepinephrine. Dietary peppers contain 3-methoxy-4-hydroxybenzylamine (MHBA), a compound that can interfere with the internal standard used in some assays for metanephrines.

Table 11–12. Factors potentially causing misleading catecholamine or metanephrine results: high pressure liquid chromatography with electrochemical detection (HPLC-ECD).*

Drugs	Foods	Conditions
Acetaminophen[3]	Bananas[1]	Amyotrophic lateral sclerosis[1]
Aldomet[3]	Caffeine[1]	Brain lesions[1]
Amphetamines[1]	Coffee[3]	Carcinoid[1]
Bronchodilators[1]	Peppers[3]	Eclampsia[1]
Buspirone[3]		Emotion (severe)[1]
Captopril[3]		Exercise (vigorous)[1]
Cocaine[1]		Guillain-Barré syndrome[1]
Contrast media		Hypoglycemia[1]
(meglumine		Lead poisoning[1]
acetrizoate,		Myocardial infarction (acute)[1]
meglumine		Pain (severe)[1]
diatrizoate)[4]		Porphyria (acute)[1]
Cimetidine[3]		Psychosis (acute)[1]
Codeine[3]		Quadriplegia[1]
Decongestants[1]		Renal failure[2]
Ephedrine[1]		
Fenfluramine[2]		
Isoproterenol[1]		
Levodopa[3]		
Labetalol[1,3]		
Mandelamine[3]		
Metoclopramide[3]		
Nitroglycerin[1]		
Viloxazine[3]		

*Reproduced, with permission, from Tierney LM Jr., McPhee SJ, Papadakis MA (editors). *Current Medical Diagnosis & Treatment 2003*. McGraw Hill, 2003.
[1]Increases catecholamine excretion.
[2]Decreases catecholamine excretion
[3]May cause confounding peaks on HPLC chromatograms.
[4]May decrease urine metanephrine excretion.

C. DISEASES

Any severe stress can elicit increased production of catecholamines and metanephrines. Diseases causing reduced catecholamine production (Table 11–12) include malnutrition and quadriplegia. Urinary excretion of catecholamines and metanephrines is reduced in renal failure.

Differential Diagnosis of Pheochromocytoma (Table 11–13)

Pheochromocytomas have such protean manifestations that many conditions enter into the differential diagnosis. **Essential hypertension** is extremely common, and

Table 11–13. Differential diagnosis of pheochromocytoma.

Acute intermittent porphyria
Autonomic epilepsy
Cardiac arrhythmias
Clonidine withdrawal
Coronary vasospasm
Encephalitis
Erythromelalgia
Essential hypertension
Hypertensive crisis associated with–
    Cerebrovascular accidents
    Surgery
    Acute pulmonary edema
    Severe pain
    Hypertensive crisis of MAO inhibitors
Hypoglycemia
Hypogonadal hot flushes
Lead poisoning
Mastocytosis
Migraine and cluster headache
Renal artery stenosis
Sympathomimetic drug ingestion
Tabetic crisis
Thyrotoxicosis
Toxemia (eclampsia) of pregnancy

it is not practical to screen for pheochromocytoma in all patients with elevated blood pressure. However, pheochromocytoma should enter the differential diagnosis for any hypertensive patient having blood pressures above 180 mm Hg systolic and for any hypertensive patient who has one of the following symptoms: headaches, palpitations, sweating episodes, or unexplained bouts of abdominal or chest pains.

Anxiety (panic) attacks begin abruptly and can be associated with tachycardia, tachypnea, and chest discomfort, symptoms that are commonly seen with pheochromocytomas. However, patients with panic attacks are more likely to have a precipitating social situation, tend to be exhausted for more than 2 hours following an attack, live in dread of the next attack, and often change their activities to avoid situations that might trigger anxiety.

Renal artery stenosis and **renal parenchymal disease** can cause increased secretion of renin resulting in severe hypertension. However, a detectable serum renin level does not exclude pheochromocytoma, since catecholamines can stimulate renin secretion and pheochromocytomas can secrete renin ectopically. Furthermore, large pheochromocytomas and paragangliomas arising near the renal hilum can occlude the renal artery, causing concomitant renovascular hypertension.

Hypogonadism can cause vasomotor instability in both women and men; attacks of flushing, sweating, and palpitations can mimic symptoms seen with pheochromocytoma. **Factitious symptoms** may be caused by surreptitious self-administration of various drugs. **Hyperthyroidism** can cause heat intolerance, sweating, palpitations, and systolic hypertension with a widened pulse pressure. **Carcinoid syndrome** causes flushing during attacks but usually without pallor, hypertension, palpitations, or diaphoresis.

The differential diagnosis also includes intracranial lesions, preeclampsia-eclampsia, clonidine withdrawal, hypertensive crisis due to MAO inhibitors, cardiac arrhythmias, unstable angina, hypoglycemia, vascular or cluster headaches, autonomic epilepsy, mastocytosis, acute intermittent porphyria, lead poisoning, encephalitis, and tabetic crisis.

Patients with **erythromelalgia** can have episodic hypertension, but it is associated with flushing of the face and legs during the attack; patients with pheochromocytoma have facial pallor during attacks. With erythromelalgia, patients have painful erythema and swelling in the legs that is relieved by application of ice; such symptoms are not characteristic of pheochromocytoma.

Patients who have **intermittent bizarre symptoms** may have their blood pressure and pulse checked during a symptomatic episode with a home blood pressure meter or an ambulatory blood pressure monitor. Those who are normotensive during an attack are not likely to have a pheochromocytoma.

Pheochromocytomas often present with abdominal pain and vomiting. Such symptoms are similar to those of an **intra-abdominal emergency,** particularly in the presence of leukocytosis and fever, which can also be seen with pheochromocytomas. Abdominal pain usually prompts a CT scan of the abdomen, which will generally show the pheochromocytoma or paraganglioma. Even after detection on CT scan, pheochromocytomas and juxtarenal paragangliomas may be mistaken for **renal carcinoma.** Large left-sided pheochromocytomas are often mistaken for **carcinoma of the tail of the pancreas.**

Neuroblastomas are poorly differentiated malignancies and are the most common solid tumor of childhood. Neuroblastomas may develop in the adrenal gland or in sympathetic nerve ganglia near the cervical or thoracic vertebrae or in the pelvis. They metastasize to bones, lymph nodes, liver, and skin. Cutaneous metastases may present as widespread bluish nodules such that these young patients have been called "blueberry muffin children." When such nodules are rubbed they tend to blanch, with a ring of surrounding erythema. Neuroblastomas usually present with pain and are often visualized on MRI as "dumbbell lesions" in

the neural foramina. About 85% of affected children secrete excessive catecholamines—but rarely in sufficient amounts to cause symptomatic hypotension or the paroxysms typical of pheochromocytomas. Neuroblastomas concentrate ^{123}I-MIBG but can be distinguished from paragangliomas by clinical and histological criteria.

Localization Studies for Pheochromocytoma

A. METAIODOBENZYLGUANIDINE (MIBG) SCANNING

Benzylguanidine is a derivative of guanethidine; it is a false neurotransmitter that was initially developed as therapy for hypertension. It was ineffective as an antihypertensive drug but was found to selectively accumulate in cells that store catecholamines in proportion to the concentration of neurosecretory granules. Scintigraphy using ^{123}I-MIBG or ^{131}I-MIBG is useful for determining whether an adrenal mass is a pheochromocytoma, for imaging occult paragangliomas, and for confirming whether a certain extra-adrenal mass is a paraganglioma or neuroblastoma. MIBG scanning is useful also for screening patients for metastases. Interestingly, MIBG uptake does occur in apparently nonfunctioning pheochromocytomas.

The isotope that is preferable for precise imaging is ^{123}I-MIBG, since ^{123}I has a more useful photon flux and lower-energy gamma emissions than ^{131}I, allowing for clearer images and single photon emission computed tomography (SPECT). Additional advantages of ^{123}I include its shorter half-life and reduced heavy particle emissions, resulting in less overall radiation exposure to the patient. ^{123}I-MIBG SPECT scanning is more sensitive than ^{123}I-MIBG planar imaging for detecting small metastases and has the advantage of being able to do the scanning on the day following injection of the isotope. However, most centers use ^{131}I-MIBG, since it has a longer half-life than ^{123}I-MIBG and is commercially available. SPECT scanning with radiolabeled MIBG can be combined with simultaneous CT imaging on the same ("Hawkeye") scanner; the resultant combined images can help distinguish whether a given mass has taken up MIBG.

The overall sensitivity of ^{123}I-MIBG for pheochromocytomas is about 85%; it is more sensitive for pheochromocytomas that are benign, unilateral, adrenal, capsule-invasive, and sporadic. Scanning with ^{123}I-MIBG is less sensitive for bilateral, malignant, extra-adrenal, noninvasive, and MEN 2a or 2b-related or von Hippel-Lindau disease-related pheochromocytomas.

To block the thyroid's uptake of free radioiodine, saturated solution of potassium iodide, 5 drops orally three times daily, is given before the injection and daily for several days afterward. The ^{123}I-MIBG is given intravenously, and scanning may be performed between 1 and 3 days thereafter.

1. False-negative MIBG scans are seen in about 15% of cases of either benign or malignant pheochromocytoma. False-negative scans can occur in patients who have taken certain drugs—eg, tricyclic antidepressants or cyclobenzaprine—within 6 weeks. Other drugs that can cause false-negative scans when taken within 2 weeks include amphetamines, phenylpropanolamine, haloperidol, phenothiazines, thiothixene, reserpine, nasal decongestants, cocaine, and diet pills. Labetalol reduces MIBG uptake, but the scan can still be done, albeit with suboptimal sensitivity (Table 11–14).

2. False-positive MIBG scans occur infrequently. Uptake in the normal adrenal medulla and renal pelvis and bladder is commonly seen on day 1 and must be - distinguished from tumor uptake. The salivary glands are typically visualized since they are richly innervated. The heart and liver normally take up some ^{123}I-MIBG. Urine contamination with ^{123}I-MIBG can also cause a false-positive scan. Some isotope is excreted in the stool, and intracolonic collections can be mistaken for tumor. When there is doubt about whether an area of uptake is a tumor, scanning can be repeated on days 2 and 3, preceded by a laxative if required.

B. COMPUTED TOMOGRAPHY (FIGURES 11–9, 11–10)

After a pheochromocytoma has been diagnosed by clinical and biochemical criteria, hypertension must first be controlled (see below), since intravenous contrast can precipitate a hypertensive crisis. The pheochromocytoma must then be localized. The first step in locating a pheochromocytoma is to perform a CT scan of the entire abdomen from the diaphragm through the pelvis; thin-section cuts should be obtained through the adrenals.

If urine samples for metanephrines are to be collected within 72 hours following the CT scan, it is important that diatrizoate sodium and not meglumine diatrizoate or acetate be used as the iodinated contrast agent since the former does not interfere with the

Table 11–14. Factors inhibiting MIBG uptake by pheochromocytomas.

Inhibitors of type I catecholamine uptake: cocaine, tricyclic drugs, labetalol (2–6 weeks)
Stimulants of catecholamine discharge: reserpine (2 weeks)
Displacement of catecholamines from intracellular stores and competition with uptake of MIBG: all amphetamines; nasal decongestants, oral or nasal (2 weeks)
Others: Phenothiazines, haloperidol, thiothixene (2 weeks)

metanephrine assay. Glucagon should not be used during a CT scan to locate a pheochromocytoma since it may provoke a hypertensive crisis.

If no mass is discovered, a ^{123}I-MIBG scan may be obtained or the CT scan may be extended into the chest and thoracic spine in search of a paraganglioma—or both procedures may be employed. The great majority of pheochromocytomas are over 2 cm in diameter, well within the resolution capacity of the CT scan. The overall sensitivity of CT scanning for an adrenal pheochromocytoma is about 90%—and over 95% for pheochromocytomas that are over 0.5 cm in diameter. However, CT scanning is less sensitive for the detection of small adrenal pheochromocytomas or adrenal medullary hyperplasia; this becomes an important issue in patients with MEN 2 or von Hippel-Lindau disease. CT is also less sensitive for detecting extra-adrenal paragangliomas, small metastases, and early recurrent tumors in the adrenal surgical bed.

C. MAGNETIC RESONANCE IMAGING (MRI)

MRI does not require intravenous iodinated contrast, thereby minimizing the risk of hypertensive crisis. MRI is the scanning technique of choice during pregnancy because it avoids radiation to the fetus. It can help determine whether an adrenal mass is a pheochromocytoma when biochemical studies are inconclusive. The T2-weighted signal is hyperintense relative to the liver in about 75% of cases. However, some adrenal adenomas may have the same appearance, so the MRI scan lacks true specificity. MRI of the abdomen has a sensitivity of about 95% for adrenal pheochromocytomas over 0.5 cm in diameter. Like CT scanning, MRI is less sensitive for the detection of extra-adrenal paragangliomas, metastatic disease, and recurrent small tumors in the adrenal surgical bed. MRI can visualize and confirm metastases to bone suspected on ^{123}I-MIBG imaging.

D. POSITRON EMISSION TOMOGRAPHY (PET)

PET employs certain isotopes that emit positrons during their decay. Positrons are antimatter, so positron-electron collisions occur immediately and produce energy, emitting gamma photons traveling in precisely opposite directions (180 degrees out of phase). In the PET scanner, sensitive gamma detectors surround the patient; simultaneous activation of two gamma detectors indicates that the source is located directly between them. Multiple such detections of this nature allow three-dimensional CT of tumors, which can accurately determine their location and volume. Deoxyglucose is taken up by tissues with active metabolism, including tumors; for PET scanning, it may be tagged with [82]Rb or [18]F (fluorodeoxyglucose, FDG). [^{18}F]FDG PET scanning can be useful for localizing metastases from a

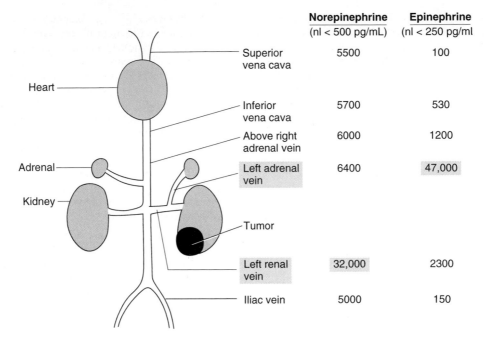

	Norepinephrine (nl < 500 pg/mL)	Epinephrine (nl < 250 pg/ml
Superior vena cava	5500	100
Inferior vena cava	5700	530
Above right adrenal vein	6000	1200
Left adrenal vein	6400	47,000
Tumor		
Left renal vein	32,000	2300
Iliac vein	5000	150

Figure 11–10. Plasma norepinephrine and epinephrine levels in samples of blood from venous sampling. Note that the level of epinephrine is very high in the left adrenal vein sample, distinguishing it from the drainage of the tumor, which secretes mainly norepinephrine into the left renal vein. Note the relatively normal peripheral levels of epinephrine (as seen in the iliac vein or the superior vena cava). Such sampling is rarely required.

malignant pheochromocytoma. However, [18F]FDG PET scanning detects other tumors besides pheochromocytoma; it localizes in other tissues having a high metabolic rate, including areas of inflammation, shivering muscles, or other tumors; and it is thus less specific for pheochromocytoma than is 123I-MIBG scanning.

PET scanning may also be performed using 6-[18F] fluorodopamine, a technique currently undergoing clinical investigation. It is more specific for paraganglioma and metastatic pheochromocytoma than is [18F]FDG, since dopamine is a substrate for the norepinephrine transporter in tumor tissue.

PET scanning can be done almost immediately, which gives it some advantage over MIBG scanning, which must be delayed for 24–48 hours after the injection to allow dissipation of background radiation. PET -scanning does not require pretreatment with iodine to protect the thyroid, as is necessary with MIBG scanning. However, PET scanning is very expensive and has not been directly compared with 123I-MIBG or 131I-MIBG scanning for sensitivity and specificity. The isotope 18F has a half-life of just 2 hours and must be produced in a cyclotron, so [18F]FDG scanning is practical only at medical centers having a cyclotron nearby.

E. Somatostatin Receptor Imaging (SRI)

Scanning with 111In-labeled octreotide (SRI) has a sensitivity of only 25% for adrenal pheochromocytomas. However, SRI detects 87% of pheochromocytoma metastases and is also a sensitive technique for detecting paragangliomas of the head and neck (chemodectomas). SRI also detects some metastases not visible on MIBG scanning, and vice versa. SRI has been reported to detect a cardiac paraganglioma that was not visible on MIBG scanning. When paragangliomas or metastases are suspected, SRI may be useful, particularly when MIBG scanning is negative.

Adrenal Percutaneous Fine-Needle Aspiration Biopsy

Most pheochromocytomas can be readily diagnosed on the basis of their clinical, biochemical, and radiologic presentation. Fine-needle aspiration biopsy (FNAB) is not usually required for the diagnosis of a pheochromocytoma. However, some pheochromocytomas are discovered incidentally on abdominal CT or ultrasound and may be clinically or biochemically silent. Without preparatory α-adrenergic blockade, biopsy of pheochromocytomas has produced hypertensive crisis as well as hemorrhage, resulting in death. Therefore, all patients with an adrenal mass require testing for pheochromocytoma before a biopsy is even considered. When a pheochromocytoma is biopsied, the cytology can be misinterpreted as a different primary malignancy or a metastasis from another malignancy; this potential for confusion is due to the fact that pheochromocytomas are rare tumors and have pleomorphic and hyperchromic nuclei. Large left-sided pheochromocytomas have been misdiagnosed as carcinoma of the tail of the pancreas based upon CT scanning and biopsy.

Preoperative Medical Management

Patients need to be treated with oral antihypertensives in order to be relatively stable hemodynamically prior to surgery. Patients receiving increasing doses of antihypertensive medications should have daily measurements of blood pressure and pulse rate in the lying, sitting, and standing positions. Additionally, patients are taught to determine their own blood pressure and pulse rate during any paroxysmal symptoms. Prolonged preoperative preparation for longer than 7 days is no more effective for preventing intraoperative hypertension than are shorter preparation times of 4–7 days. In fact, some hypertensive patients have been admitted emergently for hypertension control and hydration, stabilized, and operated on successfully with intravenous infusion of a vasodilator drug (eg, nicardipine, nitroprusside, nitroglycerin; see below).

A. Calcium Channel Blockers

Calcium channel blockers are excellent antihypertensive agents for patients with pheochromocytomas and are preferred in many centers. Patients tend to tolerate calcium channel blockers better than alpha-blockers. Perioperative fluid requirements have been lower among patients who were pretreated with calcium channel blockers instead of alpha-blockers. In a French series, 70 patients with pheochromocytoma were successfully prepared for surgery using oral calcium channel blockers (usually nicardipine). Nicardipine may be given in doses of 20–40 mg orally every 8 hours; nicardipine is also available as a sustained-release preparation that may be given in doses of 30–60 mg orally every 12 hours. Nifedipine is a similar calcium channel blocker that is administered as a slow-release preparation in doses of 30–60 mg orally once or twice daily. For hypertensive paroxysms, nifedipine 10 mg (chewed pierced capsule) is usually a fast and effective treatment. Chewed nifedipine is generally safe for use by patients with pheochromocytoma, who may self-administer the drug at home during paroxysms but only with close blood pressure monitoring. Nifedipine causes a reduction in mitotic index and proliferation of pheochromocytoma cells in vitro; its potential clinical usefulness to reduce tumor growth has not been studied. In one small study, nifedipine therapy appeared to improve the uptake of MIBG into pheochromocytomas in four of eight patients at scanning doses. Another reported therapeutic option is sustained-release verapamil, 120–240 mg orally once daily.

B. Alpha-Adrenergic Blockers

Alpha-adrenergic blockers have historically been used for most patients with pheochromocytoma in preparation for surgical resection. Patients who are normotensive are also usually treated (carefully) preoperatively. Phenoxybenzamine (10 mg capsules) is an oral nonselective alpha-blocker that is the most commonly used alpha-blocking agent; it is given orally in a starting dose of 10 mg daily and increased by 10 mg every 3–5 days until the blood pressure is < 140/90 mm Hg. Phenoxybenzamine does not block the synthesis of catecholamines; in fact, the synthesis of catecholamines and metanephrines tends to increase during alpha blockade. Therapy with phenoxybenzamine increases the heart rate but decreases the frequency of ventricular arrhythmias. Patients are encouraged to hydrate themselves well. Patients must be monitored daily for symptomatic orthostatic hypotension. Certain adverse effects are common, including dry mouth, headache, diplopia, inhibition of ejaculation, and nasal congestion. Patients must be cautioned not to use nasal decongestants if urinary catecholamines or ^{123}I-MIBG scanning is planned, but antihistamines are acceptable. Phenoxybenzamine crosses the placenta and accumulates to levels that are 60% higher in the fetus than in the maternal circulation; this can cause hypotension and respiratory depression in the newborn for several days following birth. Most patients require 30–60 mg/d, but the dosage is sometimes escalated to as high as 140 mg/d. Excessive alpha blockade with phenoxybenzamine is undesirable since it worsens postoperative hypotension. Furthermore, excessive alpha blockade may deny a critical surgical indicator, ie, a drop in blood pressure after complete resection of the tumor and aggravation of hypertension during palpation of the abdomen in case of multiple tumors or metastases. Doxazosin is another alpha-blocker with demonstrated effectiveness in the medical management of pheochromocytomas when given orally in doses of 2–16 mg daily. Alternatively, a short-acting selective alpha-blocker (eg, **prazosin**) appears to cause less reflex tachycardia and less postoperative hypotension. The starting dose of prazosin is 0.5 mg/d, increasing up to 10 mg twice daily if necessary.

C. Angiotensin-Converting Enzyme (ACE) Inhibitors

ACE inhibitors have successfully treated hypertension in patients with pheochromocytomas but not as the sole agent. Catecholamines stimulate renin production. In turn, renin stimulates the production of angiotensin I, which is converted by ACE to angiotensin II; this can be blocked by ACE inhibitors. Furthermore, pheochromocytomas have been demonstrated to have ACE binding sites. Similarly, **angiotensin receptor blockers (ARBs)** have been successfully added to multidrug antihypertensive therapy. ACE inhibitors are contraindicated in pregnancy, since their use in the second and third trimesters has been associated with fetal malformations, including skull hypoplasia, renal failure, limb and craniofacial deformation, lung hypoplasia, intrauterine growth retardation, patent ductus arteriosus, and death.

D. Beta-Adrenergic Blockers

These agents are generally not prescribed for patients with pheochromocytomas until treatment has been started with antihypertensive medications such as α-adrenergic blockers or calcium channel blockers. Beta-adrenergic blockade should then be used for treatment of β-adrenergic symptoms such as flushing, pounding heart, or tachycardia. It is important to institute alpha blockade first, since blocking vasodilating β_2 receptors without also blocking vasoconstricting α_1 receptors can lead to hypertensive crisis if serum norepinephrine levels are high. Even **labetalol**, a mixed alpha- and beta-blocker, has been reported to cause an unexpected temporary exacerbation of hypertension. Metoprolol is effective. **Propranolol,** 10–40 mg orally four times daily, is occasionally required. Propranolol crosses the placenta and can cause intrauterine growth retardation. Newborns of mothers taking propranolol at delivery exhibit bradycardia, respiratory depression, and hypoglycemia.

E. Metyrosine (α-Methylparatyrosine)

Metyrosine inhibits the enzyme tyrosine hydroxylase, which catalyzes the first reaction in catecholamine biosynthesis. Because of its potential side effects, it is usually used only to treat hypertension in patients with metastatic pheochromocytoma. However, it can be useful as an adjunct with antihypertensive medications to treat patients with uncontrolled hypertension prior to surgery. Metyrosine is administered orally as 250 mg capsules, beginning with one every 6 hours; the dose is titrated upward every 3–4 days according to blood pressure response and side effects. The maximum dosage is 4 g/d. Catecholamine excretion is usually reduced by 35–80%. Preoperative treatment with metyrosine tends to reduce intraoperative hypertension and arrhythmias;

however, postoperative hypotension is likely to be more severe for several days. Side effects of metyrosine include sedation, psychiatric disturbance, extrapyramidal symptoms, and potentiation of sedatives and phenothiazines. Crystalluria and urolithiasis can occur, so adequate hydration is mandatory. Metyrosine does not inhibit MIBG uptake by the tumor, allowing concurrent ^{123}I-MIBG scanning or high-dose ^{131}I-MIBG treatment.

F. Octreotide

Octreotide has not been formally studied or approved for use in patients with pheochromocytoma. However, octreotide, 100 μg subcutaneously three times daily, has been reported to reduce hypertensive episodes and catecholamine excretion in a man with pheochromocytoma whose hypertensive paroxysms were uncontrolled using other means. Octreotide therapy has been observed to reduce bone pain in a woman with a malignant paraganglioma whose skeletal metastases were avid for ^{111}In-labeled octreotide. Octreotide therapy is usually begun at a dose of 50 μg injected subcutaneously every 8 hours. Side effects are common and may include nausea, vomiting, abdominal pain, and dizziness. If the drug is tolerated, the dose can be titrated upward to a maximum of 1500 μg daily; monthly injections of octreotide LAR may be considered.

G. Other Therapies

Patients with pheochromocytomas may have recurrent fevers caused by tumoral release of interleukin-6 (IL-6). Symptomatic relief may be obtained with nonsteroidal anti-inflammatory drugs such as naproxen.

Surgical Management of Pheochromocytoma

A. Preoperative Preparation

Prior to surgery, patients should be reasonably normotensive on medication (see above) and should be well hydrated. It is ideal for patients to be admitted for administration of intravenous fluids at least 1 day prior to surgery. Patients may predonate blood for autologous transfusion. The transfusion of 2 units of blood within 12 hours before surgery reduces the risk of postoperative hypotension.

Blood pressure must be monitored continuously during surgery. This requires placement of an arterial line, preferably in a large artery that is not prone to spasm (eg, femoral artery). A central venous pressure (CVP) line helps to determine the volume of fluid replacement. For certain high-risk patients with congestive heart failure or coronary artery disease, a pulmonary artery (Swan-Ganz) line is inserted preoperatively to further optimize fluid replacement. Constant electrocardiographic monitoring is mandatory. Severe hypertension can occur—even in "fully blocked" patients—upon bladder catheterization, intubation, or surgical incision. During laparoscopic surgery, catecholamine release is typically stimulated by pneumoperitoneum and by tumor manipulation. However, laparoscopic procedures cause less fluctuation of catecholamine levels and blood pressure than do open surgeries. All antihypertensive medications that might be required should be available and in the operating room well in advance.

B. Anesthesia

Anesthetic agents such as intravenous propofol, enflurane, isoflurane, sufentanil, alfentanil, and nitrous oxide appear to be safe and effective. Muscle relaxants with the least hypertensive effect should be employed (eg, vecuronium). Intraoperative hypertension can be managed by increasing the depth of anesthesia and by intravenous vasodilators for blood pressures over 160/90 mm Hg. Serum catecholamine levels drop sharply after adrenal vein ligation, and profound hypotension can occur suddenly after resection of a pheochromocytoma. Therefore, it is prudent to stop the vasodilator infusion just prior to adrenal vein ligation.

C. Antihypertensive and Antiarrhythmic Drugs

1. Nicardipine is a calcium channel blocker that is an effective antihypertensive agent when administered as an intravenous infusion in doses of 2–6 $\mu g/kg/min$. Nicardipine was successfully used as the sole intraoperative vasodilating agent in one French series of 70 patients and in another series of 19 patients.

2. Sodium nitroprusside, given by intravenous infusion, is an effective drug for managing hypertensive episodes; advantages include widespread familiarity with its use and its short duration of action. The usual dose of nitroprusside is 0.3–10 $\mu g/kg/min$. High infusion rates should not be given for prolonged periods; long-duration (over 6 hours) nitroprusside infusion rates above 2 $\mu g/kg/min$ cause cyanide accumulation to toxic concentrations. Coadministration of sodium thiosulfate (1 g/100 mg nitroprusside) prevents cyanide accumulation.

3. Nitroglycerin, given by intravenous infusion, is effective therapy for perioperative hypertension; the required dosage range is 5–100 $\mu g/min$. Since nitroglycerin adheres to polyvinyl chloride tubing, non-PVC infusion sets must be used. Nitroglycerin infusions may cause headache and hypotension. Methemoglobinemia has occurred during prolonged high-dose infusions and is manifested by cyanosis in the presence of a normal arterial PO_2. The therapy for methemoglobinemia consists of immediately stopping the nitroglycerin and giving methylene blue, 1–2 mg/kg intravenously.

4. Phentolamine mesylate is a short-acting α-adrenergic blocker having an intravenous half-life of 19 minutes. It can be given intravenously in bolus doses of 5–15 mg (1–3 mg for children) for blood pressure control. Phentolamine may also be given by intravenous infusion at a rate of 0.5–1 mg/min. Side effects include hypotension, tachycardia, cardiac arrhythmias, nasal stuffiness, nausea, and vomiting.

5. Magnesium, given intravenously, has been reported to be effective in managing hypertension during resection of a pheochromocytoma during pregnancy.

6. Lidocaine may be used to treat cardiac ventricular arrhythmias; doses of 50–100 mg are given intravenously.

7. Atrial tachyarrhythmias may be treated with intravenous atenolol in 1-mg boluses or by constant infusion of esmolol, a short-acting beta-blocker.

8. Drugs to avoid include labetalol, atropine, and diazoxide. Labetalol is not recommended for preoperative or intraoperative management of pheochromocytomas since it aggravates postresection hypotension as a consequence of its long half-life. It can also paradoxically initially aggravate hypertension, since its beta-blocking effect may occur initially, allowing a brief period of unopposed alpha receptor stimulation. Labetalol also inhibits MIBG uptake and causes misleading elevations in urinary catecholamine determinations in certain assays.

Atropine should not be used as preoperative medication for patients with pheochromocytomas since it can precipitate arrhythmias and severe hypertension. Diazoxide is not recommended because intravenous boluses can cause profound hypotension.

D. Operative Management

Perioperative mortality is about 2.4% overall, but morbidity rates of up to 24% have been reported. Surgical complications do occur and include splenectomy, which is more common with open abdominal exploration than with laparoscopic surgery. Reported surgical complication rates have been higher in patients with severe hypertension and in patients having reoperations. Surgical morbidity and mortality risks can be minimized by adequate preoperative preparation, accurate tumor localization, and meticulous intraoperative care.

1. Laparoscopy—Most pheochromocytomas can be resected by laparoscopy, which has become the procedure of choice for removing most adrenal neoplasms that are under 6 cm in diameter. Adrenal laparoscopic surgery is usually performed through four subcostal ports of 10–12 mm. Laparoscopic surgery is widely used now that preoperative localization of the tumor is possible. However, tumors that are invasive or over 6 cm in diameter are more difficult to resect laparoscopically and may require open surgery. For larger pheochromocytomas, a lateral laparoscopic approach can be used, since it affords greater opportunity to explore the abdomen and inspect the liver for metastases. For patients with small adrenal pheochromocytomas and for those who have had prior abdominal surgery, a posterior laparoscopic approach may be preferred.

The laparoscope allows unsurpassed magnified views of the pheochromocytoma and its vasculature. Pheochromocytomas are "bagged" to reduce the risk of fragmentation and spread of tumor cells within the peritoneum or at the port site. Larger tumors can be removed through laparoscopic incisions that can be widened for the surgeon's hand (laparoscopic-assisted adrenalectomy). With laparoscopic surgery, hypotensive episodes are less frequent and less severe. Laparoscopic adrenalectomy has other advantages also compared with open adrenalectomy: less postoperative pain, faster return to oral foods, and shorter hospital stays (median 3 days versus 7 days). This approach is the least invasive for the patient, who can usually begin eating and ambulating the next day. The laparoscopic approach may also be used during pregnancy. The technique has also been used successfully for certain extra-adrenal paragangliomas. Surgical mortality is under 3% at referral centers.

2. Needlescopic adrenalectomy—This procedure uses three subcostal ports of 2–5 mm, with a larger umbilical port for tumor removal. In one series of 15 patients, this technique reduced surgical times and recovery time compared with the standard laparoscopic approach. However, extensive prior surgical experience with laparoscopy is required.

3. Adrenal cortex-sparing surgery—All patients undergoing bilateral total adrenalectomies require lifelong glucocorticoid and mineralocorticoid hormone replacement. In order to avoid adrenal insufficiency, patients with benign familial or bilateral pheochromocytomas have had successful selective laparoscopic resection of small pheochromocytomas, sparing the adrenal cortex. Such adrenal-sparing surgery has unfortunately resulted in a pheochromocytoma recurrence rate of about 24%.

4. Open laparotomy—Open laparotomy is indicated for patients with particularly large pheochromocytomas or for those with intra-abdominal metastases that require debulking. An open anterior midline or subcostal approach usually yields adequate exposure.

E. Therapy of Shock Occurring After Pheochromocytoma Resection

Severe shock and cardiovascular collapse can occur immediately following ligation of the adrenal vein during resection of a pheochromocytoma, particularly in patients having norepinephrine-secreting tumors. Such hypotension may be due to desensitization of α_1-adrenergic receptors, persistence of antihypertensives, and low plasma volume. Preoperative preparation with calcium channel blockers or alpha blockade plus intravenous hydration or blood transfusions reduces the risk of shock. Intravenous antihypertensives are held just prior to ligation of the adrenal vein. Treatment of shock consists of large volumes of intravenous saline or colloid. Intravenous norepinephrine is sometimes required in very high doses.

F. Intravenous Dextrose

Immediately following removal of a pheochromocytoma, intravenous 5% dextrose should be infused at a constant rate of about 100 mL/h to prevent the postoperative hypoglycemia that is otherwise frequently encountered.

Pregnancy & Pheochromocytoma

During the first 6 months of pregnancy, it is often possible to treat a woman with alpha blockade followed by laparoscopic resection of the tumor. If a pheochromocytoma is not discovered until the last trimester, treatment consists of alpha blockade followed by elective cesarean delivery as early as feasible. Intravenous magnesium is also useful. The tumor is resected after delivery.

Phenoxybenzamine crosses the placenta and accumulates in the fetus. After 26 days of maternal phenoxybenzamine therapy, cord blood levels in the newborn are 60% higher than the mother's serum levels. Therefore, some perinatal depression and hypotension may occur in newborns of mothers receiving phenoxybenzamine. For maternal treatment near term, a short-acting selective alpha-blocker (eg, prazosin) would have an obvious theoretical advantage over long-acting alpha-blockers; chronic use increases the risk of fetal demise. The starting dose of prazosin is 0.5 mg/d orally, increasing up to 10 mg orally twice daily if necessary. Nifedipine is tolerated and preferred.

If possible, beta blockade should not be used at all during pregnancy. Propranolol crosses the placenta and can cause intrauterine growth restriction. Newborns of mothers taking propranolol at delivery exhibit bradycardia, respiratory depression, and hypoglycemia. Therefore, during cesarean delivery, serious atrial tachyarrhythmias should be controlled by a short infusion of esmolol, a beta blocker with a very short half-life.

Malignant Pheochromocytoma & Paraganglioma

Metastases are evident at the time of diagnosis in about 10% of patients with an adrenal pheochromocytoma. Another 5% are found to have metastatic disease within

5–20 years. Patients with MEN have been found to have a higher risk that a pheochromocytoma will be malignant. Paragangliomas are commonly malignant (30–50%).

Metastases can often be detected at the time of initial discovery of the pheochromocytoma or paraganglioma. Metastases are usually evident on the initial CT or MIBG procedure. Neither histopathologic examination nor endocrine testing can reliably determine whether a given pheochromocytoma is benign or malignant. The risk of malignancy is higher under the following circumstances: extra-adrenal location, larger size (6 cm or more in diameter), confluent tumor necrosis, vascular invasion, or extensive local invasion. Tumors having a high c-*myc* mRNA expression are also more likely to be malignant. In one series, 50% of patients with malignant pheochromocytoma were found to have high serum levels of neuron-specific enolase (NSE), but in none of 13 patients in another series with benign pheochromocytomas was there high NSE.

Serum neuropeptide Y (NPY) levels tend to be higher in malignant than in benign pheochromocytomas, but NPY has not proved helpful in making the diagnosis of malignancy. Malignancy is really determined only by the presence of metastases, which may be detected on whole-body ^{123}I-MIBG, ^{111}In-octreotide, PET, or CT scanning of the abdomen, pelvis, and chest. Patients must be followed closely after resection of an apparently benign pheochromocytoma, since metastases may require 20 years or more to become apparent. Urinary norepinephrine or normetanephrines and serum CgA usually fall into the normal range by 2 weeks following successful resection of a single benign pheochromocytoma. However, normal postoperative tests are not reliable indicators of benignancy, since small or nonsecretory metastases may still be present.

The differential diagnosis for apparent metastases includes benign paragangliomas, multicentric paragangliomas, second pheochromocytomas, intraperitoneal seeding during surgery, and false-positive ^{123}I-MIBG scanning. Malignant pheochromocytomas typically metastasize to bones, lymph nodes, liver, the contralateral adrenal, the lungs, and sometimes to brain or muscle (Table 11–15). The bones most frequently involved include vertebrae, pelvis and ischium, clavicles, and proximal femurs and humeri; metastases to the cranium occur frequently, having a predilection for the frontal bone. Prevertebral paragangliomas may destroy adjacent vertebrae, and spinal cord compression may occur. The 5-year survival for patients with metastatic disease is about 50%. However, patients with multiple pulmonary metastases generally have a poorer prognosis.

It is usually best to surgically resect the primary tumor as well as large metastases. CT scans may not vi-

Table 11–15. Distribution of metastases in 41 cases of malignant pheochromocytoma.[1]

	Autopsy Cases (n = 26)	Nonautopsy Cases (n = 15)	Percentage
Skeleton	12	6	44
Liver	12	3	37
Lymph node	11	4	37
Lungs	9	2	27
Central nervous system	4	0	10
Pleura	4	0	10
Kidneys	2	0	5
Pancreas	1	0	2
Omentum	1	0	2

[1]Reproduced, with permission, from Schönebeck J: Scand J Urol Nephrol 1969;3:66.

sualize small malignant intra-abdominal metastases that are visualized with preoperative ^{123}I-MIBG scanning. In such cases, following preoperative injection of ^{123}I-MIBG, the surgeon may be able to locate small tumors with the intraoperative use of a portable gamma probe. Hypertension must be adequately controlled.

Chemotherapy has been administered to patients with metastatic pheochromocytomas or paragangliomas. One reported chemotherapy regimen uses cyclophosphamide, vincristine, and dacarbazine (CVD); this chemotherapy regimen, given to 12 patients every 21 days, caused complete or partial remissions in 57%. For metastatic paraganglioma, a regimen of cyclophosphamide, doxorubicin, and dacarbazine has caused partial remission or stabilization in most patients. However, tumors usually relapse after cessation of chemotherapy. Chemotherapy has successfully caused temporary clearing of bone marrow metastases in preparation for stem cell harvest before therapy with high-dose ^{131}I-MIBG (see below).

External beam radiation therapy is administered to symptomatic metastases in the spine, long bones, or central nervous system. When administered to patients with symptomatic spinal or cranial metastases, radiation therapy can reduce pain and produce neurologic improvement. However, pheochromocytomas are relatively resistant to conventional radiation therapy. Radiation therapy to large primary tumors or intra-abdominal metastases is not advisable, since it is usually ineffective and causes morbidity such as radiation enteritis and a proclivity to later surgical complications such as wound dehiscence, infections, and fistulas. Therefore, surgical debulking of large abdominal or thoracic tumors (or other therapies) is usually preferable to radiation therapy.

^{131}I-MIBG treatment was first given to patients with malignant pheochromocytomas in 1983 at the University of Michigan. Subsequently, many other patients have been treated with this agent. Most treatment protocols employ repeated doses up to 200 mCi (7.4 GBq). Uptake occurs in many nonfunctioning pheochromocytomas and metastases, and such treatment can therefore be effective for such nonfunctioning tumors if scanning demonstrates that they are avid for MIBG. Following therapy with ^{131}I-MIBG, once background radiation has dissipated, a posttreatment whole body scan is obtained.

High-dose ^{131}I-MIBG is being given to patients with metastatic pheochromocytomas under a phase II treatment protocol at the University of California San Francisco. Precautions that must be taken before therapy include bone marrow biopsy to ensure absence of tumor in the marrow; granulocyte colony-stimulating factor-stimulated stem cell leukapheresis is then performed and cells cryopreserved for use in the event of prolonged marrow suppression. Patients are medicated with potassium iodide and potassium perchlorate to reduce the risk of thyroid damage that could be caused by any free ^{131}I generated through metabolism of ^{131}I-MIBG. The patient receives an intravenous infusion of ^{131}I-MIBG at a dose of up to 18 mCi/kg to a maximum of 800 mCi (29.6 GBq) over about 2 hours. Patients remain hospitalized until the emitted gamma radiation declines to acceptable levels, which usually requires about 5–7 days.

Most patients receiving ^{131}I-MIBG therapy achieve partial remission, stable disease, or symptomatic relief. Complete remissions are uncommon and have usually occurred in patients with a light tumor burden. Therapy with high-dose ^{131}I-MIBG appears to improve 5-year survival. High doses tend to cause temporary nausea; long-term risks include bone marrow suppression, infertility, and a projected slight increase in the lifetime risk of second malignancies. Repeated treatments may be required.

Prognosis

The mortality rate for patients undergoing pheochromocytoma resection has dropped to under 3% thanks to better medical preparation and surgical techniques. Laparoscopic surgical techniques reduced perioperative morbidity and have shortened the length of hospitalization. However, even after complete resection of the pheochromocytoma, hypertension persists or recurs in 25%. Recurrent hypertension is an indication for reevaluation for pheochromocytoma.

Patients with benign pheochromocytomas have a 5-year survival rate of 96%. Risk factors for death from pheochromocytoma include tumor size over 5 cm, metastatic disease, and local tumor invasion. Patients with metastatic pheochromocytomas have a 5-year survival rate of only 44%; those with diffuse pulmonary metastases have an even poorer prognosis. The survival of patients with metastatic disease can be improved by intensive blood pressure control and aggressive resection of the primary tumor and metastases. Metastatic and recurrent pheochromocytomas and paragangliomas vary greatly in their aggressiveness. Some metastatic or recurrent tumors are indolent or slow-growing, and prolonged survival has been reported. The symptoms and survival rate for patients with MIBG-avid metastases may also be improved with ^{131}I-MIBG therapy.

Pheochromocytoma Follow-Up

All patients with pheochromocytomas require close follow-up. Persistent symptoms or hypertension can signify lack of cure and possibly metastatic disease. About 10% of pheochromocytomas have metastasized at the time of diagnosis or soon postoperatively. However, occult metastatic disease is detected up to 20 years later in another 5%. Other patients develop multiple recurrent intra-abdominal tumors probably caused by tumor seeding that may occur spontaneously from the original tumor or during surgery.

Patients are followed with 24-hour urine collections for fractionated catecholamines, metanephrines, and creatinine. The first postoperative urine collection for fractionated catecholamines, metanephrines, and creatinine is obtained at least 2 weeks after surgery since catecholamine excretion often remains high for up to 10 days after successful surgery (see above). Quarterly urine collections are obtained during the first year following surgery, then annually or semiannually for at least 5 years. Serum CgA is a useful tumor marker for patients with pheochromocytomas whose renal function is normal; elevated and rising levels of CgA usually indicate tumor recurrence or metastases. Nonfunctioning tumors may later develop functioning metastases. Lifetime medical follow-up is required.

Weekly home blood pressure monitoring is recommended for the first year postoperatively and monthly afterward. A rising blood pressure or recurrence of symptoms should trigger a full work-up for recurrent or metastatic pheochromocytoma.

A ^{123}I-MIBG scan is recommended for all patients—but especially for those in whom there is any doubt about complete resection of the pheochromocytoma and for any patients with paraganglioma or multiple tumors. The first postoperative scan is usually obtained several months after surgery. Follow-up ^{123}I-MIBG scanning is particularly useful for patients with malignant or nonsecreting pheochromocytomas.

REFERENCES

Historical

Fränkel F: Ein Fall von doppelseitigem, völlig latent verlaufenen Nebennierentumor und gleichzeitiger Nephritis mit Veränderungen am Circulationsapparat und Retinitis. Virchows Arch Pathol Anat Physiol 1886;103:244.

Manasse P: Zur Histologie and Histogenese der primären Nierengeschwülste. Virchows Arch Pathol Anat 1896;145:113.

Rabin CB: Chromaffin cell tumor of the supra-renal medulla (Pheochromocytoma). Arch Pathol 1929;7:228.

Strömbeck JP, Hedberg TP: Tumor of the suprarenal medulla associated with paroxysmal hypertension. Report of case preoperatively diagnosed and cured by extirpation after capsular incision. Acta Chir Scand 1939;82:177.

Welbourn RB: Early surgical history of phaeochromocytoma. Br J Surg 1987;74:594. [PMID: 3304519]

Adrenal Medulla Physiology

Cavadas C et al: NPY regulates catecholamine secretion from human adrenal chromaffin cells. J Clin Endocrinol Metab 2001;86:5956. [PMID: 11739470]

Grazzini E et al: Vasopressin receptors in human adrenal medulla and pheochromocytoma. J Clin Endocrinol Metab 1999;84:2195. [PMID: 10372731]

Hoffman BB: Adrenoreceptor-activating and other sympathomimetic drugs. In: Katzung BG (editor): *Basic and Clinical Pharmacology,* 8th ed. McGraw Hill, 2001.

Jensen TB et al: Library of sequence-specific radioimmunoassays for human chromogranin A. Clin Chem 1999;45:549. [PMID: 10102916]

Kapas S, Hinson JP: Adrenomedullin in the adrenal. Microsc Res Tech 2002;57:91. [PMID: 11921359]

Kennedy B et al: Nonadrenal epinephrine-forming enzymes in humans. Characteristics, distribution, regulation, and relationship to epinephrine levels. J Clin Invest 1995;95:2896. [PMID: 7769131]

Liggett SB: Polymorphisms of the beta$_2$-adrenergic receptor. N Engl J Med 2002;346:536. [PMID: 11844862]

Munakata M et al: Clinical significance of blood pressure response triggered by a doctor's visit in patients with essential hypertension. Hypertens Res 2002;25:343. [PMID: 12135311]

O'Connor DT et al: Early decline in the catecholamine release-inhibitory peptide catestatin in humans at genetic risk of hypertension. J Hypertens 2002;20:1335. [PMID: 12131530]

Satoh F et al: Adrenomedullin in human brain, adrenal glands and tumor tissues of pheochromocytoma, ganglioneuroblastoma and neuroblastoma. J Clin Endocrinol Metab 1995;80:1750. [PMID: 7745031]

Shimosawa T et al: Proadrenomedullin NH$_2$-terminal 20 peptide, a new product of the adrenomedullin gene, inhibits norepinephrine overflow from nerve endings. J Clin Invest 1995;96:1672. [PMID: 7657838]

Vincent S, Robertson D: The broader view: catecholamine abnormalities. Clin Auton Res 2002;12:I44. [PMID: 12102462]

Adrenergic Insufficiency

Low PA et al: Efficacy of midodrine for neurogenic orthostatic hypotension. Reply. JAMA 1997;278:388. [PMID: 11536812]

Robertson D et al: Isolated failure of autonomic noradrenergic neurotransmission. Evidence for impaired beta-hydroxylation of dopamine. N Engl J Med 1986;314:1494. [PMID: 3010116]

Pheochromocytoma & Paranglioma Reviews

Bravo EL: Pheochromocytoma. Cardiol Rev 2002;10:44. [PMID: 11790269]

Case Records of the Massachusetts General Hospital: Paraganglioma of the posterior mediastinum. N Engl J Med 2001;344:1314.

Ein SH et al: Pediatric pheochromocytoma. A 36-year review. Pediatr Surg Int 1997;12:595. [PMID: 9354733]

Fitzgerald PJ et al: Intracardiac pheochromocytoma with dual coronary blood supply: case report and literature review. Cardiovasc Surg 1995;3:557. [PMID: 7872191]

Kebebew E, Duh QY: Benign and malignant pheochromocytoma: diagnosis, treatment, and follow-up. Surg Oncol Clin N Am 1998;7:765. [PMID: 9735133]

Loh KC et al: Phaeochromocytoma: a ten year survey. Q J Med 1997;90:51. [PMID: 9093589]

Lucon AM et al: Pheochromocytoma: study of 50 cases. J Urol 1997;157:1208. [PMID: 9120903]

Manger WM, Gifford RW: Pheochromocytoma. J Clin Hypertens 2002;4:62. [PMID: 11821644]

Manger WM, Gifford RW Jr: *Clinical and Experimental Pheochromocytoma,* 2nd ed. Blackwell, 1996.

Pacak K et al: Recent advances in genetics, diagnosis, localization, and treatment of pheochromocytoma. Ann Intern Med 2001;134:315. [PMID: 11182843]

O'Riordain DS et al: Clinical spectrum and outcome of functional extraadrenal paraganglioma. World J Surg 1996;20:916. [PMID: 8678971]

Werbel SS, Ober KP: Pheochromocytoma. Update on diagnosis, localization, and management. Med Clin North Am 1995;79:131. [PMID: 7808088]

Pheochromocytoma Pathology & Physiology

DeS Senanayake P et al: Production, characterization, and expression of neuropeptide Y by human pheochromocytoma. J Clinical Investigation 1995;96:2503. [PMID: 7593641]

Dishy V et al: The effect of common polymorphisms of the β$_2$-adrenergic receptor on agonist-mediated vascular desensitization. N Engl J Med 2001;345:1030. [PMID: 11557915]

Eisenhofer G et al: Plasma metanephrines are markers of pheochromocytoma produced by catechol-O-methyltransferase within tumors. J Clin Endocrinol Metab 1998;83:2175. [PMID: 9626157]

Eurin J et al: Release of neuropeptide Y and hemodynamic changes during surgical removal of human pheochromocytoma. Regulatory Peptides 2000;86:95. [PMID: 10672908]

Fried G et al: Multiple neuropeptide immunoreactivities in a renin-producing human paraganglioma. Cancer 1994;74:142. [PMID: 7911735]

Grouzmann E et al: Disappearance rate of catecholamines, total metanephrines, and neuropeptide Y from the plasma of patients after resection of pheochromocytoma. Clin Chem 2001 Jun;47:1075. [PMID: 11375294]

Higashi Y et al: Excess norepinephrine impairs both endothelium-dependent and -independent vasodilation in patients with pheochromocytoma. Hypertension 2002;39:513. [PMID: 11882600]

Januszewicz W et al: Alterations in plasma neuropeptide Y immunoreactivity and catecholamine levels during surgical removal of pheochromocytoma. J Hypertens 1998;16:543. [PMID: 11800059]

Kirby BD et al: Normotensive pheochromocytoma. Pharmacologic, paraneoplastic and anesthetic considerations. West J Med 1983;139:221. [PMID: 6636736]

Lack EE: Adrenal medullary hyperplasia and pheochromocytoma. In: *Pathology of the Adrenal Glands.* Lack EE (editor). Churchill Livingstone, 1990.

Linnoila RI et al: Histopathology of benign versus malignant sympathoadrenal paragangliomas: Clinicopathologic study of 120 cases including unusual histologic features. Hum Pathol 1990;21:1168. [PMID: 2172151]

Liu J et al: Expression patterns of the c-*myc* gene in adrenocortical tumors and pheochromocytomas. J Endocrinol 1997;152:175. [PMID: 9071974]

Loh KC et al: Hypercalcemia in malignant paraganglioma due to parathyroid hormone-related protein. Horm Res 1998;50:217.

Lonergan GJ et al: From the archives of the AFIP: Neuroblastoma, ganglioneuroblastoma, and ganglioneuroma: Radiologic-pathologic correlation. Radiographics 2002;22:911. [PMID: 12110723]

Lumachi F et al: Extraadrenal and multiple pheochromocytomas. Are there really any differences in pathophysiology and outcome? J Exp Clin Cancer Res 1998;17:303. [PMID: 9894766]

Meunier JP et al: Cardiac pheochromocytoma. Ann Thorac Surg 2001;71:712. [PMID: 11235739]

Munakata M et al: Altered sympathetic and vagal modulations of the cardiovascular system in patients with pheochromocytoma: their relations to orthostatic hypotension. Am J Hypertens 1999;12:572. [PMID: 10371366]

Paleologos TS et al: Paraganglioma of the cauda equina: a case presenting features of increased intracranial pressure. J Spinal Disord 1998;11:362. [PMID: 9726310]

Platts JK et al: Death from phaeochromocytoma: lessons from a post-mortem survey. J R Coll Physicians Lond 1995;29:299. [PMID: 7473324]

Pommier RF et al: Comparison of adrenal and extraadrenal pheochromocytomas. Surgery 1993;114:1160. [PMID: 8256223]

Sutton MG et al: Prevalence of clinically unsuspected pheochromocytoma. Review of a 50-year autopsy series. Mayo Clin Proc 1981;56:354. [PMID: 6453259]

Genetic Aspects of Pheochromocytomas

Brandi ML et al: Consensus: Guidelines for diagnosis and therapy of MEN Type 1 and 2. J Clin Endocrinol Metab 2001;86:5658. [PMID: 11739416]

Eisenhofer G et al: Plasma normetanephrine and metanephrine for detecting pheochromocytoma in von Hippel-Lindau disease and multiple endocrine neoplasia type 2. N Engl J Med 1999;340:1872. [PMID: 10369850]

Eisenhofer G et al: Pheochromocytomas in von Hippel-Lindau syndrome and multiple endocrine neoplasia type 2 display distinct biochemical and clinical phenotypes. J Clin Endocrinol Metab 2001;86:1999. [PMID: 11344198]

Januszewicz A et al: Incidence and clinical relevance of *RET* proto-oncogene germline mutations in pheochromocytoma patients. J Hypertens 2000;18:1019. [PMID: 10953992]

Koch CA et al: Somatic *VHL* gene deletion and point mutation in MEN 2A-associated pheochromocytoma. Oncogene 2002;21:479. [PMID: 11821960]

Koch CA et al: Pheochromocytoma in von Hippel-Lindau disease: distinct histopathologic phenotype compared to pheochromocytoma in multiple endocrine neoplasia type 2. Endocr Pathol 2002;13:17. [PMID: 12114747]

Koch CA et al: Genetic aspects of pheochromocytoma. Endocr Regul 2001;35:43. [PMID: 11308996]

Neumann HP et al: Germ-line mutations in nonsyndromic pheochromocytoma. N Engl J Med 2002;346:1459. [PMID: 12000816]

Richard S et al: Pheochromocytoma as the first manifestation of von Hippel-Lindau disease. Surgery 1994;116:1076. [PMID: 7985090]

Diagnostic Tests for Pheochromocytoma

Baguet JP et al: Metastatic phaeochromocytoma: risks of diagnostic needle puncture and treatment by arterial embolisation. J Hum Hypertens 2001;15:209. [PMID: 11317207]

d'Herbomez M et al: Chromogranin A assay and ^{131}I-MIBG scintigraphy for diagnosis and follow-up of pheochromocytoma. J Nucl Med 2001;42:993. [PMID: 11438617]

Feldman JM: Falsely elevated urinary excretion of catecholamines and metanephrines in patients receiving labetalol therapy. J Clin Pharmacol 1987;27:288. [PMID: 3680586]

Ferrari L et al: The biological characteristics of chromogranin A and its role as a circulating marker in neuroendocrine tumours. Anticancer Res 1999;19:3415. [PMID: 10629629]

Giampaolo B et al: Chromogranin "A" in normal subjects, essential hypertensives and adrenalectomized patients. Clin Endocrinol (Oxf) 2002;57:41. [PMID: 12100068]

Giovanella L, Ceriani L: Serum chromogranin-alpha immunoradiometric assay in the diagnosis of pheochromocytoma. Int J Biol Markers 2002;17:130. [PMID: 12113580]

Goldstein DS et al: Dihydrocaffeic acid: a common contaminant in the liquid chromatographic-electrochemical measurement of plasma catecholamines in man. J Chromatogr 1984;311:148. [PMID: 6520156]

Heron E et al: The urinary metanephrine-to-creatinine ratio for the diagnosis of pheochromocytoma (see comments). Ann Intern Med 1996;125:300. [PMID: 8678394]

Lenders JW et al: Biochemical diagnosis of pheochromocytoma: which test is best? JAMA 2002;287:1427. [PMID: 11903030]

Lenz T et al: Diagnosis of pheochromocytoma Clin Lab 2002;48:5. [PMID: 11833676]

Lumachi F et al: Fine-needle aspiration cytology of adrenal masses in noncancer patients: clinicoradiologic and histologic correlations in functioning and nonfunctioning tumors. Cancer 2001;93:323. [PMID: 11668467]

McCorkell SJ, Niles NL: Fine-needle aspiration of catecholamine-producing adrenal masses: A possibly fatal mistake. AJR Am J Roentgenol 1985;145:113. [PMID: 3873829]

Peaston RT et al: Overnight excretion of urinary catecholamines and metabolites in the detection of pheochromocytoma. J Clin Endocrinol Metab 1996;81:1378. [PMID: 8636337]

Stuerenburg HJ et al: Plasma concentrations of 5-HT, 5-HIAA, norepinephrine, epinephrine and dopamine in ecstasy users. Neuroendocrinol Lett 2002;23:259. [PMID: 12080289]

Stridsberg M, Husebye ES: Chromogranin A and chromogranin B are sensitive circulating markers for phaeochromocytoma (see comments). Eur J Endocrinol 1997;136:67. [PMID: 9037129]

Weise M et al: Utility of plasma free metanephrines for detecting childhood pheochromocytoma. J Clin Endocrinol Metab 2002;87:1955. [PMID: 11994324]

Yanaihara H et al: Application of region-specific immunoassay for chromogranin A: substantial clue for detection and measurement of chromogranin A in human plasma. Regul Pept 1999;80:83. [PMID: 10235638]

Localizing Scans for Pheochromocytoma

Hoegerle S et al: Pheochromocytomas: detection with 18F DOPA whole body PET—initial results. Radiology 2002;222:507. [PMID: 11818620]

Jalil ND et al: Effectiveness and limits of preoperative imaging studies for the localization of pheochromocytomas and paragangliomas: a review of 282 cases. French Association of Surgery (AFC), and The French Association of Endocrine Surgeons (AFCE). Eur J Surg 1998;164:23. [PMID: 9537705]

Kaltsas G et al: Comparison of somatostatin analog and meta-iodobenzylguanidine radionuclides in the diagnosis and localization of advanced neuroendocrine tumors. J Clin Endocrinol Metab 2001;86:895. [PMID: 11158063]

Kaltsas GA et al: The value of radiolabelled MIBG and octreotide in the diagnosis and management of neuroendocrine tumours. Ann Oncol 2001;12(Suppl 2):S47. [PMID: 11762352]

Khafagi FA et al: Labetalol reduces iodine-131 MIBG uptake by pheochromocytoma and normal tissues. J Nucl Med 1989;30:481. [PMID: 2738677]

Khafagi FA et al: Phaeochromocytoma and functioning paraganglioma in childhood and adolescence: role of iodine 131

metaiodobenzylguanidine. Eur J Nucl Med 1991;18:191. [PMID: 1645665]

Lin JC et al: Cardiac pheochromocytoma: resection after diagnosis by 111-indium octreotide scan. Annals of Thoracic Surgery 1999;67:555. [PMID: 10193931]

Neumann DR et al: Malignant pheochromocytoma of the anterior mediastinum: PET findings with (^{18}F)FDG and ^{82}Rb. J Comput Assist Tomogr 1996;20:312. [PMID: 8606245]

Pacak K et al: 6-[^{18}F]fluorodopamine positron emission tomographic (PET) scanning for diagnostic localization of pheochromocytoma. Hypertension 20001;38:6. [PMID: 11463751]

Pacak K et al: A "pheo" lurks: novel approaches for locating occult pheochromocytoma. J Clin Endocrinol Metab 2001;86:3641. [PMID: 11502790]

Roelants V et al: Iodine-131-MIBG scintigraphy in adults: interpretation revisited? J Nucl Med 1998;39:1007. [PMID: 9627334]

Shapiro B, Gross MD: Radiochemistry, biochemistry, and kinetics of ^{131}I-metaiodobenzylguanidine (MIBG) and ^{123}I-MIBG: clinical implications of the use of ^{123}I-MIBG. Med Pediatr Oncol 1987;15:170. [PMID: 3309602]

Shulkin BL, Shapiro B: Current concepts on the diagnostic use of MIBG in children. J Nucl Med 1998;39:678. [PMID: 9544682]

Sone H et al: Radioiodinated metaiodobenzylguanidine scintigraphy for pheochromocytoma. A false-positive case of adrenocortical adenoma and literature review. Horm Res 1996;46:138. [PMID: 8894669]

van der Harst E et al: [^{123}I]metaiodobenzylguanidine and [^{111}In]octreotide uptake in benign and malignant pheochromocytomas. J Clin Endocrinol Metab 2001;86:685. [PMID: 11158032]

Zagar I et al: Meta-(^{131}I)iodobenzylguanidine in the scintigraphic evaluation of neural crest tumors. Q J Nucl Med 1995;39 (Suppl 1):13. [PMID: 9002742]

Incidental Adrenal Tumors

Aron DC: The adrenal incidentaloma: disease of modern technology and public health problem. Rev Endocr Metab Disord 2001;2:335. [PMID: 11705137]

Barzon L, Boscaro M: Diagnosis and management of adrenal incidentalomas. J Urol 2000;163:398. [PMID: 10647642]

Cook DM: Adrenal mass. Endocrinol Metab Clin North Am 1997;26:829. [PMID: 9429862]

Medical Therapy for Pheochromocytoma

Combemale F et al: Exclusive use of calcium channel blockers and cardioselective beta-blockers in the pre- and peri-operative management of pheochromocytoma. 70 cases. Ann Chir 1998;52:341. [PMID: 9752467]

Dabrowska B et al: Influence of alpha-adrenergic blockade on ventricular arrhythmias, QTc interval and heart rate variability in phaeochromocytoma. J Hum Hypertens 1995;9:925. [PMID: 8583473]

Johanning RJ et al: A retrospective study of sodium nitroprusside use and assessment of the potential risk of cyanide poisoning. Pharmacotherapy 1995;15:773. [PMID: 8602386]

Koriyama N et al: Control of catecholamine release and blood pressure with octreotide in a patient with pheochromocytoma: a case report with in vitro studies. Horm Res 2000;53:46. [PMID: 10965221]

Starikova AM et al: Nifedipine-induced morphological differentiation of rat pheochromocytoma cells. Neuroscience 1998;86:611. [PMID: 9881873]

Steinsapir J et al: Metyrosine and pheochromocytoma. Arch Intern Med 1997;157:901. [PMID: 9129550]

Adrenal Surgery

Baghai M et al: Pheochromocytomas and paragangliomas in von Hippel-Lindau disease: a role for laparoscopic and cortical-sparing surgery. Arch Surg 2002;137:682. [PMID: 12049539]

Berends FJ et al: Safe retroperitoneal endoscopic resection of pheochromocytomas. World J Surg 2002;26:527. [PMID: 12098038]

Colson P et al: Haemodynamic heterogeneity and treatment with the calcium channel blocker nicardipine during phaeochromocytoma surgery. Acta Anaesthesiol Scand 1998;42:1114. [PMID: 9809099]

Demeure MJ et al: Laparoscopic removal of a right adrenal pheochromocytoma in a pregnant woman. J Laparoendosc Adv Surg Tech A 1998;8:315. [PMID: 9820725]

Duh QY: Editorial: Evolving surgical management for patients with pheochromocytoma. J Clin Endocrinol Metab 2001;86:1477. [PMID: 11297570]

Duh QY et al: Laparoscopic adrenalectomy. Comparison of the lateral and posterior approaches. Arch Surg 1996;131:870. [PMID: 8712912]

Gill IS et al: Needlescopic adrenalectomy—the initial series: comparison with conventional laparoscopic adrenalectomy. Urology 1998;52:180. [PMID: 9697779]

Grant CS: Pheochromocytoma. In: *Textbook of Endocrine Surgery*, Clark OH, Duh Q-Y (editors). Saunders, 1997.

Joris JL et al: Hemodynamic changes and catecholamine release during laparoscopic adrenalectomy for pheochromocytoma. Anesth Analg 1999;88:16. [PMID: 9895059]

Korman JE et al: Comparison of laparoscopic and open adrenalectomy. Am Surg 1997;63:908. [PMID: 9322671]

Kozlowski PM et al: Laparoscopic management of bladder pheochromocytoma. Urology 2001;57:365. [PMID: 11182363]

Kreienmeyer J: Total intravenous anesthesia with propofol and sufentanil for resection of pheochromocytoma. Anaesthesiol Reanim 1997;22:80. [PMID: 9324368]

Lehnert H et al: Intraoperative localization of malignant pheochromocytoma by ^{123}I-metaiodobenzylguanidine single probe measurement. Klin Wochenschr 1988;66:61. [PMID: 3347006]

Munro J et al: Calcium channel blockade and uncontrolled blood pressure during phaeochromocytoma surgery. Can J Anaesth 1995;42:228. [PMID: 7743576]

Neumann HP et al: Preserved adrenocortical function after laparoscopic bilateral adrenal sparing surgery for hereditary pheochromocytoma. J Clin Endocrinol Metab 1999;84:2606. [PMID: 10443647]

Newell KA et al: Plasma catecholamine changes during excision of pheochromocytoma. Surgery 1988;104:1064. [PMID: 3194833]

O'Riordan JA: Pheochromocytomas and anesthesia. Int Anesthesiol Clin 1997;35:99. [PMID: 9444533]

Plouin P-F et al: Factors associated with perioperative morbidity and mortality in patients with pheochromocytoma: analysis of 165 operations at a single center. J Clin Endocrinol Metab 2001;86:1480. [PMID: 11287571]

Sprung J et al: Anesthetic aspects of laparoscopic and open adrenalectomy for pheochromocytoma. Urology 2000;55:339. [PMID: 10699606]

Tagaya N et al: Laparoscopic resection of a functional paraganglioma in the organ of Zuckerkandl. Surg Endosc 2002;16:219. [PMID: 11961657]

Winfield HN et al: Technique of laparoscopic adrenalectomy. Urol Clin North Am 1997;24:459. [PMID: 9126244]

Pheochromocytoma in Pregnancy

Ahlawat SK et al: Pheochromocytoma associated with pregnancy: case report and review of the literature. Obstet Gynecol Surg 1999;54:728. [PMID: 10546277]

Hamilton A et al: Anesthesia for phaeochromocytoma in pregnancy. Can J Anaesth 1997;44:654. [PMID: 9187786]

Rosenthal T, Oparil S: The effect of antihypertensive drugs on the fetus. J Hum Hypertens 2002;16:293. [PMID: 12082488]

Santeiro ML et al: Phenoxybenzamine placental transfer during the third trimester. Ann Pharmacother 1996;30:1249. [PMID: 8913406]

Malignant Pheochromocytoma

Averbuch SD et al: Malignant pheochromocytoma: effective treatment with a combination of cyclophosphamide, vincristine, and dacarbazine. Ann Intern Med 1988;109:267. [PMID: 3395037]

Fernandez-Llamazares J et al: Functioning metastases of a nonfunctioning paraganglioma. J Surg Oncol 1988;37:213. [PMID: 3352278]

Grouzmann E et al: Neuropeptide Y and neuron-specific enolase levels in benign and malignant pheochromocytoma. Cancer 1990;66:1833. [PMID: 2208039]

Loh KC, Fitzgerald PA et al: The treatment of malignant pheochromocytoma with iodine-131 metaiodobenzylguanidine (131-I MIBG): a comprehensive review of 116 reported patients. J Endocrinol Invest 1997;20:648. [PMID: 9492103]

Mukherjee JJ et al: Treatment of metastatic carcinoid tumours, phaeochromocytoma, paraganglioma and medullary carcinoma of the thyroid with ^{131}I-meta-iodobenzylguanidine (^{131}I-mIBG). Clin Endocrinol 2001;55:47. [PMID: 11453952]

Patel SR et al: A 15-year experience with chemotherapy of patients with paraganglioma. Cancer 1995;76:1476. [PMID: 8620426]

Rao F et al: Malignant pheochromocytoma. Chromaffin granule transmitters and response to treatment. Hypertension 2000;36:1045. [PMID: 11116123]

Sisson JC et al: Radiopharmaceutical treatment of malignant pheochromocytoma. J Nucl Med 1984;24:197. [PMID: 6726430]

Tsuchimochi S et al: Metastatic pulmonary pheochromocytomas: positive I-123 SPECT with negative I-131 MIBG and equivocal I-123 MIBG planar imaging. Clin Nucl Med 1997; 22:687. [PMID: 9343724]

Tanaka S et al: Malignant pheochromocytoma with hepatic metastasis diagnosed 20 years after resection of the primary adrenal lesion. Intern Med 1993;32:789. [PMID: 8012074]

Troncone L, Rufini V: Nuclear medicine therapy of pheochromocytoma and paraganglioma. Q J Nucl Med 1999;43:344. [PMID: 10731785]

Yu L et al: Radiation therapy of metastatic pheochromocytoma: case report and review of the literature. Am J Clin Oncol 1996;19:389. [PMID: 8677912]

Testes

12

Glenn D. Braunstein, MD

ACTH	Adrenocorticotropic hormone	**ICSI**	Intracyloplasmic sperm injection
cAMP	Cyclic adenosine monophosphate	**IVF**	In vitro fertilization
DHEA	Dehydroepiandrosterone acetate	**LH**	Luteinizing hormone
DHT	Dihydrotestosterone	**mRNA**	Messenger ribonucleic acid
FSH	Follicle-stimulating hormone	**PRL**	Prolactin
GnRH	Gonadotropin-releasing hormone	**SHBG**	Sex hormone-binding globulin
hCG	Human chorionic gonadotropin		

The testes contain two major components which are structurally separate and serve different functions. The **Leydig cells,** or **interstitial cells,** comprise the major endocrine component. The primary secretory product of these cells, testosterone, is responsible either directly or indirectly for embryonic differentiation along male lines of the external and internal genitalia, male secondary sexual development at puberty, and maintenance of libido and potency in the adult male. The **seminiferous tubules** comprise the bulk of the testes and are responsible for the production of approximately 30 million spermatozoa per day during male reproductive life (puberty to death).

Both of these testicular components are interrelated, and both require an intact hypothalamic-pituitary axis for initiation and maintenance of their function. In addition, several accessory genital structures are required for the functional maturation and transport of spermatozoa. Thus, disorders of the testes, hypothalamus, pituitary, or accessory structures may result in abnormalities of androgen or gamete production, infertility, or a combination of these problems.

■ ANATOMY & STRUCTURE-FUNCTION RELATIONSHIPS (FIGURE 12–1)

TESTES

The adult testis is a prolate spheroid with a mean volume of 18.6 ± 4.8 mL. The average length is 4.6 cm

(range, 3.6–5.5 cm), and the average width is 2.6 cm (range, 2.1–3.2 cm). The testes are located within the scrotum, which not only serves as a protective envelope but also helps to maintain the testicular temperature approximately 2 °C (3.6 °F) below abdominal temperature. Three layers of membranes—visceral tunica vaginalis, tunica albuginea, and tunica vasculosa—comprise the testicular capsule. Extensions of the tunica albuginea into the testicle as fibrous septa result in the formation of approximately 250 pyramidal lobules each of which contains coiled seminiferous tubules. Within each testis there are almost 200 m of seminiferous tubules, and these structures account for 80–90% of the testicular mass. The approximately 350 million androgen-producing Leydig cells, as well as the blood and lymphatic vessels, nerves, and fibroblasts, are interspersed between the seminiferous tubules.

The blood supply to the testes is derived chiefly from the testicular arteries, which are branches of the internal spermatic arteries. After traversing a complicated capillary network, blood enters multiple testicular veins that form an anastomotic network, the pampiniform plexus. The pampiniform plexuses coalesce to form the internal spermatic veins. The right spermatic vein drains directly into the vena cava; the left enters the renal vein.

The seminiferous tubules in the adult average 165 μm in diameter and are composed of Sertoli cells and germinal cells. The Sertoli cells line the basement membrane and form tight junctions with other Sertoli cells. These tight junctions prevent the passage of proteins from the interstitial space into the lumens of the seminiferous tubules, thus establishing a "blood-testis barrier." Through extension of cytoplasmic processes, the

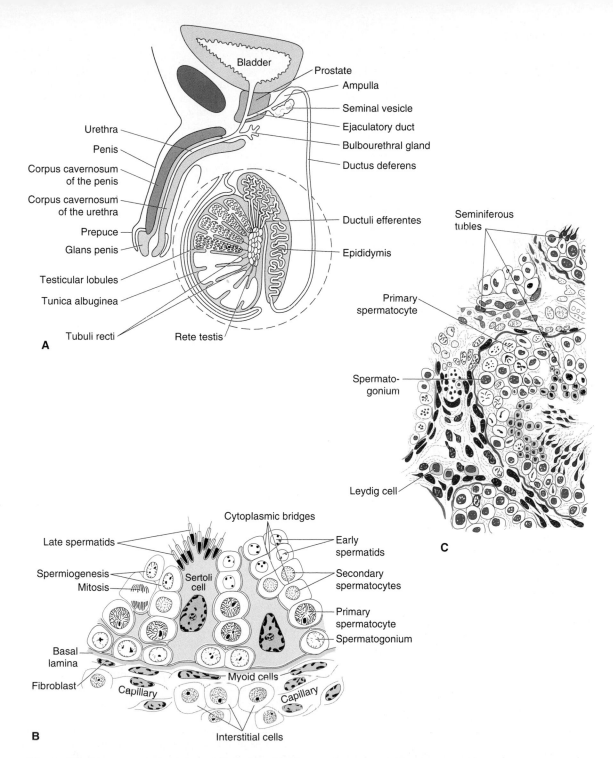

Figure 12–1. Male genital system. *A:* The testis and the epididymis are in different scales from the other parts of the reproductive system. Observe the communication between the testicular lobules. *B:* Structural organization of the human seminiferous tubule and interstitial tissue. This figure does not show the lymphatic vessels frequently found in the connective tissue. (*A* and *B* reproduced, with permission, from Junqueira LC, Carneiro J, Kelley RO: *Basic Histology,* 9th ed. McGraw-Hill, 1999.) *C:* Section of human testis. (*C* reproduced, with permission, from Ganong WF: *Review of Medical Physiology,* 20th ed. McGraw-Hill, 2001.)

Sertoli cells surround developing germ cells and provide an environment essential for germ cell differentiation. In addition, these cells have been shown to be responsible for the movement of germ cells from the base of the tubule toward the lumen and for the release of mature sperm into the lumen. These cells also actively phagocytose damaged germ cells and residual bodies, which are portions of the germ cell cytoplasm not used in the formation of spermatozoa. Finally, in response to follicle-stimulating hormone (FSH) or testosterone, the Sertoli cells secrete androgen-binding protein, a molecule with high affinity for androgens. This substance, which enters the tubular lumen, provides a high concentration of testosterone to the developing germinal cells during the process of spermatogenesis.

More than a dozen different types of germ cells have been described in males. Broadly, they can be classified as spermatogonia, primary spermatocytes, secondary spermatocytes, spermatids, and spermatozoa. Spermatogenesis occurs in an orderly fashion, with the spermatocytes being derived from the spermatogonia via mitotic division. Through meiotic (or reduction) division, the spermatids are formed; they contain a haploid number of chromosomes (23). The interval from the beginning of spermatogenesis to release of mature spermatozoa into the tubular lumen is approximately 74 days. Although there is little variation in the duration of the spermatogenic cycle, a cross section of a seminiferous tubule will demonstrate several stages of germ cell development.

ACCESSORY STRUCTURES

The seminiferous tubules empty into a highly convoluted anastomotic network of ducts called the rete testis. Spermatozoa are then transported through efferent ductules and into a single duct, the epididymis, by testicular fluid pressure, ciliary motion, and contraction of the efferent ductules. During the approximately 12 days required for transit through the epididymis, spermatozoa undergo morphologic and functional changes essential to confer upon the gametes the capacity for fertilizing an ovum. The epididymis also serves as a reservoir for sperm. Spermatozoa stored in the epididymis enter the vas deferens, a muscular duct 35–50 cm long that propels its contents by peristaltic motion into the ejaculatory duct.

In addition to the spermatozoa and the secretory products of the testes, retia testis, and epididymides, the ejaculatory ducts receive fluid from the seminal vesicles. These paired structures, 10–20 cm long, are composed of alveolar glands, connective tissue, and muscle. They are the source of seminal plasma fructose, which provides nourishment to the spermatozoa. In addition, the seminal vesicles secrete phosphorylcholine, ergothioneine, ascorbic acid, flavins, and prostaglandins. About 60% of the total volume of seminal fluid is derived from the seminal vesicles.

The ejaculatory ducts terminate in the prostatic urethra. There additional fluid (approximately 20% of total volume) is added by the prostate, a tubuloalveolar gland with a fibromuscular stroma that weighs about 20 g and measures $4 \times 2 \times 3$ cm. The constituents of the prostate fluid include spermine, citric acid, cholesterol, phospholipids, fibrinolysin, fibrinogenase, zinc, acid phosphatase, and prostate-specific antigen, a 34-kDa kallikrein-like serine protease. Fluid is also added to the seminal plasma by the bulbourethral (Cowper) glands and urethral (Littre) glands during its transit through the penile urethra.

■ PHYSIOLOGY OF THE MALE REPRODUCTIVE SYSTEM

GONADAL STEROIDS (FIGURE 12–2)

The three steroids of primary importance in male reproductive function are testosterone, dihydrotestosterone, and estradiol. From a quantitative standpoint, the most important androgen is testosterone. Over 95% of the testosterone is secreted by the testicular Leydig cells. In addition to testosterone, the testes secrete small amounts of the potent androgen dihydrotestosterone and the weak androgens dehydroepiandrosterone (DHEA) and androstenedione. The Leydig cells also secrete small quantities of estradiol, estrone, pregnenolone, progesterone, 17α-hydroxypregnenolone, and 17α-hydroxyprogesterone. The steps in testicular androgen biosynthesis are illustrated in Figure 12–2.

Dihydrotestosterone and estradiol are derived not only by direct secretion from the testes but also by conversion in peripheral tissues of androgen and estrogen precursors secreted by both the testes and the adrenals. Thus, about 80% of the circulating concentrations of these two steroids is derived from such peripheral conversion. Table 12–1 summarizes the approximate contributions of the testes, adrenals, and peripheral tissues to the circulating levels of several sex steroid hormones in men.

In the blood, androgens and estrogens exist in either a free (unbound) state or bound to serum proteins. Although about 38% of testosterone is bound to albumin, the major binding protein is **sex hormone-binding**

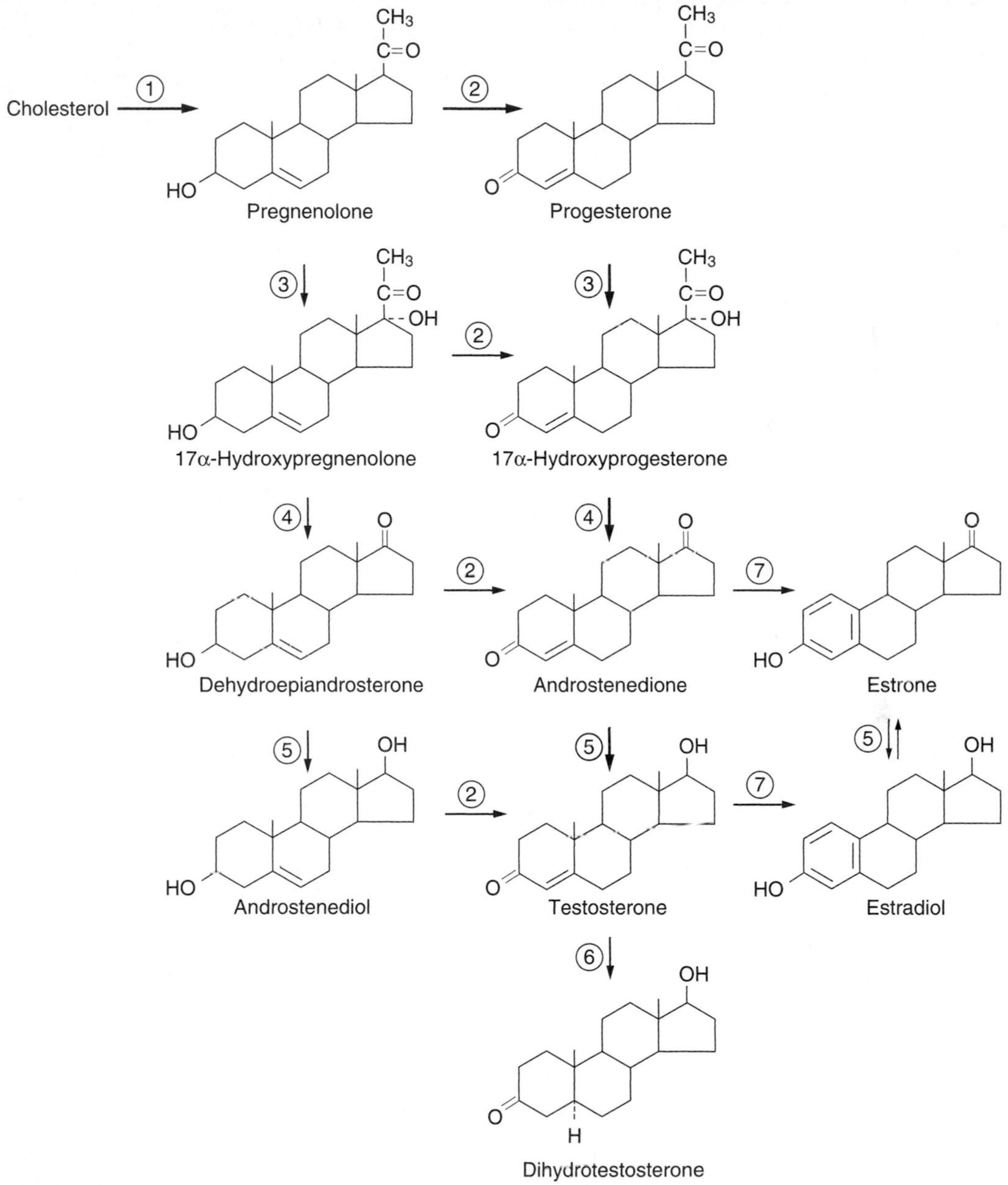

Figure 12–2. Pathways for testicular androgen and estrogen biosynthesis. Heavy arrows indicate major pathways. Circled numbers represent enzymes as follows: ①, 20,22-desmolase (P450scc); ②, 3β-hydroxysteroid dehydrogenase and Δ^5,Δ^4-isomerase; ③, 17-hydroxylase (P-450c17); ④, 17,20-desmolase (P450c17); ⑤, 17-ketoreductase; ⑥, 5α-reductase; ⑦, aromatase. (See also Figures 9–4, 13–4, and 14–13.)

Table 12–1. Relative contributions (approximate percentages) of the testes, adrenals, and peripheral tissues to circulating levels of sex steroids in men.

	Testicular Secretion	Adrenal Secretion	Peripheral Conversion of Precursors
Testosterone	< 95	< 1	< 5
Dihydrotestosterone	< 20	< 1	80
Estradiol	< 20	< 1	80
Estrone	< 2	< 1	98
DHEA sulfate	< 10	90	...

globulin (SHBG), which binds 60% of the testosterone. This glycosylated dimeric protein is homologous to, yet distinct from, the androgen-binding protein secreted by the Sertoli cells. SHBG is synthesized in the liver, with the gene located on the short arm of chromosome 17. The serum concentrations of this protein are increased by estrogen, tamoxifen, phenytoin, or thyroid hormone administration and by hyperthyroidism and cirrhosis and are decreased by exogenous androgens, glucocorticoids, or growth hormone and by hypothyroidism, acromegaly, and obesity. About 2% of the circulating testosterone is not bound to serum proteins and is able to enter cells and exert its metabolic effects. In addition, some of the protein-bound testosterone may dissociate from the protein and enter target tissues; thus, the amount of bioavailable testosterone may be greater than just the amount of non-protein-bound testosterone.

As noted below, testosterone may be converted to dihydrotestosterone within specific androgen target tissues. Most circulating testosterone is converted primarily by the liver into various metabolites such as androsterone and etiocholanolone, which, after conjugation with glucuronic or sulfuric acid, are excreted in the urine as 17-ketosteroids. However, it should be noted that only 20–30% of the urinary 17-ketosteroids are derived from testosterone metabolism. The majority of the 17-ketosteroids are formed from the metabolism of adrenal steroids. Therefore, 17-ketosteroid determinations do not reliably reflect testicular steroid secretion.

Testosterone leaves the circulation and rapidly traverses the cell membrane (Figure 12–3). In most androgen target cells, testosterone is enzymatically converted to the more potent androgen dihydrotestosterone by the microsomal isoenzyme 5α-reductase-2, which has a pH optimum of 5.5. Another isoenzyme, 5α-reductase-1, has a pH optimum near 8.0 and may involve androgen action in the skin, but it is not active in the uro-

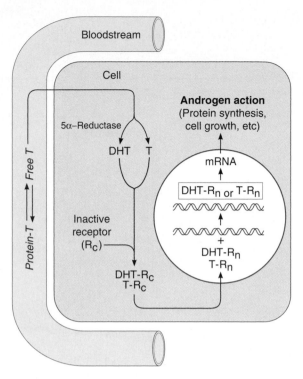

Figure 12–3. Mechanisms of androgen action. (T, testosterone; DHT, dihydrotestosterone; R_n, activated nuclear receptor; mRNA, messenger RNA; R_c, inactive receptor.)

genital tract. Dihydrotestosterone as well as testosterone then binds to the same specific intracellular receptor protein (R_c in Figure 12–3) that is distinct from both androgen-binding protein and SHBG. The genes that encode for this protein are located on the X chromosome. The androgen receptor, a phosphoprotein of about 110 kDa, is a member of the steroid-thyroid hormone nuclear superfamily. It is synthesized in the cytoplasm and is associated with several heat shock proteins. When testosterone or dihydrotestosterone binds to the carboxyl terminal androgen-binding portion of the receptor, the heat shock proteins dissociate and conformational changes in the receptor take place that allow it to be translocated into the nucleus (R_n in Figure 12–3). Some studies suggest that androgen binding to the receptor takes place only in the nucleus and not in the cytoplasm. In the nucleus, the androgen-androgen receptor complex binds to DNA through the DNA-binding domain of the receptor, which allows the polymorphic transactivating domain of the receptor to initiate transcriptional activity. This results in the synthesis of messenger RNA (mRNA), which is eventually transported to the cytoplasm, where it directs new protein synthesis and other changes that together constitute androgen action.

A variety of biologic effects of androgens have been defined in males. As discussed in Chapter 14, they are essential for appropriate differentiation of the internal and external male genital system during fetal development. During puberty, androgen-mediated growth of the scrotum, epididymis, vas deferens, seminal vesicles, prostate, and penis occurs. The functional integrity of these organs requires androgens. Androgens stimulate skeletal muscle growth and growth of the larynx, which results in deepening of the voice; and of the epiphysial cartilaginous plates, which results in the pubertal growth spurt. Both ambisexual (pubic and axillary) hair growth and sexual (beard, mustache, chest, abdomen, and back) hair growth are stimulated, as is sebaceous gland activity. Other effects include stimulation of erythropoiesis and social behavioral changes.

CONTROL OF TESTICULAR FUNCTION

Hypothalamic-Pituitary-Leydig Cell Axis (Figure 12–4)

The hypothalamus synthesizes a decapeptide, go-nadotropin-releasing hormone (GnRH), and secretes it in pulses every 90–120 minutes into the hypothalamo-hypophysial portal blood. After reaching the anterior pituitary, GnRH binds to the gonadotrophs and stimulates the release of both luteinizing hormone (LH) and, to a lesser extent, FSH into the general circulation. LH is taken up by the Leydig cells, where it binds to specific membrane receptors. The LH receptor is a G protein-coupled receptor containing seven transmembrane domains with a serine and threonine-rich cytoplasmic region containing a phosphorylation site and a 350- to 400-amino-acid extracellular hormone-binding domain. The binding of LH to the receptor leads to activation of adenylyl cyclase and generation of cAMP and other messengers that ultimately result in the secretion of androgens. In turn, the elevation of androgens inhibits the secretion of LH from the anterior pituitary through a direct action on the pituitary and an inhibitory effect at the hypothalamic level. Both the hypothalamus and the pituitary have androgen and estrogen receptors. Experimentally, pure androgens such as dihydrotestosterone (DHT) reduce LH pulse frequency, while estradiol reduces LH pulse amplitude. However, the major inhibitory effect of androgen on the hypothalamus appears to be mediated principally by estradiol, which may be derived locally through the aromatization of testosterone. Leydig cells also secrete small quantities of oxytocin, renin, corticotropin-releasing factor, insulin-like growth factor I, transforming

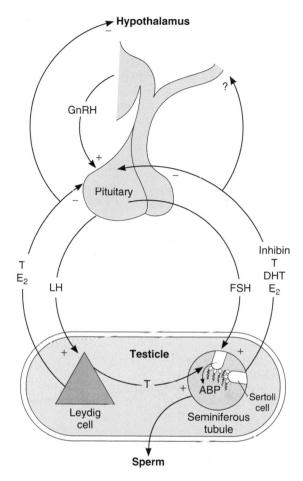

Figure 12–4. Hypothalamic-pituitary-testicular axis. (GnRH, gonadotropin-releasing hormone; LH, luteinizing hormone; FSH, follicle-stimulating hormone; T, testosterone; DHT, dihydrotestosterone; ABP, androgen-binding protein; E_2, estradiol; +, positive influence; –, negative influence.)

growth factors α and β, interleukin 1, lipotropin, β-endorphin, dynorphin, angiotensin, inhibin, gastrin-releasing peptide, stem cell factor, substance P, and prostaglandins, which may be important for paracrine regulation of testicular function.

Hypothalamic-Pituitary-Seminiferous Tubular Axis (Figure 12–4)

After stimulation by GnRH, the gonadotrophs secrete FSH into the systemic circulation. This glycoprotein hormone binds to specific receptors in the Sertoli cells and stimulates the production of androgen-binding protein. FSH is necessary for the initiation of spermatogenesis. However, full maturation of the spermatozoa appears to require not only an FSH effect but also testosterone. Indeed, the major action of FSH on spermatogenesis may be via the stimulation of androgen-binding protein production, which allows a high intratubular concentration of testosterone to be maintained.

In addition to androgen-binding protein, the Sertoli cell secretes several other substances including GnRH-like peptide, insulin-like growth factor-1, transferrin, plasminogen activator, ceruloplasmin, müllerian duct inhibitory factor, H-Y antigen, and inhibin. At least three genes have been found to direct inhibin synthesis. Two forms of inhibin have been identified, inhibin A and inhibin B. Both are 32-kDa proteins composed of the same alpha subunit cross-linked with different beta subunits, and each can selectively inhibit FSH release from the pituitary without affecting LH release. FSH directly stimulates the Sertoli cells to secrete inhibin. There is a reciprocal relationship between serum inhibin B and FSH levels, and inhibin B is therefore probably a physiologic regulator of pituitary FSH secretion, possibly together with the gonadal steroids. Inhibin levels decline with advancing age.

Two additional inhibin-related proteins that have been identified in porcine follicular fluid may also be present in the testes. These factors, designated follicle regulatory protein and activin, are composed of inhibin beta subunit dimers and can selectively stimulate pituitary FSH secretion in vitro. They are structurally similar to transforming growth factor β (TGFβ), which can also stimulate pituitary FSH release. The physiologic role, if any, that follicle regulatory protein, activin, and TGFβ have in the regulation of FSH secretion is unknown.

■ EVALUATION OF MALE GONADAL FUNCTION

CLINICAL EVALUATION

Clinical Presentation

The clinical presentation of patients with deficient testosterone production or action depends upon the age at onset of hypogonadism. Androgen deficiency during the second to third months of fetal development results in varying degrees of ambiguity of the genitalia and male pseudohermaphroditism. If the deficiency develops during the third trimester, defects in testicular descent leading to cryptorchidism as well as

micropenis may occur. These topics are covered in Chapters 14 and 15.

Prepubertal androgen deficiency leads to poor secondary sexual development and eunuchoid skeletal proportions. The penis fails to enlarge, the testes remain small, and the scrotum does not develop the marked rugae characteristic of puberty. The voice remains high-pitched and the muscle mass does not develop fully, resulting in less than normal strength and endurance. The lack of appropriate stimulation of sexual hair growth results in sparse axillary and pubic hair (which receive some stimulation from adrenal androgens) and absent or very sparse facial, chest, upper abdominal, and back hair. Although the androgen-mediated pubertal growth spurt will fail to take place, the epiphysial plates of the long bones will continue to grow under the influence of insulin-like growth factor-I and other growth factors. Thus, the long bones of the upper and lower extremities will grow out of proportion to the axial skeleton. Healthy white men have an average upper segment (crown to pubis) to lower segment (pubis to floor) ratio of > 1, whereas prepubertal hypogonadism results in a ratio of < 1. Similarly, the ratio of total arm span to total height averages 0.96 in white men. Because of the relatively greater growth in the upper extremities, the arm span of eunuchoid individuals exceeds height by 5 cm or more.

If testosterone deficiency develops after puberty, the patient may complain of decreased libido, erectile dysfunction, and low energy. Patients with mild androgen deficiency or androgen deficiency of recent onset may not note a decrease in facial or body hair growth; it appears that although adult androgen levels must be achieved to *stimulate* male sexual hair growth, relatively low levels of androgens are required to *maintain* sexual hair growth. With long-standing hypogonadism, the growth of facial hair will diminish, and the frequency of shaving may also decrease (Figure 12–5). In addition, fine wrinkles may appear in the corners of the mouth and eyes and, together with the sparse beard growth, result in the classic hypogonadal facies.

Genital Examination

Adequate assessment of the genitalia is essential in the evaluation of male hypogonadism. The examination should be performed in a warm room in order to relax the dartos muscle of the scrotum. The penis should be examined for the presence of hypospadias, epispadias, and chordee (abnormal angulation of the penis due to a fibrotic plaque), which may interfere with fertility. The fully stretched dorsal penile length should be measured in the flaccid state from the pubopenile skin junction to the tip of the glans. The normal range in

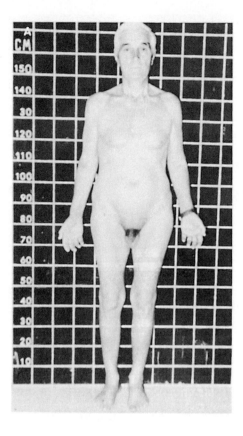
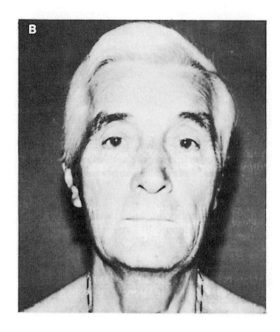

Figure 12–5. A: Hypogonadal habitus. Note absence of body and facial hair as well as feminine body distribution. ***B:*** Hypogonadal facies. Note absence of facial hair and fine wrinkles around the corners of the eyes and lips.

adults is 12–16 cm (10th and 90th percentiles, respectively).

Assessment of testicular volume is also vital to the evaluation of hypogonadism. Careful measurement of the longitudinal and transverse axes of the testes may be made and testicular volume (V) calculated from the formula for a prolate spheroid: $V = 0.52 \times length \times width^2$. The mean volume for an adult testis is 18.6 ± 4.8 mL. Alternatively, volume may be estimated with the Prader orchidometer, which consists of a series of plastic ellipsoids ranging in volume from 1 mL to 25 mL (Figure 12–6). Each testis is compared with the appropriate ellipsoid. Adults normally have volumes greater than 15 mL by this method.

Since 80–90% of testicular volume is composed of seminiferous tubules, decrease in volume indicates lack of tubular development or regression of tubular size. The consistency of the testicle should be noted. Small,

firm testes are characteristic of hyalinization or fibrosis, as may occur in Klinefelter's syndrome. Small, rubbery testes are normally found in prepubertal males; in an adult, they are indicative of deficient gonadotropin stimulation. Testes with a mushy or soft consistency are characteristically found in individuals with postpubertal testicular atrophy.

The epididymis and vas deferens should also be examined. One of the most important parts of the examination is evaluation for the presence of varicocele resulting from incompetence of the internal spermatic vein. As will be discussed later, this is an important and potentially correctable cause of male infertility. The patient should be examined in the upright position while performing the Valsalva maneuver. The examiner should carefully palpate the spermatic cords above the testes. A varicocele can be felt as an impulse along the posterior portion of the cord. About 85% of

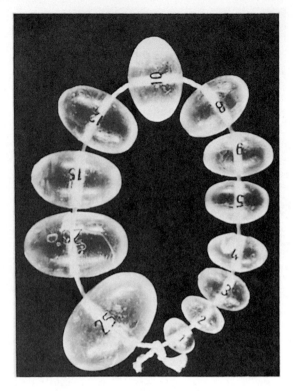

Figure 12–6. Prader orchidometer.

varicoceles are located on the left side, and 15% are bilateral.

LABORATORY TESTS OF TESTICULAR FUNCTION

Semen Analysis

With some exceptions, a normal semen analysis excludes gonadal dysfunction. However, a single abnormal semen analysis is not a sufficient basis for a diagnosis of disturbance of testicular function, since marked variations in several of the parameters may be seen in normal individuals: At least three semen samples must be examined over a 2- to 3-month interval in order to evaluate this facet of male gonadal function. As noted above, approximately 3 months are required for completion of the spermatogenic cycle and movement of the mature spermatozoa through the ductal system. Therefore, when an abnormal semen sample is produced, one must question the patient about prior fever, trauma, drug exposure, and other factors that may temporarily damage spermatogenesis.

The semen should be collected by masturbation after 1–3 days of sexual abstinence and examined within 2 hours after collection. Normal semen has a volume of 2–5 mL, with 20×10^6 or more sperms per milliliter. Over half of the spermatozoa should exhibit progressive motility, and 30% or more should have normal morphology.

Steroid Measurements

Each of the gonadal steroids may be measured by immunoassay. Although single determinations may distinguish between normal individuals and patients with severe hypogonadism, mild defects in androgen production may be missed. In normal individuals, there are frequent, rapid pulsatile changes in serum testosterone concentration as well as a slight nocturnal elevation. Therefore, at least three separate blood samples should be collected at 20- to 40-minute intervals during the morning for testosterone measurement. The testosterone may be measured in each of the serum samples, or equal aliquots of each of the three serum samples may be combined, mixed, and subjected to testosterone analysis. The latter procedure provides a savings in cost as well as a mean serum testosterone concentration that takes into account the pulsatile release of testosterone.

Androgen and estrogen immunoassays measure total serum steroid concentrations. This is the sum of the free, biologically active hormone and the protein-bound moiety. Although in most circumstances it is not necessary to determine the actual quantity of free steroid hormones, in some situations alterations in the binding protein concentration may occur. Lowered concentrations of SHBG are seen in patients with hypothyroidism, obesity, and acromegaly. In these circumstances, the free testosterone concentration should be directly measured, since it may be normal when the total serum testosterone level is decreased. The normal male serum concentrations of gonadal steroids collected in the basal state are given in Table 12–2.

Table 12–2. Normal ranges for gonadal steroids, pituitary gonadotropins, and prolactin in men.

	Ranges
Testosterone, total	260–1000 ng/dL (9.0–34.7 nmol/L)
Testosterone, free	50–210 pg/mL (173–729 pmol/L)
Dihydrotestosterone	27–75 ng/dL (0.9–2.6 nmol/L)
Androstenedione	50–200 ng/dL (1.7–6.9 nmol/L)
Estradiol	15–40 pg/mL (55–150 pmol/L)
Estrone	15–65 pg/mL (55.5–240 pmol/L)
FSH	1.5–14 mIU/mL (1.5–14 IU/L)
LH	1.5–5.6 mIU/mL (1.5–5.6 IU/L)
PRL	3–14.7 ng/mL (130–640 nmol/L)

Gonadotropin & Prolactin Measurements

LH and, to a lesser extent, FSH are released in pulsatile fashion throughout the day. Therefore, as with testosterone, at least three blood samples should be obtained at 20- to 40-minute intervals during the day. FSH and LH may be measured in each of the samples or in a single pooled specimen. Although many laboratories give a numerical value for the lower limits of normal for gonadotropins, some normal males have concentrations of FSH and LH undetectable by presently available immunoassay techniques. Furthermore, the concentrations of gonadotropins measured in one laboratory may not be directly comparable to those measured in another because of differences in the reference preparations used. The primary use of basal FSH and LH concentrations is to distinguish between hypergonadotropic hypogonadism, in which either or both of the gonadotropins are elevated, and hypogonadotropic hypogonadism, in which the gonadotropins are low or inappropriately normal in the presence of decreased androgen production.

Elevations of serum prolactin (PRL) inhibit the normal release of pituitary gonadotropins (shown by a reduced LH pulse frequency), probably through an effect on the hypothalamus. Thus, serum PRL measurements should be performed in any patient with hypogonadotropic hypogonadism. Serum PRL concentrations are generally stable throughout the day; therefore, measurement of this hormone in a single sample is usually sufficient. However, the patient should abstain from eating for 3 hours before the blood sample is obtained, since a protein meal may acutely stimulate the release of PRL from the pituitary. The normal ranges for serum PRL and gonadotropins are shown in Table 12–2.

Dynamic Tests

A. CHORIONIC GONADOTROPIN STIMULATION TEST

Human chorionic gonadotropin (hCG) is a glycoprotein hormone with biologic actions similar to those of LH. Following an injection of chorionic gonadotropin, this hormone binds to the LH receptors on the Leydig cells and stimulates the synthesis and secretion of testicular steroids. Therefore, the Leydig cells may be directly assessed by the intramuscular injection of 4000 IU of chorionic gonadotropin daily for 4 days. A normal response is a doubling of the testosterone level following the last injection. Alternatively, a single intramuscular dose of chorionic gonadotropin (5000 IU/1.7 m^2 in adults or 100 IU/kg in children) may be given, with blood samples taken for testosterone measurements 72 and 96 hours later. Patients with primary gonadal disease will have a diminished response following administration of chorionic gonadotropin, while patients with

Leydig cell failure secondary to pituitary or hypothalamic disease will have a qualitatively normal response.

B. CLOMIPHENE CITRATE STIMULATION TEST

Clomiphene citrate is a nonsteroid compound with weak estrogenic activity. It binds to estrogen receptors in various tissues, including the hypothalamus. By preventing the more potent estrogen estradiol from occupying these receptors, the hypothalamus in effect "sees" less estradiol. As noted above, most if not all of the hypothalamic-pituitary feedback control by testicular androgens is mediated by estradiol, which is derived from the peripheral conversion of androgens. The apparent estradiol deficiency leads to an increase of GnRH release the net result of which is stimulation of the gonadotrophs to secrete increased quantities of LH and FSH.

The test is performed by giving clomiphene citrate, 100 mg orally twice daily for 10 days. Three blood samples are collected at 20-minute intervals (see comments above, under Steroid Measurements) 1 day before the drug is administered and again on days 9 and 10 of drug administration. LH, FSH, and testosterone should be measured in pooled aliquots from each of these samples. Healthy men have a 50–250% increase in LH, a 30–200% increase in FSH, and a 30–220% increase in testosterone on day 10 of the test. Patients with pituitary or hypothalamic disease do not show a normal increment in LH or FSH.

C. GONADOTROPIN-RELEASING HORMONE TEST

The decapeptide GnRH (gonadorelin) directly stimulates the gonadotrophs of the anterior pituitary to secrete LH and FSH. It was expected that measurement of LH and FSH following the administration of GnRH would be useful in distinguishing between hypothalamic and pituitary lesions, but this has not proved to be the case. Patients with destructive lesions of the pituitary and those with long-standing hypogonadism due to hypothalamic disorders may not show a response to a GnRH test. However, if the releasing factor is administered by repeated injections every 60–120 minutes or by a programmable pulsatile infusion pump for 7–14 days, patients with hypothalamic lesions may have their pituitary responsiveness to GnRH restored, whereas patients with pituitary insufficiency do not. Conversely, a normal LH and FSH response to GnRH in a hypogonadal male does not eliminate hypopituitarism as the cause of the gonadal failure, since patients with mild hypogonadotropic hypogonadism may demonstrate a normal response.

The test is performed by administering 100 μg of gonadorelin by rapid intravenous bolus. Blood is drawn at −15, 0, 15, 30, 45, 60, 90, 120, and 180 minutes for LH and FSH measurements. Normal adult males have a two- to fivefold increase in LH over baseline concentrations and an approximately twofold rise of FSH. However, some normal males fail to have an increase in FSH following GnRH. Patients with primary testicular disease may respond with exaggerated increases in LH and FSH. If seminiferous tubule damage alone is present, abnormal FSH rise and normal LH response may be seen.

Testicular Biopsy

Testicular biopsy in hypogonadal men is primarily indicated in patients with normal-sized testes and azoospermia in order to distinguish between spermatogenic failure and ductal obstruction. Although germinal aplasia, hypoplasia, maturation arrest, and other abnormalities of spermatogenesis may be diagnosed by examination of testicular tissue in oligospermic males, knowledge of the type of defect does not alter therapy. Therefore, testicular biopsy is not usually indicted for evaluation of mild to moderate oligospermia.

Evaluation for Male Hypogonadism

Figure 12–7 outlines an approach to the diagnosis of male gonadal disorders. Semen analysis and determination of the basal concentrations of testosterone, FSH, and LH allow the clinician to distinguish patients with primary gonadal failure who have poor semen characteristics, low or normal testosterone, and elevated FSH or LH from those with secondary gonadal failure and abnormal semen analysis, decreased testosterone, and low or inappropriately normal gonadotropins.

In patients with elevations of gonadotropins resulting from primary testicular disease, chromosomal analysis will help to differentiate between genetic abnormalities and acquired testicular defects. Since no therapy exists that will restore spermatogenesis in an individual with severe testicular damage, androgen replacement is the treatment of choice. Patients with isolated seminiferous tubule failure may have normal or elevated FSH concentrations in association with normal LH and testosterone levels and usually severe oligospermia. Patients with azoospermia require evaluation for the possible presence of ductal obstruction, since this defect may be surgically correctable. Fructose is added to seminal plasma by the seminal vesicles, and an absence of fructose indicates that the seminal vesicles are absent or bilaterally obstructed. The combination of a poor semen analysis with low testosterone, FSH, and LH is indicative of a hypothalamic or pituitary defect. Such patients need further evaluation of anterior and posterior pituitary gland function with appropriate pituitary function tests, as well as neuroradiologic and neuro-ophthalmologic studies (Chapter 5).

■ PHARMACOLOGY OF DRUGS USED TO TREAT MALE GONADAL DISORDERS

ANDROGENS

A variety of drugs are available for the treatment of androgen deficiency. Preparations for sublingual or oral administration such as methyltestosterone, oxymetholone, and fluoxymesterone have the advantage of ease of administration but the disadvantage of erratic absorption, potential for cholestatic jaundice, and decreased effectiveness when compared to the intramuscular preparations. Testosterone propionate is a short-acting androgen. Its main use is in initiating therapy in older men, whose prostate glands may be exquisitely sensitive to testosterone. A dose of 50 mg two or three times per week is adequate. Obstructive symptoms due to benign prostatic hypertrophy following therapy with this androgen usually resolve rapidly because of its short duration of action.

Androgen deficiency may be treated with testosterone enanthate or cyclopentylpropionate (cypionate) given intramuscularly. Unlike the oral androgen preparations, both of these agents are capable of completely virilizing the patients. Therapy may be initiated with 200 mg intramuscularly every 1–2 weeks for 1–2 years. After adequate virilization has been achieved, the androgen effect may be maintained by doses of 100–200 mg every 2–3 weeks. Testosterone pellets may be implanted subcutaneously for a longer duration of effect. However, this therapy has not enjoyed much popularity. Transdermal delivery via membranes impregnated with testosterone is another method of replacement therapy. One variety (Testoderm) is placed on the scrotum. The patches, which are placed daily, provide physiologic levels of testosterone that closely mimic the normal diurnal testosterone fluctuation. Elevated serum concentrations of dihydrotestosterone—a finding of unknown clinical significance—have been noted in patients using these patches. Another type of transdermal patch (Androderm; Testoderm TTS) can be placed on the skin of the back, shoulder, or abdomen and provides normal androgen concentrations without elevation in dihydrotestosterone. A testosterone gel (Andro Gel 1%; Testim 1%) that is applied daily to the abdomen, shoulders, or upper arms also results in physiologic concentrations of testosterone.

Androgens, both oral and intramuscular, have been used (illegally) by some athletes to increase muscle mass and strength. Although this may achieve the anticipated result in some individuals, adverse effects include

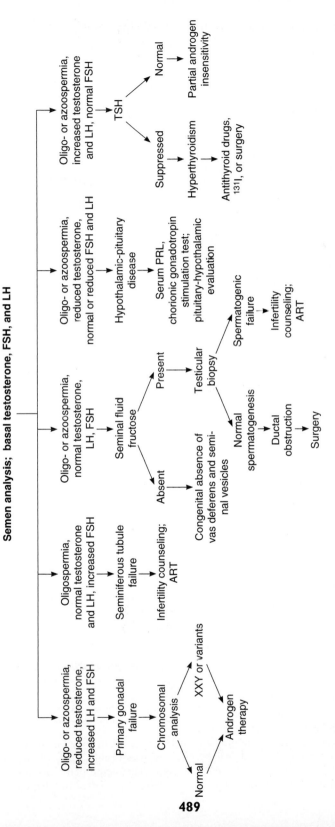

489

Figure 12-7. Scheme for evaluation of clinical hypogonadism. (ART, assisted reproductive technologies such as in vitro fertilization and sperm injection into ova.)

oligospermia and testicular atrophy—in addition to some of the complications noted below.

Androgen therapy is contraindicated in patients with prostatic carcinoma. About 1–2% of patients receiving oral methyltestosterone or fluoxymesterone develop intrahepatic cholestatic jaundice that resolves when the drug is discontinued. Rarely, these methylated or halogenated androgens have been associated with benign and malignant hepatocellular tumors.

Androgen therapy may also cause premature fusion of the epiphyses in an adolescent, and this may result in some loss of potential height. Therefore, androgen therapy is usually withheld until a hypogonadal male reaches 13 years of age. Sodium and water retention may induce hypertension or congestive heart failure in susceptible individuals. Since androgens stimulate erythropoietin production, erythrocytosis may occur during therapy. This is not usually clinically significant. Inhibition of spermatogenesis is mediated through suppression of gonadotropins by the androgens. Gynecomastia may develop during initiation of androgen therapy but usually resolves with continued administration of the drug. Sleep apnea may be precipitated. Priapism, acne, and aggressive behavior are dose-related adverse effects and generally disappear after reduction of dosage. Androgens decrease the production of thyroxine-binding globulin and corticosteroid-binding globulin by the liver. Therefore, total serum thyroxine and cortisol concentrations may be decreased though the free hormone concentrations remain normal. High-density lipoprotein concentrations may also be reduced.

GONADOTROPINS

In patients with hypogonadism due to inadequate gonadotropin secretion, spermatogenesis and virilization may be induced by exogenous gonadotropin injections. Since the gonadotropins are proteins with short half-lives, they must be administered parenterally two or three times a week.

The expense and inconvenience of this type of therapy preclude its routine use for the treatment of androgen deficiency. The two major indications for exogenous gonadotropins are treatment of cryptorchidism (see below) and induction of spermatogenesis in hypogonadal males who wish to father children.

To induce spermatogenesis, 2000 IU of chorionic gonadotropin may be given intramuscularly three times a week for 9–12 months. In some individuals with partial gonadotropin deficiencies, this may induce adequate spermatogenesis. In patients with more severe deficiencies, menotropins, available in vials containing 75 IU each of FSH and LH, or highly purified urinary FSH (urofollitropin) or FSH produced by recombinant DNA technology (follitropin beta), each containing 75 IU of FSH, is added to chorionic gonadotropin therapy after 9–12 months and is administered in a dosage of one vial intramuscularly three times a week.

Adverse reactions with such therapy are minimal. Acne, gynecomastia, or prostatic enlargement may be noted as a result of excessive Leydig cell stimulation. Reduction of the chorionic gonadotropin dosage or a decrease in the frequency of chorionic gonadotropin injections generally results in resolution of the problem.

GONADOTROPIN-RELEASING HORMONE

GnRH (gonadorelin acetate), administered in pulses every 60–120 minutes by portable infusion pumps, effectively stimulates the endogenous release of LH and FSH in hypogonadotropic hypogonadal patients. This therapy does not currently appear to offer any major advantage over the use of exogenous gonadotropins for induction of spermatogenesis or the use of testosterone enanthate or cypionate for virilization. A long-acting analog of GnRH, leuprolide acetate, is available for the treatment of prostatic carcinoma. Daily subcutaneous administration of 1 mg or monthly intramuscular injections of 7.5 mg of a depot preparation—22.5 mg for 3 months or 30 mg for 4 months results in desensitization of the pituitary GnRH receptors, which reduces LH and FSH levels and so ultimately testosterone concentrations. Similar results are produced with a subcutaneous injection of the depot form of the GnRH analog goserelin. With these therapies, initial remission rates for prostatic carcinoma are similar to those found with orchiectomy or treatment with diethylstilbestrol (about 70%). In patients with benign prostatic hypertrophy, prostate size has been reduced with this therapy. Another potent intranasally administered GnRH analog, nafarelin acetate, is available for the treatment of endometriosis and central precocious puberty. Central precocious puberty also may be treated with leuprolide acetate and another analog, histrelin acetate. Long-acting GnRH agonists combined with testosterone have been studied as a possible male contraceptive, but they do not uniformly induce azoospermia.

■ CLINICAL MALE GONADAL DISORDERS

Hypogonadism may be subdivided into three general categories (Table 12–3). A thorough discussion of the hypothalamic-pituitary disorders that cause hypogonadism is presented in Chapters 5 and 15. The defects

Table 12–3. Classification of male hypogonadism.

Hypothalamic-pituitary disorders
Panhypopituitarism
Isolated LH deficiency (fertile eunuch)
Isolated FSH deficiency
LH and FSH deficiency
  a. With normal sense of smell
  b. With hyposmia or anosmia (Kallmann's syndrome)
  c. With complex neurologic syndromes
    Prader-Willi syndrome
    Laurence-Moon Biedl syndrome
    Möbius' syndrome
    Lowe's syndrome
    Cerebellar ataxia
Biologically inactive LH
Hyperprolactinemia
Gonadal abnormalities
Klinefelter's syndrome
Other chromosomal defects (XX male, XY/XXY, XX/XXY, XXXY, XXXXY, XXYY, XYY)
Bilateral anorchia (vanishing testes syndrome)
Leydig cell aplasia
Cryptorchidism
Noonan's syndrome
Myotonic dystrophy
Adult seminiferous tubule failure
Adult Leydig cell failure
Defects in androgen biosynthesis
Defects in androgen action
Complete androgen insensitivity (testicular feminization)
Incomplete androgen insensitivity

in androgen biosynthesis and androgen action are described in Chapter 14. The following section emphasizes the primary gonadal abnormalities.

KLINEFELTER'S SYNDROME (XXY SEMINIFEROUS TUBULE DYSGENESIS)

Klinefelter's syndrome is the most common genetic cause of male hypogonadism, occurring in one of 500 male births. An extra X chromosome is present in about 0.2% of male conceptions and 0.1% of live-born males. Sex chromosome surveys of mentally retarded males have revealed an extra X chromosome in 0.45–2.5% of such individuals. Patients with an XXY genotype have classic Klinefelter's syndrome; those with an XXXY, XXXXY, or XXYY genotype or with XXY/chromosomal mosaicism are considered to have variant forms of the syndrome.

Etiology & Pathophysiology

The XXY genotype is usually due to maternal meiotic nondisjunction, which results in an egg with two X chromosomes. The frequency of meiotic errors correlates positively with maternal age. Meiotic nondisjunction may also occur during spermatogenesis.

At birth there are generally no physical stigmas of Klinefelter's syndrome, and during childhood there are no specific signs or symptoms. The chromosomal defect is expressed chiefly during puberty. As the gonadotropins increase, the seminiferous tubules do not enlarge but rather undergo fibrosis and hyalinization, which results in small, firm testes. Obliteration of the seminiferous tubules results in azoospermia.

In addition to dysgenesis of the seminiferous tubules, the Leydig cells are also abnormal. They are present in clumps and appear to be hyperplastic upon initial examination of a testicular biopsy. However, the Leydig cell mass is not increased, and the apparent hyperplasia is actually due to the marked reduction in tubular volume. Despite the normal mass of tissue, the Leydig cells are functionally abnormal. The testosterone production rate is reduced, and there is a compensatory elevation in serum LH. Stimulation of the Leydig cells with exogenous chorionic gonadotropin results in a subnormal rise in testosterone. The clinical manifestations of androgen deficiency vary considerably from patient to patient. Thus, some individuals have virtually no secondary sexual developmental changes, whereas others are indistinguishable from healthy individuals.

The elevated LH concentrations also stimulate the Leydig cells to secrete increased quantities of estradiol and estradiol precursors. The relatively high estradiol:testosterone ratio is responsible for the variable degrees of feminization and gynecomastia seen in these patients. The elevated estradiol also stimulates the liver to produce SHBG. This may result in total serum testosterone concentrations that are within the low normal range for adult males. However, the free testosterone level may be lower than normal.

The pathogenesis of the eunuchoid proportions, personality, and intellectual deficits and associated medical disorders is presently unclear.

Testicular Pathology

Most of the seminiferous tubules are fibrotic and hyalinized, although occasional Sertoli cells and spermatogonia may be present in some sections. Absence of elastic fibers in the tunica propria is indicative of the dysgenetic nature of the tubules. The Leydig cells are arranged in clumps and appear hyperplastic, although the total mass is normal.

Clinical Features
(Figure 12–8)

A. SYMPTOMS AND SIGNS

There are usually no symptoms before puberty other than poor school performance in some affected individuals. Puberty may be delayed, but not usually by more than 1–2 years. During puberty, the penis and scrotum undergo varying degrees of development, with some individuals appearing normal. Most patients (80%) have diminished facial and torso hair growth. The major complaint is often persistent gynecomastia, which is clinically present in over half of patients. The testes are uniformly small (< 2 cm in longest axis, and < 4 mL in volume) and firm as a result of fibrosis and hyalinization. Other complaints include infertility or insufficient libido and po-

tency. The patient may have difficulty putting into words his embarrassment in situations where he must disrobe in the presence of other men, and the subnormal development of the external genitalia along with gynecomastia may lead to feelings of inadequacy that may be partly responsible for the dyssocial behavior some patients exhibit. Osteopenia may be severe in patients with long-standing androgen deficiencies.

Patients with Klinefelter's syndrome have abnormal skeletal proportions that are not truly eunuchoid. Growth of the lower extremities is relatively greater than that of the trunk and upper extremities; therefore, pubis-to-floor height is greater than crown-to-pubis height, and span is less than total height. Thus, the abnormal skeletal proportions are not the result of androgen deficiency per se (which results in span greater than height).

Intellectual impairment is noted in many patients with Klinefelter's syndrome, but the true proportion of affected individuals with subnormal intelligence is not known. Dyssocial behavior is common (see above). Patients generally show want of ambition, difficulties in maintaining permanent employment, and a tendency to ramble in conversations.

Several clinical and genotypic variants of Klinefelter's syndrome have been described. In addition to small testes with seminiferous tubular hyalinization, azoospermia, deficient secondary sexual development, and elevated gonadotropins, patients with three or more X chromosomes uniformly have severe mental retardation. The presence of more than one Y chromosome tends to be associated with aggressive antisocial behavior and macronodular acne. Skeletal deformities such as radioulnar synostosis, flexion deformities of the elbows, and clinodactyly are more commonly seen in Klinefelter variants. Patients with sex chromosome mosaicism (XX/XXY) may have only a few of the Klinefelter stigmas. These patients may have normal testicular size and may be fertile if their testes contain the XY genotype.

Medical disorders found to be associated with Klinefelter's syndrome with more than chance frequency include chronic pulmonary disease (emphysema, chronic bronchitis), varicose veins, extragonadal germ cell tumors, cerebrovascular disease, glucose intolerance, primary hypothyroidism, and taurodontism—with early tooth decay. There is a 20-fold increased risk of breast cancer.

B. LABORATORY FINDINGS

Serum testosterone is low or normal; FSH and LH concentrations are elevated. Azoospermia is present. The buccal smear is chromatin-positive (> 20% of cells having a Barr body), and chromosomal analysis reveals a 47,XXY karyotype.

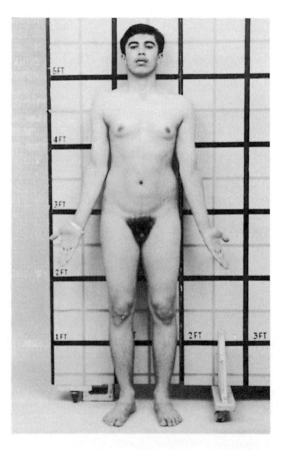

Figure 12–8. Klinefelter's syndrome in a 20-year-old man. Note relatively increased lower/upper body segment ratio, gynecomastia, small penis, and sparse body hair with a female pubic hair pattern.

Differential Diagnosis

Klinefelter's syndrome should be distinguished from other causes of hypogonadism. Small, firm testes should suggest Klinefelter's syndrome. Hypothalamic-pituitary hypogonadism may be associated with small, rubbery testes if puberty has not occurred or atrophic testes if normal puberty has occurred. The consistency of the testes in Klinefelter's syndrome is also different from that noted in acquired forms of adult seminiferous tubular damage. The elevated gonadotropins place the site of the lesion at the testicular level, and chromosomal analysis confirms the diagnosis. Chromosomal analysis is also required to differentiate classic Klinefelter's syndrome from the variant forms.

Treatment

A. MEDICAL TREATMENT

Androgen deficiency should be treated with testosterone replacement. Patients with personality defects should be virilized gradually to decrease the risk of aggressive behavior. Testosterone enanthate or cypionate, 100 mg intramuscularly, may be given every 2–4 weeks initially and increased to 200 mg every 2 weeks if well tolerated. Patients with low normal androgen levels may not require androgen replacement therapy.

B. SURGICAL TREATMENT

If gynecomastia presents a cosmetic problem, mastectomy may be performed.

Course & Prognosis

Patients generally feel better after androgen replacement therapy has begun. However, the personality defects do not improve, and these patients often require long-term psychiatric counseling. Life expectancy is not affected.

BILATERAL ANORCHIA (VANISHING TESTES SYNDROME)

Approximately 3% of phenotypic boys undergoing surgery to correct unilateral or bilateral cryptorchidism are found to have absence of one testis, and in about 1% of cryptorchid males both testes are absent. Thus, bilateral anorchia is found in approximately one out of every 20,000 males.

Etiology & Pathophysiology

Functional testicular tissue must be present during the first 14–16 weeks of embryonic development in order for wolffian duct growth and müllerian duct regression to occur and for the external genitalia to differentiate along male lines. Absence of testicular function before this time will result in varying degrees of male pseudohermaphroditism with ambiguous genitalia. Prenatal testicular injury occurring after 16 weeks of gestation as a result of trauma, vascular insufficiency, infection, or other mechanisms may result in loss of testicular tissue in an otherwise normal phenotypic male; hence the term "vanishing testes syndrome."

Testicular Pathology

In most instances, no recognizable testicular tissue has been identified despite extensive dissections. Wolffian duct structures are generally normal, and the vas deferens and testicular vessels may terminate blindly or in a mass of connective tissue in the inguinal canal or scrotum.

Clinical Features

A. SYMPTOMS AND SIGNS

At birth, patients appear to be normal phenotypic males with bilateral cryptorchidism. Growth and development are normal until secondary sexual development fails to occur at puberty. The penis remains small; pubic and axillary hair does not fully develop despite the presence of adrenal androgens; and the scrotum remains empty. If the patient does not receive androgens, eunuchoid proportions develop. Gynecomastia does not occur.

An occasional patient will undergo partial spontaneous virilization at puberty. Although anatomically no testicular tissue has been identified in such patients, catheterization studies have demonstrated higher testosterone concentrations in venous blood obtained from the spermatic veins than in the peripheral venous circulation. This suggests that functional Leydig cells are present in some patients, although they are not associated with testicular germinal epithelium or stroma.

B. LABORATORY FINDINGS

Serum testosterone concentrations are generally quite low, and both LH and FSH are markedly elevated. Serum testosterone concentrations do not rise following a chorionic gonadotropin stimulation test. Serum müllerian duct inhibitory factor levels are low. Chromosomal analysis discloses a 46,XY karyotype.

C. IMAGING STUDIES

Testicular artery arteriograms and spermatic venograms show vessels that taper and end in the inguinal canal or scrotum without an associated gonad.

D. SPECIAL EXAMINATIONS

Thorough inguinal and abdominal laparoscopic examination or retroperitoneal examination at laparotomy may locate the testes. If testicular vessels and the vas deferens are identified and found to terminate blindly together, it may be assumed that the testis is absent.

Differential Diagnosis

Bilateral cryptorchidism must be differentiated from congenital bilateral anorchia. A normal serum testosterone concentration that rises following stimulation with chorionic gonadotropin is indicative of functional Leydig cells and probable bilateral cryptorchidism. Elevated serum LH and FSH and a low testosterone that fails to rise after administration of exogenous chorionic gonadotropin indicate bilateral absence of functional testicular tissue.

Treatment

Androgen replacement therapy is discussed in the section on pharmacology (see Androgens, above).

Implantation of testicular prostheses for cosmetic purposes may be beneficial after the scrotum has enlarged in response to androgen therapy.

LEYDIG CELL APLASIA

Defective development of testicular Leydig cells is a rare cause of male pseudohermaphroditism with ambiguous genitalia.

Etiology & Pathophysiology

Testes are present in the inguinal canal and contain prepubertal-appearing tubules with Sertoli cells and spermatogonia without germinal cell maturation. The interstitial tissue has a loose myxoid appearance with an absence of Leydig cells. The syndrome is caused by inactivating mutations in the LH receptor that alters receptor signal transduction. The presence of a vas deferens and epididymis in these patients indicates that the local concentration of testosterone was high enough during embryogenesis to result in differentiation of the wolffian duct structures. However, the ambiguity of the genitalia indicates that the androgen concentration in these patients was insufficient to bring about full virilization of the external genitalia. The absence of müllerian duct structures is compatible with normal fetal secretion of müllerian duct inhibitory factor from the Sertoli cells.

Clinical Features

A. SYMPTOMS AND SIGNS

These patients may present in infancy with variable degrees of genital ambiguity, including a bifid scrotum, clitoral phallus, urogenital sinus, and blind vaginal pouch. Alternatively, they may appear as normal phenotypic females and escape detection until adolescence, when they present with primary amenorrhea, with or without normal breast development. The gonads are generally located in the inguinal canal. Axillary and pubic hair, although present, may be sparse. Mild defects may result in Leydig cell hypoplasia, a disorder whose clinical manifestations include micropenis, hypospadias, and variable suppression of fertility.

B. LABORATORY FINDINGS

Serum gonadotropins are elevated, and testosterone levels are below normal limits for a male and within the low normal range for females. There is no increase in testosterone following chorionic gonadotropin administration.

Differential Diagnosis

Leydig cell aplasia should be differentiated from the vanishing testes syndrome, from testosterone biosynthetic defects, from disorders of androgen action, and from 5α-reductase deficiency. The differential diagnostic features of these disorders are discussed in Chapter 14.

Treatment

Patients with Leydig cell aplasia respond well to the exogenous administration of testosterone, and it would be anticipated that they would be fully virilized and even develop some degree of spermatogenesis with exogenous testosterone administration. However, since the few patients that have been reported have been discovered either late in childhood or as adolescents and have been raised as females, it would be inappropriate to attempt a gender reversal at such a late period. Removal of the cryptorchid testes and feminization with exogenous estrogens would appear to be the most prudent course of therapy.

CRYPTORCHIDISM

Cryptorchidism is unilateral or bilateral absence of the testes from the scrotum because of failure of normal testicular descent from the genital ridge through the external inguinal ring. About 5% of full-term male infants have cryptorchidism. In most cases of cryptorchidism noted at birth, spontaneous testicular descent occurs during the first year of life, reducing the incidence to 0.2–0.8% by 1 year of age. Approximately 0.75% of adult males are cryptorchid. Unilateral cryptorchidism is five to ten times more common than bilateral cryptorchidism.

Almost 50% of cryptorchid testes are located at the external inguinal ring or in a high scrotal position; 19%

lie within the inguinal canal between the internal and external inguinal rings (canalicular); 9% are intra-abdominal; and 23% are ectopic, ie, located away from the normal pathway of descent from the abdominal cavity to the scrotum. Most ectopic testes are found in a superficial inguinal pouch above the external inguinal ring.

Etiology & Pathophysiology

Testicular descent usually occurs between the twelfth week of fetal development and birth. Both mechanical and hormonal factors appear to be important for this process: Cryptorchidism is common in patients with congenital defects in androgen synthesis or action and in patients with congenital gonadotropin deficiency, and experimental studies have demonstrated that dihydrotestosterone is required for normal testicular descent. These observations suggest that prenatal androgen deficiency may be of etiologic importance in the development of cryptorchidism.

It is not known whether pathologic changes in the testes are due to the effects of cryptorchidism or to intrinsic abnormalities in the gonad. Experimental studies in animals have shown that an increase in the temperature of the testes by 1.5–2 °C (2.7–3.6 °F) (the temperature differential between the abdomen and scrotum) results in depression of spermatogenesis. Serial testicular biopsies in cryptorchid patients have demonstrated partial reversal of the histologic abnormalities following surgical correction, suggesting that the extrascrotal environment is partly responsible for the observed pathologic abnormalities.

An intrinsic abnormality in the testes in patients with unilateral cryptorchidism is suggested by the observation that such patients are at increased risk for development of germ cell neoplasms in the scrotal testis. Similarly, the observation that adults with unilateral cryptorchidism surgically corrected before puberty had low sperm counts, high basal serum LH and FSH concentrations, and an exaggerated FSH response to GnRH suggests either that both testes are intrinsically abnormal or that the cryptorchid gonad somehow suppresses the function of the scrotal testis.

Pathology

Histologic studies on cryptorchid testes have demonstrated a decrease in the size of the seminiferous tubules and number of spermatogonia and an increase in peritubular tissue. The Leydig cells usually appear normal. It is unclear at what age these changes first appear. Abnormalities have been detected as early as 6 months. It is well established that the longer a testis remains cryptorchid, the more likely it is to show pathologic changes. More severe changes are generally found in intra-abdominal testes than in canalicular testes.

Clinical Features

A. SYMPTOMS AND SIGNS

There are usually no symptoms unless a complication such as testicular torsion, trauma, or malignant degeneration occurs. School-age children may have gender identity problems. Adults may complain of infertility, especially if they have a history of bilateral cryptorchidism.

Absence of one or both testes is the cardinal clinical finding. This may be associated with a small scrotum (bilateral cryptorchidism) or hemiscrotum (unilateral cryptorchidism). Signs of androgen deficiency are not present.

B. LABORATORY FINDINGS

Basal or stimulated serum FSH, LH, and testosterone concentrations are not helpful in evaluating prepubertal unilaterally cryptorchid males. However, serum FSH and LH concentrations and the testosterone response to exogenous chorionic gonadotropin are useful in differentiating cryptorchid patients from those with congenital anorchia. The latter have high basal gonadotropins, low serum testosterone, and absent or diminished testosterone rise following chorionic gonadotropin stimulation.

Postpubertal adults may have oligospermia, elevated basal serum FSH and LH concentrations, and an exaggerated FSH increase following GnRH stimulation. Such abnormalities are more prevalent in patients with a history of bilateral cryptorchidism than with unilateral cryptorchidism.

C. IMAGING STUDIES

Intravenous urography will disclose an associated abnormality of the upper urinary tract in 10% of cases—horseshoe kidney, renal hypoplasia, ureteral duplication, hydroureter, and hydronephrosis.

Differential Diagnosis

Retractile testis (pseudocryptorchidism) is due to a hyperactive cremasteric reflex, which draws the testicle into the inguinal canal. Cold temperature, fear, and genital manipulation commonly activate the reflex, which is most prominent between the ages of 5 and 6 years. The child should be examined with warm hands in a warm room. The testis can usually be "milked" into the scrotum with gentle pressure over the lower abdomen in the direction of the inguinal canal.

Bilateral anorchia is associated with elevated gonadotropins, decreased testosterone, and an absent or subnormal response to stimulation with chorionic gonadotropin.

The virilizing forms of congenital adrenal hyperplasia may result in prenatal fusion of the labial-scrotal folds and clitoral hypertrophy (Chapter 14). Severely affected females have the appearance of phenotypic males with bilateral cryptorchidism. Because of the potentially disastrous consequences (acute adrenal insufficiency) if this diagnosis is missed, a chromosomal analysis should be performed on bilaterally cryptorchid phenotypic male infants.

Complications & Sequelae

A. HERNIA

Approximately 90% of cryptorchid males have associated ipsilateral inguinal hernia resulting from failure of the processus vaginalis to close. This is rarely symptomatic.

B. TORSION

Because of the abnormal connection between the cryptorchid testis and its supporting tissues, torsion may occur. This should be suspected in any patient with abdominal or pelvic pain and an ipsilateral empty scrotum.

C. TRAUMA

Testes that lie above the pubic tubercle are particularly susceptible to traumatic injury.

D. NEOPLASMS

A cryptorchid testis is 20–30 times more likely to undergo malignant degeneration than are normal testes. The incidence of such tumors is greater in patients with intra-abdominal testes than in patients with canalicular testes. Seminomas are the neoplasms most commonly associated with maldescended testes. Because of the increased risk of neoplasia, many urologists recommend orchiectomy for a unilaterally undescended testicle in a patient first seen during or after puberty. Patients who present with bilateral cryptorchidism after puberty should have bilateral orchiopexy and testicular biopsies to preserve testicular endocrine function and to make palpation for detection of neoplasia easier.

E. INFERTILITY

Over 75% of untreated bilaterally cryptorchid males are infertile. About 30–50% of bilaterally cryptorchid patients who undergo prepubertal orchiopexy have been found to be fertile. About half of patients with untreated unilateral cryptorchidism are infertile, whereas infertility is found in less than one-fourth of such patients whose cryptorchidism is surgically repaired before puberty.

Prevention

Although cryptorchidism cannot be prevented, the complications can. It is clear that the adverse changes that take place in the testes are related in part to the location of the maldescended testis and the duration of the cryptorchidism. Most testes that are undescended at birth enter the scrotum during the first year of life. However, it is rare for a cryptorchid testis to descend spontaneously after the age of 1 year. Since adverse histologic changes have been noted around the age of 2 years, hormonal or surgical correction should be undertaken at or before that time.

Treatment

A. MEDICAL:

1. Intramuscular chorionic gonadotropin therapy—Because growth of the vas deferens and testicular descent are at least partially dependent upon androgens, stimulation of endogenous testosterone secretion by chorionic gonadotropin may correct the cryptorchidism. Cryptorchidism is corrected in less than 25% of patients treated with a course of chorionic gonadotropin, and recent studies suggest that patients with conditions that respond to hormonal therapy may actually have retractile testes rather than true cryptorchidism. Nevertheless, this therapy should be tried prior to orchiopexy, since it is innocuous and may avoid the need for surgery. For bilateral cryptorchidism, give a short course of chorionic gonadotropin consisting of 3300 units intramuscularly every other day over a 5-day period (three injections). For unilateral cryptorchidism, give 500 units intramuscularly three times a week for 6½ weeks (20 injections).

2. Intranasal GnRH therapy—GnRH given three times a day for 28 days by nasal spray has been shown to be as effective as chorionic gonadotropin injections in correcting cryptorchidism in some patients. This therapy is not approved for treatment of cryptorchidism in the USA.

B. SURGICAL TREATMENT

Several procedures have been devised to place the maldescended testis into the scrotum (orchiopexy). The operation may be performed in one or two stages. Inguinal hernia should be repaired if present.

NOONAN'S SYNDROME (MALE TURNER'S SYNDROME)

Phenotypic and genotypic males with many of the physical stigmas of classic Turner's syndrome have been described under a variety of names, including Noonan's syndrome and male Turner's syndrome. It may occur sporadically or may be familial, inherited in an autosomal dominant fashion with variable penetrance. Approximately half of the patients have a mutation in the *PTPN11* gene on chromosome 12. A number of pathologic features have been noted, including reduced seminiferous tubular size with or without sclerosis, diminished or absent germ cells, and Leydig cell hyperplasia.

Clinical Features

A. SYMPTOMS AND SIGNS

The most common clinical features are short stature, webbed neck, hypertelorism, cubitus valgus, and bleeding diathesis. Other somatic defects are variably observed in these patients. Congenital cardiac anomalies are common and involve primarily the right side of the heart—in contrast to patients with XO gonadal dysgenesis.

Cryptorchidism is frequently present. Although some affected individuals are fertile, with normal testes, most have small testes and mild to moderate hypogonadism.

B. LABORATORY FINDINGS

Serum testosterone concentrations are usually low or low normal, and serum gonadotropins are high. The karyotype is 46,XY.

Differential Diagnosis

The clinical features of Noonan's syndrome are sufficiently distinct so that confusion with other causes of hypogonadism is usually not a problem. However, a rare individual with XY/XO mosaicism may have similar somatic anomalies requiring chromosomal analysis for differentiation.

Treatment

If the patient is hypogonadal, androgen replacement therapy is indicated.

MYOTONIC DYSTROPHY

Myotonic dystrophy type 1 is one of the familial forms of muscular dystrophy. There are two types of myotonic dystrophy, but 80% of affected males with myotonic dystrophy type 1 have some degree of primary testicular failure.

The disorder is transmitted in an autosomal dominant fashion, with marked variability in expression. The underlying lesion is an expansion CTG repeat of the 3′ untranslated region of a gene that encodes a serine-threonine protein kinase located on chromosome 19.

Testicular histology varies from moderate derangement of spermatogenesis with germinal cell arrest to regional hyalinization and fibrosis of the seminiferous tubules. The Leydig cells are usually preserved and may appear in clumps.

The testes are normal in affected prepubertal individuals, and puberty generally proceeds normally. Testosterone secretion is normal, and secondary sexual characteristics develop. After puberty, seminiferous tubular atrophy results in a decrease in testicular size and change of consistency from firm to soft or mushy. Infertility is a consequence of disrupted spermatogenesis. If testicular hyalinization and fibrosis are extensive, Leydig cell function may also be impaired.

Clinical Features

A. SYMPTOMS AND SIGNS

The disease usually becomes apparent in adulthood. Progressive weakness and atrophy of the facial, neck, hand, and lower extremity muscles is commonly observed. Severe atrophy of the temporalis muscles, ptosis due to weakness of the levator muscles of the eye with compensatory wrinkling of the forehead muscles, and frontal baldness comprise the myopathic facies characteristic of the disorder. Myotonia is present in several muscle groups and is characterized by inability to relax the muscle normally after a strong contraction.

Testicular atrophy is not noted until adulthood, and most patients develop and maintain normal facial and body hair growth and libido. Gynecomastia is usually not present.

Associated features include mental retardation, cataracts, cranial hyperostosis, diabetes mellitus, and primary hypothyroidism.

B. LABORATORY FINDINGS

Serum testosterone is normal to slightly decreased. FSH is uniformly elevated in patients with atrophic testes. LH is also frequently elevated, even in patients with normal serum testosterone levels. Leydig cell reserve is generally diminished, with subnormal increases in serum testosterone following stimulation with chorionic gonadotropin. An excessive rise in FSH and, to a lesser extent, LH is found following GnRH stimulation.

Differential Diagnosis

Myotonic dystrophy type 1 should be distinguished from proximal myotonic myopathy, and myotonic dystrophy type 2. All may be associated with primary hypogonadism but have different clinical features and do not exhibit myotonic dystrophy type 1 mutations.

Treatment

There is no therapy that will prevent progressive muscular atrophy in this disorder. Testosterone replacement therapy is not indicated unless the serum testosterone levels are subnormal.

ADULT SEMINIFEROUS TUBULE FAILURE

Adult seminiferous tubule failure encompasses a spectrum of pathologic alterations of the seminiferous tubules that results in hypospermatogenesis, germinal cell arrest, germinal cell aplasia, and tubular hyalinization. Almost half of infertile males exhibit some degree of isolated seminiferous tubule failure.

Etiology, Pathology, & Pathophysiology

Etiologic factors in seminiferous tubule failure include mumps or gonococcal orchitis, leprosy, cryptorchidism, irradiation, uremia, alcoholism, paraplegia, lead poisoning, and therapy with antineoplastic agents such as cyclophosphamide, chlorambucil, vincristine, methotrexate, and procarbazine. Vascular insufficiency resulting from spermatic artery damage during herniorrhaphy, testicular torsion, or sickle cell anemia may also selectively damage the tubules. Similar pathologic changes may be found in oligospermic patients with varicoceles. In many patients, no etiologic factors can be identified, and the condition is referred to as "idiopathic."

The rapidly dividing germinal epithelium is more susceptible to injury than are the Sertoli or Leydig cells. Thus, pressure necrosis (eg, mumps or gonococcal orchitis), increased testicular temperature (eg, cryptorchidism and perhaps varicocele and paraplegia), and the direct cytotoxic effects of irradiation, alcohol, lead, and chemotherapeutic agents primarily injure the germ cells. Although the Sertoli and Leydig cells appear to be morphologically normal, severe testicular injury may result in functional alterations in these cells.

Several different lesions may be found in testicular biopsy specimens. The pathologic process may involve the entire testes or may appear in patches. The least severe lesion is hypospermatogenesis, in which all stages of spermatogenesis are present but there is a decrease in the number of germinal epithelial cells. Some degree of peritubular fibrosis may be present. Cessation of development at the primary spermatocyte or spermatogonial stage of the spermatogenic cycle is classified as germinal cell arrest. More severely affected testes may demonstrate a complete absence of germ cells with maintenance or morphologically normal Sertoli cells (Sertoli cell only syndrome). The most severe lesion is fibrosis or hyalinization of the tubules. This latter pattern may be indistinguishable from that seen in Klinefelter's syndrome.

Irrespective of the etiologic factors involved in damage to the germinal epithelium, the alterations in spermatogenesis result in oligospermia. If the damage is severe, as in the Sertoli cell only syndrome or tubular hyalinization, azoospermia may be present. Since testicular volume consists chiefly of tubules, some degree of testicular atrophy is often present in these patients. Some patients have elevations in basal serum FSH concentrations and demonstrate a hyperresponsive FSH rise following GnRH, suggesting that the Sertoli cells are functionally abnormal despite their normal histologic appearance.

Clinical Features

A. SYMPTOMS AND SIGNS

Infertility is usually the only complaint. Mild to moderate testicular atrophy may be present. Careful examination should be made for the presence of varicocele by palpating the spermatic cord during Valsalva's maneuver with the patient in the upright position. The patients are fully virilized, and gynecomastia is not present.

B. LABORATORY FINDINGS

Semen analysis shows oligospermia or azoospermia, and serum testosterone and LH concentrations are normal. Basal serum FSH levels may be normal or high, and an excessive FSH rise following GnRH may be present.

Differential Diagnosis

Patients with hypothalamic or pituitary disorders may have oligospermia or azoospermia and testicular atrophy. The serum FSH and LH concentrations are often in the low normal range, and the testosterone level is usually (not always) diminished. The presence of neurologic and ophthalmologic abnormalities, diabetes insipidus, anterior pituitary trophic hormone deficiencies, or an elevated serum PRL concentration distinguishes these patients from those with primary seminiferous tubule failure. Other causes of primary testicular failure are associated either with clinical signs and symptoms of androgen deficiency or with enough somatic abnormalities to allow differentiation from isolated seminiferous tubule failure.

Prevention

In many instances, damage to the seminiferous tubules cannot be prevented. Early correction of cryptorchidism, adequate shielding of the testes during diagnostic radiologic procedures or radiotherapy, and limitation of the total dose of chemotherapeutic agents may prevent or ameliorate the adverse effects.

Treatment

A. MEDICAL

Attempts to treat oligospermia and infertility medically have included testosterone rebound therapy, low-dose testosterone, exogenous gonadotropins, thyroid hormone therapy, vitamins, and clomiphene citrate. None of these agents have been found to be uniformly beneficial, and several may actually lead to a decrease in the sperm count.

B. SURGICAL

Some of the pathologic changes in the testes have been reversed by early orchiopexy in cryptorchid individuals. If a varicocele is found in an oligospermic, infertile male, it should be ligated.

Course & Prognosis

Patients who have received up to 300 cGy of testicular irradiation may show partial or full recovery of spermatogenesis months to years following exposure. The prognosis for recovery is better for individuals who receive the irradiation over a short interval than for those who are exposed over several weeks.

Recovery of spermatogenesis may also occur months to years following administration of chemotherapeutic agents. The most important factor determining prognosis is the total dose of chemotherapy administered.

Improvement in the quality of the semen is found in 60–80% of patients following successful repair of varicocele. Restoration of fertility has been reported in about half of such patients.

The prognosis for spontaneous improvement of idiopathic oligospermia due to infection or infarction is poor.

ADULT LEYDIG CELL FAILURE (ANDROPAUSE)

In contrast to the menopause in women, men do not experience an abrupt decline or cessation of gonadal function. However, a gradual diminution of testicular function does occur in many men as part of the aging process (see Chapter 25). It is not known how many men develop symptoms directly attributable to this phenomenon.

Etiology, Pathology, & Pathophysiology

After age 50, there is a gradual decrease in the total serum testosterone concentration, although the actual values remain within the normal range. The levels of free testosterone decrease to a greater extent because of an increase in SHBG. The testosterone production rate declines, and Leydig cell responsiveness to hCG also decreases. A gradual compensatory increase in serum LH levels has also been noted. Aging also is associated with alterations in the hypothalamic-pituitary portion of the axis.

Histologic studies of the aging testes have shown patchy degenerative changes in the seminiferous tubules with a reduction in number and volume of Leydig cells. The pathologic changes are first noted in the regions most remote from the arterial blood supply. Thus, microvascular insufficiency may be the etiologic basis for the histologic tubular changes and the decrease in Leydig cell function noted with aging. In addition, virtually all of the conditions that cause adult seminiferous tubule failure may lead to Leydig cell dysfunction if testicular injury is severe enough.

Clinical Features

A. SYMPTOMS AND SIGNS

A great many symptoms have been attributed to the male climacteric (andropause), including decreased libido and potency, emotional instability, fatigue, decreased strength, decreased concentrating ability, vasomotor instability (palpitations, hot flushes, diaphoresis), and a variety of diffuse aches and pains. There are usually no associated signs unless the testicular injury is severe. In such patients, a decrease in testicular volume and consistency may be present as well as gynecomastia.

B. LABORATORY FINDINGS

Serum testosterone may be low or low normal; serum LH concentration is usually high normal or slightly high. Oligospermia is usually present. Bone mineral density may be decreased.

C. SPECIAL EXAMINATIONS

Because many men with complaints compatible with Leydig cell failure have testosterone and LH concentrations within the normal adult range, a diagnostic trial of testosterone therapy may be attempted. The test is best performed double-blind over an 8-week period. During the first or last 4 weeks, the patient receives testosterone enanthate, 200 mg intramuscularly per week; during the other 4-week period, placebo injections are administered. The patient is interviewed by the physician 2 weeks after the last course of injections. After the interview, the code is broken; if the patient notes amelioration of symptoms during the period of androgen administration but not during the placebo period, the diagnosis of adult Leydig cell failure is substantiated. If the patient experiences no subjective improvement following testosterone, of if improvement is noted following both placebo and testosterone injections, Leydig cell failure is effectively ruled out.

Differential Diagnosis

Erectile dysfunction from vascular, neurologic, or psychologic causes must be distinguished from Leydig cell failure. A therapeutic trial of androgen therapy will not help erectile dysfunction that is not due to androgen deficiency.

Treatment

Androgen replacement therapy is the treatment of choice for both symptomatic and asymptomatic Leydig cell failure. This results in increases in lean body mass, bone mineral density, hemoglobin, libido, strength, and sense of well being and decreases in total and HDL cholesterol and urine hydroxyproline.

MALE INFERTILITY

About 15% of married couples are unable to produce offspring. Male factors are responsible in about 40% of cases, female factors in about 40%, and couple factors in 20%.

Etiology & Pathophysiology

In order for conception to occur, spermatogenesis must be normal, the sperm must complete its maturation during transport through patent ducts, adequate amounts of seminal plasma must be added to provide volume and nutritional elements, and the male must be able to deposit the semen near the female's cervix. Any defect in this pathway can result in infertility due to a male factor problem. The spermatozoa must also be able to penetrate the cervical mucus and reach the uterine tubes, where conception takes place. These latter events may fail to occur if there are female reproductive tract disorders or abnormalities of sperm motility or fertilizing capacity.

Table 12–4 lists the identified causes of male infertility. Disturbances in the function of the hypothalamus, pituitary, adrenals, or thyroid are found in approximately 4% of males evaluated for infertility. Sex chromosome abnormalities, cryptorchidism, adult seminiferous tubule failure, and other forms of primary testicular failure are found in 15% of infertile males. Congenital or acquired ductal problems are found in approximately 6% of such patients, and poor coital technique, sexual dysfunction, ejaculatory disturbances, and anatomic abnormalities such as hypospadias are causative factors in 4–5% of patients evaluated for infertility. Idiopathic infertility, in which no cause can be identified with certainty, accounts for approximately

Table 12–4. Causes of male infertility.

Endocrine
  Hypothalamic-pituitary disorders
  Testicular disorders
  Defects of androgen action
  Hyperthyroidism
  Hypothyroidism
  Adrenal insufficiency
  Congenital adrenal hyperplasia

Systemic illness

Defects in spermatogenesis
  Immotile cilia syndrome
  Drug-induced
  Adult seminiferous tubule failure

Ductal obstruction
  Congenital
  Acquired

Seminal vesicle disease

Prostatic disease

Varicocele

Retrograde ejaculation

Antibodies to sperm or seminal plasma

Anatomic defects of the penis

Poor coital technique

Sexual dysfunction

Idiopathic

35% of patients. Some of these patients may have mild forms of androgen receptor defects, microdeletions of the Y chromosome, or mutations in the cystic fibrosis gene. Autoimmune disturbances that lead to sperm agglutination and immobilization causes infertility in only a small fraction of patients. Varicoceles are found in 25–40% of patients classified as having idiopathic infertility. The significance of this finding is uncertain, since 8–20% of males in the general population have varicoceles.

Clinical Features

A. SYMPTOMS AND SIGNS

The clinical features of the hypothalamic-pituitary, thyroid, adrenal, testicular, and sexual dysfunctional disorders have been discussed in preceding sections of this chapter. Evaluation for the presence of varicocele has also been described.

Patients with immotile cilia syndrome have associated mucociliary transport defects in the lower airways that result in chronic pulmonary obstructive disease. Some patients with this disorder also have Kartagener's syndrome, with sinusitis, bronchiectasis, and situs inversus. Infections of the epididymis or vas deferens may be asymptomatic or associated with scrotal pain that may radiate to the flank, fever, epididymal swelling and tenderness, and urethral discharge. The presence of thickened, enlarged epididymis and vas is indicative of chronic epididymitis. Chronic prostatitis is usually asymptomatic, although a perineal aching sensation or low back pain may be described. A boggy or indurated prostate may be found on rectal palpation. A careful examination for the presence of penile anatomic abnormalities such as chordee, hypospadias, or epispadias should be made, since these defects may prevent the deposit of sperms in the vagina.

B. Laboratory Findings

A carefully collected and performed semen analysis is mandatory. A normal report indicates normal endocrine function and spermatogenesis and an intact transport system. Semen analysis should be followed by a postcoital test, which consists of examining a cervical mucus sample obtained within 2 hours after intercourse. The presence of large numbers of motile spermatozoa in mucus obtained from the internal os of the cervix rules out the male factor as a cause of infertility. If a postcoital test reveals necrospermia (dead sperms), asthenospermia (slow-moving sperms), or agglutination of sperms, examination of the female partner for the presence of sperm-immobilizing antibodies or cervical mucus abnormalities should be carried out.

If semen analysis shows abnormalities, at least two more specimens should be obtained at monthly intervals. Persistent oligospermia or azoospermia should be evaluated by studies outlined in Figure 12–7.

The female partner should be thoroughly examined to verify patency of the uterus and uterine tubes, normal ovulation, and normal cervical mucus. This examination must be done even in the presence of a male factor abnormality, since infertility is due to a combination of male and female factors in about 20% of cases.

Treatment

A. Endocrine Disorders

Correction of hyperthyroidism, hypothyroidism, adrenal insufficiency, and congenital adrenal hyperplasia generally restores fertility. Patients with hypogonadotropic hypogonadism may have spermatogenesis initiated with gonadotropin therapy. Chorionic gonadotropin (2000 units intramuscularly three times per week) with urofollitropin or follitropin beta (75 units intramuscularly three times per week) added after

12–18 months if sperms do not appear in the ejaculate, will restore spermatogenesis in most hypogonadotropic men. The sperm count following such therapy usually does not exceed 10 million/mL but may still allow impregnation. Patients with isolated deficiency of LH may respond to chorionic gonadotropin alone. There is no effective therapy for adult seminiferous tubule failure not associated with varicocele or cryptorchidism. However, if the oligospermia is mild (10–20 million/mL), cup insemination of the female partner with concentrates of semen may be tried. In vitro fertilization and other assisted reproductive techniques, including direct injection of a spermatozoon into an egg (intracytoplasmic sperm injection; ICSI), are increasingly being utilized as a method for achieving pregnancy in couples in which the male is oligospermic.

B. Defects of Spermatogenesis

There is no treatment for immotile cilia syndrome or for chromosomal abnormalities associated with defective spermatogenesis. Drugs that interfere with spermatogenesis should be discontinued. These include the antimetabolites, phenytoin, marijuana, alcohol, monoamine oxidase inhibitors, sulfasalazine, and nitrofurantoin. Discontinuing use of these agents may be accompanied by restoration of normal sperm density. In some patients with maturation arrest, severe hypospermatogenesis or incomplete Sertoli cell only, retrieval of sperms through testicular aspiration or testicular biopsy followed by IVF or ICSI have resulted in pregnancies.

C. Ductal Obstruction

Localized obstruction of the vas deferens may be treated by vasovasotomy. Sperm are detected in the ejaculate of 60–80% of patients following this procedure. However, the subsequent fertility rate is only 30–35%; the presence of antisperm antibodies that agglutinate or immobilize sperms probably accounts for the high failure rate.

Epididymovasostomy may be performed for epididymal obstruction. Sperm in the postoperative ejaculate have been found in approximately half of patients treated with this procedure, but subsequent fertility has been demonstrated in only 20% of cases.

D. Genital Tract Infections

Acute prostatitis may be treated with daily sitz baths, prostatic massage, and antibiotics. A combination of trimethoprim (400 mg) and sulfamethoxazole (2000 mg), twice a day for 10 days followed by the same dosage once a day for another 20 days, has been used with some success. Acute epididymitis may respond to injections of local anesthetic into the spermatic cord just above the testicle. Appropriate antibiotic therapy should also be given. The prognosis for fertility following severe bilateral chronic epididymitis or extensive scarring from acute epididymitis is poor.

E. VARICOCELE

The presence of varicocele in an infertile male with oligospermia is an indication for surgical ligation of the incompetent spermatic veins. Improvement in the semen is noted in 60–80% of treated patients, and about half are subsequently fertile.

F. RETROGRADE EJACULATION

Ejaculation of semen into the urinary bladder may occur following disruption of the internal bladder sphincter or with neuropathic disorders such as diabetic autonomic neuropathy. Normal ejaculation has been restored in a few patients with the latter problem following administration of phenylpropanolamine, 15 mg orally twice daily in timed-release capsules. Sperm can also be recovered from the bladder following masturbation for the purpose of direct insemination of the female partner.

G. ANTIBODIES TO SPERM OR SEMINAL PLASMA

Antibodies in the female genital tract that agglutinate or immobilize sperms may be difficult to treat. Older methods such as condom therapy or administration of glucocorticoids have not been uniformly successful. Currently, intrauterine insemination with washed spermatozoa, in vitro fertilization, and gamete intrafallopian transfer are considered the most effective treatments.

H. ANATOMIC DEFECTS OF THE PENIS

Patients with hypospadias, epispadias, or severe chordee may collect semen by masturbation for use in insemination.

I. POOR COITAL TECHNIQUE

Couples should be counseled not to use vaginal lubricants or postcoital douches. In order to maximize the sperm count in cases of borderline oligospermia, intercourse should not be more frequent than every other day. Exposure of the cervix to the seminal plasma is increased by having the woman lie supine with her knees bent up for 20 minutes after intercourse.

Course & Prognosis

The prognosis for fertility depends upon the underlying cause. It is good for patients with nontesticular endocrine abnormalities, varicoceles, retrograde ejaculation, and anatomic defects of the penis. If fertility cannot be restored, the couple should be counseled regarding artificial donor insemination, in vitro fertilization, or adoption.

ERECTILE DYSFUNCTION (IMPOTENCE)

Erectile dysfunction is the inability to achieve or maintain an erection of sufficient duration and firmness to complete satisfactory sexual activity in more than 25% of attempts. It may occur with or without associated disturbances of libido or ejaculation. Approximately 5% of men are completely impotent by age 40, and 15% by age 70. Some degree of erectile dysfunction is present in about 50% of men between ages 40 and 70.

Etiology & Pathophysiology

Penile erection occurs when blood flow to the penile erectile tissue (corpora cavernosa and spongiosum) increases as a result of dilation of the urethral artery, the artery of the bulb of the penis, the deep artery of the penis, and the dorsal artery of the penis following psychogenic or sensory stimuli transmitted to the limbic system and then to the thoracolumbar and sacral autonomic nervous system. The relaxation of the cavernosal arterial and cavernosal trabecular sinusoidal smooth muscles occurs following stimulation of the sacral parasympathetic (S2–4) nerves, which results in the release of acetylcholine, vasoactive intestinal peptide, and an endothelial cell-derived nitric oxide, which activates guanylyl cyclase. As the sinusoids become engorged, the subtunical venous plexus is compressed against the tunica albuginea, preventing egress of blood from the penis. Contraction of the bulbocavernosus muscle through stimulation of the somatic portion of the S2–4 pudendal nerves further increases the intracavernosal pressure. These processes result in the distention, engorgement, and rigidity of the penis that constitute erection.

Broadly speaking, erectile dysfunction may be divided into psychogenic and organic causes. Major epidemiologic factors that have been associated with erectile dysfunction include diabetes, hypertension, depression, smoking, aging, low HDL cholesterol, and a low serum DHEA sulfate level. Table 12–5 lists various pathologic conditions and drugs that may be associated with erectile dysfunction.

Most organic causes of erectile dysfunction result from disturbances in the neurologic pathways essential for the initiation and maintenance of erection or in the blood supply to the penis. Many of the endocrine disorders, systemic illnesses, and drugs associated with erectile dysfunction affect libido, the autonomic pathways essential for erection, or the blood flow to the penis.

Table 12–5. Organic causes of erectile dysfunction.

Neurologic
  Anterior temporal lobe lesions
  Spinal cord lesions
  Autonomic neuropathy
Vascular
  Leriche's syndrome
  Pelvic vascular insufficiency
  Sickle cell disease
  Venous leaks
  ?Aging
Endocrine
  Diabetes mellitus
  Hypogonadism
  Hyperprolactinemia
  Adrenal insufficiency
  Feminizing tumors
  Hypothyroidsm
  Hyperthroidism
Urogenital
  Trauma
  Castration
  Priapism
  Peyronie's disease
Systemic illness
  Cardiac insufficiency
  Cirrhosis
  Uremia
  Respiratory insufficiency
  Lead poisoning
Postoperative
  Aortoilliac or aortofemoral reconstruction
  Lumbar sympathectomy
  Perineal prostatectomy
  Retroperitoneal dissection
Drugs
  Endocrinologic
    Antiandrogens
    Estrogens
    5α-Reductase inhibitors
    GnRH agonists
  Antihypertensives
  Diuretics
  Psychotropic agents
  Tranquilizers
  Monoamine oxidase inhibitors
  Tricyclic antidepressants
    Other
    Tobacco
    Alcohol
    Opioids
    H_2-receptor antagonists
    Gemfibrozil
    Amphetamines
    Cocaine

Venous incompetence because of anatomic defects in the corpora cavernosa or subtunical venous plexus is being recognized with increasing frequency. Local urogenital disorders such as Peyronie's disease (idiopathic fibrosis of the covering sheath of the corpus cavernosum) may mechanically interfere with erection. In some patients, the cause of erectile dysfunction is multifactorial. For example, some degree of erectile dysfunction is reported by over 50% of men with diabetes mellitus. The basis of the erectile dysfunction is usually autonomic neuropathy. However, vascular insufficiency, antihypertensive medication, uremia, and depression may also cause or contribute to the problem in diabetics.

Clinical Features

A. SYMPTOMS AND SIGNS

Patients may complain of constant or episodic inability to initiate or maintain an erection, decreased penile turgidity, decreased libido, or a combination of these difficulties. Besides the specific sexual dysfunction symptoms, symptoms and signs of a more pervasive emotional or psychiatric problem may be elicited. If an underlying neurologic, vascular, or systemic disorder is the cause of erectile dysfunction, additional symptoms and signs referable to the anatomic or metabolic disturbances may be present. A history of claudication of the buttocks or lower extremities should direct attention toward arterial insufficiency.

The differentiation between psychogenic and organic erectile dysfunction can usually be made on the basis of the history. Even though the patient may be selectively unable to obtain or maintain a satisfactory erection to complete sexual intercourse, a history of repeated normal erections at other times is indicative of psychogenic erectile dysfunction. Thus, a history of erections that occur nocturnally, during masturbation, or during foreplay or with other sexual partners eliminates significant neurologic, vascular, or endocrine causes of erectile dysfunction. Patients with psychogenic erectile dysfunction often note a sudden onset of sexual dysfunction concurrently with a significant event in their lives such as loss of a friend or relative, an extramarital affair, or the loss of a job.

Patients with organic erectile dysfunction generally note a more gradual and global loss of potency. Initially, such individuals may be able to achieve erections with strong sexual stimuli, but ultimately they may be unable to achieve a fully turgid erection under any circumstances. In contrast to patients with psychogenic erectile dysfunction, patients with organic erectile dysfunction generally maintain a normal libido. However, patients with systemic illness may have a concurrent diminution of libido and potency. Hypogonadism should be suspected in a patient who has never had an erection (primary erectile dysfunction).

During the physical examination, the patient's secondary sexual characteristics should be assessed and examination performed for gynecomastia, discordant or diminished femoral pulses, reduced testicular volume or consistency, penile plaques, and evidence of peripheral or autonomic neuropathy. The bulbocavernosus reflex tests the integrity of the S2–4 nerves. It is performed by inserting a finger into the patient's rectum while squeezing his glans penis. Contraction of the anal musculature represents a normal response.

B. LABORATORY FINDINGS AND SPECIAL EXAMINATIONS

Serum testosterone measurements may uncover a mild and otherwise asymptomatic androgen deficiency. If the testosterone level is low, serum PRL should be measured since hyperprolactinemia—whether drug-induced or due to a pituitary or hypothalamic lesion—may inhibit androgen production. Because diabetes mellitus is a relatively common cause of erectile dysfunction and because erectile dysfunction may be the presenting symptom of diabetes, fasting and 2-hour postprandial blood glucose measurements should be ordered.

In a patient with a normal physical examination and screening blood tests, many clinicians elect to begin with a therapeutic trial of 50 mg of oral sildenafil (Viagra), a type 5 phosphodiesterase inhibitor that potentiates the effects of nitric oxide by inhibiting the breakdown of cyclic guanosine monophosphate. This should be tried only if the patient is not taking nitrates, has not had a myocardial infarction in the last 6 months, and does not have unstable angina, hypotension, severe congestive heart failure, or retinitis pigmentosa.

The integrity of the neurologic pathways and the ability of the blood vessels to deliver a sufficient amount of blood to the penis for erection to occur may be objectively examined by placement of a strain gauge behind the glans penis and at the base of the penis at the time the patient retires for sleep. The occurrence of nocturnal penile tumescence can thus be recorded. Healthy men and those with psychogenic erectile dysfunction have three to five erections a night associated with rapid eye movement (REM) sleep. Absence or reduced frequency of nocturnal tumescence indicates an organic lesion. Penile rigidity as well as tumescence can be evaluated with an ambulatory monitor called Rigi-Scan. The vascular integrity of the penis may be examined by Doppler ultrasonography with spectral analysis following intracorporeal injection of a vasoactive drug.

This method allows detection of venous leaks with a sensitivity of 55–100% and specificity of 69–88%. Arterial problems are also detected with a sensitivity of 82–100% and specificity of 64–96%. The choice of other laboratory tests such as cavernosometry, cavernosography, or arteriography depends upon associated organic symptoms or signs.

Treatment

Discontinuation of an offending drug usually results in a return of potency. Similarly, effective therapy of an underlying systemic or endocrine disorder may cure the erectile dysfunction. For psychogenic erectile dysfunction, simple reassurance and explanation, formal psychotherapy, and various forms of behavioral therapy have a reported 40–70% success rate. Sildenafil taken about 1 hour before anticipated intercourse is approximately 70–80% effective in patients with a wide variety of causes of erectile dysfunction, including psychogenic ones. This agent is absolutely contraindicated in men receiving oral or transdermal nitrates for vascular disease. Side effects include headache (16%) and visual disturbances (3%).

Vasoactive drugs including prostaglandin E_1, papaverine hydrochloride, and phentolamine mesylate, either alone or in combination, may induce an erection following intracavernous injection. Of these, the only FDA-approved agent is prostaglandin E_1 (alprostadil), which needs to be individualized within the dosage range of 2.5–60 μg per injection. In clinical studies, up to 90% of men with erectile dysfunction developed erections with intracavernosal injections. Side effects include penile pain (33% of patients), hematoma (3%), penile fibrosis (3%), and priapism (0.4%). Intraurethral insertion of a 1.4 mm pellet containing alprostadil leads to satisfactory erections in two-thirds of patients, with effect beginning within 10 minutes and lasting 30–60 minutes). The major side effects are penile pain (36%), urethral pain (13%), and dizziness (4%).

Devices have been developed that use suction to induce penile engorgement and constrictive bands to maintain the ensuing erection. Erections are achieved in 90% of patients with an approximately 70% couple satisfaction rate. Alternatively, a surgically implanted semirigid or inflatable penile prosthesis provides satisfactory results in 85–90% of cases, but the device must be replaced every 5–10 years.

Repair of venous leaks and microsurgical revascularization of arterial lesions have had variable success rates. Patients with permanent erectile dysfunction due to organic lesions that cannot be corrected should be counseled in noncoital sensate focus techniques.

GYNECOMASTIA

Gynecomastia is common during the neonatal period and is present in about 70% of pubertal males (Chapter 15). Clinically apparent gynecomastia has been noted at autopsy in almost 1% of adult males, and 40% of autopsied males have histologic evidence of gynecomastia.

Etiology & Pathophysiology

The causes of gynecomastia are listed in Table 12–6. Several mechanisms have been proposed to account for this disorder. All involve a relative imbalance between estrogen and androgen concentrations or action at the mammary gland level. Decrease in free testosterone may be due to primary gonadal disease or an increase in SHBG as is found in hyperthyroidism and some forms of liver disease (eg, alcoholic cirrhosis). Decreased androgen action in patients with the androgen insensitivity syndromes results in unopposed estrogen action on the breast glandular tissue. Acute or chronic excessive stimulation of the Leydig cells by pituitary gonadotropins alters the steroidogenic pathways and favors excessive estrogen and estrogen precursor secretion relative to testosterone production. This mechanism may be responsible for the gynecomastia found with hypergonadotropic states such as Klinefelter's syndrome and adult Leydig cell failure. The rise of gonadotropins during puberty may lead to an estrogen-androgen imbalance by similar mechanisms. Patients who are malnourished or have systemic illness may develop gynecomastia during refeeding or treatment of the underlying disorder. Malnourishment and chronic illness are accompanied by a reduction in gonadotropin secretion, and during recovery the gonadotropins rise and may stimulate excessive Leydig cell production of estrogens relative to testosterone.

Table 12–6. Causes of gynecomastia.

Physiologic	*Psychoactive agents*
Neonatal	Diazepam
Pubertal	Haloperidol
Involutional	Phenothiazines
Drug-induced	Tricyclic antidepressants
Hormones	*Drugs of abuse*
Androgens and anabolic steroids	Alcohol
Chorionic gonadotropin	Amphetamines
Estrogens and estrogen agonists	Heroin
Growth hormone	Marijuana
Antiandrogens or inhibitors of androgen synthesis	*Other*
Cyproterone	Phenytoin
Flutamide	Penicillamine
Antibiotics	**Endocrine**
Isoniazid	Primary hypogonadism with Leydig cell damage
Ketoconazole	Hyperprolactinemia
Metronidazole	Hyperthyroidism
Antiulcer medications	Androgen receptor disorders
Cimetidine	Excessive aromatase activity
Omeprazole	**Systemic diseases**
Ranitidine	Hepatic cirrhosis
Cancer chemotherapeutic agents (especially alkylating agents)	Uremia
Cardiovascular drugs	Recovery from malnourishment
Amiodarone	**Neoplasms**
Captopril	Testicular germ cell or Leydig cell tumors
Digitoxin	Feminizing adrenocortical adenoma or carcinoma
Enalapril	hCG-secreting nontrophoblastic neoplasms
Methyldopa	**Idiopathic**
Nifedipine	
Reserpine	
Spironolactone	
Verapamil	

Excessive stimulation of Leydig cells may also occur in patients with hCG-producing trophoblastic or non-trophoblastic tumors. In addition, some of these tumors are able to convert estrogen precursors into estradiol. Feminizing adrenocortical and Leydig cell neoplasms may directly secrete excessive quantities of estrogens. The mechanisms by which PRL-secreting pituitary tumors and hyperprolactinemia produce gynecomastia are unclear. Elevated serum PRL levels may lower testosterone production and diminish the peripheral actions of testosterone, which may result in an excessive estrogen effect on the breast that is not counteracted by androgens.

Drugs such as phenothiazines, methyldopa, and reserpine may induce gynecomastia through elevations of PRL. Other drugs may reduce androgen production (eg, spironolactone), peripherally antagonize androgen action (spironolactone, cimetidine), or interact with breast estrogen receptors (spironolactone, digitoxin, phytoestrogens in marijuana).

Finally, it has been proposed that patients with idiopathic and familial gynecomastia have breast glandular tissue that is inordinately sensitive to normal circulating levels of estrogen or excessively converts estrogen precursors to estrogens.

Pathology

Three histologic patterns of gynecomastia have been recognized. The florid pattern consists of an increase in the number of budding ducts, proliferation of the ductal epithelium, periductal edema, and a cellular fibroblastic stroma. The fibrous type has dilated ducts, minimal duct epithelial proliferation, no periductal edema, and a virtually acellular fibrous stroma. An intermediate pattern contains features of both types.

Although it has been proposed that different causes of gynecomastia are associated with either the florid or the fibrous pattern, it appears that the duration of gynecomastia is the most important factor in determining the pathologic picture. Approximately 75% of patients with gynecomastia of 4 months' duration or less exhibit the florid pattern, while 90% of patients with gynecomastia lasting a year or more have the fibrous type. Between 4 months and 1 year, 60% of patients have the intermediate pattern.

Clinical Features

A. Symptoms and Signs

The principal complaint is unilateral or bilateral concentric enlargement of breast glandular tissue. Nipple or breast pain is present in one-fourth of patients and objective tenderness in about 40%. A complaint of nipple discharge can be elicited in 4% of cases. Histologic examination has demonstrated that gynecomastia is almost always bilateral, although grossly it may be detected only on one side. The patient will often complain of discomfort in one breast despite obvious bilateral gynecomastia. Breast or nipple discomfort generally lasts less than 1 year. Chronic gynecomastia is usually asymptomatic, with the major complaint being the cosmetic one.

Symptoms and signs of underlying disorders may be present. Gynecomastia may be the earliest manifestation of an hCG-secreting testicular tumor; therefore, it is mandatory that careful examination of the testes be performed in any patient with gynecomastia. Enlargement, asymmetry, and induration of a testis may be noted in such patients.

B. Laboratory Findings

Once pubertal and drug-induced gynecomastia have been excluded, a biochemical screen for liver and renal abnormalities should be performed. If those are normal, then serum hCG, LH, testosterone, and estradiol levels should be measured. The interpretation of the results is outlined in Figure 12–9.

Differential Diagnosis

Gynecomastia should be differentiated from lipomas, neurofibromas, carcinoma of the breast, and obesity. Breast lipomas, neurofibromas, and carcinoma are usually unilateral, painless, and eccentric, whereas gynecomastia characteristically begins in the subareolar areas and enlarges concentrically. The differentiation between gynecomastia and enlarged breasts due to obesity may be difficult. The patient should be supine. Examination is performed by spreading the thumb and index fingers and gently palpating the breasts during slow apposition of the fingers toward the nipple. In this manner, a concentric ridge of tissue can be felt in patients with gynecomastia but not in obese patients without glandular tissue enlargement. The examination may be facilitated by applying soap and water to the breasts.

Complications & Sequelae

There are no complications other than possible psychologic damage from the cosmetic defect. Patients with gynecomastia may have a slightly increased risk of development of breast carcinoma.

Treatment

A. Medical Treatment

The underlying disease should be corrected if possible, and offending drugs should be discontinued. Antiestrogens, such as tamoxifen, and aromatase inhibitors have

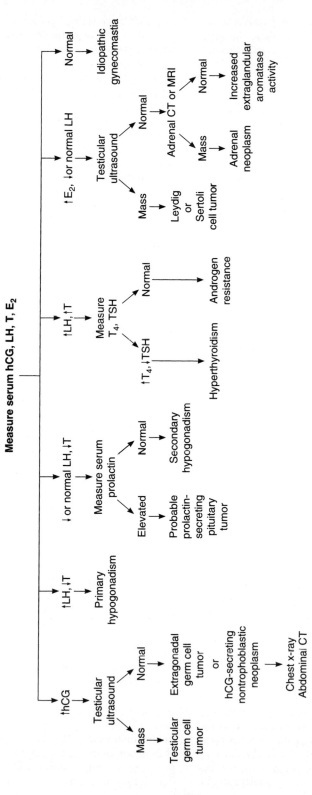

Figure 12–9. Diagnostic evaluation for endocrine causes of gynecomastia. (hCG, human chorionic gonadotropin; LH, luteinizing hormone; T, testosterone; E₂, estradiol; T₄, thyroxine; TSH, thyrotropic hormone.) (Reproduced, with permission, from Braunstein GD: Gynecomastia. N Engl J Med 1993;328:490.)

been found useful for relieving pain and reversing gynecomastia in a few patients. Whether these therapies will be useful in most patients with gynecomastia remains to be seen.

B. SURGICAL TREATMENT

Reduction mammoplasty should be considered for cosmetic reasons in any patient with long-standing gynecomastia that is in the fibrotic stage.

C. RADIOLOGIC TREATMENT

Patients with prostatic carcinoma may receive low-dose radiation therapy (900 cGy or less) to the breasts before initiation of estrogen therapy. This may prevent or diminish the gynecomastia that usually results from such therapy. Radiotherapy should not be given to other patients with gynecomastia.

Course & Prognosis

Pubertal gynecomastia usually regresses spontaneously over 1–2 years. Patients who develop drug-induced gynecomastia generally have complete or near-complete regression of the breast changes if the drug is discontinued during the early florid stage. Once gynecomastia from any cause has reached the fibrotic stage, little or no spontaneous regression occurs.

TESTICULAR TUMORS

Testicular neoplasms account for 1–2% of all male-related malignant neoplasms and 4–10% of all genitourinary neoplasms. They are the second most frequent type of cancer in men between 20 and 34 years of age. The incidence is 2–3 per 100,000 men in the USA and 4–6 per 100,000 men in Denmark. The incidence is lower in nonwhite than in white populations. Ninety-five percent of testicular tumors are of germ cell origin; 5% are composed of stromal or Leydig cell neoplasms.

Etiology & Pathophysiology

The cause of testicular tumors is not known. Predisposing factors include testicular maldescent and dysgenesis. About 4–12% of testicular tumors are found in association with cryptorchidism, and such a testicle has a 20- to 30-fold greater risk of developing a neoplasm than does a normally descended one. Almost 20% of testicular tumors associated with cryptorchidism arise in the contralateral scrotal testis, suggesting that testicular dysgenesis may be of etiologic importance in the development of germ cell neoplasms. Although trauma is frequently cited as an etiologic factor in testicular tumors,

no causal relationship has been established. What is more likely is that testicular trauma serves to call the patient's attention to the presence of a testicular mass. In a few cases a genetic component is present and is associated with mutations in chromosome Xq27.

Bilateral gynecomastia is uncommon in patients who present with testicular cancer. It is generally associated with production of hCG by the trophoblastic elements in the tumor. The hCG stimulates the Leydig cells to produce excessive estrogens relative to androgen production, resulting in estrogen-androgen imbalance and gynecomastia. In addition, the trophoblastic tissue in some of the tumors may convert estrogen precursors to estrogens.

Pathology

A. GERM CELL TUMORS

Seminomas account for 33–50% of all germ cell tumors. They are composed of round cells with abundant cytoplasm, prominent nuclei, and large nucleoli. The cells are arranged in cords and nests and have a thin delicate network of stromal connective tissue. Embryonal cell neoplasms comprise 20–33% of germ cell tumors. These tumors have multiple histologic patterns composed of cuboidal pleomorphic cells. One distinct pattern of cellular arrangement is the endodermal sinus tumor (yolk sac tumor), the most frequent germ cell neoplasm found in infants. Immunohistochemical techniques have localized alpha-fetoprotein to the embryonal cells. About 10% of germ cell tumors are teratomas, which are composed of well-differentiated cells derived from all three germ layers. When one or more of the teratoid elements are malignant or are mixed with embryonal carcinoma cells, the term teratocarcinoma is applied. These tumors account for one-tenth to one-third of germ cell neoplasms. Choriocarcinoma is the rarest form of germ cell tumor (2%) and is composed of masses of large, polymorphic, multinucleated syncytiotrophoblastic cells. Although pure choriocarcinoma is rare, many testicular tumors contain an occasional trophoblastic giant cell. Immunohistochemical techniques have shown that these cells are the source of hCG in such tumors.

B. LEYDIG CELL TUMORS

Leydig cell (interstitial cell) tumors are rare. Most are benign and are composed of sheets of oval to polygonal cells arranged in lobules separated from one another by thin strands of connective tissue. Malignant Leydig cell tumor disseminates by both lymphatic and venous channels, with initial metastatic deposits being found in the regional lymph nodes, followed by metastases to liver, lung, and bone.

Clinical Features

A. SYMPTOMS AND SIGNS

1. Germ cell tumors—Testicular tumors usually present as painless enlargement of a testicle with an associated feeling of fullness or heaviness in the scrotum. Thus, about 80% of patients note a testicular swelling or mass, whereas only 25% complain of testicular pain or tenderness. About 6–25% of patients give a history of testicular trauma that brought the testicular mass to their attention. Gynecomastia may be present initially in 2–4% of patients and develops subsequently in another 10%. About 5–10% of patients present with symptoms of distant metastatic disease, including backache, skeletal pains, gastrointestinal and abdominal pains, inguinal adenopathy, and neurologic dysfunction.

A testicular mass or generalized enlargement of the testis is often present on examination. In 5–10% of patients, a coexisting hydrocele may be present. In the presence of metastatic disease, supraclavicular and retroperitoneal lymph node enlargement may be present.

2. Leydig cell tumors—In children, Leydig cell tumors of the testes may produce sexual precocity, with rapid skeletal growth and development of secondary sexual characteristics. Adults with such tumors usually present with a testicular mass and occasionally gynecomastia. Decreased libido may also be present in such patients.

B. LABORATORY FINDINGS

1. Germ cell tumors—The tumor markers hCG and alpha-fetoprotein should be measured in every male presenting with a testicular mass. hCG is found in the sera of 5–10% of males with seminoma, over half of patients with teratocarcinoma or embryonal cell carcinoma, and all patients with choriocarcinoma. hCG should be measured by the beta subunit or other hCG-specific immunoassay method. Elevated serum immunoreactive alpha-fetoprotein concentrations are found in almost 70% of patients with nonseminomatous forms of germ cell neoplasms. Both markers are elevated in over 50% of patients with nonseminomatous germ cell tumors, and at least one of the markers is elevated in 85% of such patients. These markers can also be used to monitor the results of therapy.

2. Leydig cell tumors—Urinary 17-ketosteroids and serum DHEA sulfate concentrations are increased. Both urinary and serum estrogen levels may also be increased. Serum testosterone concentrations tend to be low or within the normal adult range.

C. IMAGING STUDIES

Staging of testicular tumors requires chest and abdominal CT scans and other radiologic procedures depending on the type of tumor and the symptoms.

Differential Diagnosis

Testicular tumors are sometimes misdiagnosed as epididymitis or epididymo-orchitis. An inflammatory reaction of the epididymis often involves the vas deferens. Therefore, both the vas and the epididymis will be thickened and tender on examination during the acute disease. Pyuria and fever also help to differentiate between epididymitis and testicular tumor. Because hydrocele may coexist with testicular tumor, the testes should be carefully examined following aspiration of the hydrocele.

Other conditions that can cause confusion with testicular tumors include inguinal hernia, hematocele, hematoma, torsion, spermatocele, varicocele, and (rarely) sarcoidosis, tuberculosis, and syphilitic gumma. Ultrasonic examination of the scrotum may help distinguish between testicular tumors and extratesticular disease such as acute or chronic epididymitis, spermatocele, or hydrocele.

Benign Leydig cell tumors of the testes must be differentiated from adrenal rest tumors in patients with congenital adrenal hyperplasia. Since the testes and the adrenals are derived from the same embryologic source, ectopic adrenal tissue may be found to migrate with the testes. This tissue can enlarge under the influence of ACTH in patients with congenital adrenal hyperplasia or Cushing's disease. Adrenal rest tumors tend to be bilateral, whereas patients with Leydig cell tumors generally have unilateral disease. Both may be associated with elevated urine 17-ketosteroids and elevated serum DHEA sulfate concentrations. Elevated serum and urinary estrogen concentrations are found with both disorders. However, patients with congenital adrenal hyperplasia or Cushing's disease will have a decrease in 17-ketosteroids, DHEA sulfate, and estrogen concentrations, as well as a decrease in tumor size, following administration of dexamethasone.

Treatment

A. GERM CELL TUMORS

Seminomas are quite radiosensitive, and disease localized to the testes is usually treated with orchiectomy and 2000–4000 cGy of conventional radiotherapy delivered to the ipsilateral inguinal-iliac and bilateral para-aortic lymph nodes to the level of the diaphragm. For disease that has spread to the lymph nodes below the diaphragm, additional whole abdominal radiotherapy and prophylactic mediastinal and supraclavicular lymph node irradiation are usually given. Widely disseminated disease is generally treated with a combination of radiotherapy and chemotherapy, especially with alkylating agents.

Nonseminomatous tumors are treated with orchiectomy, retroperitoneal lymph node dissection, and, if necessary, radiotherapy or chemotherapy (or both). Although many chemotherapeutic agents have been used, combinations of etoposide, bleomycin, and cisplatin currently appear to produce the best overall results. Patients with nonseminomatous tumors treated by these means should be monitored with serial measurements of serum hCG and alpha-fetoprotein.

B. LEYDIG CELL TUMORS

Benign Leydig cell tumors of the testes are treated by unilateral orchiectomy. Objective remissions of malignant Leydig cell tumors have been noted following treatment with mitotane.

Course & Prognosis

A. GERM CELL TUMORS

In patients with seminoma confined to the testicle, the 5-year survival rates after orchiectomy and radiotherapy are 98–100%. Disease in the lymph nodes below the diaphragm also has an excellent prognosis, with 5-year survival rates of 80–85%. Disease above the diaphragm and disseminated disease have 5-year survival rates as low as 18%.

In patients with nonseminomatous germ cell tumors, aggressive surgery and combination chemotherapy have raised the 5-year survival rates from less than 20% to 60–90%.

B. LEYDIG CELL TUMORS

Removal of a benign Leydig cell tumor is accompanied by regression of precocious puberty in children or feminization in adults. The prognosis for malignant Leydig cell tumor is poor, with most patients surviving less than 2 years from the time of diagnosis.

REFERENCES

Physiology

Josso N, di Clemente N, Gouedard L: Anti-Mullerian hormone and its receptors. Mol Cell Endocrinol 2001;179:25. [PMID: 11420127]

Themmen APN, Huhtaniemi IT: Mutations of gonadotropins and gonadotropin receptors: elucidating the physiology and pathophysiology of pituitary-gonadal function. Endocr Rev 2000;21:551. [PMID: 11041448]

Androgen Therapy

Report of National Institute on Aging Advisory Panel on Testosterone Replacement in Men. J Clin Endocrinol Metab 2001;86:4611. [PMID: 11600511]

Vermeulen A: Androgen replacement therapy in the aging male—a critical evaluation. J Clin Endocriol Metab 2001;86:2380. [PMID:11397827]

Hypogonadism

Docimo SG, Silver RI, Cromie W: The undescended testicle: diagnosis and management. Am Fam Phys 2000;62:2037. [PMID: 11087186]

Loy CJ, Yong EL: Sex, infertility and the molecular biology of the androgen receptor. Curr Opin Obstet Gynecol 2001;13:315. [PMID: 11396657]

Meola G: Clinical and genetic heterogeneity in myotonic dystrophies. Muscle Nerve 2000;23:1789. [PMID: 11102902]

Smyth CM: Diagnosis and treatment of Klinefelter syndrome. Hosp Pract 1999;34:111. [PMID: 10901753]

Infertility

Khorram O et al: Reproductive technologies for male infertility. J Clin Endocrinol Metab 2001;86:2373. [PMID: 11397826]

Oehninger S: Strategies for the infertile male. Semin Reprod Med 2001;19:231. [PMID: 11679904]

Sharlip ID et al: Best practice policies for male infertility. Fert Steril 2002;77:873. [PMID: 12009338] (Also available at http://shop.auanet.org/timssnet/products/best_practice/index.cfm; and at http://www.asrm.org/Media/Practice/practice.html.)

Erectile Dysfunction

Kandeel FR, Koussa VKT, Swerdloff RS: Male sexual function and its disorders: physiology, pathophysiology, clinical investigation, and treatment. Endocr Rev 2001;22:342. [PMID: 11399748]

Lue TF: Drug therapy: erectile dysfunction. N Engl J Med 2000; 342:1802. [PMID:10853004]

Gynecomastia

Braunstein GD: Aromatase and gynecomastia. Endocr Relat Cancer 1999;6:315. [PMID: 10731125]

Gruntmanis U, Braunstein GD: Treatment of gynecomastia. Curr Opin Invest Drugs 2001;2:643. [PMID: 11569940]

Testicular Cancer

Dearnaley DP, Huddart RA, Horwich A: Managing testicular cancer. BMJ 2001;322:1583. [PMID: 11431302]

Female Reproductive Endocrinology & Infertility

13

Mitchell Rosen, MD, & Marcelle I. Cedars, MD

ACTH	Adrenocorticotropic hormone	IVF	In vitro fertilization
AIS	Androgen insensitivity syndrome	LDL	Low-density lipoprotein
AMH	Anti-müllerian hormone	LH	Luteinizing hormone
ART	Assisted reproductive therapy	MBH	Medial basal hypothalamus
BBT	Basal body temperature	MMP	Matrix metalloproteinase
BMD	Bone mineral density	MPA	Medroxyprogesterone acetate
cAMP	Cyclic adenosine monophosphate	MRI	Magnetic resonance imaging
CRH	Corticotropin-releasing hormone	OMI	Oocyte maturation inhibitor
DHEA	Dehydroepiandrosenedione	PCOS	Polycystic ovarian syndrome
DHEAS	Dehydroepiandrosenedione sulfate	PG	Prostaglandin
EGF	Epidermal growth factor	PID	Pelvic inflammatory disease
FSH	Follicle-stimulating hormone	PIT-1	Transcription factor for pituitary hormone
GH	Growth hormone	POF	Premature ovarian failure
GnRH	Gonadotropin-releasing hormone	PRL	Prolactin
hCG	Human chorionic gonadotropin	PROP-1	Transcription factor for pituitary hormone
HDL	High-density lipoprotein		
HPO	Hypothalamic-pituitary-ovarian (axis)	REM	Rapid eye movement
HRT	Hormone replacement therapy	SERMs	Selective estrogen receptor modulators
HSD	Hydroxysteroid dehydrogenase	SHBG	Sex hormone binding globulin
IGF	Insulin-like growth factor	SRY	Sex-determining region of the Y gene
IGFBP	Insulin-like growth factor binding protein	StAR	Steroidogenic acute regulatory protein
		TGF	Transforming growth factor
IUD	Intrauterine device	TSH	Thyroid-stimulating hormone
IUI	Intrauterine insemination	VEGF	Vascular endothelial growth factor

EMBRYOLOGY & ANATOMY

No gene has yet been identified that generates an ovary from an undifferentiated gonad. It is only in the absence of the sex-determining region of the Y gene *(SRY)* that the gonad will develop into an ovary. (For more details, refer to the discussion of sexual differentiation in Chapter 14.) Primordial germ cells originate in the yolk sac endoderm (hindgut) and migrate through the dorsal mesentery into the gonadal ridge, which is located lateral to the dorsal mesentery of the gut and me-

dial to the mesonephros (Figure 13–1). Prior to migration, the germ cells divide mitotically. Once migration starts, mitosis is inhibited until the germ cells reach the gonadal ridge in the sixth week of gestation. Failure of primordial germ cells to develop or to migrate into the gonadal ridge results in failure of ovarian development.

When the germ cells reach the gonadal ridge, mitosis resumes, with primordial germ cells subsequently developing into oogonia (premeiotic germ cells). At 10–12 weeks of gestation, some oogonia leave the mitotic pool and begin meiosis, where they arrest in

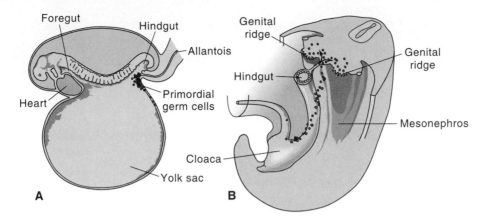

Figure 13–1. A: Schematic drawing of a 3-week-old embryo showing the primordial germ cells in the wall of the yolk sac, close to the attachment of the allantois. **B:** Drawing to show the migrational path of the primordial germ cells along the wall of the hindgut and the dorsal mesentery into the genital ridge. (Reproduced, with permission, from Langman J, Sadler TW: *Langman's Medical Embryology*, 8th ed. Lippincott Williams and Wilkins, 2000.)

prophase I (dictyotene stage). These arrested germ cells are now called primary oocytes. By 16 weeks, primordial follicles are first identified, making a clear distinction for gonadal differentiation into an ovary. At approximately 20 weeks of gestation, a peak of 6–7 million germ cells (two-thirds of them primary oocytes and one-third oogonia) are present in the ovaries. During the second half of gestation, the rate of mitosis rapidly decreases and the rate of oogonial and follicular atresia increases. Those oogonia that are not transformed into primary oocytes will undergo atresia before birth. This results in a reduction in the number of germ cells, resulting in a total of 1–2 million germ cells at birth. No germ cell mitosis occurs after birth, while follicular atresia continues, with the result that the average girl entering puberty has only 300,000–400,000 germ cells.

The ovary is organized into an outer cortex and an inner medulla. The germ cells are located within the cortex. Along the outer surface of the cortex is the germinal epithelium. This cell layer is composed of cuboidal cells resting on a basement membrane and forms a continuous layer with the peritoneum. Even though it is called the germinal epithelium, there are no germ cells within this layer. During embryonic development, the epithelial cells proliferate and enter the underlying tissue of the ovary to form cortical cords. When the primordial germ cells arrive at the genital ridge, they are incorporated into these cortical cords. At the same time the germ cells migrate from the yolk sac, the stromal cells of the ovary (granulosa and interstitial cells) migrate from the mesonephric tubules into the gonad. **Primordial follicles** form within the cortical cords. They are composed of a primary oocyte and one layer of granulosa cells with its basement membrane. Oocytes not surrounded by granulosa cells are lost, probably by apoptosis. It is this finite follicle population that represents the pool of germ cells which will ultimately be available to enter the follicular cycle.

During fetal development, the gonad is held in place by the suspensory ligament at the upper pole and the gubernaculum at the lower pole. The final location of the gonad is dependent on hormone production. In the presence of testosterone, the gubernaculum grows while the suspensory ligament regresses. As the gubernaculum continues to grow, the gonad (testis) descends into the scrotum. In contrast, when testosterone is absent, the suspensory ligament remains and the gubernaculum regresses. This process will maintain the gonad (ovary) in the pelvis.

The remainder of the female internal reproductive organs are formed from the paramesonephric (müllerian) ducts. In the absence of antimüllerian hormone (AMH), the paramesonephric system develops into the uterine (fallopian) tubes, the uterus, the cervix, and the upper third of the vagina. Unlike wolffian duct differentiation, the development of the female reproductive tract is not dependent on hormone production. (For more details, refer to the discussion of sexual differentiation in Chapter 14.) Briefly, the müllerian buds are formed lateral to the wolffian ducts and the gonadal ridge after 37 days of gestation (Figure 13–2). These

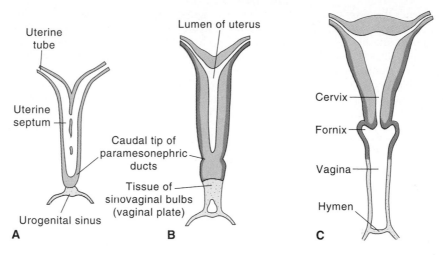

Figure 13–2. Schematic drawing showing the formation of the uterus and vagina. **A:** At 9 weeks. Note the disappearance of the uterine septum. **B:** At the end of the third month. Note the tissue of the sinovaginal bulbs. **C:** Newborn. The upper portion of the vagina and the fornices are formed by vacuolization of the paramesonephric tissue and the lower portion by vacuolization of the sinovaginal bulbs. (Reproduced, with permission, from Langman J, Sadler TW: *Langman's Medical Embryology*, 8th ed. Lippincott Williams and Wilkins, 2000.)

buds elongate, canalize, and extend caudally and medially. The adjacent paired müllerian ducts abut and eventually fuse in the midline as they reach the müllerian tubercle. The intervening septum resorbs after 10 weeks of gestation, resulting in a single uterine cavity. The most cranial parts of the müllerian ducts remain unfused and form the uterine tubes, which remain patent with the coelom (future peritoneal cavity). The caudal segments stimulate solid cords to extend from the müllerian tubercle to the sinovaginal bulbs from the posterior aspect of the urogenital sinus. In turn, the sinovaginal bulbs extend cranially and fuse with the vaginal cords, forming the vaginal plate. The vagina is subsequently formed by canalization of the vaginal plate. It is ultimately the cervix and the upper third of the vagina that are derived from the müllerian structures, while the remaining lower two-thirds is formed from the urogenital sinus.

The uterus is composed of endometrium (innermost lining), myometrium, and serosa. The adult uterus is a pear-shaped hollow organ. The cervical portion extends approximately 2 cm into the vagina, and the remaining corpus extends approximately 6 cm into the abdomen. The normal adult uterus weighs 40–80 g.

The uterus is located in the pelvis and rests on the pelvic floor. Seventy to 80 percent of the time, the uterine position is anteflexed (cervical-uterine corpus angle) and anteverted (cervical-vaginal angle). Therefore, when a woman is standing, the corpus of the uterus is

horizontal and resting on top of the bladder. The uterus has several paired ligaments that develop from thickenings of the peritoneum and serve to maintain this anatomic position. The cardinal ligament (Mackenrodt) is the main supporting ligament. It attaches to the lateral margins of the cervix at the upper vagina and extends to the lateral pelvic wall. The remaining ligaments—uterosacral, round, and broad—have a lesser role in supporting the uterus.

The uterine artery originates from the anterior division of the internal iliac artery (hypogastric), enters the cardinal ligament, and supplies the uterus. The uterine artery divides into a descending branch and an ascending branch known as the vaginal and arcuate arteries, respectively. The arcuate arteries anastomose with each other and form a vascular network around the uterus. The radial arteries branch off from the arcuate network and penetrate the uterus to supply the myometrium. Smaller basal branches and spiral arteries supply the endometrium.

The ovary is suspended in the pelvis and has three associated ligaments. The average adult ovary is 2.5–5 × 2.5 × 1 cm in size and weighs 3–8 g. The position of the ovary is variable, but in a nulliparous woman it is often located in a peritoneal depression on the pelvic sidewalls between the ureter and external iliac vein. The suspensory (infundibulopelvic) ligament attaches to the cranial pole of the ovary and extends to the pelvic brim.

This ligament suspends the ovary in the pelvis and contains the ovarian vessels, lymphatics, and nerves. The utero-ovarian ligament attaches to the inferior pole of the ovary and extends to the uterus. The mesovarium connects the anterior portion of the ovary to the posterior leaf of the broad ligament. The blood supply of the ovary originates from the abdominal aorta, passes through the suspensory ligament, and enters the mesovarium to form an anastomotic network with branches from the uterine artery. The ovarian artery enters the ovarian hilum and branches into spiral arteries that enter the medulla and extend to the ovarian cortex. Other branches from the anastomotic network, located in the mesovarium, supply the uterine tubes.

OVARIAN STEROIDOGENESIS

The ovaries are not only the store for germ cells—they also produce and secrete hormones that are vital for reproduction and the development of secondary sexual characteristics. The next section will briefly discuss the biosynthesis of ovarian hormones. (See also Figures 9–4, 12–2, and 14–14.)

In the ovary, the major source of hormone production is the maturing follicle. The components of the follicle are the theca cells, the granulosa cells, and the primary oocyte. The theca cells produce androgens, and the granulosa cells produce estrogens. The other stromal cells that contribute to androgen production can be divided into two populations of cells: the secondary interstitial cells (derived from theca) and the hilum cells. These cells are the major ones involved in ovarian hormone production during menopause (see below).

The ovarian hormones are derived from cholesterol. Steroidogenic cells acquire the cholesterol substrate from one of three sources. The most common source is plasma lipoprotein carrying cholesterol, primarily in the form of low-density lipoprotein (LDL). Other minor sources include de novo synthesis from acetate and liberation from stored lipid droplets (cholesterol esters). Stimulation of ovarian cells by trophic hormones such as follicle-stimulating hormone (FSH) and luteinizing hormone (LH) facilitate uptake of cholesterol by increasing the number of LDL receptors on the cell surface. The LDL particle is subsequently internalized and degraded in the lysosome. The free cholesterol that is liberated from the lysosome is delivered to the mitochondria by an unknown mechanism, possibly via microfilaments and microtubules. The cholesterol is then translocated into the mitochondria by the steroidogenic acute regulatory protein (StAR).

The initial step that commits cholesterol to steroid synthesis is the cholesterol side chain cleavage enzyme reaction (P450scc) (Figure 13–3). This reaction converts cholesterol to pregnenolone, the precursor of steroid hormones, and takes place in the mitochondria. Acute alterations in steroid production result from changes in delivery of cholesterol to P450scc, while long-term changes in steroid synthesis involve alterations in gene expression.

Once pregnenolone is formed, the hormone secreted is dependent on the synthesizing endocrine organ and cell type. For example, the main sources of sex steroids in the female come from the adrenal gland and the ovary. The specific type of hormone secreted is dependent on the cell type. In the adrenal gland there are three zones: zona glomerulosa, zona fasciculata, and zona reticularis. The cells in the different zones start with the same hormone precursor but differ in their secretory products. The glomerulosa produces mainly aldosterone, while cortisol and androgen are produced by the zona fasciculata and zona reticularis, respectively. The major androgen produced by the adrenal is DHEAS. Differences in enzymatic activity among cells in the various zones are what regulate hormone production. The zona reticularis and zona fasciculata lack 11β-hydroxylase, which is necessary for aldosterone synthesis (Figure 13–3; and see Chapters 9 and 10). The zona glomerulosa lacks 17-hydroxylase and 17,20-lyase (CYP17), which are necessary for sex steroid synthesis.

Ovarian cells similarly secrete different hormones due to differential enzyme activity. The theca interstitial and secondary interstitial cells lack aromatase and hence are the androgen producers in the ovarian cortex. The granulosa cells, on the other hand, lack CYP17 and therefore secrete estrogens—mainly estradiol in the proliferative phase and progesterone in the luteal phase. Differences in androgen secretion between the adrenal and ovary can be explained by the relative activity of type II 3β-hydroxysteroid dehydrogenase and δ⁵-isomerase (3β-HSD). Both organs can produce all the androgens, but the lack of activity of 3β-HSD, at least during the reproductive years, contributes to adrenal DHEA production. In contrast, ovarian 3β-HSD activity can be stimulated by gonadotrophs, leading to androstenedione and testosterone production.

PHYSIOLOGY OF THE MENSTRUAL CYCLE

The menstrual cycle is regulated by complex interactions between the hypothalamic-pituitary-ovarian (HPO) axis and the uterus. Briefly, the hypothalamus secretes gonadotropin-releasing hormone (GnRH), which stimulates the pituitary to release FSH and LH. These gonadotropins then trigger the ovary to release an oocyte that is capable of fertilization. Concurrently, the ovary secretes hormones, which act on the endometrial lining of the uterus to prepare for implantation. In addition,

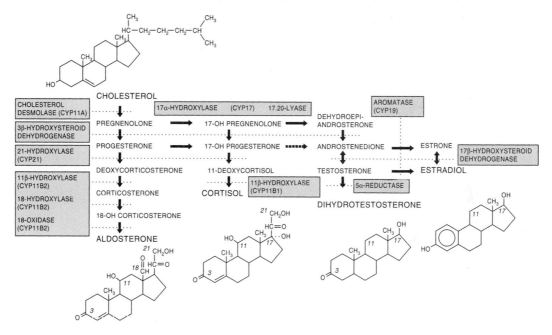

Figure 13–3. Pathways of steroid biosynthesis. The pathways for synthesis of progesterone and mineralocorticoids (aldosterone), glucocorticoids (cortisol), androgens (testosterone and dihydrotestosterone), and estrogens (estradiol) are arranged left to right. The enzymatic activities catalyzing each bioconversion are written in the boxes. For those activities mediated by specific cytochrome P450, the systematic name of the enzyme ("CYP" followed by a number) is listed in parentheses. CYPB2 and CYP17 have multiple activities. The planar structures of cholesterol, aldosterone, cortisol, dihydrotestosterone, and estradiol are placed near the corresponding labels. (Reproduced, with permission, from White PC, Speiser PW: Congenital adrenal hyperplasia due to 21-hydroxylase deficiency. Endocr Rev 2000;21:245.)

the ovarian hormones feed back to the hypothalamus and pituitary, regulating the secretion of gonadotropins during the phases of the menstrual cycle. This complex interaction will be discussed in greater detail below. The hormonal changes associated with menstruation are summarized in Figure 13–4.

The Hypothalamic-Pituitary Axis

GnRH-secreting neurons originate in the olfactory placode and migrate to the arcuate nucleus of the medial basal hypothalamus (MBH). These neurons project to the median eminence and secrete GnRH, with inherent rhythmic behavior ("pulse generator"). GnRH is composed of ten amino acids and has a short half-life of 2–4 minutes. The pulsatile frequency of GnRH secretion regulates gonadotropin synthesis and the secretion of pituitary gonadotropes. (See Chapter 5.)

During the late luteal-follicular phase, the slower pulsatile release of GnRH—every 90–120 minutes—favors FSH secretion. In response to FSH, the maturing

follicle in the ovary secretes estradiol. This hormone is involved in a negative feedback loop that directly inhibits the release of FSH. Estradiol is involved in a positive feedback loop that increases the frequency of GnRH to every 60 minutes during the follicular phase and acts directly on the pituitary to stimulate LH secretion. LH stimulates the ovary to further increase estradiol production (see two-cell theory, below). Although at this point there is no acute change in GnRH pulsatility, estradiol and other regulatory factors (see below) augment pituitary sensitivity to GnRH. This increased sensitivity results in a rapid elevation of LH production—the LH surge—which stimulates ovulation. After ovulation, the ruptured follicle (corpus luteum) secretes progesterone. This hormone is involved in a negative feedback loop via increased endogenous opioid activity—and possibly directly—to decrease the GnRH pulsatility to every 3–5 hours, favoring FSH synthesis during the luteal-follicular transition. As progesterone levels fall again, GnRH pulsatility increases, favoring FSH release.

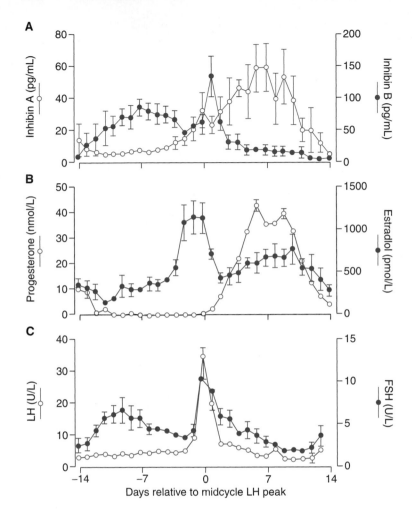

Figure 13–4. The endocrinology of the luteal–follicular transition in women. Data are mean ± SE of daily serum concentrations of FSH, LH, estradiol, progesterone, and immunoreactive inhibin in women with normal cycles. Note the secondary rise in plasma FSH in the late luteal phase (~ 2 days before menses). (Reproduced with permission from Erickson GF: *Ovarian Anatomy and Physiology. Lobo R* [ed]. Academic Press, 2000.)

Role of the Pituitary

Gonadotropes are located in the adenohypophysis and make up approximately 10% of the cells in the pituitary. These cells synthesize and secrete FSH and LH. Pituitary hormones belong to a family of glycoproteins that include thyroid-stimulating hormone (TSH) and human chorionic gonadotropin (hCG) and therefore contain carbohydrate moieties. Gonadotropins are functional as heterodimers and are composed of an alpha subunit and a beta subunit. The alpha subunit amino acid sequence is identical for all of the glycoproteins, while the beta subunit is characterized by different amino acids and confers unique specificity on the glycoprotein.

The differential gene expression that leads to the production and release of gonadotropins by cells in the pituitary is regulated by GnRH and ovarian hormones through feedback loops. Slower GnRH secretion en-

hances FSH beta subunit expression and favors LH secretion. In turn, rapid GnRH pulses stimulate LH beta subunit expression while promoting FSH release. Thus, ovarian steroid modification of hypothalamic GnRH pulsatility controls pituitary gonadotrophin production.

An intrapituitary network involves several factors that play a role in regulating gonadotropin synthesis and secretion. The gonadotropes produce and secrete peptides that are in the transforming growth factor (TGF) family. Activin is a local regulatory protein that is involved in gonadotrope expression. Slow pulses of GnRH enhance activin synthesis, which subsequently enhances FSH transcription. Follistatin, another TGF-related protein that binds to activin, is stimulated by rapid pulses of GnRH. This decreases the bioavailability of activin and consequently reduces FSH synthesis. In addition to these local modifiers, ovarian transforming growth factors such as inhibin also modulate the expression of gonadotropins (see below).

Role of the Ovary

The ovary is intimately involved in regulating the menstrual cycle via steroid feedback to alter gonadotropin secretion. In addition, the ovary contains an intraovarian network involving factors that are synthesized locally and have a paracrine and autocrine role in the modulation of gonadotropin activity. The intraovarian regulators include the insulin-like growth factor (IGF) family, the transforming growth factor (TGF) superfamily, and the epidermal growth factor (EGF) family. Furthermore, it is these factors that assist in the coordination of follicular development and ovulation.

The menstrual cycle of the ovary includes a follicular phase and a luteal phase. The follicular phase is characterized by growth of the dominant follicle and ovulation. It typically lasts 10–14 days. It is, however, this phase that is variable in duration and most often accounts for the variability in menstrual cycle length in ovulatory women. The luteal phase starts after ovulation and is the period when the ovary secretes hormones that are essential to accommodate conceptus implantation. This phase is relatively constant and averages 14 days (range, 12–15 days) in duration. The next section will describe the two phases in some detail.

Primordial follicles are the fundamental reproductive units that comprise the pool of resting oocytes. Morphologically, they are composed of a primary oocyte that is surrounded by a single layer of squamous granulosa cells and a basement membrane. They have no blood supply. These primordial follicles develop between the sixth and ninth months of gestation and harbor the complete supply of ovarian follicles.

Prior to ovulation, it is essential for primordial follicles to leave the pool of nongrowing follicles and enter the growth phase. The exact mechanisms controlling the initial recruitment are largely unknown. The resting follicular pool is probably controlled by inhibitory factors. These follicles may remain quiescent for many months or years. This initial recruitment is a continuous process that begins once the germ pool is created and ends with follicular exhaustion. This complex process is gonadotropin-independent. Several studies have suggested that the intraovarian network— especially members of the TGF superfamily—is involved in primordial follicle recruitment. It is the decrease of inhibitory influences and the increase in stimulators that initiate recruitment. Several other factors have been described to date, and many more will be identified in the future. The ongoing search for these growth factors and hormones will ultimately elucidate the physiology of primordial follicle recruitment. There is a finite number of germ cells, and each successive recruitment further depletes the germ pool. Any abnormality that alters the number of germ cells or accelerates recruitment could perhaps lead to early ovarian follicular depletion and, therefore, early reproductive failure. (See section on infertility, below.)

Primary follicle development is the first stage of follicular growth (Figure 13–5). Primary follicles differ from primordial follicles in several ways. The oocyte begins to grow. As growth progresses, the zona pellucida is formed. This is a thick layer of glycoprotein that is most likely synthesized by the oocyte. It completely surrounds the oocyte and is formed between the oocyte and the granulosa cell layer. It serves a number of biologic functions that are critical for conception. Finally, the granulosa cells undergo a morphologic change from squamous to cuboidal. This stage of development may last 150 days.

The progression to a **secondary follicle** includes attainment of maximal oocyte growth (120 μm in diameter), proliferation of granulosa cells, and acquisition of theca cells. The exact mechanism involved in acquiring theca cells is not completely understood but is thought to be derived from the surrounding ovarian mesenchyme (stromal fibroblasts) as the developing follicle migrates to the medulla. It is the development of this layer that gives rise to the theca interna and theca externa. With theca cell development, these follicles gain an independent blood supply, although the granulosa cell layer remains avascular. In addition, the granulosa cells in the secondary follicle develop FSH, estrogen, and androgen receptors. This phase of follicular development may take as long as 120 days, probably because of the long doubling time (> 250 hours) of granulosa cells.

Further follicular development leads to the **tertiary follicle** or **early antral phase.** This phase is characterized by the formation of an antrum or cavity in the follicle. The antral fluid contains steroids, proteins, electrolytes, proteoglycans, and an ultrafiltrate that forms from diffusion through the basal lamina. Other changes in this phase include further theca cell differentiation. Subpopulations of thecal interstitial cells develop within the theca interna, acquire LH receptors, and are capable of steroidogenesis. The granulosa cells begin to differentiate into distinct cell layers. Starting from the basal lamina, the cells can be stratified into the membrana, periantral, cumulus oophorus, and corona radiata layers. This developmental process is influenced by FSH and unidentified signals originating from the oocyte. In addition, the granulosa cells—most likely in response to FSH—start producing activin, a member of the TGF family. Activin is composed of two types of beta subunits, βA and βB, which are held together by disulfide bonds. It is the combination of these subunits that generates the various activins (activin A [βA,βA], AB [βA,βB], or BB [βB,βB]). Activin most likely does not have an endocrine role given the fact that serum

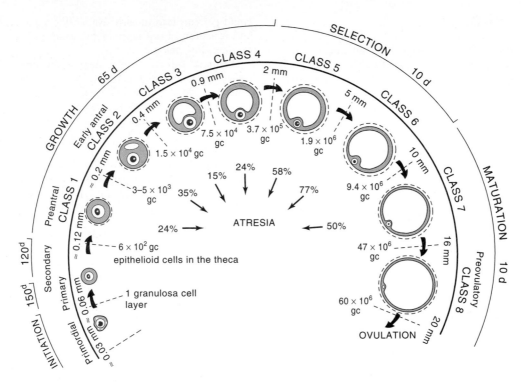

Figure 13–5. The chronology of folliculogenesis in the human ovary. Folliculogenesis is divided into two major periods, preantral (gonadotropin independent) and antral (FSH dependent). In the preantral period, a recruited primordial follicle develops into the primary/secondary (class 1) and early tertiary (class 2) stages, at which time cavitation or antrum formation begins. The antral period includes the small graafian (0.9–5 mm, classes 4 and 5), medium graafian (6–10 mm, class 6), large graafian (10–15 mm, class 7), and preovulatory (16–20 mm, class 8) follicles. Time required for completion of preantral and antral periods is approximately 300 and 40 days, respectively. Number of granulosa cells (gc), follicle diameter (mm), and atresia (%) are indicated. (Reproduced, with permission, from Gougeon A: Regulation of ovarian follicular development in primates: facts and hypotheses. Endo Rev 1996;17:121.)

levels of activin do not change throughout the menstrual cycle. Activin's primary activity is within the ovary, where it plays an autocrine role by enhancing FSH receptor gene expression in the granulosa cells and accelerating folliculogenesis.

Follicular growth during the early antral phase occurs at a slow and constant pace. The follicle achieves a diameter of 400 µm. FSH-stimulated mitosis of granulosa cells is the major contributor of follicular growth at this stage. Until this point, follicular growth and survival are largely independent of gonadotropins. In fact, prepubertal females and women taking oral contraceptives may have follicles arrested at various phases up until this point. It is at this phase in follicular development that FSH is critical for growth and survival. If FSH does not rescue these follicles, they undergo atresia.

The morphologic follicular unit, consisting of theca cells and granulosa cells, is also a functional hormonal unit capable of substantial estrogen production. The stimulation of granulosa cells by FSH increases their expression of P450 aromatase. In addition, the granulosa cells produce a third subunit of the TGF family—α—which combines with other β subunits to create a heterodimer known as inhibin A (αβA) or inhibin B (αβB). Given that the predominant β peptide expressed in the follicular phase is βB, inhibin B is the dominant inhibin produced. This hormone peaks in the early follicular phase and is involved in a negative feedback loop that inhibits pituitary expression of FSH. The thecal interstitial cells, under the influence of LH, increase levels of LH receptors on the cell surface and augment the enzyme activity of StAR, 3β-HSD, and

P450c17 to acutely increase androgen production. The maximal expression of these enzymes occurs just prior to ovulation. The androgens—mainly androstenedione—diffuse through the basal lamina of the follicle and are the precursors that interstitial cells and granulosa cells utilize for maximal estrogen production (**two-cell theory;** see Figure 13–6). This interaction between the two cell types is essential given that theca cells lack aromatase, while granulosa cells are deficient in P450c17. The estrogen produced then acts on the follicle to increase levels of FSH receptors on the granulosa cells. This promotes granulosa cell proliferation and subsequently plays a very important role in selection of the dominant follicle.

The next stage of follicular development is the antral growth phase. It is characterized by rapid growth (1–2 mm/d) and is gonadotropin-dependent. In response to FSH, the antral follicle rapidly grows to a diameter of 20 mm, primarily as a result of accumulation of antral fluid. The theca interna continues to differentiate into interstitial cells that produce increasing amounts of androstenedione for aromatization to estradiol. The granulosa cell layers have continued to differentiate from each other. The membrana layer, through the action of FSH, acquires LH receptors. This differs from the cumulus layer, which lacks LH receptors. The final progression to a mature graafian follicle is a selection process that in most cases generates one dominant follicle destined for ovulation.

The selection process begins in the midluteal phase of the previous cycle. The rise in estrogen level that is generated by the preovulatory follicle augments FSH activity within the follicle while exerting negative feedback on the pituitary release of FSH. The decrease in pituitary release of FSH results in withdrawal of gonadotropin support from the smaller antral follicles, promoting their atresia. The dominant follicle continues to grow despite decreasing levels of FSH by accumulating a greater mass of granulosa cells with more FSH receptors. Increased vascularity of the theca cells allows preferential FSH delivery to the dominant follicle despite waning FSH levels. Increased estrogen levels in the follicle facilitate FSH induction of LH receptors on the granulosa cells, allowing the follicle to respond to the ovulatory surge of LH levels. Without estrogen, LH receptors do not develop on the granulosa cells.

A positive feedback loop involving estrogens stimulates the pituitary and results in an LH surge. This surge results in the resumption of meiosis I in the oocyte with release of a polar body just prior to ovulation. Evidence suggests that the granulosa membrana cells secrete an oocyte maturation inhibitor (OMI) which interacts with the cumulus to block the progression of meiosis during most of folliculogenesis. It is theorized that OMI exerts its inhibitory influence by stimulating the cumulus to increase cAMP production, which diffuses into the oocyte and halts meiotic maturation. The LH surge overcomes the arrest of meiosis by inhibiting OMI secretion, thereby decreasing cAMP levels and increasing intracellular calcium, allowing the resumption of meiosis (see Figure 13–7).

With the LH surge, progesterone production increases, and this may be responsible at least in part for the midcyle peak in FSH. The FSH peak stimulates the production of an adequate number of LH receptors on the granulosa cells for luteinization. FSH, LH, and progesterone induce expression of proteolytic enzymes that degrade the collagen in the follicular wall, thereby making it prone to rupture. Prostaglandin production increases and may in part be responsible for contraction of smooth muscle cells on the ovary, aiding the extrusion of the oocyte.

The LH surge lasts approximately 48–50 hours. Thirty-six hours after onset of the LH surge, ovulation

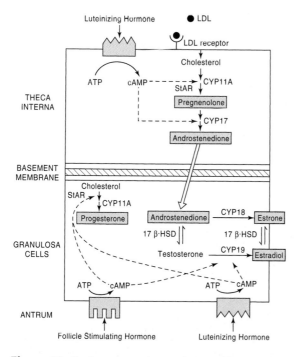

Figure 13–6. Gonadotropin regulation of follicular estrogen biosynthesis in the two-cell, two-gonadotropin model. ATP, adenosine triphosphate; cAMP, cyclic adenosine monophosphate; CYP, P450scc; CYP17, P450c17; CYP19, P450arom; 17β-HSD, 17-β-hydroxysteroid dehydrogenase; LDL, low-density lipoprotein; StAR: steroidogenic acute regulatory protein. (Reproduced, with permission, from DeGroot LJ et al [editors]: *Endocrinology*, 4th ed. Saunders, 2001.)

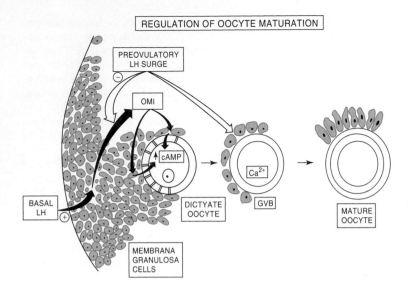

Figure 13–7. Current concepts of control of meiotic maturation. (Reproduced, with permission, from Felig P, Frohman LA [editors]: Endocrinology and Metabolism, 4th ed. McGraw-Hill, 2001.)

occurs. The feedback signal to terminate the LH surge is not known. Perhaps the rise in progesterone production results in a negative feedback loop and inhibits pituitary LH secretion by decreasing the pulsatility of GnRH. In addition, just prior to ovulation LH downregulates its own receptors, which decreases the activity of the functional hormonal unit (two-cell theory). As a result, estradiol production decreases.

Following ovulation and in response to LH, the granulosa cells (membrana) and thecal interstitial cells that remain in the ovulated follicle differentiate into granulosa lutein and theca lutein cells, respectively, to form the corpus luteum. In addition, LH induces the granulosa lutein cells to produce vascular endothelial growth factor (VEGF), which plays an important role in developing the corpus luteum vascularization. This neovascularization penetrates the basement membrane and provides the granulosa lutein cells with LDL for progesterone biosynthesis. After ovulation, the luteal cells up-regulate their LH receptors by an unknown mechanism. This is critical in that it allows basal levels of LH to maintain the corpus luteum. Rescue of the corpus luteum with human chorionic gonadotropin (hCG) from the developing conceptus works through the LH receptor, which is vital for embryonic life. In response to LH and hCG, the luteal cells increase their expression of P450scc and 3β-hydroxysteroid dehydrogenase (HSD) to increase the production of progesterone, 17α-progesterone, androstenedione, estradiol, and inhibin A. The secretion of progesterone and estradiol is episodic and correlates with the LH pulses. FSH has minimal influence on progesterone production but continues to stimulate estrogen production during the luteal phase. The progesterone levels continue to rise

and reach a peak on approximately day 8 of the luteal phase. The luteal phase lasts approximately 14 days.

The corpus luteum starts to undergo luteolysis (programmed cell death) approximately 9 days after ovulation. The mechanism of luteal regression is not completely known. Once luteolysis begins, there is a rapid decline in progesterone levels. A number of studies suggest that estrogen has a role in luteolysis. It has been shown that direct injection of estrogen into the ovary containing a corpus luteum induces luteolysis and a fall in progesterone levels. Experimental data suggest that there is increased aromatase activity in the corpus luteum just prior to luteolysis. The rise in aromatase activity is secondary to gonadotropin (FSH and LH) stimulation, but later in the luteal phase FSH probably plays a more important role. Consequently, estrogen production increases, and this decreases 3β-HSD activity. This may result in a decline in progesterone levels and lead to luteolysis. Furthermore, local modifiers such as oxytocin, which is secreted by luteal cells, have been shown to modulate progesterone synthesis. Other evidence supports prostaglandin's role in luteolysis. Experimental data suggest that prostaglandin $F_{2\alpha}$, which is secreted from the uterus or ovary during the luteal phase, stimulates the synthesis of cytokines such as tumor necrosis factor; this causes apoptosis and therefore may be linked to corpus luteum degeneration.

The process of luteolysis is known to involve proteolytic enzymes. Evidence suggests that matrix metalloproteinase (MMP) activity is increased during luteolysis. hCG is a known modulator of MMP activity. This may play an important role in early pregnancy, when hCG rescues the corpus luteum and prevents luteal regression. However, in the absence of pregnancy, the corpus luteum regresses, resulting in a decrease in progesterone, estradiol, and inhibin A levels. The decrease in these hormones allows for increased GnRH pulsatility and FSH secretion. The rise in FSH will rescue another cohort of follicles and initiate the next menstrual cycle.

Role of the Uterus

The sole function of the uterus is to accommodate and support a fetus. Furthermore, it is the endometrium, the lining of the uterine cavity, that differentiates during the menstrual cycle so that it can support and nourish the conceptus. Histologically, the endometrium is made up of an epithelium composed of glands and a stroma that contains stromal fibroblasts and extracellular matrix. The endometrium is divided into two layers based on morphology: the basalis layer and the functionalis layer. The basalis layer lies adjacent to the myometrium and contains glands and supporting vasculature. It provides the components necessary to develop the functionalis layer. The functionalis is the dynamic layer that is regenerated every cycle. More specifically, it is this layer that can accommodate implantation of the blastocyst.

During the menstrual cycle, the endometrium responds to hormones secreted from the ovaries. Somewhat like the other endocrine organs, it contains a network of local factors that modulate hormonal activity. The endometrial phases are coordinated with ovulatory phases. During the follicular phase, the endometrium goes through the proliferative phase. It begins with the onset of menses and ends at ovulation. During the luteal phase, the endometrium undergoes the secretory phase. It starts at ovulation and ends just before menses. If implantation does not occur, a degenerative phase follows the secretory phase within the endometrium. It is this phase that results in menstruation. The next section will discuss the phases of the endometrium in more detail.

During the follicular phase, the ovary secretes estrogen, which stimulates the glands in the basalis to initiate formation of the functionalis layer. Estrogen promotes growth by enhancing gene expression of cytokines and a variety of growth factors, including EGF, TGFα, and IGF. These factors provide a microenvironment within the endometrium to modulate the effects of hormones. At the beginning of the menstrual cycle, the endometrium is thin and is usually less than 2 mm in total thickness. The endometrial glands are straight and narrow and extend from the basalis toward the surface of the endometrial cavity. As the epithelium and the underlying stroma develop, they acquire estrogen and progesterone receptors. The spiral blood vessels from the basalis layer extend through the stroma to maintain blood supply to the epithelium. Ultimately, the lining (functionalis) surrounds the entire uterine cavity and achieves a thickness of 3–5 mm in

height (total thickness 6–10 mm). This phase is known as the proliferative phase.

After ovulation, the ovary secretes progesterone, which inhibits further endometrial proliferation. This mechanism may be mediated by antagonizing estrogen effects. Progesterone down-regulates estrogen receptors in the epithelium and mediates estradiol metabolism within the endometrium by stimulating 17β-HSD activity and converting estradiol into a weaker estrogen known as estrone. During the luteal phase, the glandular epithelium accumulates glycogen and begins to secrete glycopeptides and proteins—along with a transudate from plasma—into the endometrial cavity. It is this fluid that provides nourishment to the free-floating blastocyst. Progesterone also stimulates differentiation of the endometrium and causes characteristic histologic changes. The glands become progressively more tortuous, and the spiral vessels coil and acquire a corkscrew appearance. The underlying stroma becomes very edematous as a result of increased capillary permeability and the cells begin to appear large and polyhedral, with each cell developing an independent basement membrane. This process is termed predecidualization. These cells are very active and respond to hormonal signals. They produce prostaglandins along with other factors that play an important role in menstruation, implantation, and pregnancy. This phase is known as the secretory phase.

If there is no embryo implantation, the endometrium undergoes the degenerative phase. Estrogen and progesterone withdrawal promotes prostaglandin production—$PGF_{2\alpha}$ and PGE_2. These prostaglandins stimulate progressive vasoconstriction and relaxation of the spiral vessels. These vasomotor reactions lead to endometrial ischemia and reperfusion injury. Eventually there is hemorrhage within the endometrium with subsequent hematoma formation. The progesterone withdrawal triggers MMP activity, which facilitates degradation of the extracellular matrix. As ischemia and degradation progress, the functionalis becomes necrotic and sloughs away as menstruum consisting of endometrial tissue and blood. The amount of blood lost in normal menses ranges from 25 mL to 60 mL. Although $PGF_{2\alpha}$ is a potent stimulus for myometrial contractility and limits postpartum bleeding, it has minimal impact on cessation of menstrual bleeding. The major mechanisms responsible for limiting blood loss involve the formation of thrombin-platelet plugs and estrogen-induced healing of the basalis layer by reepithelialization of the endometrium, which begins in the early follicular phase of the next menstrual cycle.

If conception takes place, implantation can occur in the endometrium during the midsecretory (midluteal) phase, at which time it is of sufficient thickness and full of sustenance. The syncytiotrophoblast subsequently secretes hCG, which rescues the corpus luteum and maintains progesterone secretion, essential for complete endometrial decidual development.

In summary, the ovary has two phases during the menstrual cycle: the follicular phase and the luteal phase. The endometrium has three phases and is synchronized by the ovary. The complex feedback loops between the ovary and the hypothalamic-pituitary axis regulate the menstrual cycle. During the follicular phase, the ovary secretes estradiol, which stimulates the endometrium to undergo the proliferative phase. After ovulation (luteal phase), the ovary secretes estrogen and progesterone, which maintains the endometrial lining and promotes the secretory phase. In a nonpregnant cycle, luteolysis occurs, resulting in cessation of hormone production. This hormone withdrawal results in the degenerative phase and the onset of menses.

■ MENSTRUAL DISTURBANCES

Amenorrhea

Amenorrhea can be defined as either the absence of menarche by age 16 or no menses for more than three cycles in an individual who has previously had cyclic menses. The definition, though arbitrary, nonetheless gives a general guideline to the clinician for further evaluation. Although amenorrhea does not cause harm, in the absence of pregnancy it may be a sign of genetic, endocrine and/or anatomic abnormalities. If the outflow tract is intact, amenorrhea is most likely the result of disruption in the hypothalamic-pituitary-ovarian (HPO) axis. These aberrations can affect any level of control in the menstrual cycle and thus result in menstrual abnormalities.

Amenorrhea was formerly classified as primary or secondary depending on whether or not the individual had experienced menses in the past. This classification may lead to misdiagnosis of the cause of amenorrhea. Although primary amenorrhea is more often associated with genetic and anatomic abnormalities, each individual should be assessed by means of the history and clinical findings, including the presence or absence of secondary sexual characteristics (see Table 13–1). The causes of amenorrhea will be grouped according to the level of involvement in the regulatory systems that govern normal menstrual activity, ie, hypothalamic, pituitary, ovarian, and uterine amenorrhea.

HYPOTHALAMIC AMENORRHEA

Isolated GnRH Deficiency

The hypothalamus is the source of GnRH, which directs the synthesis and secretion of pituitary gonadotropins.

Dysfunction at this level leads to hypogonadotropic hypogonadism or eugonadotropic hypogonadism. Disorders of GnRH production can result in a wide range of clinical manifestations. The individual's appearance will be dependent upon the age at onset and the degree of dysfunction.

Isolated GnRH deficiency results in hypogonadotropic hypogonadism. Female patients present with amenorrhea, and females and males present with absent or incomplete pubertal development secondary to absent or diminished sex steroids (estradiol in females, testosterone in males). They have normal stature with a eunuchoidal body habitus. Since the adrenal glands are unaffected by the absence of GnRH, body hair distribution is not affected.

A. GENETIC ORIGIN

Several genetic lesions associated with GnRH deficiency have been described. The best-characterized form of GnRH deficiency is Kallmann's syndrome, which involves the *Kal-1* gene. This gene normally codes for anosmin, an adhesion molecule that appears to be involved in the migration of GnRH and olfactory neurons from the olfactory placode to the hypothalamus. The *Kal-1* gene is located on the short arm of the X chromosome. Most cases of Kallmann's syndrome are sporadic, though the disorder has also been observed to have a familial pattern, and most often it occurs by X-linked recessive inheritance. Autosomal recessive and dominant patterns have been reported but are much less common. When mutations exist in the *Kal-1* gene, there may be associated defects, including anosmia and, less frequently, midline facial defects, renal anomalies, and neurologic deficiency. The disorder affects both sexes, but because of the X-linked inheritance pattern it is more common in boys. Unlike males, the specific genetic mutations in the *Kal-1* gene in females with hypogonadotropic hypogonadism have not been identified, suggesting that there may be other genetic mutations that cause this disorder. Several studies have shown that females with presumed Kallmann's syndrome demonstrate variable responses to exogenous GnRH administration, which suggests a GnRH receptor defect. In fact, mutations in the GnRH receptor have been identified in both sexes and are inherited in an autosomal recessive fashion.

Management of hypogonadotropic hypogonadism involves scheduled hormone replacement therapy to stimulate the development of secondary sexual characteristics and increase bone mineral density. If pregnancy is desired, treatment involves the administration of pulsatile GnRH or gonadotropin treatment. This will be discussed further later in this chapter in the section on infertility.

Table 13–1. Assessment of patients with amenorrhea.[1]

I. **Absent breast development; uterus present**
   A. Gonadal failure
      1. Gonadal agenesis
      2. Gonadal dysgenesis
         a. 45,X (Turner's syndrome)
         b. 46,X abnormal X (eg, short- or long-arm deletion)
         c. Mosaicism (eg, X/XX, X/XX/XXX)
         d. 46,XX or 46,XY (Swyer syndrome) gonadal dysgenesis
   B. Defects in estrogen biosynthesis (46, XX)
      1. 17,20-Lyase deficiency
      2. CYP 17α deficiency
   C. Hypothalamic failure secondary to inadequate GnRH release
      1. Insufficient GnRH secretion
         a. FHA
         b. Anorexia nervosa and bulimia
         c. CNS neoplasm (craniopharyngioma, gliomas)
         d. Excessive exercise
         e. Constitutional delay
      2. Inadequate GnRH synthesis (Kallman's syndrome)
      3. Developmental anatomic abnormalities in central nervous system
   D. Pituitary failure
      1. Isolated gonadotropin insufficiency
      2. GnRH resistance
      2. Pituitary tumors (hyperprolactinemia)
      3. Pituitary insufficiency
         a. Infections (mumps, encephalitis)
         b. Newborn kernicterus
      4. Prepubertal hypothyroidism
II. **Breast development; uterus absent**
   A. Androgen resistance (androgen insensitivity syndrome)
   B. Congenital absence of uterus (utero-vaginal agenesis)
III. **Absent breast development; uterus absent**
   A. Defects in testosterone biosynthesis (46,XY)
      1. 17,20-Lyase deficiency
      2. CYP17α deficiency
      3. 17β-Hydroxysteroid dehydrogenase deficiency
   B. Testicular regression syndrome (46,XY)

IV. **Breast development; uterus present**
   A. Pregnancy
   B. Hypothalamic etiology
      1. FHA
      2. Anorexia nervosa and bulimia
      3. Psychogenic (depression)
      4. CNS neoplasm
      5. Chronic disease
   C. Pituitary etiology
      1. Pituitary tumors (hyperprolactinemia)
      2. Pituitary insufficiency
         a. Hypotensive event (Sheehan's syndrome)
         b. Infections
         c. Autoimmune destruction
         d. Iatrogenic (surgery, radiation)
   D. Ovarian etiology
      1. POF
         a. Mosaicism (46,XX/XO,XX/XY)
         b. Autoimmune destruction
         c. Iatrogenic (radiation, chemotherapy)
         d. Fragile X syndrome
         e. Infections
      2. Resistant ovarian syndrome (Savage's syndrome)
   E. Chronic estrogenized anovulation
      1. Hyperandrogenic
         a. PCOS
         b. NCAH
         c. Cushing's syndrome
         d. Androgen secreting tumors
      2. Other
         a. Adrenal insufficiency
         b. Thyroid disorders
   F. Outflow tract
      1. Congenital abnormalities
         a. Transvaginal septum
         b. Imperforate hymen
      2. Asherman's syndrome

B. ENDOCRINE CAUSES

1. Functional hypothalamic amenorrhea—Functional hypothalamic amenorrhea is one of the most common types of amenorrhea and accounts for 15–35% of cases. It is an endocrine disorder, though the exact mechanism has not been definitively determined. It is characterized by dysfunctional release of GnRH (decrease in pulse frequency and amplitude) leading to low or low-normal serum levels of FSH and LH and resulting in anovulation. The ratio of serum FSH and LH in these patients is often equivalent to that of a prepubertal female with a relative FSH dominance.

The adipocyte hormone leptin has been implicated in the development of this disorder. Leptin is an important nutritional satiety factor, but it is also necessary for maturation of the reproductive system. The potential link to the reproductive system is thought to be through leptin receptors, which have been identified in the hypothalamus and gonadotropes. This is supported by the observation that leptin can stimulate GnRH pulsatility and gonadotropin secretion. Several studies suggest that women with functional hypothalamic amenorrhea have lower serum leptin levels in comparison with eumenorrheic controls. This relative deficiency may lead to dysfunctional release of GnRH and subsequent development of functional hypothalamic amenorrhea.

Abnormal activation of the hypothalamic-pituitary-adrenal axis is associated with functional hypothalamic amenorrhea as evidenced by small increases in serum cortisol levels. The inciting event may be excessive production of corticotropin-releasing hormone (CRH), which has been shown to decrease the pulse frequency of GnRH and increase cortisol levels in vivo. In contrast, another study suggests that although acute elevations of CRH can suppress GnRH release, this suppression cannot be maintained with CRH alone.

The cause of functional hypothalamic amenorrhea often remains unclear, but the associated hypercortisolemia suggests that it is preceded by psychologic stress, strenuous exercise, or poor nutrition. There is support for the concept that these factors may act synergistically to further suppress GnRH drive. In fact, patients with functional hypothalamic amenorrhea resulting from psychologic stress are usually high achievers who have dysfunctional coping mechanisms when dealing with daily stress. The severity of hypothalamic suppression is reflected by the clinical manifestations. The significant interpatient variability in the degree of psychologic or metabolic stress required to induce a menstrual disturbance explains the heterogeneity of clinical presentations, ranging from luteal phase defects to anovulation with erratic bleeding to amenorrhea.

Functional hypothalamic amenorrhea is reversible. Interestingly, the factors that have predicted the rate of recovery are body mass index and basal cortisol levels. When patients recover, ovulation is preceded by return of cortisol levels to baseline. Some experts have shown that cognitive behavioral therapy, teaching the patient how to cope with stress—and nutritional consultation—reverse this condition. Complete reversal may be less likely if the functional insult occurs during the period of peripubertal maturation of the HPO axis.

Many of these patients are hypoestrogenic but do not have symptoms. However, the estrogen status should still be evaluated given the strong correlation between hypoestrogenemia and the development of osteoporosis. Estrogen status can be determined by means of the progesterone withdrawal test or by measurement of serum estradiol. If there is no withdrawal, hormone replacement therapy (HRT) with combination contraceptive hormones—or traditional HRT—should be instituted. If withdrawal bleeding occurs, any cyclic progestin-containing therapy will be adequate to combat unopposed estrogen and the development of endometrial hyperplasia.

2. Amenorrhea in the female athlete—Hypothalamic dysfunction has been observed in female athletes. Competitors in events such as gymnastics, ballet, marathon running, and diving can show menstrual irregularities ranging from luteal phase defects to amenorrhea. The **female athletic triad** as defined by the American College of Sports Medicine is characterized by disordered eating, amenorrhea, and osteoporosis. The associated nutritional deficiencies can lead to impaired growth and delayed sexual maturation. The neuroendocrine abnormalities are similar to those of women with functional hypothalamic amenorrhea.

These patients have very low body fat, often below the tenth percentile. There is evidence that a negative correlation between body fat and menstrual irregularities exists. In addition, there appears to be a critical body fat level that must be present in order to have a functioning reproductive system. Several studies have shown that these amenorrheic athletes have significantly lower serum leptin levels, which further supports leptin's role as a mediator between nutritional status and the reproductive system. The strenuous exercise these athletes engage in amplifies the effects of the associated nutritional deficiency. This synergism causes severe suppression of GnRH, leading to the low estradiol levels.

Amenorrhea alone is not harmful. However, low serum estradiol over a period of time may lead to osteoporosis and delayed puberty. An analysis of estrogen status may be obtained with measurement of serum estradiol levels or with the progestin withdrawal test (see above). If estrogen is low, a bone mineral density scan should be performed. All patients diagnosed with female athletic triad need combination contraceptive therapy or hormone replacement.

3. Amenorrhea associated with eating disorders—**Anorexia nervosa** is a disorder characterized by relentless dieting in pursuit of a thin body habitus. Approximately 95% of cases occur in females, and the onset is chiefly in adolescence. The clinical features include extreme weight loss leading to a body weight less than 85% of normal for age and height, a distorted body image, and intense fear of gaining weight. These patients usually have a preoccupation with food and are hyperactive, with an obsessive-compulsive personality. The associated symptoms include hypothermia, mild bradycardia, dry skin, constipation, and symptoms of hypoestrogenemia. Furthermore, as part of the diagnostic criteria they must experience at least 3 months of no menses.

The dysfunction in the neuroendocrine system is similar to but often more severe than that described in association with functional hypothalamic amenorrhea. The severe reduction in GnRH pulsatility leads to suppression of FSH and LH secretion, possibly to undetectable levels, and results in anovulation and low serum estradiol levels. Given the severe psychologic and metabolic stress experienced by these individuals, the hypothalamic-pituitary-adrenal axis is activated. The circadian rhythm of adrenal secretion is maintained, but both cortisol production and plasma cortisol levels are persistently elevated secondary to increased pituitary secretion of ACTH. Serum leptin levels in these individuals are significantly lower than normal healthy controls and correlate with percentage of body fat and body weight. A rise in leptin levels in response to dietary treatment is associated with a subsequent rise in gonadotropin levels. This further suggests leptin's role as a potential link between energy stores and the reproductive system.

The self-induced starvation state associated with anorexia nervosa leads to additional endocrine abnormalities not observed in other causes of hypothalamic amenorrhea. For instance, thyroid hormone metabolism is altered. TSH and T_4 levels are in the low normal range, but T_3 levels are usually below normal. This is attributable to decreased peripheral conversion of T_4 to T_3 and increased conversion of T_4 to the metabolically inactive thyroid hormone, reverse T_3—a change that often resembles other states of starvation. This may be a protective mechanism in that the relative hypothyroid state attempts to reduce basal metabolic function in response to a highly catabolic state.

Bulimia occurs in about half of anorectic patients and is defined as binge eating followed by self-induced purging. Not all bulimics have low body weight—in fact, normal-weight bulimic individuals are much more common. These patients also have a variety of neuroendocrine aberrations—often to a lesser degree than those with anorexia—which also lead to menstrual disturbances. Leptin levels are lower than in matched controls but not as low as in individuals with anorexia nervosa. They also have neurotransmitter abnormalities—notably low serotonin levels—which might help explain the often coexisting psychologic difficulties.

Anorexia nervosa is a life-threatening illness with a significant mortality rate due to its metabolic consequences. Anorexic patients should be considered for inpatient therapy and management with a multidisciplinary approach that includes nutritional counseling and psychotherapy. Force-feeding may be necessary in some patients. If weight gain cannot be achieved with oral intake, meals may need to be supplemented by enteral or parenteral feeding. Because anorexia nervosa is a hypoestrogenic state and there is a high potential for the development of osteoporosis, all patients should receive hormone therapy either in the form of hormone replacement or combination contraceptive pills.

In summary, the hypothalamic amenorrhea endocrine syndromes are probably a continuum of disordered eating and nutritional deficiencies resulting in increasingly severe abnormalities in the reproductive system. Furthermore, the age at onset impacts the potential complications of these disorders. If low estradiol levels are present before age 20, bone mineralization may be profoundly affected since this period is critical for building peak bone mass. In addition, if these conditions occur prior to puberty, it may result in stunted growth and delayed development of secondary sexual characteristics.

C. ANATOMIC CAUSES

There are numerous anatomic abnormalities within the central nervous system that can result in a menstrual disturbance. These include developmental defects, brain tumors and infiltrative disorders. The most common anatomic lesion associated with delayed puberty and amenorrhea is a craniopharyngioma. It is derived from Rathke's pouch, and extends into the hypothalamus, pituitary and third ventricle. The symptoms include headaches, visual loss and hypoestrogenism.

Infiltrative disorders that involve the hypothalamus are uncommon. This rare manifestation can result from systemic diseases including sarcoidosis, histiocytosis, hemochromatosis, and lymphoma. These diseases do not initially present with amenorrhea. However, in the presence of these diseases, the hypothalamus may be affected, so they should be part of the differential diagnosis of amenorrhea.

PITUITARY AMENORRHEA

There are a few genetic mutations affecting the pituitary that cause amenorrhea. Rare autosomal recessive mutations may cause deficiencies in FSH, LH, TSH, prolactin, and GH. The clinical manifestations may include delayed puberty, a hypoestrogenic state, and infertility.

A. GENETIC CAUSES

A deficiency in FSH and LH may be a result of GnRH receptor gene mutations. Such mutations are primarily compound heterozygous mutations that affect GnRH receptor-dependent signal transduction. The phenotype of these individuals is similar to that of those with isolated GnRH deficiency. In fact, some investigators speculate that these receptor mutations may be the cause of isolated GnRH deficiency in women, given that no mutations have yet been identified in the ligand or *Kal-1* gene. The estimated prevalence of GnRH receptor mutations in women with hypothalamic amenorrhea is 2%. In a family with other affected females, the prevalence is 7%.

Other rare genetic defects have been associated with amenorrheic women. Mutations in the *FSHβ* gene have been reported. These have an autosomal recessive pattern of inheritance and lead to low serum FSH and estradiol levels and high plasma LH levels. The clinical features include minimal development of secondary sexual characteristics and amenorrhea with no history of menses. Combined hormone deficiencies have also been described. Mutations in PROP-1, a pituitary transcription factor, lead to deficiencies in gonadotropins, TSH, prolactin, and GH. These patients present with stunted growth, hypothyroidism, and delayed puberty in addition to amenorrhea.

B. Endocrine Causes

Hyperprolactinemia is one of the most common causes of amenorrhea, accounting for 15–30% of cases. In the absence of pregnancy or postpartum lactation, persistently elevated prolactin is almost always associated with a hypothalamic-pituitary disorder. Normal prolactin secretion is regulated by several stimulatory and inhibitory factors (see Chapter 5). Prolactin secretion is primarily under tonic inhibition by dopamine, so that any interference with dopamine synthesis or transport from the hypothalamus may result in elevated prolactin levels. In addition to menstrual disturbances, individuals with hyperprolactinemia may present with galactorrhea. In fact, hyperprolactinemia is a common cause of galactorrhea, and up to 80% of patients with amenorrhea and galactorrhea have elevated prolactin levels. Other associated symptoms include headaches, visual field defects, infertility, and osteopenia.

The mechanism whereby hyperprolactinemia causes amenorrhea is not completely known. Studies have shown that prolactin can affect the reproductive system in several ways. Prolactin receptors have been identified on GnRH neurons and may directly suppress GnRH secretion. Others have postulated that elevated prolactin levels inhibit GnRH pulsatility indirectly by increasing other neuromodulators such as endogenous opioids. There is also evidence that GnRH receptors on the pituitary may be down-regulated in the presence of hyperprolactinemia. Furthermore, prolactin may affect the ovaries by altering ovarian progesterone secretion and estrogen synthesis. The best data now available suggest that hyperprolactinemia causes amenorrhea primarily by suppression of GnRH secretion.

Approximately half of patients with elevated prolactin levels have radiologic evidence of a pituitary tumor. The most common type is a prolactin-secreting tumor (prolactinoma), accounting for 40–50% of pituitary tumors. Prolactinomas are mainly composed of lactotrophs; however, these tumors may rarely be mixed with other cell types present in the pituitary. The most common of these mixed tumors secretes both GH and PRL.

The diagnosis of a pituitary adenoma is usually made by examination of the pituitary with MRI. These tumors are categorized into two groups based on their dimensions—microadenomas are those less than 10 mm in diameter, and macroadenomas are the larger ones. These tumors are usually located in the lateral wings of the anterior pituitary. Rarely, a microadenoma will infiltrate the surrounding tissue, including the dura, cavernous sinus, or adjacent skull base. A macroadenoma may expand farther and grow out of the sella to impinge on surrounding structures, including cranial nerve areas such as the optic chiasm; or may extend into the sphenoid sinus. As a result, macroadenomas are more frequently associated with severe headaches, visual field defects, and ophthalmoplegia. The incidence of a microadenoma progressing to a macroadenoma is relatively low, only 3–7%. During pregnancy the risk of a microprolactinoma enlarging is also low, but in the presence of a macroprolactinoma the chance of tumor growth is up to 25%.

Some investigators have found a correlation between pituitary adenoma size and serum prolactin levels. If the serum prolactin level was less than 100 ng/mL, a microprolactinoma was more likely, whereas if the level was greater than 100 ng/mL a macroprolactinoma was more often present. Although this correlation has been reported, the evidence supporting it is not strong. In fact, low prolactin levels may be associated with other pituitary tumors such as nonfunctioning macroadenomas. These "nonfunctioning" tumors may synthesize glycoproteins such as FSH, LH, or their free alpha and beta subunits. Rarely, functioning tumors may arise from other pituitary cells, resulting in excessive hormone secretion. If a macroadenoma is present, measurement of IGF-I, alpha subunit, TSH, and 24-hour urinary cortisol will exclude other functioning adenomas or pituitary insufficiency.

Other tumors of nonpituitary origin may also result in delayed puberty and amenorrhea. The most common of these, is a craniopharyngioma. Although it is most commonly located in the suprasellar region, anatomically, these tumors originate from the anterior surface of the pituitary and can disort the infundibulum of the pituitary. This tumor has not been shown to produce hormones, but because it may compress the infundibulum, it can interfere with the tonic inhibition or prolactin and result in mildly elevated prolactin levels.

Hyperprolactinemia in a patient with amenorrhea is defined as a prolactin level greater than 20 ng/mL, though the limit of normal may vary between laboratories. Normal prolactin release follows a sleep-circadian rhythm, but prolactin may also be secreted in response to stress, physical exercise, breast stimulation, or a meal. Therefore, prolactin should be measured in the mid morning hours and in the fasting state. Other causes of mildly elevated prolactin include medications such as oral contraceptives, neuroleptics, tricyclic antidepressants, metoclopramide, methyldopa, and verapamil. Hyperprolactinemia has also been observed in several chronic diseases, including cirrhosis and renal disease. Furthermore, inflammatory diseases such as sarcoidosis and histiocytosis can infiltrate the hypothalamus or pituitary and result in hyperprolactinemia. Elevated prolactin levels may be a physiologic response. During pregnancy, prolactin levels may be two to four times baseline. With postpartum breast-feeding, the prolactin level should be below 100 ng/mL after 7 days and below 50 ng/mL after 3 months. If a woman is not breast-feeding, prolactin levels should return to baseline by 7 days postpartum (see Table 5–8).

Persistently elevated prolactin levels may also be present in primary hypothyroidism. Approximately 40% of patients with primary hypothyroidism present with a minimal increase in prolactin (25–30 ng/mL), and 10% present with even higher serum levels. Individuals with primary hypothyroidism have an increase in thyrotroph-releasing hormone (TRH) from the hypothalamus, which stimulates TSH and prolactin release and leads to hyperprolactinemia. Patients with long-standing primary hypothyroidism may eventually manifest profound pituitary enlargement due to hypertrophy of thyrotrophs. This mass effect with elevated prolactin levels mimics a prolactinoma. Therefore, all patients with hyperprolactinemia should have their thyroid function investigated to exclude hypothyroidism as the cause.

Prolactinomas are the most common cause of persistent hyperprolactinemia. All patients with elevated prolactin levels should have the test repeated. In addition to blood tests, a careful clinical and pharmacologic history and physical examination should be performed to exclude other causes of hyperprolactinemia. If elevated prolactin levels persist or if any measurement is found to be above 100 ng/mL, MRI of the hypothalamic-pituitary region should be performed. If a microadenoma is observed, the diagnosis of microprolactinoma can be made. If a macroadenoma is observed, other pituitary hormones should be measured to exclude other functioning adenomas or hypopituitarism. All patients diagnosed with macroadenoma should have a visual field examination.

The treatment of choice for prolactinoma is dopamine agonist therapy. These drugs (bromocriptine, cabergoline, pergolide, quinagolide) are very effective at lowering prolactin levels, resolving symptoms, and stimulating tumor shrinkage. Treatment will result in a rapid reduction in prolactin levels in 60–100% of cases. Following diminution of prolactin levels, 60–100% of women resume ovulatory menses within 6 weeks, and galactorrhea disappears within 1–3 months after starting treatment. Reduction in tumor size is usu-ally evident after 2–3 months of drug therapy, but it may occur within days after initiation of treatment. The extrasellar portion of the tumor appears to be particularly sensitive to drug therapy, which explains the improvement in symptoms such as visual impairment or ophthalmoplegia with drug therapy. In patients diagnosed with a microadenoma that is manifested only as a menstrual disturbance, observation should be considered. These individuals may be offered oral contraceptives to control the bleeding pattern or to protect bone from estrogen deficiency. However, the long-term sequelae of persistently elevated prolactin levels are unknown. If dopamine agonist treatment is initiated for a microadenoma, therapy may be continued long-term. If the tumor responds, the dose may be tapered and stopped after menopause. In contrast, individuals with a macroadenoma should take dopamine agonist therapy indefinitely. All patients diagnosed with a prolactinoma should have follow-up imaging, determination of serum prolactin levels, and visual field examinations.

An alternative to medical management of pituitary tumors is transsphenoidal surgery, after which resolution of symptoms may be immediate. However, the success and recurrence rates vary and are dependent on the size of the tumor and the depth of invasion. The larger and more invasive the tumor is, the less chance there is for complete resection and the greater the chance for recurrence. In general, the success rate of surgery for a microadenoma may be up to 70% and for a macroadenoma less than 40%. Overall, the recurrence rate with surgery is approximately 50%. Surgery is a good alternative for resistant tumors or for patients intolerant of medical treatment. Since non-prolactin-secreting pituitary tumors often do not respond well to medical therapy, operation is the treatment of choice for these tumors as well. The risks of surgery include infection, diabetes insipidus, and panhypopituitarism. Complete pituitary testing should be performed prior to surgery.

C. ANATOMIC CAUSES

1. Pituitary destruction—Amenorrhea may be the result of not only pituitary neoplasms, but also pituitary destruction. Similar infiltrative disorders that can involve the hypothalamus can affect the pituitary, and is slightly more vulnerable. Other disorders that cause pituitary insufficiency may be situational. A rare autoimmune disease, lymphocytic hypophysitis can cause pituitary destruction during the puerperium and ultimately results in panhypopituitarism. Pituitary necrosis may also occur secondary to a hypotensive event. Typically, 80–90% of the pituitary must be damaged before pituitary failure ensues and the robust blood supply to the pituitary makes this an uncommon event. If pituitary ischemia and necrosis are related to postpartum hemorrhage, it is known as Sheehan's syndrome, otherwise, it is called Simmond's disease. Since this type of injury typically affects the entire pituitary, most often more than one or all the pituitary hormones may be deficient. Observation has suggested that hormone loss follows a pattern, starting with the gonadotropins, followed by GH and PRL. Fortunately, ACTH and TSH are the last to be lost, since they are vital.

OVARIAN AMENORRHEA

The physiologic period in a woman's life when there is permanent cessation of menstruation and regression of ovarian function is known as menopause (see below). The cause of ovarian failure is thought to be depletion of ovarian follicles. The median age at menopause is 51.1 years. Premature menopause is defined as ovarian failure prior to age 40, which is reported to occur in 1% of the population. The etiology of premature ovarian failure may have a genetic basis. Several mutations that affect gonadal function have been identified and include defects in hormone receptors and steroid synthesis. Other potential causes include autoimmune ovarian destruction, iatrogenic ovarian injury, and idiopathic ovarian failure. The most severe form of premature ovarian failure presents with absent secondary sexual characteristics and is most often due to gonadal agenesis or dysgenesis (see Chapter 14). Less severe forms may result only in diminished reproductive capacity.

The other ovarian cause of amenorrhea is repetitive ovulation failure or anovulation. Other than menopause, it is the most common cause of amenorrhea. Chronic anovulation may be secondary to disorders of the hypothalamic-pituitary axis and has been previously discussed. Anovulation may also be due to systemic disorders. The causes of ovarian failure and anovulation due to peripheral disorders will be discussed below.

Ovarian failure is diagnosed based on the clinical picture of amenorrhea and the demonstration of elevated FSH (> 40 IU/L). This may occur at any time from embryonic development onward. If it occurs prior to age 40, it is called premature ovarian failure. The presence or absence of secondary sexual characteristics is evidence of whether ovarian activity was present in the past. The most common cause of hypergonadotropic amenorrhea in the absence of sexual characteristics is abnormal gonadal development, which occurs in more than half of these individuals. When the gonad fails to develop, this is known as **gonadal agenesis.** The karyotype of these individuals is 46,XX, and the cause of failure is usually unknown. If streak gonads are present, this indicates at least partial gonadal development and is called **gonadal dysgenesis.** The karyotype of these individuals may be normal, but it is more likely that there will be alterations in sex chromosomes (see Chapter 14).

Premature Ovarian Failure

A. GENETIC ORIGIN OF PREMATURE OVARIAN FAILURE

Two intact X chromosomes are necessary for the maintenance of oocytes during embryogenesis, and the loss of or any alteration in the sex chromosome leads to accelerated follicular loss. This implies that two intact alleles are required for the normal function of some genes on the X chromosome. Turner's syndrome is a classic example of complete absence of one X chromosome. It manifests as short stature, sexual infantilism, amenorrhea, and ovarian dysgenesis. This is a well-recognized condition that occurs in 1:2000–1:5000 females at birth. Turner's syndrome is associated with a number of other phenotypic abnormalities, including a webbed neck, broad chest, low hairline, and cardiovascular and renal defects. It is interesting that fewer than half of patients with Turner's syndrome have a single cell line with the karyotype 45,X. The majority of patients actually present with a mosaic karyotype such as 45,X/46,XX. These patients have varying degrees of the Turner syndrome phenotype and may display some secondary sexual development or may have a history of menstrual function. Some pregnancies have been reported.

Another mosaic pattern that has been associated with Turner's syndrome is the 45,X/46,XY karyotype. This chromosomal anomaly has been termed **mixed gonadal dysgenesis.** These patients may have some functional testicular tissue and present with varying degrees of genital ambiguity. If enough testicular tissue is present to produce antimüllerian hormone (AMH), these patients may also present with abnormalities of the internal genitalia. An extreme case of this would be a patient with 46,XX/46,XY karyotype who has both ovarian tissue and testicular tissue along with wolffian and müllerian structures internally. These patients are **true hermaphrodites.**

Patients with gonadal dysgenesis may be phenotypically normal and the abnormality may be manifested only as delayed pubertal development and amenorrhea. They probably have normal müllerian structures and streak gonads. These individuals can display an array of karyotypes, including 46,XY (Swyer's syndrome). Patients with a male karyotype but a female phenotype presumably underwent testicular failure prior to internal or external genitalia differentiation. If a dysgenetic gonad contains a Y chromosome or a fragment of the Y chromosome, there is a 10–30% risk for future gonadal malignancy, and gonadal extirpation is indicated at the time of diagnosis.

Premature ovarian failure may also be defined as ovarian failure before age 40 but after puberty. Since complete absence of an X chromosome results in a dysgenetic gonad, candidate genes for premature ovarian failure are probably those that escape X inactivation. In mammals, X inactivation occurs in all cells in order to provide dosage compensation for X-linked genes between males and females (Lyon hypothesis). Further observation has illustrated that terminal deletions in Xp lead to the classic stigmas of Turner's syndrome while deletions in Xp or Xq present with varying degrees of early reproductive failure. However, most of the genes involved in folliculogenesis appear to be located on the long arm of the X chromosome. Several regions on the X chromosome, including POF 1 and POF 2, have been evaluated with knockout models in animals and have shown varying effects on ovarian development (Figure 13–8).

Limited observations have found that deletions occurring closer to the centromere manifest a more severe phenotype that includes disruption of pubertal development. In contrast, deletions that occur in the distal regions tend to present with early reproductive aging and infertility. An example of a distal mutation on the long arm is the *FMR1* gene (fragile X gene). An association has been described between the *FMR1* permutation state and premature ovarian failure. The prevalence of *FMR1* gene permutations approximates 2–3% of patients who present with sporadic premature ovarian failure and may be as high as 15% in familial cases. Although a number of genes on the X chromosome have demonstrated involvement in ovarian physiology, the majority of premature ovarian failure patients have no identifiable mutations on the X chromosome.

Autosomal recessive genes that have shown contributions to premature ovarian failure are very rare. FSH receptor mutations have been identified in humans with premature ovarian failure. These individuals present with a phenotype that ranges from absent secondary sexual development to normal development and early reproductive failure. The prevalence of FSH receptor mutations varies but is most common in the Finnish population (1% carriers). This mutation has not been observed in North America. An inactivated LH receptor has been identified in patients with normal puberty and amenorrhea but is quite rare. Mutations in genes involved in steroidogenesis have also been associated with premature ovarian failure. These enzymes include CYP17α and aromatase. Patients with CYP17α mutations may have a 46,XX or 46,XY karyotype. They have a similar phenotype except that those with 46,XY have absent müllerian structures since AMH is produced from their testes. Individuals with aromatase deficiency present with sexual ambiguity and clitoromegaly. Several other autosomal genetic mutations have been discovered that may have a role in ovarian physiology. However, at this time, most cases of premature ovarian failure with normal pubertal development have not been associated with any specific genetic mutation (see Chapter 14).

B. Autoimmune Origin of Premature Ovarian Failure

Autoimmune ovarian destruction is another potential cause of premature ovarian failure. This diagnosis is difficult to make unless it presents with one of the autoimmune polyglandular syndromes (see Chapter 4). The circumstantial evidence supporting the diagnosis is found in the high incidence of concomitant autoimmune disease—20% or more in patients with premature ovarian failure. The strongest association is with autoimmune thyroid disease. In addition, 10–20% of individuals with autoimmune adrenal disease experience premature ovarian failure. Conversely, 2–10% of patients with idiopathic premature ovarian failure develop adrenal insufficiency.

Premature ovarian failure patients are often diagnosed as having autoimmune disease if autoimmune antibodies are identified. Thyroid antibodies are most frequently screened. If abnormal, thyroid function should be evaluated. All patients with suspected autoimmune premature ovarian insufficiency should be screened regularly for adrenal insufficiency.

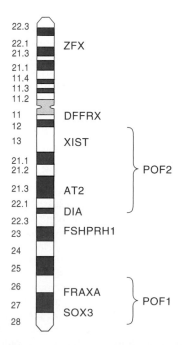

Figure 13–8. Candidate genes on the X chromosome for premature ovarian failure (POF). (Reproduced, with permission, from Davison RM, Davis CJ, Conway GS: The X chromosome and ovarian failure. Clin Endocrinol 1999;51:673.)

C. IATROGENIC CAUSES OF PREMATURE OVARIAN FAILURE

Iatrogenic causes of premature ovarian failure include radiation therapy, chemotherapy, and ovarian insults resulting from torsion or surgery. The risk of premature ovarian failure following radiation and chemotherapy is proportionate to the patient's age. If the radiation dose is higher than 800 Gy, all women experience ovarian failure. Chemotherapy alone may induce temporary or permanent ovarian failure. In general, younger individuals with chemotherapy-induced ovarian injury are more likely to recover.

D. RESISTANT OVARY SYNDROME

A rare cause of hypergonadotropic amenorrhea associated with numerous unstimulated ovarian follicles is the resistant ovary syndrome. These patients classically have no history of ovulatory dysfunction and present with secondary sexual characteristics and symptoms suggestive of estrogen deficiency. This diagnosis was established in an era when ovarian biopsy was used to determine the cause of menstrual disturbances. However, the definition of resistant ovary syndrome is not universally accepted. In fact, in the original series, cases were included in which patients had demonstrated ovulatory function in the past but later developed a clinical picture suggestive of ovarian resistance. This pattern is more typical of ovarian aging and follicular depletion.

The cause is not known. Histologic features of ovarian biopsy demonstrate that there is no plasma cell or lymphocytic infiltration, indicating that it is not caused by autoimmune destruction. The presence of numerous follicles indicates that premature ovarian failure is not due to follicular depletion. Several studies have looked at gonadotropins, FSH receptors, and antibodies that serve as blockers to the gonadotropin receptors, and the literature to date is inconclusive about the cause.

A certain diagnosis can only be established with ovarian biopsy. However, current recommendations for management of amenorrhea do not include surgery to make a diagnosis. The diagnosis is therefore one of exclusion. In the absence of autoimmune disease and of any history of ovulation, karyotyping should be performed to exclude chromosomal abnormalities. In patients with normal karyotypes, the diagnosis of premature ovarian failure and resistant ovary syndrome will be hard to make without biopsy. Improvements in ultrasound technology may make it possible to differentiate these entities by the measurement of ovarian volumes and antral follicle counts.

E. SUMMARY

In over half of patients with premature ovarian failure, no specific cause can be identified. The age defining premature ovarian failure is somewhat arbitrary. By definition, menopause is preceded by reproductive failure. It is thought that the time interval between menopause and the end of fertility may be approximately 10 years, and we know that approximately 10% of women reach menopause by 46 years of age and 1% by 40 years. Therefore, women who experience menopause at 45 years of age probably encounter a decline in reproductive potential or even reproductive failure at 35 years of age. This has obvious implications for women who are delaying childbearing. Several studies have described a significant association between the menopausal ages of mothers and daughters, twins, and sisters. A number of studies have identified new genes that are involved in ovarian physiology. It is hoped that these investigations will help in the treatment of subfertility and result in a reduction in infertility. At a minimum, they may allow better prospective individual prediction of reproductive risk.

ANOVULATION

Chronic anovulation may be defined as repetitive ovulation failure, which differs from ovarian failure in that viable oocytes remain in the ovary. Anovulation is the most common cause of amenorrhea during the reproductive years. There are several causes; those associated with hypothalamic and pituitary disorders have previously been mentioned and will not be considered in this section. Other conditions that cause anovulation include the peripheral endocrinopathies. These disorders result in a hormonal imbalance—mainly elevated androgens or estrogens—and lead to inappropriate feedback mechanisms and ovulatory failure. The peripheral endocrine disorders will be discussed below in greater detail.

Polycystic Ovarian Syndrome

Hyperandrogenic anovulation accounts for over 30% of cases of amenorrhea. Most often it is due to polycystic ovarian syndrome (PCOS). The reported prevalence of PCOS depends on the criteria used to define it. Although there is considerable controversy over the definition, most investigators have focused on the 1990 NIH-NICHD diagnostic criteria (see Table 13–2). That definition includes ovulatory dysfunction, with evidence of hyperandrogenism either clinically or by laboratory testing, in the absence of identifiable causes of hyperandrogenism. Using these criteria, the prevalence of unexplained hyperandrogenic chronic anovulation approximates 4–6%, and it is considered the most common endocrine disorder in women of reproductive age. In fact, PCOS is responsible for over 20% of all cases of amenorrhea and up to 75% of all cases of anovulatory infertility.

Table 13–2. Diagnostic criteria for polycystic ovary syndrome (PCOS)—percentage of participants agreeing at 1990 NICHD PCOS Conference.[1]

Definite or Probable	Possible
Hyperandrogenemia, 64%	Insulin resistance, 69%
Exclusion of other causes, 60%	Perimenarchal onset, 62%
Exclusion of CAH, 59%	Elevated LH/FSH, 55%
Menstrual dysfunction, 52%	Polycystic ovary by ultrasound, 52%
Clinical hyperandrogenism, 48%	Clinical hyperandrogenism, 52%
	Menstrual dysfunction, 45%

[1]Reproduced, with permission, from Dunaif A: Insulin resistance and the polycystic ovary syndrome: mechanism and implications for pathogenesis. Endocr Rev 1997;18:774.

The clinical manifestations of PCOS are oligomenorrhea or amenorrhea with symptoms suggestive of hyperandrogenism such as acne or hirsutism. Approximately 50% of women diagnosed with PCOS are obese, and most have polycystic ovaries present on sonography (see below). Underlying these features are numerous biochemical abnormalities that have been associated with this syndrome, including elevated circulating total testosterone, free testosterone, DHEAS, and insulin as well as decreased sex hormone binding globulin (SHBG) and an elevated LH/FSH ratio. However, these abnormalities are not present in all PCOS patients. In fact, only 40% of women who present with only hirsutism have elevated total testosterone levels, and 30–70% have elevated DHEAS levels. Similarly, the LH/FSH ratio is not a reliable diagnostic test. Although elevated LH/FSH ratios are common findings in thin women, in obese PCOS patients the ratio is within the normal range about half of the time. Hyperinsulinemia has recently been hypothesized to play a major role in the pathogenesis of PCOS (see below). The prevalence of insulin resistance may approximate 50–60%, compared with 10–25% observed in the general population. However, insulin resistance is difficult to measure. Part of the difficulty is that there is no universally agreed upon definition of insulin resistance and the laboratory tests are not standardized. Furthermore, baseline insulin levels vary depending on the population and body weight. For example, up to 60% of ovulatory obese patients have demonstrated some form of insulin resistance. Nonetheless, there is good evidence that a subset of normal-weight women and obese women with PCOS have a greater degree of insulin resistance and compensatory hyperinsulinemia compared with weight-matched controls.

A. DIAGNOSIS OF PCOS

The diagnosis of PCOS is typically based on clinical features, though additional information may be obtained with biochemical testing and sonographic examination. In most situations, however, measurement of serum androgen levels should play only a limited role in the evaluation. Most patients who have hyperandrogenemia present with obvious clinical manifestations, and the presence of normal androgen levels in a patient with hirsutism or acne does not exclude the diagnosis of PCOS. However, there are subsets of amenorrheic patients who are hyperandrogenemic without clinical manifestations, most likely as a result of relative insensitivity to circulating androgens. It is in these patients that assessing androgen levels may be of value in determining the cause of amenorrhea. More commonly, androgens such as DHEAS and testosterone are measured to exclude other causes of hyperandrogenic anovulation such as nonclassic adrenal hyperplasia and androgen-secreting tumors (see below).

In Europe (particularly in England), sonography is used to identify morphologic evidence of PCOS. Polycystic ovaries tend to be enlarged and are characterized by the presence of ten or more cysts that are between 2 mm and 8 mm in diameter and arranged along the subcapsular edge of the ovary in a "string of pearls" fashion. Even so, the finding of polycystic ovaries does not establish the diagnosis of PCOS. In fact, over 80% of hirsute women with normal menses demonstrate polycystic ovaries. Polycystic ovaries are common in any woman with hyperandrogenism presenting with acne, seborrhea, or male pattern alopecia independent of menstrual disturbances. Furthermore, over 20% of normal women have this ovarian morphologic feature. Thus, the finding of polycystic ovaries alone is not diagnostic of polycystic ovarian syndrome as understood in the USA, and ovarian morphology is not a useful marker for defining the cause of chronic anovulation.

B. MECHANISM OF ANOVULATION

The mechanism of anovulation in PCOS remains unclear. It is evident that the population of preantral follicles is increased and that follicular development is arrested. It is also known that the development of preantral follicles is not primarily under hormonal control. Evidence supports the components of the intraovarian network as regulators of antral follicle development. It is known that many of the accumulated follicles in PCOS remain steroidogenically competent and are capable of producing estrogen and progesterone. In fact, it is interesting that women with PCOS produce both androgens and estrogen in excess (estrone). Under normal conditions, follicles respond to LH after they reach approximately 10 mm in diameter. However, polycystic ovarian follicles acquire responsiveness to LH at a much smaller diameter, which may lead to inappropriate terminal differentiation of granulosa cells and result in disorganized follicular development. The elevated LH levels and relative hyperinsulinemia that exist in some PCOS patients may synergistically potentiate disordered folliculogenesis. Although hyperandrogenism is part of the diagnostic criteria for PCOS, its direct impact on folliculogenesis is not clear. It is conceivable that androgens contribute to the effects of LH and insulin on follicular maturation. It is also possible that the excess estrogens may result in a negative feedback loop to inhibit FSH release and prevent further follicular development.

A fundamental abnormality in PCOS is excess androgen production. Both the adrenal glands and the ovaries contribute to circulating androgens. The relative strengths of androgens are listed in Table 13–3.

During the reproductive years, both the ovaries and the adrenals contribute up to 25% of the circulating testosterone by direct secretion. The remaining 50% arises from peripheral conversion of androstenedione, which is produced equally by the adrenal gland and the ovary. This differs from males, in whom only 5% of the circulating testosterone is derived from androstenedione. It is also estimated that androstenedione conversion contributes to the increased circulating estrogen levels. This weaker androgen is peripherally converted to estrone by adipose tissue, hair follicles, and the liver. Furthermore, it is estimated that over 60% of the most potent androgen, dihydrotestosterone, is derived from androstenedione in women. DHEAS is the major androgen produced by the adrenal gland. It is responsible for over 95% of the circulating DHEAS levels. Although it is the most abundant androgen circulating in the body, it contributes minimally to serum testosterone levels (Figure 13–3).

Androgen production within the ovary is mainly by the thecal interstitial cells that surround the follicle and to a lesser extent the secondary interstitial cells located in the stroma. The CYP17α complex is thought to be the key enzyme in biosynthesis of ovarian androgens. Under normal conditions, a large proportion of the androgens produced by the theca cells diffuse into the granulosa cell layer of the follicle where they are rapidly converted to estrogen as shown in Figures 13–6 and 13–9 (two-cell theory). The intrinsic control of androgen production in the ovary is modulated by intraovarian factors and hormones (see section on ovarian steroidogenesis at the beginning of this chapter). It is the dysregulation of hormone production that is most likely responsible for PCOS.

Several studies have shown that women with PCOS have an exaggerated ovarian androgen response to various stimuli. To illustrate: hyperstimulation of 17-hydroxyprogesterone levels was noted when women diagnosed with PCOS were given a GnRH agonist or hCG, suggesting increased CYP17α activity. This study is supported by in vitro studies in which measurement of steroids in cultured human theca cells from polycystic ovaries revealed concentrations of androstenedione, 17α-hydroxyprogesterone, and progesterone that were respectively twentyfold, tenfold, and fivefold higher than levels in control cells. Additional studies have found increased expression of the genes encoding CYP17α hydroxylase, P450scc, the LH receptor, and StAR. These findings reflect a global enhancement of steroidogenesis. This situation is compounded by the hypertrophy of theca cells that is present in women with PCOS.

Several studies have evaluated the intraovarian modulators as participants in the pathogenesis of PCOS. IGF-binding proteins (BPs), especially BP2 and BP4, are found to be increased in the follicular fluid of PCOS ovaries. They may act locally to decrease free IGF-I and thus decrease the effects of FSH on the oocyte and granulosa cells. Inhibin also is a likely candidate since a large proportion of women with PCOS have relative FSH suppression. However, studies have not shown consistent results, suggesting that if inhibin is involved, the effect is minimal. Follistatin, the activin-binding protein, was in the past thought to play an important role in the development of PCOS. It was initially implicated because activin functions to inhibit androgen production and enhance FSH expression. However, current studies do not demonstrate a significant association between abnormalities in follistatin and PCOS.

The adrenal gland may be significantly involved in the pathogenesis of some cases of PCOS. The connection seems plausible since adrenal androgens can be converted to more potent androgens in the ovary. Furthermore, a significant portion of women with congenital adrenal hyperplasia have polycystic ovaries (see below). Several studies have shown that DHEAS is ele-

Table 13–3. Relative androgenic activity of androgens.[1]

Steroid	Activity
Dihydrotestosterone	300
Testosterone	100
Androstenedione	10
DHEA, DHEAS	5

[1]Reproduced, with permission, from Yen SSC, Jaffe RB, Barbieri RL (editors). *Reproductive Endocrinology.* Saunders, 1999.

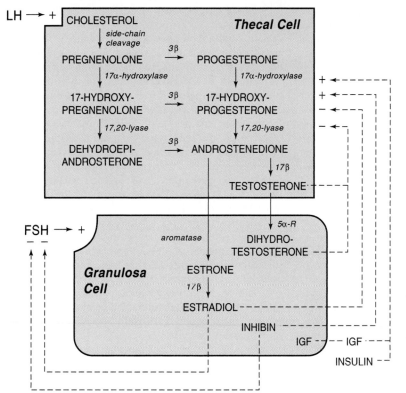

Figure 13–9. Major steroid pathways in the ovary according to the two-cell hypothesis of ovarian function. (Reproduced, with permission, from Ehrmann DA, Barnes RB, Rosenfeld RL: Polycystic ovary syndrome as a form of functional ovarian hyperandrogenism due to dysregulation of androgen secretion. Endocr Rev 1995;16:322.)

vated in 25–60% of patients with PCOS. It has also been reported that there is an increased response of androstenedione and 17α-hydroxyprogesterone to exogenous ACTH. These findings suggest an underlying abnormality in the CYP17α expressed in the adrenal gland as well as in the ovary. However, there are minimal data to support CYP17α dysfunction in the adrenal gland. It has also been shown that ovarian steroids can stimulate adrenal androgen production; however, additional findings suggest that the ovary is not the primary cause of adrenal hyperresponsiveness. The critical role played by adrenal androgens during the pubertal transition has not been fully investigated as a potential contributor to the development of PCOS.

Hyperinsulinemia

A relationship between insulin and hyperandrogenism has been postulated based on several observations. Various case reports have shown that acanthosis nigricans—hyperpigmentation of skin in the intertriginous areas—is associated with severe insulin resistance. A number of these patients also presented with hyperandrogenism and anovulation. The relationship was substantiated when it was observed that the degree of hyperinsuline-

mia was correlated with the degree of hyperandrogenism. Further studies revealed that hyperinsulinemia is frequently identified in women with PCOS. It has been shown that the cause of hyperinsulinemia is insulin resistance and that the dysfunction lies in the postbinding signaling pathway. The frequency and degree of hyperinsulinemia in women with PCOS is amplified in the presence of obesity. Although many women with PCOS exhibit insulin resistance, some do not. However, insulin resistance is also observed in some thin PCOS patients.

Insulin may cause hyperandrogenism in several different ways, though the exact mechanism has not been well defined. It is suggested that insulin has a stimulatory effect on CYP17α. There is evidence from in vitro models that insulin may act directly on the ovary. It has been shown that the ovary possesses insulin receptors and IGF-I receptors. In addition, several studies have reported that insulin stimulates ovarian estrogen, androgen, and progesterone secretion and that its effect is greatly enhanced by the addition of gonadotropins. Administration of an insulin-sensitizing agent (eg, metformin or a thiazolidinedione) to obese women with PCOS leads to a substantial reduction in 17α-hydroxyprogesterone levels, reflecting decreased CYP17α activity. However, clinical studies in which insulin infusions were administered to normal women failed to demonstrate increased testosterone production, and there were no changes in androgen levels when normal women were given insulin-sensitizing agents. These observations suggest that insulin's effect on androgen production is more likely a modifier rather than a predisposing agent.

The relationship between insulin and adrenal androgen production is less clear. Some studies have shown that insulin increases secretion of 17α-hydroxyprogesterone and DHEAS in response to ACTH. Other studies have shown that DHEAS decreases after acute insulin infusions are administered to normal men and women. Furthermore, when insulin-sensitizing agents were administered to women with PCOS, a decrease in DHEAS was observed. Although there is less evidence to support the association of insulin and adrenal androgen production, if there is an insulin effect it is as a modulator of adrenal secretory activity.

Insulin may indirectly affect androgen levels. Several studies have reported that insulin directly inhibits SHBG production. There is an inverse correlation between insulin levels and SHBG, so that decreasing insulin levels would decrease the circulating bioavailable androgen level (via increases in SHBG). It has also been shown that insulin decreases insulin-like growth factor binding protein-1 (IGFBP-1). This would increase free IGF-I, which could modulate ovarian androgen production in a fashion similar to insulin. Although these indirect mechanisms may play a role, the literature suggests that insulin acts directly to augment androgen production. However, it appears that a dysregulation in steroidogenesis must also exist in order for insulin to cause hyperandrogenism.

There is increasing evidence for a strong genetic component in the etiology of PCOS. Several candidate genes have been investigated, including genes involved in steroidogenesis and carbohydrate metabolism, but none have been conclusively linked with the disease. PCOS is heterogeneous clinically, raising the possibility of different genetic causes and a variable environmental contribution to the syndrome.

Increasing attention is being directed to the possibility that PCOS begins before adolescence. In fact, the initial insult may begin in utero, where there is ample exposure to androgens derived from the fetal adrenal and ovary. This hormonal environment may reprogram the ovary and alter steroidogenesis in a manner that predisposes to PCOS. The phenotypic expression of PCOS would then be determined by environmental factors such as diet and exercise.

The various biochemical abnormalities associated with PCOS have led to studies investigating metabolic sequelae of this syndrome. Long-term health problems such as the development of cardiovascular disease and diabetes have been linked to PCOS. However, there are limited studies looking at whether women with PCOS actually experience increased cardiovascular events. Several observational studies have demonstrated that women with PCOS have alterations in their lipid profiles, including increased triglycerides and LDL and decreased HDL compared with weight-matched controls. Furthermore, the degree of dyslipidemia has been correlated with the magnitude of insulin resistance. The fact that insulin resistance occurs with greater frequency in women with PCOS suggests that they are at higher risk for the development of diabetes mellitus. It is known that up to 30–40% of women with PCOS have impaired glucose tolerance, though it is most often seen in patients who are obese. Limited retrospective studies have suggested that women with PCOS have an increased frequency of developing type 2 diabetes. In summary, as demonstrated by surrogate markers, the available data show that these patients have increased risk factors for cardiovascular events and diabetes. Long-term prospective studies will be required to determine if these patients are really at risk for increased mortality and morbidity.

The fact that hyperinsulinemia underlies many of the potential adverse sequelae raises a question about whether insulin resistance should be assessed in all patients diagnosed with PCOS. However, the potential impact of hyperinsulinemia is unknown. Furthermore, there is no universal laboratory criterion or standardization for establishing the diagnosis of insulin resistance, which raises doubts about whether any potential adverse sequelae can be prevented if insulin resistance is identified. Further data are necessary prior to widespread use of medications such as metformin or a thiazolidinedione to reduce insulin resistance in patients with PCOS and to determine (1) if these patients are indeed at risk for cardiovascular events, (2) if hyperinsulinemia is an independent risk factor, and (3) whether long-term treatment with any insulin-sensitizing agent will decrease the potential sequelae.

C. ADDITIONAL RISKS ASSOCIATED WITH ANOVULATION

Another concern is that women who are anovulatory do not produce a significant amount of progesterone. This leads to an unopposed estrogen environment on the uterine lining, which is a significant risk factor for development of endometrial cancer. In fact, an association has been found between endometrial cancer and PCOS. There is also some evidence to suggest an association of PCOS with both breast cancer and ovarian cancer, but PCOS has not been conclusively shown to be an independent risk factor for either disease.

D. Treatment

The treatment of PCOS should be directed toward prevention of potential malignant endometrial sequelae and the patient's symptoms. Combination oral contraceptives have been shown to promote a significant reduction in endometrial cancer in the general population. It makes sense to think that a similar benefit would accrue to women with PCOS since the ovarian stimulation is minimized and the progestin would counteract the estrogenic environment. Oral contraceptives also improve menstrual irregularities, and combination oral contraceptives improve hirsutism and acne in PCOS. The mechanism is not completely known, but oral contraceptives decrease the amount of bioavailable androgens via increased SHBG production and by ovarian suppression. It has also been shown that progestins can inhibit 5α-reductase activity, which further decreases the production of dihydrotestosterone, the major androgen that stimulates hair growth. The maximal effect is evident after 6 months of treatment (the hair cycle length is estimated to be 4 months). If hirsutism is severe or if oral contraceptives alone are not effective, the addition of spironolactone may be beneficial. Spironolactone is an antimineralocorticoid agent that inhibits androgen biosynthesis in the adrenal and ovary, inhibits 5α-reductase, and is a competitive inhibitor of the androgen receptor. Side effects are minimal and include diuresis in the first few days, dyspepsia, breast tenderness, and abnormal bleeding which can be alleviated with concomitant use of oral contraceptives. Because oral contraceptives and spironolactone act by different mechanisms, the combined effect is synergistic. Long-acting GnRH agonists and 5α-reductase inhibitors (finasteride) have been used for refractory cases with some success.

ADRENAL CAUSES OF AMENORRHEA

Androgen Excess

A. Congenital Adrenal Hyperplasia

Congenital adrenal hyperplasia is another disorder that may cause hyperandrogenism. It presents with a wide range of clinical forms, ranging from severe—which may be classified as "classic," "salt-wasting," or "simple virilizing"—to milder forms known as "acquired," "adult-onset," "nonclassic," or "late-onset" congenital hyperplasia. The clinical manifestations reflect the severity of the enzymatic defect. Severe or classic forms are discussed in Chapter 14 and will not be considered here. This section will discuss the nonclassic forms, ranging in prevalence from 1% to 10% depending on the ethnicity of the patient. The clinical features are similar to those of patients diagnosed with PCOS and

include menstrual irregularities, hyperandrogenism, infertility, and polycystic ovaries.

The adrenal gland consists of a cortex and a medulla. The cortex is divided into three functional zones based on location and the principal hormone secreted (see Chapter 9). The zona glomerulosa is the outermost zone and lies adjacent to the adrenal capsule. It is primarily responsible for aldosterone production. The zona fasciculata lies immediately below the glomerulosa. It principally secretes glucocorticoids, though it is capable of producing androgens. The zona reticularis is located beneath the zona fasciculata and overlies the adrenal medulla. It is this zone that principally secretes androgens. Both the zona fasciculata and the zona reticularis are regulated by ACTH. It is the secretory activity of these two zones that results in nonclassic adrenal hyperplasia.

Congenital adrenal hyperplasia is an inherited autosomal recessive disorder that is caused by mutations of genes involved with adrenal steroidogenesis. The mutations mostly occur in the 21-hydroxylase genes *(P450c21A and P450c21B)* and rarely in the 3β-hydroxysteroid dehydrogenase gene or 11β-hydroxylase genes *(P450c11B and P450c11AS)*. In classic forms, the enzymatic defects are severe and result in cortisol deficiency diagnosed at birth. Owing to the cortisol deficiency, there is corticotropin excess and hyperstimulation of the adrenal gland. The adrenal precursors produced proximal to the enzymatic defect accumulate and are converted in the periphery to more potent androgens, resulting in symptoms of hyperandrogenism. However, most patients with nonclassic adrenal hyperplasia do not demonstrate deficient cortisol production or excess ACTH. It is suggested that most of the androgen excess in nonclassic adrenal hyperplasia arises as a consequence of subtle alterations in enzyme kinetics. Furthermore, some studies report a generalized adrenocortical hyperactivity rather than deficient enzyme activity.

The diagnosis can be established by measuring early morning basal 17-hydroxyprogesterone levels. Levels greater than 800 ng/dL (24.24 pmol/L) are diagnostic of 21-hydroxylase deficiency. However, the elevation in 17-hydroxyprogesterone is often not impressive and does not differ from that observed in PCOS. If the basal 17-hydroxyprogesterone levels are greater than 200 ng/dL (6.06 pmol/L) and less than 800 ng/dL (24.2 pmol/L), a provocative test with ACTH (250 μg intravenously) should be performed. If 17-hydroxyprogesterone levels are greater than 1000 ng/dL (30.30 pmol/L) 1 hour after administration of ACTH, the diagnosis of 21-hydroxylase deficiency can be made. (Elimination of a false elevation in 17-hydroxyprogesterone due to ovulation must be excluded by simultaneous measurement of progesterone.) The other rare enzymatic defects that result in nonclassic adrenal hyperplasia can similarly be tested with measurements of steroid products proximal to the blockade following provocative testing.

Treatment of nonclassic adrenal hyperplasia is similar to that of PCOS, raising a question about whether an etiologic diagnosis is necessary. It is certainly an expense, leading to no change in management except in regard to infertility treatment (see below). Diagnosis may also be advisable in the woman with adrenal hyperplasia who intends future childbearing for genetic counseling and to prepare for in utero treatment should an affected fetus be identified by amniocentesis. While some experts suggest dexamethasone treatment for symptoms of hyperandrogenism, studies show inconsistent results, and there is concern about the consequent adrenal suppression.

B. Cushing's Syndrome

Chronic glucocorticoid excess, whatever its cause, leads to the constellation of symptoms and physical features known as Cushing's syndrome. The most common cause is iatrogenic as a result of glucocorticoid treatment. However, an ACTH-secreting microadenoma (Cushing's disease) accounts for more than 70% of cases of endogenous hypercortisolism. Less common causes include primary adrenal disease (tumors or hyperplasia) and ectopic (not hypothalamic-pituitary) ACTH-producing or CRH-producing tumors. Patients with Cushing's syndrome have a range of clinical manifestations that vary with age at onset and etiology. This section will discuss the adult clinical presentation briefly. For a more detailed discussion, see Chapter 9.

Cushing's syndrome (noniatrogenic) is rare and occurs in approximately 2.6 per million individuals. It may be responsible for less than 1% of those individuals who present with hirsutism. Although it is uncommon, it can present similarly to PCOS and congenital adrenal hyperplasia and needs to be considered in the differential diagnosis of hyperandrogenism and anovulation. Patients with corticotropin excess typically have additional clinical features suggestive of glucocorticoid or mineralocorticoid hypersecretion. The most common features include obesity with increased centripetal fat, moon facies, muscle weakness, and striae. Other manifestations may include diabetes, hypertension, and osteoporosis. Women with primary tumors tend to have a rapid onset of symptoms and often manifest with severe hyperandrogenism (frank virilization) which includes male pattern baldness, deepening voice, clitoromegaly, and defeminization.

Hirsutism or acne is present in about 60–70% of women with Cushing's syndrome. However, the exact mechanism of hyperandrogenic effects is not completely known. It is evident that excess corticotropin causes hyperstimulation of the zona fasciculata and zona reticularis and results in hypersecretion of cortisol and androgens. It is also known that adrenal tumors may selectively overproduce androgens.

Menstrual irregularities occur in over 80% of patients with Cushing's syndrome. The exact cause of anovulation is unclear. It has already been observed that hyperandrogenemia may have a significant impact on ovulation. However, several studies have shown that glucocorticoids can also suppress the hypothalamic-pituitary axis. Thus, the elevated glucocorticoids may be an additional factor in the pathophysiology of anovulation associated with this syndrome. (See Chapters 5 and 9 for the diagnosis and treatment of Cushing's syndrome.)

C. Androgen-Secreting Tumor

If there is a rapid onset of androgenic symptoms, an androgen-secreting adrenal tumor should be suspected. Elevated testosterone (> 200 ng/dL; 6.9 nmol/L) and DHEAS (> 700 ng/mL; 19 μmol/L) levels should raise the suspicion of a tumor. However, more than 50% of adrenal androgen-secreting tumors have testosterone levels below 200 ng/dL (6.9 nmol/L). Furthermore, the majority of patients with high testosterone levels do not have tumors. Measurement of levels of DHEAS in these patients yields similar inconsistencies. This suggests that laboratory tests have limited value in screening for androgen-secreting tumors, and a better predictor is a clinical history and physical examination. Additional symptoms include weight loss, anorexia, bloating, and back pain. If suspicion is high, an abdominal CT scan will confirm the diagnosis. The treatment involves surgical resection, mitotane (adrenolytic), and steroid synthesis inhibitors.

Androgen-secreting tumors can also originate from the ovary. The incidence approximates 1:500–1:1000 hyperandrogenic patients. Testosterone levels > 200 ng/dL (6.9 nmol/L) arouse the suspicion, though in 20% of patients with ovarian androgen-producing tumors, testosterone levels are below this value. Again, the best screening procedures are the clinical history and physical examination. In the absence of cushingoid features, adrenal and ovarian tumors present similarly. Ovarian tumors often have unilateral ovarian enlargement that can be palpated on pelvic examination. Ultrasonography often confirms the diagnosis. In selected cases, selective venous sampling may be performed if CT-scan or sonography cannot identify the source of androgen production.

Anovulation Unrelated to Excess Sex Steroid Production

A. Adrenal Insufficiency

Adrenocortical insufficiency may be categorized as primary or secondary. Primary adrenal insufficiency (Addison's disease) is caused by destruction of cortical tissue. Secondary adrenal insufficiency is due to defects in the hypothalamic-pituitary axis resulting in a deficiency in ACTH. Both types lead to cortisol deficiency, which is life-threatening.

The main cause of primary adrenal failure is autoimmune destruction confined to the adrenal cortex. In fact, in the industrialized world, it accounts for more than 60% of cases of primary adrenocortical deficiency. The symptoms are typically those of chronic insufficiency and include weakness, fatigue, menstrual disturbances, and gastrointestinal symptoms such as nausea, abdominal pain, and diarrhea. Additional signs may include weight loss, hypotension, and pigmentary changes of the skin and mucous membranes. These symptoms may appear insidiously with a mean duration of approximately 3 years. Symptoms usually wax and wane until there is complete decompensation.

Autoimmune adrenal failure may occur as an isolated event, but estimates link more than 70% to a polyglandular failure syndrome. This syndrome has two subtypes: type I and type II. Type I is an illness of childhood that consists of hypoparathyroidism, chronic mucocutaneous candidiasis, celiac disease, and ovarian failure in addition to adrenal failure. It is associated with a mutation in the autoimmune regulator gene *(AIRE)* and has a recessive pattern of inheritance. Type II (Schmidt's syndrome) is an adult form of autoimmune adrenal insufficiency. The most common age at onset is the third decade. The most common manifestations include type 1 diabetes mellitus, myasthenia gravis, thyroiditis, ovarian failure, and adrenal insufficiency. Susceptibility to this disorder seems to be inherited as a dominant trait in linkage dysequilibrium with the HLA-B region of chromosome 6. The pathogenesis of adrenal insufficiency involves autoantibodies that are directed toward enzymes involved with steroidogenesis. Several studies suggest that the antigens in this disorder include 17α-hydroxylase, 21-hydroxylase, and P450scc. Detection of antibodies directed at these enzymes is helpful in making the diagnosis of autoimmune adrenal failure (see Chapter 4).

Worldwide, infection—especially tuberculosis—is the most common cause of primary adrenal failure. The adrenal cortex and medulla are involved and may be completely replaced by caseating granulomas. This phenomenon is always associated with other evidence of a tuberculous infection. Fungal, viral, and bacterial pathogens are less common causes.

The most common cause of secondary adrenal insufficiency is adrenal suppression after exogenous glucocorticoid administration. Less common settings are post treatment of Cushing's disease, hypothalamic-pituitary lesions, and hypopituitarism (Sheehan's syndrome). These patients more commonly present with symptoms suggestive of acute adrenal insufficiency. The clinical features include abdominal pain, hypotension, fever, severe volume depletion, and possibly profound shock.

Menstrual disturbances are a frequent presentation in patients with adrenal insufficiency. Autoimmune adrenal insufficiency is often accompanied by gonadal failure. In the polyglandular syndromes, premature ovarian failure develops in type I 50% of the time and in type II 10% of the time. It has been shown that antibodies—particularly to CYP17α and P450scc—are associated with premature ovarian failure. The other causes of adrenal failure are associated with menstrual disorders more than 25% of the time. The cause of anovulation is not certainly known, but chronic illness itself is probably responsible.

Diagnosis and treatment are discussed in Chapter 9. The screening process includes blood chemistries and basal cortisol levels. The diagnosis is confirmed with provocative tests using exogenous ACTH.

B. THYROID DISORDERS

Thyroid disorders result from altered thyroid hormone secretion. The prevalence of overt thyroid dysfunction is 1–2% in women of reproductive age. Thyroid disorders can develop secondary to an insult in the hypothalamus, pituitary, or thyroid, the latter being most common. In order to understand the pathophysiology of these disorders, it is important to be familiar with the normal physiologic regulation (see Chapter 7). This section will briefly review the common causes of hyperthyroidism and hypothyroidism, their manifestations after the onset of puberty, and their impact on reproductive function.

1. Hyperthyroidism—Hyperthyroidism is the clinical syndrome associated with excessive thyroid hormone activity. The clinical presentation of hyperthyroidism (thyrotoxicosis) depends on the age at onset and the degree of thyrotoxicosis. The clinical manifestations can involve most organ systems, and the presentation ranges from asymptomatic to thyroid storm. The typical features include nervousness, malaise, palpitations, heat intolerance, weight loss, and inability to concentrate. Additional features may involve the eyes and include lid lag, proptosis, and ophthalmoplegia. The reproductive abnormalities include menstrual abnormalities, infertility, and spontaneous abortions.

The most common variety of hyperthyroidism is due to autoimmune disease that affects intrinsic thyroid function (Graves' disease). Antibodies bind to the TSH receptor and stimulate the thyroid gland to secrete increased amounts of thyroid hormone. Less common causes include subacute thyroiditis, toxic multinodular goiter, and struma ovarii.

Excess thyroid hormone has an impact on sex-steroids. It stimulates hepatic production of SHBG. As a result, total serum estradiol, estrone, testosterone, and dihydrotestosterone are increased, yet free levels of these hormones remain within the normal range. The metabolic clearance pathways appear to be altered, which can be explained in part by the increased binding. The conversion rates of androstenedione to estrogen and testosterone are increased. The significance of the alterations in metabolism has not been determined.

Menstrual irregularities frequently occur in hyperthyroid states. The exact mechanism is unclear. Altered levels of TRH and TSH do not appear to have a significant impact on the HPO axis. The LH surge may be impaired, though studies have shown that hyperthyroid patients have normal FSH and LH responses to exogenous GnRH. It is possible that the weight loss and psychologic disturbances associated with this disease may contribute to the menstrual abnormalities. It is interesting to note that endometrial biopsies of many amenorrheic patients with hyperthyroidism have demonstrated a secretory endometrium, indicating that many of these women remain ovulatory. Menstrual abnormalities return to normal with treatment.

2. Hypothyroidism—Hypothyroidism—a more common disorder than hyperthyroidism in women of reproductive age—results from inadequate thyroid hormone production. The manifestations can involve almost any organ system, and the presentation can range from asymptomatic to myxedema coma. The common symptoms include lethargy, memory defects, cold intolerance, dry skin, hair loss or occasionally excess hair growth, deepening of the voice, nausea, and constipation. Physical findings include somnolence, bradycardia, mild hypertension, dry skin, periorbital puffiness, nonpitting edema of the hands, face, and ankles, and decreased tendon reflexes. Reproductive abnormalities include menstrual disorders, infertility, and spontaneous abortions.

The most common cause is autoimmune destruction of the thyroid (Hashimoto's thyroiditis). It is mediated by humoral and cell-mediated processes. The antibodies are directed toward thyroglobulin (anti-Tg) and thyroid microsomal peroxidase (thyroperoxidase antibody). Histologic specimens show lymphocytic infiltration. Other causes include ablative therapy of the thyroid gland (post surgery or radioactive iodine), end-stage Graves' disease, and transient thyroiditis (viral, drug-induced, postpartum).

Inadequate thyroid levels influence the metabolism of sex-steroids. The production of SHBG is decreased. As a result, serum estradiol and testosterone concentrations are decreased but free hormone levels remain within normal range. However, the metabolism of these steroids is altered and differs from that found in individuals with hyperthyroidism. The significance of the metabolites formed in consequence is not known.

The mechanism underlying menstrual abnormalities in hypothyroidism is incompletely understood. Since primary hypothyroidism is associated with elevated serum prolactin in up to one-third of patients, it is plausible that the hyperprolactinemia is a contributing factor (see Chapter 5). However, menstrual abnormalities are also observed in the absence of elevated prolactin. Alterations in FSH and LH levels have been investigated, and studies have shown inconclusive results, although several studies suggest that the midcycle surge is absent. Menstrual function returns to normal with replacement therapy.

Thyroid dysfunction often presents with nonspecific symptoms, which often delays the diagnosis. If only menstrual abnormalities are present, it is prudent to screen for thyroid abnormalities. Most cases will be detected by TSH assays. Confirmation is obtained with a repeat TSH level and serum thyroid hormone levels.

OUTFLOW TRACT DISORDERS

The true prevalence of müllerian tract abnormalities is not known. It is reported in as many as 4–5% of women. The reproductive consequences depend on the type of abnormality identified. A septate uterus is the most common defect described. These patients often present with infertility or obstetric complications. Other abnormalities include unicornous, bicornous, and didelphic uteri. These abnormalities present most commonly with reproductive or obstetric complications. Müllerian agenesis, androgen insensitivity syndrome, and congenital outflow obstruction defects are abnormalities that present with primary amenorrhea with no history of menses. In the following section these two abnormalities are discussed in greater detail.

A. Müllerian Agenesis

Müllerian agenesis (Mayer-Rokitansky-Küster-Hauser syndrome) is the second most common cause of primary amenorrhea. It is a congenital condition that occurs in one in 5000 female births. These individuals have normal ovarian development, normal endocrine function, and normal female sexual development. The physical findings are a shortened or absent vagina in addition to absence of the uterus, though small masses resembling a rudimentary uterus may be noted (see the section on embryology at the beginning of this chapter). About one-third of patients have renal abnormalities, and several have had bone abnormalities and eighth nerve deafness. These individuals have a 46,XX karyotype.

The exact cause has not been identified. It is known that regression of müllerian structures in males is controlled by AMH, which is secreted by the Sertoli cells of the testis. One hypothesis assigns the underlying defect to an activating mutation of either the *AMH* gene or its receptor. The genes for both AMH and AMH receptor have been investigated, but no mutations have yet been identified with this syndrome.

B. ANDROGEN INSENSITIVITY SYNDROME

Androgen insensitivity syndrome (AIS) presents in somewhat the same way as müllerian agenesis. The presentation differs in that individuals with complete AIS have minimal sexual hair. These patients have a male karyotype with a mutation of the androgen receptor on the X chromosome. They have normal testicular development and endocrine function. However, since the internal and external male sexual structures need testosterone for development, they are absent. This results in a female phenotype. Since the testis still secretes AMH, müllerian regression does occur. Secondary sexual characteristics (female) develop as a result of peripheral conversion of testosterone to estradiol, effectively resulting in unopposed estrogen stimulation.

The diagnosis of either disorder is entertained when pelvic examination reveals a short or absent vagina and no uterus on rectal examination. Confirmation of absent uterus can be obtained with ultrasound, MRI, or laparoscopy. These two disorders can usually be differentiated based on physical examination since patients with AIS have no pubic hair. However, the differential diagnosis becomes more difficult when patients have incomplete AIS. A testosterone level and karyotype can easily differentiate the two syndromes.

For further discussion, refer to Chapter 14.

C. CONGENITAL OUTFLOW OBSTRUCTION

Transvaginal septum and imperforate hymen are typical obstructive abnormalities. These patients usually present with cyclic lower abdominal pain and amenorrhea. The physical findings are a shortened or absent vagina. However, this syndrome differs from müllerian agenesis in that the pelvic organs are present. Behind either defect is old blood that has not escaped with menses. The differential diagnosis is sometimes difficult, though bulging of the introitus suggests imperforate hymen since the defect is thinner than a transvaginal septum.

The embryologic formations of the transvaginal septum and imperforate hymen are similar but not identical. Transvaginal septum is due to failure of complete canalization of the vaginal plate (see the section on embryology at the beginning of this chapter). The septum can vary in thickness and can be located at any level in the vagina. The hymen represents the junction of the sinovaginal bulbs and urogenital sinus. Typically, the hymen is perforated during fetal development. The hymen is thin and is always at the junction of the vestibule and vagina. It is important to distinguish these defects because the surgical correction procedures are different and require different levels of expertise.

D. ASHERMAN'S SYNDROME

Intrauterine adhesions or synechiae (Asherman's syndrome) are an acquired condition that may obliterate the endometrial cavity. These patients usually present with a range of menstrual disturbances, infertility, and recurrent spontaneous abortions. The most frequent symptom is amenorrhea.

Intrauterine adhesions result from damage to the endometrial basal layer. A common antecedent factor is a surgical procedure within the uterine cavity, and most often it is endometrial curettage that occurs shortly after pregnancy. The concurrent presence of infection or heavy bleeding increases the risk. Endometrial tuberculosis and septic abortion are rare causes.

The diagnosis is entertained after demonstrating no withdrawal bleeding after administration of estrogen and progesterone. Confirmation is made with a hysterosalpingogram, saline sonogram, or hysteroscopy. Treatment involves lysis of adhesions and hormonal therapy.

■ MENOPAUSE

The ovary is unique in that the woman's age at which it ceases to function appears to have remained constant despite the increase in longevity experienced by women over the last century. Because the loss of ovarian function has a profound impact on the hormonal milieu in women and the subsequent risk for the development of disease resulting from the loss of estrogen production, improving our understanding of reproductive aging is critical for optimal female health.

Human follicles begin development in the fourth gestational month. Approximately 1000–2000 germ cells migrate to the gonadal ridge and multiply, reaching a total of six to seven million around the fifth month of intrauterine life. At this point, multiplication stops and follicle loss begins, declining to approximately 1 million by birth. In the human male, the germ cells become quiescent and maintain their stem cell identity. In contrast, in the human female, between weeks 12 and 18, the germ cells enter meiosis and differentiate. Thus, in the female, all germ stem cells have differentiated prior to birth. In the adult woman, the germ cells may remain quiescent, may be recruited for further development and ovulation, or may be destroyed by apoptosis. Over time, the population of oocytes will be depleted (without regeneration) through recruitment and apoptosis until less than a thousand oocytes remain and menopause ensues. Approximately 90% of women experience menopause with a mean age of 51.2 years. The remainder experience menopause prior to age 46 years (often termed early menopause), with 1% of women experiencing menopause before age 40 years (premature menopause; premature ovarian failure).

Understanding ovarian aging has been quite difficult. The variability in definitions has made comparisons from study to study difficult. The participants in the recent Stages of Reproductive Aging Workshop (STRAW) study developed criteria for staging female reproductive aging. They utilized menstrual cyclicity and early follicular FSH levels as the primary determinants for this staging system. Five stages precede the final menstrual period and two stages follow it. Stages −5 to −3 include the reproductive interval; stages −2 to −1 are termed the menopausal transition; and stages +1 and +2 are the postmenopause (Figure 13–10). The menopausal transition begins with increased variability in menstrual cyclicity (> 7 days) in women with elevated FSH levels. This stage ends with the final menstrual period, which cannot be recognized until after 12 months of amenorrhea. Early postmenopause is defined as the first 5 years following the final menstrual period. Late postmenopause is variable in length, beginning 5 years after the final menstrual period and continuing until death.

While this system is said to include endocrinologic aspects of ovarian aging, it still depends largely on menstrual cyclicity as a key indicator of ovarian age. The system includes measurement of FSH; however, by the time FSH is elevated, even in the face of cyclic menstrual cycles, oocyte depletion has already proceeded to such an extent that fertility (as a marker of reproductive aging) is significantly diminished. Evidence suggests that genetic and environmental factors influence both age at menopause and the decline in fertility, though the specific nature of these relationships is poorly characterized. Premature menopause can be due to failure to attain adequate follicle numbers in utero or to accelerated depletion thereafter. Potentially, either of these causes could be affected by genetic and environmental factors. The timing of menopause has a consistent impact on overall health with respect to osteoporosis, cardiovascular disease, and cancer risk. Over the next decade, it is estimated that more than 40 million women in the USA will enter menopause.

OOCYTE DEPLETION

As discussed above, the leading theory regarding the onset of menopause relates to a critical threshold in oocyte number. The theory that menopause is primarily triggered by ovarian aging is supported by the coincident occurrence of follicular depletion, elevation of gonadotropins, and menstrual irregularity with ultimate cessation.

Faddy et al (1992) developed a mathematical model to predict the rate of follicular decline (Figure 13–11). These workers utilized existing data to construct a model that ultimately showed a biexponential decline with an acceleration in oocyte loss when the remaining oocyte number equaled approximately 25,000. In their model, this occurred at 37.5 years of age. At this point, the rate of follicular atresia accelerates. In the absence of this acceleration, the model suggests that menopause would be delayed until age 71. The cause of this accel-

Stages:	−5	−4	−3	−2	−1	0	+1	+2
Terminology:	Reproductive			Menopausal transition			Postmenopause	
	Early	Peak	Late	Early	Late*		Early*	Late
				Perimenopause				
Duration of stage:	Variable			Variable		ⓐ 1 yr	ⓑ 4 yrs	Until demise
Menstrual cycles:	Variable to regular	Regular		variable cycle length (> 7 days different from normal)	≥ 2 skipped cycles and an interval of amenorrhea (≥ 60 days)	Amen x 12 mos	none	
Endocrine:	Normal FSH		↑ FSH	↑ FSH			↑ FSH	

*Stages most likely to be characterized by vasomotor symptoms   ↑ = elevated

Figure 13–10. **Stages of reproductive aging.** (Reproduced, with permission, from Soules MR et al: Stages of Reproductive Aging Workshop [STRAW]. J Womens Health Gend Based Med 2001;10:843.)

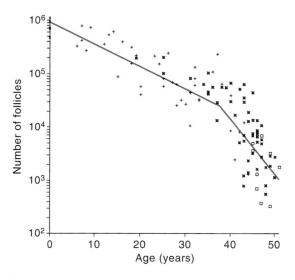

Figure 13–11. Bi-exponential model of declining follicle numbers in pairs of human ovaries from neonatal age to 51 years old. Data were obtained from the studies of Block (+, n=6; + n=43), Richardson et al. (1987) (squares, n=9) and Gougeon (unpublished) (*, n=52). (Reproduced, with permission, from Faddy MJ et al: Accelerated disappearance of ovarian follicles in mid-life: implications for forecasting menopause. Hum Reprod 1992;7:1342.)

erated depletion is not well defined. It is also clear—if the factor predicting the rate of decline is follicle number and not age—that other factors which might account for a diminished follicle number (genetic risk and possible toxic exposure) would lead to an earlier rate of accelerated decline and an earlier age at menopause.

ENDOCRINE SYSTEM CHANGES WITH AGING

The entire endocrine system changes with advancing age. The somatotrophic axis begins to decline in the fourth decade, prior to the decline in ovarian function. This decline is accelerated in the face of ovarian failure and may act to accelerate the decline in ovarian function. However, pituitary concentrations of growth hormone as well as ACTH and TSH remain constant into the ninth decade. While the thyroid gland undergoes progressive fibrosis with age and concentrations of T_3 decline by 25–40%, elderly patients still remain euthyroid. B cell function also undergoes degeneration with aging such that by age 65 years, 50% of subjects have abnormal glucose tolerance tests. Frank diabetes is rare, however, occurring in only 7% of the population. The

female reproductive system, on the other hand, undergoes complete failure at a relatively early age.

As noted above, in the late fourth decade, FSH levels begin to rise even in the face of continued cyclic menses. The most likely cause is a decrease in functional granulosa cells from the oocyte pool with a decrease in inhibin B negative feedback, permitting a monotropic rise in FSH. Early on, there is also a decline in luteal phase progesterone levels. As ovarian aging progresses, estradiol levels may be quite variable, with chaotic patterns and occasionally very high or very low levels. This dramatic variability may lead to an increase in symptomatology during the perimenopausal years (stages −2 to −1). As peripheral gonadotropins rise, LH pulsatile patterns become abnormal. There is an increase in pulse frequency, with a decrease in GnRH inhibition by opioids.

Estrogens

The main circulating estrogen during the premenopausal years is 17β-estradiol. Levels of this hormone are controlled by the developing follicle and resultant corpus luteum. The fact that oophorectomy will reduce peripheral estradiol levels from 120 pg/mL (440 pmol/L) to 18 pg/mL (66.1 pmol/L) suggests that over 95% of circulating estradiol is derived from the ovary. Other sources of estrogen include estrone and the peripheral conversion of testosterone to estradiol. Very small amounts are secreted by the adrenal gland. As the two-cell theory (see above) requires aromatization of theca-produced androgens in the granulosa cell, follicular exhaustion is associated with gradual declines in estradiol concentrations.

The predominant estrogen in the postmenopausal woman is estrone, with a biologic potency approximately one-third that of estradiol. Estrone is derived largely from peripheral conversion of androstenedione. Extraglandular aromatase is found in liver, fat, and certain hypothalamic nuclei. This activity increases with aging and increased fat content (also an age-related change). Estrone and estradiol production rates during the postmenopausal years are 40 μg/d and 6 μg/d, respectively. This compares with 80–500 μg/d for estradiol during the reproductive years. Essentially all estradiol in postmenopausal women is derived from conversion of estrone.

Androgens

Dehydroepiandrosterone sulfate (DHEAS) levels decrease in both men and women with aging. The decline is greater in women and may be due to the relative estrogen deprivation. Changes in DHEAS levels have been associated with alterations in body composition with aging. Androstenedione is the predominant androgen during the reproductive years, and production declines from 1500 pg/mL to 800 pg/mL in postmenopausal women. The postmenopausal ovary contributes only 20% to circulating androstenedione levels. Testosterone levels also decline postmenopausally, but not to the same extent as estradiol levels. Postmenopausal testosterone is derived from the ovary (25%), from the adrenal gland (25%), and—by extraglandular conversion—from androstenedione (50%). The postmenopausal ovary produces a larger percentage of testosterone (50%) than does the premenopausal ovary.

MENOPAUSAL CONSEQUENCES

Given the endocrinologic changes associated with aging, many symptoms appearing in the aging female may be due to estrogen deficiency or diminished androgen or growth hormone secretion. Disorders that are definitely due to estrogen deprivation include vasomotor symptoms and urogenital atrophy. Osteoporosis is thought to be due largely to estrogen deficiency, but this may be exacerbated by the relative decline in growth hormone levels. The same may be said for the hormone-related increase in the prevalence of atherosclerotic cardiovascular disease and psychosocial symptoms, including insomnia, fatigue, short-term memory changes, and possibly depression. Both DHEAS and growth hormone may impact on these phenomena as well.

Vasomotor Symptoms

Vasomotor symptoms (hot flushes) are experienced with greatest frequency during stages −1 and +1, with about 75–85% of women complaining of this symptom. While 80% of U.S. women have symptoms lasting for at least a year, only 25% of women are still symptomatic at 5 years after the final menstrual period. Studies of hot flushes with external monitoring of skin temperature and resistance have shown a frequency of approximately 54 ± 10 minutes. In sleep studies, hot flush frequency has been shown to interrupt REM sleep and may contribute to some of the psychosocial complaints. Hot flushes are temporarily correlated with pulses of LH—but exogenous LH does not induce a flush, suggesting that there is some central mediator leading to both the flush and the elevation in LH.

Estrogen is the drug of choice for the treatment of vasomotor symptoms. Other drugs have been tried in women for whom estrogen is contraindicated, though none have the efficacy associated with estrogen replacement. These alternatives include transdermal clonidine, ergot alkaloids, and, more recently, selective serotonin reuptake inhibitors. High-dose progestins may also produce some relief.

Genital Atrophy

The vagina, vulva, urethra, and bladder trigone not only share embryonic proximity but all contain estrogen receptors. Atrophy begins (again) in stage −2 to −1. The most common symptoms include itching and vaginal thinning, with decreased distensibility and reduced secretions, leading to vaginal dryness and pain with intercourse. This and the change in pH with resultant changes in vaginal flora increase the incidence of vaginal and urinary tract infections. Estrogen is the treatment of choice, and treatment must continue for at least 1–3 months for symptomatic improvement to be noted. The systemic dosage necessary for vaginal protection is somewhat higher than that needed for bone protection (see below), and local therapy by means of creams or vaginal rings may thus be advisable to limit systemic absorption. It should be noted, however, that vaginal absorption of steroids is quite efficient once estrogenization and revascularization have occurred. If the goal is to limit systemic absorption, slow-release rings may be superior to estrogen creams.

Vaginal estrogen will frequently improve symptoms of urinary frequency, dysuria, urgency, and postvoid dribbling. Its direct effect to improve stress incontinence is less clear.

Osteoporosis

Osteoporosis is a condition in which bone loss has been sufficient to allow mechanical fracture with limited stress. The risk for development of osteoporosis is dependent on the peak bone density attained in early childhood (stressing the importance of bone building in the young) and the rate of loss (accelerated with estrogen deficiency). Primary or "senile" osteoporosis usually affects women between the ages of 55 and 70 years. The most common sites include the vertebrae and the long bones of the arms and legs. Secondary osteoporosis is caused by a specific disease (such as hyperparathyroidism) or medication usage (such as glucocorticoids) (see Chapter 8).

Menopausal bone loss begins before the final menstrual period during stage −1. Postmenopausal osteoporosis causes over 1.3 million fractures annually in the USA. Most of the more than 250,000 hip fractures are due to primary osteoporosis, and—given that 15% of patients die within a year after a hip fracture and 75% of patients lose their independence—the social costs, not to mention the financial costs, are great.

Bone loss following natural menopause is approximately 1–2% per year compared with 3.9% per year following oophorectomy. A woman's genetic background, lifestyle, dietary habits, and coexisting disease will also impact the development of osteoporosis. Cigarette smoking, caffeine usage, and alcohol consumption also negatively impact bone loss, while weight-bearing activity appears to have a positive influence. See Chapter 8 for a detailed discussion of bone mineral metabolism.

A. TREATMENT

1. Estrogen therapy—Estrogen therapy acts via inhibition in bone resorption. Both bone mineral density and fracture rate are improved with estrogen therapy. However, with cessation of estrogen therapy, there is a rapid and progressive loss of bone mineral content. By 4 years after therapy, bone density is no different from that of patients who were never treated with estrogen. While estrogen is approved for prevention of osteoporosis, there is also some support for its usage in treatment. Dosages of 0.625 mg of conjugated estrogens orally daily—and, more recently, as low as 0.3 mg—have been shown to slow bone loss and provide adequate protection against the development of osteoporosis. Higher dosages may be required to treat existing disease.

2. Alternative therapies for osteoporosis—

   a. Calcitonin—Calcitonin is a hormone normally secreted by the thyroid gland. Calcitonin (salmon) is available as a nasal spray, specifically developed to decrease local side effects caused by subcutaneous injection. While few studies have been performed and no data are available regarding reduction in hip fracture, it does seem to be especially beneficial for women with a recent and still painful vertebral fracture. Intranasal calcitonin has also been shown to improve spinal bone density and decrease the vertebral fracture rate in established osteoporosis. The increase in bone density appears to peak in as little as 12–18 months. This may be due to down-regulation of the calcitonin receptors and the development of neutralizing antibodies. It also appears that some patients do not respond to this therapy, and those nonresponders cannot be prospectively identified.

   b. Bisphosphonates—These compounds are analogs of pyrophosphates that have an affinity for a hydroxyapatite in bone. The basic structure of bisphosphonates allows a large number of manipulations of the basic molecule, producing different types of bisphosphonates that vary considerably in their potency on bone. The first bisphosphonate to be used was etidronate, and on a scale of potency it is the weakest agent. In order of increasing potency appeared pamidronate, alendronate, and risedronate. Etidronate, if given continuously for more than 6 months, impairs mineralization of bone and may cause osteomalacia. There have been occasional reports of pamidronate also causing impaired mineralization of bone. However, continuous administration of alendronate or risedronate has not caused these changes.

Alendronate has been evaluated more extensively than calcitonin and has reduced fracture rates in patients with osteoporosis. Alendronate has been shown to inhibit markers of bone remodeling and increase bone mineral density at the lumbar spine, hip, and total body. Alendronate is taken orally; the recommended daily dose of 10 mg, however, must be taken according to a very strict dosing schedule (in the morning on an empty stomach, with the patient required to remain upright for 30 minutes thereafter). The medication has very poor bioavailability (approximately 1%), and for that reason these instructions must be meticulously obeyed. Alendronate also has a propensity for causing irritation of the esophagus and stomach, especially in women with preexisting esophageal reflux or gastric or duodenal disease. A newer formulation allows for once-weekly administration, and efforts are continuing to develop a once-yearly formulation. Risedronate is equally effective in lower dosage.

Increases in bone density with alendronate are greater than with calcitonin and equal to what is seen with HRT. The escape phenomenon seen with calcitonin is also not seen with alendronate.

The final question concerning alendronate has to do with the near-permanent changes in bone that occur with the incorporation of this agent into the bone matrix. While short-term fracture data appear favorable, the long-term effects of these agents and the ability of alendronate-treated bone to heal (eg, following hip fracture) are not known.

   c. SERMs—Raloxifene is the first of a new generation of compounds known as selective estrogen receptor modulators (SERMs). We will begin to see an explosion in the development of these agents. They may represent a new alternative for breast cancer patients or for long-term use in osteoporotic patients. These new agents act as selective estrogen receptor agonists in some tissues (bone and heart) and antagonists in others (breast and uterus and possibly brain). Data with raloxifene are now available and suggest good preservation of bone density, albeit less than that seen with alendronate or HRT, and fracture data support a protective effect.

It is believed that the differential effect of estrogens and antiestrogens is related to the transcriptional activation of specific estrogen response elements. Two different domains of the estrogen receptor (AF-1 and AF-2) appear to be responsible for this transcriptional activation. Estrogens and antiestrogens appear to act via different domains, leading to their differential effects. Both appear to act to maintain bone density—at least partially—via regulation of the gene for transforming growth factor β.

   d. Calcium and vitamin D—These are important components of all three antiresorptive agents. Decreased ability to absorb calcium among older women is due in part to impaired vitamin D activation and effect. Older women may have limited exposure to sunlight, and their dietary vitamin D intake may be lower than that of younger women.

Daily intake of 1500 mg of calcium and 400–800 IU of vitamin D per day is probably sufficient to reduce the risk of fragility fractures by about 10%.

Atherosclerotic Cardiovascular Disease

Cardiovascular disease is the number one killer of both men and women in Western societies. This is largely attributed to age and lifestyle. Lifestyle modifications are known to decrease the incidence. For women, cardiovascular disease is largely a disease of the postmenopause. Women will now spend more than a third of their lives in the postmenopausal years, and preventive measures are thus of paramount importance. There has been a large body of observational evidence to support a protective effect of estrogen replacement therapy on cardiovascular disease. Observational data, however, are limited by the confounding variables of patient self-selection. Animal and in vitro studies as well as assessment of surrogate markers in women have also shown a positive effect of estrogen and hormone replacement therapy (HRT) against cardiovascular disease development. However, recent randomized, controlled studies have failed to support a protective role for HRT.

HRT was first evaluated in secondary prevention trials. The HERS trial evaluated the use of daily HRT (0.625 mg conjugated estrogens plus 2.5 mg medroxyprogesterone acetate) in 2763 postmenopausal women with a mean age of 66.7 years and pre-existing vascular disease. The study failed to demonstrate any overall difference in vascular events. This occurred despite improvements in lipid parameters in those patients receiving HRT. The Estrogen Replacement and Atherosclerosis (ERA) Trial, published in 2000, compared 3.2 years of treatment with estrogen, combined estrogen and progestin, and placebo in postmenopausal women aged 42–80 years. This, again, was a secondary prevention trial and also failed to demonstrate a significant difference in the rate of progression of coronary atherosclerosis between the three groups. The importance of this study was the inclusion of an estrogen-only arm.

The Women's Health Initiative (WHI) is the first large randomized study to look at primary prevention of cardiovascular disease. The combined HRT regimen utilized in the HERS trial was also utilized for this study. The study was recently stopped when interim analysis demonstrated an unacceptable risk profile for the HRT arm. There was an increase in the incidence in breast cancer (an increase of eight cases per 10,000 women) with no cardiovascular protection (and potentially increased cardiovascular risk). There was, in fact,

an increase in blood clots, strokes, and coronary heart disease. The risk of stroke and clot continued for the 5 years of study, while most of the coronary heart disease was limited to the first year of treatment. There were, however, documented decreases in the risk of fracture and colon cancer.

The WHI study did not address the effect of hormone treatment on hot flushes and vaginal atrophy. Clearly, there are alternatives for the treatment of osteoporosis and cardiovascular disease that are superior if prevention is the sole reason for HRT. Every woman should discuss with her caregiver the optimal management for her as an individual. This should take into account the medical and family history as well as symptomatology. It can be uniformly recommended, however, that menopausal women maintain appropriate nutrition, weight reduction, and exercise along with moderation in alcohol and caffeine intake and cessation of smoking.

■ INFERTILITY

Infertility is defined as the inability of a couple to conceive after 1 year of frequent unprotected intercourse without contraception. This definition is based on observational data showing that over 90% of couples achieve pregnancy after 1 year of unprotected coitus. Using this definition, a 1995 survey reported that approximately 7% of married couples of reproductive age experienced infertility. However, the diagnosis of infertility does not mean that they cannot conceive—a more precise diagnosis term would be "subfertility," or a diminished capacity to conceive. The actual probability of the fertility potential of a population may be better assessed with variables that can quantify a monthly cycle rate. The concepts that have been used for quantitative analysis are fecundability and fecundity. Fecundability is defined as the probability of achieving a pregnancy within one menstrual cycle, and in normal couples the chance of conception after 1 month is approximately 25%. Fecundity is a related concept that is defined as the ability to achieve a live birth within one menstrual cycle.

In the United States, demands for infertility treatment have dramatically increased. The 1995 National Survey of Family Growth reported that 9.3 million women received infertility treatment in their lifetime compared with 6.8 million in 1988. This rise in treatment is due not only to increased public awareness—it also reflects the significant demographic, societal, and economic changes in our society. These include the aging of the "baby boom" generation, which has increased the size of the reproductive age population. Perhaps more important is the increased use of contraception and postponement of childbearing until the last 2 decades of a woman's reproductive life. Approximately 20% of women in the United States now have their first child after 35 years of age.

Age alone has a significant impact on fertility and affects a woman many years before the onset of menopause. One factor is the age-dependent loss of ovarian follicles (see above). A 38-year-old woman has 25% of the fecundability of a woman under 30 years of age. Another age-related subfertility factor is that the spontaneous abortion rate increases with advancing age. The overall incidence of clinical abortion increases from 10% in women under age 30 to more than 40% in women over 40. The increased pregnancy loss can be largely attributed to abnormalities in the aging oocyte; older follicles have an increased rate of meiotic dysfunction, resulting in higher rates of chromosomal abnormalities.

The main causes of female subfertility can be classified in the following way: (1) ovulatory defects, (2) pelvic disorders, and (3) male factors. These factors account for 80–85% of couples diagnosed with infertility. They are not mutually exclusive—about 15% of couples have more than one cause of subfertility. In approximately 20% of couples, the cause remains unknown and is classified as unexplained infertility. This section will briefly discuss the causes of subfertility and review the diagnosis and management.

DIAGNOSIS OF INFERTILITY

Ovulatory Defects

Ovulatory disorders are responsible for 25% of cases of infertility. Ovulatory status can be obtained from the history. If a woman experiences cyclic, predictable menses at monthly intervals, ovulation can be predicted 98% of the time. This is not an invariable rule, however, and irregular menstrual cycles are not a sure sign of anovulation.

The only way to confirm ovulation is by achieving pregnancy. However, a variety of methods can indicate that ovulation has occurred. For example, a thermal shift occurs around the time of ovulation. Prior to ovulation, morning basal body temperature (BBT) is below 98 °F (36.7 °C), and after ovulation the temperature increases at least 0.4 °F (0.2 °C) for at least 10–13 days. This rise in temperature reflects the progesterone that is secreted from the corpus luteum, which consequently raises the hypothalamic set-point for BBT. The temperature rise occurs approximately 2 days after ovulation because of the time and "dose" required for the progesterone effect at the hypothalamus. BBT can therefore not be utilized to prospectively predict ovulation.

Measurements of midluteal serum progesterone concentration can also be performed to document the oc-

currence of ovulation. If this level is greater than 3 µg/L (9.5 nmol/L), it is a strong indication that ovulation has occurred. An endometrial biopsy can confirm ovulation. It is performed during the luteal phase and gives a qualitative assessment of ovulation since the duration of progesterone exposure produces predictable endometrial histology. Lastly, a sonographic examination documenting a decrease in follicle size—or disappearance altogether of the previously developed follicle—is suggestive of ovulation. All of these methods indicate that ovulation has occurred. There are only a few ways to predict that ovulation is going to occur. The most common way is to detect the LH surge. Ovulation typically occurs 34–36 hours after the onset of the LH surge.

Although ovulation may occur, some women may have a luteal-phase defect. This is characterized by an inadequate quantity or duration of progesterone secretion by the corpus luteum. There is a distinct window of time for implantation. The theory is that the progesterone deficiency desynchronizes ovulation (egg) and implantation (endometrium). However, the incidence of luteal phase defects is difficult to assess because the definition is not standardized. Typically, the diagnosis is established by luteal phase endometrial dating; if the histologic development of the endometrium lags more than 2 days beyond the day of the cycle, it is diagnostic of a luteal phase defect. However, up to 30% of women with normal cycles meet this criterion. Another method involves measuring midluteal progesterone levels. If progesterone is less than 10 ng/mL, it suggests a luteal phase defect. This is not reliable because progesterone is intermittently secreted, and the serum progesterone level can change from 1 hour to the next in the same individual. Furthermore, the lack of valid tests questions the existence of luteal phase defects and its association with subfertility. Lastly, as empiric treatment for unexplained infertility has developed, delaying treatment (see below: superovulation with IUI) for exact diagnoses has less importance. More sophisticated testing of endometrial proteins required for implantation (eg, integrins, glycodelin) may revive enthusiasm for making a specific diagnosis in the future.

The cause of ovulatory dysfunction has been previously discussed. All anovulatory patients should have determination of prolactin and TSH levels- and, if necessary, androgen levels—to identify the cause of the ovulatory disturbance. Treatment should be directed toward the cause, which is discussed in greater detail below. It could be argued that all patients should have evaluation of early follicular cycle (days 2–4) FSH, LH, and estradiol to assess ovarian "reserve" (age).

Pelvic Disorders

Pelvic disorders account for over 30% of couples with the diagnosis of infertility. Uterine tube damage and adhesion formation are responsible for most pelvic pathologic processes causing infertility, while endometriosis is the primary pelvic disorder causing subfertility. The causes of tubal damage and adhesions include postinfectious state (pelvic inflammatory disease [PID], endometriosis, and a history of pelvic surgery (especially surgery for ruptured appendicitis).

Pelvic inflammatory disease is defined as infection of upper genital tract structures and is usually caused by a sexually transmitted disease. The known initiating organisms are chlamydiae and *Neisseria gonorrhoeae*. The symptoms are variable but usually include lower abdominal pain, nausea, and vaginal discharge. However, in up to 30% of chlamydial infections, PID may be clinically inapparent and may remain undiagnosed until presenting with subfertility.

Endometriosis is the presence of endometrial glands and stroma outside of the uterus. There may be no manifestations other than infertility, or symptoms may progress to include severe pelvic pain, dysmenorrhea, and dyspareunia. The diagnosis is suspected if findings on surgical exploration show characteristic lesions. Lesions can be staged according to published criteria. Diagnosis is confirmed with biopsy of the peritoneal lesions. The disease occurs in approximately 3–10% of reproductive age women and may be responsible for up to 25–35% of the female factors responsible for subfertility.

The pathogenesis of endometriosis is not completely known. A prominent theory (Sampson) involves retrograde menstruation. It is well established that menses can flow through the uterine tubes into the abdominal cavity. In fact, this phenomenon is thought to occur in almost all menstruating women. There is good evidence that the endometrial tissue subsequently invades and proliferates into the peritoneum. It is theorized that the immune system should normally dispose of the tissue and that altered immunity may result in implantation of this endometrial tissue outside the uterus in those women who subsequently develop endometriosis.

There is a strong association between adhesive disease and endometriosis. In these cases, the cause of subfertility is a result of distorted anatomy and consequently altered function. However, in mild cases of endometriosis, where only peritoneal lesions are identified and no anatomic distortion exists, the cause of infertility remains uncertain and controversial. There is evidence that the peritoneal fluid is altered in the presence of endometrial tissue with increased macrophages and inflammatory mediators. Several studies suggest that inflammatory changes result in adverse effects on folliculogenesis, ovum transport, fertilization, and implantation.

Tubal damage can be diagnosed with a hysterosalpingogram or surgical exploration. Hysterosalpingography involves the introduction of radiopaque contrast media into the pelvis through the cervix and then fluo-roscopy, revealing an outline of contrast in the uterine cavity, uterine tubes, and peritoneal cavity. The diagnosis of pelvic endometriosis can only be made by surgery, and most often the surgical procedure is laparoscopy. Diagnostic laparoscopy is usually done when there is a high suspicion of endometriosis based on the clinical history or adhesive disease based on a history of PID or pelvic surgery. Laparoscopy may also be performed if all other tests are normal and the couple continues not to achieve a pregnancy.

Male Factor Causes

The male factor contributes in 40–50% of cases of diagnosed infertility, and all evaluations should include the male partner. The diagnostic test for male factor infertility is the semen analysis. While this is a largely descriptive test (volume; sperm count, motility, and morphology), there is some correlation with pregnancy outcome. This should be used solely as a screening test. To understand the pathophysiology of male factor, it is important to review the physiology of spermatogenesis and the anatomy of the male reproductive tract as described in Chapter 12.

Unexplained Infertility

Approximately 15–20% of the couples diagnosed with infertility have no identifiable cause after a full investigation. The term "unexplained" implies that there is a potential explanation for the subfertility but the cause has not yet been identified. The cause may be subtle abnormalities in folliculogenesis, sperm-ovum interactions, or defective implantation.

Several studies have evaluated the natural history of unexplained infertility. It is estimated that fecundity in younger couples (female partner under the age of 40) with unexplained infertility is 3–5% compared with 20–25% in the age-matched couples with normal fertility. Treatment involves methods that increase fecundability and are discussed later.

MANAGEMENT OF THE INFERTILE COUPLE

It is important to remember that in most couples there is a chance for spontaneous conception. Recent studies estimate the average probability for live birth without treatment at 25–40% during the 3 years after the first infertility consultation. This translates into a cycle fecundity rate of 0.7–1% per month. The presence of endometriosis, abnormal sperm, or tubal disease independently reduced the chance of spontaneous pregnancy and live birth by approximately 50% for each variable. Infertility for more than 3 years, female age over 30 years, and primary infertility were important negative prognostic factors.

Evaluation should focus on known causes of infertility or subfertility: ovulatory defects, pelvic disorders (tubal disease, endometriosis), and male factor issues.

Ovulatory Disorders

Treatment should be diagnosis-specific, if possible. For the female, this means that the cause of any ovulatory defect should be determined and specific treatment then instituted. This will enhance outcome and decrease the risk of complications (spontaneous abortion and multiple gestation). This treatment might include the use of dopamine agonists (hyperprolactinemia), thyroid replacement (hypothyroidism), pulsatile gonadotropin-releasing hormone (hypogonadotropic hypogonadism), or clomiphene citrate (for PCOS). The most common cause of anovulation is inappropriate feedback such as in PCOS. Ovulation in PCOS patients can be induced with clomiphene citrate, which is a nonsteroidal agonist-antagonist of estrogen that blocks the hypothalamic-pituitary axis from feedback by circulating estrogens. As a result, there is increased gonadotropin release to stimulate follicular recruitment and ovulation. In addition, since PCOS has recently been associated with insulin resistance, insulin sensitizers such as metformin have been used to enhance ovulatory response in women with PCOS.

Pelvic Disorders

In general, adhesive tubal lesions should be treated surgically. However the location and extent of disease should be evaluated. Patients with distal tubal occlusion—unless it is very mild—are most often better served by assisted reproduction (IVF). Other possible causes of infertility should also be examined. If a patient has a history of documented tubal disease in addition to other abnormalities (ovulatory dysfunction or male factor infertility) or if they are over 35, the likelihood for successful surgical management decreases by approximately 50% and consideration for avoiding surgery and moving directly to assisted reproduction is paramount. The exception to this rule is documentation of hydrosalpinges on ultrasound. The presence of hydrosalpinges that retain fluid when nondistended (ie, not seen only with hysterosalpingography) leads to a significant reduction in outcome with assisted reproductive therapy (ART). Prior removal or proximal occlusion of the tube to prevent "contamination" of the uterine cavity should be performed before ART is offered.

There are conflicting data in the literature concerning the appropriate treatment for mild endometriosis. A well-designed randomized trial from Canada evaluated the effect of surgical treatment on pregnancy outcome for patients diagnosed with mild endometriosis without anatomic distortion. It showed that pregnancy rates at 9 months post laparoscopy were 27% in the surgically treated group compared with 18% in the untreated group. Severe endometriosis (disease that alters the pelvic anatomy or involves the ovary with endometriomas) should be surgically treated to restore normal pelvic anatomy. There appears to be no advantage to medical therapy for endometriosis in women seeking fertility.

Male Factor Infertility

Male factor infertility is discussed in Chapter 12. Like female partner treatment, therapy if possible should be targeted toward the cause of subfertility. Obstructive disease may be treated surgically. A prominent varicocele with a "stress" pattern on semen analysis (decreased motility with increased abnormal morphology) may suggest a need for surgical repair. Any endocrinologic abnormalities (while less common in the male) should be treated (eg, prolactinoma). Unfortunately, beyond this point, most treatments require a combined approach very similar to that discussed below for unexplained infertility.

Unexplained Infertility

The treatment of unexplained infertility can be frustrating for the physician and the patients because the recommendations for therapy are not targeted toward a specific diagnosis. Although there are very limited evidence-based data to guide treatment, therapy should be directed toward increasing the fecundability rate. The two main treatments are superovulation plus intrauterine insemination (IUI) and in vitro fertilization (IVF).

Superovulation methods are designed to qualitatively improve the cycle and to hyperstimulate the ovary with rescue of more follicles (quantitative improvement). Administration of clomiphene citrate or of gonadotropins alone can be used for superovulation. However, higher success rates are observed when superovulation is combined with intrauterine insemination (IUI) of washed sperm (Table 13–4). In vitro fertilization provides a higher fecundability rate. However, these procedures are significantly more costly and more invasive, and they should only be used after a trial (three or four cycles) of superovulation and IUI has failed. With older patients, aggressive therapy should be considered earlier in the treatment effort.

■ CONTRACEPTION

Approximately 50% of all pregnancies in the USA are unplanned. In adolescents and in women of older reproductive age, the unplanned pregnancy rate is higher,

Table 13–4. Pregnancy rates after treatment for unexplained infertility. Aggregate data for each treatment.[1]

Treatment	No. of Studies	No. (%) of Pregnancies per Initiated Cycle	Percent of Quality-Adjusted Pregnancies per Initiated Cycle
Control groups	11	64/3,539 (1.8)	1.3
Control groups, randomized studies	6	23/597 (3.8)	4.1
IUI	9	15/378 (4)	3.8
Clomiphene citrate	3	37/617 (6)	5.6
Clomiphene citrate + IUI	5	21/315 (6.7)	8.3
hMG	13	139/1806 (7.7)	7.7
hMG + IUI	14	207/1133 (18)	17.1
IVF	9	378/683 (22.5)	20.7
GIFT	9	158/607 (26.0)	27.0

[1]Reproduced, with permission, from Guzick DS et al: Efficacy of treatment of unexplained infertility. Fertil Steril 1998;70:207. GIFT = gamete intrafollicular transfer; hMG = human menopausal gonadotrophin; IVF = in vitro fertilization; IUI = intrauterine insemination.

approaching 82% and 77%, respectively. This equates to 3.5 million unplanned pregnancies in the USA per year. With the advent of oral contraceptives, women were able to postpone childbearing. However, approximately 50% of unplanned pregnancies are due to contraceptive failures. Possible causes of failure include lack of education, poor compliance, and side effect profiles. In this section we discuss the different methods of hormonal contraception. We shall discuss also the target population for the various modalities of contraception and their mechanisms, side effects, and ways to decrease failure rates. At the end of the section, emergency contraception will be briefly discussed.

ORAL CONTRACEPTIVES

Combination

In the United States, oral contraceptive pills are the most widely used method for contraception. There are two types of oral contraception: combination pills and progestin-only pills. The various hormones used in birth control pills are illustrated in Figure 13–12.

The development of oral contraceptive agents began with the isolation of progesterone. However, progesterone was very expensive and difficult to isolate. Ethisterone, a derivative of an androgen, was found to have progestin activity and was much easier to isolate than progesterone. With removal of carbon 19, the progestational activity was increased and the new compound was termed norethindrone. When this hormone was administered to women, ovulation was inhibited. During the process of norethindrone purification, an estrogen contaminant was found. When this contaminant was removed, women would experience breakthrough

bleeding. The estrogen was added back, thereby creating the first-generation combination birth control pill, which was FDA-approved in 1960.

Oral contraceptives can be divided into generations based on dose and type of hormone. The first-generation birth control pills contained more than 50 μg of ethinyl estradiol or mestranol and a progestin. The adverse events associated with high-dose estrogen, such as coronary thrombosis, led to development of the second-generation pill, which contained less than 50 μg of ethinyl estradiol and progestins other than levonorgestrel derivatives. Next, attention was directed toward the progestin, which was thought to have adverse androgenic effects such as affecting lipid profiles and glucose tolerance. This led to the development of third-generation pills that contain both a lower dose of estrogen (20–30 μg of ethinyl estradiol) and newer progestins (gonanes: desogestrel or norgestimate). Indeed, studies have shown a reduction in metabolic changes associated with these progestins, but limited data are available to demonstrate any actual reduction of cardiovascular events. Another recently developed progestin, drospirenone, has antimineralocorticoid and antiandrogenic activity in addition to its pharmacologic progestational effects. As an analog of spironolactone rather than androgen, it competitively binds to aldosterone receptors, and it may counteract the estrogen stimulation of the renin-angiotensin system, resulting in more weight stability and less water retention. A new combination oral contraceptive, Yasmin, which contains 3 mg drospirenone and 30 μg ethinyl estradiol, has recently been approved by the FDA and will be prescribed for women with hyperandrogenism or other side effects attributable to oral contraceptives. However, the relative antiandrogenic activity of drospirenone is small com-

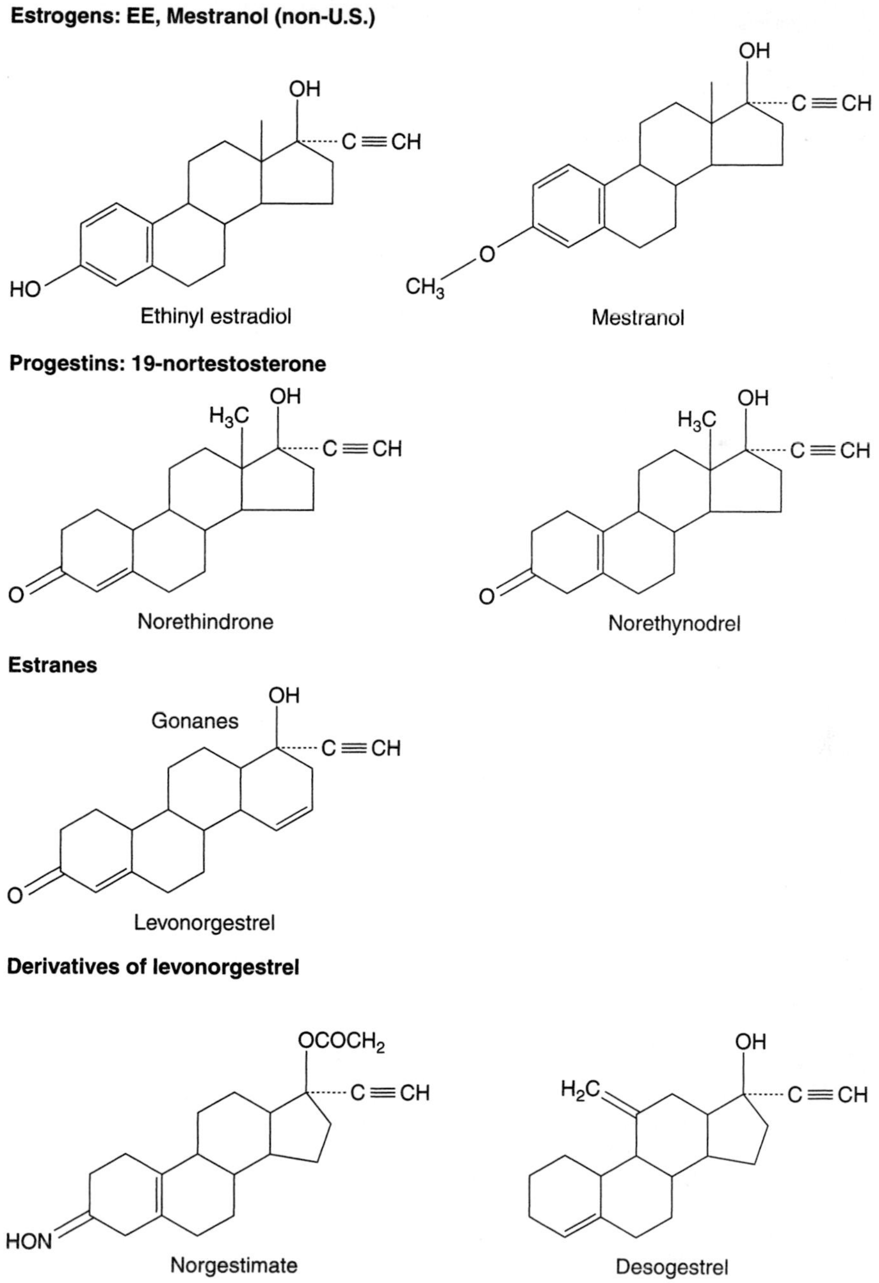
Estrogens: EE, Mestranol (non-U.S.)
OH
C≡CH
HO
Ethinyl estradiol
OH
C≡CH
O
CH3
Mestranol
Progestins: 19-nortestosterone
OH
H3C
C≡CH
O
Norethindrone
OH
H3C
C≡CH
O
Norethynodrel
Estranes
OH
Gonanes
C≡CH
O
Levonorgestrel
Derivatives of levonorgestrel
OCOCH2
C≡CH
HON
Norgestimate
OH
H2C
C≡CH
Desogestrel

Figure 13–12. Oral contraceptive pill hormonal components. All are synthetic steroids.

Pregnanes

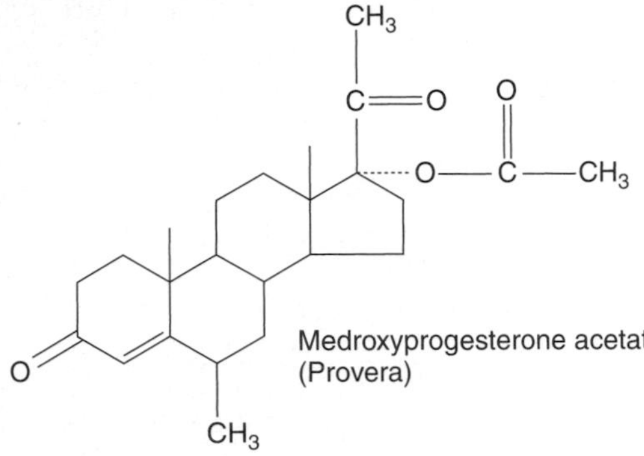

Medroxyprogesterone acetate
(Provera)

Endogenous hormones

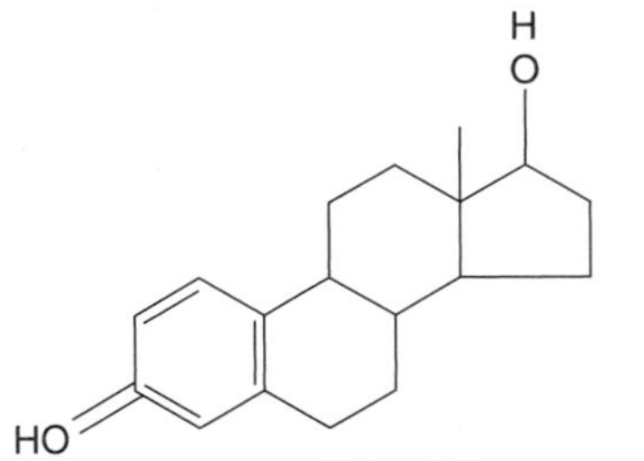

Estradiol

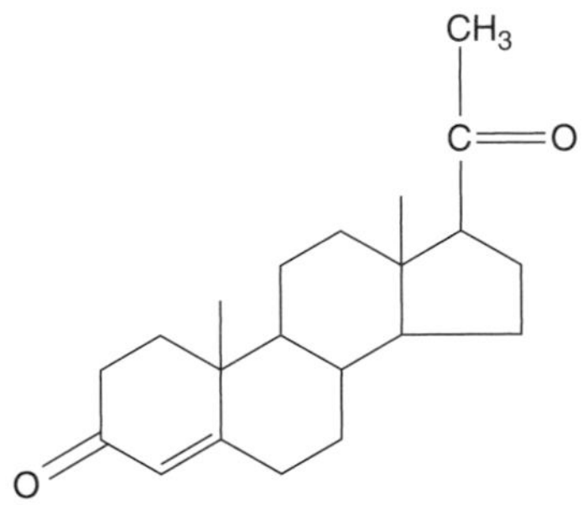

Progesterone

Figure 13–12. Continued

pared with cyproterone acetate or the therapeutic dose of spironolactone used for the treatment of hirsutism.

Contraceptives can be classified also on formulas or schedules of administration. The theory behind phasic preparations was to further decrease the amount of total progestin administered in an attempt to reduce metabolic changes attributed to the progestin, thereby decreasing adverse effects. The traditional monophasic pill (eg, Loestrin) contains 30 μg of ethinyl estradiol and 1.5 mg of norethindrone. This dose is given every day for 3 weeks with a 1-week hormone-free interval. The progestin dose remains constant throughout the cycle. The second type is the biphasic pill (eg, Ortho-Novum 10/11), which contains 35 μg of ethinyl estradiol and either 0.5 mg or 1 mg of norethindrone. The 0.5 mg of norethindrone is administered in the first 10 days of the month and the 1 mg is administered for the following 11 days. The last 7 days of the cycle are free of hormone. With this combination, there was a theoretical increase in breakthrough bleeding and an increased pregnancy rate. A meta-analysis revealed no difference, but limited data were available.

Because of concerns that this regimen might result in both breakthrough bleeding and pregnancies, an-

other phasic formulation was developed. The triphasic pills (eg, Triphasil, Ortho-Novum 7/7/7) contain 0.5, 0.75, and 1 mg norethindrone combined with 35 μg ethinyl estradiol. Theoretically, this formulation improves cycle control. There are several other regimens, some of which alter estrogen doses to simulate the estrogen cyclic rhythm (Triphasil-30, 40, 30 μg ethinyl estradiol) and possibly decrease breakthrough bleeding. A meta-analysis comparing biphasic versus triphasic pills revealed that triphasic pills significantly improved cycle control. However, the progestins in each pill tested were different, and this could account for better cycle control rather than the phasic formulation. An additional meta-analysis was performed on triphasic versus monophasic pills to assess cycle control and metabolic effects. This analysis revealed no difference between the formulations. Therefore, there is little scientific rationale for prescribing phasic preparations in preference to the monophasic pill.

The pharmacologic activity of progestins is based on the progestational activity and bioavailability of each progestin as well as the dose. The relative potencies of the different progestins are levonorgestrel > norgestrel > norethindrone. The active estrogen component of oral contraceptives is ethinyl estradiol (even if mestranol is administered).

When the hormones are administered for 21 days of the cycle, there is enough progestin to inhibit rapid follicle growth for about 7 more days. Figure 13–13 demonstrates that during the steroid-free interval there is no rise in estrogen, indicating no follicular maturation. It is likely that pills missed after this time are responsible for some of the unintended pregnancies. Therefore, it is important that this interval not be extended.

Pharmacologic doses of progestin inhibit ovulation by suppressing GnRH pulsatility and possibly inhibiting release of pituitary LH. Progestins also impair implantation and produce thick, scanty cervical mucus that retards sperm penetration. These latter methods play a minor role in the mechanism of oral contraception.

Ethinyl estradiol helps prevent the selection of a dominant follicle by suppressing pituitary FSH. In addition to FSH suppression, ethinyl estradiol provides stability to the endometrium, decreasing breakthrough bleeding. It also up-regulates the progesterone receptor and decreases clearance, thereby potentiating the activity of the progestin.

Traditionally, a pill is administered daily for 3 weeks out of 4, preferably at the same time each day (more

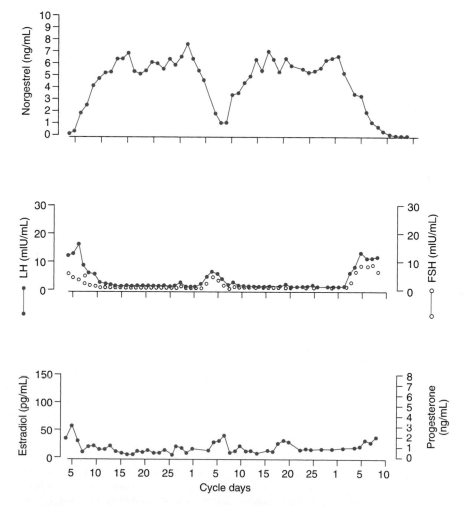

Figure 13–13. Progestin activity on steroidogenesis and ovulation. (Reproduced, with permission, from Brenner PF et al: Serum levels of d-norgestrel, luteinizing hormone, follicle-stimulating hormone, estradiol and progesterone in women during and following ingestion of combination oral contraceptives containing dl-norgestrel. Am J Obstet Gynecol 1997;129:133.)

critical with progestin-only pills). This regimen was designed to mimic the menstrual cycle with monthly withdrawal bleeding. The conventional start date is on the first Sunday after menses (first day of menses for triphasics). An alternative method is to start at the time of the clinic visit regardless of the day of the menstrual cycle with a backup method for 7 days ("Quick-Start"). This method has the advantage of immediate contraception without adverse bleeding events. In addition, with the "Quick-Start" method, women are more likely to start the second pack of oral contraceptives, suggesting increased compliance. During the 28-day regimen, there is a 1-week steroid-free interval. If the steroid-free interval is prolonged beyond the 7-day window, ovulation is possible. Therefore, this is a critical time not to neglect taking pills. On the other hand, a woman may continue to take the hormone pills and skip the steroid-free interval to avoid monthly bleeding. A randomized trial comparing continuous oral contraception with the traditional cyclic method revealed a significantly greater incidence of erratic bleeding with (overall) the same number of days of bleeding, albeit a smaller amount of bleeding. New formulations have been developed for those who do not desire cyclic bleeding. This regimen involves 84 days of continuous hormone administration followed by a steroid-free interval of 1 week. This can easily be done with the traditionally packaged oral contraceptive pills.

A routine for daily administration improves adherence and contraceptive efficacy. Failure to take the pill at the same time every day and not understanding the package insert are associated with missing two or more pills during the cycle. In order to decrease failure rates, women should understand that if they forget to take the pill, they must use barrier prophylaxis.

Postpartum women who are not breast-feeding may begin combination oral contraceptives 3 weeks after delivery. For women who are breast-feeding, it is advised that institution of combination oral contraceptives be delayed until 3 months postpartum. The recommendation for this delay is due to decreased milk letdown secondary to estrogen but may be waived once lactation is well established.

Noncompliance increases the incidence of unwanted pregnancies. Appropriate use of birth control is achieved 32–85% of the time in the general population. Teenagers have at most a 50% continuation rate, and 25% of pill users discontinue the practice in the first year. The efficacy of the oral contraceptive under conditions of perfect use is 0.1 failures per 100 woman-years (or 0.1 per 100 users). With typical use, the failure rate is 3%, with first-year failure rates approaching 7.3–8.5%. Side effects contribute to noncompliance. The most common side effect is breakthrough bleeding. Other unwanted symptoms include bloating, breast tenderness, nausea, and possibly headaches, weight gain, and depression. Some studies suggest that altering estrogen doses may improve symptoms. Failure rates may also be associated with concomitant use of drugs (eg, rifampin, hydantoins) that accelerate hormone metabolism.

Other Benefits

There are noncontraceptive benefits to the pill. These include reduced monthly blood loss (less iron deficiency) and less dysmenorrhea as well as reduced benign breast disease and mastalgia. Oral contraceptives also reduce the incidence of PID and ectopic pregnancies. Other significant benefits include a reduction in risk of ovarian cancer, endometrial cancer, and colorectal cancer. Oral contraceptive use also has cosmetic benefits where it can improve excess hair growth and acne (see PCOS). It is not unusual for the pill to be administered for noncontraceptive problems.

Potential Risks

In general, oral contraceptives have proved to be safe for most women, but the possibility of adverse effects has received much attention. Unfortunately, the literature is full of conflicting reports. Data concerning controversial adverse effects will be discussed in the following section.

While estrogen in combination oral contraceptives tends to increase triglycerides and total cholesterol, these levels are still within the normal range, and they appear to increase HDL and decrease LDL. Progestins attenuate these effects, which suggests an adverse metabolic milieu. Although it is known that low HDL/LDL ratios are associated with cardiovascular events, the importance of lipid changes associated with birth control pills is unknown. To date there is no strong evidence of an increased incidence of myocardial infarctions in healthy nonsmoking oral contraceptive users. In patients with other cardiovascular risk factors such as hypertension—at least in Europe—there is an up to twelvefold increased risk of cardiovascular events. Women who are over 35 years of age and smoke are at increased risk for cardiovascular events. This risk is amplified with use of the birth control pill. If more than 15 cigarettes per day are consumed, there is a RR of 3.3 for a cardiovascular event compared with a RR of 20.8 with concomitant use of oral contraceptives. However, if a woman smokes fewer than 15 cigarettes per day, there is a 2.0 RR of a cardiovascular event compared with 3.5 RR with concomitant contraceptive use. Former smokers after 1 year have no significant increased risk. First-generation oral contraceptives (> 50 μg ethinyl estradiol) imposed a 5.8 RR of stroke (ischemic or hemorrhagic). With low-dose agents (< 50 μg ethinyl estradiol), there appears to be no significant increased risk of stroke among healthy normotensive nonsmoking women. Hypertensive women have a 10.2–14.2 RR of hemorrhagic stroke. Since the potential exists for adverse outcomes, women taking oral contraceptives should be screened regularly for cardiovascular risk factors to ensure safe administration.

The risk of deep vein thrombosis and pulmonary embolism is increased twofold to threefold with administration of the pill. The mechanism by which oral contraceptives enhance venous thrombosis is unknown, but there may be estrogen-related changes in coagulation parameters. These include increased clotting factors and activation of platelets and a decrease in protein S and fibrinolytic activity. However, these changes in measured serum clotting factors do not predict the occurrence of deep vein thrombosis. Genetic thrombophilias increase the risk of venous thrombosis. The prevalence of factor V Leiden in the general population is 5%. The incidence of deep vein thrombosis among this population is 60 per 100,000 per year, and with use of oral contraceptives the incidence approaches 280–300 per 100,000 per year. The baseline incidence of deep vein thrombosis in women is approximately 3 per 100,000 per year, while with current oral contraceptive uses it is 9.6–21.1 per 100,000 per year. For comparison, during pregnancy, the incidence of deep vein thrombosis is 60 per 100,000 per year. Older age (40–44) increases the incidence twofold to threefold but does not affect the relative risk. There is no evidence that smoking has an effect on deep vein thrombosis incidence with oral contraceptive use. At this time, universal screening for thrombophilias is not cost-effective. However, any history of deep vein thrombosis warrants a workup for thrombophilias.

The association of oral contraceptives and cancer risk has been evaluated for breast, cervical, and liver cancer. Observational studies investigating a possible association between oral contraceptive use and breast cancer have reported conflicting results. The most recent information is that oral contraceptive usage (current or past users) has no impact on the incidence of breast cancer—RR 1.0 (CI 95% 0.8–1.3)—among women 35–64 years of age. Several observational studies have linked oral contraceptive use with invasive cervical cancer, though it is not clear if this association is causally related. A recent study investigating the association between oral contraception use and cervical cancer revealed a nearly threefold increased risk among human papillomavirus carriers with 5–9 years of use (RR 2.82; 95% CI 1.46–5.42). This evidence suggests that women taking oral contraceptives should be screened yearly with Pap smears to prevent cervical cancer. In the 1980s there was an association between hep-

atocellular carcinoma in women under 50 years of age and oral contraceptive use. With further investigation there appears to be no increased risk of hepatic cancer with the use of oral contraceptives.

After discontinuation of oral contraceptives, the activity of the HPO axis gradually returns to a precontraceptive state. After a 2- to 4-week prolongation of the follicular phase, the LH peak is observed, which suggests that the suppressive effects of the oral contraceptive have dissipated and that cyclic menses will resume.

Contraindications to oral contraceptive administration are summarized in Table 13–5.

Progestin Only

Progestin-only pills (Ortho Micronor, Nor-QD, 0.35 mg norethindrone; Ovrette, 0.075 mg levonorgestrel) are also available for contraception. The target population for administration of progestin-only contraception includes women with contraindications to estrogen, breast-feeding mothers, and older women.

The circulating levels of progestin following ingestion of progestin-only pills (minipill) are 25–50% of that following ingestion of estrogen-progestin oral contraceptive pills. Serum levels that peak 2 hours after administration are followed by rapid elimination (see graphs in Figure 13–14). The peak levels of norethindrone and levonorgestrel vary (4–14 ng/mL and 0.9–2 ng/mL, respectively), but 24 hours after pill ingestion, serum levels are 0.2–1.6 ng/mL and 0.2–0.5 ng/mL, respectively. Thus, there is no accumulation of progestin over time. Progestin-only administration results in lower steady state levels and a shorter half-life compared with concomitant administration with estrogen.

Owing to the lower levels of progestin in the progestin-only pill, there is less influence on the inhibition of ovulation and more impact of thickening cervical mucus ("hostile environment") inhibiting sperm penetration. Sperms that are able to penetrate have decreased mobility. Progestins also alter the endometrial

Table 13–5. Contraindications to combination oral contraceptive use.

Pregnancy
History of thromboembolic disease
Smoking and age ≥ 35 years
Hepatoma
Breast cancer
Endometrial cancer
History of cerebrovascular or cardiovascular disease
Undiagnosed vaginal bleeding
First-degree relative with history of thromboembolic disease
Uncontrolled hypertension

A. Norethindrone

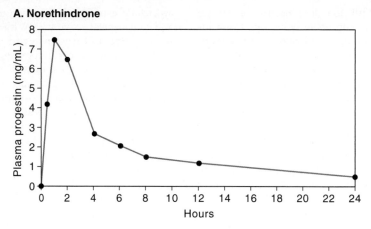

B. Levonorgestrel

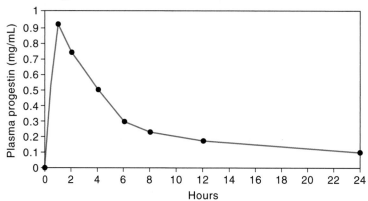

Figure 13–14. Progestin-only pill serum levels. (Reproduced, with permission, from McCann MF, Potter LS: Progestin-only oral contraception: a comprehensive review. Contraception 1994;50[6 Suppl 1]:S1.)

lining (inhibition of progesterone receptor synthesis and reduction in endometrial glandular development, preventing implantation) and perhaps inhibit the motility (number and motility of the cilia) of the uterine tube. LH peaks—as well as FSH peaks—are suppressed compared with pretreatment levels. The change in cervical mucus takes place 2–4 hours after the first dose. However, after 24 hours, thinning of the cervical mucus is evident, allowing unimpaired sperm penetration. This is why it is critical to take the progestin-only pills at the same time every day.

The progestin-only pill should be started on the first day of menses. This pill should be taken at the same time every day. If administration is 3 hours late, a backup method should be used for 48 hours. If a pill is missed, a backup method should be used for 48 hours. If two or more pills are missed, a backup method should be used for 48 hours (due to rapid resumption of the

cervical mucus effect). If there is no menses in 4 weeks, one should obtain a pregnancy test. Progestin-only pills may be administered immediately postpartum.

The efficacy of progestin-only pills under conditions of perfect use is 0.3–3.1 failures per 100 woman-years (failure rates of 1.1–9.6% in the first year) or 0.5 per 100 users. This efficacy rate is achieved only with careful compliance. The typical use is associated with a greater than 5% failure rate. Failure rates were lowest in women over 38½ years of age and those who were breast-feeding. The efficacy may also be influenced by body weight and by concomitant use of anticonvulsants. The major disadvantage is that the pill must be administered at the same time every day. As a result of even slight flexibility in the schedule, there is increased contraceptive failure.

The risks associated with progestin-only pills are minimal. Various studies have revealed no significant impact on lipids, carbohydrate metabolism, blood pressure, or the incidence of myocardial infarction and stroke. Furthermore, no adverse coagulation parameters have been associated with its use. There are almost no data on the association of progestin-only pills and endometrial, ovarian, cervical, or breast cancer. The major side effect is breakthrough bleeding (40–60%). Other side effects include acne and persistent ovarian cysts. With discontinuation of the pill, menses resume with no impact on subsequent pregnancy rates or future fertility.

CONTRACEPTION: LONG-ACTING CONTRACEPTIVES

The high rate of unintended pregnancies has led to the development of long-acting reversible contraceptive modalities. Interest in long-acting methods is increasing because they offer convenience, obviate problems of compliance, and therefore offer higher efficacy. Most long-acting systems contain either combination or progestin-only hormones. The effectiveness of these hormones is prolonged, mostly due to the sustained system that results in a gradual release. The modes of administration include injectables, transdermal patches, subdermal rods, vaginal rings, and intrauterine devices. The various types of long-acting contraceptives are discussed below.

Injectable Contraceptives

A. PROGESTIN ONLY

Injectable progestins that contain medroxyprogesterone acetate (Depo-Provera) are beneficial when women have contraindications to estrogen, use antiepileptics, are mentally handicapped, or have poor compliance. Furthermore, there is good evidence that its use is safe in the presence of coronary artery disease, congestive heart failure, diabetes, tobacco use, and a history of venous thromboembolism.

Other uses of medroxyprogesterone acetate include treatment of metastatic endometrial or renal carcinoma.

Although most other long-acting contraceptives are sustained-release formulations, Depo-Provera (150 mg medroxyprogesterone acetate) is provided as an aqueous microcrystalline suspension that gradually declines throughout the cycle (see Figure 13–15). Pharmacologic levels (> 0.5 ng/mL) are achieved within the first 24 hours and peak (at 2 ng/mL) within the first week after the injection. Serum concentrations are maintained at 1 ng/mL for approximately 3 months. Interestingly, estrogen concentration is in the early to mid follicular level (below 100 pg/mL) and persists for 4 months after the last injection. The serum concentration of medroxyprogesterone acetate decreases to 0.2 ng/mL during the last 5–6 months (ovulation occurs

when levels are < 0.1 ng/mL). However, one study observed progesterone levels to rise after 3½ months.

The mechanism of action depends on the higher peaks of hormone to mainly inhibit ovulation (LH surge). Like other progestins, medroxyprogesterone acetate increases cervical mucus viscosity, alters the endometrium, and decreases the motility of the uterine tubes and uterus. FSH levels are minimally suppressed with Depo-Provera.

The manufacturer's recommendation is to administer the agent every 3 months, starting within 5 days of menses with a grace period of 1 week. The agent is injected deeply into the upper outer quadrant of the buttock or deltoid without massage to ensure slow release. If the grace period exceeds 1 week, a pregnancy test should be performed. If the subject is postpartum and not breast-feeding, Depo-Provera should be given within 3 weeks after delivery and if lactating within 6 weeks (see Table 13–6).

Since compliance is not an issue, the failure rate is minimal at 0 to 0.7 per 100 woman-years (0.3 per 100 users). Weight and use of concurrent medications do not affect the efficacy. However, continuation rates are poor at 50–60% because of the side effect profile. The major dissatisfaction that leads to discontinuation is breakthrough bleeding, which approaches 50–70% in the first year of use. Other side effects include weight gain (2.1 kg per year), dizziness, abdominal pain, anxiety, and possibly depression. Another disadvantage with the use of Depo-Provera is a delay in fertility after discontinuation. Ovulation returns when serum levels are less than 0.1 ng/mL. The time from discontinuation to ovulation is prolonged. Only 50% of patients ovulate at 6 months after discontinuing the medication, and although this agent does not cause infertility, achieving pregnancy may be delayed for more than 1 year. (The length of time for release at the injection site is unpredictable.) After the first year, 60% of women become amenorrheic, and at 5 years the incidence of amenorrhea approaches 80%, which can be considered a potential benefit. Other benefits with use of medroxyprogesterone acetate include prevention of iron deficiency anemia, ectopic pregnancy, PID, and endometrial cancer. In addition, Depo-Provera is a recommended contraceptive for women with sickle cell disease (decreased crisis) and seizure disorders (raises seizure threshold). Other therapeutic uses include dysmenorrhea and endometrial hyperplasia or cancer.

1. Potential Risks—One major concern with use of Depo-Provera is the development of osteopenia, with possible advancement to osteoporosis later in life. Several observational studies have evaluated the potential impact on bone. A prospective trial revealed that current users, after 12 months of use, experience a mean bone mineral density (BMD) loss of 2.74%. However,

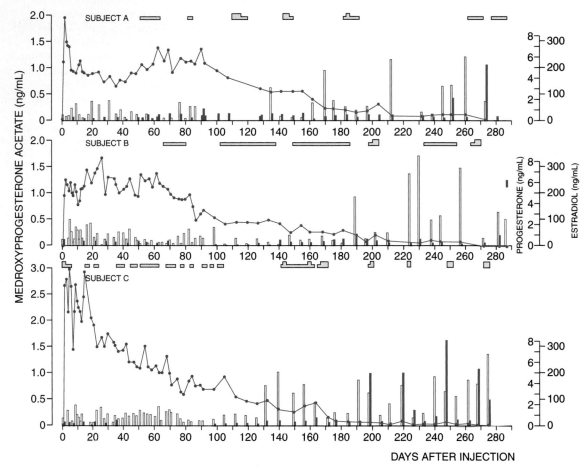

Figure 13–15. MPA levels following injection of Depo-Provera. (Reproduced, with permission, from Ortiz A et al: Serum medroxyprogesterone acetate [MPA] and ovarian function following intramuscular injection of depo-MPA. J Clin Endocrinol Metab 1977;44:32.)

on examining former users 30 months later, it was found that mean BMD was similar to that of nonusers, indicating that the loss is reversible and of minimal clinical importance. An ongoing multicenter study assessing bone density in users versus nonusers should clarify the impact of Depo-Provera on bone. BMD in adolescents has also been investigated because of this critical time of bone mineralization. A small prospective study revealed that BMD was decreased by 1.5–3.1% after 1 and 2 years of use, compared with an increased BMD of 9.3% and 9.5% in Norplant users and controls, respectively. This is a potential concern and has also led to a prospective multicenter study investigating the use of Depo-Provera in adolescents. Although one possible cause is less exposure to estrogen, an alternative and perhaps not exclusive theory involves medrox-

yprogesterone-dependent glucocorticoid activity that impairs osteoblast differentiation. Other potential risks include an adverse lipid profile (increase in LDL, decrease in HDL) and a slightly increased risk of breast cancer. The association of breast cancer with use of Depo-Provera is minimal within the first 4 years of use, with no risk after 5 years of use. Paradoxically, medroxyprogesterone has been used for treatment of metastatic breast cancer.

B. Combination

The development of monthly combination injectables (Lunelle) has responded to the erratic bleeding associated with Depo-Provera (see Figure 13–16). The cycle control is similar to what is achieved with combined oral contraceptives. The monthly withdrawal bleeding

Table 13–6. Scheduling for injectable contraceptives.[1]

Method	DMPA	MPA/E₂C
First injection		
Spontaneous menstrual cycle	Within 5 days of menses onset	Within 5 days of menses onset
Spontaneous or elective first-trimester abortion	Within 7 days	Within 7 days
Term delivery	Within 3 weeks postpartum if not lactating; within 6 weeks postpartum if lactating	Between 21 and 28 days postpartum if not lactating
Switching from combination OCs	While administered active pills or within 7 days after administering the pill pack's last active tablet	While administered active pills or within 7 days after administering the pill pack's last active tablet
Switching from DMPA	—	Within 13 weeks after last DMPA injection
Switching from MPA/E₂C	Within 33 days after previous injection	—
Switching from levonorgestrel implant	Any time within 5 years of implant insertion; use of a condom back-up is recommended for 1 week	Any time within 5 years of implant insertion; use of a condom backup is recommended for 1 week
Switching from Copper T 380A IUD	First injection should occur before IUD removal and within 10 years after IUD insertion; a condom should be used as a back-up if the first injection is not administered within 5 days of menses onset	First injection should occur before IUD removal and within 10 years after IUD insertion; a condom should be used as a back-up if the first injection is not administered within 5 days of menses onset
Subsequent injections		
Injection interval	Every 12 weeks or 3 months; earlier reinjections are acceptable	Every 28 days or 4 weeks or monthly; reinjection earlier than 23 days may impair cycle control
Grace period	2 weeks (14 weeks from last injection); after 1 week manufacturer recommends pregnancy testing before repeat injection	± 5 days (23–33 days from last injection); thereafter, pregnancy testing needed before repeat injection

DMPA = depot medroxyprogesterone acetate; MPA/E₂C = medroxyprogesterone acetate and estradiol cypionate; OCs = oral contraceptives; IUD = intrauterine device.
[1]Reproduced, with permission, from Kaunitz AM: Injectable long-acting contraceptives. Clin Obstet Gynecol 2001;44:73.

occurs 2 weeks after the injection. The target populations are adolescents and women who have difficulty with compliance. Lunelle is an aqueous solution containing 25 mg of medroxyprogesterone acetate and 5 mg of estradiol cypionate per 0.5 mL. In women who receive repeated administration of Lunelle, peak estradiol levels occur approximately 2 days after the third injection and are 247 pg/mL (similar to peak ovulatory levels). The estradiol level returns to baseline 14 days after the last injection (100 pg/mL); the drop in estradiol is associated with menstrual bleeding (2–3 weeks after the last injection). Peak medroxyprogesterone acetate (MPA) levels (2.17 ng/mL) occur at 3½ days after the third monthly injection. The mean MPA level is 1.25 ng/mL. The level at day 28 of the cycle is 0.44–0.47 ng/mL (level needed for contraceptive effect is 0.1–0.2 ng/mL).The earliest return of ovulation seen in women with multiple injections has been 60 days after the last dose. The mechanism of action is similar to that of combined oral contraceptives.

Lunelle is administered intramuscularly in the buttock or deltoid every month. The first injection should be given within the first 5 days of the menstrual cycle (see Table 13–6). Even though pharmacokinetic analysis reveals a delay in ovulation, the manufacturer recommends a 5-day grace period. The failure rate is 0.1 per 100 woman-years. Neither body weight nor use of concomitant drugs appears to affect the efficacy. Although this contraceptive has the advantages of the oral contraceptives and is associated with better compliance, the continuation rate is only 55%. This may be due to its side effect profile, which is similar to that of the combined oral contraceptives with the addition of monthly injections.

1. Potential Risks—There are limited data on potential risks. The risk potential is probably similar to that of the combined oral contraceptives, with a potentially lower incidence of deep vein thrombosis secondary to the absence of the first-pass effect. Upon discontinua-

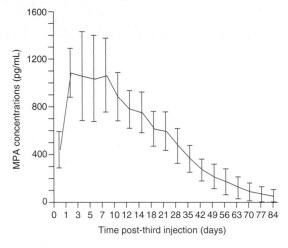

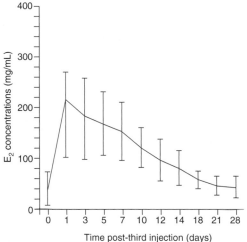

Figure 13–16. Serum MPA and estradiol levels following Lunelle injection. (Reproduced, with permission, from Rahimmy MH, Ryan KK, Hopkins NK: Lunelle monthly contraceptive injection [medroxyprogesterone acetate and estradiol cypionate injectable suspension]: steady-state pharmacokinetics of MPA and E_2 in surgically sterile women. Contraception 1999;60;209.)

tion of Lunelle, achieving pregnancy may be delayed for as long as to 3–10 months after the last injection.

Subdermal Implants

The Norplant package consists of six capsules (34 mm in length, 2.4 mm in diameter), with each capsule providing 36 mg of levonorgestrel (total 216 mg). The target population is women who have contraindications to or adverse side effects from estrogen, women who are postpartum or breast-feeding, and adolescent mothers.

This method provides long-term continuous contraception (approved for 5 years) that is rapidly reversible. The advantages, side effects, risks, and contraindications are similar to those of oral progestins. The major disadvantage—not present with use of oral progestins—is the surgical insertion and removal of the rods. A newer system, Norplant II, contains two rods (4 cm in length, 3.4 cm in diameter) and releases 50 μg/d of norgestrel (approved for 3 years). The two-rod system has the same mechanism of action and side effect profile as its predecessor. However, it is much easier and faster to insert and remove than the capsules.

Within the first 24 hours, serum concentrations of levonorgestrel are 0.4–0.5 ng/mL. The capsules release 85 μg of levonorgestrel per 24 hours for the first year (equivalent to the daily dose of progestin-only pills) and then 50 μg for the remaining 5 years. The mean serum levels of progestin after the first 6 months are 0.25–0.6 ng/mL, slightly decreased at 5 years to 0.17–0.35 ng/mL). A levonorgestrel concentration below 0.2 ng/mL is associated with increased pregnancy rates. The site of implantation (leg, forearm, and arm) does not affect circulating progestin levels. Even though progestin levels are sufficient to prevent ovulation within the first 24 hours, the manufacturer recommends use of a backup method for 3 days after insertion. Upon removal, the progestin levels rapidly decline and undetectable serum levels are achieved after 96 hours. As a result, most women ovulate within 1 month after removal of the implants.

There are several ways in which Norplant provides contraception. In the first 2 years, the levonorgestrel concentration is high enough to suppress the LH surge—most likely at the hypothalamic level—and thereby inhibits ovulation. However, given the low concentrations of progestin, there is no real effect on FSH. The estradiol levels approximate those in ovulatory women. In addition, there are irregular serum peaks (often prolonged) and declines in serum estrogen levels that may contribute to erratic bleeding. By 5 years, more than 50% of the cycles are ovulatory. However, ovulatory cycles while using Norplant have been associated with luteal phase insufficiency. Other mechanisms of contraception are similar to oral progestins and include thickening of the cervical mucus, alterations of the endometrium, and changes in tubal and uterine motility.

The failure rate is 0.2–2.1 failures per 100 woman-years (0.9 per 100 users). Like oral progestins, body weight affects circulating levels and may result in more failures in the fourth or fifth year of use. Similar to oral progestins, the incidence of ectopic pregnancy among failures is increased to 20% (overall incidence is 0.28–1.3 per 1000 woman-years). The continuation rate (discontinuation rate of 10–15% per year) is age-dependent and ranges from 33% to 78%. Menstrual disturbances are the most frequent side effect, approaching 40–80% especially in the first 2 years. Although the incidence of abnormal uterine bleeding is similar to the experience with Depo-Provera, a significant difference between these methods is that Norplant provides only a 10% amenorrhea rate at 5 years. Other side effects reported include headache (30% indication for removal) and possibly weight gain, mood changes, anxiety, and depression—as well as ovarian cyst formation (eightfold increase), breast tenderness, acne, galactorrhea (if insertion occurs upon discontinuation of lactation), possible hair loss, and pain or other adverse reactions at the insertion site (0.8% of cases at discontinuation).

Transdermal Patch

The transdermal patch (Ortho Evra) is another approach to contraception. The thin 20 cm^2 patch is composed of a protective layer, a middle (medicated) layer, and a release liner that is removed prior to application. The system delivers 150 µg of norelgestromin (active metabolite of norgestimate) and 20 µg of ethinyl estradiol per day to the systemic circulation. The target population is similar to that described above for Lunelle. One advantage of this system over Lunelle is that there are no monthly injections and as a result there is greater autonomy for the patient. The patch is applied once a week for 3 consecutive weeks, followed by a patch-free week for monthly withdrawal bleeding. The patch should be changed on the same day each week. The mechanism of action, contraindications, and side effects are similar to what has been described in the section on oral contraceptives.

With use of the transdermal patch, the peak ethinyl estradiol and norelgestromin levels are 50–60 pg/mL and 0.7–0.8 ng/mL, respectively. Because of this unique delivery system, hormone levels achieve a steady state condition throughout the cycle (see below and Figure 13–17). After the seventh day of application, there are adequate hormone levels to inhibit ovulation for 2 more days. With each consecutive patch, there is minimal accumulation of norelgestromin or ethinyl estradiol. The amount of hormone delivered is not affected by the environment, activity, or site of application (abdomen, buttock, arm, torso). The adhesive is very reliable in a variety of conditions, including exercise, swimming, humidity, saunas, and bathing. Complete detachment occurs in 1.8% of cases and partial detachment in 2.9% of cases.

The failure rate is 0.7 per 100 woman-years under conditions of perfect use. Body weight has not been shown to affect the efficacy. The compliance with perfect use ranges from 88.1–91% among all age groups. This is significantly different from what is achieved with oral contraceptives (67–85%), especially with women under 20 years of age. The side effect profile is

similar to that of oral contraceptives except that there is slightly more breakthrough bleeding with the transdermal patch in the first 1–2 months (up to 12.2% versus 8.1%) and less breast tenderness (6.1% versus 18.8%). The incidence of skin reaction was 17.4%, characterized as mild in 92%, resulting in discontinuation in under 2%.

Vaginal Rings

Since the early 1900s, the vagina has been recognized as a place where steroids can be rapidly absorbed into the circulation. A study in the 1960s revealed that silicone rubber pessaries containing sex steroids would release the drug at a continuous rate. These studies led to the development of contraceptive vaginal rings.

Similar to oral contraceptives, there are combination and progestin-only formulations. Several progestin-only rings have been introduced since the 1970s. However, they were associated with significant menstrual disturbances. More recently, combination types have been developed. The most recent (2002) FDA-approved vaginal ring is a combination type called the NuvaRing.

The NuvaRing is made of ethylene vinyl acetate that provides 0.015 mg of ethinyl estradiol and 0.120 mg of etonogestrel per day. Maximum serum concentrations are achieved within 1 week after placement. The ring is designed to be used for 21 days and then removed for 1 full week to permit withdrawal bleeding. This device is capable of inhibiting ovulation within 3 days after insertion. After removal, the time to ovulation is 19 days. The mechanism of action, contraindications, and risks are similar to those of oral contraceptives. However, when assessing systemic exposure, use of the vaginal ring allows for 50% of the total exposure to ethinyl estradiol (15 µg in the ring compared with a 30 µg ethinyl estradiol-containing oral contraceptive).

The failure rate is similar to that reported with oral contraceptives. The continuation rate was 85.6–90%. Irregular bleeding was minimal (5.5%), and overall the device was well tolerated with an associated 2.5% discontinuation rate. Side effects are similar to those of oral contraceptives, but cycle control appears to be improved. The reported incidence of vaginal discharge is 23%, versus 14.5% with use of oral contraceptives. The ring does not appear to interfere with intercourse (1–2% of partners reported discomfort); however, the device can be removed for 2–3 hours during intercourse without changing efficacy.

Intrauterine Devices

Intrauterine devices (IUDs) are another modality of contraception that has been used clinically since the 1960s. Historically, these devices were made of plastic (polyethylene) impregnated with barium sulfate to make

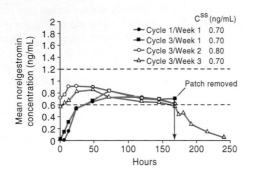
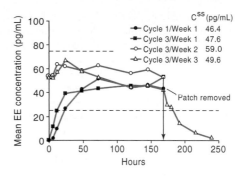
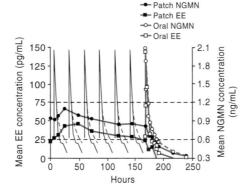

Figure 13–17. Comparative serum steroid levels of norelgestromin (NGMN) and ethinyl estradiol (EE) following patch administration. (Reproduced, with permission, from Abrams LS et al: Multiple-dose pharmacokinetics of a contraceptive patch in healthy women participants. Contraception 2001;64:287.)

them radiopaque. Several other devices were subsequently developed, including the Dalkon Shield. After the introduction of the Dalkon Shield, an increase in pelvic infections was observed secondary to its multifilament tail. Furthermore, tubal infertility and septic abortions were increasing, and massive litigation was the result. Consequently, even though the modern IUD has negligible associated risk, the use of IUDs in the United States is minimal—less than 1% of married women.

Currently two types of IUDs are used in the United States: the copper and the hormone-containing devices. The most recent FDA-approved intrauterine system contains levonorgestrel (Mirena) and is approved for 5 years of use. Several studies have demonstrated that these devices are unlike the Dalkon shield, and are very safe and efficacious. The target population is women who desire highly effective contraception that is long-term and rapidly reversible.

The copper (TCu-380A) IUD is a T-shaped device. The mechanism of action is mostly spermicidal due to the sterile inflammatory reaction that is created sec-

ondary to a foreign body in the uterus. The abundance of white blood cells that are present as a result kills the spermatozoa by phagocytosis. The amount of dissolution of copper is less than the daily amount ingested in the diet. However, with release of copper, salts are created that alter the endometrium and cervical mucus. Sperm transport is significantly impaired, limiting access to the oviducts.

There are two hormone-containing intrauterine devices: the progesterone-releasing device (Progestasert) and the levonorgestrel-releasing device (Mirena). The Progestasert contains progesterone and is released at a rate of 65 mg/d (approved for 1 year). This diffuses into the endometrial cavity, resulting in decidualization and atrophy of the endometrium. Serum progesterone levels do not change with the use of Progestasert. The main mechanism of action is to impair implantation. Mirena contains 52 mg of levonorgestrel and is gradually released at a rate of 20 µg/d (approved for 5 years). Unlike Progestasert, systemic absorption of levonorgestrel inhibits ovulation about half the time. Although women may continue to have cyclic menses, over 40% have impaired follicular growth, with up to 23% developing luteinized unruptured follicles. Other mechanisms of action are similar to those described for Progestasert and the progestin-only pills. Mirena has the added advantage of significantly decreasing menstrual flow and has been used to treat menorrhagia.

The IUD should be placed within 7 days after onset of the menstrual cycle or at any time postpartum. The protection begins immediately after insertion. The failure rates after the first year of use are for copper IUD 0.5–0.8%, Progestasert 1.3–1.6%, and Mirena 0.1–0.2%. The expulsion rate is approximately 10%. If a woman becomes pregnant with an IUD in place, the incidence of an ectopic pregnancy is 4.5–25%, with higher rates associated with use of Progestasert. The incidence of ectopic pregnancies with IUDs varies depending on the type of device. With Progestasert, the ectopic rate is slightly higher (6.80 per 1000 woman-years), most likely because its mechanism of action is limited to inhibiting implantation in the endometrium—in contrast to the copper or levonorgestrel IUD (0.2–0.4 per 1000 woman-years), both of which also interfere with conception.

The continuation rate range for the current IUDs is 40–66.2% (Mirena). The side effects of the copper IUD include dysmenorrhea and menorrhagia. The most common adverse effect associated with the hormone-containing devices is erratic bleeding, albeit significantly less bleeding. In fact, 40% experienced amenorrhea at 6 months and 50% at 12 months. The incidence of spotting in the first 6 months was 25% but decreased to 11% after 2 years. Other side effects of levonorgestrel that have been reported include depression, headaches, and acne. There is a tendency to develop ovarian cysts early after insertion with the levonorgestrel-containing device that resolves after 4 months of use.

The nominal risks associated with IUD use include pelvic infection (within 1 month after insertion), lost IUD (ie, perforation into the abdominal cavity; 1:3000), and miscarriage. There is no association between IUD use and uterine or cervical cancer.

Contraindications to IUD use are active genital infection and unexplained bleeding.

EMERGENCY CONTRACEPTION

Postcoital contraception is a method that may be used by a woman who believes her contraceptive method has failed or who has had unprotected intercourse and feels that she may be at risk for an unintended pregnancy. The first study to evaluate the efficacy of emergency contraception with hormones was in 1963. Subsequently, several studies have been performed with various contraceptives that paved the way for more widespread use. In 1997, the FDA approved the use of high-dose oral contraceptives for postcoital contraception. Since then, pharmaceutical companies have marketed specific packaging for the use of emergency contraception. Other methods, including mifepristone (RU-486) and the IUD have also been effective for postcoital contraception.

Similar to the formulas of oral contraception, there are both combination and progestin-only types of emergency contraception. The combination method (Yuzpe regimen) entails administration of two doses of two tablets (Ovral: 50 μg ethinyl estradiol, 0.5 mg norgestrel) 12 hours apart (total: 200 μg ethinyl estradiol, 2 mg norgestrel). Other oral contraceptives may be used with adjustment in the number of pills for equivalence (ie, two doses of four tablets: any second-generation oral contraceptive 12 hours apart). The specific medication (Preven) that is FDA-approved and marketed for postcoital contraception contains two doses of four tablets (ethinyl estradiol 50 μg, levonorgestrel 0.25 mg) 12 hours apart. The progestin-only method involves two doses of ten pills (Ovrette 0.075 mg) 12 hours apart (Plan A). The marketed form (Plan B) contains two doses of one tablet (levonorgestrel 0.75 mg) 12 hours apart.

Following a single oral dose of 0.75 mg of levonorgestrel, the serum concentration peak (5–10 ng/mL) was at 2 hours with a rapid decline during the first 24 hours. The mechanism of action is uncertain, but levonorgestrel most likely inhibits ovulation and alters the endometrium to prevent implantation. Studies have shown decreased sperm recovery from the uterine cavity, possibly due to thickened cervical mucus, or the alkalinization of the intrauterine environment. Others have shown that decreased factors such as integrins can alter endometrial receptivity. The mode of action most likely depends on the timing of intercourse relative to ovulation and to the administration of emergency contraception.

Maximum efficacy is achieved if the first dose is administered within 72 hours after intercourse and repeated in 12 hours. The failure rate with combination formulas is 2–3% and with progestin only 1%. Emergency contraception effectively reduces the rate of unintended pregnancies from 8% to 2%, a 75% reduction. However, with increasing time since unprotected intercourse, the efficacy changes from 0.4% to 1.2% to 2.7% for the first, second, or third 24-hour period after unprotected intercourse. For maximum efficacy, emergency contraception may be prescribed in advance so women will already have the correct dosing. No increase in risk-taking behavior has been noted with this strategy.

Significant nausea or emesis (51.7%) is associated with use of emergency contraception, though substantially less with progestin-only formulations. An antiemetic should be administered 1 hour before each treatment. If a patient vomits within 1 hour after ingestion, additional pills need to be administered.

Contraindications to emergency contraception with the combination regimen are possibly the same as those described for oral contraceptives; for progestin-only pills, there are no contraindications. Emergency contraception should be an optional function of the rape management protocol.

REFERENCES

Embryology and Anatomy

Ahmed SF, Hughes IA: The genetics of male under-masculinization. Clin Endocrinol (Oxf) 2002;56:1. [PMID: 11849240]

McElreavey K, Fellous M: Sex determination and the Y chromosome. Am J Med Genet 1999;89:76. [PMID:10727993]

Oocyte Development

Erickson GF: The ovary: Basic principles and concepts. In: *Endocrinology and Metabolism,* 4th ed. Felig P, Frohman LA (editors). McGraw-Hill, 2001.

Gougeon A: Regulation of ovarian follicular development in primates: facts and hypotheses. Endocr Rev 1996;17:121. [PMID: 8706629]

Suh CS, Sonntag B, Erickson GF: The ovarian life cycle: a contemporary view. Rev Endocr Metab Disord 2002;3:5. [PMID: 11883105]

Teixeira J, Maheswaran S, Donahoe PK: Müllerian inhibiting substance: an instructive developmental hormone with diagnostic and possible therapeutic applications. Endocr Rev 2001;22:657. [PMID: 11588147]

Ovarian Steroidogenesis

Strauss JF, Hsueh AJ: Ovarian hormone synthesis. In: DeGroot LJ et al (editors). *Endocrinology,* 4th ed. Saunders, 2001.

Menstrual Cycle

Chabbert-Buffet N, Bouchard P: The normal human menstrual cycle. Rev Endocr Metab Disord 2002;3:173. [PMID: 12215712]

McGee EA, Hsueh AJW: Initial and cyclic recruitment of ovarian follicles. Endocr Rev 2000;21:200. [PMID: 10782364]

Amenorrhea

Marcus MD, Loucks TL, Berga SL: Psychological correlates of functional hypothalamic amenorrhea. Fertil Steril 2001;76:310. [PMID: 11476768].

Marshall JC, Eagleson CA, McCartney CR: Hypothalamic dysfunction. Mol Cell Endocrinol 2001;183:29. [PMID: 11604221]

Seminara SB, Hayes FJ, Crowley WF Jr: Gonadotropin-releasing hormone deficiency in the human (idiopathic hypogonadotropic hypogonadism and Kallmann's syndrome):

Pathophysiological and genetic considerations. Endocr Rev 1998;19:521. [PMID: 9793755]

Ovarian Failure

Christin-Maitre S et al: Genes and premature ovarian failure. Mol Cell Endocrinol 1998;145:75. [PMID: 9933102]

Davison RM, Davis CJ, Conway GS: The X chromosome and ovarian failure. Clin Endocrinol 1999;51:573. [PMID: 10619970.

Hoek A, Shoemaker J, Drexhage HA: Premature ovarian failure and ovarian autoimmunity. Endocr Rev 1997;18:107. [PMID: 9034788]

Layman LC: Human gene mutations causing infertility. J Med Genet 2002;3:153. [PMID: 11897813]

Anovulation Due to Polycystic Ovarian Syndrome

Abbott DH, Dumesic DA, Franks S: Developmental origin of polycystic ovary syndrome—A hypothesis. J Endocrinol 2002;174:1. [PMID: 12098657]

Dunaif A: Insulin resistance and the polycystic ovary syndrome: mechanism and implications for pathogenesis. Endocr Rev 1997;18:774. [PMID: 9408743]

Ehrmann DA, Barnes RB, Rosenfield RL: Polycystic ovary syndrome as a form of functional ovarian hyperandrogenism due to dysregulation of androgen secretion. Endocr Rev 1995;16:322. [PMID: 7671850]

Ibanez L et al: Premature adrenarche—normal variant or forerunner of adult disease? Endocr Rev 2000;21:671. [PMID: 11133068]

Legro RS: Polycystic ovary syndrome: the new millennium. Mol Cell Endocrinol 2001;184:87. [PMID: 11694344]

Nestler JE, Jakubowicz DJ: Decreases in ovarian cytochrome P450c17α activity and serum free testosterone after reduction of insulin secretion in polycystic ovarian syndrome N Engl J Med 1996;335:617. [PMID:]8687515]

Poretsky L et al: The insulin-related ovarian regulatory system in health and disease. Endocr Rev 1999;20:535. [PMID: 10453357]

Anovulation Due to Adrenal Disorders

Betterle C et al: Autoimmune adrenal insufficiency and autoimmune polyendocrine syndromes: autoantibodies, autoantigens, and their applicability in diagnosis and disease prediction. Endocr Rev 2002;23:327. [PMID: 12050123]

Newell-Price J et al: The diagnosis and differential diagnosis of Cushing's syndrome and pseudo-Cushing's states. Endocr Rev 1998;19:647. [PMID: 9793762]

White PC, Speiser PW: Congenital adrenal hyperplasia due to 21-hydroxylase deficiency. Endocr Rev 2000;21:245. [PMID: 10857554]

Müllerian Anomalies

Homer HA, Li T-C, Cooke ID: The septate uterus: a review of management and reproductive outcome. Fertil Steril 2000;73:1. [PMID: 10632403]

Raga F et al: Reproductive impact of congenital Müllerian anomalies. Hum Reprod 1997;12:2277. [PMID: 9402295]

Menopause: General References

Faddy MJ et al: Accelerated disappearance of ovarian follicles in mid-life: implications for forecasting menopause. Hum Reprod 1992;7:1342. [PMID: 1291557]

Nelson HD et al: Postmenopausal hormone replacement therapy: scientific review. JAMA 2002;288:872. [PMID: 12186605]

Nair GV, Herrington DM: The ERA trial: Findings and implications for the future. Climacteric 2000;3:227. [PMID: 11910581]

Prior J: Perimenopause: the complex endocrinology of the menopausal transition. Endocr Rev 1998;19:397. [PMID: 9715373]

Soules MR et al: Stages of Reproductive Aging Workshop (STRAW). J Womens Health Gend Based Med 2001; 10:843. [PMID: 11747678]

Menopause Due to Cardiovascular Disease

Barrett-Connor E et al: Raloxifene and cardiovascular events in osteoporotic postmenopausal women: four-year results from the MORE (Multiple Outcomes of Raloxifene Evaluation) randomized trial. JAMA 2002;287:847. [PMID: 11851576]

Grady D et al: Cardiovascular disease outcomes during 6.8 years of hormone therapy: Heart and Estrogen/progestin Replacement Study follow-up (HERS II). JAMA 2002;288:49. [PMID: 12090862]

Hulley S et al: Randomized trial of estrogen plus progestin for secondary prevention of coronary heart disease in postmenopausal women. Heart and Estrogen/progestin Replacement Study (HERS) Research Group. JAMA 1998;280:605. [PMID: 9718051]

Postmenopausal hormone replacement therapy for primary prevention of chronic conditions: recommendations and rationale. Ann Intern Med 2002;137:834. [PMID: 12435221]

Rossouw JE et al: Risks and benefits of estrogen plus progestin in healthy postmenopausal women: principal results from the Women's Health Initiative randomized controlled trial. JAMA 2002;288:321. [PMID: 12117397]

Menopause: Osteoporosis

Meta-analyses of therapies for postmenopausal osteoporosis. Endocr Rev 2002;23:495. [PMID: 12202463]

Menopause: Selective Estrogen Receptor Modulators

Cosman F, Lindsay R: Selective estrogen receptor modulators: clinical spectrum. Endocr Rev 1999;20:418. [PMID: 10368777]

Miller CP: SERMs: Evolutionary chemistry, revolutionary biology. Curr Phar Des 2002;8:2089. [PMID: 12171520]

Hormone Replacement and Alzheimer's Disease

Fillit HM: The role of hormone replacement therapy in the prevention of Alzheimer disease. Arch Intern Med 2002;162:1934. [PMID: 12230415]

Infertility

Cedars, MI: Infertility in obstetrics and gynecology: a longitudinal approach. In: *Gynecology and Obstetrics: A Longitudinal Approach.* Moore TR et al (editors). Churchill Livingstone, 1993.

Collins JA et al: Treatment-independent pregnancy among infertile couples. N Engl J Med 1983;309:1201. [PMID: 6633567]

Guzick DS et al: Efficacy of treatment for unexplained infertility. Fertil Steril 1998;70:207. [PMID: 9696208]

te Velde ER, Dorland M, Broekmans FJ: Age at menopause as a marker of reproductive ageing. Maturitas 1998;30:119. [PMID: 9871906]

Contraception

Abma JC et al: Centers for Disease Control and Prevention, National Center for Health Statistics. Fertility, family planning, and women's health: new data from the 1995 National Survey of Family Growth, Report No. 19, Series 23, 1997.

Abrams LS et al: Multiple-dose pharmacokinetics of a contraceptive patch in healthy women participants. Contraception 2001;64:287. [PMID: 1777488]

Archer DF: New contraceptive options. Clin Obstet Gynecol 2001;44:122. [PMID: 11219241]

Brenner PF et al: Serum levels of d-norgestrel, luteinizing hormone, follicle-stimulating hormone, estradiol, and progesterone in women during and following ingestion of combination oral contraceptives containing dl-norgestrel. Am J Obstet Gynecol 1977;129:133. [PMID: 900174]

Burkman RT et al: Current perspectives on oral contraceptive use. Am J Obstet Gynecol 2001;185(2 Suppl):S4. [PMID: 11521117]

Cedars MI: Infertility in obstetrics and gynecology: a longitudinal aproach. In: *Gynecology and Obstetrics: A Longitudinal Approach.* Moore TR et al (editors). Churchill Livingstone, 1993.

Croxatto HB et al: Mechanism of action of hormonal preparations used for emergency contraception: a review of the literature. Contraception 2001;63:111. [PMID: 11868982]

Kaunitz AM: Injectable long-acting contraceptives. Clin Obstet Gynecol 2001;44:73. [PMID: 11219248]

Marchbanks PA et al: Oral contraceptives and the risk of breast cancer. N Engl J Med 2002;346:2025. [PMID: 12087137]

McCann MF, Potter LS: Progestin-only oral contraception: a comprehensive review. Contraception 1994;50(6 Suppl):S1. [PMID: 10226677]

Ortiz A et al: Serum medroxyprogesterone acetate (MPA) and ovarian function following intramuscular injection of depo-MPA. J Clin Endocrinol Metab 1977;44:32. [PMID: 833262]

Rahimy MH, Ryan KK, Hopkins NK: Lunelle monthly contraceptive injection (medroxyprogesterone acetate and estradiol cypionate injectable suspension): steady-state pharmacokinetics of MPA and E_2 in surgically sterile women. Contraception 1999;60;209. [PMID: 10640167]

Abnormalities of Sexual Determination & Differentiation

14

Felix A. Conte, MD, & Melvin M. Grumbach, MD

ACTH	Adrenocorticotropic hormone		**hCG**	Human chorionic gonadotropin
AHC	Adrenal hypoplasia congenita		**HMG**	High mobility group
AMH	Anti-müllerian hormone		**IGF**	Insulin-like growth factor
CAH	Congential adrenal hyperplasia		**LH**	Luteinizing hormone
CMPD1	Campomelic dysplasia		**PAR**	Pseudoautosomal region
DAX1	DSS-AHC-critical region on the X chromosome gene 1		**RFLP**	Restriction fragment length polymorphism
DAZ	Deleted in azoospermia		**SF-1**	Steroidogenic factor-1
DHEA	Dehydroepiandrosterone		**SHBG**	Sex hormone-binding globulin
DHT	Dihydrotestosterone		**SOX-9**	SRY-like HMG box-9
DMD	Duchenne muscular dystrophy		*SRY*	Sex-determining region Y
DMRT1	Double sex Mab3-related transcription factor gene 1		**StAR**	Steroidogenic acute regulatory protein
			TGF	Transforming growth factor
DSS	Dosage-sensitive sex reversal		**WAGR**	Wilms tumor-aniridia-genital anomalies-mental retardation syndrome
FISH	Fluorescent in situ hybridization			
FSH	Follicle-stimulating hormone		*WNT4*	Human homolog of drosophila wingless gene
GH	Growth hormone			
GK	Glycerol kinase		*WT-1*	Wilms tumor repressor gene
GM-CSF	Granulocyte-macrophage colony-stimulating factor		**XIC**	X inactivation center
			XIST	X-inactive specific transcripts
GnRH	Gonadotropin-releasing hormone		**ZFY**	Zinc finger Y

Advances in molecular genetics, experimental embryology, steroid biochemistry, and methods of evaluation of the interaction between the hypothalamus, pituitary, and gonads have helped to clarify problems of sexual determination and differentiation. Anomalies may occur at any stage of intrauterine development of the hypothalamus, pituitary, gonads, and genitalia and lead to gross ambisexual development or to subtle abnormalities that do not become manifest until sexual maturity is achieved.

NORMAL SEX DIFFERENTIATION

Chromosomal Sex

The normal human diploid cell contains 22 autosomal pairs of chromosomes and two sex chromosomes (two X, or one X and one Y). When arranged serially and numbered according to size and centromeric position, they are known as a karyotype. Advances in the techniques of staining chromosomes (Figure 14–1) permit positive identification of each chromosome by its

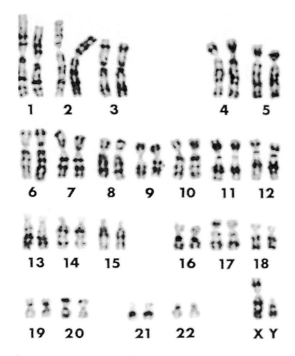

Figure 14–1. A normal 46,XY karyotype stained with Giemsa's stain to produce G bands. Note that each chromosome has a specific banding pattern. (Reproduced, with permission, from Grumbach MM, Hughes IA, Conte FA: Disorders of sex differentiation. In: Larsen PR et al [editors]: *Williams Textbook of Endocrinology,* 10th ed. Saunders, 2002.)

unique "banding" pattern. Bands can be produced in the region of the centromere (C bands), with the fluorescent dye quinacrine (Q bands), and with Giemsa stain (G bands). Fluorescent banding (Figure 14–2) is particularly useful because the Y chromosome stains so brightly that it can be identified easily in both interphase and metaphase cells. A technique called fluorescence in situ hybridization has been particularly useful in identifying "marker" chromosomes, especially deleted sex chromosomes that are not readily identifiable by standard banding techniques. High-resolution chromosome banding and "painting techniques" provide precise identification of each chromosome. The standard nomenclature for describing the human karyotype is shown in Table 14–1. A complete clone map of the euchromatic region of the Y chromosome has been described. This is the first map of this type for a human chromosome, and it spans about 35 million base pairs.

Studies in animals as well as humans with abnormalities of sexual differentiation indicate that the sex chromosomes (the X and Y chromosomes) and the autosomes carry genes that influence sex determination and differentiation by causing the bipotential gonad to develop either as a testis or as an ovary. Two intact and normally functioning X chromosomes, in the absence of a Y chromosome (and the genes for testicular organogenesis), lead to the formation of an ovary, whereas a Y chromosome or the presence of the male-determining region on the short arm of the Y chromosome—the **testis-determining factor**—will lead to testicular organogenesis.

In humans, there is a marked discrepancy in size between the X and Y chromosomes. Gene dosage compensation is achieved in all persons with two or more X chromosomes in their genetic constitution by partial inactivation of all X chromosomes except one. This phenomenon is thought to be a random process that occurs in each cell in the late blastocyst stage of embryonic development during which either the maternally or the paternally derived X chromosome undergoes heterochromatinization. The result of this process is formation of an X chromatin body (Barr body) in the interphase cells of persons having two or more X chromosomes (Figure 14–3). A gene termed *XIST* (X inactive specific transcripts) is located in the region of the putative X inactivation center at Xq13.2 on the paracentromeric region of the long arm of the X chromosome. *XIST* is expressed only by the inactive X chromosome. The *XIST* gene encodes a large RNA that appears to "coat" the X chromosome and facilitate inactivation of genes on the X chromosome.

The distal portion of the short arm of the X chromosome escapes inactivation and has a short (2.5-megabase) segment homologous to a segment on the distal portion of the short arm of the Y chromosome. This segment is called the **pseudoautosomal region;** it is these two limited regions of the X and Y that pair during meiosis, undergo obligatory chiasm formation, and allow for exchange of DNA between these specific regions of the X and Y chromosomes. At least seven genes have been localized to the pseudoautosomal region on the short arm of the X and Y chromosomes. Among these are *MIC2,* a gene coding for a cell surface antigen recognized by the monoclonal antibody, 12E7; the gene for the granulocyte-macrophage colony-stimulating factor (GM-CSF) receptor; the human interleukin-3 receptor; a gene whose deletion results in the neurocognitive defects observed in Turner's syndrome; and a gene for short stature, *PHOG/SHOX.* This gene is expressed in bone and is associated with idiopathic short stature as well as dyschondrosteosis (Leri-Weill syndrome) in heterozygotes. Homozygous mutations of this gene are associated with a more severe form of short stature, Langer mesomelic dwarfism. A pseudoautosomal region has also been described for the distal ends of the long arms of the X and Y chromosomes (Figures 14–4 and 14–5).

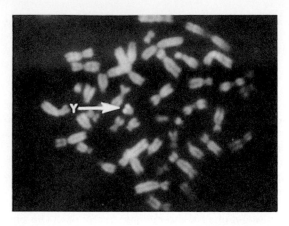 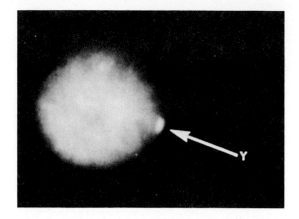

Figure 14–2. Metaphase chromosomes stained with quinacrine and examined through a fluorescence microscope. Note the bright fluorescence of the distal arms of the Y chromosome, which can also be seen in interphase cells ("Y body" at right). (Reproduced, with permission, from Grumbach MM, Hughes IA, Conte FA: Disorders of sex differentiation. In: Larsen PR et al [editors]: *Williams Textbook of Endocrinology,* 10th ed. Saunders, 2002.)

In buccal mucosal smears of 46,XX females, a sex chromatin body is evident in 20–30% of the interphase nuclei examined, whereas in normal 46,XY males, a comparable sex chromatin body is absent. In patients with more than two X chromosomes, the maximum number of sex chromatin bodies in any diploid nucleus is one less than the total number of X chromosomes. Using sex chromatin and Y fluorescent staining, one can determine indirectly the sex chromosome complement of an individual (Table 14–2). FISH analysis for

SRY (Y chromosome) and the pericentric region of the X can rapidly identify the sex chromosome constitution in interphase as well as metaphase cells (Figure 14–6).

Sex Determination (*SRY* Is the Testis-Determining Factor)

In studies of 46,XX males with very small Y-to-X translocations, a gene was localized to the region just proximal to the pseudoautosomal boundary of the Y

Table 14–1. Nomenclature for describing the human karyotype pertinent to designating sex chromosome abnormalities.[1]

Paris Conference	Description	Former Nomenclature
46,XX	Normal female karyotype	XX
46,XY	Normal male karyotype	XY
47,XXY	Karyotype with 47 chromosomes including an extra Y chromosome	XXY
45,X	Monosomy X	XO
45,X/46,XY	Mosaic karyotype composed of 45,X and 46,XY cell lines	XO/XY
p	Short arm	p
q	Long arm	q
46,X,del (X) (p21)	Deletion of the short arm of the X distal to band Xp21	XXp–
46,X,del (X) (q21)	Deletion of the long arm of the X distal to band Xq21	XXq–
46,X,i(Xq10)	Isochromosome of the long arm of X; q10 = centromeric band	XXqi
46,Xr(X)(p22q25)	Ring X chromosome with breaks at p22 and q25	XXr
46,XY,der(7)t(Y;7)(q11;q13)	Translocation of the distal fluorescent portion of the Y chromosome to the long arm of chromosome 7	46,XYt (Yq–7q+)

[1]Reproduced, with permission, from Grumbach MM, Hughes IA, Conte FA: Disorders of sex differentiation. In: Larsen PR et al (editors): *Williams Textbook of Endocrinology,* 10th ed. Saunders, 2002.

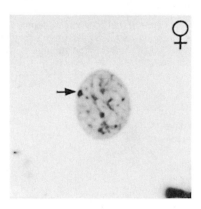

Figure 14–3. X chromatin (Barr) body in the nucleus of a buccal mucosal cell from a normal 46,XX female. (Reproduced, with permission, from Grumbach MM, Hughes IA, Conte FA: Disorders of sex differentiation. In: Larsen PR et al [editors]: *Williams Textbook of Endocrinology*, 10th ed. Saunders, 2002.)

chromosome (Figure 14–5). This gene has been cloned, expressed, and named sex-determining region Y (*SRY*). *Sry* (the mouse analog of the human *SRY* gene) is expressed in the embryonic genital ridge of the mouse between days 10.5 and 12.5, just before and during the time at which testis differentiation first occurs. Furthermore, deletions or mutations of the human *SRY* gene occur in about 15–20% of 46,XY females with complete XY gonadal dysgenesis. The most compelling evidence that *SRY* is the testis-determining factor is that transfection of the *Sry* gene into 46,XX mouse embryos results in transgenic 46,XX mice with testes and male sex differentiation.

The *SRY* gene encodes a DNA-binding protein that has an 80-amino-acid domain similar to that found in high mobility group (HMG) proteins. This domain binds to DNA in a sequence-specific manner (A/TAA-CAAT). It bends the DNA and is thus thought to facilitate interaction between DNA-bound proteins to affect the transcription of "downstream genes." The mechanism of action of SRY and its downstream targets have not yet been defined, although *SOX9* is a candidate downstream gene. At least four cellular roles for the SRY protein have been defined. They include induction of Sertoli cell differentiation, migration of mesonephric cells into the genital ridge, proliferation of cells in the genital ridge, and the development of male-specific vasculature in the gonad with recruitment of a large number of endothelial cells from the mesonephros. Most of the mutations thus far described in 46,XY females with gonadal dysgenesis have occurred in the nucleotides of the *SRY* gene encoding the

DNA binding region (the HMG box) of the SRY protein.

A number of genes are involved in the testis-determining cascade. Heterozygous mutations and deletions of the Wilms tumor gene (*WT1*) located on 11p13 result in urogenital malformations as well as Wilms tumors. Knockout of the *WT1* gene in mice results in apoptosis of the metanephric blastema with the resultant absence of the kidneys and gonads. Thus, *WT1*, a transcriptional regulator, appears to act on metanephric blastema early in urogenital development. Heterozygous mutations in humans result in the Denys-Drash and Frasier syndromes.

SF-1 (steroidogenic factor-1) is an orphan nuclear receptor involved in transcriptional regulation. It is expressed in both the female and male urogenital ridges as well as in steroidogenic tissues, where it is required for the synthesis of testosterone, and in Sertoli cells, where it regulates the antimüllerian hormone gene. SF-1 is encoded by the mammalian homolog of the drosophila gene *Ftz-f1*. Knockout of the gene encoding SF-1 in mice results in apoptosis of the cells of the genital ridge that give rise to the adrenals and gonads and thus lack of gonadal and adrenal gland morphogenesis in both males and females. This gene thus appears to play a critical role in the formation of all steroid-secreting glands, ie, the adrenals, testes, and ovaries. WT1 and SF1 are both active early in the development of the genital ridge and in the determination of both the ovaries and the testes.

XY gonadal dysgenesis with resulting female differentiation in 46,XY patients with intact *SRY* function has been reported in individuals with duplications of Xp21, a locus that contains the *DAX1* gene. A mutation or deletion of *DAX1*, which encodes a transcriptional factor, results in X-linked congenital adrenal hypoplasia (AHC) and hypogonadotropic hypogonadism. Deletion or mutation of the *DAX1* gene in 46,XY individuals has not resulted in an abnormality of testicular differentiation in humans. Similarly, duplication of the *DAX1* gene appears not to affect ovarian morphogenesis and function in 46,XX females. Duplication or deletion of the *Dax1* (mouse homolog) gene in 46,XY mice has caused sex reversal when tested against weak alleles of *Sry*. Thus, it appears that duplication of *DAX1* is responsible for dosage-sensitive sex reversal in human XY individuals. It has been suggested that *DAX1* is an "antitestis" factor rather than an ovary-determining gene. This hypothesis is supported by the finding that null mutations of the *Dax1* locus in the female mouse do not affect ovarian differentiation or fertility (Figure 14–7).

Campomelic dysplasia is a skeletal dysplasia associated with sex reversal due to gonadal dysgenesis in 46,XY individuals. The gene for campomelic dysplasia (*CMPD1*) has been localized to 17q24.3–q25.1. Muta-

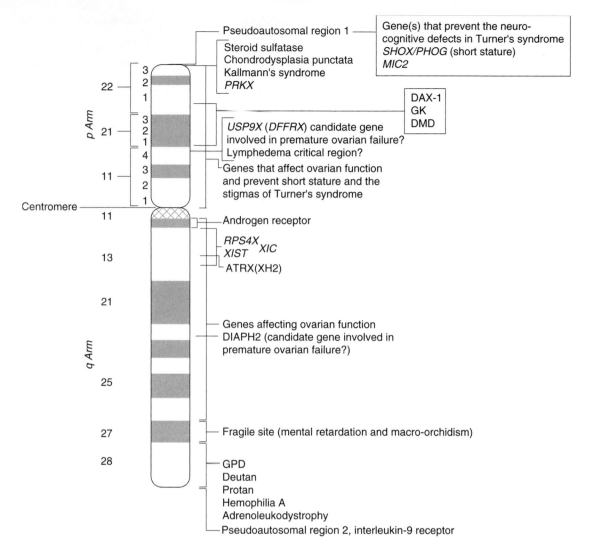

Figure 14–4. Diagrammatic representation of G-banded X chromosome. Selected X-linked genes are shown. (*PHOG,* pseudoautosomal homeobox osteogenic gene; *SHOX,* short-stature homeobox gene; *MIC2,* a cell surface antigen recognized by monoclonal antibody 12E7; *PRKX,* a member of the cAMP-dependent serine-threonine protein kinase gene family (illegitimate X-Y interchange occurs most frequently between *PRKX* and *PRKY*); *DAX1, DSS-AHC*-critical region on the X chromosome gene 1; GK, glycerol kinase; DMD, Duchenne's muscular dystrophy; *USP9X,* human x-linked homolog of the drosophila fat facets-related gene *(DFFRX); RPS4X,* ribosomal protein S4; *XIST,* Xi-specific transcripts; XIC, X-inactivation center; ATRX, α-thalassemia, X-linked mental retardation; *DIAPH2,* human homolog of the drosophila diaphanous gene.) (Reproduced with permission from Grumbach MM, Hughes IA, Conte FA. Disorders of sex differentiation. In Larsen PR et al (editors): *Williams Textbook of Endocrinology,* 10th ed. Saunders, 2002.)

tions in one allele of the *SOX9* gene, a gene related to *SRY* (called a *SOX* gene because it has an SRY HMG box that is more than 60% homologous to that of SRY), can result in both *CMPD1* and XY gonadal dysgenesis with sex reversal. Duplication of the *SOX9* gene both in humans and mice results in sex reversal in XX

individuals who are *SRY*-negative. Hence, it appears that *SOX9* is the only critical gene needed "downstream" of *SRY* for male sex determination. XY individuals with 9p– and 10q– deletions exhibit gonadal dysgenesis and male pseudohermaphroditism. Haploinsufficiency of *DMRT1*—a gene related to "double sex" in drosophila

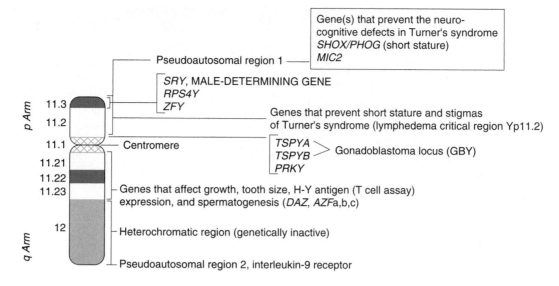

Figure 14–5. Diagrammatic representation of a G-banded Y chromosome. *SHOX/PHOG*, short stature homeobox gene/pseudoautosomal homeobox osteogenic gene; *MIC2*, gene for a cell surface antigen recognized by monoclonal antibody 12E7; *SRY*, sex-determining region Y; *RPS4Y*, ribosomal protein S4; *ZFY*, zinc finger Y; *TSPYA,B*, members of the testes-specific factor gene family; *PRKY*, a member of the cAMP-dependent serine-threonine protein kinase gene family; *DAZ*, deleted in azoospermia; *AZF*, azoospermic factor. (Reproduced with permission from Grumbach MM, Hughes IA, Conte FA. Disorders of sex differentiation. In Larsen PR et al [editors]: *Williams Textbook of Endocrinology*, 10th ed. Saunders, 2002.)

Table 14–2. Sex chromosome complement correlated with X chromatin and Y bodies in somatic interphase nuclei.[1]

Sex Chromosomes	Maximum Number in Diploid Somatic Nuclei	
	X Bodies	**Y Bodies**
45,X	0	0
46,XX	1	0
46,XY	0	1
47,XXX	2	0
47,XXY	1	1
47,XYY	0	2
48,XXXX	3	0
48,XXXY	2	1
48,XXYY	1	2
49,XXXXX	4	0
49,XXXXY	3	1
49,XXXYY	2	2

[1]The maximum number of X chromatin bodies in diploid somatic nuclei is one less than the number of Xs, whereas the maximum number of Y fluorescent bodies is equivalent to the number of Ys in the chromosome constitution. (Reproduced with permission from Grumbach MM, Hughes IA, Conte FA: Disorders of sex differentiation. In Larsen PR et al (editors). *Williams Textbook of Endocrinology*, 10th ed. Saunders, 2002.)

and "Mab3" in *C elegans*— is a candidate for the abnormality in testis development noted in patients with 9p–. No gene has as yet been identified on 10q to account for sex reversal in these patients. Recently, an XY female with a duplication of chromosome region 1p31–35 was described containing a duplication of the *WNT4* gene. Studies indicated that testis development was inhibited as a result of up-regulation of *DAX1* by the WNT4 duplication, resulting in inhibition of SF1 and SOX9 up-regulation in the developing testes and sex reversal. *WNT4* is expressed in the ovary and is thought to be an essential signal for ovarian determination along with germ cells and unknown other genes (Figure 14–7A).

TESTICULAR & OVARIAN DIFFERENTIATION

Until the 12-mm stage (approximately 42 days of gestation), the embryonic gonads of males and females are indistinguishable. By 42 days, 300–1300 primordial germ cells have seeded the undifferentiated gonad from their extragonadal origin in the yolk sac dorsal endoderm. These large cells are the progenitors of oogonia and spermatogonia; lack of these cells is incompatible

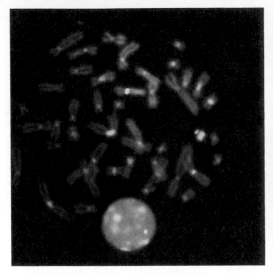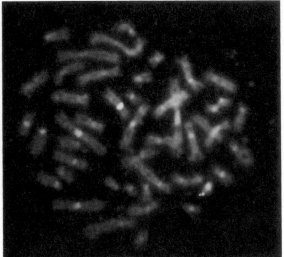

Figure 14–6. FISH analyses for *SRY* in 46, XY interphase cells and metaphase chromosomes. The *SRY* probe (red) localizes to the distal short arm of the Y chromosome (Yp11.3). Another probe (blue) localizes the centromere region of the X chromosome. Both probes are visible in an interphase nucleus. (Courtesy of Dr. Philip Cotter, Oakland Children's Hospital; and Helen Jenks, U.C. Davis Medical Center. Reprinted with permission from Grumbach MM, Hughes IA, Conte IA: Disorders of sex differentiation. In Larsen PR et al. (editors) *Williams Textbook of Endocrinology,* 10th ed. Saunders, 2002.)

with further ovarian differentiation but not testicular differentiation. Under the influence of *SRY* and other genes that encode male sex determination (Figure 14–7B), the gonad will begin to differentiate as a testis at 43–50 days of gestation. Leydig cells are apparent by about 60 days, and differentiation of male external genitalia occurs by 65–77 days of gestation.

In the gonad destined to be an ovary, the lack of differentiation persists. At 77–84 days—long after differentiation of the testis in the male fetus—a significant number of germ cells enter meiotic prophase to characterize the transition of oogonia into oocytes, which marks the onset of ovarian differentiation from the undifferentiated gonads. Primordial follicles (small oocytes surrounded by a single layer of flat granulosa cells and a basement membrane) are evident after 90 days. Preantral follicles are seen after 6 months, and fully developed oocytes with fluid-filled cavities and multiple layers of granulosa cells are present at birth. As opposed to the testes, there is little evidence of hormone production by the fetal ovaries (Figure 14–8).

Differentiation of Genital Ducts (Figure 14–9)

By the seventh week of intrauterine life, the fetus is equipped with the primordia of both male and female genital ducts. The müllerian ducts, if allowed to persist,

form the uterine (fallopian) tubes, the corpus and cervix of the uterus, and the upper third of the vagina. The wolffian ducts, on the other hand, have the potential for differentiating into the epididymis, vas deferens, seminal vesicles, and ejaculatory ducts of the male. In the presence of a functional testis, the müllerian ducts undergo apoptosis under the influence of antimüllerian hormone (AMH), a dimeric glycoprotein secreted by fetal Sertoli cells. This hormone acts "locally" to cause müllerian duct repression ipsilaterally.

The gene for AMH encodes a 560-amino-acid protein whose carboxyl terminal domain shows marked homology with transforming growth factor (TGF)-β and the B chain of inhibin and activin. The gene has been localized on the short arm of chromosome 19. AMH is secreted by human fetal and postnatal Sertoli cells until 8–10 years of age and can be used as a marker for the presence of these cells. SF-1, an orphan nuclear receptor, in combination with WT1, SOX9, and GATA4 (Figure 14–6), has been shown to regulate AMH gene expression. The human AMH receptor gene has been cloned and mapped to the q13 band of chromosome 12. The receptor has been identified as being similar to other type II receptors of the TGF-β family.

The differentiation of the wolffian duct is mediated by testosterone secretion from the testis. SF-1 regulates steroidogenesis by the Leydig cell in the testes by binding to the promoter of the genes encoding P450scc and P450c17. In the presence of an ovary or in the absence

A

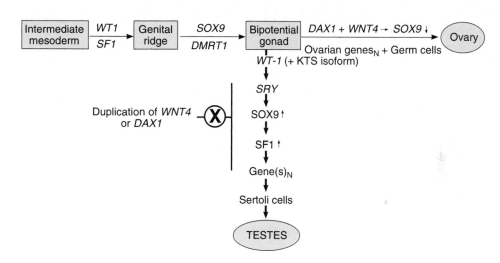

B

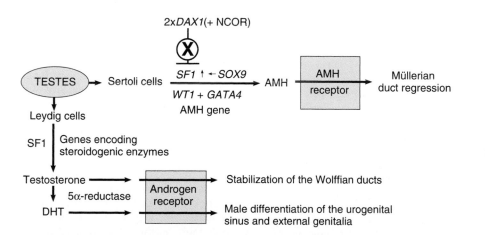

Figure 14–7. **A:** Hypothetical diagrammatic representation of the cascade of genes involved in testes determination in humans shown as a linear pathway rather than a "combinational network." *WT1,* Wilms tumor suppressor, *SF1,* steroidogenic factor-1; *DAX1, DSS-AHC*-critical region on the X chromosome gene 1; a double dose of *DAX1* inhibits the up-regulation of *SOX9* and *SF1* and results in inhibition of testes determination; *WNT4,* human gene related to the drosophila "wingless gene." Duplication of *WNT4* up-regulates *DAX1* and prevents testes determination. *SOX9,* autosomal gene containing an SRY-like HMG box; AMH, antimüllerian hormone; GATA4, a transcription factor. *SRY*-regulated homeobox gene 9; *DMRT1,* double sex (drosophila) Mab3 *(C elegans)*-related transcription factor. **B:** Hypothetical diagrammatic cascade of genes involved in sex differentiation. (Reproduced with permission from Grumbach MM, Hughes IA, Conte FA. Disorders of Sex Differentiation. In: Larsen PR [editors]: *Williams Textbook of Endocrinology,* 10th ed. Saunders, 2002.)

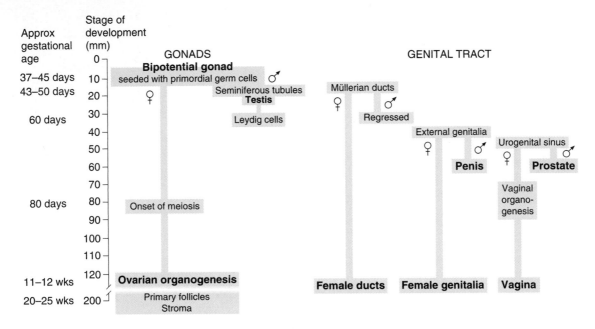

Figure 14–8. Schematic sequence of sexual differentiation in the human fetus. Note that testicular differentiation precedes all other forms of differentiation. (Reproduced, with permission, from Grumbach MM, Conte FA: Disorders of sex differentiation. In: Larsen PR et al [editors]: *Williams Textbook of Endocrinology*, 10th ed. Saunders, 2002.)

of a functional fetal testis, müllerian duct differentiation occurs, and the wolffian ducts involute.

Differentiation of External Genitalia (Figure 14–10)

Up to the eighth week of fetal life, the external genitalia of both sexes are identical and have the capacity to differentiate into the genitalia of either sex. Female sex differentiation will occur in the presence of an ovary or streak gonads or if no gonad is present (Figure 14–11). Differentiation of the external genitalia along male lines depends on the action of testosterone and particularly dihydrotestosterone, the 5α-reduced metabolite of testosterone. In the male fetus, testosterone is secreted by the Leydig cells, perhaps autonomously at first and thereafter under the influence of human chorionic gonadotropin (hCG), and then by stimulation from fetal pituitary luteinizing hormone (LH). Masculinization of the external genitalia and urogenital sinus of the fetus results from the action of dihydrotestosterone, which is converted from testosterone in the target cells by the enzyme 5α-reductase. Dihydrotestosterone (as well as testosterone) is bound to a specific protein receptor in the nucleus of the target cell. The transformed steroid-receptor complex dimerizes and binds with high affinity to specific DNA domains, initiating DNA-directed, RNA-mediated transcription. This results in androgen-induced proteins that lead to differentiation and growth of the cell. The gene that encodes the intracellular androgen-binding protein has been localized to the paracentromeric portion of the long arm of the X chromosome (Figure 14–5). Thus, an X-linked gene controls the androgen response of all somatic cell types by specifying the androgen receptor protein.

As in the case of the genital ducts, there is an inherent tendency for the external genitalia and urogenital sinus to develop along female lines. Differentiation of the external genitalia along male lines requires androgenic stimulation early in fetal life. The testosterone metabolite dihydrotestosterone and its specific nuclear receptor must be present to effect masculinization of the external genitalia of the fetus. Dihydrotestosterone stimulates growth of the genital tubercle, fusion of the urethral folds, and descent of the labioscrotal swellings to form the penis and scrotum. Androgens also inhibit descent and growth of the vesicovaginal septum and differentiation of the vagina. There is a critical period for action of the androgen. After about the 12th week of gestation, fusion of the labioscrotal folds will not occur even under intense androgen stimulation, though phallic growth can be induced. Incomplete masculinization of the male fetus results from (1) impairment in the synthesis or secretion of fetal testosterone or in its conversion to dihydrotestosterone, (2) deficient or defective androgen receptor activity, or (3) defective pro-

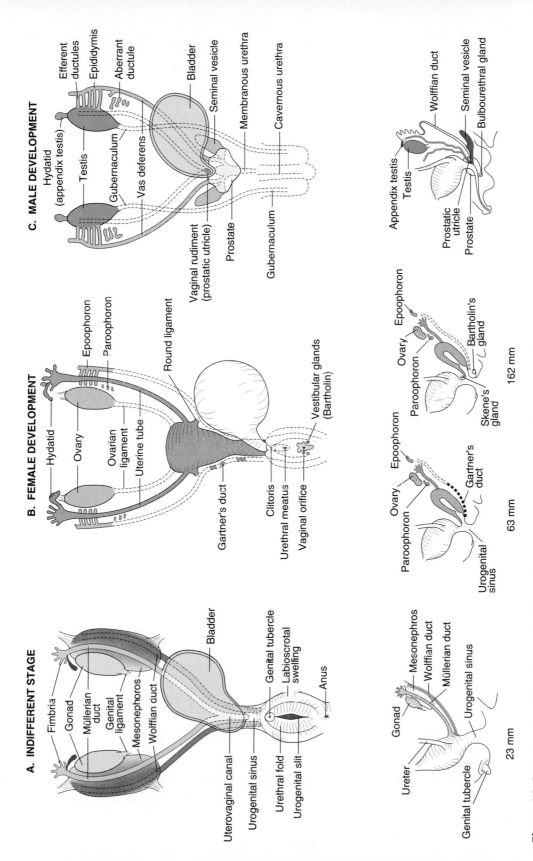

Figure 14–9. Embryonic differentiation of male and female genital ducts from wolffian and müllerian primordia. **A:** Indifferent stage showing large mesonephric body. **B:** Female development. Remnants of the mesonephros and wolffian ducts are now termed the epoophoron, paroophoron, and Gartner's duct. **C:** Male ducts before descent into the scrotum. The only müllerian remnant is the testicular appendix. The prostatic utricle (vagina masculina) is derived from the urogenital sinus. (Redrawn from Corning and Wilkins.)

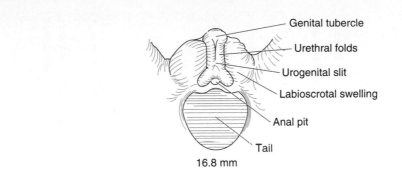

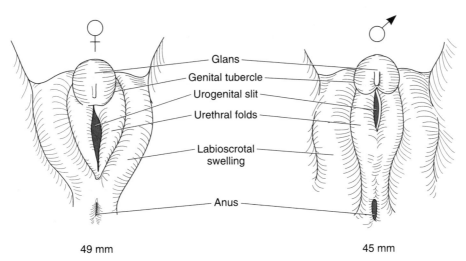

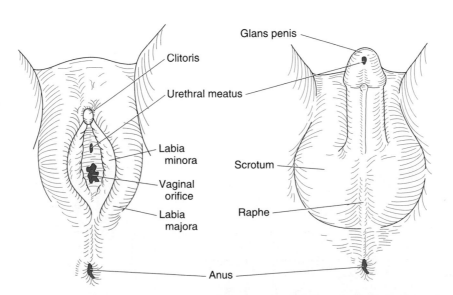

Figure 14–10. Differentiation of male and female external genitalia from bipotential primordia. (Reproduced, with permission, from Grumbach MM, Hughes IA, Conte FA: Disorders of sex differentiation. In: Larsen PR et al [editors]: *Williams Textbook of Endocrinology*, 10th ed. Saunders, 2002.)

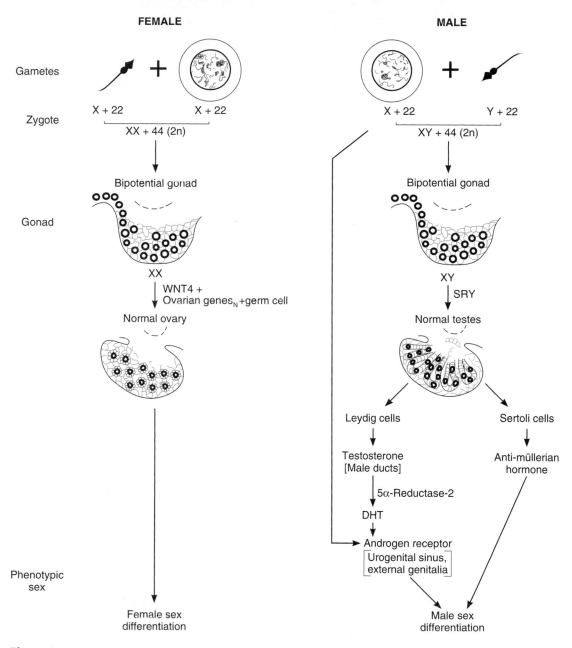

Figure 14–11. Diagrammatic summation of human sexual differentiation. DHT, dihydrotestosterone. (Reproduced, with permission, from Grumbach MM, Hughes IA, Conte FA: Disorders of sex differentiation. In: Larsen PR et al [editors]: *Williams Textbook of Endocrinology,* 10th ed. Saunders, 2002.)

duction and local action of antimüllerian hormone. Exposure of the female fetus to abnormal amounts of androgens from either endogenous or exogenous sources, especially before the 12th week of gestation, can result in virilization of the external genitalia.

PSYCHOSEXUAL DIFFERENTIATION

Psychosexual differentiation may be classified into four broad categories: (1) gender identity, defined as the identification of self as either male or female; (2) gender role, ie, those aspects of behavior in which males and females differ from one another in one's culture at this time; (3) gender orientation, the choice of sexual partner; and (4) cognitive differences.

Over the past 30 years, the prevailing dogma has been that newborns are born psychosexually neutral and that gender identity is imprinted postnatally by words, attitudes, and comparisons of one's body with that of others. Recently, this hypothesis has been rigorously challenged by Diamond and Sigmundson as well as Reiner. Their studies, among others, suggest that prenatal exposure to androgen and the presence of genes on the Y chromosome can influence gender identity in the patient with ambiguous genitalia. Gender identity has been hypothesized to be established by 12–18 months of age; however, it appears to be more plastic than previously thought. If, at puberty, discordant secondary sexual characteristics are allowed to mature, some individuals, especially those with 5α-reductase deficiency, 45,X/46,XY mosaicism, or 17β-hydroxysteroid dehydrogenase-3 deficiency, have had doubts about their gender identity and have chosen to change their assigned sex from female to male. However, there are 46,XY individuals who have had normal testicular function and androgen responsiveness in fetal life and have been assigned female gender which has been well accepted over time. This suggests that androgens have a "facultative" and not a "deterministic" role in gender identity. Thus, it is obvious that both genes and hormones (Nature) and environment (Nurture) are critical factors in the development and maintenance of gender identity. Further studies on patients with ambiguous genitalia and, in particular, long-term outcomes of gender identity, gender role, and sexual activity in intersex patients are necessary before the relative roles of nature and nurture can be resolved.

ABNORMAL SEX DIFFERENTIATION

Classification of Errors in Sex Differentiation (Table 14–3)

Disorders of sexual differentiation are the result of abnormalities in complex processes that originate in ge-

netic information on the X and Y chromosomes as well as on the autosomes. A true hermaphrodite is defined as a person who possesses both ovarian and testicular tissue. A male pseudohermaphrodite is one whose gonads are exclusively testes but whose genital ducts or external genitalia (or both) exhibit incomplete masculinization. A female pseudohermaphrodite is a person whose gonadal tissue is exclusively ovarian but whose genital development exhibits ambiguous or male appearance.

SEMINIFEROUS TUBULE DYSGENESIS: CHROMATIN-POSITIVE KLINEFELTER'S SYNDROME & ITS VARIANTS

Klinefelter's syndrome is one of the most common forms of primary hypogonadism and infertility in males. The invariable clinical features in adults are a male phenotype, firm testes less than 3 cm in length, and azoospermia. Gynecomastia is common. Affected patients usually have a 47,XXY sex chromosome constitution and an X chromatin-positive buccal smear, though subjects with a variety of sex chromosome constitutions, including mosaicism, have been described. Virtually all of these variants have in common the presence of at least two X chromosomes and a Y chromosome, except for the rare group in which only an XX sex chromosome complement is found.

Surveys of the prevalence of 47,XXY fetuses by karyotype analysis of unselected newborn infants indicate an incidence of about 1:800 newborn males. Prepubertally, the disorder is characterized by small undescended testes, disproportionately long legs, personality and behavioral disorders, and a lower mean verbal IQ score when compared with that of control subjects but no significant difference in full-scale IQ. Severe mental retardation requiring special schooling is uncommon. Gynecomastia and other signs of androgen deficiency such as diminished facial and body hair, a small phallus, poor muscular development, and a eunuchoid body habitus occur postpubertally in affected patients. Adult males with a 47,XXY karyotype tend to be taller than average, with adult height close to the 75th percentile, mainly because of the disproportionate length of their legs. Untreated adult males, especially those with subnormal sex steroid levels, are at increased risk for the development of osteoporosis. They also have an increased incidence of mild diabetes mellitus, varicose veins, stasis dermatitis, cerebrovascular disease, chronic pulmonary disease, and carcinoma of the breast; the incidence of breast carcinoma in patients with Klinefelter's syndrome is 20 times higher than that in normal men. Patients with Klinefelter's syndrome often have a delay in the onset of adolescence. There is an increased risk for developing malig-

Table 14–3. Classification of anomalous sexual development.[1]

I. Disorders of gonadal differentiation
  A. Seminiferous tubule dysgenesis (Klinefelter's syndrome)
  B. Syndrome of gonadal dysgenesis and its variants (Turner's syndrome)
  C. Complete and incomplete forms of XX and XY gonadal dysgenesis
  D. True hermaphroditism
II. Female pseudohermaphroditism
  A. Congenital virilizing adrenal hyperplasia
  B. P450 aromatase deficiency
  C. Androgens and synthetic progestins transferred from maternal circulation
  D. Associated with malformations of intestine and urinary tract (non-androgen-induced female pseudohermaphroditism)
  E. Glucocorticoid receptor gene mutation
  F. Other teratologic factors
III. Male pseudohermaphroditism
  A. Testicular unresponsiveness to hCG and LH (Leydig cell agenesis or hypoplasia)
  B. Inborn errors of testosterone biosynthesis
    1. Enzyme defects affecting synthesis of both corticosteroids and testosterone (variants of congenital adrenal hyperplasia)
      a. StAR deficiency (congenital lipoid adrenal hyperplasia): side-chain (P450scc) cleavage deficiency
      b. 3β-Hydroxysteroid dehydrogenase deficiency
      c. P450c17 (17α-hydroxylase) deficiency
      d. Smith-Lemli-Opitz syndrome: 7-dehydrocholesterol reductase deficiency
    2. Enzyme defects primarily affecting testosterone biosynthesis by the testes
      a. P450c17 (17,20-lyase) deficiency
      b. 17β-Hydroxysteroid oxidoreductase deficiency
  C. Defects in androgen-dependent target tissues
	1. End-organ resistance to androgenic hormones (androgen receptor and postreceptor defects)
	      a. Syndrome of complete androgen resistance and its variants (testicular feminization and its variant forms)
	      b. Syndrome of partial androgen resistance and its variants (Reifenstein's syndrome)
	      c. Androgen resistance in infertile men
	      d. Androgen resistance in fertile men
	    2. Defects in testosterone metabolism by peripheral tissues
	      a. 5α-Reductase-2 deficiency (pseudovaginal perineoscrotal hypospadias)
	  D. Dysgenetic male pseudohermaphroditism
	    1. XY gonadal dysgenesis (incomplete)
	    2. XO/XY mosaicism, SRY mutation structurally abnormal Y chromosome, Xp+, 9p–, 10q–
	    3. Denys-Drash Frasier syndrome (*WT-1* mutation)
	    4. WAGR (*WT-1* deletion)
	    5. Campomelic dysplasia (*SOX9* mutation)
	    6. *SF1* mutation
	    7. *WNT-4* duplication
	    8. ATRX syndrome (XH2 mutation)
	    9. Testicular regression syndrome
	  E. Defects in synthesis, secretion, or response to AMH
	    1. Female genital ducts in otherwise normal men—"herniae uteri inguinale"; persistent müllerian duct syndrome
	  F. Environmental chemicals
	IV. Unclassified forms of abnormal sexual development
	  A. In males
	    1. Hypospadias
	    2. Ambiguous external genitalia in 46,XY males with multiple congenital anomalies
	  B. In females
	    1. Absence or anomalous development of the vagina, uterus, and uterine tubes (Rokitansky-Küster syndrome)

[1]Modified from Grumbach MM, Conte FA: Abnormalities of sex differentiation. In: *Williams Textbook of Endocrinology,* 9th ed. Wilson JD et al (editors). Saunders, 1998.

nant extragonadal germ cell tumors, including central nervous system germinomas and mediastinal tumors, which may be hCG-secreting and cause sexual precocity in the prepubertal patient.

The testicular lesion is progressive and gonadotropin-dependent. It is characterized in the adult by extensive seminiferous tubular hyalinization and fibrosis, absent or severely deficient spermatogenesis, and pseudoadenomatous clumping of the Leydig cells. Although hyalinization of the tubules is usually extensive, it varies considerably from patient to patient and even between testes in the same patient. Azoospermia is the rule, and patients who have been reported to be fertile invariably have been 46,XY/47,XXY mosaics. Recently,

the technique of intracytoplasmic sperm injection (ICSI) has been utilized with some success for achieving fertility in patients with Klinefelter's syndrome. It is likely that success is achieved only in those patients who are mosaics with a 46,XY cell line in their gonads.

Nondisjunction during the first or second meiotic division of gametogenesis plays an important role in the genesis of a 47,XXY karyotype. Fifty-three percent of cases appear to result from paternal nondisjunction at the first meiotic division, 34% from meiotic nondisjunction during the first maternal meiotic division, and 9% from nondisjunction at the second meiotic division. Only 3% of patients appear to have arisen from postzygotic mitotic nondisjunction.

The diagnosis of Klinefelter's syndrome is suggested by the classic phenotype and hormonal changes. It is confirmed by the finding of an X chromatin-positive buccal smear and demonstration of a 47,XXY karyotype in blood, skin, or gonads. After puberty, levels of serum gonadotropins (especially follicle-stimulating hormone [FSH]) are raised. The testosterone production rate, the total and free levels of testosterone, and the metabolic clearance rates of testosterone and estradiol tend to be low, while plasma estradiol levels are relatively normal or high. Testicular biopsy reveals the classic findings of hyalinization of the seminiferous tubules, severe deficiency of spermatogonia, and pseudoadenomatous clumping of Leydig cells.

Treatment of patients with Klinefelter's syndrome is directed toward androgen replacement, especially in patients in whom puberty is delayed or fails to progress or in those who have subnormal testosterone levels for age and developmental stage. Testosterone therapy may help to enhance secondary sexual characteristics and sexual performance, prevent osteoporosis, prevent or cause regression of gynecomastia, and improve general well-being in most patients. If testosterone deficiency and/or elevated gonadotropins are present, testosterone therapy early in adolescence should commence with 50 mg of testosterone enanthate in oil intramuscularly every 4 weeks, gradually increasing to the adult replacement dose of 200 mg every 2 weeks after a bone age of 14½ years. Thereafter, transdermal testosterone therapy (testosterone patch) may be used for adult replacement. A marked decrease in gynecomastia may result from testosterone therapy; however, once advanced, gynecomastia may not be amenable to hormone therapy but can be surgically corrected if it is severe or psychologically disturbing to the patient. Early diagnosis, support, and appropriate counseling will improve the overall prognosis.

Variants of Chromatin-Positive Seminiferous Tubule Dysgenesis

A. Variants of Klinefelter's Syndrome

Variants of Klinefelter's syndrome include 46,XY/47,XXY mosaics as well as patients with multiple X and Y chromosomes. With increasing numbers of X chromosomes in the genome, both mental retardation and other developmental anomalies such as radioulnar synostosis become prevalent.

B. 46,XX Males

Phenotypic males with a 46,XX karyotype have been described since 1964; the incidence of 46,XX males is approximately 1:20,000 births. In general, these individuals have a male phenotype, male psychosocial gender identity, and testes with histologic features similar to those observed in patients with a 47,XXY karyotype. At least 10% of patients have hypospadias or ambiguous external genitalia. XX males have normal body proportions and a mean final height that is shorter than that of patients with an XXY sex chromosome constitution or normal males but taller than that of normal females. As in XXY patients, testosterone levels are low or low normal, gonadotropins are elevated, and spermatogenesis is impaired postpubertally. Gynecomastia is present in approximately one-third of cases.

The presence of testes and male sexual differentiation in 46,XX individuals has been a perplexing problem. However, the paradox has been clarified by the use of recombinant DNA studies. Males with a 46,XX karyotype have been shown by genetic linkage studies and X chromosome restriction fragment length polymorphisms (RFLPs) to possess one X chromosome from each of their parents. Approximately 80% of XX males have a Y chromosome-specific DNA segment from the distal portion of the Y short arm translocated to the distal portion of the short arm of the paternal X chromosome. This translocated segment is heterologous in length but always includes the *SRY* gene, which encodes testis-determining factor as well as the pseudoautosomal region of the Y chromosome. The site of translocation in 30–40% of 46,XX males involves *PRKX/PRKY*, a novel protein kinase gene, with homologs on the X and Y chromosome. Thus, in 80% of XX males, an abnormal X–Y terminal exchange during paternal meiosis has resulted in two products: an X chromosome with an *SRY* gene and a Y chromosome deficient in this gene (the latter would result in a female with XY gonadal dysgenesis). Fewer than 20% of XX males tested have been shown to lack Y chromosome-specific DNA sequences, including the *SRY* gene and the pseudoautosomal region of the Y chromosome. These XX, Y DNA-negative males tend to have hypospadias and may have relatives with true hermaphroditism.

The finding of XX males who lack any evidence of Y chromosome-specific genes suggests that testicular determination—and, thus, male differentiation—can occur in the absence of a gene or genes from the Y chromosome. This could be a result of (1) mutation or duplication of a "downstream" autosomal gene involved in male sex determination, eg, *SOX9*; or (2) mutation, deletion, or aberrant inactivation of a gene sequence on the X chromosome, critical to testis determination and differentiation; or (3) circumscribed Y chromosome mosaicism (eg, occurring only in the gonads). Further studies will be necessary to elucidate the pathogenesis of male sex determination and differentiation in those 46,XX males who lack ascertainable Y-to-X chromosome translocations.

SYNDROME OF GONADAL DYSGENESIS: TURNER'S SYNDROME & ITS VARIANTS

Turner's Syndrome: 45,X Gonadal Dysgenesis

One in 5000 newborn females has a 45,X sex chromosome constitution. It has been estimated that 99% of 45,X fetuses do not survive beyond 28 weeks of gestation, and 15% of all first-trimester abortuses have a 45,X karyotype. In about 70–80% of instances, the origin of the normal X chromosome is maternal. Patients with a 45,X karyotype represent approximately 50% of all patients with X chromosome abnormalities. The cardinal features of 45,X gonadal dysgenesis are a variety of somatic anomalies, sexual infantilism at puberty secondary to gonadal dysgenesis, and short stature. Patients with a 45,X karyotype can be recognized in infancy, usually because of lymphedema of the extremities and loose skin folds over the nape of the neck. In later life, the typical patient is often recognizable by her distinctive facies in which micrognathia, epicanthal folds, prominent low-set ears, a fish-like mouth, and ptosis are present to varying degrees. The chest is shield-like and the neck is short, broad, and webbed (40% of patients). Additional anomalies associated with Turner's syndrome include coarctation of the aorta (10%), hypertension, renal abnormalities (50%), pigmented nevi, cubitus valgus, a tendency to keloid formation, puffiness of the dorsum of the hands and feet, short fourth metacarpals and metatarsals, Madelung deformity of the wrist, scoliosis, and recurrent otitis media, which may lead to conductive hearing loss. Routine intravenous urography or renal sonography is indicated for all patients to rule out a surgically correctable renal abnormality. The most common renal anomalies are rotation of the kidney, duplication of the renal pelvis and ureter, and hydronephrosis secondary to ureteropelvic obstruction. Complete absence of the kidney or gross renal ectopia has been reported. The internal ducts as well as the external genitalia of these patients are invariably female except in rare patients with a 45,X karyotype, in whom a Y-to-autosome or Y-to-X chromosome translocation has been found.

Short stature is an invariable feature of the syndrome of gonadal dysgenesis. Mean final height in 45,X patients is 143 cm, with a range of 133–153 cm. Short stature found in patients with the syndrome of gonadal dysgenesis is not due to a deficiency of growth hormone, insulin-like growth factor I, sex steroids, or thyroid hormone. It is related, at least in part, to haploinsufficiency of the *PHOG/SHOX* gene in the pseudoautosomal region of the X and Y chromosome. (See earlier section.) Nevertheless, administration of high-dose biosynthetic human growth hormone results in an increase in final height.

Gonadal dysgenesis is another feature of patients with a 45,X chromosome constitution. The gonads are typically streak-like and usually contain only fibrous stroma arranged in whorls. Longitudinal studies of both basal and gonadotropin-releasing hormone (GnRH)-evoked gonadotropin secretion in patients with gonadal dysgenesis indicate a lack of feedback inhibition of the hypothalamic-pituitary axis by the dysgenetic gonads in affected infants and children (Figure 14–12). Thus, plasma and urinary gonadotropin levels, particularly FSH levels, are high during early infancy and after 9–10 years of age. Since ovarian function is impaired, puberty does not usually ensue spontaneously; hence, sexual infantilism is a hallmark of this syndrome. Rarely, patients with a 45,X karyotype may undergo spontaneous pubertal maturation, menarche, and pregnancy.

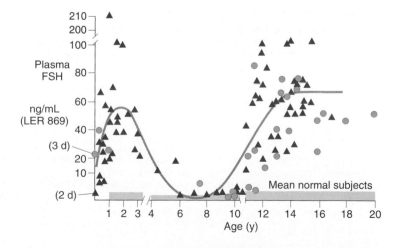

Figure 14–12. Diphasic variation in basal levels of plasma follicle-stimulating hormone (FSH) (ng/mL-LER 869) in patients with a 45,X karyotype (solid triangles) and patients with structural abnormalities of the X chromosome and mosaics (solid circles). Note that mean basal levels of plasma FSH in patients with gonadal dysgenesis are in the castrate range before 4 years and after 10 years of age. (Reproduced, with permission, from Conte FA, Grumbach MM, Kaplan SL: A diphasic pattern of gonadotropin secretion in patients with the syndrome of gonadal dysgenesis. J Clin Endocrinol Metab 1975;40:670.)

A variety of disorders are associated with this syndrome, including obesity, osteoporosis, diabetes mellitus, Hashimoto's thyroiditis, rheumatoid arthritis, inflammatory bowel disease, intestinal telangiectasia with bleeding, chronic liver disease, sensorineural hearing loss, and anorexia nervosa. Because an increased prevalence of bicuspid aortic valve, coarctation of the aorta, and aortic dilation with aneurysm formation and rupture has been reported in patients with Turner's syndrome, screening and periodic echocardiography are indicated in all patients with a 45,X cell line.

Phenotypic females with the following features should have a karyotype analysis: (1) short stature (> 2.5 SD below the mean value for age); (2) somatic anomalies associated with the syndrome of gonadal dysgenesis; and (3) delayed adolescence with an increased level of plasma FSH.

Therapy should be directed toward maximizing final height and inducing secondary sexual characteristics and menarche at an age commensurate with that of normal peers. The results of clinical trials suggest that patients treated with recombinant growth hormone (0.375 mg/kg/wk divided into seven once-daily doses), with or without oxandrolone (0.0625 mg/kg/d by mouth), had an increase in growth rate that was sustained and resulted in a mean 8–10 cm increase in height after 3–7 years of therapy. However, beginning growth hormone therapy earlier (when the child's height is less than −2 SD from the mean) will result in a greater gain in height and allow for the administration of estrogen replacement at an age commensurate with normal puberty. Before initiation of growth hormone therapy, a thorough analysis of the costs, benefits, and possible side effects must be discussed with the parents and the child. Long-term studies with low-dose estrogen therapy have not demonstrated a positive effect on final height in girls with Turner's syndrome. No synergistic effect of combined estrogen and growth hormone therapy on final height has been found. In patients who have been treated with growth hormone and have achieved an acceptable height and in those who have refused growth hormone therapy, estrogen replacement therapy is usually initiated after 12–13 years of age. Conjugated estrogens (0.3 mg or less) or ethinyl estradiol (5 μg) are given orally for the first 21 days of the calendar month. Thereafter, the dose of estrogen is gradually increased over the next several years to 0.6–1.25 mg of conjugated estrogens or 10 μg of ethinyl estradiol daily for the first 21 days of the month. The minimum dose of estrogen necessary to maintain secondary sexual characteristics and menses and prevent osteoporosis should be administered. After the first year of estrogen therapy, medroxyprogesterone acetate, 5 mg, or a comparable progestin is given on the tenth to twenty-first days of the month to ensure physiologic menses and to reduce the risk of endometrial carcinoma, which is associated with unopposed estrogen stimulation.

X Chromatin-Positive Variants of the Syndrome of Gonadal Dysgenesis

Patients with structural abnormalities of the X chromosome (deletions and additions) and sex chromosome mosaicism with a 45,X cell line may manifest the somatic as well as the gonadal features of the syndrome of gonadal dysgenesis (Table 14–4). Evidence suggests that genes on both the long and short arms of the X chromosome control gonadal differentiation, whereas genes pri-

Table 14–4. Relationship of structural abnormalities of the X and Y to clinical manifestations of the syndrome of gonadal dysgenesis.[1]

Type of Sex Chromosome Abnormality	Karyotype	Phenotype	Sexual Infantilism	Short Stature	Somatic Anomalies of Turner's Syndrome
Loss of an X or Y	45,X	Female	+	+	+
Deletion of short arm of an X[2]	46,XXqi	Female	+ (occ. ±)	+	+
	46,XXp–	Female	+, ±, or –	+	+ (–)
Deletion of long arm of an X[2]	46,XXq–	Female	+	–	–
Deletion of ends of both arms of an X[3]	46,XXr	Female	– or +	+	+ or (±)
Deletion of short arm of Y	46,XYp–	Female	+	+	+

[1]Reproduced, with permission, from Grumbach MM, Conte FA: Disorders of sex differentiation. In: Wilson JD et al (editors): *Williams Textbook of Endocrinology,* 9th ed. Saunders, 1998.
[2]In Xp– and Xq–, the extent and site of the deleted segment are variable. Xqi = Isochromosome for long arm of an X; Xp– = deletion of short arm of an X; Xq– = deletion of long arm of an X; Xr = ring chromosome derived from an X.
[3]Patients with small ring X chromosomes can have mental retardation and somatic abnormalities not usually associated with the Turner phenotype owing to noninactivation of genes on the small ring X chromosome.

marily on the short arms of the X prevent the short stature and somatic anomalies that are seen in 45,X patients (Figure 14–4). In general, 45,X/46,XX mosaicism will modify the 45,X phenotype toward normal and can even result in normal gonadal function. Some patients with a 45,X/46,Xr(X) karyotype may manifest mental retardation and congenital anomalies not usually associated with Turner's syndrome. Recent data indicate that these abnormalities are related to lack of inactivation of small ring X chromosomes and, hence, functional disomy for genes on the ring X chromosome and the normal X chromosome.

X Chromatin-Negative Variants of the Syndrome of Gonadal Dysgenesis

These patients usually have mosaicism with a 45,X and a Y-bearing cell line—45,X/46,XY; 45,X/47,XXY; 45,X/46,XY/47,XYY—or perhaps a structurally abnormal Y chromosome. They range from phenotypic females with the features of Turner's syndrome through patients with ambiguous genitalia to completely virilized males with few stigmas of Turner's syndrome. The variations in gonadal differentiation range from bilateral streaks to bilateral dysgenetic testes to apparently "normal" testes, and there may be asymmetric development, ie, a streak on one side and a dysgenetic testicle or, rarely, a normal testis on the other side—sometimes called **mixed gonadal dysgenesis.** The development of the external genitalia and of the internal ducts correlates with the degree of testicular differentiation and, presumably, the capacity of the fetal testes to secrete antimüllerian hormone and testosterone.

The risk of development of gonadal tumors is greatly increased in patients with 45,X/46,XY mosaicism and streak or dysgenetic gonads; hence, prophylactic removal of streak gonads or dysgenetic undescended testes in this syndrome is indicated. Breast development at or after the age of puberty in these patients is commonly associated with a gonadal neoplasm, usually a gonadoblastoma. Pelvic sonography, computed tomography scanning, or magnetic resonance imaging (MRI) may be useful in screening for neoplasms in these patients. Gonadoblastomas are calcified and so may be visible even on a plain film of the abdomen.

The diagnosis of 45,X/46,XY mosaicism can be established by the demonstration of both 45,X and 46,XY cells in blood, skin, or gonadal tissue. In some mosaics, a marker chromosome is found that is cytogenetically indistinguishable as X or Y. In these cases, either fluorescence in situ hybridization or molecular analyses with X- and Y-specific probes is indicated to definitively determine the origin of the marker chromosome, since gonadoblastomas have been reported in pa-

tients with deleted Y chromosomes—even those with deletions of the *SRY* gene. The decision regarding the sex of rearing should be based on the age at diagnosis and the potential for normal function of the external genitalia. Most patients with 45,X/46,XY mosaicism ascertained by amniocentesis have normal male genitalia and normal testicular histology. Thus, the ambiguity of the genitalia invariably described in patients with 45,X/46,XY mosaicism is due to ascertainment bias. We have observed a short 30-year-old male with documented 45,X/46,XY mosaicism who has normal male genitalia and is fertile.

In phenotypic female XO/XY patients assigned a female gender role, the dysgenetic gonads should be removed. Estrogen therapy should be initiated at the age of puberty, as in patients with a 45,X karyotype (see above). In affected infants who are assigned a male gender role, all gonadal tissue except that which appears functionally and histologically normal and is in the scrotum should be removed. Removal of the müllerian structures and repair of hypospadias are also indicated. At puberty, depending on the functional integrity of the retained gonads, androgen replacement therapy may be indicated in doses similar to those prescribed for patients with the incomplete form of XY gonadal dysgenesis. In patients with retained scrotal testes, frequent clinical examinations and ultrasonography is indicated. A gonadal biopsy is indicated postpubertally to rule out the possibility of carcinoma in situ, a premalignant lesion (see below).

In infants and children with 45,X/46,XY mosaicism who have normal genitalia and normal testicular integrity as assessed by gonadotropin levels and pelvic MRI, gonadal biopsy may be deferred until adolescence. If biopsy and sonography show no evidence of carcinoma in situ, a second biopsy at 20 years of age is recommended. The risk of gonadal malignancies in males with 45,X/46,XY mosaicism who have normal male genitalia and histologically and functionally normal testes in the scrotum is still to be ascertained.

46,XX & 46,XY Gonadal Dysgenesis

The terms XX and XY gonadal dysgenesis have been applied to 46,XX or 46,XY patients who have bilateral streak gonads, a female phenotype, and no somatic stigmas of Turner's syndrome. After the age of puberty, these patients exhibit sexual infantilism, castrate levels of plasma and urinary gonadotropins, normal or tall stature, and eunuchoid proportions.

46,XX Gonadal Dysgenesis

Familial and sporadic cases of XX gonadal dysgenesis have been reported with an incidence as high as 1:8300 females in Finland. Pedigree analysis of familial cases is consistent with autosomal recessive inheritance.

Analysis of familial cases in Finland revealed that a locus on chromosome 2p was linked to XX gonadal dysgenesis in females. The gene for the FSH receptor has been localized to chromosome 2p. Analysis of this gene revealed a mutation in exon 7 of the FSH receptor that segregated with XX gonadal dysgenesis. This mutation affected the extracellular ligand-binding domain of the FSH receptor and reduced the binding capacity of the receptor and consequently signal transduction, resulting in variable ovarian function, including "streak ovaries" and hypergonadotropic hypogonadism in some XX females at puberty. Further studies in Western Europe and the United States of females with 46,XX gonadal dysgenesis have been negative for FSH receptor gene mutations, suggesting that a mutation in this gene is rare and that other causes for this phenotype are more common. Preliminary data suggest that males homozygous for this mutation are phenotypically normal, with spermatogenesis varying from normal to absent.

Studies of familial cohorts have revealed apparent marked heterogeneity in pathogenesis. Siblings, one with a 46,XX karyotype and the other with a 46,XY karyotype, both with gonadal "agenesis," have been reported, supporting the involvement of an autosomal gene in this family. However, in view of the normal phenotype in XY males observed with a mutation in the FSH receptor, it seems unlikely that these patients have an FSH receptor defect. Rather, they may have a mutation in an autosomal recessive gene involved in gonadal determination. In one family, four affected women had an inherited interstitial deletion of the long arm of the X chromosome involving the q21–q27 region. This region seems to contain a gene or genes critical to ovarian development and function. In three families, XX gonadal dysgenesis was associated with deafness of the sensorineural type. In several affected groups of siblings, a spectrum of clinical findings occurred, eg, varying degrees of ovarian function, including breast development and menses followed by secondary amenorrhea. Recently, haploinsufficiency of *FOXL2,* a gene on chromosome 3q23, has been shown to cause autosomal dominant blepharophimosis-ptosis-epicanthus inversus syndrome (BPES type 1) and XX gonadal dysgenesis. In contrast to Turner's syndrome, stature is normal. The diagnosis of 46,XX gonadal dysgenesis should be suspected in phenotypic females with sexual infantilism and normal müllerian structures who lack the somatic stigmas of the syndrome of gonadal dysgenesis (Turner's syndrome). Karyotype analysis reveals only 46,XX cells. As in Turner's syndrome, gonadotropin levels are high, estrogen levels are low, and treatment consists of cyclic estrogen and progesterone replacement.

Sporadic cases of XX gonadal dysgenesis, similar to familial cases, may represent a heterogeneous group of patients from a pathogenetic point of view. XX gonadal dysgenesis should be distinguished from ovarian failure due to infections such as mumps, antibodies to gonadotropin receptors, biologically inactive FSH, gonadotropin-insensitive ovaries, and galactosemia as well as errors in steroid (estrogen) biosynthesis. In the latter group, ultrasound or MRI should reveal polycystic ovaries.

46,XY Gonadal Dysgenesis

46,XY gonadal dysgenesis occurs both sporadically and in familial aggregates. Patients with the complete form of this syndrome have female external genitalia, normal or tall stature, bilateral streak gonads, müllerian duct development, sexual infantilism, eunuchoid habitus, and a 46,XY karyotype. Clitoromegaly is quite common, and, in familial cases, a continuum of involvement ranging from the complete syndrome to ambiguity of the external genitalia has been described. The phenotypic difference between the complete and incomplete forms of XY gonadal dysgenesis is due to the degree of differentiation of testicular tissue and the functional capacity of the fetal testis to produce testosterone and antimüllerian hormone. Early in infancy and after the age of puberty, plasma and urinary gonadotropin levels are markedly elevated.

Analysis of familial and sporadic cases of 46,XY gonadal dysgenesis indicates that about 15–20% of patients have a mutation in the HMG box of the *SRY* gene that affects DNA binding or bending by the SRY protein. So far, all patients in whom mutations have been detected have had "complete" gonadal dysgenesis. Patients with large deletions of the short arm of the Y chromosome may have, in addition to gonadal dysgenesis, stigmas of Turner's syndrome. Mutations outside the HMG box region of the *SRY* gene as well as in X-linked or autosomal genes may be responsible for those patients in whom no molecular abnormality has as yet been found. A mutation in the HMG box of the *SRY* gene has been described in normal 46,XY fathers and their "daughters" with 46,XY gonadal dysgenesis. These familial cohorts suggest that these mutations and modifier genes may affect either the level or the timing of *SRY* expression and in this manner result in either normal or abnormal testicular differentiation.

More than 20 patients with 46,XY gonadal dysgenesis have been reported with a duplication of the Xp21.2 → p22.11 region of the X chromosome. This region contains a gene, *DAX1*. Deletion or mutation of *DAX1* in males causes adrenal hypoplasia congenita and hypogonadotropic hypogonadism. The finding that 46,XY males with adrenal hypoplasia and hypogonadotropic hypogonadism have normal sex differentiation suggests that *DAX1* is not required for testicular differentiation; duplicating *DAX1*, however, impairs testis differentiation. Thus, *DAX1* appears to be an antitestis gene. (See earlier section.)

XY gonadal dysgenesis associated with campomelic dysplasia is due to a mutation of one allele of an *SRY*-related gene, *SOX9* on chromosome 17. In addition, XY gonadal dysgenesis has been associated with 9p– (DMRT1) and 10q– deletions, as well as duplication of 1p32-36 (WNT4).

Therapy for patients with 46,XY gonadal dysgenesis who have female external genitalia involves prophylactic gonadectomy at diagnosis and estrogen substitution at puberty. In the incomplete form of XY gonadal dysgenesis, assignment of a male gender role and treatment with testosterone to augment phallic size in infancy must be considered. Prophylactic gonadectomy must be considered, since fertility is unlikely and there is an increased risk of malignant transformation of the dysgenetic gonads in these patients. Biopsy of all retained gonads should be done pre- and postpubertally in order to detect early malignant changes (carcinoma in situ). In affected individuals raised as males, prosthetic testes should be implanted at the time of gonadectomy, and androgen substitution therapy is instituted at the age of puberty. Testosterone enanthate in oil (or another long-acting testosterone ester) is used, beginning with 50 mg intramuscularly every 4 weeks and gradually increasing after a bone age of 14½ years to a full replacement dose of 200 mg intramuscularly every 2 weeks.

TRUE HERMAPHRODITISM

In true hermaphroditism, both ovarian and testicular tissue are present in one or both gonads. Differentiation of the internal and external genitalia is highly variable. The external genitalia may simulate those of a male or female, but most often they are ambiguous. Cryptorchidism and hypospadias are common. A testis or ovotestis, if present, is located in the labioscrotal folds in one-third of patients, in the inguinal canal in one-third, and in the abdomen in the remainder. A uterus is usually present, though it may be hypoplastic or unicornuate. The differentiation of the genital ducts usually follows that of the ipsilateral gonad. The ovotestis is the most common gonad found in true hermaphrodites (60%), followed by the ovary and, least commonly, by the testis. At puberty, breast development is usual in untreated patients, and menses occur in over 50% of cases. Whereas the ovary or the ovarian portion of an ovotestis may function normally, the testis or testicular portion of an ovotestis is almost always dysgenetic.

Sixty percent of true hermaphrodites have been reported to have a 46,XX karyotype, 20% 46,XY, and about 20% have chromosome mosaicism or 46,XX/46,XY chimerism. 46,XX true hermaphroditism appears to be a genetically heterogeneous entity. A small proportion of 46,XX true hermaphrodites, including some in family cohorts with 46,XX males, have been reported to be *SRY*-positive. Hence, Y-to-X and Y-to-autosome translocations, hidden sex chromosome mosaicism, or chimerism can explain the pathogenesis in these patients. The majority of 46,XX true hermaphrodites, however, are *SRY*-negative. A number of families have been reported that had both *SRY*-negative 46,XX males and 46,XX true hermaphrodites. This latter observation suggests a common genetic pathogenesis in these patients. Possible genetic mechanisms to explain *SRY*-negative true hermaphroditism include (1) mutation of a downstream autosomal gene or modifier genes involved in testicular determination; (2) mutation, deletion, duplication, or anomalous inactivation of an X-linked locus involved in testis determination; or (3) circumscribed chimerism or mosaicism that occurred only in the gonads.

The diagnosis of true hermaphroditism should be considered in all patients with ambiguous genitalia. The finding of a 46,XX/46,XY karyotype or a bilobate gonad compatible with an ovotestis in the inguinal region or labioscrotal folds suggests the diagnosis. Basal plasma testosterone levels are elevated above 40 ng/dL in affected patients under 6 months of age, and testosterone levels increase after hCG stimulation. The estradiol response to human menopausal gonadotropins has been shown to be a reliable test for differentiating infants with true hermaphroditism from those with other disorders of sexual differentiation. If all other forms of male and female pseudohermaphroditism have been excluded, laparotomy and histologic confirmation of both ovarian and testicular tissue establish the diagnosis. The management of true hermaphroditism is contingent upon the age at diagnosis and a careful assessment of the functional capacity of the gonads, genital ducts, and external genitalia. In general, 46,XX true hermaphrodites should be raised as females, with the possible exception of the well-virilized patient in whom no uterus is found.

Gonadal Neoplasms in Dysgenetic Gonads

While gonadal tumors are rare in patients with 47,XXY Klinefelter's syndrome and 45,X gonadal dysgenesis, the prevalence of gonadal neoplasms is greatly increased in patients with certain types of dysgenetic gonads. The frequency is increased in 45,X/46,XY mosaicism, especially in those with female or ambiguous genitalia; in patients with a structurally abnormal Y chromosome;

and in those with XY gonadal dysgenesis, either with a female phenotype or with ambiguous genitalia. Gonadoblastomas, germinomas, seminomas, and teratomas are found most frequently. Prophylactic gonadectomy is advised in these patients as well as in those with Turner's syndrome who manifest signs of virilization, regardless of karyotype. The significance of hidden mosaicism in patients with Turner's syndrome for Y chromosomal DNA determined by recombinant DNA technology is controversial at present with respect to the risk of gonadal neoplasms. Gonadoblastomas have been reported in patients with marker chromosomes of Y origin lacking the *SRY* gene. The testis should be preserved in patients who are to be raised as males only if it is histologically and functionally normal and is or can be situated in the scrotum. The fact that a testis is palpable in the scrotum does not preclude malignant degeneration and tumor dissemination, as seminomas tend to metastasize at an early stage before a mass is obvious. If a testis is preserved in the scrotum in a patient with 45,X/46,XY mosaicism or in rare cases of true hermaphroditism, it is prudent to follow the patient closely with sonography or pelvic MRI and a biopsy postpubertally in order to monitor for the development of a premalignant or malignant lesion.

FEMALE PSEUDOHERMAPHRODITISM

Affected individuals have normal ovaries and müllerian derivatives associated with ambiguous external genitalia. In the absence of testes, a female fetus will be masculinized if subjected to increased circulating levels of androgens derived from a fetal or maternal source. The degree of masculinization depends upon the stage of differentiation at the time of exposure (Figure 14–13). After 12 weeks of gestation, androgens will produce only clitoral hypertrophy. Rarely, ambiguous genitalia that superficially resemble those produced by androgens are the result of other teratogenic factors.

Congenital Adrenal Hyperplasia (Figure 14–14)

Congenital adrenal hyperplasia is responsible for most cases of female pseudohermaphroditism and around 50% of all cases of ambiguous genitalia. There are five major types of congenital adrenal hyperplasia, all transmitted as autosomal recessive disorders. The common denominator of all six types is a defect in the synthesis of cortisol that results in an increase in ACTH and consequently in adrenal hyperplasia. Both males and females can be affected, but males are rarely diagnosed at birth unless they have ambiguous genitalia, are salt losers and manifest adrenal crises, are identified during newborn screening, or are known to be at risk because they have an affected sibling. Defects in 21-hydroxylation and 11β-hydroxylation are confined to the adrenal gland and produce virilization. Defects in 3β-hydroxysteroid dehydrogenase type II, 17α-hydroxylase (17,20-lyase), and StAR (steroidogenic acute regulatory protein) and P450scc (side chain cleavage) have in common blocks in cortisol and sex steroid synthesis in both the adrenals and the gonads. The latter types produce chiefly incomplete masculinization in the male and little or no virilization in the female (Table 14–5). Consequently, these will be discussed primarily as forms of male pseudohermaphroditism.

P450c21 Hydroxylase Deficiency

21-Hydroxylase activity is mediated by P450c21, a microsomal cytochrome P450 enzyme. A deficiency of

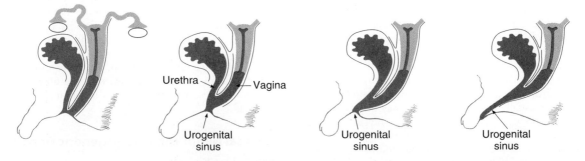

Figure 14–13. Female pseudohermaphroditism induced by prenatal exposure to androgens. Exposure after the 12th fetal week leads only to clitoral hypertrophy (diagram at left). Exposure at progressively earlier stages of differentiation (depicted from left to right in drawings) leads to retention of the urogenital sinus and labioscrotal fusion. If exposure occurs sufficiently early, the labia will fuse to form a penile urethra. (Reproduced, with permission, from Grumbach MM, Ducharme J: The effects of androgens on fetal sexual development: Androgen-induced female pseudohermaphroditism. Fertil Steril 1960;11:757.)

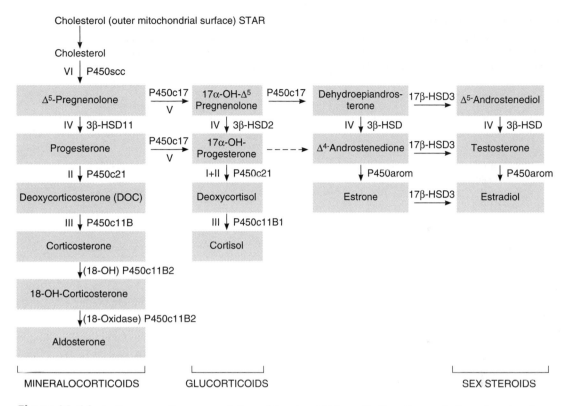

Figure 14–14. A diagrammatic representation of the steroid biosynthetic pathways in the adrenal and gonads. I–VI correspond to enzymes whose deficiency results in congenital adrenal hyperplasia. (OH, hydroxy or hydroxylase; 3β-HSD, 3β-hydroxysteroid dehydrogenase and Δ⁵-isomerase; 17β-HSD3, 17β-hydroxysteroid dehydrogenase 3; P450scc, cholesterol side-chain cleavage, previously termed 20,22 desmolase; P450c21, 21-hydroxylase; P450c17, 17-hydroxylase; P450arom, aromatase. P450c17 also mediates 17,20-lyase activity; P450c11B2 (aldosterone synthase) mediates 18-hydroxylase and 18-oxidase reactions; P450c11B1 mediates 11-hydroxylation of deoxycortisol to cortisol and DOC to corticosterone. The dashed arrow indicates that this reaction may not occur in humans. (Modified and reproduced, with permission, from Conte FA, Grumbach MM. Pathogenesis, classification, diagnosis, and treatment of anomalies of sex. In: DeGroot L [editor]: *Endocrinology*. Grune & Stratton, 1989.)

this enzyme results in the most common type of adrenal hyperplasia, with an overall prevalence of 1:14,000 live births in Caucasians. Over 95% of patients with congenital adrenal hyperplasia have 21-hydroxylase deficiency. The locus for the gene that encodes 21-hydroxylation is on the short arm of chromosome 6, close to the locus for C4 (complement) between HLA-B and HLA-D. DNA analysis has detected two genes, designated *P450c21A* and *P450c21B*, in this region in tandem with the two genes for complement, *C4A* and *C4B*. *P450c21A* is a nonfunctional "pseudogene," ie, it is missing critical sequences and does not encode a functional 21-hydroxylase. Seventy-five percent of patients with "classic" P450c21 deficiency have point mutations that change a small portion of the *P450c21B* to

a sequence similar to that in the nonfunctional *P450c21A* gene—hence a "microgene conversion." Approximately 15% of severely affected *21-OH* genes have a deletion extending from exon 3 to exon 8 of the *P450c21A* pseudogene to a similar region of the *21-OHB* gene, resulting in a nonfunctional fusion *21-OHA/21-OHB* gene. The remainder have gene deletions and macrogene conversions. Recent work has demonstrated that classic salt-wasting 21-hydroxylase deficiency is associated with a mutation, deletion, or gene conversion that abolishes or severely reduces 21-hydroxylase activity. Most patients with 21-hydroxylase deficiency are compound heterozygotes, ie, they have a different genetic lesion in each of their *P450c21B* allelic genes. The phenotypic spectrum observed—salt loss,

Table 14–5. Clinical manifestations of the various types of congenital adrenal hyperplasia.[1]

Enzymatic Defect	StAR[2]		3β-Hydroxysteroid Dehydrogenase		P450c17 (17α-Hydroxylase)		P450c11 (11β-Hydroxylase)		P450c21 (21α-Hydroxylase)		P450scc[3]	
Chromosomal	XX	XY	XX	XY	XX	XY	XX	XY	XX	XY	XX	XY
External genitalia (at birth)	Female	Female	Female (w/wo clitoromegaly)	Ambiguous	Female	Female or ambiguous	Ambiguous[4]	Male	Ambiguous[4]	Male	Female	Ambiguous
Postnatal virilization	Normal female puberty, secondary amenorrhea	Sexual infantilism at puberty	+ or –	Mild to moderate	– (Sexual infantilism at puberty)		+		+		Normal female	(?) Sexual infantilism at puberty
Addisonian crises	+		+ or –		–		–		+ in 80%		+	
Hypertension	–		–		+		+		–		–	

[1]Reproduced, with permission, from Grumbach MM, Hughes IA, Conte FA: Disorders of sex differentiation. In: Larsen PR et al (editors): *Williams Textbook of Endocrinology,* 10th ed. Saunders, 2002.
[2]StAR = steroidogenic acute regulatory protein. StAR deficiency leads to secondary P450scc deficiency
[3]Only one patient, a 46,XY with a heterozygous mutation, has been reported. A null mutation in this enzyme would not be compatible with survival since the placenta requires P450scc to make progesterone.
[4]Normal female in late-onset and "cryptic" forms.

simple virilization, or late onset of virilization—is a consequence of the degree of enzymatic deficiency. The latter is determined by the functionally less severely mutated *P450c21B* allele. The gene for P450c21 (21-hydroxylase) deficiency is not only closely linked to the HLA supergene complex, but certain specific HLA subtypes are found to be statistically increased in patients with 21-hydroxylase deficiency. These include Bw51 in the simple virilizing form, Bw47 in the salt-losing form, and B14 in the nonclassic form.

A. P450c21 Hydroxylase Deficiency
with Virilization

This defect in P450c21 (21-hydroxylase) activity results in impaired cortisol synthesis, increased ACTH levels, and increased adrenal androgen precursor and androgen secretion. Its incidence is 1:50,000 persons, and it accounts for about 20% of individuals with P450c21 hydroxylase deficiency. Before 12 weeks of gestation, high fetal androgen levels lead to a varying degree of labioscrotal fusion and clitoral enlargement in the female fetus; exposure to androgen after 12 weeks induces clitoromegaly alone. In the male fetus, no abnormalities in the external genitalia are evident at birth, but the phallus may be enlarged. These patients produce sufficient amounts of aldosterone to prevent the signs and symptoms of mineralocorticoid deficiency,

though they may have a defect in mineralocorticoid synthesis as evidenced by an elevated plasma renin level. Virilization continues after birth in untreated patients. This results in rapid growth and bone maturation as well as the physical signs of excess androgen secretion (eg, acne, seborrhea, increased muscular development, premature development of pubic or axillary hair, and phallic enlargement). True (central) precocious puberty can occur following initiation of glucocorticoid therapy in affected children with peripubertal bone ages.

Mild defects in P450c21 (21-hydroxylase) activity have been reported. Patients can be symptomatic (late-onset or nonclassic) or asymptomatic ("cryptic" form). These mild forms of P450c21 hydroxylase deficiency are HLA-linked, as is "classic" P450c21 hydroxylase deficiency; however, they occur much more frequently than the classic form of the disease. It has been postulated that "nonclassic" P450c21 hydroxylase deficiency is the most common autosomal recessive disorder, affecting about one in 100 persons of all ethnic groups but having an incidence two to three times higher in Hispanics and Ashkenazic Jews. Females with late-onset P450c21 hydroxylase deficiency have normal female genitalia at birth and do not have an electrolyte abnormality. Mild virilization occurs later in childhood and adolescence, resulting in the premature development of pubic or axillary hair, slight clitoral enlargement, menstrual irregularities, acne, hirsutism, polycystic ovary syndrome, and an advanced bone age. Affected males have normal male genitalia at birth, rapid growth, and advanced skeletal maturation. Later in childhood, they exhibit premature growth of pubic or axillary hair, sexual precocity with inappropriately small testes, and increased muscular development. While tall as children, they end up as short adults due to advanced bone maturation and premature epiphysial fusion. Asymptomatic individuals who have the same biochemical abnormalities as patients with mild forms of P450c21 hydroxylase deficiency have been detected by hormonal testing of families in which there is at least one member with symptoms.

B. P450c21 Hydroxylase Deficiency with Virilization and Salt Loss

The salt-losing variant of P450c21 hydroxylase deficiency accounts for about 80% of patients with classic 21-hydroxylase deficiency and involves a more severe deficit of P450c21 hydroxylase, which leads to impaired secretion of both cortisol and aldosterone. This results in electrolyte and fluid losses after the fifth day of life and, as a consequence, hyponatremia, hyperkalemia, acidosis, dehydration, and vascular collapse. Rarely, this can occur later at 6–12 weeks, usually associated with a concomitant physiologic stress. Masculinization of the external genitalia of affected females tends to be more severe than that found in patients with simple P450c21 hydroxylase deficiency. Affected males may have macrogenitosomia. Recently, patients with 21-hydroxylase and 11β-hydroxylase deficiency have been shown to have adrenomedullary hypofunction secondary to low intraadrenal concentrations of cortisol and developmental defects in formation of the adrenal medulla.

The diagnosis of P450c21 hydroxylase deficiency should always be considered (1) in patients with ambiguous genitalia who have a 46,XX karyotype (and are thus female pseudohermaphrodites); (2) in apparent cryptorchid males; (3) in any infant who presents with shock, hypoglycemia, and chemical findings compatible with adrenal insufficiency; and (4) in males or females with signs of virilization before puberty, including premature adrenarche. In the past, the diagnosis of P450c21 hydroxylase deficiency was based on the finding of elevated levels of 17-ketosteroids and pregnanetriol in the urine. Although still valid and useful, urinary steroid determinations have been replaced by the simpler and more cost-effective measurement of plasma 17-hydroxyprogesterone, androstenedione, and testosterone levels.

The concentration of plasma 17-hydroxyprogesterone is elevated in umbilical cord blood but rapidly decreases into the range of 100–200 ng/dL (3–6 nmol/L) by 24 hours after delivery. In premature infants and in stressed full-term newborns, the levels of 17-hydrox-

yprogesterone are higher than those observed in nonstressed full-term infants. In patients with P450c21 hydroxylase deficiency, the 17-hydroxyprogesterone values usually are greater than 5000 ng/dL (150 nmol/L), depending on the age of the patient and the severity of P450c21 hydroxylase deficiency. Patients with mild P450c21 hydroxylase deficiency, ie, late-onset and cryptic forms, may have borderline basal 17-hydroxyprogesterone values, but they can be distinguished from heterozygotes by the magnitude of the 17-hydroxyprogesterone response to the parenteral administration of ACTH as demonstrated by New and coworkers.

Salt losers may be ascertained clinically or by chemical evidence of hyponatremia and hyperkalemia on a regular infant diet. In these patients, aldosterone levels in both plasma and urine are low in relation to the serum sodium concentration, while plasma renin activity is elevated. Breast milk and many infant formulas have a low concentration of sodium.

HLA typing, measurement of amniotic fluid 17-hydroxyprogesterone levels, and chorionic villus biopsy with HLA typing and gene analysis have been used in the prenatal diagnosis of affected fetuses. Data indicate that prenatal therapy with dexamethasone given to the mother early in pregnancy can lessen the genital ambiguity seen in affected newborn females; however, the use of this therapy is controversial. While the immediate effects of maternal dexamethasone therapy on reducing masculinization of the female external genitalia may be striking, long-term studies are needed to exclude late untoward effects. (See Consensus statement on 21-hydroxylase deficiency from the Lawson Wilkins Pediatric Endocrine Society and the European Society for Paediatric Endocrinology. J Clin Endocrinol Metab 2002;87:4048. [PMID: 12213842])

Heterozygosity has been ascertained by HLA typing in informative families, by the use of ACTH-induced rises in plasma 17-hydroxyprogesterone levels and by genetic analysis. Measurement of plasma 17-hydroxyprogesterone levels using heel-stick capillary blood specimens blotted onto paper has been shown to be a useful and valid screening tool for the diagnosis of 21-hydroxylase deficiency in newborn infants.

C. P450c11 Hydroxylase Deficiency

Classic P450c11 hydroxylase deficiency (virilization with hypertension) is rare; however, it is the second most common form of congenital adrenal hyperplasia, representing 5–8% of all cases. It occurs in 1:100,000 births in persons of European ancestry. However, in Middle Eastern people, it is much more common. In the classic patient, a defect in 11-hydroxylation leads to decreased cortisol levels with a consequent increase in ACTH and the hypersecretion of 11-deoxycorticosterone and 11-deoxycortisol in addition to adrenal androgens. Marked heterogeneity in the clinical and hormonal manifestations of this defect has been described, including mild, late-onset, and even "cryptic" forms. Patients with this form of adrenal hyperplasia classically exhibit virilization secondary to increased androgen production and hypertension related to increased 11-deoxycorticosterone secretion. Plasma renin activity is either normal or suppressed. The hypertension is not invariable; it occurs in approximately two-thirds of patients and may be associated with hypokalemic alkalosis.

Two P450c11 hydroxylase genes have been localized to the long arm of chromosome 8: $P450c11\beta1$ and $P450c11\beta2$. Similar to 21-hydroxylase, these two genes are 95% homologous. $P450c11\beta1$ encodes the enzyme for 11-hydroxylation and is expressed in the zona fasciculata and zona reticularis and is ACTH-dependent. It primarily mediates 11-hydroxylation of 11-deoxycortisol to cortisol and deoxycorticosterone (DOC) to corticosterone. It has about one-twelfth the capacity of P450c11β2 for 18-hydroxylation and does not oxidize 18-hydroxycorticosterone to aldosterone. $P450c11\beta2$ encodes the angiotensin-dependent isozyme aldosterone synthase and is only expressed in the zona glomerulosa, where it mediates 11-hydroxylation, 18-hydroxylation, and 18-oxidation. Mutations, deletions, and gene duplications can produce a wide variety of clinical manifestations from virilization and hypertension ($P450c11\beta1$ deficiency) to isolated salt wasting (P450c11β2 [aldosterone synthase] deficiency) to glucocorticoid-remedial hypertension (due to fusion of the ACTH-dependent regulatory region of the 11-hydroxylase gene with the coding region of aldosterone synthase). Both genes encoding P450c11β1 and P450c11β2 are located on chromosome 8 and thus are not linked to HLA. ACTH stimulation tests have thus far failed to demonstrate a consistent biochemical abnormality in obligate heterozygotes.

The diagnosis of P450c11β-hydroxylase deficiency can be confirmed by demonstration of elevated basal or ACTH-induced plasma levels of 11-deoxycortisol and 11-deoxycorticosterone, at least three times higher than the 95th percentile for age, and increased excretion of their metabolites in urine (mainly tetrahydro-11-deoxycortisol).

D. TYPE IV—3β-HYDROXYSTEROID DEHYDROGENASE DEFICIENCY

Male or female pseudohermaphroditism and adrenal insufficiency are discussed below.

E. TYPE V—P450C17 DEFICIENCY

Male pseudohermaphroditism, sexual infantilism, hypertension, and hypokalemic alkalosis are discussed below.

F. TYPE VI—STAR DEFICIENCY

Congenital lipoid adrenal hyperplasia, male pseudohermaphroditism, sexual infantilism, and adrenal insufficiency are discussed below.

Treatment

Treatment of patients with adrenal hyperplasia may be divided into acute and chronic phases. In acute adrenal crises, a deficiency of both cortisol and aldosterone results in hypoglycemia, hyponatremia, hyperkalemia, hypovolemia, acidosis, and shock. If the patient is hypoglycemic, an intravenous bolus of glucose, 0.25–0.5 g/kg (maximum 25 g), should be administered. If the patient is in shock, an infusion of normal saline (20 mL/kg) may be given over the first hour; thereafter, replacement of glucose, fluid, and electrolytes is calculated on the basis of deficits and standard maintenance requirements. Hydrocortisone sodium succinate, 50 mg/m^2, should be given as a bolus and another 50–100 mg/m^2 added to the infusion fluid over the first 24 hours of therapy. If hyponatremia and hyperkalemia are present, 0.05–0.1 mg of fludrocortisone by mouth may be given along with the intravenous saline and hydrocortisone. Since hydrocortisone has mineralocorticoid activity, it may suffice to correct the electrolyte abnormality along with the saline. In extreme cases of hyponatremia, hyperkalemia, and acidosis, sodium bicarbonate and a cation exchange resin (eg, sodium polystyrene sulfonate) may be needed.

Once the patient is stabilized and a definitive diagnosis has been arrived at by means of appropriate steroid studies, the patient should receive maintenance doses of glucocorticoids to permit normal growth, development, and bone maturation (hydrocortisone, approximately 10–15 mg/m^2/d by mouth in three divided doses). The dose of hydrocortisone must be titrated in each patient, depending on steroid hormone levels in plasma and urine, linear growth, bone maturation, and clinical signs of steroid overdose or of virilization. Salt losers need treatment with mineralocorticoid (fludrocortisone, 0.05–0.2 mg/d by mouth) and added dietary salt (1–3 g/d) in infancy. The dose of mineralocorticoid should be adjusted so that the electrolytes and blood pressure, as well as the plasma renin activity, are in the normal range. Recently, as a result of the difficulty of "optimally" treating these patients, several novel therapies have been suggested. These include adrenalectomy in patients with null mutations of $P450c21$, growth hormone to augment final height, and the use of physiologic doses of hydrocortisone (8 mg/m^2), fludrocortisone, flutamide, an androgen receptor blocker, and an aromatase inhibitor in combination.

Patients with ambiguous external genitalia should have plastic repair. Clitoral recession or clitoroplasty—

not clitoridectomy!—is indicated. Of major importance to the family with an affected child is the assurance that the child will grow and develop into a normal adult. In patients with the most common form of adrenal hyperplasia—21-hydroxylase deficiency—fertility in males and feminization, menstruation, and fertility in females can be expected with adequate treatment. Long-term psychologic guidance and support by the physician for the patient and family are essential.

Adrenal rests in the testes of males with P450c21 hydroxylase deficiency (especially salt losers) may enlarge under the stimulus of ACTH and be mistaken for testicular neoplasms. These adrenal rests are often bilateral and are made up of cells that appear indistinguishable from Leydig cells histologically except that they lack Reinke crystalloids. The rests are usually seen in noncompliant or undertreated patients. To prevent this complication as well as the risk of adrenal crisis, pituitary basophil hyperplasia, and adrenal carcinoma, continuous treatment with a glucocorticoid (and, if indicated, a mineralocorticoid) is recommended even in adult males.

P450 AROMATASE DEFICIENCY

A new form of androgen-induced female pseudohermaphroditism has been defined that is due to aromatase deficiency. Mutations in the gene encoding P450arom result in defective placental conversion of C_{19} steroids to estrogens, leading to exposure of the fetus to excessive amounts of testosterone and masculinization of the external genitalia of the female fetus. Virilization of the mother during gestation can also occur. At puberty, defective aromatase activity in the gonads leads to pubertal failure, hypergonadotropic hypogonadism, polycystic ovaries, mild virilization, tall stature, and osteoporosis. A striking delay in bone age occurs despite increased concentrations of plasma testosterone, supporting the concept that estrogens rather than androgens are the major sex steroids affecting bone maturation, bone turnover, and epiphyseal fusion in females as well as males. The diagnosis of aromatase deficiency is suggested by the finding of the above clinical picture and elevated plasma androstenedione and testosterone levels in the face of low estrogen levels.

Glucocorticoid Receptor Gene Mutation

Glucocorticoid resistance due to a homozygous mutation in the gene encoding the glucocorticoid receptor has recently been reported to induce female pseudohermaphroditism. Glucocorticoid resistance results in an increase in ACTH levels with a consequent increase in cortisol, mineralocorticoids, and adrenal androgens. The latter steroids induce virilization, which in the female infant results in female pseudohermaphroditism.

MATERNAL ANDROGENS & PROGESTOGENS

Masculinization of the external genitalia of a female infant can occur if the mother is given testosterone, other androgenic steroids, or certain synthetic progestational agents during pregnancy. After the 12th week of gestation, exposure results in clitoromegaly alone. Norethindrone, ethisterone, norethynodrel, and medroxyprogesterone acetate have all been implicated in masculinization of the female fetus. Nonadrenal female pseudohermaphroditism can occur as a consequence of maternal ingestion of danazol, the 2,3-*d*-isoxazol derivative of 17α-ethinyl testosterone. In rare instances, masculinization of a female fetus is due to a virilizing maternal ovarian or adrenal tumor, congenital virilizing adrenal hyperplasia in the mother, or a luteoma of pregnancy. The fetus is protected from excess androgen exposure by the ability of the fetal-placental unit to aromatize androgens to estrogens, especially after the first trimester.

The diagnosis of female pseudohermaphroditism arising from transplacental passage of androgenic steroids is based on exclusion of other forms of female pseudohermaphroditism and a history of drug exposure. Surgical correction of the genitalia, if needed, is the only therapy necessary.

Nonadrenal female pseudohermaphroditism can be associated with imperforate anus, renal anomalies, and other malformations of the lower intestine and urinary tract. Sporadic as well as familial cases have been reported.

MALE PSEUDOHERMAPHRODITISM

Male pseudohermaphrodites have gonads that are testes, but the genital ducts or external genitalia, or both, are not completely masculinized. Male pseudohermaphroditism can result from deficient testosterone secretion as a consequence of (1) defective testicular differentiation (testicular dysgenesis), (2) impaired secretion of testosterone or antimüllerian hormone, (3) failure of target tissue response to testosterone and dihydrotestosterone or antimüllerian hormone, and (4) failure of conversion of testosterone to dihydrotestosterone.

Testicular Unresponsiveness to hCG & LH

Male sexual differentiation is dependent upon the production of testosterone by fetal Leydig cells. Leydig cell testosterone secretion is under the influence of placental hCG during the critical period of male sexual differentiation and, thereafter, fetal pituitary LH during gestation.

The finding of normal male sexual differentiation in XY males with anencephaly, apituitarism, or congenital hypothalamic hypopituitarism suggests that male sex differentiation in the human occurs independently of the secretion of fetal pituitary gonadotropins.

Absence, hypoplasia, or unresponsiveness of Leydig cells to hCG LH results in deficient testosterone production and, consequently, male pseudohermaphroditism. The extent of the genital ambiguity is a function of the degree of testosterone deficiency, and the phenotype has ranged from extreme forms with female external genitalia to milder forms with micropenis and to males with normal male genitalia and hypergonadotropic hypogonadism at puberty. A small number of patients with absent, hypoplastic, or unresponsive Leydig cells due to a mutation in the gene encoding the LH-hCG receptor have been reported as well as an animal model, the "vet" rat. In most of the patients thus far reported, the defect resulted in female-appearing genitalia and a short blind-ending vagina. Müllerian duct regression was complete. Basal gonadotropin levels as well as GnRH-evoked responses were elevated in postpubertal patients. Plasma 17α-hydroxyprogesterone, androstenedione, and testosterone levels were low, and hCG elicited little or no response in testosterone or its precursors. In two siblings with the extreme phenotype of this syndrome, a homozygous missense mutation in exon 11 of the LH receptor gene was found. This mutation resulted in an alanine-to-proline change in the sixth transmembrane domain of the LH receptor and a nonfunctional receptor. Other inactivating mutations of the LH receptor gene have been described in unrelated families with LH resistance. These mutations have resulted in a variable degree of hCG-LH resistance and a variable phenotype in the affected XY individual. Recent studies in patients with the clinical and chemical features of Leydig cell hypoplasia have demonstrated that the causes of the syndrome are heterogeneous, and it may result from mutations outside the coding region of the LH-hCG receptor or in other Leydig cell-specific genes. Treatment depends on the age at diagnosis and the extent of masculinization. A female sex assignment has usually been chosen in patients with female external genitalia. In patients with predominantly male external genitalia, testosterone will augment phallic development and virilize the patient at puberty.

Inborn Errors of Testosterone Biosynthesis

Figure 14–15 demonstrates the major pathways in testosterone biosynthesis in the gonads; each step is associated with an inherited defect that results in testosterone deficiency and, consequently, male pseudohermaphroditism. Steps 1, 2, and 3 are enzymatic deficiencies that occur in both the adrenals and gonads and result in defective synthesis of both corticosteroids and testosterone. Thus, they represent forms of congenital adrenal hyperplasia.

A. StAR Deficiency and Congenital Lipoid Adrenal Hyperplasia

Male pseudohermaphroditism, sexual infantilism, and adrenal insufficiency is a very early defect in the synthesis of all steroids affecting the conversion of cholesterol to Δ^5-pregnenolone and results in severe adrenal and gonadal deficiency. The *P450scc* gene has been isolated, cloned, and localized to chromosome 15. However, thus far, molecular analysis of this gene has revealed only one patient in whom a heterozygous mutation (haploinsufficiency) was found. This patient was a hyperpigmented 4-year-old 46,XY male pseudohermaphrodite with clitoromegaly, no labial fusion, a blind vaginal pouch, and late-onset adrenal insufficiency. Mutations in a steroidogenic acute regulatory (StAR) protein that is necessary for the transport of cholesterol from the outer to the inner mitochondrial membrane, the site of P450scc, have been identified in all other patients with the clinical syndrome of congenital lipoid adrenal hyperplasia. StAR is expressed in the adrenals and gonads but not in the placenta; hence, placental synthesis of progesterone, which is required to maintain pregnancy in humans, is apparently not affected. A homozygous null mutation in the *P450scc* gene resulting in a deficit of side-chain cleavage enzymatic activity most likely would be lethal, as it is essential for progesterone synthesis by the human fetoplacental unit.

Affected males usually have female or, rarely, ambiguous external genitalia with a blind vaginal pouch and hypoplastic male genital ducts but no müllerian derivatives; the genitalia of affected females are normal, and ovarian function occurs at puberty but subsequently subsides, secondary to the accumulation of cholesterol in the functioning ovaries with subsequent organ failure. Large lipid-laden adrenals that displace the kidneys downward may be demonstrated by intravenous urography, abdominal ultrasonography, or computed tomography scan. Death in early infancy from adrenal insufficiency is not uncommon. The diagnosis is confirmed by the lack of or low levels of all C_{21}, C_{19}, and C_{18} steroids in plasma and urine and an absent response to ACTH and hCG stimulation. Treatment involves replacement with appropriate doses of glucocorticoids and mineralocorticoids, prophylactic orchiectomy in affected 46,XY patients raised as females, and estrogen replacement at puberty.

B. 3β-Hydroxysteroid Dehydrogenase and Δ^5-Isomerase 2 Deficiency

3β-Hydroxysteroid dehydrogenase type 2 Δ^5-isomerase deficiency is an early defect in steroid synthesis that re-

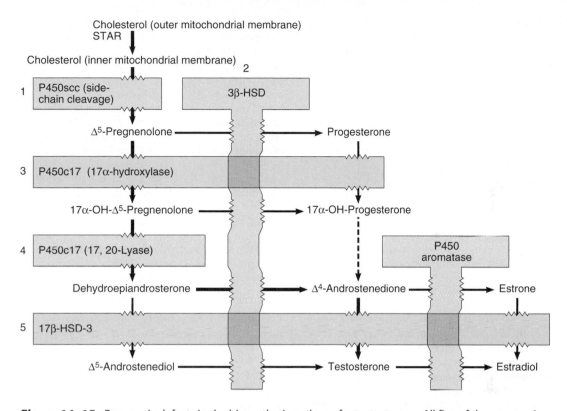

Figure 14–15. Enzymatic defects in the biosynthetic pathway for testosterone. All five of the enzymatic defects cause male pseudohermaphroditism in affected males. Although all of the blocks affect gonadal steroidogenesis, those at steps 1, 2, and 3 are associated with major abnormalities in the biosynthesis of glucocorticoids and mineralocorticoids in the adrenal. All reported patients except one with apparent P450scc deficiency have a mutation in StAR (steroidogenic acute regulatory protein), a protein necessary for the transport of cholesterol from the outer to the inner mitochondrial membrane, where P450scc resides. OH, hydroxy; 3β-HSD, 3β-hydroxysteroid dehydrogenase; 17β-HSD, 17β-hydroxysteroid dehydrogenase-3. Chemical names for enzymes are shown with traditional names in parentheses. (Modified and reproduced, with permission, from Conte FA, Grumbach MM. Pathogenesis, classification, diagnosis, and treatment of anomalies of sex. In: DeGroot L [editor]: *Endocrinology.* Grune & Stratton, 1989.)

sults in inability of the adrenals and gonads to convert 3β-hydroxy-Δ^5 steroids to 3-keto-Δ^4 steroids. Deficiency leads to male or female pseudohermaphroditism and adrenal insufficiency. This enzyme is encoded for by a gene on the short arm of chromosome number 1. Recent data indicate that there are two highly homologous genes encoding 3β-hydroxysteroid dehydrogenase on chromosome 1. The type 1 3β-hydroxysteroid dehydrogenase gene is expressed in the placenta and peripheral tissues, while type 2 is expressed in the adrenals and gonads. 3β-Hydroxysteroid dehydrogenase is not a cytochrome P450 enzyme, and it requires NAD$^+$ as a cofactor. Mutations causing frame shifts, stops, and missense have been reported in the type 2 gene in affected

patients. This defect in its complete form results in a severe deficiency of aldosterone, cortisol, testosterone, and estradiol secretion. Males with this defect are incompletely masculinized, and females have normal female genitalia or mild clitoromegaly. Salt loss and adrenal crises usually occur in early infancy in affected patients. Affected males may experience normal male puberty but often have prominent gynecomastia. Patients with a mild non-salt-losing form of 3β-hydroxysteroid dehydrogenase type 2 deficiency have been described as well as late-onset patients presenting with only premature pubarche. These patients were shown to have elevated Δ^5 steroids as well as mutations in the 3β-hydroxysteroid type 2 gene.

The diagnosis of 3β-hydroxysteroid dehydrogenase deficiency is based on finding elevated concentrations of Δ^5-pregnenolone, Δ^5-17α-hydroxypregnenolone, dehydroepiandrosterone (DHEA) and its sulfate, and other 3β-hydroxy-Δ^5 steroids in the plasma and urine of patients with a consistent clinical picture. 3-keto-Δ^4 steroids, ie, 17-hydroxyprogesterone and androstenedione, may be elevated owing to peripheral conversion of 3β-hydroxy-Δ^5 to 3-keto-Δ^4 steroids by the enzyme encoded by the type 1 gene. The diagnosis of 3β-hydroxysteroid dehydrogenase deficiency may be facilitated by detecting abnormal levels of serum Δ^5-17α-hydroxypregnenolone and DHEA and its sulfates as well as abnormal ratios of Δ^5 to Δ^4 steroids after intravenous administration of 0.25 mg of synthetic ACTH. After ACTH stimulation, 17-hydroxypregnenolone levels are > 5.3 SD above the mean for unaffected individuals in affected infants, > 35 SD above the mean in prepubertal children, and > 21 SD above the mean in adults. The 17-hydroxypregnenolone/cortisol ratio is > 6.4 SD above the mean in infants, > 23 SD above the mean in prepubertal children, and > 221 SD above the mean in adults (see Lutfallah et al). It can be confirmed by detecting a mutation in the type II β-hydroxysteroid dehydrogenase Δ^5 isomerase gene. Suppression of the increased plasma and urinary 3β-hydroxy-Δ^5 steroids by the administration of dexamethasone distinguishes 3β-hydroxysteroid dehydrogenase deficiency from a virilizing adrenal tumor. Treatment of this condition is similar to that of other forms of adrenal hyperplasia (see above).

C. P450c17 Deficiency, 17α-Hydroxylase Deficiency

A defect in 17α-hydroxylation in the zona fasciculata of the adrenal and in the gonads results in impaired synthesis of 17-hydroxyprogesterone and 17-hydroxypregnenolone and, consequently, cortisol and sex steroids. The secretion of large amounts of corticosterone and DOC leads to hypertension, hypokalemia, and alkalosis. Increased DOC secretion with resultant hypertension produces suppression of renin and, consequently, decreased aldosterone secretion. Clinically, this results in male pseudohermaphroditism, sexual infantilism, hypertension, and hypokalemic alkalosis.

A single gene on chromosome 10 encodes both adrenal and testicular P450c17 hydroxylase as well as 17,20-lyase activity. This enzyme catalyzes the 17-hydroxylation of pregnenolone and progesterone to 17-hydroxypregnenolone and 17-hydroxyprogesterone as well as the scission (lyase) of 17-hydroxypregnenolone to the C_{19} steroid—dehydroepiandrosterone—in the adrenal cortex and gonads. Mutations affecting 17-hydroxylase activity have included stop codons, frame shifts, deletions, and missense substitutions.

The clinical manifestations result from the adrenal and gonadal defect. Affected XX females have normal development of the internal ducts and external genitalia but manifest sexual infantilism with elevated gonadotropin concentrations at puberty. Affected males with less than 25% 17α-hydroxylase activity have impaired testosterone synthesis by the fetal testes, which results in female or ambiguous genitalia. At adolescence, sexual infantilism, low renin hypertension, and often hypokalemia are the hallmarks of this defect.

The diagnosis of 17-hydroxylase deficiency should be suspected in XY males with female or ambiguous genitalia or XX females with sexual infantilism who also manifest hypertension associated with hypokalemic alkalosis. High levels of progesterone, Δ^5-pregnenolone, DOC, corticosterone, and 18-hydroxycorticosterone in plasma and increased excretion of their urinary metabolites establish the diagnosis. Plasma renin activity and aldosterone secretion are diminished in these patients.

D. Smith-Lemli-Opitz Syndrome

The phenotypic spectrum of this syndrome typically includes microcephaly, mental retardation, ptosis, micrognathia, severe hypospadias, micropenis, growth failure, and, rarely, adrenal insufficiency. The genitalia in affected 46,XY males may range from normal male to female. The syndrome is caused by a mutation in the gene sterol Δ-7-reductase, *DHCR7*, causing deficiency of cholesterol. The diagnosis is made by the clinical features and confirmed by demonstration of low levels of cholesterol and increased levels of 7-dehydrocholesterol. *Note: The following errors affect testosterone and estrogen biosynthesis in the gonads primarily.*

E. P450c17 Deficiency (17,20-Lyase Deficiency)

The enzyme encoded by the *P450c17* gene mediates both the 17-hydroxylation of pregnenolone and progesterone to 17-hydroxypregnenolone and 17-hydroxyprogesterone and the scission of the $C_{17,20}$ bond of 17-hydroxypregnenolone to yield DHEA. In the human, the scission of 17-hydroxyprogesterone to androstenedione occurs at a low level. Rare patients are reported to have a defect primarily in the scission of the C_{21} steroids to C_{19} steroids, which results in a defect in testosterone synthesis and subsequently pseudohermaphroditism in the male and impaired sex steroid synthesis and secretion in the affected 46,XX female. Two male pseudohermaphrodites from consanguineous marriages who had micropenis, perineal hypospadias, bifid scrotum, a blind vaginal pouch, and cryptorchidism have recently been studied. The administration of hCG resulted in a marked rise in plasma 17-hydroxyprogesterone with a paucity of response in plasma DHEA, androstenedione, and testosterone consistent with a diagnosis of isolated 17,20-lyase deficiency. Analyses of the *P450c17* gene in these patients demonstrated one to be homozygous for an $Arg^{347} \rightarrow$ His mutation and the other to have an $Arg^{358} \rightarrow$ Gln mutation. Both of these mutations result in a specific decrease in 17,20-lyase activity of the product encoded by the *P450c17* gene.

Patients with 17,20-lyase deficiency have low circulating levels of testosterone, androstenedione, DHEA, and estradiol. The diagnosis can be confirmed by demonstration of an increased ratio of 17-hydroxy C_{21} steroids to C_{19} steroids (testosterone, DHEA, Δ^5-androstenediol, and androstenedione) after stimulation with ACTH or hCG and by DNA analysis of the *P450c17* gene.

F. 17β-HYDROXYSTEROID DEHYDROGENASE-3 DEFICIENCY

There are at least six isoenzymes that mediate the 17β-hydroxysteroid dehydrogenase reaction in humans. The last step in testosterone and estradiol biosynthesis by the gonads involves the reduction of androstenedione to testosterone and estrone to estradiol by 17-hydroxysteroid oxidoreductase-3, an NADPH-dependent microsomal enzyme. This gene is located on chromosome 9q22 and is expressed primarily in the testes. Mutations in this gene have been described in male pseudohermaphrodites. At birth, males with a deficiency of the enzyme 17-hydroxysteroid dehydrogenase-3 have predominantly female or mildly ambiguous external genitalia resulting from testosterone deficiency during male differentiation. They have male duct development, absent müllerian structures with a blind vaginal pouch, and inguinal or intra-abdominal testes. The finding of wolffian ducts associated with female external genitalia in these patients is as yet not fully explained. At puberty, progressive virilization with clitoral hypertrophy occurs as a result of peripheral extraglandular conversion of androstenedione to testosterone by 17β-hydroxysteroid dehydrogenase-5. This is often associated with the concurrent development of gynecomastia. Plasma gonadotropin, androstenedione, and estrone levels are elevated, whereas testosterone and estradiol concentration are relatively low. A putative late-onset form of 17-hydroxysteroid oxidoreductase-3 deficiency has been reported in a small number of postadolescent males with gynecomastia and normal male genitalia.

Analysis of 17 patients with classic 17β-hydroxysteroid dehydrogenase-3 deficiency, including four from San Francisco, has revealed 14 mutations in the 17β-hydroxysteroid oxidoreductase-3 gene. Twelve patients had homozygous mutations, four were compound heterozygotes, and one was a presumed heterozygote. In a large cohort from the Gaza Strip, an $Arg^{80} \rightarrow$ Gln mutation was found with partial (15–20%) enzymatic activity.

17-Hydroxysteroid dehydrogenase-3 deficiency should be included in the differential diagnosis of (1) male pseudohermaphrodites with absent müllerian derivatives who have no abnormality in glucocorticoid or mineralocorticoid synthesis; and (2) male pseudohermaphrodites who virilize at puberty, especially if they also exhibit gynecomastia. The diagnosis of 17-hydroxysteroid dehydrogenase-3 deficiency is confirmed by the demonstration of inappropriately high plasma levels of estrone and androstenedione and increased ratios of plasma androstenedione to testosterone and estrone to estradiol before and after stimulation with hCG.

Management of the patients, as of those with other forms of male pseudohermaphroditism, depends on the age at diagnosis and the degree of ambiguity of the external genitalia. In the patient assigned a male gender identity, plastic repair of the genitalia and testosterone augmentation of phallic growth prepubertally as well as testosterone replacement therapy at puberty are indicated. In patients reared as females (the usual case), the appropriate treatment is castration, followed by estrogen replacement therapy at puberty. Affected females have no abnormalities in phenotype or gonadal function, since 17β-hydroxysteroid dehydrogenase-3 is not expressed in the ovary.

Defects in Androgen-Dependent Target Tissues

The complex mechanism of action of steroid hormones at the cellular level has recently been clarified (Figure 14–16; see also Chapter 12 and Figure 12–3).

Free testosterone enters the target cells and undergoes 5α reduction to dihydrotestosterone. Dihydrotestosterone binds to the intracellular androgen receptor, inducing a conformational change that facilitates the release of heat shock protein, nuclear transport, dimerization, and binding to the specific hormone response elements of DNA. It initiates transcription, translation, and protein synthesis that leads to androgenic actions. A lack of androgen effect at the end organ and, consequently, male pseudohermaphroditism may result from abnormalities in 5α-reductase activity, transformation of the steroid-receptor complex, receptor binding of dihydrotestosterone, receptor-ligand complex binding to DNA, transcription, exportation, or translation.

End-Organ Resistance to Androgenic Hormones (Androgen Receptor Defects)

A. SYNDROME OF COMPLETE ANDROGEN RESISTANCE (INSENSITIVITY) AND ITS VARIANTS (TESTICULAR FEMINIZATION)

The syndrome of complete androgen resistance (testicular feminization) is characterized by a 46,XY karyotype, bilateral testes, absent or hypoplastic wolffian

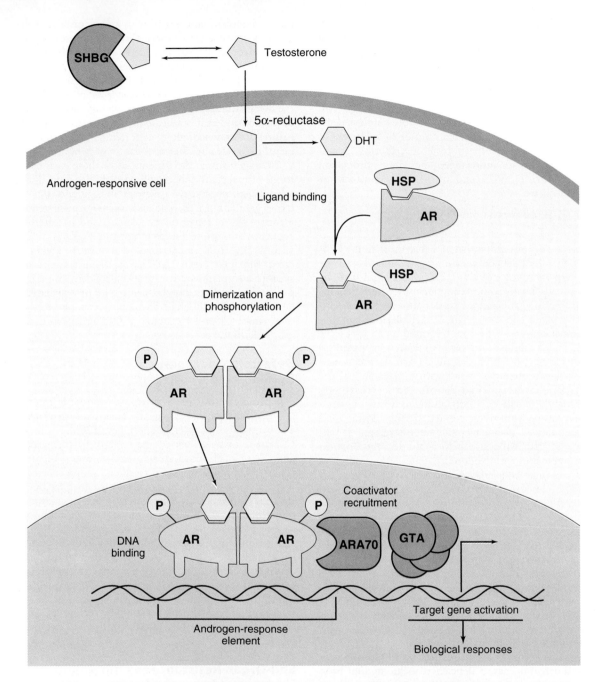

Figure 14–16. Diagrammatic representation of the putative mechanism of action of testosterone on target cells. Testosterone (T) enters the cells, where it is either 5α-reduced to dihydrotestosterone (DHT) or aromatized to estradiol (E₂). Dihydrotestosterone binds to the androgen receptor (AR) in the cytoplasm and "activates" it with the release of heat shock proteins (HSP). The activated AR complex is then translocated to the nucleus, where it binds as a dimer to specific hormone response elements of the DNA and along with coactivators initiates transcription, translation, and protein synthesis, with consequent androgenic effects. (Redrawn and modified from Feldman D: The development of androgen-independent prostate cancer. Nat Rev Cancer 2001;1:34.)

ducts, female-appearing external genitalia with a hypoplastic clitoris and labia minora, a blind vaginal pouch, and absent or rudimentary müllerian derivatives (33%). At puberty, female secondary sexual characteristics develop, but menarche does not ensue. Pubic and axillary hair is usually sparse and in one-third of patients is totally absent. Affected patients are taller than average females (mean height 162.3 cm). Some patients have a variant form of this syndrome and exhibit slight clitoral enlargement. These patients may exhibit mild virilization in addition to the development of breasts and a female habitus.

Androgen resistance during embryogenesis prevents masculinization of the external genitalia and differentiation of the wolffian ducts. Secretion of antimüllerian hormone by the fetal Sertoli cells leads to regression of the müllerian ducts. Thus, affected patients are born with female external genitalia and a blind vaginal pouch. At puberty, androgen resistance results in augmented LH secretion with subsequent increases in testosterone and estradiol. Estradiol arises from peripheral conversion of testosterone and androstenedione as well as from direct secretion by the testes. Androgen resistance coupled with increased testicular estradiol secretion and conversion of androgens to estrogens result in the development of female secondary sexual characteristics at puberty. The timing of the pubertal growth spurt is similar to that in unaffected girls.

The androgen receptor gene is located on the X chromosome between Xq11 and Xq13. The gene is composed of eight exons, numbered 1 through 8. Exon 1 encodes the amino terminal end of the androgen receptor protein and is thought to play a role in transcription. Exons 2 and 3 encode the DNA-binding zinc finger of the androgen receptor protein. The 5' portion of exon 4 is called the hinge region and plays a role in nuclear targeting. Exons 5–8 specify the carboxyl terminal portion of the androgen receptor, which is the androgen binding domain (Figure 14–17).

Patients with complete androgen resistance have been found to be heterogeneous with respect to dihydrotestosterone binding to the androgen receptor. Receptor-negative and receptor-positive individuals with qualitative defects such as thermolability, instability, and impaired binding affinity as well as individuals with presumed normal binding have been described. Analysis of the androgen receptor gene has shed light on the pathogenesis of the heterogeneity in receptor studies found in patients with complete androgen resistance. Patients with the receptor-negative form of complete androgen resistance have been found to have primarily point mutations or substitutions in exons 5–8, which encode the androgen-binding domain of the receptor. Most of the mutations are familial in nature. Other defects such as deletions, mutations in a splice

donor site, and point mutations causing premature termination codons are less common in this group of patients. Mutations in exon 3 (which encodes the DNA-binding segment of the androgen receptor) are associated with normal binding of androgen to the receptor but inability of the ligand-receptor complex to bind to DNA and thus to initiate mRNA transcription. These mutations result in receptor-positive complete androgen resistance. The phenotype of the affected patient does not correlate as well with the receptor studies as it does with the transcriptional activity of the ligand-androgen receptor complex. Other factors that play a role in genotype-phenotype variations include somatic mosaicism, coregulator proteins, and other "modifier" genes.

The diagnosis of complete androgen resistance can be suspected from the clinical features. Before puberty, the presence of testis-like masses in the inguinal canal or labia in a phenotypic female suggests the diagnosis. Postpubertally, the patients present with primary amenorrhea, normal breast development, and absent or sparse pubic or axillary hair. Pelvic examination or ultrasound confirms the absence of a cervix and uterus.

The complete and incomplete forms (Reifenstein's syndrome) of androgen resistance must be distinguished from other forms of male pseudohermaphroditism due to androgen deficiency or to 5α-reductase deficiency. Unfortunately, there is no readily available, rapid in vivo or in vitro assay for androgen sensitivity. The diagnosis is suggested by the clinical picture, the family history, and the presence of elevated basal and hCG-induced testosterone levels with normal levels of dihydrotestosterone. A lack of decrease in sex hormone-binding globulin levels after a short course of the anabolic steroid stanozolol has been suggested as a biologic test for androgen resistance. However, few or no confirmatory data on this assay have yet been reported. Also, one would expect that some patients with incomplete androgen resistance might respond to this test in somewhat the same way as normal individuals. It has been suggested that an elevated antimüllerian hormone level is a marker of androgen resistance and androgen deficiency. Abnormalities in androgen binding and mutational analysis as well as studies of transactivation are all diagnostic, but they are time-consuming, labor-intensive, and not universally available. In the infant with ambiguous genitalia in whom the sex of rearing is in question, we have used a trial of testosterone enanthate in oil, 25 mg intramuscularly every four weeks for 3 months, as a predictive test of androgen responsiveness and future phallic growth before assigning a sex of rearing.

Therapy of patients with complete androgen resistance involves affirmation and reinforcement of their female gender identity. Castration, either before or after

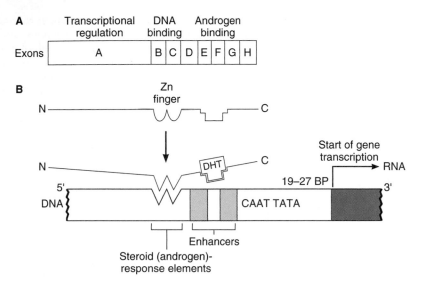

Figure 14–17. A: Diagrammatic representation of the androgen receptor gene divided into its eight exons. Exon A encodes the amino terminal domain and regulates transcription. Exons B and C encode two zinc fingers. Exons E–H encode the androgen-binding domain of the receptor. ***B:*** The organization of a steroid-responsive gene. Ligand binding activates the receptor, and it binds to the steroid response elements of the gene (as a dimer; not shown). Steroid-independent enhancers as well as a CAAT and a TATA box are present. Gene transcription begins 19–27 base pairs downstream of the TATA box. (Reproduced, with permission, from Grumbach MM, Conte FA: Disorders of sex differentiation. In: Larsen PR et al [editors]: *Williams Textbook of Endocrinology,* 10th ed. Saunders, 2002.)

puberty, is indicated because of the increased risk of gonadal neoplasms with age. Estrogen replacement therapy is required at the age of puberty in orchidectomized patients. In most cases, vaginal reconstructive surgery is not required.

B. Syndrome of Incomplete Androgen Resistance (Insensitivity) and Its Variants (Reifenstein's Syndrome)

Patients with incomplete androgen resistance manifest a wide spectrum of phenotypes as far as the degree of masculinization is concerned. The external genitalia at birth can range from ambiguous, with a blind vaginal pouch, to hypoplastic male genitalia. There is variability of masculinization of affected males even within kinships. Müllerian duct derivatives are absent and wolffian duct derivatives are present, but they are usually hypoplastic. At puberty, virilization recapitulates that seen in utero and is generally poor; pubic and axillary hair as well as gynecomastia are usually present. The most common phenotype postpubertally is the

male with perineoscrotal hypospadias and gynecomastia. Axillary and pubic hair are normal. The testes remain small and exhibit azoospermia as a consequence of germinal cell arrest. As in the case of patients with complete androgen resistance, there are elevated levels of plasma LH, testosterone, and estradiol. However, the degree of feminization in these patients despite high estradiol levels is less than that found in the syndrome of complete androgen resistance.

Androgen receptor studies in these patients have usually shown quantitative or qualitative abnormalities in androgen binding. It would be expected that mutations which lead to partial reduction of androgen action would result in incomplete virilization. As previously noted, the best correlation to phenotype is the degree of impairment of transcriptional activity of the ligand-androgen receptor complex. A wide variety of androgen receptor gene mutations can result in the same phenotype, and a specific mutation may not always be associated with the same phenotype in all affected patients. In general, point mutations that result in more conservative amino acid substitutions are more likely to result in partial rather than complete androgen resistance.

Androgen Resistance in Men with Normal Male Genitalia

Partial androgen resistance has been described in a group of infertile men who have a normal male phenotype but may exhibit gynecomastia. Unlike other patients with androgen resistance, some of these patients have normal plasma LH and testosterone levels. Infertility in otherwise normal men may be the only clinical manifestation of androgen resistance. However, infertility may not always be associated with androgen resistance. A family has been described in which there were five males with gynecomastia, all of them with a small phallus. Plasma testosterone levels were elevated, and a subtle qualitative abnormality in ligand binding was noted. Fertility was documented in four of the five males. These patients represent the mildest form of androgen resistance presently documented.

Defects in Testosterone Metabolism by Peripheral Tissues; 5α-Reductase-2 Deficiency (Pseudovaginal Perineoscrotal Hypospadias)

The defective conversion of testosterone to dihydrotestosterone produces a unique form of male pseudohermaphroditism (Figure 14–18). Phenotypically, these patients may vary from those with a microphallus to patients with pseudovaginal perineoscrotal hypospadias. At birth, in the most severely affected patients, ambiguous external genitalia are manifested by a small hypospadiac phallus bound down in chordee, a bifid scrotum, and a urogenital sinus that opens onto the perineum. A blind vaginal pouch is present, opening either into the urogenital sinus or onto the urethra, immediately behind the urethral orifice. The testes are either inguinal or labial. Müllerian structures are absent, and the wolffian structures are well-differentiated. At puberty, affected males virilize; the voice deepens, muscle mass increases, and the phallus enlarges. The bifid scrotum becomes rugose and pigmented. The testes enlarge and descend into the labioscrotal folds, and spermatogenesis may ensue. Gynecomastia is notably absent in these patients. Of note is the absence of acne and the presence of temporal hair recession and hirsutism. A remarkable feature of this form of male pseudohermaphroditism in some cultural isolates has been the reported change in gender identity from female to male at puberty.

After the onset of puberty, patients with 5α-reductase-2 deficiency have normal to elevated testosterone levels and slightly elevated plasma concentrations of LH. As expected, plasma dihydrotestosterone is low, and the testosterone-dihydrotestosterone ratio is abnormally high. Apparently, lack of 5α reduction of testosterone to dihydrotestosterone in utero during the critical phases of male sex differentiation results in incomplete masculinization of the urogenital sinus and external genitalia, while testosterone-dependent wolffian structures are normally developed. Partial and mild forms of 5α-reductase deficiency have been described. These patients can present with hypospadias or microphallus (or both). Three male siblings in a Swedish kindred who were compound heterozygotes for 5α-reductase-2 deficiency had hypospadias repair in infancy, and two were demonstrably fertile.

5α-Reductase-2 deficiency is transmitted as an autosomal recessive trait, and the enzymatic defect exhibits genetic heterogeneity. There are two classes of affected individuals: those with absent enzyme activity and those with a measurable but unstable enzyme. Two genes catalyze the conversion of testosterone to dihydrotestosterone, and they are termed type 1 and type 2. The type I enzyme is not expressed in the fetus but is expressed in skin, especially from puberty onward. The type 2 isoenzyme is the enzyme found in fetal genital skin, male accessory glands, and the prostate. In patients with 5α-reductase deficiency, the isozyme with a

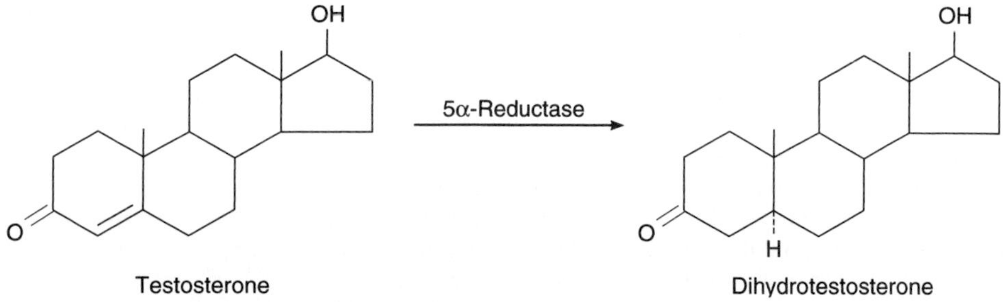

Figure 14–18. Metabolism of testosterone.

pH 5.5 optimum is deficient (type 2). The gene encoding this enzyme contains five exons and is localized to chromosome 2, band p23. A variety of mutations are reported, including deletions, nonsense, splicing defects, and the more common missense mutations. Two-thirds of patients are homozygous for a single mutation, while the remainder are compound heterozygotes. It has been suggested that the marked virilization noted at puberty as opposed to its absence in utero may be the result of the expression and function of the type 1 gene at puberty and, consequently, the generation of sufficient amounts of dihydrotestosterone by peripheral conversion to induce phallic growth and other signs of masculinization.

5α-Reductase-2 deficiency should be suspected in male pseudohermaphrodites with a blind vaginal pouch and in males with hypospadias or microphallus. The diagnosis can be confirmed by demonstration of an abnormally high plasma testosterone-dihydrotestosterone ratio, either under basal conditions or after hCG stimulation. Other confirmatory findings, especially in newborns, include an increased 5β:5α ratio of urinary C_{19} and C_{21} steroid metabolites. One can also examine the level of 5α-reductase activity in cultures of genital skin and the degree of conversion of infused labeled testosterone to dihydrotestosterone in vivo.

The early diagnosis of this condition is particularly critical. In view of the natural history of this disorder, a male gender assignment is indicated, and dihydrotestosterone (if available) or high-dose testosterone therapy should be initiated in order to augment phallic size. Repair of hypospadias should be performed in infancy or early childhood. In patients who are diagnosed after infancy in whom gender identity is unequivocally female after the age of puberty, genitoplasty, prophylactic orchiectomy and estrogen substitution therapy is still the treatment of choice.

Dysgenetic Male Pseudohermaphroditism (Ambiguous Genitalia Due to Dysgenetic Gonads)

Defective gonadogenesis of the testes results in ambiguous development of the genital ducts, urogenital sinus, and external genitalia. Patients with 45,X/46,XY mosaicism, structural abnormalities of the Y chromosome, and forms of XY gonadal dysgenesis manifest defective gonadogenesis and thus defective virilization. These disorders are classified under disorders of gonadal differentiation but are included also as a subgroup of male pseudohermaphroditism. 46,XY gonadal dysgenesis has been associated with deletion and mutation of the *SRY* gene on the Y chromosome, duplication of the *DAX1 (AHC)* gene of the X chromosome, and chromosome 9p− *(DMRT1, 2)* or 10q− deletions. In addition

SOX9, DHCR7, and XH2 mutations and WNT4 duplications result in dysgenetic male pseudohermaphroditism (see pp. 566–569).

Male pseudohermaphroditism can occur in association with early-onset degenerative renal disease and hypertension as well as with Wilms' tumor (Denys-Drash syndrome) and late-onset renal disease and an increased incidence of gonadoblastoma formation in streak gonads (Frasier syndrome). In Denys-Drash syndrome, both the kidneys and the testes are dysgenetic, and a predisposition for renal neoplasms exists. Patients with the Wilms tumor-aniridia-genital anomalies-mental retardation (WAGR) syndrome have been described. These patients exhibit various forms of ambiguous or hypoplastic male genitalia, including bifid scrotum, hypospadias, and cryptorchidism. Recent data indicate that the Denys-Drash, Frasier, and WAGR syndromes are due to heterozygous mutations in coding exons—mostly exon 9 (Denys-Drash)—or heterozygous mutations in the donor splice site of intron 9, leading to a reversal of the +KTS/−KTS (lysine-threonine-serine) ratio of WT1 proteins (Denys-Drash) or deletions (WAGR) involving the Wilms tumor repressor gene *WT1* on chromosome 11.

A mutation in the gene encoding SF-1 has recently been reported in a 46,XY patient. Similar to the mouse "knockout," the patient had female sex differentiation including müllerian derivatives and severe, neonatal onset adrenal insufficiency. In the human, however, the mutation was heterozygous (present in only one allele of the *SF-1* gene) and gonadotropin secretion was preserved (as opposed to the deficiency of gonadotropins observed in the homozygous Sf-1 "knockout" mouse). This illuminating patient demonstrates that SF-1 plays a critical role in adrenal and gonadal development and function in humans. Subsequently, a female heterozygote and a male with a homozygous *SF-1* mutation have been described. The heterozygote parents and siblings of the latter case had normal adrenal and gonadal function.

Testicular Regression Syndrome (Vanishing Testes Syndrome; XY Agonadism; Rudimentary Testes Syndrome; Congenital Anorchia)

Cessation of testicular function during the critical phases of male sex differentiation can lead to various clinical syndromes depending on when testicular function ceases. At one end of the clinical spectrum of these heterogeneous conditions are the XY patients in whom testicular deficiency occurred before 8 weeks of gestation, which results in female differentiation of the internal and external genitalia—so-called XY gonadal dysgenesis.

At the other end of the spectrum are the patients with "anorchia" or "vanishing testes" in which the testes are lost later in gestation. These patients have perfectly normal male differentiation of their internal and external structures, but gonadal tissue is absent. The diagnosis of anorchia should be considered in all cryptorchid males. Administration of chorionic gonadotropin, 1000–2000 units/m^2 injected intramuscularly every other day for 2 weeks (total of seven injections), is a useful test of Leydig cell function. In the presence of normal Leydig cell function, there is a rise in serum testosterone from concentrations of less than 20 ng/dL (0.69 nmol/L) to over 200 ng/dL (6.9 nmol/L) in prepubertal males. In infants under 4 years of age and children over 10 years of age, plasma FSH levels are a sensitive index of gonadal integrity. The gonadotropin response to a 100 µg intravenous injection of GnRH can also be used to diagnose the absence of gonadal feedback on the hypothalamus and pituitary. In agonadal children, GnRH elicits a rise in LH and FSH levels that is greater than that achieved in prepubertal children with normal gonadal function. Patients with high gonadotropin levels and no testosterone response to chorionic gonadotropin usually lack recognizable testicular tissue at surgery. Recent data indicate that both antimüllerian hormone and inhibin levels are useful in ascertaining the absence of functioning Sertoli cells and, hence, presumed anorchia.

Persistent Müllerian Duct Syndrome (Defects in the Synthesis, Secretion, or Response to Antimüllerian Hormone)

Patients have been described in whom normal male development of the external genitalia has occurred but in whom the müllerian ducts persist. The retention of müllerian structures can be ascribed to failure of the Sertoli cells to synthesize antimüllerian hormone and to an end-organ defect in the response of the duct to antimüllerian hormone. This condition is transmitted as an autosomal recessive trait. The gene for antimüllerian hormone has been cloned and mapped to chromosome 19, and mutations in the antimüllerian gene have been reported. More recently, the gene encoding the antimüllerian receptor has been isolated, and patients with mutations in the AMH receptor have been described. In these patients müllerian ducts are present despite the presence of normal to high levels of AMH in plasma. Therapy involves removal of the müllerian structures.

Environmental Chemicals

An increase in disorders of development and function of the urogenital tract in males has been noted over the past 50 years. It has been hypothesized that this increased incidence of reproductive abnormalities observed in human males is related to increasing exposure in utero to "estrogens" found in the diet both naturally and as a result of chemical contamination. It has been demonstrated that *p,p'*-DDE (dichlorodiphenyldichloroethylene)—the major and persistent DDT metabolite—binds to the androgen receptor and inhibits androgen action in developing rodents. Further studies on the levels as well as the risks to humans of environmental chemicals and other endocrine disruptors are necessary before abnormalities of the reproductive tract can be ascribed to these agents.

UNCLASSIFIED FORMS OF ABNORMAL SEXUAL DEVELOPMENT IN MALES

Hypospadias

Hypospadias occurs as an isolated finding in 1:300 newborn males. It is often associated with ventral contraction and bowing of the penis, called chordee. Deficient virilization of the external genitalia of the male fetus implies subnormal Leydig cell function in utero, end-organ resistance, or an inappropriate temporal correlation of the rise in fetal plasma testosterone and the critical period for tissue response. Although in most patients there is little reason to suspect these mechanisms, recent reports in a small number of patients have suggested that simple hypospadias can be associated with an abnormality (or competitive inhibition) of the androgen receptor, the nuclear localization of the ligand-receptor complex, an aberration in the maturation of the hypothalamic-pituitary-gonadal axis, and 5α-reductase deficiency. Further studies are necessary to determine the prevalence and role of these abnormalities in the pathogenesis of simple hypospadias. Nonendocrine factors that affect differentiation of the primordia may be found in a variety of genetic syndromes. A study of 100 patients with hypospadias reported one patient to be an XX female with congenital adrenal hyperplasia; five had sex chromosome abnormalities; and one had the incomplete form of XY gonadal dysgenesis. Nine affected males were the product of pregnancies in which the mother had taken progestational compounds during the first trimester. Thus, a presumed pathogenetic mechanism was found in 15% of patients.

Micropenis

Microphallus without hypospadias—micropenis—can result from a heterogeneous group of disorders, but by far the most common cause is fetal testosterone deficiency; more rarely, 5α-reductase deficiency or mild defects in the androgen receptor are implicated (Table

Table 14–6. Etiology of micropenis.[1]

I. Deficient testosterone secretion
  A. Hypogonadotropic hypogonadism
    1. Isolated, including Kallman's syndrome
    2. Associated with other pituitary hormone deficiencies
    3. Prader-Willi syndrome
    4. Laurence-Moon-Biedl syndrome
    5. Bardet-Biedl syndrome
    6. Rudd's syndrome
  B. Primary hypogonadism
    1. Anorchia
    2. Klinefelter's and poly X syndromes
    3. Gonadal dysgensis (incomplete form)
    4. LH receptor defects (incomplete forms)
    5. Genetic defects in testosterone steroidogenesis (incomplete forms)
    6. Noonan's syndrome
    7. Trisomy 21
    8. Robinow's syndrome
II. Defects in testosterone action
  A. GH/IGF-1 deficiency
  B. Androgen receptor defects (incomplete forms)
  C. 5α-Reductase deficiency (incomplete forms)
  D. Fetal hydantoin syndrome
III. Developmental anomalies
  A. Aphallia
  B. Cloacal exstrophy
IV. Idiopathic
V. Associated with other congential malformation

[1]Source: Bin Abbas VB et al: Congenital hypogonadotropic hypogonadism and micropenis: Effect of testosterone treatment on adult penile size—Why sex reversal is not indicated. J Pediatr 1999;134:570.

Table 14–7. Normal values for stretched penile length.

Age	Length (cm) (mean ± SD)
Newborn: 30 weeks[1]	2.5 ± 0.4
Newborn: full-term[1]	3.5 ± 0.4
0–5 months[2]	3.9 ± 0.8
6–12 months[2]	4.3 ± 0.8
1–2 years[2]	4.7 ± 0.8
2–3 years[2]	5.1 ± 0.9
3–4 years[2]	5.5 ± 0.9
5–6 years[2]	6.0 ± 0.9
10–11 years	6.4 ± 1.1
Adult[3]	12.4 ± 2.7

[1]Data from Feldman and Smith (1975); see Tuladhar et al (1998) for the normal range of penile length in preterm infants between 24 and 36 weeks of gestational age.
[2]Data from Schonfeld and Beebe (1942).
[3]Data from Wessels et al (1996).
Source: Bin Abbas B et al: Congenital hypogonadotrophic hypogonadism and micropenis: Effect of testosterone treatment on adult penile size—Why sex reversal is not indicated. J Pediatr 1999;134:79.

14–6). In the human male fetus, testosterone synthesis by the fetal Leydig cell during the critical period of male differentiation (8–12 weeks) is under the influence of placental hCG. After midgestation, fetal pituitary LH modulates fetal testosterone synthesis by the Leydig cell and, consequently, affects the growth of the differentiated penis. Thus, males with congenital hypopituitarism as well as isolated gonadotropin deficiency and "late" fetal testicular failure can present with normal male differentiation and micropenis at birth (penis < 2.5 cm in length) (Table 14–7). Patients with hypothalamic hypopituitarism or pituitary aplasia may also have midline craniofacial defects, hypoglycemia, and giant cell hepatitis. After appropriate evaluation of anterior pituitary function (ie, determination of the plasma concentration of growth hormone, ACTH, cortisol, thyroid-stimulating hormone, thyroxine, and gonadotropins), stabilization of the patient with hormone

replacement should be achieved. Thereafter, all patients with micropenis should receive a trial of testosterone therapy before definitive gender assignment is made. Patients with fetal testosterone deficiency as a cause of micropenis—whether due to gonadotropin deficiency or to a primary testicular disorder—respond to 25–50 mg of testosterone enanthate intramuscularly monthly for 3 months with a mean increase of 2 cm in penile length (Figure 14–19). A long-term study of eight males with micropenis due to congenital hypogonadotropic hypogonadism who were followed in our clinic revealed that fetal deficiency of gonadotropins and testosterone did not prevent the penis from responding to testosterone in infancy and at the age of puberty. Final penile length for all patients who were treated with one or more short courses of repository testosterone in infancy or childhood and with replacement doses of testosterone in adolescence was in the normal adult range. Furthermore, these patients had a male gender identity, erections, ejaculation, and orgasm (Table 14–8). We found no clinical, psychologic, or physiologic indications to support conversion of males with micropenis secondary to diminished testosterone secretion during gestation to females.

Complete absence of the phallus is a rare anomaly. The urethra may open on the perineum or into the rectum. Assignment of a female gender, castration, and plastic repair of the genitalia and urethra has been the approach followed in the past; however, this course is being seriously questioned by some investigators.

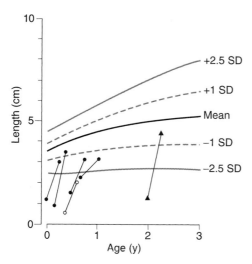

Figure 14–19. The response in phallic length to a 3-month course of testosterone in six patients with microphallus. Patients were under 2 years of age. Each patient was given 25 mg of testosterone enanthate in oil intramuscularly monthly for 3 months. Lines set off with solid triangles and open circles indicate two patients who subsequently underwent a second course of testosterone therapy. (Reproduced, with permission, from Burstein S, Grumbach MM, Kaplan SL: Early determination of androgen-responsiveness is important in the management of microphallus. Lancet 1979;2:983.)

UNCLASSIFIED FORMS OF ABNORMAL SEXUAL DEVELOPMENT IN FEMALES

Congenital absence of the vagina occurs in 1:5000 female births. It can be associated with müllerian derivatives that vary from normal to absent. Ovarian function is usually normal. Therapy may involve plastic repair of the vagina.

Müllerian agenesis may be associated with renal aplasia (an absent kidney) and cervicothoracic somite dysplasia ("MURCS").

MANAGEMENT OF PATIENTS WITH INTERSEX PROBLEMS

The evaluation and management of the patient with ambiguous genitalia are best undertaken by a team consisting of an endocrinologist, a psychiatrist or psychologist, a pediatrician or internist, a surgeon, a urologist, and a social worker. The goal of management of patients with ambiguous genitalia is to establish an etiologic diagnosis promptly and, with the informed consent of the parents, assign a sex of rearing that is most compatible with the prospect for a well-adjusted life and sexual adequacy. Steps in the diagnosis of intersexuality are set forth in Figures 14–20 and 14–21.

Repeated, lucid, simple, comprehensive discussions with the parents about the cause of their child's "atypical" genitalia, the natural history of other patients with

Table 14–8. Treatment of eight males with micropenis secondary to congenital hypogonadotropic hypogonadism, followed from infancy or childhood to maturity (ages 18–27 years).[1]

Characteristics of Patients	Group I	Group II
Age at start of testosterone	4 months to 2 years	6–13 years
Mean penile length and range	1.1 cm (–4 SD) (range 0.5–1.5 cm)	2.7 cm (–3.4 SD) (range 1.5–3.5 cm)
Mean penile length and range after 3 months of testosterone	3.3 cm (–1.6 SD) (range 2.5–4 cm)	4.8 cm (–1.4 SD) (range 2.5–7.5 cm)
Age of replacement testosterone	13–15 years	13–15 years
Mean final adult penile length	10.3 cm (–0.8 SD) (range 8–12 cm)	10.3 cm (–0.8 SD) (range 8.5–14 cm)

[1]Four patients were treated with testosterone before 2 years of age (group I) and four were treated between 6 and 13 years of age (group II). All patients received one or more courses of three intramuscular injections of testosterone enanthate (25 or 50 mg) at 4-week intervals in infancy or childhood to induce penile growth. At the age of puberty, the dose was gradually increased to adult replacement doses. Final adult penile length in both groups was 10.3 cm ± 2.7 cm with a range of 8–14 cm, which was within the normal range for mean adult stretched penile length in white men.
Source: Bin Abbas B et al: Congenital hypogonadotrophic hypogonadism and micropenis: Effect of testosterone treatment on adult penile size—Why sex reversal is not indicated. J Pediatr 1999;134:79.

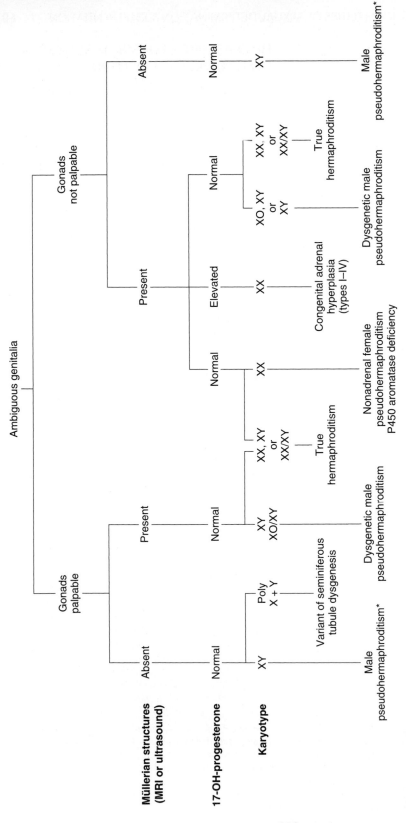

Figure 14–20. Steps in the differential diagnosis of ambiguous genitalia.

similar pathophysiology, prognosis, and the possible hormonal and surgical options available is critical to their coming to an informed decision on the sex rearing of their child. This discussion must take into account the parental anxieties, religious views, social mores, cultural factors, and, most important, the level of understanding of the parents. Parents of intersexed children as well as the patient need the ongoing support of psychiatrists or psychologists who have knowledge of the pathogenesis of abnormalities of sex differentiation and who understand the complexities of intersexuality, gender behavior, and gender identity.

There is a great deal of discussion and controversy involving the management of infants with intersexuality. Advances in biochemistry, genetics, and endocrinology have increased our knowledge and understanding of the pathogenesis of abnormalities of sex determination and differentiation. It is now possible to make a specific diagnosis in the majority of patients with ambiguous genitalia. This information, coupled with phallic response to testosterone, advances in surgical reconstruction, strikes a note of optimism. Further, we now recognize that genes, hormones, and the environment are critical factors determining gender identity. Androgens in utero are facultative but not determinative in their effect on gender identity in patients with intersexuality. However, there are large gaps in long-term outcome data in many of these disorders. All of these considerations lead us to the following recommendations for newborns with abnormalities of sex determination and differentiation.

We recommend male sex assignment in 46,XY male pseudohermaphrodites except for those with complete androgen resistance or those who have completely female external genitalia due to Leydig cell unresponsiveness to hCG and LH and rare errors in testosterone biosynthesis, where extensive discussion with the family is especially warranted. In some societies, the social, cultural, and economic benefits of a male gender identity are more compelling than phallic adequacy and are a prevailing—if not the most important—factor in the parental decision about the sex of rearing.

All female pseudohermaphrodites, including those affected infants with complete masculinization of the external genitalia, should be reared as females.

Reassignment of sex in infancy and childhood is always a difficult psychosocial problem for the patient, the parents, and the physicians involved. While easier in infancy than after 1 year of age, it should only be undertaken after deliberation and with provision for long-term medical and psychiatric supervision and counseling.

It is desirable to initiate plastic repair of the external genitalia by 6 months of age. In children raised as females, the clitoris should be salvaged by clitoroplasty. All surgical procedures should strive to preserve the functional capacity of all genital structures. This consideration should outweigh cosmetic appearance. Reconstruction of a vagina, if necessary, can be deferred until adolescence if a surgeon experienced in genitoplasty is not available. Hypospadias repair is best performed at 6 months to 1 year of age.

Removal of rudimentary gonads in children with Y chromosome material and gonadal dysgenesis should be performed at the time of initial repair of the external genitalia, because gonadoblastomas, seminomas, and germinomas can occur during the first decade. However, histologically and presumably functionally "normal" scrotal testes should be retained in male pseudohermaphrodites assigned a male identity—especially those with 45,X/46,XY mosaicism.

In a patient with complete androgen resistance, the gonads may be left in situ (provided they are not situated in the labia majora) to provide estrogen until late adolescence. The patient may then undergo prophylactic castration, having had her female identity reinforced by normal feminization at puberty. However, it is reasonable to remove the gonads prepubertally, especially if herniorrhaphy is necessary. In this circumstance, sex steroid replacement therapy at the time of puberty is indicated.

In patients with incomplete androgen resistance reared as females or in patients with errors of testosterone biosynthesis in whom some degree of masculinization occurs at puberty, gonadectomy should be performed before puberty.

Cyclic estrogen and progestin are used in individuals reared as females in whom a uterus is present. In males, virilization is achieved by the administration of a repository preparation of testosterone.

In all patients, continuing endocrinologic and psychologic support are critical aspects of follow-up and should be available throughout infancy, childhood, and adolescence. Patients should have progressive, step-by-step, age-appropriate discussion about their diagnosis, its pathophysiology, their quality of life, and their potential for fertility. Disclosure is critical. However, in those mature adult intersex patients who are well-adjusted and happy with their lives and their "assigned" gender identity, disclosure should be on a "need to know" basis. The patient (when possible) and the parents should be involved in decisions about surgery and sex hormone replacement.

In sum, the physician and the consortium concerned with the diagnosis, selection of sex of rearing, and management of the infant with intersexuality must be prepared to address the complex ethical, cultural, social, religious, clinical, and surgical issues presented by the intersex patient in order to maximize the patient's potential for a well-adjusted, normal life. This task is complicated now by the lack of complete outcome data.

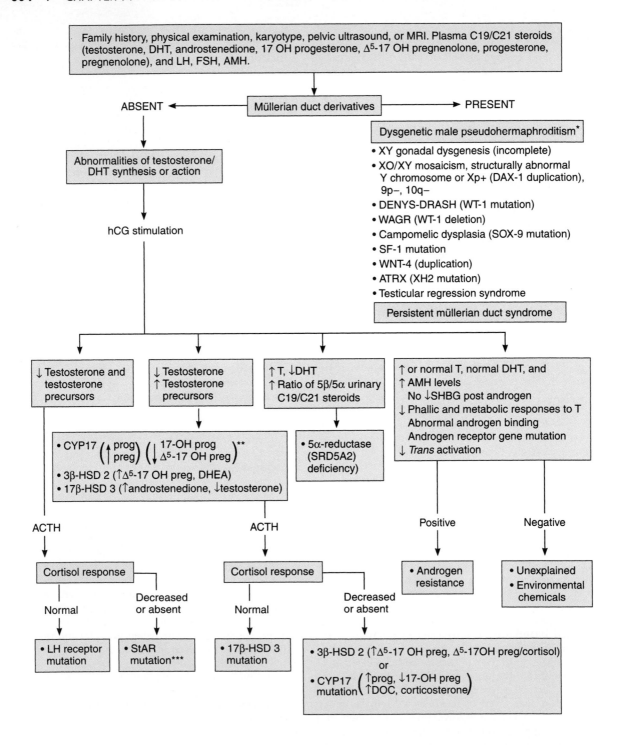

Figure 14–21. Steps in the diagnosis of male pseudohermaphroditism in infancy and childhood. Step 1 involves initial workup and provisional diagnosis (see Figure 14–20). Step 2 (this figure) is utilized in selected cases. (Reproduced, with permission, from Grumbach MM, Hughes IA, Conte FA: Disorders of sex differentiation. In: Larsen PR et al [editors]: *Williams Textbook of Endocrinology,* 10th ed. Saunders, 2002.)

*Patients with dysgenetic male pseudohermaphroditism may manifest varying degrees of testicular dysgenesis with consequent testosterone/DHT or AMH deficiency (or both). Therefore, not all patients may manifest either ambiguous genitalia or the presence of müllerian ducts.

**CYP17 (P450c17) catalyzes the 17-hydroxylation of progesterone and pregnenolone to 17-hydroxyprogesterone and Δ^5-17-hydroxypregnenolone as well as the scission (lyase) of 17-hydroxypregnenolone to DHEA. Patients with 17,20-lyase deficiency have elevated levels of 17-hydroxyprogesterone and Δ^5-17-hydroxypregnenolone in relation to androstenedione and DHEA either before or after hCG stimulation.

***The StAR (steroidogenic acute regulatory) protein is involved in the transport of cholesterol from the outer to the inner mitochondrial membrane, where the enzyme P450scc resides. Patients with a mutation in the gene for this protein have a markedly diminished ability to convert cholesterol to Δ5-17-hydroxypregnenolone, though their P450scc enzymatic activity is intact, and they manifest congenital lipoid adrenal hyperplasia. WAGR, Wilms' tumor, aniridia, genital anomalies, and mental retardation; SF-1, steroidogenic factor-1; CYP17, 17α-hydroxylase/17,20-lyase; 3β-HSD 2, 3β-hydroxysteroid dehydrogenase/Δ^5-isomerase; 17β-HSD 3, 17β-hydroxysteroid dehydrogenase (oxidoreductase); T, testosterone; DHT, dihydrotestosterone; AMH, antimüllerian hormone; SHBG, sex hormone-binding globulin; DHEA, dehydroepiandrosterone.

REFERENCES

Achermann JC et al: A mutation in the gene encoding steroidogenic factor-1 causes XY sex reversal and adrenal failure in humans. Nat Genet 1999;22:125.

Aittomaki K et al: Mutation in the follicle-stimulating hormone receptor gene causes hereditary hypergonadotropic ovarian failure. Cell 1995;82:959.

Andersson S et al: Molecular genetics and pathophysiology of 17β-hydroxysteroid dehydrogenase 3 deficiency. J Clin Endocrinol Metab 1996;81:130.

Avner P, Heard E: X-chromosome inactivation: counting, choice and initiation. Nat Rev Genet 2001;2:59. [PMID 11253071]

Beau I et al: A novel phenotype related to partial loss of function: Mutations of the follicle stimulating hormone receptor. J Clin Invest 1998;102:1352.

Bin Abbas B et al: Congenital hypogonadotropic hypogonadism and micropenis: Effects of testosterone treatment on adult penile size—Why sex reversal is not indicated. J Pediatr 1999; 134:599.

Bose HS et al: The physiology and genetics of congenital lipoid adrenal hyperplasia. N Engl J Med 1996;335:1870.

Canning CA, Lovell-Badge R: Sry and sex determination: how lazy can it be? Trends Genet 2002;18:111. [PMID 1858826]

Cerame BI et al: Prenatal diagnosis and treatment of 11β-hydroxylase deficiency congenital adrenal hyperplasia resulting in normal female genitalia. J Clin Endocrinol Metab 1999; 84:3129.

Chu J et al: Male fertility is compatible with an Arg[840] Cys substitution in the AR in a large Chinese family affected with divergent phenotypes of the androgen insensitivity syndrome. J Clin Endocrinol Metab 2002;87:347. [PMID 11788673]

Clarkson MJ, Harley VR: Sex with two SOX on: SRY and SOX9 in testes development. Trends Endocrine Metab 2002;13:106. [PMID11893523]

Conte FA et al: A syndrome of female pseudohermaphroditism, hypergonadotropic hypogonadism, and multicystic ovaries associated with missense mutations in the gene encoding aromatase (P450arom). J Clin Endocrinol Metab 1994;78:1287.

Conte FA, Grumbach MM: Diagnosis and management of ambiguous external genitalia. Endocrinologist 2003. [In press.]

Diamond M, Sigmundson HK: Sex reassignment at birth. Long-term review and clinical implications. Arch Pediatr Adolesc Med 1997;151:298.

Donahoue PA et al: Congenital adrenal hyperplasia. In: *The Metabolic and Molecular Bases of Inherited Disease,* 7th ed. Scriver CR et al (editors). McGraw-Hill, 1995.

Donahoue PA et al: Congential adrenal hyperplasia. In: Scriver CR et al (editors): *The Metabolic and Molecular Bases of Inherited Disease,* 8th ed. McGraw-Hill, 2001.

El'Sheikh M et al: Turner's syndrome in adulthood. Endocr Rev 2002;23:120. [PMID 11844747]

Evans JA et al: Agenesis of the penis: patterns of associated malformations. Am J Med Genet 1999;84:47.

Feldman KW, Smith DW: Fetal phallic growth and penile standards for newborn male infants. J Pediatr 1975;86:395.

Ferguson-Smith MA, Goodfellow PN: SRY and primary sex reversal syndromes. In: Scriver CR et al (editors): *The Metabolic and Molecular Bases of Inherited Disease,* 7th ed. McGraw-Hill, 1995.

Geller DH et al: The genetic and functional basis of isolated 17,20-lyase deficiency. Nat Genet 1997;17:201.

Griffen JE, Wilson JD: The androgen resistance syndromes: Steroid 5α reductase 2 deficiency, testicular feminization, and related syndromes. In: Scriver CR et al (editors): *The Metabolic and Molecular Bases of Inherited Disease,* 8th ed. McGraw-Hill, 2001.

Grumbach MM, Auchus R: Estrogen consequences and implications of human mutations in synthesis and action. J Clin Endocrinol Metab 1999;84:4677. [PMID 10599737]

Grumbach MM, Hughes IA, Conte FA: Disorders of sex differentiaiton. In: *Williams Textbook of Endocrinology,* 10th ed. Larsen PR et al (editors). Saunders, 2002.

Hadjiathanasiou CG et al: True hermaphroditism: Genetic variants and clinical management. J Pediatr 1994;125:738.

Harada N et al: Biochemical and molecular genetic analyses on placental aromatase (P450arom) deficiency. J Biol Chem 1992; 267:4781.

Hastie N: Life, sex and WT1 isoforms—3 amino acids make a difference. Cell 2001;106:3911. [PMID 11525724]

Hughes IA et al: Developmental aspects of androgen action. Mol Cell Endocrinol 2001;185:33. [PMID 11738792]

Imbeaud S et al: A 27 base-pair deletion of the anti-müllerian Type II receptor gene is the most common cause of the persistent müllerian duct syndrome. Hum Mol Genet 1996;5:1269.

Imbeaud S et al: Insensitivity to anti-müllerian hormone due to a mutation in the human anti-müllerian hormone receptor. Nat Genet 1995;11:382.

Jimenez R, Burgos M: Mammalian sex determination: Joining pieces of the genetic puzzle. Bioessays 1998;20:696.

Jordan BK et al: Familial mutation in testes-determining gene SRY shared by XY female and normal father. J Clin Endocrinol Metab 2002;87:3428. [PMID 12107262]

Jordan BK et al: Up-regulation of WNT-4 signaling and dosage-sensitive sex reversal in humans. Am J Hum Genet 2001;68: 1102. [PMID 11351829]

Koopman P et al: Male development of chromosomally female mice transgenic for SRY. Nature 1991;351:17.

Kreidberg JA et al: WT-1 is required in early kidney development. Cell 1993;74:679.

Kuhnle U et al: The impact of culture on sex assignment and gender development in intersex patients. Perspect Biol Med 2002;45:85. [PMID 11796934]

Latronico AC et al: A homozygous microdeletion in helix 7 of the luteinizing hormone receptor associated with familial testicular and ovarian resistance is due to both decreased cell surface expression and impaired effector activation by the cell surface receptor. Mol Endocrinol 1998;123:442.

Lo JC et al: Normal female infants born of mothers with classic congenital adrenal hyperplasia due to 21-hydroxylase deficiency. J Clin Endocrinol Metab 1999;84:930.

Lutfallah C et al: Newly proposed hormonal criteria via genotypic proof for type II 3beta-hydroxysteroid dehydrogenase deficiency. J Clin Endocrinol Metab 2002;87:2611. [PMID 12050224]

Mendez JP et al: A reliable endocrine test with human menopausal gonadotropins for diagnosis of true hermaphroditism in early infancy. J Clin Endocrinol Metab 1998;83:3523.

Mendonca BB et al: Female pseudohermaphrodism caused by a novel homozygous missense mutation of the GR gene. J Clin Endocrinol Metab 2002;87:1805. [PMID 11932321]

Mendonca BB et al: Male pseudohermaphrodism due to 17 beta-hydroxysteroid dehydrogenase 3 deficiency. Diagnosis, psychological evaluation, and management. Medicine (Baltimore) 2000;79:299. [PMID 11039078]

Meyer-Bahlburg HFL: Gender assignment in intersexuality. J Hum Psychol Hum Sexuality 1998;10:1.

Miller WL: Prenatal treatment of congenital adrenal hyperplasia: A promising experimental therapy of unproven safety. Trends Endocrinol Metab 1998;9:290.

Moghrabi N, Andersson S: 17β-Hydroxysteroid dehydrogenases: Physiologic roles in health and disease. Trends Endocrinol Metab 1998;9:265.

Morel Y et al: Aetiological diagnosis of male sex ambiguity. A collaborative study. Eur J Pediatr 2002;161:49. [PMID 11808880]

Morishima A et al: Aromatase deficiency in male and female siblings caused by a novel mutation and the physiological role of estrogens. J Clin Endocrinol Metab 1995;80:3689.

Muller J et al: Management of males with 45,X/46,XY gonadal dysgenesis. Horm Res 1999;52:11. [PMID 10640893]

Nachtigall MW et al: Wilms tumor 1 and Dax-1 modulate the orphan nuclear receptor SF-1 in sex-specific gene expression. Cell 1998;93:445.

New MI et al: Prenatal diagnosis for congenital adrenal hyperplasia in 532 pregnancies. J Clin Endocrinol Metab 2001;86:5651. [PMID 11739415]

Oberfield SW et al: Clitoral size in full term infants. Am J Perinat 1989;4:453. [PMID 31125757]

Ozisk G et al: The role of SF1 in adrenal and reproductive function: insights from naturally occurring mutations in humans. Mol Genet Metab 2002;76:85. [PMID 12083805]

Pontiggia A et al: Sex-reversing mutations affect the architecture of SRY-DNA complexes. EMBO J 1994;13:6115.

Quigley CA et al: Androgen receptor defects: Historical, clinical and molecular properties. Endocr Rev 1995;6:271.

Rao E et al: Pseudoautosomal deletions encompassing a novel homeobox gene cause growth failure in idiopathic short stature and Turner syndrome. Nat Genet 1997;16:54.

Raymond CS et al: A region of human chromosome 9p required for testis development contains two genes related to known sexual regulators. Hum Mol Genet 1999;8:989.

Reiner WG: Sex assignment in the neonate with intersex or inadequate genitalia. Arch Pediatr Adolesc Med 1997;151:1044.

Rey R: Endocrine, paracrine and cellular regulation of postnatal anti-müllerian hormone secretion by Sertoli cells. Trends Endocrinol Metab 1998;9:271.

Richter-Unruh A et al: Leydig cell hypoplasia: Cases with new mutations, new polymorphisms and cases without mutations in the luteinizing hormone receptor gene. Clin Endocrinol 2002;56:103. [PMID 11849253]

Russell DW, Wilson JD: Steroid 5α-reductase: Two genes/two enzymes. Annu Rev Biochem 1994;63:25.

Schonfeld WA, Beebe GW: Normal growth and variation in male genitalia from birth to maturity. J Urol 1942;64:759.

Short RV (editor): *The Genetics and Biology of Sex Determination.* Novartis Foundation Symposium 244-2002. Wiley, 2002.

Slijper FM et al: Long term psychological evaluation of intersex children. Arch Sex Behav 1998;27:125.

Speiser P (editor): Congenital adrenal hyperplasia. Endocrinol Metab Clin North Am 2001;30:1.

Swain A et al: Dax-1 antagonizes Sry action in mammalian sex determination. Nature 1998;391:761.

Tajima T et al: Heterozygous mutation in the cholesterol side-chain cleavage enzyme (p450scc) gene in a patient with 46,XY sex reversal and adrenal insufficiency. J Clin Endocrinol Metab 2001;86:3820. [PMID 11502818]

Tillman C, Capel B: Cellular and molecular pathways regulating mammalian sex determination. Recent Prog Horm Res 2002; 57:1. [PMID 12017538]

Tuladhar R et al: Establishment of a normal range of penile length in preterm infants. J Paediatr Child Health 1998;34:471.

Van Niekerk WA: *True Hermaphroditism.* Harper & Row, 1974.

Wajnrajch MP, New MI: Defects in adrenal steroidogenesis, In: De Groot LJ, Jameson JL (editors): *Endocrinology.* Saunders, 2001.

Wessels H et al: Penile length in the flaccid and erect status: Guidelines for penile augmentation. J Urol 1996;156:995.

Wilson JD et al: Steroid 5α-reductase deficiency. Endocr Rev 1993;14:577.

Wilson JD: Androgens, androgen receptors and male gender role behavior. Horm Behav 2001;40:358. [PMID 11534997]

Wilson JD: The role of 5alpha-reduction in steroid hormone physiology. Reprod Fertil Devel 2001;13:573. [PMID 11999320]

Yu RN et al: Role of AHCH in gonadal development and gametogenesis. Nat Genet 1998;20:353.

Puberty

Dennis Styne, MD

ACTH	Adrenocorticotropic hormone		**IGF-1**	Insulin-like growth factor-1
cAMP	Cyclic adenosine monophosphate		**IRMA**	Immunoradiometric assay
DHEA	Dehydroepiandrosterone		**LH**	Luteinizing hormone
DHEAS	Dehydroepiandrosterone sulfate		**PRL**	Prolactin
FSH	Follicle-stimulating hormone		**PSA**	Prostate-specific antigen
GH	Growth hormone		**RIA**	Radioimmunoassay
GnRH	Gonadotropin-releasing hormone		**SHBG**	Sex hormone-binding globulin
hCG	Human chorionic gonadotropin		**TGF-2**	Transforming growth factor-2
hGH	Human growth hormone		**TSH**	Thyroid-stimulating hormone (thyrotropin)
ICMA	Immunochemiluminometric assay			

Puberty is best considered as one stage in the continuing process of growth and development that begins during gestation and continues until the end of reproductive life. After an interval of childhood quiescence—the juvenile pause—the hypothalamic pulse generator increases activity in the peripubertal period, just before the physical changes of puberty commence. This leads to increased secretion of pituitary gonadotropins and, subsequently, gonadal sex steroids that bring about secondary sexual development, the pubertal growth spurt, and fertility. Historical records show that the age at onset of particular stages of puberty in boys and girls in Western countries has steadily declined over the last several hundred years; this is probably due to improvements in socioeconomic conditions, nutrition, and, therefore, the general state of health during that period. However, this trend ceased during the last 5 decades in developed societies, suggesting the attainment of optimal conditions to allow puberty to begin at a genetically determined age.

Many endogenous and exogenous factors can alter age at onset of puberty. Moderate obesity may be associated with an earlier onset, while severe obesity may delay puberty. Indeed, there is evidence that the age at onset of puberty might once again be decreasing, apparently due to the increasing prevalence of obesity in young children. Chronic illness and malnutrition often delay puberty. There is a significant concordance of age at menarche between mother-daughter pairs and within ethnic populations, indicating the influence of genetic factors.

PHYSIOLOGY OF PUBERTY

Physical Changes Associated With Puberty

Descriptive standards proposed by Tanner for assessing pubertal development in males and females are in wide use. They focus attention on specific details of the examination and make it possible to objectively record subtle progression of secondary sexual development that may otherwise be overlooked. Self-assessment of pubertal development by subjects using reference pictures has been attempted, but reliability is poor. Thus, physical examination is necessary to reliably determine if puberty has begun or is proceeding.

A. FEMALE CHANGES

The first sign of puberty in the female, as noted in longitudinal studies, is an increase in growth velocity that heralds the beginning of the pubertal growth spurt; girls are not usually examined frequently enough to

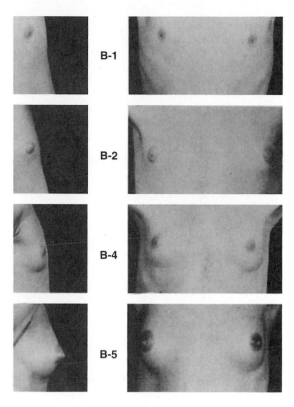

Figure 15–1. Stages of breast development, according to Marshall and Tanner. (Photographs from van Wieringen JC et al, 1971; with permission.) **Stage B1:** Preadolescent; elevation of papilla only. **Stage B2:** Breast bud stage; elevation of breast and papilla as a small mound, and enlargement of areolar diameter. **Stage B3:** Further enlargement of breast and areola, with no separation of their contours. **Stage B4:** Projection of areola and papilla to form a secondary mound above the level of the breast (not shown). **Stage B5:** Mature stage; projection of papilla only, owing to recession of the areola to the general contour of the breast.

demonstrate this change in clinical practice, so breast development is the first sign of puberty noted by most examiners. Breast development (Figure 15–1) is stimulated chiefly by ovarian estrogen secretion, though other hormones also play a part. The size and shape of the breasts may be determined by genetic and nutritional factors, but the characteristics of the stages in Figure 15–1 are similar in all females. Standards are available for the change in areolar (nipple) plateau diameter during puberty: Nipple diameter changes little from stages B1 to B3 (mean of 3–4 mm) but enlarges substantially in subsequent stages (mean of 7.4 mm at stage B4 to 10 mm at stage B5), presumably as a result of increased estrogen secretion at the time of menarche. Other features reflecting estrogen action include enlargement of the labia minora and majora, dulling of the vaginal mucosa from its prepubertal reddish hue (due to cornification of the vaginal epithelium), and production of a clear or slightly whitish vaginal secretion prior to menarche. Pubic hair development (Figure 15–2) is determined chiefly by adrenal and ovarian androgen secretion. Breast development and growth of pubic hair usually proceed at similar rates, but because

discrepancies in rates of advancement are possible, it is best to stage breast development separately from pubic hair progression.

Uterine size and shape change with pubertal development as reflected by ultrasonographic studies; with prolonged estrogen stimulation, the fundus:cervix ratio increases, leading to a bulbous form, and the uterus elongates from less than 3 cm to 5 cm or more. Ovaries enlarge with puberty from a volume of less than 1 mL to 2–10 mL. Small cysts are normally present in prepubertal girls and a "multicystic" appearance develops with puberty, but on pathologic examination there is not the polycystic appearance seen in abnormalities of puberty or during reproduction. Ultrasonographers can determine the developmental stage of the uterus and ovaries by comparing the results with established standards.

B. MALE CHANGES

The first sign of normal puberty in boys is usually an increase in the size of the testes to over 2.5 cm in the longest diameter, excluding the epididymis: this is equivalent to a testicular volume of 4 mL or more.

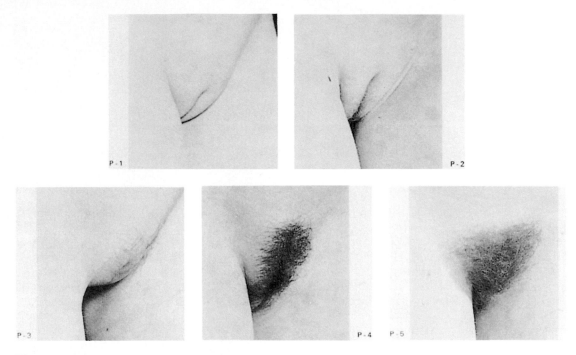

Figure 15–2. Stages of female pubic hair development, according to Marshall and Tanner. (Photographs from van Wieringen JC et al, 1971; with permission.) **Stage P1:** Preadolescent; the vellus over the area is no further developed than that over the anterior abdominal wall, ie, no pubic hair. **Stage P2:** Sparse growth of long, slightly pigmented, downy hair, straight or only slightly curled, appearing chiefly along the labia. This stage is difficult to see on photographs and is subtle. **Stage P3:** Hair is considerably darker, coarser, and curlier. The hair spreads sparsely over the superior junction of the labia majora. **Stage P4:** Hair is now adult in type, but the area covered by it is still considerably smaller than in most adults. There is no spread to the medial surface of the thighs. **Stage P5:** Hair is adult in quantity and type, distributed as an inverse triangle of the classic feminine pattern. Spread is to the medial surface of the thighs but not up the linea alba or elsewhere above the base of the inverse triangle.

Most of the increase in testicular size is due to seminiferous tubular development secondary to stimulation by FSH, with a smaller component due to Leydig cell stimulation by LH. Thus, if only Leydig cells are stimulated, as in an hCG-secreting tumor, the testis does not grow as large as in normal puberty. Pubic hair development is caused by adrenal and testicular androgen secretion and is classified separately from genital development, as noted in Figure 15–3. A longitudinal study of over 500 boys suggests adding a stage 2a to the classic five stages of pubertal development. Stage 2a indicates the absence of pubic hair in the presence of a testicular volume of 3 mL or more. Further pubertal development occurred in 82% of the subjects in stage 2a after the passage of 6 months: thus, reaching stage 2a would allow the examiner to reassure a patient that further spontaneous development is likely soon. The appear-

ance of spermatozoa in early morning urinary specimens (spermarche) occurs at a mean chronologic age of 13.4 years or a similar bone age; this usually occurs at gonadal stage 3–4 and pubic hair stage 2–4. If puberty starts at an earlier or later chronologic age, the age of spermarche changes accordingly with reference to chronologic age although spermarche occurs in such patients at the same range of gonadal or pubic hair stages. Remarkably, spermaturia is more common earlier in puberty than later, suggesting that sperm are directly released into the urine early in puberty while ejaculation may be responsible for the presence of sperm in the urines of older children.

Boys are reported with spermaturia and no secondary sexual development.

Thus, boys are reproductively mature prior to physical maturity and certainly prior to psychologic maturity.

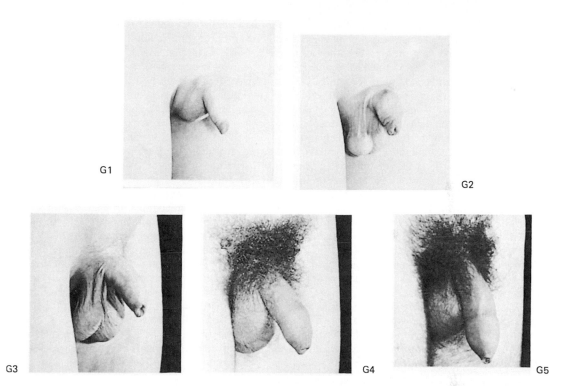

Figure 15–3. Stages of male genital development and pubic hair development, according to Marshall and Tanner. (Photographs from van Wieringen JC et al, 1971; with permission.) **Genital:** *Stage G1:* Preadolescent. Testes, scrotum, and penis are about the same size and proportion as in early childhood. *Stage G2:* The scrotum and testes have enlarged, and there is a change in the texture and some reddening of the scrotal skin. There is no enlargement of the penis. *Stage G3:* Growth of the penis has occurred, at first mainly in length but with some increase in breadth; further growth of testes and scrotum. *Stage G4:* Penis further enlarged in length and girth with development of glans. Testes and scrotum further enlarged. The scrotal skin has further darkened. *Stage G5:* Genitalia adult in size and shape. No further enlargement takes place after stage G5 is reached. **Pubic hair:** *Stage P1:* Preadolescent. The vellus is no further developed than that over the abdominal wall, ie, no pubic hair. *Stage P2:* Sparse growth of long, slightly pigmented, downy hair, straight or only slightly curled, appearing chiefly at the base of the penis. This is subtle. *Stage P3:* Hair is considerably darker, coarser, and curlier and spreads sparsely. *Stage P4:* Hair is now adult in type, but the area it covers is still considerably smaller than in most adults. There is no spread to the medial surface of the thighs. *Stage P5:* Hair is adult in quantity and type, distributed as an inverse triangle. Spread is to the medial surface of the thighs but not up the linea alba or elsewhere above the base of the inverse triangle. Most men will have further spread of pubic hair.

C. AGE AT ONSET

Ideally, the upper and lower boundaries encompassing the age at onset of puberty should be set at 2.5 SD above and below the mean. Previously, there was no comprehensive study of the start of secondary sexual development adequate to determine the lower limits of normal in United States children, so European stan-dards, primarily those of Tanner, were modified for the USA. However, a study conducted in medical offices by specially trained pediatricians studying 17,070 girls brought in for routine visits has helped establish norms for United States girls. The study revealed that 3% of white girls reach stage 2 breast development by 6 years of age and 5% by 7 years, while 6.4% of black girls had stage 2 breast development by 6 years and 15.4% by 7 years. While this was not a randomly chosen population sampled by longitudinal study, it is the largest study available. These data indicate that the diagnosis of precocious puberty is best defined as secondary sexual development starting prior to 6 years in black girls and prior to 7 years in white girls who are otherwise healthy. It is essential to use such guidelines only in healthy girls with absolutely no signs of neurologic or other disease that might pathologically advance puberty. However, recent data indicate that boys with elevated BMIs have earlier onset of puberty. There has otherwise been no change in the age at onset of puberty in boys, so 9 years is taken as the lower limit of normal pubertal development in males. The mean age at menarche in the United States is 12.8 years and has not varied since the last government study was published in 1974. White girls have menarche later (12.9 years) than black girls (12.3 years), but this 6-month difference is less than the 1-year difference in the age at onset of puberty between the two groups.

Late onset of pubertal development may indicate hypothalamic, pituitary, or gonadal failure. The time from onset of puberty to complete adult development is also of importance; delays in reaching subsequent stages may indicate any type of hypogonadism.

D. GROWTH SPURT

The striking increase in growth velocity in puberty (pubertal growth spurt) is under complex endocrine control. Hypothyroidism decreases or eliminates the pubertal growth spurt. The amplitude of growth hormone secretion increases in puberty, as does production of IGF-I; peak serum IGF-I concentrations are reached about 1 year after peak growth velocity, and serum IGF-I levels remain above normal adult levels for up to 4 years thereafter. GH and sex steroids are important in the pubertal growth spurt; when either or both are deficient, the growth spurt is decreased or absent. Sex steroids indirectly stimulate IGF-I production by increasing the secretion of GH and also directly stimulate IGF-I production in cartilage. Estrogen has recently been shown to be the most important factor in stimulating maturation of the chondrocytes and osteoblasts, ultimately leading to epiphysial fusion. A patient reported with estrogen receptor deficiency was tall, with continued growth past the age of 20 years in spite of a remarkable retardation of skeletal maturation (and decreased bone density). Patients with aromatase deficiency and therefore impaired conversion of testosterone to estrogen also demonstrate diminished advancement of bone age and decreased bone density as well as continued growth extending into the third decade. With exogenous estrogen administration, the bone age advanced and a growth spurt occurred. One

affected 46,XX individual had virilized genitalia at birth and further virilization at a pubertal age with the additional feature of multicystic ovaries. The patient, in spite of high serum testosterone concentrations, had elevated FSH and LH in the absence of estrogen production. These patients demonstrate the key role played by estrogen in advancing bone age and bringing about the cessation of growth by epiphysial fusion as well as the importance of estrogen in increasing bone density.

It is essential to realize that a pubertal growth spurt occurring in a young patient with precocious puberty may increase the growth rate sufficiently to mask the presence of coexisting GH deficiency. This situation may occur, for example, in a child with a brain tumor causing precocious puberty treated with radiation that subsequently decreases GH secretion.

In girls, the pubertal growth spurt begins in early puberty and is mostly completed by menarche. In boys, the pubertal growth spurt occurs toward the end of puberty, at an average age 2 years older than in girls. Total height attained during the growth spurt in girls is about 25 cm; in boys, it is about 28 cm. The mean adult height differential of 12 cm between men and women is due in part to heights already attained before onset of the pubertal growth spurt and in part to the height gained during the spurt.

E. CHANGES IN BODY COMPOSITION

Changes in body composition are also prominent during pubertal development. Prepubertal boys and girls start with equal lean body mass, skeletal mass, and body fat, but at maturity men have approximately 1½ times the lean body mass, skeletal mass, and muscle mass of women, while women have twice as much body fat as men. Attainment of peak values of percentage of body fat, lean body mass, and bone mineral density is earlier by several years in girls than in boys, as is the earlier peak of height velocity and velocity of weight gain in girls.

The most important phases of bone accretion occur during infancy and during puberty. Girls reach peak mineralization between 14 and 16 years of age, while boys reach a later peak at 17.5 years; both milestones occur after peak height velocity (Figure 15–4). The density of bone is determined by genes as decreased bone mass is found in familial patterns even if subjects are studied before puberty. Patients with delay in puberty for any reason will have a significant decrease in bone accretion. Moderate exercise will increase bone mass, but excessive exercise will itself delay puberty; the ultimate outcome of excessive exercise is the combination of exercise-induced amenorrhea, premature osteoporosis, and disordered eating known as the female athletic triad.

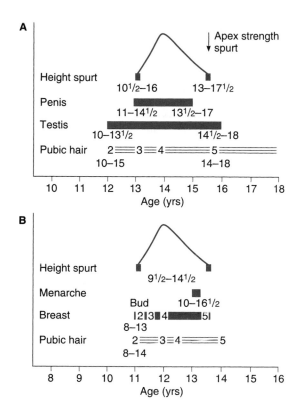

Figure 15–4. Sequence of secondary sexual development in British males **(A)** and females **(B)**. The range of ages in Britain is indicated. American boys and girls start pubertal stages earlier than British children (see text). (Reproduced, with permission, from Marshall WA, Tanner JM: Variations in the pattern of pubertal changes in boys. Arch Dis Child 1970;45:13.)

Unfortunately in the United States, only a minority of adolescents receive the recommended daily allowance of calcium, and a future epidemic of osteopenia or even osteoporosis in normal subjects who have this deficiency is a possibility. It is especially important to ensure adequate calcium intake in delayed or absent puberty and in patients treated with GnRH agonists.

F. Other Changes of Puberty

Other changes that are characteristic of puberty are mediated either directly or indirectly by the change in sex steroids. Bone density increases during normal pubertal development. Seborrheic dermatitis may appear at this age. The mouth flora changes, and periodontal disease, rare in childhood, may appear at this stage. Insulin resistance intensifies in normal adolescents as well as those with type 1 diabetes mellitus; this may be related to the increased GH levels of puberty.

Endocrine Changes from Fetal Life to Puberty

Pituitary gonadotropin secretion is controlled by the hypothalamus, which releases pulses of gonadotropin-releasing hormone (GnRH) into the pituitary-portal system to reach the anterior pituitary gland. Control of GnRH secretion is exerted by a "hypothalamic pulse generator" in the arcuate nucleus. It is sensitive to feedback control from sex steroids and inhibin, a gonadal protein product that controls the frequency and amplitude of gonadotropin secretion during development in both sexes and during the progression of the menstrual cycle in females (see Chapter 13). Individual GnRH neurons have an intrinsic pulsatility that may be the basis of the pattern of GnRH secretion.

In males, luteinizing hormone (LH) stimulates the Leydig cells to secrete testosterone, while follicle-stimulating hormone (FSH) stimulates the Sertoli cells to produce inhibin. Inhibin feeds back on the hypothalamic-pituitary axis to inhibit FSH. Inhibin is also released in a pulsatile pattern, but concentrations do not change with pubertal progression. In females, FSH stimulates the granulosa cells to produce estrogen and the follicles to secrete inhibin, while LH appears to play a minor role in the endocrine milieu until menarche, when it triggers ovulation and later stimulates the theca cells to secrete androgens (see Chapters 12 and 13).

A. Fetal Life

The concept of the continuum of development between the fetus and the adult is well illustrated by the changes that occur in the hypothalamic-pituitary-gonadal axis. Gonadotropins are demonstrable in fetal pituitary glands and serum during the first trimester. The pituitary content of gonadotropins rises to a plateau at mid gestation. Serum concentrations of LH and FSH rise to a peak at mid gestation and then gradually decrease until term. During the first half of gestation, hypothalamic GnRH content also increases, and the hypophysial-portal circulation achieves anatomic maturity. These data are compatible with a theory of early unrestrained GnRH secretion stimulating pituitary gonadotropin secretion, followed by the appearance of factors that inhibit GnRH release and decrease gonadotropin secretion after mid gestation. Since the male fetus has measurable serum testosterone concentrations but lower serum gonadotropin concentrations than the female fetus, negative feedback inhibition of gonadotropin secretion by testosterone appears operative after mid gestation.

B. CHANGES AT BIRTH

At term, serum gonadotropin concentrations are suppressed, but with postnatal clearance of high circulating estrogen concentrations, negative inhibition is reduced and postnatal peaks of serum LH and FSH are measurable for several months after birth. Serum testosterone concentrations may be increased to midpubertal levels during the several months after birth in normal males. While episodic peaks of serum gonadotropins may occur until 2 years of age, serum gonadotropin concentrations are low during later years in normal childhood. These peaks of gonadotropins and sex steroids in normal infants complicate the diagnosis of central precocious puberty at these youngest ages since it is difficult to decide whether to attribute the gonadotropin and sex steroid peaks to central precocious puberty or to normal physiology.

C. THE JUVENILE PAUSE OR THE MID CHILDHOOD NADIR OF GONADOTROPIN SECRETION

While serum gonadotropin concentrations are low in mid childhood, sensitive assays indicate that pulsatile secretion occurs and that the onset of puberty is heralded more by an increase in amplitude of secretory events than a change in frequency. Twenty-four-hour mean concentrations of LH, FSH, and testosterone rise measurably within 1 year after the development of physical pubertal changes. Patients with gonadal failure—such as those with the syndrome of gonadal dysgenesis (Turner's syndrome)—demonstrate an exaggeration of the normal pattern of gonadotropin secretion, with exceedingly high concentrations of serum LH and FSH during the first several years of life (see Chapter 14). Such patients show that negative feedback inhibition is active during childhood; without sex steroid or inhibin secretion to exert inhibition, serum gonadotropin values are greatly elevated. During mid childhood, normal individuals and patients with primary hypogonadism have lower serum gonadotropin levels than they do in the neonatal period, but the range of serum gonadotropin concentrations in hypogonadal patients during mid childhood is still higher than that found in healthy children of the same age. The decrease in serum gonadotropin concentrations in primary agonadal children during mid childhood is incompletely understood but has been attributed to an increase in the central nervous system inhibition of gonadotropin secretion during these years. Thus, the juvenile pause in normals and those with primary gonadal failure appear to be due to central nervous system restraint of GnRH secretion.

D. PERIPUBERTAL GONADOTROPIN INCREASE

Prepubertal children demonstrate a circadian rhythm of LH and FSH secretion with the rhythm of sex steroid secretion lagging behind the gonadotropin rhythm, the delay presumably due to the time necessary for biosynthesis of sex steroids. Thus, the changes that are described below which occur at puberty do not arise de novo but are based upon preexisting patterns of endocrine secretion. In the peripubertal period, endogenous GnRH secretion increases in amplitude and frequency during the early hours of sleep and serum testosterone and estrogen concentrations rise several hours later, suggesting that biosynthesis or aromatization occurs during the period of delay—a pattern that differs from the prepubertal period mainly in the increased amplitude of the secretion encountered in puberty (Figure 15–5). As puberty progresses in both sexes, the peaks of serum LH and FSH occur more often during waking hours; and, finally, in late puberty, the peaks occur at all times, eliminating the diurnal variation.

During the peripubertal period of endocrine change prior to secondary sexual development, gonadotropin secretion becomes less sensitive to negative feedback inhibition. Before this time, a small dose of exogenous sex steroids virtually eliminates gonadotropin secretion,

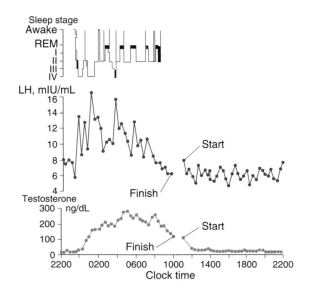

Figure 15–5. Plasma LH and testosterone measured during a 24-hour period in a 14-year-old boy in pubertal stage 2. Samples collected at night are displayed with electroencephalographic sleep stages, but there is no relationship between LH and the depth of sleep stages. (Reproduced, with permission, from Boyar RM et al: Simultaneous augmented secretion of luteinizing hormone and testosterone during sleep. J Clin Invest 1974; 54:609.)

while afterward a far larger dose is required to suppress serum FSH and LH. In prepuberty or early puberty, naltrexone, an opioid receptor antagonist, can completely suppress gonadotropin secretion as a consequence of its weak opioid effects, while after mid puberty the anti-opioid effects predominate and gonadotropin secretion increases, demonstrating an increase in resistance to opioids with pubertal development.

Most studies of gonadotropin secretion measure gonadotropin concentrations by radioimmunoassay (RIA). However, highly sensitive "sandwich" assays (immunoradiometric assay [IRMA]) and immunochemiluminometric assays (ICMA) have been developed for gonadotropin determination. They can be used to indicate the state of pubertal development based on basal samples without the necessity for GnRH testing. Elevated LH values (> 0.3 IU/L) determined by third-generation assays in random blood samples are highly predictive of elevated peak GnRH-stimulated LH and therefore indicate the onset of central precocious puberty or normal puberty. These third-generation assays further reflect the remarkable logarithmic increase in spontaneous LH secretion in the latest stages of prepuberty and earliest stages of puberty as the testicular volume increases from 1 mL to 10 mL; these increases in serum LH are far greater proportionately than those found in the last stages of pubertal development. The magnitude of increase in serum testosterone is also greater in the early stages of puberty and correlates with the increase in serum LH during this same period of early pubertal development.

E. SEX STEROID SECRETION

Sex steroid secretion is correlated with the development of gonadotropin secretion. During the postnatal period of increased episodic gonadotropin secretion, plasma concentrations of gonadal steroids are episodically elevated. This indicates the potential for secretory activity in the neonatal gonad. Later, when gonadotropin secretion decreases in mid childhood, gonadal activity decreases, but testes can still be stimulated by LH or hCG and ovaries by FSH with resulting secretion of gonadal steroids. An ultrasensitive estradiol assay demonstrates higher values of serum estradiol in prepubertal girls than prepubertal boys, indicating definite basal ovarian activity during the juvenile pause. With the onset of puberty, serum gonadal steroid concentrations progressively increase. While sex steroids are secreted in a diurnal rhythm in early puberty, they are bound to sex hormone-binding globulin, and the half-life of sex steroids is longer than that of gonadotropins. Thus, random daytime measurements of serum sex steroids are more helpful in determining pubertal status than random measurements of serum gonadotropins.

Most (97–99%) of the circulating estradiol and testosterone is associated with sex hormone-binding globulin (SHBG). The free hormone is the active fraction, but SHBG modulates the activity of the total testosterone and estradiol. Prepubertal boys and girls have equal concentrations of SHBG, but because testosterone decreases SHBG and estrogen increases SHBG, adult males have only half the concentration of SHBG than that of adult females. Thus, lower SHBG levels amplify androgen effect in men; while adult men have 20 times the amount of plasma testosterone that adult women have, adult men have 40 times the amount of free testosterone that adult women have (see Chapter 12).

F. GnRH STIMULATION

The use of intravenous GnRH has further clarified the pattern of pubertal development. When GnRH is administered to children under 2 years of age, pituitary secretion of LH and FSH increases markedly. During the juvenile pause, the period of low basal gonadotropin secretion (after age 2 until the peripubertal period), exogenous GnRH has less effect on LH release. By the peripubertal period, 100 μg of intravenous GnRH induces a greater rise in LH concentrations in boys and girls, and this response continues until adulthood. There is no significant change in the magnitude of FSH secretion after GnRH with the onset of puberty, though females at all ages release more FSH than males.

Gonadotropins are released in secretory spurts in response to endogenous GnRH, which itself is secreted episodically about every 90–120 minutes in response to a central nervous system "pulse generator." Individual GnRH-containing neurons in culture secrete GnRH in a pulsatile manner with an intrinsic rhythm. GnRH can be administered to patients in episodic boluses by a programmable pump that mimics the natural secretory episodes. A prepubertal subject without significant gonadotropin peaks will demonstrate the normal pubertal pattern of episodic secretion of gonadotropins after only a few days of such exogenously administered GnRH boluses. Hypogonadotropic patients, who in the basal state do not have normal secretory episodes of gonadotropin release, may be converted to a pattern of normal adult episodic gonadotropin secretion by this method of pulsatile GnRH administration. Varying the timing of pulsatile GnRH administration can regulate the ratio of FSH to LH just as the frequency of endogenous hypothalamic GnRH release shifts during the menstrual cycle and puberty to naturally alter this ratio. Increasing the frequency of GnRH pulses increases the LH:FSH ratio; an increased ratio is characteristic of midcycle and peripubertal dynamics. Alternatively, if GnRH is administered continuously rather than in pulses or if long-acting superactive analogs of GnRH are given, a brief period of increased gonadotropin secretion is followed by LH and FSH suppression (see below). This phenomenon is responsible for the therapeutic effects of GnRH analogs in conditions such as central precocious puberty.

G. LEPTIN AND PUBERTY

Leptin is a hormone produced in adipose cells that suppresses appetite through interaction with its receptor in the hypothalamus. Leptin plays a major role in pubertal development in mice and rats. Genetically leptin-deficient mice (ob/ob) will not initiate puberty. Leptin replacement promotes pubertal development in this mouse, and leptin administration will cause an immature normal mouse to progress through puberty. A leptin-deficient human at 9 years of age had a bone age of 13 years but no significant gonadotropin pulses and no physical evidence of pubertal development. With leptin treatment, gonadotropin peaks appeared, implying that puberty would follow. This and other data suggested that leptin might be the elusive factor which triggers the onset of puberty. Puberty and menarche occur at a younger age in obese children, and leptin seemed likely candidate to account for this phenomenon.

However, leptin does not appear to trigger the onset of puberty in normal adolescents; leptin may accompany pubertal changes rather than cause them. Leptin increases in girls during puberty in synchrony with the increase in fat mass, while leptin decreases in boys, with increased lean body mass and decreased fat mass. Thus, leptin levels vary with body composition and not with sex. Leptin appears to be a necessary component of pubertal development in human beings but not a major stimulant to this development.

Ovulation & Menarche

The last stage in hypothalamic-pituitary development is the onset of positive feedback, leading to ovulation and menarche. The ovary contains a paracrine system that regulates follicular atresia or development; it is only in the last stages of puberty that gonadotropins come into play in the maturation of the follicle. After mid puberty, estrogen in the right amount at the right time can stimulate gonadotropin release just as it can suppress gonadotropin secretion in other situations. The frequency of pulsatile GnRH release increases during the late follicular phase of the normal menstrual cycle and raises the ratio of LH to FSH secretion. This stimulates the ovary to produce estrogen and leads to the midcycle LH surge that causes ovulation. Administration of pulsatile GnRH by programmable pump can be used to bring about fertility in patients with hypothalamic GnRH deficiency by mimicking this natural pattern. However, even if the midcycle surge of gonadotropins is present, ovulation may not occur during the first menstrual cycles; 90% of menstrual cycles are anovulatory in the first year after menarche, and it is not until 4–5 years after menarche that the percentage of anovulatory cycles decreases to less than 20%. However, some of the first cycles after menarche may be ovulatory.

Thus, just as boys are reproductively mature prior to physical maturity, girls may become fertile and even pregnant prior to physical or emotional maturity.

Adrenarche

While the hypothalamic-pituitary axis has been well characterized in recent years, our understanding of the mechanism of control of adrenal androgen secretion is still somewhat rudimentary. The adrenal cortex normally secretes the weak androgens dehydroepiandrosterone (DHEA), its sulfate, dehydroepiandrosterone sulfate (DHEAS), and androstenedione in increasing amounts beginning at about 6–7 years of age in girls and 7–8 years of age in boys (Table 15–1). A continued rise in adrenal androgen secretion persists until late puberty. Thus, adrenarche (the secretion of adrenal androgens) occurs years before gonadarche (the secretion of

Table 15–1. Serum third-generation gonadotropins and sex steroids in puberty.[1]

Tanner Stage	Boys				Girls			
	LH (IU/L)	FSH (IU/L)	Testosterone (ng/dL)	DHEAS (μg/dL)	LH (IU/L)	FSH (IU/L)	Estradiol (pg/mL)	DHEAS (μg/dL)
I	0.02–0.42	0.22–1.92	2–24	5–265	0.01–0.21	0.50–2.41	5–10	5–125
II	0.26–4.84	0.72–4.60	5–70	15–380	0.27–4.12	1.73–4.68	5–115	15–150
III	0.64–3.74	1.24–10.37	15–280	60–505	0.17–4.12	2.53–7.04	5–180	20–535
IV	0.55–7.15	1.70–10.35	105–545	65–560	0.72–15.01	1.26–7.37	25–345	35–485
V	1.54–7.00	1.54–9.24	265–800	165–500	0.30–29.38	1.02–9.24	25–410	75–530

[1]Reproduced, with permission, from Fisher DA: *The Quest Diagnostics Manual: Endocrinology Test Selection and Interpretation*, 2nd ed. Quest Diagnostics, 1998.

gonadal sex steroids). The observation that patients with Addison's disease, who do not secrete adrenal androgens, and patients with premature adrenarche, who secrete increased amounts of adrenal androgens at an early age, usually enter gonadarche at a normal age suggests that age at adrenarche does not significantly influence age at gonadarche. Furthermore, patients treated with a GnRH agonist to suppress gonadotropin secretion progress through adrenarche despite their suppressed gonadarche. Measurements of urinary 17-ketosteroids reflect principally adrenal androgen secretion and not secretion of testosterone or its metabolites. Thus, urinary 17-ketosteroid levels rise considerably at adrenarche but need not do so at gonadarche.

Miscellaneous Metabolic Changes

The onset of puberty is associated with many changes in laboratory values that are either directly or indirectly caused by the rise of sex steroid concentrations. Thus, in boys, hematocrit rises and HDL concentrations fall as a consequence of increasing testosterone. In both boys and girls, alkaline phosphatase rises during the pubertal growth spurt. Serum IGF-I concentrations rise with the growth spurt, but IGF-I is more closely correlated with sex steroid concentration than with growth rate. IGF-I levels peak 1 year after peak growth velocity is reached and remain elevated for 4 years thereafter even though growth rate is decreasing. Prostate-specific antigen (PSA) is measurable after the onset of puberty in boys and provides another biochemical indication of pubertal onset.

DELAYED PUBERTY OR ABSENT PUBERTY (SEXUAL INFANTILISM)

Any girl of 13 or boy of 14 years of age without signs of pubertal development falls more than 2.5 SD above the mean and is considered to have delayed puberty (Table 15–2). By this definition, 0.6% of the healthy population are classified as having **constitutional delay** in growth and adolescence. These normal patients need reassurance rather than treatment and will ultimately progress through the normal stages of puberty, albeit later than their peers. The examining physician must make the sometimes difficult decision about which patients older than these guidelines are constitutionally delayed and which have organic disease.

Constitutional Delay in Growth & Adolescence

A patient with delayed onset of secondary sexual development whose stature is shorter than that of age-

Table 15–2. Classification of delayed puberty.

Constitutional delay in growth and adolescence
Hypogonadotropic hypogonadism
  Central nervous system disorders
    Tumors
    Other acquired disorders
    Congenital disorders
  Isolated gonadotropin deficiency
  Kallmann's syndrome
  Gonadotropin deficiency with normal sense of smell
  Multiple pituitary hormonal deficiencies
  Miscellaneous disorders
    Prader-Willi syndrome
    Laurence-Moon, Bardet-Biedl syndromes
    Chronic disease
    Weight loss
    Anorexia nervosa
    Increased physical activity in female athletes
    Hypothyroidism
Hypergonadotropic hypogonadism
  Males
    Klinefelter's syndrome
    Other forms of primary testicular failure
    Anorchia or cryptorchism
  Females
    Turner's syndrome
    Other forms of primary ovarian failure
  Pseudo-Turner syndrome
  Noonan's syndrome
  XX and XY gonadal dysgenesis

matched peers but who consistently maintains a normal growth velocity for bone age and whose skeletal development is delayed more than 2 SD from the mean is likely to have constitutional delay in puberty (Figure 15–6). These patients are at the older end of the distribution curve of age at onset of puberty. A family history of a similar pattern of development in a parent or sibling supports the diagnosis. The subject is usually thin as well. Studies suggest that disproportionately poor growth of the spine in constitutional delay in growth and adolescence relative to increased growth of the legs leads to a noticeable disproportion (lowering) of the upper to lower segment ratio; the disproportion is said to be an indicator of greater final height attainment in this group. In many cases, even if they show no physical signs of puberty at the time of examination, the initial elevation of gonadal sex steroids has already begun, and their basal LH concentrations measured by ultrasensitive third-generation assays or their plasma LH response to intravenous GnRH is pubertal. These results suggest that secondary sexual development will commence within a period of months. However, in

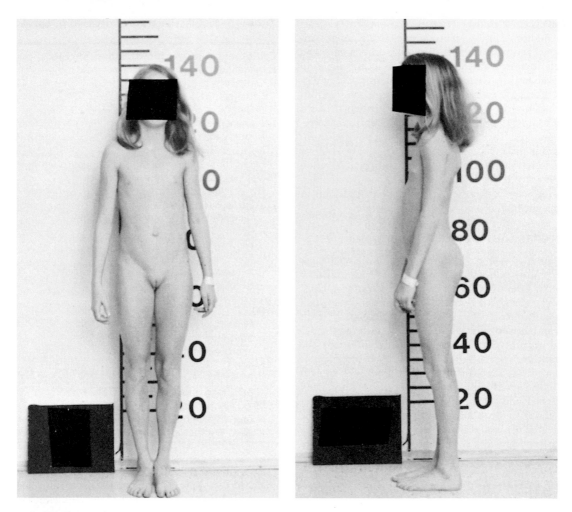

Figure 15–6. 13⁴/₁₂-year-old girl with constitutional delay in growth and puberty. History revealed a normal growth rate but short stature at all ages. Physical examination revealed a height of 138 cm (–4.5 SD) and a weight of 28.6 kg (–3 SD). The patient had recently developed early stage 2 breast development, with 1 cm of glandular tissue on the right breast and 2 cm on the left breast. The vaginal mucosa was dulled, and there was no pubic hair. Karyotype was 46,XX. Bone age was 10 years. After administration of GnRH, LH and FSH rose in a pubertal pattern. Estradiol was 40 pg/mL. She has since spontaneously progressed through further pubertal development. (Reproduced, with permission, from Styne DM, Kaplan SL: Pediatr Clin North Am 1979;26:123.)

some cases, observation for endocrine or physical signs of puberty must continue for a period of months or years before the diagnosis is made. Generally, signs of puberty will appear after the patient reaches a skeletal age of 11 years (girls) or 12 years (boys), but there is great variation. Patients with constitutional delay in adolescence will almost always manifest secondary sexual development by 18 years of chronologic age, though

there is one reported case of spontaneous puberty occurring at 25 years of age. This patient may have had Kallmann's syndrome. Reports of patients with Kallmann's syndrome and others with constitutional delay in puberty within one family suggest a possible relationship between the two conditions. See below and Chapter 5. Adrenarche is characteristically delayed—along with gonadarche—in constitutional delay in puberty.

Hypogonadotropic Hypogonadism

The absent or decreased ability of the hypothalamus to secrete GnRH or of the pituitary gland to secrete LH and FSH leads to hypogonadotropic hypogonadism. This classification denotes an irreversible condition requiring replacement therapy. If the pituitary deficiency is limited to gonadotropins, patients are usually close to normal height for age until the age of the pubertal growth spurt, in contrast to the shorter patients with constitutional delay. Bone age is usually not delayed in childhood but does not progress normally after the patient reaches the age at which sex steroid secretion ordinarily stimulates maturation of the skeleton. However, if GH deficiency accompanies gonadotropin deficiency, severe short stature will result.

A. CENTRAL NERVOUS SYSTEM DISORDERS

1. Tumors—A tumor involving the hypothalamus or pituitary gland can interfere with hypothalamic-pituitary-gonadal function as well as the control of GH, ACTH, TSH, PRL, and vasopressin secretion. Thus, delayed puberty may be a manifestation of a central nervous system tumor accompanied by any or all of the following: GH deficiency, secondary hypothyroidism, secondary adrenal insufficiency, hyperprolactinemia, and diabetes insipidus. The combination of anterior and posterior pituitary deficiencies acquired after birth makes it imperative that a hypothalamic-pituitary tumor be considered as the cause.

Craniopharyngioma is the most common type of hypothalamic-pituitary tumor leading to delay or absence of pubertal development. This neoplasm originates in Rathke's pouch but may develop into a suprasellar tumor. The peak age incidence of craniopharyngioma is between 6 and 14 years. Presenting symptoms may include headache, visual deficiency, growth failure, polyuria, and polydipsia; presenting signs may include visual defects, optic atrophy, or papilledema. Clinical manifestations may reflect gonadotropin, thyroid, and GH deficiency. Laboratory evaluation may reveal any type of anterior or posterior pituitary deficiencies. Bone age is often retarded at the time of presentation.

Calcification in the suprasellar region is the hallmark of craniopharyngiomas; 80% of cases will have calcifications on lateral skull x-ray, and a higher percentage will show this on CT scan (but calcifications will not be seen on MRI). The tumor often presents a cystic appearance on CT or MRI scan and at the time of surgery may contain dark, cholesterol-laden fluid. The rate of growth of craniopharyngiomas is quite variable—some are indolent and some are quite aggressive. Small intrasellar tumors may be resected by transsphe-noidal surgery; larger ones require partial resection and radiation therapy (see Chapter 5).

Extrasellar tumors that involve the hypothalamus and produce sexual infantilism include germinomas, gliomas (sometimes with neurofibromatosis), and astrocytomas (see Chapter 5). Intrasellar tumors such as chromophobe adenomas are quite rare in children compared to adults. Hyperprolactinemia—with or without a diagnosed microadenoma or galactorrhea—may delay the onset or progression of puberty; with therapy to decrease prolactin concentrations, puberty progresses.

2. Other acquired central nervous system disorders—Other acquired central nervous system disorders may lead to hypothalamic-pituitary dysfunction. Granulomatous diseases such as Hand-Schüller-Christian disease or histiocytosis X, when involving the hypothalamus, most frequently lead to diabetes insipidus, but any other hypothalamic defect may also occur including gonadotropin deficiency. Tuberculous or sarcoid granulomas, other postinfectious inflammatory lesions, vascular lesions, and trauma more rarely cause hypogonadotropic hypogonadism.

3. Developmental defects—Developmental defects of the central nervous system may cause hypogonadotropic hypogonadism or other types of hypothalamic dysfunction. Cleft palate or other midline anomalies may also be associated with hypothalamic dysfunction. Optic dysplasia is associated with small, hypoplastic optic disks and, in some patients, absence of the septum pellucidum on pneumoencephalography, CT scanning, or MRI; associated hypothalamic deficiencies are often present. (See Chapter 5.) Optic hypoplasia or dysplasia must be differentiated from optic atrophy; optic atrophy implies an acquired condition and may indicate a hypothalamic-pituitary tumor. Both anterior and posterior pituitary deficiencies may occur with congenital midline defects or acquired defects. Early onset of such a combination suggests a congenital defect, while late onset more strongly indicates a neoplasm.

4. Radiation therapy—Central nervous system radiation therapy involving the hypothalamic-pituitary area can lead to hypogonadotropic hypogonadism with onset at 6–18 months (or longer) after treatment. Growth hormone is more frequently affected than gonadotropin secretion, and growth hormone deficiency occurs with exposure to as little as an 18-Gy dose. Other hypothalamic deficiencies such as gonadotropin deficiency, hypothyroidism, and hyperprolactinemia occur more often with higher doses of radiation.

B. ISOLATED HORMONAL DEFICIENCY

Patients who have isolated deficiency of gonadotropins but normal GH secretion tend to be of normal height for age until the teenage years but will lack a pubertal growth spurt. They have eunuchoid proportions of increased span for height and decreased upper to lower segment ratios. Their skeletal development will be delayed for chronologic age during the teenage years, and they will continue to grow after an age when normal adolescents stop growing.

Kallmann's syndrome 1 is the most common form of isolated gonadotropin deficiency (Figure 15–7). Gonadotropin deficiency in these patients is associated with hypoplasia or aplasia of the olfactory lobes and hyposmia or anosmia; remarkably, they may not notice that they have no sense of smell, though olfactory testing will reveal it. GnRH-containing neurons fail to migrate from the olfactory placode (where they originate) to the medial basal hypothalamus in Kallmann's syndrome. This is a familial syndrome of variable manifestations in which anosmia may occur with or without hypogonadism in a given member of a kindred. X-linked Kallmann's syndrome is due to gene deletions in the region of Xp22.3, causing the absence of the *KAL* gene, which appears to code for an adhesion molecule. There is an association of Kallmann's syndrome with X-linked ichthyosis due to steroid sulfatase deficiency, mental retardation, and chondrodysplasia punctata. Associated abnormalities in Kallmann's syndrome may affect the kidneys and bones, and patients may have undescended testes, gynecomastia, and obesity. Mirror hand move-

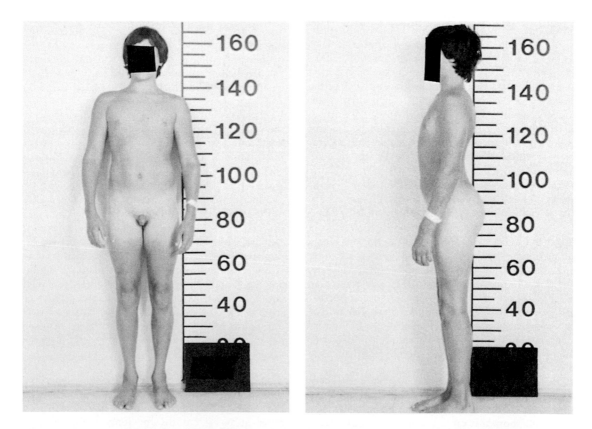

Figure 15–7. Boy, 15^{10}/$_{12}$ years old, with Kallmann's syndrome. His testes were originally undescended, but they descended into the scrotum after human chorionic gonadotropin treatment was given. His height was 163.9 cm (–1.5 SD), and the US:LS ratio was 0.86 (eunuchoid). The penis was 6.3 × 1.8 cm. Each testis was 1 × 2 cm. Plasma LH was not detectable and rose little after administration of 100 μg of GnRH; FSH rose minimally. Testosterone did not change from 17 ng/dL. He had no ability to smell standard odors. (Reproduced, with permission, from Styne DM, Grumbach MM: *Reproductive Endocrinology.* Yen SSC, Jaffe RB [editors]. Saunders, 1978.)

ments (bimanual synkinesia) is reported, with MRI evidence of abnormal development of the corticospinal tract. Ultimate height is normal, though patients are delayed in reaching adult height. Kallman's syndrome 2 is inherited in an autosomal dominant pattern. Kallman's syndrome 3 exhibits an autosomal recessive pattern.

Other cases of hypogonadotropic hypogonadism may occur sporadically or via an autosomal recessive pattern without anosmia. X-linked congenital adrenal hypoplasia is associated with hypogonadotropic hypogonadism; glycerol kinase deficiency and muscular dystrophy have been linked to this syndrome. The gene locus is at Xp21.3-p21.2 and involves a mutation in the *DAX1* gene in many but not all patients. An autosomal recessive form of congenital adrenal hypoplasia is reported. Some hypogonadal patients lack only LH secretion and have spermatogenesis without testosterone production (fertile eunuch syndrome); others lack only FSH. (See Chapters 12 and 13.)

C. Idiopathic Hypopituitary Dwarfism

Patients with congenital GH deficiency have early onset of growth failure (Figure 15–8); this feature distinguishes them from patients with GH deficiency due to hypothalamic tumors, who usually have late onset of growth failure. Even without associated gonadotropin deficiency, untreated GH-deficient patients often have delayed onset of puberty associated with their delayed bone ages. With appropriate hGH therapy, however, onset of puberty occurs at a normal age. Patients who have combined GH and gonadotropin deficiency do not undergo puberty even when bone age reaches the pubertal stage. Idiopathic hypopituitarism is usually sporadic but may follow an autosomal recessive or X-linked inheritance pattern. Birth injury or breech delivery is a common feature of the neonatal history of patients with idiopathic hypopituitarism (breech delivery being more common in the history of affected males).

The syndrome of microphallus (due to congenital gonadotropin or GH deficiency) and neonatal hypoglycemic seizures (due to congenital ACTH deficiency or GH deficiency) must be diagnosed and treated early to avoid central nervous system damage. Patients with this syndrome will not undergo spontaneous pubertal development. Testosterone in low doses (testosterone enanthate, 25 mg intramuscularly every month for three doses) can increase the size of the penis in infants diagnosed with congenital hypopituitarism without significantly advancing the bone age. Males with isolated GH deficiency can also have microphallus; the penis will enlarge to some degree with hGH therapy in these patients. It is important to note that microphallus due to hypopituitarism may be treated with testosterone, and sex reversal need not be considered (see Chapter 14).

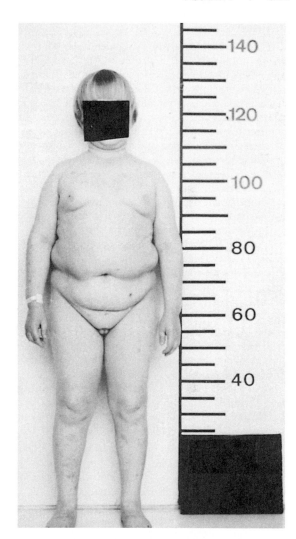

Figure 15–8. Twenty-year-old male with congenital deficiency of GRF, GnRH, TRF, and CRF. Height was 8 SD below the mean, and the phallus was 2 × 1 cm. Bone age was 10 years, and the sella turcica was small on lateral skull x-ray. LH rose minimally from a low basal value after administration of 100 µg of GnRH. Testosterone was virtually undetectable and did not rise after administration of GnRH. (Reproduced, with permission, from Styne DM, Grumbach MM: *Reproductive Endocrinology.* Yen SSC, Jaffe RB [editors]. Saunders, 1978.)

D. MISCELLANEOUS DISORDERS

1. Prader-Willi syndrome—Prader-Willi syndrome occurs sporadically and is associated with fetal and infantile hypotonia, short stature; poor feeding in infancy but insatiable hunger later, leading to massive obesity; characteristic facies with almond-shaped eyes, small hands and feet after infancy, mental retardation, and emotional instability in patients of either sex; delayed menarche in females; and micropenis and cryptorchism in males. Osteoporosis is common in these patients during the teenage years, but sex steroid replacement, when indicated, may help. Behavioral modification may improve the usual pattern of rampant weight gain. Patients have deletion or translocation of chromosome 15q11–13 derived from the father; if an abnormality in this area derives from the mother, Angelman syndrome results. Fluorescent in situ hybridization for this area of the chromosome is available from laboratories for diagnosis. (See Chapter 6.)

2. Laurence-Moon and Bardet-Biedl syndromes— These autosomal recessive conditions are characterized by obesity, short stature, mental retardation, and retinitis pigmentosa. Hypogonadotropic hypogonadism and primary hypogonadism have variously been reported in affected patients. A distinction between Bardet-Biedl (gene locus 16q21) and Laurence-Moon syndromes may be made, with the latter demonstrating polydactyly and obesity and the former being characterized by paraplegia. (See Chapter 6.)

3. Chronic disease and malnutrition—A delay in sexual maturation may be due to chronic disease or malnutrition. For example, children with intractable asthma have delayed pubertal development leading to short stature during the teenage years, though they ultimately reach an appropriate height. Children with other chronic diseases may not fare so well in long-term follow-up; eg, HIV infection in adolescence causes poor growth and pubertal progression. Weight loss to less than 80% of ideal weight caused by disease or voluntary dieting may result in gonadotropin deficiency; weight gain toward the ideal usually restores gonadotropin function.

Chronic disease may have effects on sexual maturation separate from nutritional state. For example, there is a high incidence of hypothalamic hypogonadism in thalassemia major even with regular transfusion and chelation therapy.

4. Anorexia nervosa—Anorexia nervosa involves weight loss associated with significant psychologic disorder. This condition usually affects girls who develop a disturbed body image and exhibit typical behavior such as avoidance of food and induction of regurgitation after ingestion. Weight loss may be so severe as to cause fatal complications such as immune dysfunction, fluid and electrolyte imbalance, or circulatory collapse. Primary or secondary amenorrhea is a classic finding in these patients and has been correlated with the degree of weight loss, though there is evidence that patients with anorexia nervosa may cease to menstruate before their substantial weight loss is exhibited. Other endocrine abnormalities in anorexia nervosa include elevated serum growth hormone and decreased IGF-I (these are characteristic of any type of starvation), decreased serum triiodothyronine, decreased serum 1,25-dihydroxyvitamin D_3 and elevated 24,25-hydroxyvitamin D_3 levels. Weight gain to the normal range for height, however, does not ensure immediate resumption of menses. There is an increased incidence of anorexia nervosa in ballet dancers or ballet students; the incidence of scoliosis and mitral valve insufficiency is also increased in these patients. Functional amenorrhea may also occur in women of normal weight, some of whom demonstrate evidence of psychologic stress. Decreased LH response to GnRH administration, impaired monthly cycles of gonadotropin secretion, and retention of a diurnal rhythm of gonadotropin secretion are found in anorexia nervosa patients, patterns which indicate a reversion to an earlier stage of endocrine puberty.

5. Increased physical activity—Girls who regularly participate in strenuous athletics, ballet dancing, etc, may have delayed thelarche, delayed menarche, and irregular or absent menstrual periods. This effect is not always related to less than ideal weight, since such amenorrheic patients may resume menses while temporarily bedridden. Increased physical activity and not decreased weight appears to be the cause of the amenorrhea. Statistical analysis of mothers' ages at menarche and the type of sport pursued by their daughters indicates that late maturation of some gymnasts may be referable to a familial tendency to late menarche, suggesting that gymnastic activity may not be the primary cause of late menarche. On the other hand there are disturbing studies indicating that intensive gymnastics training at an early age leads to a decrease in ultimate stature.

6. Hypothyroidism—Hypothyroidism can delay all aspects of growth and maturation, including puberty and menarche. Galactorrhea may occur in severe primary hypothyroidism due to concomitant elevation of serum prolactin. With thyroxine therapy, catch-up growth and resumed pubertal development and menses will occur. Conversely, severe primary hypothyroidism may be associated with precocious puberty and galactorrhea (due to elevated serum prolactin) in some patients (Van Wyk-Grumbach syndrome). There is evidence that excessive TSH can stimulate FSH receptors, leading to estrogen secretion and breast development.

Hypergonadotropic Hypogonadism

Primary gonadal failure is heralded by elevated gonadotropin concentration due to the absence of negative feedback effects of gonadal sex steroids. The most common causes of hypergonadotropic hypogonadism are associated with chromosomal and somatic abnormalities, but isolated gonadal failure can also present with delayed puberty without other physical findings. When hypergonadotropic hypogonadism is present in patients with a Y chromosome or a fragment of a Y chromosome (genetic males or conditions noted below), testicular dysgenesis must be considered in the differential diagnosis. The risk of testicular cancer rises in testicular dysgenesis. (Testicular cancer in normal boys is rare; for example, the incidence in Scandinavia is 0.5 per 100,000 in childhood.)

A. Syndrome of Seminiferous Tubule Dysgenesis (Klinefelter's Syndrome)

(See Chapters 12 and 14.) The most common form of primary testicular failure is Klinefelter's syndrome (47,XXY karyotype), with an incidence of 1:1000 males. Before puberty, patients with Klinefelter's syndrome have decreased upper segment:lower segment ratios, small testes, and an increased incidence of developmental delay and personality disorders. Onset of puberty is not usually delayed, because Leydig cell function is characteristically less affected than seminiferous tubule function in this condition and testosterone is adequate to stimulate pubertal development. Serum gonadotropin levels rise to castrate concentrations after the onset of puberty; the testes become firm and are rarely larger than 3.5 cm in diameter. After the onset of puberty, there are histologic changes of seminiferous tubule hyalinization and fibrosis, adenomatous changes of the Leydig cells, and impaired spermatogenesis. Gynecomastia is common, and variable degrees of male secondary sexual development are found.

Other forms of male hypergonadotropic hypogonadism are found with 46,XX/47,XXY, 48,XXYY, 48,XXXY, and 49,XXXXY karyotypes. Phenotypic males are described with 46,XX karyotypes and some physical features of Klinefelter's syndrome (see Chapter 14).

B. Other Forms of Primary Testicular Failure

Patients surviving treatment for malignant diseases form a growing category of testicular failure. Chemotherapy—primarily with alkylating agents—or radiation therapy directed to the gonads may lead to gonadal failure; injury is more likely if treatment is given during puberty than if it occurs in the prepubertal period, but even prepubertal therapy leads to risk. Normal pubertal development may occur in boys treated prepubertally with polychemotherapy, though they demonstrated elevated peak serum LH and elevated basal and peak serum FSH after GnRH as well as a high incidence of decreased or absent sperm counts; this indicates that prepubertal status does not protect a child against testicular damage from chemotherapy and that normal physical development may hide significant endocrine and reproductive damage.

The "Sertoli cell only" syndrome (germinal cell aplasia) is a congenital form of testicular failure manifested by azoospermia and elevated FSH concentrations but generally normal secondary sexual characteristics, normal testosterone concentrations, and no other anomalies. A gene at Yq11.23, the azoospermia factor (AZF), appears to play a role in the production of spermatocytes. Patients with Down's syndrome may have elevated LH and FSH levels even in the presence of normal testosterone levels, suggesting some element of primary gonadal failure.

C. Cryptorchism or Anorchia

Phenotypic males with a 46,XY karyotype but no palpable testes have either cryptorchism or anorchia. Cryptorchid males should produce a rise in testosterone levels > 2 ng/mL 72 hours after intramuscular administration of 3000 units/m^2 of chorionic gonadotropin, and the testes may descend during 2 weeks of treatment with chorionic gonadotropin given three times a week. Patients with increased plasma testosterone levels in response to chorionic gonadotropin administration but without testicular descent have cryptorchism; their testes should be brought into the scrotum by surgery to decrease the likelihood of further testicular damage due to the elevated intra-abdominal temperature and to guard against the possibility of undetected tumor formation. Cryptorchid testes may demonstrate congenital abnormalities and may not function normally even if brought into the scrotum early in life. Furthermore, the descended testis in a unilaterally cryptorchid boy may itself show abnormal histologic features; such patients have a 69% incidence of decreased sperm counts. Thus, unilateral cryptorchid patients can be infertile even if they received early treatment of their unilateral cryptorchism. In addition, patients undergoing orchiopexy may sustain subtle damage to the vas deferens, leading to the later production of antibodies to sperm that may result in infertility.

It is important to determine if any testicular tissue is present in a boy with no palpable testes, since unnoticed malignant degeneration of the tissue is a possibility. The diagnosis of anorchia due to the testicular regression syndrome may be pursued by ultrasound or MRI, laparotomy or laparoscopic examination, or by the endocrine evaluation noted above. Except for the absence of testes, patients with anorchia have normal infantile male genital development, including wolffian duct formation and müllerian duct regression. The testes were presumably present in these patients early in fetal life during sexual differentiation but degenerated after the 13th week of gestation for unknown reasons (also called the "vanishing testes syndrome") (see Chapter 12). The presence of antimüllerian factor in a young child indicates the presence of testicular tissue, although during puberty antimüllerian factor becomes nondetectable and this test cannot be employed at that stage. The presence of normal basal gonadotropin levels in a prepubertal boy without palpable testes suggests the presence of testicular tissue even if the testosterone response to hCG is low, while the presence of elevated gonadotropin levels without any testosterone response to hCG suggests anorchia.

D. Syndrome of Gonadal Dysgenesis (Turner's Syndrome)

(See Chapters 13 and 14.) 45,X gonadal dysgenesis is associated with short stature, female phenotype with sexual infantilism, and a chromatin-negative buccal smear. (We do not recommend routinely ordering a buccal smear since it is difficult for some laboratories to perform the test reliably.) Patients have "streak" gonads consisting of fibrous tissue without germ cells. Other classic but variable phenotypic features include micrognathia, "fish" mouth (downturned corners of the mouth), ptosis, low-set or deformed ears, a broad shield-like chest with the appearance of widely spaced nipples, hypoplastic areolae, a short neck with low hairline and webbing of the neck (pterygium colli), short fourth metacarpals, cubitus valgus, structural anomalies of the kidney, extensive nevi, hypoplastic nails, and vascular anomalies of the left side of the heart (most commonly coarctation of the aorta associated with hypertension). The medical history of patients with the syndrome of gonadal dysgenesis will often reveal small size at birth, lymphedema of the extremities most prominent in the newborn period, and loose posterior cervical skin folds. (The terms "Bonnevie-Ullrich syndrome" and "infant Turner's syndrome" are applied to this neonatal appearance.) Affected patients often have a history of frequent otitis media with conductive hearing loss. Intelligence is normal, but there is often impaired spatial orientation. Patients have no pubertal growth spurt and reach a mean final height of 143 cm. Short stature is a classic feature of Turner's syndrome but not of other forms of hypergonadotropic hypogonadism that occur without karyotype abnormalities. The short stature is linked to the absence of the *SHOX* homeobox gene of the pseudoautosomal region of the X chromosome (Xpter–p22.32). GH function is usually normal in Turner's syndrome. However, exogenous hGH treatment improves growth rate and increases adult stature in affected girls (see Chapter 14). Pubic hair may appear late and is usually sparse in distribution owing to the absence of any ovarian secretions; thus, adrenarche progresses in Turner's syndrome even in the absence of gonadarche. Autoimmune thyroid disease (usually hypothyroidism) is common in Turner's syndrome, and determination of thyroid function and thyroid antibody levels is important in evaluation of these patients.

Serum gonadotropin concentrations in Turner's syndrome are extremely high between birth and age 4 years. They decrease toward the normal range in prepubertal patients in the juvenile pause and then rise again to castrate levels after age 10 years. (See Chapter 14.)

Sex chromatin-positive variants of gonadal dysgenesis include 45,X/46,XX, 45,X/47,XXX, and 45,X/46, XX/47,XXX mosaicism with chromatin-positive buccal smears. Patients with these karyotypes may resemble patients with the classic syndrome of gonadal dysgenesis, or they may have fewer manifestations and normal or nearly normal female phenotypes. Streak gonad formation is not invariable; some patients have had secondary sexual development, and menarche and rare pregnancies have been reported.

Sex chromatin-negative variants of the syndrome of gonadal dysgenesis have karyotypes with 45,X/46,XY mosaicism. Physical features vary; some patients have the features of classic Turner's syndrome, while others may have ambiguous genitalia or even the features of phenotypic males. Gonads are dysgenetic but vary from streak gonads to functioning testes. These patients are at risk for gonadoblastoma formation. Since gonadoblastomas may secrete androgens or estrogens, patients with gonadoblastoma may virilize or feminize as though they had functioning gonads, confusing the clinical picture. Gonadoblastomas may demonstrate calcification on abdominal x-ray. Malignant germ cell tumors may arise in dysgenetic testes, and orchiectomy is generally indicated. In some mosaic patients with one intact X chromosome and one chromosomal fragment, it is difficult to determine whether the fragment is derived from an X chromosome or a Y chromosome. PCR techniques to search for specific sequences may be helpful if a karyotype reveals no Y chromosomal material.

Patients with Turner's syndrome have benefited from in vitro fertilization techniques. After exogenous hormonal preparation, a fertilized ovum (possibly a sister's ovum fertilized by the patient's male partner, or an extra fertilized ovum from another couple undergoing in vitro fertilization) can be introduced into the patient's uterus, and the pregnancy is then brought to term by exogenous hormone administration.

E. Other Forms of Primary Ovarian Failure

Ovaries appear to be more resistant to damage from the chemotherapy used in the treatment of malignant disease than are testes. Nonetheless, ovarian failure can occur with medical therapy. Damage is common if the ovaries are not surgically "tacked" out of the path of the beam or shielded by lead in abdominal radiation therapy. Normal gonadal function after chemotherapy does not guarantee normal function later. Late-onset gonadal failure has been described after chemotherapy. Premature menopause has also been described in otherwise healthy girls owing to the presence of antiovarian antibodies; patients with Addison's disease may have autoimmune oophoritis as well as adrenal failure. A sex steroid biosynthetic defect due to 17α-hydroxylase deficiency (P450c17) will be manifested as sexual infantilism and primary amenorrhea in a phenotypic female (regardless of genotype) with hypokalemia and hypertension. The patient with 17α-hydroxylase deficiency may have ovaries or testes and still present as a phenotypic female.

F. PSEUDO-TURNER SYNDROME (NOONAN'S SYNDROME, ULLRICH'S SYNDROME, MALE TURNER'S SYNDROME)

Pseudo-Turner syndrome is associated with manifestations of Turner's syndrome such as webbed neck, ptosis, short stature, cubitus valgus, and lymphedema, but other clinical findings such as a normal karyotype, triangular facies, pectus excavatum, right-sided heart disease, and an increased incidence of mental retardation differentiate these patients from those with Turner's syndrome. Males may have undescended testes and variable degrees of germinal cell and Leydig cell dysfunction. Pseudo-Turner syndrome follows an autosomal dominant pattern of inheritance with incomplete penetrance (gene locus 12q24).

G. FAMILIAL AND SPORADIC FORMS OF 46,XX OR 46,XY GONADAL DYSGENESIS

These forms of gonadal dysgenesis are characterized by structurally normal chromosomes and streak gonads or partially functioning gonads. They do not have the physical features of Turner's syndrome. If there is some gonadal function, 46,XY gonadal dysgenesis may present with ambiguous genitalia or virilization at puberty. If no gonadal function is present, patients appear as phenotypic sexually infantile females. Patients with 46,XY gonadal dysgenesis and dysgenetic testes should undergo gonadectomy to eliminate the possibility of malignant germ cell tumor formation.

H. PRIMARY AMENORRHEA ASSOCIATED WITH NORMAL SECONDARY SEXUAL DEVELOPMENT

If a structural anomaly of the uterus or vagina interferes with the onset of menses but the endocrine milieu remains normal, the patient presents with primary amenorrhea in the presence of normal breast and pubic hair development. A transverse vaginal septum will seal the uterine cavity from the vaginal orifice, leading to the retention of menstrual flow—as may an imperforate hymen. The Rokitansky-Küster-Hauser syndrome combines congenital absence of the vagina with abnormal development of the uterus, ranging from a rudimentary bicornuate uterus that may not open into the vaginal canal to a virtually normal uterus; surgical repair may be possible in patients with minimal anatomic abnormalities, and fertility has been reported. Associated abnormalities include major urinary tract anomalies and spinal or other skeletal disorders. The rarest anatomic abnormality in this group is absence of the uterine cervix in the presence of a functional uterus.

Male pseudohermaphroditism is an alternative cause of primary amenorrhea if a patient has achieved thelarche. The syndrome of complete androgen resistance leads to female external genitalia and phenotype without axillary or pubic hair development in the presence of pubertal breast development (syndrome of testicular feminization; see Chapter 14).

Differential Diagnosis of Delayed Puberty (Table 15–3)

Patients who do not begin secondary sexual development by age 13 (girls) or age 14 (boys) and patients who do not progress through development on a timely basis (girls should menstruate within 5 years after breast budding; boys should reach stage 5 pubertal development 4½ years after onset) should be evaluated for hypogonadism. The yield of diagnosable conditions is quite low in children younger than these ages, but many patients and families will request evaluation well before these limits. Without significant signs or symptoms of disorders discussed above, it is best to resist evaluation and offer support until these ages in most cases.

If the diagnosis is not obvious on the basis of physical or historical features, the differential diagnostic process begins with determination of whether plasma gonadotropins are (1) elevated owing to primary gonadal failure or (2) decreased owing to secondary or tertiary hypogonadism or constitutional delayed puberty. A patient with constitutional delay may have a characteristic history of short stature for age with normal growth velocity for bone age and a family history of delayed but spontaneous puberty. The patient's mother may have had late onset of menses, or the father may have begun to shave late or continued growing after high school. Not all patients with constitutional delay are so classic, and gonadotropin-deficient patients may have some features similar to those of constitutional delay in adolescence. Indeed, patients with Kallmann's

Table 15–3. Differential diagnosis of delayed puberty.

	Serum Gonadotropins	Serum Gonadal Steroids	Miscellaneous
Constitutional delay in growth and adolescence	Prepubertal (low)	Low	Patient usually has short stature for chronologic age but appropriate height and growth rate for bone age. Both adrenarche and gonadarche are delayed.
Hypogonadotropic hypogonadism	Prepubertal (low)	Low	Patient may have anosmia (Kallmann's syndrome) or other associated pituitary hormone deficiencies. If gonadotropin deficiency is isolated, the patient usually has normal height and growth rates but lacks a pubertal growth spurt. Adrenarche may occur at a normal stage in spite of absent gonadarche (serum DHEAS may be pubertal).
Hypergonadotropic hypogonadism	Elevated	Low	Patient may have abnormal karyotype and stigmas of Turner's syndrome or Klinefelter's syndrome.

syndrome and others with constitutional delay are occasionally found in the same kindred.

Laboratory evaluation is sometimes helpful but not always. A single third-generation determination of serum LH concentration in the pubertal range suggests that puberty is progressing. Determination of the rise in LH after administration of GnRH is helpful in differential diagnosis; secondary sexual development usually follows within months after conversion to a pubertal LH response to GnRH. An appropriate LH rise following administration of a superactive GnRH agonist is proposed as another useful indicator of normal pubertal progression. Frequent nighttime sampling (every 20 minutes through an indwelling catheter) to determine the amplitude of peaks of LH secretion during sleep is an alternative to GnRH testing but quite cumbersome. Unfortunately, the results of GnRH infusions or nighttime sampling are not always straightforward. Patients may have pubertal responses to exogenous GnRH but may not spontaneously secrete adequate gonadotropins to allow secondary sexual development. In females with amenorrhea, the frequency and amplitude of gonadotropin secretion may not change to allow monthly menstrual cycles. The retention of a diurnal rhythm of gonadotropin secretion (normal in early puberty) into late puberty is a pattern linked to inadequate pubertal progression. In males, a morning serum testosterone concentration over 50 ng/dL indicates the likelihood of pubertal development within 6 months. Other methods of differential diagnosis between constitutional delay and hypogonadotropic hypogonadism have been proposed but are complex or are not definitive.

Clinical observation for signs of pubertal development and laboratory evaluation for the onset of rising levels of sex steroids may have to continue until the patient is 18 years of age before the diagnosis is definite. In most cases, if spontaneous pubertal development is not noted by 18 years of age, the diagnosis is gonadotropin deficiency. Of course, the presence of neurologic impairment or other endocrine deficiency should immediately lead to investigation for central nervous system tumor or congenital defect in a patient with delayed puberty. CT or MRI scanning will be helpful in this situation.

Treatment of Delayed Puberty

A. CONSTITUTIONAL DELAY IN GROWTH AND ADOLESCENCE

1. Psychologic support—Teenagers who are so embarrassed about short stature and lack of secondary sexual development as to have significant psychologic problems may require special help if they have passed the ages of 13 years for girls or 14 years for boys. Patients with constitutional delay in growth and adolescence should be counseled that normal pubertal development will occur spontaneously. Peer pressure and teasing can be oppressive. While the majority of these patients will do quite well, severe depression must be treated appropriately, since short patients with pubertal delay have become suicidal. In some cases it helps to excuse the patient from physical education class, as the lack of development is most apparent in the locker room. In general, boys feel more stress than girls when puberty is delayed.

2. Sex steroids—The following treatment can be given: (1) for girls, a 3-month course of conjugated estrogen (0.3 mg) or ethinyl estradiol (5–10 μg) given orally each day; (2) for boys, a 3-month course of testosterone enanthate or cypionate (100 mg) given intramuscularly once every 28 days for three doses. This treatment will elicit noticeable secondary sexual development and a slight increase in stature. The low doses recommended do not advance bone age and will not significantly change final height. Such low-dose sex steroid treatment has been claimed to promote spontaneous pubertal development after sex steroid therapy is discontinued, but responding individuals may include those boys who are on the brink of further pubertal development and are therefore most likely to achieve a growth response to androgen therapy. A short course of therapy may improve patients' psychologic outlook and allow them to await spontaneous pubertal development with greater confidence. Continuous gonadal steroid replacement in these patients is not indicated, as it will advance bone age and lead to epiphysial fusion and a decrease in ultimate stature; however, after a 3- to 6-month break to observe spontaneous development, another course of therapy may be offered if no pubertal progression occurs.

B. PERMANENT HYPOGONADISM

Once a patient has been diagnosed as having delayed puberty due to permanent primary or secondary hypogonadism, replacement therapy must be considered.

Males with hypogonadism may be treated with testosterone enanthate or cypionate intramuscularly every month, gradually increasing the dosage from 100 mg to 300 mg every 28 days. Frequent erections or priapism may occur if the higher dose is used initially. Oral halogenated testosterone and methylated testosterone are not recommended because of the risk of hepatocellular carcinoma or cholestatic jaundice. A testosterone patch or gel provides an alternative to intramuscular testosterone enanthate.

Testosterone therapy may not cause adequate pubic hair development, but patients with secondary or tertiary hypogonadism may benefit from hCG administration with increased pubic hair growth resulting from endogenous androgen secretion in addition to the exogenous testosterone.

Therapy with oxandrolone has been suggested as a method of increasing secondary sexual development and increasing growth without advancing skeletal development; such claims have not been sufficiently well documented to justify a preference for oxandrolone therapy over low-dose depot testosterone. Furthermore, testosterone, which can be aromatized, increases the generally low endogenous growth hormone secretion in constitutional delayed puberty to normal, while oxandrolone, which cannot be aromatized, does not increase growth hormone secretion (see Chapter 12).

Females may be treated with ethinyl estradiol (increasing from 5 μg/d to 10–20 μg/d depending upon clinical results) or conjugated estrogens (0.3 or 0.625 mg/d) on days 1–21 of the month. Ten milligrams of medroxyprogesterone acetate are then added on days 12–21 after physical signs of estrogen effect are noted

and breakthrough bleeding occurs (and always within 6 months after initiating estrogen). Neither hormone is administered from day 22 to the end of the month to allow regular withdrawal bleeding (see Chapter 13). Later, the patient may be switched to sequential oral contraceptives. Gynecologic examinations should be performed yearly.

Hypothalamic hypogonadism may be treated with GnRH pulses by programmable pump, and fertility may be achieved. Likewise, in the absence of a functional pituitary gland, hCG and menotropins (human postmenopausal gonadotropin) may be administered in pulses. These techniques are cumbersome and best reserved for the time when fertility is desired.

C. COEXISTING GH DEFICIENCY

The treatment of patients with coexisting GH deficiency requires consideration of their bone age and amount of growth left before epiphysial fusion; if they have not yet received adequate treatment with growth hormone, sex steroid therapy may be kept in the lower range or even delayed to optimize final adult height. The goal is to allow appropriate pubertal changes to support psychologic development and to allow the synergistic effects of combined sex steroids and GH without fusing the epiphyses prematurely.

Constitutional delayed puberty may be associated with decreased growth hormone secretion in 24-hour profiles of spontaneous secretion or in stimulated testing. Growth hormone secretion increases when pubertal gonadal steroid secretion rises, so decreased GH secretion in this condition should be considered temporary. Growth hormone therapy is not proved to increase final height in patients with constitutional delay in puberty and normal height predictions; studies have shown an increased growth rate in the first year of such therapy, with a decreasing growth rate thereafter. Nonetheless, true growth hormone-deficient patients may have delayed puberty due to the growth hormone deficiency or to coexisting gonadotropin deficiency. Therefore, deciding whether a pubertal patient has temporary or a permanent GH deficiency can be difficult; previous observation may indicate a long history characteristic of constitutional delay in adolescence, while a recent decrease in growth rate may suggest the onset of a brain tumor or other cause of hypopituitarism.

D. THE SYNDROME OF GONADAL DYSGENESIS

In the past, patients with the syndrome of gonadal dysgenesis were frequently not given estrogen replacement until after age 13 years, for fear of compromising final height. It has now been demonstrated that low-dose estrogen therapy (5–10 μg of ethinyl estradiol orally) can be administered to allow feminization and improve psychologic status at 12–13 years of age without decreasing final height in these patients. Low-dose estrogen will increase growth velocity, while high-dose estrogen suppresses it. Even if growth velocity is increased, however, final height is not increased with such estrogen treatment. Treatment of Turner's syndrome with GH successfully increases adult stature (see Chapter 14).

E. BONE MASS

After infancy, most bone mass accrues during the second decade, and disorders of puberty may affect the process. Delayed puberty in boys causes decreased cross sectional bone density when the subjects are tested as adults. A range of defects in girls such as anorexia nervosa, athletics-induced delayed puberty, and Turner's syndrome also cause decreased bone density. The use of testosterone in boys and estrogen and progesterone in girls is helpful in increasing bone mass but has not been demonstrated to result in normal adult bone mass. Appropriate ingestion of dairy products containing calcium or calcium supplementation should be encouraged in hypogonadal or constitutionally delayed patients as well as in normal children; unfortunately, however, no long-term follow-up is yet available to prove the efficacy of this therapy.

PRECOCIOUS PUBERTY (SEXUAL PRECOCITY)

The appearance of secondary sexual development before the age of 7 years in Caucasian girls and 6 years in African-American girls and 9 years in boys of either race constitutes precocious sexual development (Table 15–4). When the cause is premature activation of the hypothalamic-pituitary axis, the diagnosis is central (**complete or true**) **precocious puberty;** if ectopic gonadotropin secretion occurs in boys or autonomous sex steroid secretion occurs in either sex, the diagnosis is **incomplete precocious puberty.** In all forms of sexual precocity, there is an increase in growth velocity, somatic development, and skeletal maturation. When unchecked, this rapid epiphysial development may lead to tall stature during the early phases of the disorder but to short final stature because of early epiphysial fusion. This is the paradox of the tall child growing up to become a short adult. Plasma IGF-I values may be elevated for age but more appropriate for pubertal stage in the untreated state.

Central (Complete or True) Precocious Puberty (Figure 15–9)

A. CONSTITUTIONAL CENTRAL (COMPLETE OR TRUE) PRECOCIOUS PUBERTY

Children who demonstrate isosexual precocity at an age more than 2.5 SD below the mean may simply represent the lower reaches of the distribution curve of age at

Table 15–4. Classification of precocious puberty.

Central (complete or true) isosexual precocious puberty
  Constitutional
  Idiopathic
  Central nervous system disorders
  Following androgen exposure
Incomplete isosexual precocious puberty
  Males
    Gonadotropin-secreting tumors
    Excessive androgen production
    Premature Leydig and germinal cell maturation
  Females
    Ovarian cysts
    Estrogen-secreting neoplasms
    Severe hypothyroidism
  Males and females
    McCune-Albright syndrome
Sexual precocity due to gonadotropin or sex steroid
  exposure
Variation in pubertal development
  Premature thelarche
  Premature menarche
  Premature pubarche
  Adolescent gynecomastia

onset of puberty; often there is a familial tendency toward early puberty. True precocious puberty is rarely reported to be due to an autosomal dominant or (in males) X-linked autosomal dominant trait.

B. IDIOPATHIC CENTRAL (COMPLETE OR TRUE) ISOSEXUAL PRECOCIOUS PUBERTY

Affected children with no familial tendency toward early development and no organic disease may be considered to have idiopathic central isosexual precocious puberty. Electroencephalographic abnormalities or other evidence of neurologic dysfunction such as epilepsy or developmental delay may be found in these patients. Pubertal development may follow the normal course or may wax and wane. Serum gonadotropin and sex steroid concentrations and response to GnRH are similar to those found in normal pubertal subjects. In idiopathic central precocious puberty, as in all forms of true isosexual precocity, testicular enlargement in boys should be the first sign; in girls, breast development or, rarely, pubic hair appearance may be first. Girls present with idiopathic central precocious puberty more commonly than boys. Children with precocious puberty have a tendency toward obesity based upon elevated BMI in the untreated state.

C. CENTRAL NERVOUS SYSTEM DISORDERS

1. Tumors—Central nervous system tumor as a cause of central precocious puberty is more common in boys

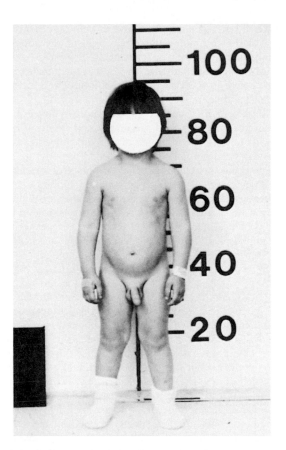

Figure 15–9. Boy 2⁵/₁₂ years of age with idiopathic true precocious puberty. By 10 months of age, he had pubic hair and phallic and testicular enlargement. At 1 year of age, his height was 4 SD above the mean; the phallus was 10 × 3.5 cm; each testis was 2.5 × 1.5 cm. Plasma LH was pubertal and rose in an adult pattern after administration of 100 μg of GnRH. Plasma testosterone was 416 ng/dL. At the time of the photograph, he had been treated with medroxyprogesterone acetate (to suppress LH and FSH secretion) for 1½ years, with reduction of his rapid growth rate and decreased gonadotropin and testosterone secretion. His height was 95.2 cm (> 2 SD above mean height for his age); plasma testosterone was 7 ng/dL, and after 100 μg of GnRH, plasma LH rose only slightly, demonstrating suppression. (Reproduced, with permission, from Styne, DM, Grumbach MM: *Reproductive Endocrinology.* Yen SSC, Jaffe RB [editors]. Saunders, 1978.)

than in girls. Optic gliomas or hypothalamic gliomas, astrocytomas, ependymomas, germinomas, and other central nervous system tumors may cause precocious puberty by interfering with neural pathways that inhibit GnRH secretion, thus releasing the central nervous system restraint of gonadotropin secretion. A survey found that 46% of patients with optic gliomas and neurofibromatosis type 1 had precocious puberty, but no patients with isolated neurofibromatosis (that did not have optic gliomas) demonstrated precocious puberty. Remarkably, craniopharyngiomas, which are known to cause delayed puberty, can also trigger precocious pubertal development. Radiation therapy is often indicated in radiosensitive tumors such as germinomas and craniopharyngiomas, where complete surgical extirpation is impossible. Hamartomas of the tuber cinereum contain GnRH and neurosecretory cells such as are found in the median eminence; they may cause precocious puberty by secreting GnRH. Some hypothalamic hamartomas associated with central precocious puberty do not elaborate GnRH but instead contain TGF-α, which stimulates GnRH secretion itself. With improved methods of imaging the central nervous system, hamartomas, with their characteristic radiographic appearance, are now more frequently diagnosed in patients who were previously thought to have idiopathic precocious puberty. These tumors do not grow and so pose no increasing threat to the patients in the absence of intractable seizures. These seizures are rare in patients with pedunculated hamartomas causing central precocious puberty. Because of the location of the hamartoma, surgery is a dangerous alternative to GnRH therapy.

Tumors or other abnormalities of the central nervous system may cause growth hormone deficiency in association with central precocious puberty. This may also occur after irradiation therapy for such tumors. Such patients will grow much faster than isolated growth hormone-deficient patients but slower than children with classic precocious puberty. Often the growth hormone deficiency will be unmasked after successful treatment of precocious puberty. This combination must be considered during the diagnostic process. (See also Chapter 6.)

2. Other causes of true precocious puberty—Infectious or granulomatous conditions such as encephalitis, brain abscess, postinfectious (or postsurgical or congenital) suprasellar cysts, sarcoidosis, and tuberculous granulomas of the hypothalamus cause central precocious puberty. Suprasellar cysts and hydrocephalus cause central precocious puberty that is particularly amenable to surgical correction. Brain trauma may be followed by either precocious or delayed puberty. Radiation therapy for acute lymphoblastic leukemia of the central nervous system, or prior to bone marrow transplantation, is characteristically associated with hormonal deficiency, but an increasing number of cases are reported of precocious puberty occurring after such therapy; higher doses of radiation may be more likely to cause gonadotropin-releasing hormone deficiency, and lower doses down to 18 Gy may lead to central precocious puberty. Epilepsy and developmental delay are associated with central precocious puberty in the absence of a central nervous system anatomic abnormality.

D. Virilizing Syndromes

Patients with long-untreated virilizing adrenal hyperplasia who have advanced bone ages may manifest precocious puberty after the adrenal hyperplasia is controlled with glucocorticoid suppression. Children with virilizing tumors or those given long-term androgen therapy may follow the same pattern when the androgen source is removed. Advanced maturation of the hypothalamic-pituitary-gonadal axis appears to occur with any condition causing excessive androgen secretion and advanced skeletal age.

Incomplete Isosexual Precocious Puberty

A. Boys

Males may manifest premature sexual development in the absence of hypothalamic-pituitary maturation from either of two causes: (1) ectopic or autonomous endogenous secretion of hCG or LH or iatrogenic exogenous administration of chorionic gonadotropin, which can stimulate Leydig cell production of testosterone; or (2) autonomous endogenous secretion of androgens from the testes or adrenal glands or from iatrogenic exogenous administration of androgens. (In females, secretion of hCG will not by itself cause secondary sexual development.)

1. Gonadotropin-secreting tumors—These include hepatomas or hepatoblastomas of the liver as well as teratomas or choriocarcinoma of the mediastinum, gonads, retroperitoneum, or pineal gland and germinomas of the central nervous system. The testes are definitely enlarged but not to the degree found in central precocious puberty.

2. Autonomous androgen secretion—Secretion of androgens can occur because of inborn errors of adrenal enzyme function, as in 21-hydroxylase (P450c21) or 11β-hydroxylase (P450c11β) deficiency, virilizing adrenal carcinomas, interstitial cell tumors of the testes, or premature Leydig and germinal cell maturation. Newly recognized forms of late-onset congenital adrenal hyperplasia, generally of the 21-hydroxylase deficiency form, may occur years after birth with no congenital or neonatal manifestations of virilization.

Adrenal rest tissue may be found in the testes as a vestige of the common embryonic origin of the adrenal glands and the testes; in states of ACTH excess—primarily congenital adrenal hyperplasia—adrenal rests can enlarge (sometimes to remarkable size) and secrete adrenal androgens (see Chapter 14).

In boys with **familial gonadotropin-independent premature Leydig and germinal cell maturation,** plasma testosterone levels are in the pubertal range but plasma gonadotropin levels and the LH response to exogenous GnRH are in the prepubertal range or lower because autonomous testosterone secretion suppresses endogenous GnRH release. The cause of this sex-limited dominant condition lies in a constitutive activation of the LH receptor causing increased cyclic adenosine monophosphate (cAMP) production in the absence of LH leaving the LH receptor "on"; several mutations have been reported in the LH receptor gene in different families (eg, $Asp^{578} \rightarrow Gly$ or $Met^{571} \rightarrow Ile$). The differential diagnosis rests between testosterone-secreting tumor of the adrenal, testosterone-secreting Leydig cell neoplasm, and premature Leydig and germinal cell maturation.

If hCG secretion causes incomplete male isosexual precocity, FSH is not elevated; and since the seminiferous tubules are not stimulated, the testes do not enlarge as much as in complete sexual precocity. If incomplete sexual precocity is due to a testicular tumor, the testes may be large, asymmetric, and irregular in contour. Symmetric bilateral moderate enlargement of the testes suggests familial gonadotropin-independent premature maturation of Leydig and germinal cells, which is a sex-limited dominant condition. The testes are somewhat smaller in this condition than in true precocious puberty but are still over 2.5 cm in diameter.

B. Girls

Females with incomplete isosexual precocity have a source of excessive estrogens. In all cases of autonomous endogenous estrogen secretion or exogenous estrogen administration, serum LH and FSH levels are low.

1. Follicular cysts—If follicular cysts are large enough, they can secrete sufficient estrogen to cause breast development and even vaginal withdrawal bleeding; some girls have recurrent cysts that lead to several episodes of vaginal bleeding. Patients with cysts may have levels of serum estrogen high enough to mimic a tumor. Larger follicular cysts can twist on their pedicles and become infarcted, causing symptoms of acute abdomen in addition to the precocious estrogen effects.

2. Granulosa or theca cell tumors—These tumors of the ovaries secrete estrogen and are palpable in 80% of cases. Gonadoblastomas found in streak gonads, lipoid tumors, cystadenomas, and ovarian carcinomas are rare ovarian sources of estrogens or androgens.

3. Adrenal rest tissue—Adrenal rest tissue has long been known to cause testicular enlargement and androgen secretion in boys, particularly with the increased ACTH secretion of congenital adrenal hyperplasia. Recently, however, a girl with an ovarian adrenal rest was reported to have hypertension, precocious puberty, Cushing's syndrome, and ovarian enlargement.

4. Exogenous estrogen administration—Ingestion of estrogen-containing substances or even cutaneous absorption of estrogen can cause feminization in children. Epidemics of gynecomastia and precocious thelarche in Puerto Rico and Italy have variously been attributed to ingestion of estrogen-contaminated food, estrogens in the environment, or undetermined causes. One outbreak of gynecomastia in boys and precocious thelarche in girls in Bahrain was traced to ingestion of milk from a cow given continuous estrogen treatment by its owner to ensure uninterrupted milk production.

5. Hypothyroidism—Severe untreated hypothyroidism can be associated with sexual precocity and galactorrhea (Van Wyk-Grumbach syndrome); treatment with thyroxine will correct hypothyroidism, halt precocious puberty and galactorrhea, and lower PRL levels. The cause of this syndrome was initially postulated to be increased gonadotropin secretion associated with the massive increase in TSH secretion. However, TSH can act on FSH receptors, causing gonadotropic effects due to elevated serum TSH concentrations.

6. McCune-Albright syndrome—McCune-Albright syndrome is classically manifested as a triad of irregular café au lait spots, fibrous dysplasia of long bones with cysts, and precocious puberty. However, hyperthyroidism, adrenal nodules with Cushing's syndrome, acromegaly, hyperprolactinemia, hyperparathyroidism, hypophosphatemic hyperphosphaturic rickets, or autonomous endogenous functioning ovarian cysts are described in girls. Precocious puberty may be central or incomplete; longitudinal studies demonstrate that some patients start with incomplete precocious puberty and progress to central precocious puberty. Long-term follow-up of McCune-Albright patients reveals a high incidence of pathologic fractures and orthopedic deformities due to the bone cysts, as well as hearing impairment due to the thickening of the temporal area of the skull. Patients may have a mutation of the Arg201 in exon 8 of the gene encoding the G protein alpha subunit that stimulates cAMP formation; this mutation impairs GTPase activity of the alpha subunit and increases adenylyl cyclase activity leading to the endocrine abnormalities described above. This defect originates in somatic rather than germ cells, leading to genetic mosaicism wherever the defective gene product is expressed; thus, a wide variety of tissues are affected.

Incomplete Contrasexual Precocity in Girls

Excess androgen effect can be caused by premature adrenarche or more significant pathologic conditions such as congenital or nonclassic adrenal hyperplasia or adrenal or ovarian tumors. P450c21 adrenal hyperplasia can be diagnosed on the basis of elevated serum 17-hydroxyprogesterone concentrations in the basal or ACTH-stimulated state (other adrenal metabolites may be elevated depending upon the defect under investigation). (See Chapter 14.) Both adrenal and ovarian tumors generally secrete testosterone, while adrenal tumors secrete DHEA. Thus, the source of the tumor may be difficult to differentiate if it produces only testosterone; MRI or CT scanning may be inadequate to diagnose the tumor's organ of origin, and selective venous sampling may be needed.

Variations in Pubertal Development

A. PREMATURE THELARCHE

The term "premature thelarche" denotes unilateral or bilateral breast enlargement without other signs of androgen or estrogen secretion of puberty. Patients are usually under 3 years of age; the breast enlargement may regress within months or remain until actual pubertal development occurs at a normal age. Areolar development and vaginal mucosal signs of estrogen effect are usually absent. Premature thelarche may be caused by brief episodes of estrogen secretion from ovarian cysts. Plasma estrogen levels are usually low in this disorder, perhaps because blood samples are characteristically drawn after the initiating secretory event. However, ultrasensitive estradiol assays do show a difference in estrogen production between control girls and those with premature thelarche. Classically, premature thelarche is self-limited and does not lead to central precocious puberty. However, there are reports of progression to central precocious puberty in a minority of cases, and follow-up for such progression is indicated.

B. PREMATURE MENARCHE

In rare cases, girls may begin to menstruate at an early age without showing other signs of estrogen effect. An unproved theory suggests that they may be manifesting increased uterine sensitivity to estrogen. In most subjects, menses stop within 1–6 years, and normal pubertal progression occurs thereafter.

C. PREMATURE ADRENARCHE

The term "premature adrenarche" denotes the early appearance of pubic or axillary hair without other signs of virilization or puberty. This nonprogressive disorder is compatible with a normal age at onset of other signs of puberty. It is more common in girls than in boys and usually is found in children over 6 years of age, overlapping with the new age limits of puberty in girls. Plasma and urinary DHEAS are elevated to stage 2 pubertal levels, which are higher than normally found in this age group. Bone and height ages may be slightly advanced for chronologic age. Patients may have abnormal electroencephalographic tracings without other signs of neurologic dysfunction. The presenting symptoms of late-onset adrenal hyperplasia may be similar to those of premature adrenarche, and the differential diagnosis may require ACTH stimulation testing (see Chapter 9). Other abnormalities in ovulation and menstruation have been reported following premature thelarche. This condition may be related to ovarian hyperandrogenism (see Chapter 13). Intrauterine growth-retarded babies have a predilection to develop premature adrenarche; girls may also progress to a polycystic ovary type of condition, and boys and girls alike may develop insulin resistance.

D. Adolescent Gynecomastia

Up to seventy-five percent of boys have transient unilateral or bilateral gynecomastia, usually beginning in stage 2 or 3 of puberty and regressing about 2 years later. Serum estrogen and testosterone concentrations are normal, but the estradiol:testosterone ratio may be elevated and SHBG concentrations may be high. Reassurance is usually all that is required, but some severely affected patients with extremely prominent breast development will require reduction mammoplasty if psychologic distress is extreme.

Aromatase inhibitors are in clinical trials as medical therapy for pronounced adolescent gynecomastia.

Some pathologic conditions such as Klinefelter's and Reifenstein's syndromes and the syndrome of incomplete androgen resistance are also associated with gynecomastia; these disorders should be clearly differentiated from the gynecomastia of normal puberty in males.

Differential Diagnosis of Precocious Puberty

The history and physical examination should be directed toward one of the diagnostic possibilities discussed above. Serum gonadotropin and sex steroid concentrations are determined in order to distinguish gonadotropin-mediated secondary sexual development (serum gonadotropin and sex steroid levels elevated) from autonomous endogenous secretion or exogenous administration of gonadal steroids (serum gonadotropin levels suppressed and sex steroid levels elevated). Third-generation immunoassays can identify the onset of increased gonadotropin secretion with a single basal unstimulated serum sample. In the past, a GnRH

test was required to confirm an increase in LH secretion at puberty because of the overlap of pubertal and prepubertal values of LH in the basal state. These third-generation gonadotropin assays can be applied to urine as well as serum samples; this may eliminate the need for GnRH testing and serial serum sampling.

If serum LH concentrations measured in an assay that cross-reacts with hCG are quite high in a boy or if a pregnancy screening test (βhCG) is positive, the likely diagnosis is an extrapituitary hCG-secreting tumor. β-LH values will be suppressed. If no abdominal or thoracic source of hCG is found, MRI of the head with particular attention to the hypothalamic-pituitary area is indicated to evaluate the possibility of a germinoma of the pineal gland.

If serum sex steroid levels are very high and gonadotropin levels are low, an autonomous source of gonadal steroid secretion must be assumed. If plasma gonadotropin and sex steroid levels are in the pubertal range, the most likely diagnosis is complete precocious puberty. In such patients, third-generation LH assays or the GnRH test will confirm the diagnosis (Table 15–5).

Differentiation between premature thelarche and central precocious puberty is usually accomplished by physical examination, but determination of serum estradiol or gonadotropins may be required. The evaluation of uterine size by ultrasound may also be useful as premature thelarche causes no increase in uterine volume while central precocious puberty does; ovarian size determination is a less useful method of distinguishing between the two possibilities. As noted above, some girls initially thought to have precocious thelarche progress to complete precocious puberty, but there is no way to distinguish girls who will progress from those who will not.

The onset of true or complete precocious puberty may indicate the presence of a hypothalamic tumor. Boys more often than girls have central nervous system tumors associated with complete precocious puberty. Skull x-rays are not usually helpful, but CT or MRI scanning is indicated in children with true precocious puberty. The present generation of CT and MRI scanners can make thin cuts through the hypothalamic-pituitary area with good resolution; small hypothalamic hamartomas are now being diagnosed more frequently. Generally, MRI is preferable to CT scan because of better resolution; the use of contrast may help to evaluate possible central nervous system lesions.

Treatment of Precocious Puberty

A. Central Precocious Puberty

In the past, medical treatment of true precocious puberty involved medroxyprogesterone acetate or cypro-

Table 15–5. Differential diagnosis of precocious puberty.

	Serum Gonadotropin Concentrations	LR Response to GnRH	Serum Sex Steroid Concentrations	Gonadal Size	Miscellaneous
Central (complete or true) precocious puberty					
	Pubertal	Pubertal pattern	Pubertal values	Normal pubertal enlargement of gonads in males	MRI scan of head to rule out a central nervous system tumor
Incomplete precocious puberty					
Males					
Chorionic gonadotropin-secreting tumor	High hCG (or LH in cross-reactive assay), positive pregnancy test, but β-LH (specific assay) is low	High basal hCG or LH that does not rise with GnRH, but β-LH is low and does not rise	High or pubertal values	Slight to moderate enlargement of gonads	Hepatic tumor must be considered. MRI scan of head if hCG-secreting central nervous system tumor suspected. LH assay typically measures hCG, so both results are high while β-hCG is high and β-LH, which does not detect hCG, is low
Leydig cell tumor	Prepubertal (low)	Prepubertal or suppressed pattern	Extremely high testosterone	Irregular asymmetric enlargement of testes	
Familial gonadotropin-independent sexual precocity with premature Leydig and germ cell maturation	Prepubertal (low)	Prepubertal or suppressed pattern	Pubertal or higher values	Testes larger than 2.5 cm but smaller than expected for stage of pubertal development	Often found in sex-limited dominant patterns
Females					
Granulosa cell tumor (follicular cysts may have similar presentation)	Prepubertal (low)	Prepubertal or suppressed pattern	Extremely high estradiol	Ovarian enlargement on physical, CT, MRI, or sonographic examination	Granulosa cell tumor is usually palpable on rectal examination
Follicular cyst	Prepubertal (low)	Prepubertal or suppressed pattern of LH. FSH secretion may rise above normal range	High to extremely high estradiol	Cysts may be visible on sonogram	Withdrawal bleeding may occur when estrogen levels decrease. Cysts may recur.

terone acetate, progestational agents that reduce gonadotropin secretion by negative feedback.

However, current treatment for precocious puberty due to a central nervous system lesion is much more effective. GnRH agonists are the preferred treatment for true precocious puberty to suppress sexual maturation and decrease growth rate and skeletal maturation. Chronic administration of highly potent and long-acting analogs of GnRH has been shown to down-regulate GnRH receptors and reduce pituitary gland response to GnRH, thereby causing decreased secretion of gonadotropin and sex steroids and rapidly stopping the progression of signs of sexual precocity. In girls, pubertal enlargement of the ovaries and uterus reverts toward the prepubertal state, and the multicystic appearance of the pubertal ovary regresses as well. This suppressive effect is reversed after therapy is discontinued. GnRH agonist treatment has been successful for idiopathic precocious puberty and precocious puberty caused by hamartomas of the tuber cinereum, neoplasms of the central nervous system, or long-term androgen exposure. The GnRH agonists were originally given by daily subcutaneous injection or intranasal insufflation; the successful use of these agents in microcapsules that are injected every 4 weeks or in depot preparations has now made treatment much easier and has improved compliance. Complete suppression of gonadotropin secretion is necessary because an incompletely suppressed patient may appear to have arrested pubertal development while actually secreting low but significant levels of sex steroids. Under these conditions, bone age advances while the growth rate is decreased, leading to even shorter adult stature. Side effects have generally been limited to allergic skin reactions and elevation of immunoglobulins directed against GnRH. Significant anaphylactic reactions to an injection have been reported. Decrease in bone mineral density is a potential side effect of GnRH agonists; increased dietary calcium supplementation is necessary. The FDA has approved histrelin, a GnRH agonist administered on a daily basis, and leuprolide acetate, a long-acting GnRH agonist, administered every 28 days for the management of precocious puberty. A daily dose form of leuprolide is also available. Individual monitoring is essential to ascertain gonadotropin suppression.

Growth velocity decreases within 5 months after the start of therapy, and rapid bone age advancement decreases to a rate below the increase in chronologic age. Without therapy, final height in patients with central precocious puberty approaches 152 cm in girls and 155–164 cm in boys. The first patients treated with GnRH agonists have now reached final height: The girls have a mean height of 157 cm and the boys a mean height of 164 cm—a definite improvement over the untreated state. The worst height prognosis is in children with an early diagnosis of precocious puberty who are not treated. The best outcomes of therapy are noted when diagnosis and therapy are achieved early, and as earlier diagnosis is now made in children with central precocious puberty and earlier therapy is offered, better results are expected in the future. Menarche is reported after the discontinuation of therapy in girls, indicating a reversion to normal pubertal endocrine function following GnRH agonist treatment. The new lower age limits of normal pubertal development in girls have led clinicians to reassess the criteria used to identify appropriate candidates for therapy. Patients without significant elevation of serum estrogen, who have a predicted height appropriate for family, and who have slowly progressing variants without early menarche may achieve an appropriate final height without therapy.

Psychologic support is important for patients with sexual precocity. The somatic changes or menses will frighten some children and may make them the object of ridicule. These patients do not experience social maturation to match their physical development, though their peers, teachers, and relatives will tend to treat them as if they were older because of their large size. Thus, supportive counseling must be offered to both patient and family. Evidence indicates that children with precocious puberty are more often sexually abused, so appropriate precautions are necessary.

B. INCOMPLETE PRECOCIOUS PUBERTY

Treatment of the disorders discussed above under incomplete precocious puberty is directed toward the underlying tumor or abnormality rather than toward the signs of precocious puberty. If the primary cause is controlled, signs of sexual development will be halted in progression or may even regress.

Males with familial Leydig and germ cell maturation will not initially respond to GnRH agonist therapy, but some have improved with medroxyprogesterone acetate. Affected boys were successfully treated with ketoconazole, an antifungal agent that can block 17,20-lyase and therefore decrease testosterone production. After initial control with ketoconazole, the boys developed true precocious puberty, because prolonged exposure to androgens matured their hypothalamic-pituitary axis; treatment with a GnRH agonist then effectively halted this pubertal progression. Newer therapy involves the use of an aromatase inhibitor and an antiandrogen combination as for the treatment of McCune-Albright syndrome.

A successful therapy for McCune-Albright syndrome in girls is a combination of testolactone (an aromatase inhibitor) and spironolactone (which acts as an anti-androgen). Long-term follow-up demonstrated some decrease in menses and improvement in growth patterns and bone age advancement. Some escaped from control, necessitating the addition of a GnRH agonist, which then suppressed pubertal development. Girls with recurrent estrogen-secreting ovarian cyst formation may have a decreased incidence of cysts with medroxyprogesterone acetate therapy, and a GnRH agonist may also be effective in such cases. Surgical removal of ovarian cysts may be unnecessary if such medical therapy is first utilized.

Precocious thelarche or adrenarche requires no treatment, as both are self-limited benign conditions. No therapy has been reported for premature menarche, and none may be indicated. Severe, persistent cases of adolescent gynecomastia have been treated successfully by testolactone and dihydrotestosterone heptanoate, though surgical removal of breast tissue is often necessary. Aromatase inhibitors may ultimately be approved for this use.

REFERENCES

General

Ahmed ML et al: Longitudinal study of leptin concentrations during puberty: sex differences and relationship to changes in body composition. J Clin Endocrinol Metab 1999;84:899.

Bachrach LK et al: Bone mineral acquisition in healthy Asian, Hispanic, black, and Caucasian youth: a longitudinal study. J Clin Endocrinol Metab 1999;84:4702.

Chan GM, Hoffman K, McMurry M: Effects of dairy products on bone and body composition in pubertal girls. J Pediatr 1995;126:551.

Greulich WW, Pyle SI: *Radiographic Atlas of Skeletal Development of the Hand and Wrist,* 2nd ed. Stanford Univ Press, 1959.

Grumbach MM, Styne DM: Puberty, ontogeny, neuroendocrinology, physiology, and disorders. In: Larsen PR et al [editors]: *Williams Textbook of Endocrinology,* 10th ed. Saunders, 2002.

Grumbach MM, Auchus RJ: Estrogen: consequences and implications of human mutations in synthesis and action. J Clin Endocrinol Metab 1999;84:4677.

Harris DA et al: Somatomedin-C in normal puberty and in true precocious puberty before and after treatment with a potent luteinizing hormone-releasing hormone agonist: Evidence for an effect of estrogen and testosterone on somatomedin-C concentrations. J Clin Endocrinol Metab 1985;61:152.

Hergenroeder AC et al: Validity of self-assessment of pubertal maturation in African American and European American adolescents. J Adolesc Health 1999;24:201.

Herman-Giddens ME et al: Secondary sexual characteristics and menses in young girls seen in office practice: a study from the Pediatric Research in Office Settings network. Pediatrics 1997;99:505.

Manasco PK et al: Ontogeny of gonadotropin, testosterone, and inhibin secretion in normal boys through puberty based on overnight serial sampling. J Clin Endocrinol Metab 1995; 80:2046.

Miller WL, Styne DM: Female puberty and its disorders. In: Yen SSC, Jaffe RB, Barberi RL (editors): *Reproductive Endocrinology,* 4th ed. Saunders, 1999.

Mitamura R et al: Diurnal rhythms of luteinizing hormone, follicle-stimulating hormone, and testosterone secretion before the onset of male puberty. J Clin Endocrinol Metab 1999; 84:29.

Neely EK et al: Normal ranges for immunochemiluminometric gonadotropin assays. J Pediatr 1995;127:40.

Smith EP et al: Estrogen resistance caused by a mutation in the estrogen-receptor gene in a man. N Engl J Med 1994;331: 1056.

Styne DM: New aspects in the diagnosis and treatment of pubertal disorders. Pediatr Clin North Am 1997;44:505.

Styne DM: The testes: disorders of sexual maturation and puberty. In: *Pediatric and Adolescent Endocrinology,* 2nd ed. Sperling MA (editor). Saunders, 2002.

Vieira JG et al: Serum levels of prostate-specific antigen in normal boys throughout puberty. J Clin Endocrinol Metab 1994;78: 1185.

Physical Changes Associated with Puberty

Attie KM et al: The pubertal growth spurt in eight patients with true precocious puberty and growth hormone deficiency: Evidence for a direct role of sex steroids. J Clin Endocrinol Metab 1990;71:975.

Bayley N, Pinneau SF: Tables for predicting adult height from skeletal age: Revised for use with the Greulich-Pyle standards. J Pediatr 1952;40:423.

Marshall WA, Tanner JM: Variations in the pattern of pubertal changes in boys. Arch Dis Child 1970;45:13.

Marshall WA, Tanner JM: Variations in the pattern of pubertal changes in girls. Arch Dis Child 1969;44:291.

Van Wieringen JC et al: *Growth Diagrams 1965 Netherlands: Second National Survey on 0–24 Year Olds.* Groningen, Netherlands Institute for Preventive Medicine NO Leiden, Wolters-Noordhoff Publishing, 1971.

Delayed Puberty & Sexual Infantilism

Achermann JC et al: Mutational analysis of *DAX1* in patients with hypogonadotropic hypogonadism or pubertal delay. J Clin Endocrinol Metab 1999;84:4497.

Barrio R et al: Induction of puberty with human chorionic gonadotropin and follicle-stimulating hormone in adolescent males with hypogonadotropic hypogonadism. Fertil Steril 1999;71:244.

Curtis J et al: The endocrine outcome after surgical removal of craniopharyngiomas. Pediatr Neurosurg 1994;21(Suppl 1):24.

Gertner JM et al: Delayed somatic growth and pubertal development in human immunodeficiency virus-infected hemophiliac boys. Hemophilia Growth and Development Study. J Pediatr 1994;124:896.

Grumbach MM, Conte FA: Disorders of sexual differentiation. In: Larsen PR et al [editors]: *Williams Textbook of Endocrinology,* 10th ed. Saunders, 2002.

Osipova GR et al: PCR detection of Y-specific sequences in patients with Ullrich-Turner syndrome: clinical implications and limitations. Am J Med Genet 1998;76:283.

Rosenfeld RG et al: Growth hormone therapy of Turner's syndrome: beneficial effect on adult height. J Pediatr 1998; 132:319.

Rosenfield RL et al: Optimizing estrogen replacement treatment in Turner syndrome. Pediatrics 1998;102:486.

Seminara SB et al: X-linked adrenal hypoplasia congenita: a mutation in *DAX1* expands the phenotypic spectrum in males and females. J Clin Endocrinol Metab 1999;84:4501.

Seminara SB, Hayes FJ, Crowley WFJ: Gonadotropin-releasing hormone deficiency in the human (idiopathic hypogonadotropic hypogonadism and Kallmann's syndrome): pathophysiological and genetic considerations. Endocr Rev 1999;19:521.

Siddiqi SU et al: Premature sexual development in individuals with neurodevelopmental disabilities. Dev Med Child Neurol 1999;41:392.

Sexual Precocity

Anasti JN et al: A potential novel mechanism for precocious puberty in juvenile hypothyroidism. J Clin Endocrinol Metab 1995;80:276.

Bar A et al: Bayley-Pinneau method of height prediction in girls with central precocious puberty: Correlation with adult height. J Pediatr 1995;126:955.

Boot AM et al: Bone mineral density and body composition before and during treatment with gonadotropin-releasing hormone agonist in children with central precocious and early puberty. J Clin Endocrinol Metab 1998;83:370.

Carel JC et al: Final height after long-term treatment with triptorelin slow release for central precocious puberty: importance of statural growth after interruption of treatment. French Study Group of Decapeptyl in Precocious Puberty. J Clin Endocrinol Metab 1999;84:1973.

Feuillan PP et al: Reproductive axis after discontinuation of gonadotropin-releasing hormone analog treatment of girls with precocious puberty: long term follow-up comparing girls with hypothalamic hamartoma to those with idiopathic precocious puberty. J Clin Endocrinol Metab 1999;84:44.

Feuillan PP, Jones J, Cutler GB: Long-term testolactone therapy for precocious puberty in girls with the McCune-Albright syndrome. J Clin Endocrinol Metab 1993;77:647.

Heger S, Partsch CJ, Sippell WG: Long-term outcome after depot gonadotropin-releasing hormone agonist treatment of central precocious puberty: final height, body proportions, body composition, bone mineral density and reproductive function. J Clin Endocrinol Metab 2000;85:4583.

Ibanez L, de Zegher F, Potau N: Anovulation after precocious pubarche: early markers and time course in adolescence. J Clin Endocrinol Metab 1999;84:2691.

Klein KO et al: Estrogen levels in girls with premature thelarche compared with normal prepubertal girls as determined by an ultrasensitive recombinant cell bioassay. J Pediatr 1999;134:190.

Klein KO et al: Use of an ultrasensitive recombinant cell bioassay to determine estrogen levels in girls with precocious puberty treated with a luteinizing hormone-releasing hormone agonist. J Clin Endocrinol Metab 1998;83:2387.

Kornreich L et al: Central precocious puberty: Evaluation by neuroimaging. Pediatr Radiol 1995;25:7.

Laue L et al: Genetic heterogeneity of constitutively activating mutations of the human luteinizing hormone receptor in familial male-limited precocious puberty. Proc Natl Acad Sci U S A 1995;92:1906.

Leschek EW et al: Six-year results of spironolactone and testolactone treatment of familial male-limited precocious puberty with addition of deslorelin after central puberty onset. J Clin Endocrinol Metab 1999;84:175.

Neely EK et al: Spontaneous serum gonadotropin concentrations in the evaluation of precocious puberty. J Pediatr 1995;127:47.

Palmert MR, Malin HV, Boepple PA: Unsustained or slowly progressive puberty in young girls: initial presentation and long-term follow-up of 20 untreated patients. J Clin Endocrinol Metab 1999;84:415.

Paul D et al: Long-term effect of gonadotropin-releasing hormone agonist therapy on final and near-final height in 26 children with true precocious puberty treated at a median age of less than 5 years. J Clin Endocrinol Metab 1995;80:546.

Salardi S et al: Outcome of premature thelarche: relation to puberty and final height. Arch Dis Child 1998;79:173.

Styne DW et al: Treatment of true precocious puberty with a potent luteinizing hormone-releasing factor agonist: Effect on growth, sexual maturation, pelvic sonography, and the hypothalamic-pituitary-gonadal axis. J Clin Endocrinol Metab 1985;61:142.

The Endocrinology of Pregnancy

16

Robert N. Taylor, MD, PhD, & Dan I. Lebovic, MD, MA

ACTH	Adrenocorticotropic hormone	**hPL**	Human placental lactogen
cAMP	Cyclic adenosine monophosphate	**IGF**	Insulin-like growth factor
CBG	Corticosteroid-binding globulin	**LH**	Luteotropic hormone
CRH	Corticotropin-releasing hormone	**MRI**	Magnetic resonance imaging
CT	Computed tomography	**PDGF**	Platelet-derived growth factor
DHEA	Dehydroepiandrosterone acetate	**PRL**	Prolactin
DOC	Deoxycorticosterone	**SHBG**	Sex hormone-binding globulin
EGF	Epidermal growth factor	**TBG**	Thyroid hormone-binding globulin
FGF	Fibroblast growth factor	**TGF**	Transforming growth factor
FSH	Follicle-stimulating hormone	**TRH**	Thyrotropin-releasing hormone
GH	Growth hormone	**TSH**	Thyroid-stimulating hormone (thyrotropin)
GnRH	Gonadotropin-releasing hormone		
hCG	Human chorionic gonadotropin	**TSI**	Thyroid-stimulating immunoglobulin

Throughout pregnancy, the fetal-placental unit secretes protein and steroid hormones into the mother's bloodstream, and these apparently or actually alter the function of every endocrine gland in her body. Both clinically and in the laboratory, pregnancy can mimic hyperthyroidism, Cushing's disease, pituitary adenoma, diabetes mellitus, and polycystic ovary syndrome.

The endocrine changes associated with pregnancy are adaptive, allowing the mother to nurture the developing fetus. Although maternal reserves are usually adequate, occasionally, as in the case of gestational diabetes or hypertensive disease of pregnancy, a woman may develop overt signs of disease as a direct result of pregnancy.

Aside from creating a satisfactory maternal environment for fetal development, the placenta serves as a repository endocrine gland as well as a respiratory, alimentary, and excretory organ. Measurements of fetal-placental products in the maternal serum provide one means of assessing fetal well-being. This chapter will consider the changes in maternal endocrine function in pregnancy and during parturition as well as fetal endocrine development. The chapter concludes with a discussion of some endocrine disorders complicating pregnancy.

CONCEPTION & IMPLANTATION

Fertilization

In fertile women, ovulation occurs approximately 12–16 days after the onset of the previous menses. The ovum must be fertilized within 24–48 hours if conception is to result. For about 48 hours around ovulation, cervical mucus is copious, nonviscous, slightly alkaline, and forms a gel matrix that acts as a filter and conduit for sperm. Following intercourse, sperm that are to survive penetrate the cervical mucus within minutes and can remain viable there until the mucus character changes, approximately 24 hours following ovulation. Sperm begin appearing in the outer third of the uterine tube (the ampulla) 5–10 minutes after coitus and continue to migrate to this location from the cervix for about 24–48 hours. Of the 200×10^6 sperm that are deposited in the vaginal fornices, only approximately 200 reach the distal uterine tube. Fertilization normally occurs in the ampulla.

Implantation

Implantation in the uterus does not occur until 8–10 days after ovulation and fertilization, when the conceptus is a blastocyst. In most pregnancies, the dates of ovulation and implantation are not known. Weeks of gestation ("gestational age") are by convention calculated from the first day of the last menstrual period. Within 24 hours after implantation, or at about 3 weeks of gestation, human chorionic gonadotropin (hCG) is detectable in maternal serum. Under the influence of increasing hCG production, the corpus luteum continues to secrete steroid hormones in increasing quantities. Without effective implantation and subsequent hCG production, the corpus luteum survives for only about 14 days following ovulation.

Symptoms & Signs of Pregnancy

Breast tenderness, fatigue, nausea, absence of menstruation, softening of the uterus, and a sustained elevation of basal body temperature are all attributable to hormone production by the corpus luteum and developing placenta.

Ovarian Hormones of Pregnancy

The hormones produced by the corpus luteum include progesterone, 17-hydroxyprogesterone, and estradiol. The indispensability of the corpus luteum in early pregnancy has been demonstrated by ablation studies, in which luteectomy or oophorectomy before 42 days of gestation results in precipitous decreases in levels of serum progesterone and estradiol, followed by abortion. Exogenous progesterone will prevent abortion, proving that progesterone alone is required for maintenance of early pregnancy. After about the seventh gestational week, the corpus luteum can be removed without subsequent abortion owing to compensatory progesterone production by the placenta.

Because the placenta does not produce appreciable amounts of 17-hydroxyprogesterone, this steroid provides a marker of corpus luteum function. As shown in Figure 16–1, the serum concentrations of estrogens and total progesterone exhibit a steady increase, but the concentration of 17-hydroxyprogesterone rises and then declines to low levels that persist for the duration of the pregnancy. The decline of corpus luteum func-

tion occurs despite the continued production of hCG; in fact, corpus luteum production of 17-hydroxyprogesterone declines while hCG is still rising to maximal levels. Whether this is due to down-regulation of corpus luteal hCG receptors is not known.

Another marker of corpus luteum function is the polypeptide hormone relaxin, a protein with a molecular mass of about 6000. It is similar in its tertiary structure to insulin. Relaxin becomes detectable at about the same time as hCG begins to rise, and it maintains a maximum maternal serum concentration of about 1 ng/mL during the first trimester. The serum concentration then falls approximately 20% and is constant for the remainder of the pregnancy.

Pharmacologically, relaxin ripens the cervix, softens the pubic symphysis, and acts synergistically with progesterone to inhibit uterine contractions. A major physiologic role for relaxin in human gestation has not been established. Luteectomy after 7 weeks of gestation does not interfere with gestation in spite of undetectable relaxin levels. Extraluteal production of relaxin by the decidua and placenta has been demonstrated, however, and local effects may be exerted without alteration of systemic hormone concentrations.

FETAL-PLACENTAL-DECIDUAL UNIT

The function of the placenta is to establish effective communication between the mother and the developing fetus while maintaining the immune and genetic integrity of both individuals. Initially, the placenta functions autonomously. By the end of the first trimester, however, the fetal endocrine system is sufficiently developed to influence placental function and to provide some hormone precursors to the placenta. From this time, it is useful to consider the conceptus as the fetal-placental unit.

The fetal-placental unit will be considered in three separate but related categories: (1) as a source of secretion of protein and steroid hormones into the maternal circulation; (2) as a participant in the control of fetal endocrine function, growth, and development; and (3) as a selective barrier governing the interaction between the fetal and maternal systems.

Within 8 days after fertilization, implantation begins. The alpha-v-beta-3 integrin vitronectin receptor may serve as a link between the maternal and embryonic epithelia. The trophoblast invades the endometrium, and two layers of developing placenta can be demonstrated. Columns of invading cytotrophoblasts anchor the placenta to the endometrium. The differentiated syncytiotrophoblast, also derived from precursor cytotrophoblasts, is in direct contact with the maternal circulation. The syncytiotrophoblast is the major source of hormone production, containing the

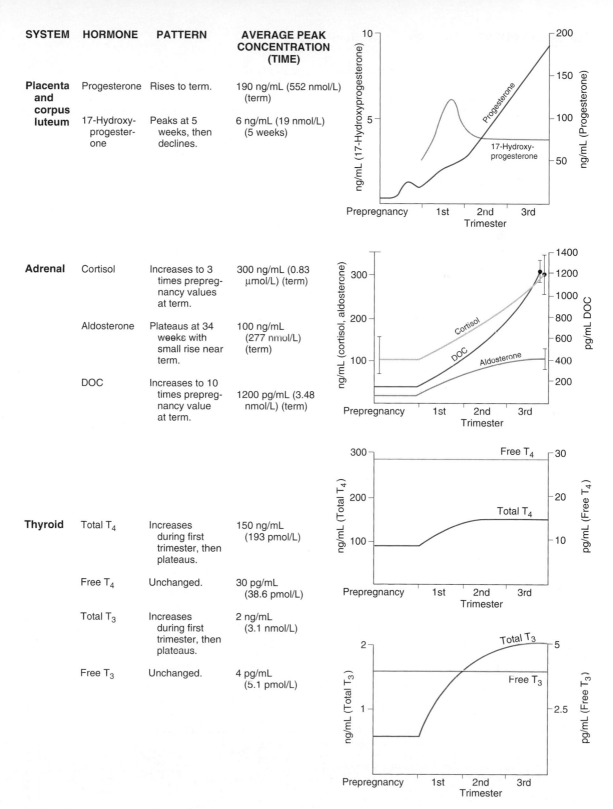

SYSTEM	HORMONE	PATTERN	AVERAGE PEAK CONCENTRATION (TIME)
Placenta and corpus luteum	Progesterone	Rises to term.	190 ng/mL (552 nmol/L) (term)
	17-Hydroxy-progester-one	Peaks at 5 weeks, then declines.	6 ng/mL (19 nmol/L) (5 weeks)
Adrenal	Cortisol	Increases to 3 times prepreg-nancy values at term.	300 ng/mL (0.83 μmol/L) (term)
	Aldosterone	Plateaus at 34 weeks with small rise near term.	100 ng/mL (277 nmol/L) (term)
	DOC	Increases to 10 times prepreg-nancy value at term.	1200 pg/mL (3.48 nmol/L) (term)
Thyroid	Total T$_4$	Increases during first trimester, then plateaus.	150 ng/mL (193 pmol/L)
	Free T$_4$	Unchanged.	30 pg/mL (38.6 pmol/L)
	Total T$_3$	Increases during first trimester, then plateaus.	2 ng/mL (3.1 nmol/L)
	Free T$_3$	Unchanged.	4 pg/mL (5.1 pmol/L)

Figure 16–1. Maternal serum hormone changes during pregnancy.

SYSTEM	HORMONE	PATTERN	AVERAGE PEAK CONCENTRATION (TIME)
Anterior pituitary	GH	Unchanged.	
	LH, FSH	Low, basal levels.	
	ACTH	Unchanged.	
	TSH	Reaches nadir during first trimester, then plateaus.	
	PRL	Rise to term.	200 ng/mL (g nmol/L) (term)
Placental proteins	hCG	Peaks at 10 weeks, then decreases to a lower plateau.	5 μg/mL (0.2 μmol/L) (end of first trimester)
	hPL	Rises with placental weight.	5–25 μg/mL (term) (0.2–1.0 μmol/L)
	CRH	Rises acutely about 20 days before delivery.	1–3 ng/mL (2–6 nmol/L) at term
Fetopla-cental estrogens	Estriol	Increases to term.	15–17 ng/mL (55–62 nmol/L) (term)
	Estradiol	Increases to term.	12–15 ng/mL (42–52 nmol/L) (term)
	Estrone	Increases to term.	5–7 ng/mL (18.5–26 nmol/L) (term)
Fetopla-cental androgens	Testos-terone	Rises to 10 times pre-pregnancy values.	2000 pg/mL (6.9 nmol/L) (term)
	DHEA	Falls during pregnancy.	5 ng/mL (17.3 nmol/L) (pre-pregnancy)
	Andro-stenedione	Small increase.	2.6 ng/mL (9.0 nmol/L) (term)

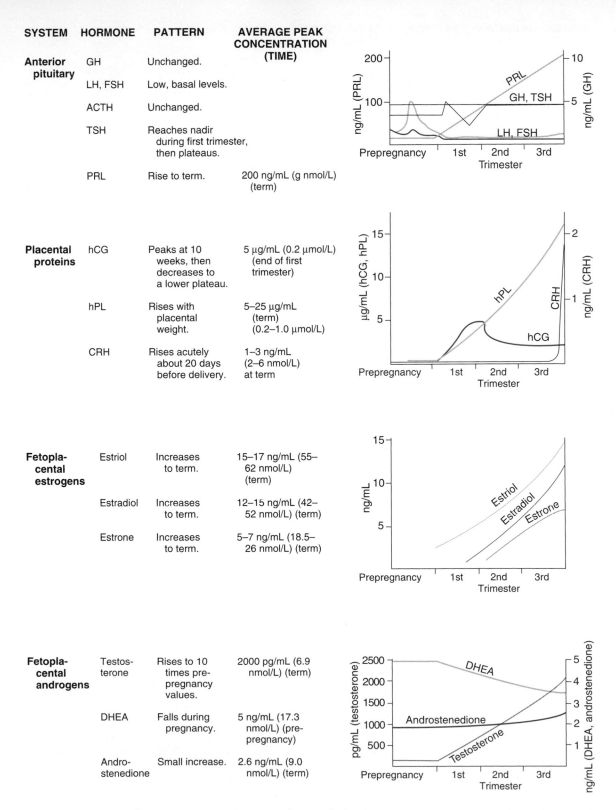

Figure 16–1 (cont'd). Maternal serum hormone changes during pregnancy.

cellular machinery needed for synthesis, packaging, and secretion of both steroid and polypeptide hormones.

The decidua is the endometrium of pregnancy. Recent investigation has shown that the decidual cells are capable of synthesizing a variety of polypeptide hormones, including prolactin (PRL), relaxin, and a variety of paracrine factors, in particular IGF-binding protein I. The role of the decidua as an endocrine organ has not been established, but its role as a source of prostaglandins during labor is certain (see Endocrine Control of Parturition, below).

Modern methods of screening for fetal chromosomal aneuploidy, particularly trisomy 21 (Down's syndrome), utilize circulating biochemical markers. Screening by maternal age alone (> 35 years) led to the prenatal identification of only about 25% of aneuploid fetuses. As an aneuploid chromosome complement affects both fetal and placental tissues, their protein and steroid products have been evaluated. A combination of alpha-fetoprotein, hCG, and unconjugated estriol concentrations, secreted into and measured in maternal serum between 15 and 18 weeks' gestation, can be used to identify fetal Down's syndrome and trisomy 18 with a detection rate of 60% over all age groups.

POLYPEPTIDE HORMONES

Human Chorionic Gonadotropin

The first marker of trophoblast differentiation and the first measurable product of the placenta is chorionic gonadotropin (hCG). hCG is a glycoprotein consisting of about 237 amino acids. It is quite similar in structure to the pituitary glycoproteins in that it consists of two chains: an alpha chain, which is species-specific; and a beta chain, which determines receptor interaction and ultimate biologic effect. The alpha chain is identical in sequence to the alpha chains of the hormonal glycoproteins TSH, FSH, and LH. The beta chain has significant sequence homology with LH but is not identical; of the 145 amino acids in β-hCG, 97 (67%) are identical to those of β-LH. In addition, the placental hormone has a carboxyl terminal segment of 30 amino acids not found in the pituitary LH molecule. Carbohydrate constitutes approximately 30% by weight of each subunit. Sialic acid alone accounts for 10% of the weight of the molecule and confers a high degree of resistance to degradation and consequently a long plasma half-life of about 24 hours.

In the early weeks of pregnancy (up to 6 weeks), the concentration of hCG doubles every 1.7–2 days, and serial measurements provide a sensitive index of early trophoblast function. Maternal plasma hCG peaks at about 100,000 mIU/mL during the tenth gestational week and then declines gradually to about 10,000 mIU/mL in the third trimester. Peak concentrations correlate temporally with the establishment of maternal blood flow in the intervillous space (Figure 16–1).

These characteristics of hCG all contribute to the possibility of diagnosing pregnancy several days before any symptoms occur or a menstrual period has been missed. Without the long plasma half-life of hCG (24 hours), the tiny mass of cells comprising the blastocyst could not produce sufficient hormone to be detected in the peripheral circulation within 24 hours of implantation. Antibodies to the unique β-carboxyl terminal segment of hCG do not cross-react significantly with any of the pituitary glycoproteins. As little as 5 mIU/mL (1 ng/mL) of hCG in plasma can be detected without interference from the higher levels of LH, FSH, and TSH.

Like its pituitary counterpart LH, hCG is luteotropic, and the corpus luteum has high-affinity receptors for hCG. The stimulation of increased amounts of progesterone production by corpus luteum cells is driven by increasing concentrations of hCG. Steroid synthesis can be demonstrated in vitro and is mediated by the cAMP system. hCG has been shown to enhance placental conversion of maternal low-density lipid cholesterol to pregnenolone and progesterone.

The concentration of hCG in the fetal circulation is less than 1% of that found in the maternal compartment. However, there is evidence that fetal hCG is an important regulator of the development of the fetal adrenal and gonad during the first trimester.

hCG is also produced by trophoblastic neoplasms such as hydatidiform mole and choriocarcinoma, and the concentration of hCG or its beta subunit is used as a tumor marker, for diagnosis, and for monitoring the success or failure of chemotherapy in these disorders. Women with very high hCG levels due to trophoblastic disease may become clinically hyperthyroid and revert to euthyroidism as hCG is reduced during chemotherapy.

Human Placental Lactogen

A second placental polypeptide hormone, also with homology to a pituitary protein, is termed placental lactogen (hPL). hPL is detectable in the early trophoblast, but detectable serum concentrations are not reached until 4–5 gestational weeks (Figure 16–1). hPL is a protein of about 190 amino acids whose primary, secondary, and tertiary structures are similar to those of growth hormone (GH). The two molecules cross-react in immunoassays and in some receptor and bioassay systems. However, hPL has only some of the biologic activities of GH. Like GH, hPL is diabetogenic, but it has minimal growth-promoting activity as measured by standard GH bioassays. hPL also shares many structural features with prolactin (PRL).

The physiologic role of hPL during pregnancy remains controversial, and normal pregnancy without detectable hPL production has been reported. Although not clearly shown to be a mammotropic agent, hPL contributes to altered maternal glucose metabolism and mobilization of free fatty acids; causes a hyperinsulinemic response to glucose loads; appears to directly stimulate pancreatic islet insulin secretion; and contributes to the peripheral insulin resistance characteristic of pregnancy. Along with prolonged fasting and insulin-induced hypoglycemia, pre-beta-HDL and apoprotein A-I are two factors that stimulate release of hPL. hPL production is roughly proportionate to placental mass. Actual production rates may reach as much as 1–1.5 g/d. The disappearance curve shows multiple components but yields a serum half-life of 15–30 minutes. Serum hPL concentration had been proposed as an indicator of the continued health of the placenta, but the range of normal values is wide, and serial determinations are necessary. hPL determinations have largely been replaced by biophysical profiles, which are more sensitive indicators of fetal jeopardy.

Other Chorionic Peptide Hormones & Growth Factors

Other chorionic peptides have been identified, but their functions have not yet been defined. One of these proteins is a glycoprotein with partial sequence and functional homology to TSH. Its existence as a separate entity from hCG has been debated in the literature, with some reports suggesting that chorionic TSH is a protein with a molecular weight of about 28,000, structurally different from hCG, with weak thyrotropic activity. Similarly, ACTH-like, lipotropin-like, and endorphin-like peptides have been isolated from placenta, but they have low biologic potency and undetermined physiologic roles. A chorionic FSH-like protein has also been isolated from placenta but has not yet been detected in plasma. Good evidence exists that the cytotrophoblast produces a human chorionic gonadotropin-releasing hormone that is biologically and immunologically indistinguishable from the hypothalamic GnRH. The release of hCG from the syncytiotrophoblast may be under the direct control of this factor, in a fashion analogous to the hypothalamic control of anterior pituitary secretion of gonadotropins. Preliminary evidence is also available for similar paracrine control of syncytiotrophoblastic release of TSH, somatostatin, and corticotropin by analogous cytotrophoblastic releasing hormones. Activin, inhibin, corti-

cotropin-releasing factor, and multiple peptide growth factors, including fibroblast growth factor (FGF), epidermal growth factor (EGF), platelet-derived growth factor (PDGF), and the insulin-like growth factors (IGFs)—and many of their cognate receptors—have all been isolated from placental tissue. Placental EGF and the related TGFα have been suggested to play a role in fetal growth.

STEROID HORMONES

In contrast to the impressive synthetic capability exhibited in the production of placental proteins, the placenta does not appear to have the capability to synthesize steroids de novo. All steroids produced by the placenta are derived from maternal or fetal precursor steroids.

No tissue, however, even remotely approaches the syncytiotrophoblast in its capacity to efficiently interconvert steroids. This activity is demonstrable even in the early blastocyst, and by the seventh gestational week, when the corpus luteum has undergone relative involution, the placenta becomes the dominant source of steroid hormones.

Progesterone

The placenta relies on maternal cholesterol as its substrate for progesterone production. Fetal death has no immediate influence on progesterone production, suggesting that the fetus is a negligible source of substrate. Enzymes in the placenta cleave the cholesterol side chain, yielding pregnenolone, which in turn is partially isomerized to progesterone; 250–350 mg of progesterone is produced daily by the third trimester, and most enters the maternal circulation. The maternal plasma concentration of progesterone rises progressively throughout pregnancy and appears to be independent of factors that normally regulate steroid synthesis and secretion (Figure 16–1). Whereas exogenous hCG increases progesterone production in pregnancy, hypophysectomy has no effect. Administration of ACTH or cortisol does not influence progesterone concentrations, nor does adrenalectomy or oophorectomy after 7 weeks.

Progesterone is necessary for establishment and maintenance of pregnancy. Insufficient corpus luteum production of progesterone may contribute to failure of implantation, and luteal phase deficiency is implicated in some cases of infertility and recurrent pregnancy loss. Furthermore, progesterone, along with nitric oxide (NO), seems to maintain uterine quiescence during pregnancy. Progesterone also may act as an immunosuppressive agent in some systems and inhibits T cell-mediated tissue rejection. Thus, high local concentrations of progesterone may contribute to immunologic tolerance by the uterus of invading embryonic trophoblast tissue.

Estrogens

Estrogen production by the placenta also depends on circulating precursors, but in this case both fetal and maternal steroids are important sources. Most of the estrogens are derived from fetal androgens, primarily dehydroepiandrosterone sulfate (DHEA sulfate). Fetal DHEA sulfate, produced mainly by the fetal adrenal, is converted by placental sulfatase to the free dehydroepiandrosterone (DHEA) and then, through enzymatic pathways common to steroid-producing tissues, to androstenedione and testosterone. These androgens are finally aromatized by the placenta to estrone and estradiol, respectively.

Placental corticotropin-releasing hormone (CRH) may be an important regulator of fetal adrenal DHEA sulfate secretion. The greater part of fetal DHEA sulfate is metabolized to produce a third estrogen: estriol. Estriol is a weak estrogen with one-tenth the potency of estrone and one-hundredth the potency of estradiol. While serum estrone and estradiol concentrations are increased during pregnancy about 50-fold over their maximal prepregnancy values, estriol increases approximately 1000-fold. The key step in estriol synthesis is 16α-hydroxylation of the steroid molecule (Figure 13–4). The substrate for the reaction is primarily fetal DHEA sulfate, and the vast majority of the production of the 16α-hydroxy-DHEA sulfate occurs in the fetal adrenal and liver, not in maternal or placental tissues. The final steps of desulfation and aromatization to estriol occur in the placenta. Maternal serum or urinary estriol measurements, unlike measurements of progesterone or hPL, reflect fetal as well as placental function. Normal estriol production, therefore, reflects the integrity of fetal circulation and metabolism as well as adequacy of the placenta. Rising serum or urinary estriol concentrations are the best available biochemical indicator of fetal well-being (Figure 16–1). 17-Hydroxysteroid dehydrogenase type II prevents fetal exposure to potent estrogens by catalyzing the conversion of estradiol to less potent estrone.

There are some circumstances in which decreased estriol production is the result of congenital derangements or iatrogenic intervention. Maternal estriol remains low in pregnancies with placental sulfatase deficiency and in cases of fetal anencephaly. In the first case, DHEA sulfate cannot be hydrolyzed; in the second, little fetal DHEA is produced because fetal adrenal stimulation by ACTH is lacking. Maternal administration of glucocorticoids inhibits fetal ACTH and lowers maternal estriol. Administration of DHEA to the mother during a healthy pregnancy increases estriol production. Antibiotic therapy can reduce estriol levels by interfering with bacterial glucuronidases and maternal reabsorption of estriol from the gut. Estetrol, an estrogen metabolite with a fourth hydroxyl at the 16 position, is unique to pregnancy.

Cases of aromatase deficiency and estrogen receptor mutations indicate that estrogen action is not mandatory for the maintenance of pregnancy. Homozygous mutant mice with disrupted estrogen receptor genes undergo apparently normal blastocyst, fetal, and placental development. This observation has been corroborated by a clinical case of a spontaneous missense mutation of the estrogen receptor in a man.

MATERNAL ADAPTATION TO PREGNANCY

As a successful "parasite," the fetal-placental unit manipulates the maternal "host" for its own gain but normally avoids imposing excessive stress that would jeopardize the "host" and thus the "parasite" itself. The prodigious production of polypeptide and steroid hormones by the fetal-placental unit directly or indirectly results in physiologic adaptations of virtually every maternal organ system. These alterations are summarized in Figure 16–2. Most of the commonly measured maternal endocrine function tests are radically changed. In some cases, true physiologic alteration has occurred; in others, the changes are due to increased production of specific serum binding proteins by the liver or to decreased serum levels of albumin. Additionally, some hormonal changes are mediated by altered clearance rates owing to increased glomerular filtration, decreased hepatic excretion of metabolites, or metabolic clearance of steroid and protein hormones by the placenta. The changes in endocrine function tests are summarized in Table 16–1. Failure to recognize normal pregnancy-induced alterations in endocrine function tests can lead to unnecessary diagnostic tests and therapy that may be seriously detrimental to mother and fetus.

Maternal Pituitary Gland

The mother's anterior pituitary gland hormones have little influence on pregnancy after implantation has occurred. The gland itself enlarges by about one-third, with the major component of this increase being hyperplasia of the lactotrophs in response to the high plasma estrogens. PRL, the product of the lactotrophs, is the only anterior pituitary hormone that rises progressively during pregnancy and peaks at the time of delivery, with contributions from both the anterior pituitary and the decidua. In spite of the high serum concentrations,

SYSTEM	PARAMETER	PATTERN
Cardiovascular	Heart rate	Gradually increases 20%.
	Blood pressure	Gradually decreases 10% by 34 weeks, then increases to prepregnancy values.
	Stroke volume	Increases to maximum at 19 weeks, then plateaus.
	Cardiac output	Rises rapidly by 20%, then gradually increases an additional 10% by 28 weeks.
	Peripheral venous distention	Progressive increase to term.
	Peripheral vascular resistance	Progressive decrease to term.
Pulmonary	Respiratory rate	Unchanged.
	Tidal volume	Increases by 30–40%.
	Expiratory reserve	Gradual decrease.
	Vital capacity	Unchanged.
	Respiratory minute volume	Increases by 40%.
Blood	Volume	Increases by 50% in second trimester.
	Hematocrit	Decreases slightly.
	Fibrinogen	Increases.
	Electrolytes	Unchanged.
Gastrointestinal	Sphincter tone	Decreases.
	Gastric emptying time	Increases.

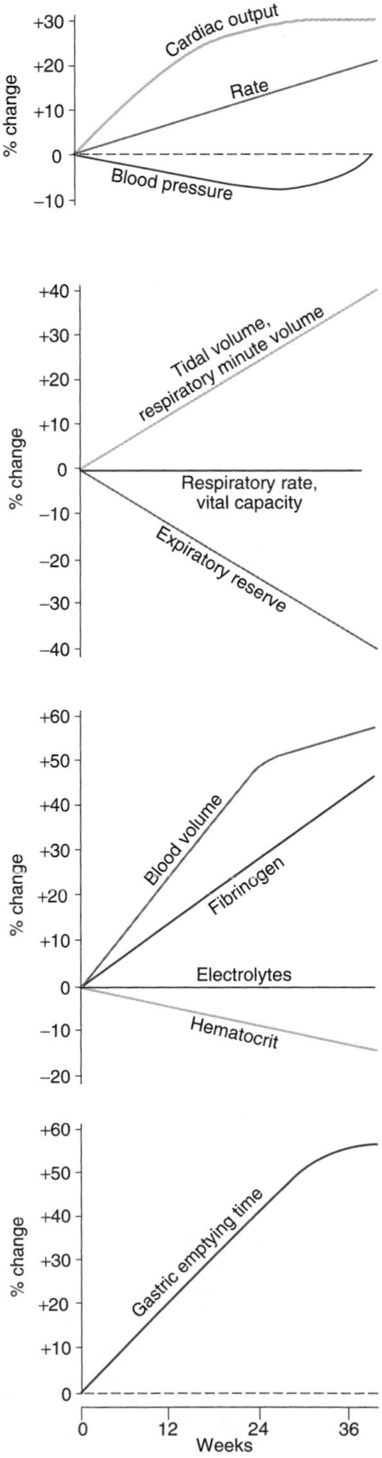

Figure 16–2. Maternal physiologic changes during pregnancy.

SYSTEM	PARAMETER	PATTERN
Renal	Renal flow	Increases 25–50%.
	Glomular filtration rate	Increases early, then plateaus.
Weight	Uterine weight	Increases from about 60–70 g to about 900–1200 g.
	Body weight	Average 11-kg (25-lb) increase.

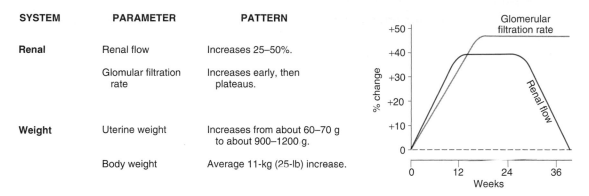

Figure 16–2 (cont'd). Maternal physiologic changes during pregnancy.

pulsatile release of PRL and nocturnal and food-induced increases persist. Hence, the normal neuroendocrine regulatory mechanisms appear to be intact in the maternal adenohypophysis. Pituitary ACTH and TSH secretion remain unchanged. Serum FSH and LH fall to the lower limits of detectability and are unresponsive to GnRH stimulation. GH concentrations are not significantly different from nonpregnant levels, but pituitary response to provocative testing is markedly altered. GH response to hypoglycemia and arginine infusion is enhanced in early pregnancy but thereafter becomes depressed. Established pregnancy can continue in the face of hypophysectomy, and in women hypophysectomized prior to pregnancy, induction of ovulation and normal pregnancy can be achieved with appropriate replacement therapy. In cases of primary pituitary hyperfunction, the fetus is not affected.

Maternal Thyroid Gland

The thyroid becomes palpably enlarged during the first trimester, and a bruit may be present. Thyroid iodide clearance and thyroidal ^{131}I uptake, which are clinically contraindicated in pregnancy, have been shown to be increased. These changes are due in large part to the increased renal clearance of iodide, which causes a relative iodine deficiency. While total serum thyroxine is elevated as a result of estrogen-stimulated increased thyroid hormone-binding globulin (TBG), free thyroxine and triiodothyronine are normal (Figure 16–1). High circulating concentrations of hCG, particularly asialo-hCG, which has weak TSH-like activity, contributes to the thyrotropic action of the placenta in early pregnancy. In fact, there is often a significant though transient biochemical hyperthyroidism associated with hCG stimulation in early gestation.

Maternal Parathyroid Gland

The net calcium requirement imposed by fetal skeletal development is estimated to be about 30 g by term. This is met by hyperplasia of the parathyroid glands and elevated serum levels of parathyroid hormone. The maternal serum calcium concentration declines to a nadir at 28–32 weeks, largely owing to the hypoalbuminemia of pregnancy. Ionized calcium is maintained at normal concentrations throughout pregnancy.

Maternal Pancreas

The nutritional demands of the fetus require alteration of maternal metabolic homeostatic control, which results in both structural and functional changes in the maternal pancreas. The size of pancreatic islets increases, and insulin-secreting β cells undergo hyperplasia. Basal levels of insulin are lower or unchanged in early pregnancy but increase during the second trimester. Thereafter, pregnancy is a hyperinsulinemic state, with resistance to the peripheral metabolic effects of insulin. The increased concentration of insulin has been shown to be a result of increased secretion rather than decreased metabolic clearance. The measured half-life for insulin is unchanged in pregnant women. The effects of pregnancy on the pancreas can be mimicked by appropriate treatment with estrogen, progesterone, hPL, and corticosteroids.

Pancreatic production of glucagon remains responsive to usual stimuli and is suppressed by glucose loading, although the degree of responsiveness has not been well evaluated.

The major role of insulin and glucagon is the intracellular transport of nutrients, specifically glucose, amino acids, and fatty acids. These concentrations are regulated during pregnancy for fetal as well as maternal

Table 16–1. Effect of pregnancy on endocrine function tests.

	Test	Result
Pituitary FSH, LH	GnRH stimulation	Unresponsive from third gestational week until puerperium
GH	Insulin tolerance test	Response increases during the first half of pregnancy and then is blunted until the puerperium
	Arginine stimulation	Hyperstimulation during the first and second trimesters, then suppression
TSH	TRH stimulation	Response unchanged
Pancreas Insulin	Glucose tolerance	Peak glucose increases, and glucose concentration remains elevated longer
	Glucose challenge	Insulin concentration increases to higher peak levels
	Arginine infusion	Insulin response is blunted in mid to late pregnancy
Adrenal Cortisol	ACTH infusion	Exaggerated cortisol and 17-hydroxycorticosterone responses
	Metyrapone	Diminished response
Mineralocorticoids	ACTH infusion	No DOC response
	Dexamethasone suppression	No DOC response

needs, and the pre- and postfeeding levels cause pancreatic responses that act to support the fetal economy. Insulin is not transported across the placenta but rather exerts its effects on transportable metabolites. During pregnancy, peak insulin secretion in response to meals is accelerated, and glucose tolerance curves are characteristically altered. Fasting glucose levels are maintained at low normal levels. Excess carbohydrate is converted to fat, and fat is readily mobilized during decreased caloric intake.

Amino acid metabolism is also altered during pregnancy at the expense of maternal needs. Because alanine, the key amino acid for gluconeogenesis, is preferentially transported to the fetus, maternal hypoglycemia leads to lipolysis.

The normal result of pregnancy, then is to reduce glucose levels modestly but to reserve glucose for fetal needs while maternal energy requirements are met increasingly by the peripheral metabolism of fatty acids. These changes in energy metabolism are beneficial to the fetus and innocuous to the mother with an adequate diet. Even modest fasting, however, causes ketosis, which is potentially injurious to the fetus.

Maternal Adrenal Cortex

A. GLUCOCORTICOIDS

Plasma cortisol concentrations increase to three times nonpregnant levels by the third trimester. Most of the increase can be accounted for by a doubling of corticosteroid-binding globulin (CBG). The increased estrogen levels of pregnancy account for the increase in CBG, which, in turn, is sufficient to account for decreased catabolism of cortisol by the liver. The result is a doubling of the half-life of plasma cortisol. The actual production of cortisol by the zona fasciculata also is increased in pregnancy. The net effect of these changes is an increase in plasma free cortisol, which is approximately doubled by late pregnancy. Whether this increase is mediated through ACTH or by other mechanisms is not known. In spite of cortisol concentrations approaching those found in Cushing's syndrome, diurnal variation in plasma cortisol is maintained. The elevated free cortisol probably contributes to the insulin resistance of pregnancy and possibly to the appearance of striae, but most signs of hypercortisolism do not occur in pregnancy. It is possible that high progesterone levels act as a glucocorticoid antagonist and prevent some cortisol effects.

B. MINERALOCORTICOIDS AND THE RENIN-ANGIOTENSIN SYSTEM

Serum aldosterone is markedly elevated in pregnancy. The increase is due to an eight- to tenfold increased production of aldosterone by the zona glomerulosa and not to increased binding or decreased clearance. The peak in aldosterone production is reached by mid pregnancy and is maintained until delivery. Renin substrate is increased owing to the influence of estrogen on hepatic synthesis, and renin also is increased.

The increases in both renin and renin substrate inevitably lead to increases in renin activity and angiotensin. In spite of these dramatic changes, normal pregnant women show few signs of hyperaldosteronism. There is no tendency to hypokalemia or hypernatremia, and blood pressure at mid pregnancy—when changes in the aldosterone-renin-angiotensin system are maximal—tends to be lower than in the nonpregnant state.

Although the quantitative aspects of this apparent paradox are not fully understood, a qualitative explanation is possible. Progesterone is an effective competitive inhibitor of mineralocorticoids in the distal renal tubules. Exogenous progesterone (but not synthetic progestins) is natriuretic and potassium-sparing in intact humans, whereas it has no effect in adrenalectomized subjects not receiving mineralocorticoids. Progesterone also blunts the response of the kidney to exogenous aldosterone—thus, the increases in renin and aldosterone may simply be an appropriate response to the high gestational levels of progesterone. The concomitant increase in angiotensin II as a result of increased plasma renin activity apparently does not normally result in hypertension, because of diminished sensitivity of the maternal vascular system to angiotensin. Even during the first trimester, exogenous angiotensin provokes less of a rise in blood pressure than in the nonpregnant state.

It is clear that the high levels of renin, angiotensin, and aldosterone in pregnant women are subject to the usual feedback controls, because they respond appropriately to changes in posture, dietary sodium, and water loading and restriction in qualitatively the same way as they do in nonpregnant women. Finally, in patients with preeclampsia, the most common form of pregnancy-related hypertension, serum renin, aldosterone, and angiotensin levels are lower than in normal pregnancy, thus ruling out any primary role for the renin-angiotensin system in this disorder. Production of the mineralocorticoid 11-deoxycorticosterone (DOC) rises throughout pregnancy, and plasma levels six to ten times normal are achieved by term. In contrast to the nonpregnant state, DOC production in pregnancy is unaffected by ACTH or glucocorticoid administration. Fetal pregnenolone-3,21-disulfate may serve as a placental precursor of maternal DOC. DOC is not elevated in hypertensive disorders of pregnancy.

C. ANDROGENS

In normal pregnancy, the maternal production of androgens is slightly increased. The most important determinant of plasma levels of specific androgens, however, appears to be whether or not the androgen binds to sex hormone-binding globulin (SHBG). Testosterone, which binds avidly to SHBG, increases to the normal male range by the end of the first trimester, but free testosterone levels are actually lower than in the nonpregnant state. Dehydroepiandrosterone sulfate (DHEA sulfate) does not bind significantly to SHBG, and plasma concentrations of DHEA sulfate actually decrease during pregnancy. The desulfation of DHEA sulfate by the placenta and the conversion of DHEA sulfate to estrogens by the fetal-placental unit also are important factors in its increased metabolic clearance.

FETAL ENDOCRINOLOGY

Because of the inaccessibility of the fetus, much of our information about fetal endocrinology is derived indirectly. Most early studies of fetal endocrinology relied upon observations of infants with congenital disorders or inferences from ablation studies or acute manipulation in experimental animals. The development of effective cell culture methods, sensitive immunoassays, and the ability to achieve stable preparations of chronically catheterized monkey fetuses have increased our understanding of the dynamics of intrauterine endocrine events.

Study of the fetal endocrine system is further complicated by the multiplicity of sources of the various hormones. The fetus is exposed to maternal and placental hormones as well as to those it produces itself. Amniotic fluid contains a variety of hormones of mixed fetal and maternal origin, and these hormones are of uncertain importance. Inferences from the behavior of adult endocrine systems are not transferable to the fetus, because target organs, receptors, modulators, and regulators develop at different times. Study of the isolated fetus, even if possible, would thus be of little physiologic relevance.

Dating of events in fetal development is usually given in "fetal weeks," which begin at the time of ovulation and fertilization. Thus, fetal age is always 2 weeks less than gestational age.

Human fetal growth is influenced by endocrine and hemodynamic factors that dictate the partitioning of nutrients between the mother and the conceptus. The main metabolic substrates for fetal and placental growth are glucose, lactate, amino acids, and lipids. A variety of placental transport proteins regulate the partitioning of these nutrients. In addition, placental hormones such as hPL, GH-variant, and IGF-I and IGF-II are secreted into the maternal and fetal circulations where they modulate energy metabolism and fetal growth.

The endocrine system is among the first to develop in fetal life. Differentiation of the gonads is crucial for normal male sexual development and reproductive potential. Primary testis differentiation begins with development of the Sertoli cells at 8 weeks' gestation. SRY is the sex-determining locus on the Y chromosome which directs the differentiation of the Sertoli cells, which are the sites of müllerian-inhibiting substance (MIS) synthesis. MIS, a member of the TGFβ family of growth factors, specifically triggers the ipsilateral resorption of the müllerian tract in males. Embryonic androgen production begins in the developing Leydig cells at about 10 weeks, coincident with the peak production of placental hCG. The ovarian counterpart in the female is smaller and less differentiated at this stage of embryonic life. Oogonia mitosis is active and steroid-producing theca cell precursors are identifiable at 20 weeks. This corresponds with peak gonadotropin levels from the fetal pituitary. Activin and inhibin peptide subunits are expressed in the midtrimester human testis but not in the midtrimester human ovary. In contrast to the male fetus, ovarian steroid production is not essential for female phenotypic development (see Chapter 14).

Fetal Anterior Pituitary Hormones

The characteristic anterior pituitary cell types are discernible as early as 8–10 fetal weeks, and all of the hormones of the adult anterior pituitary are extractable from the fetal adenohypophysis by 12 weeks. Similarly, the hypothalamic hormones thyrotropin-releasing hormone (TRH), gonadotropin-releasing hormone (GnRH), and somatostatin are present by 8–10 weeks. The direct circulatory connection between hypothalamus and pituitary develops later, with capillary invasion initially visible at about 16 weeks.

The role of the fetal pituitary in organogenesis of various target organs during the first trimester appears to be negligible. None of the pituitary hormones are released into the fetal circulation in large quantities until after 20 fetal weeks. Even growth hormone (GH) appears not to be influential, and in fact total absence of GH is consistent with normal development at birth. Development of the gonads and adrenals during the first trimester appears to be directed by hCG rather than by fetal pituitary hormones.

During the second trimester, there is a marked increase in secretion of all of the anterior pituitary hormones, which coincides with maturation of the hypophysial portal system. Observations include a marked rise in production of GH and an increase in fetal serum TSH, with a concomitant increase in fetal thyroidal iodine uptake. Gonadotropin production also increases, with the female achieving higher FSH levels in both pituitary and serum than does the male. The fetal gonadotropins do not direct the events of early gonadal development but are essential for normal development of the differentiated gonads and external genitalia. ACTH rises significantly during the second trimester and assumes an increasing role in directing the maturation of the differentiated adrenal, as shown by the anencephalic fetus, in which the fetal zone of the adrenal undergoes atrophy after 20 weeks. Fetal PRL secretion also increases after the 20th fetal week, but the functional significance of this hormone, if any, is unknown.

During the third trimester, maturation of feedback systems modulating hypothalamic release signals causes serum concentrations of all of the pituitary hormones except PRL to decline.

Fetal Posterior Pituitary Hormones

Vasopressin and oxytocin are demonstrable by 12–18 weeks in the fetal posterior pituitary gland and correlate with the development of their sites of production, the supraoptic and paraventricular nuclei, respectively. The hormone content of the gland increases toward term, with no evidence of feedback control.

During labor, umbilical artery oxytocin is higher than umbilical vein oxytocin. It has been suggested that the fetal posterior pituitary may contribute to the onset or maintenance of labor.

Fetal Thyroid Gland

The thyroid gland develops in the absence of detectable TSH. By 12 weeks the thyroid is capable of iodine-concentrating activity and thyroid hormone synthesis.

During the second trimester, TRH, TSH, and free T_4 all begin to rise. The maturation of feedback mechanisms is suggested by the subsequent plateau of TSH at about 20 fetal weeks. Fetal T_3 and reverse T_3 do not become detectable until the third trimester. The hormone produced in largest amount throughout fetal life is T_4, with the metabolically active T_3 and its inactive derivative, reverse T_3, rising in parallel to T4 during the third trimester. At birth, conversion of T_4 to T_3 becomes demonstrable.

The development of thyroid hormones occurs independently of maternal systems, and very little placental transfer of thyroid hormone occurs in physiologic concentrations. This prevents maternal thyroid disorders from affecting the fetal compartment but also prevents effective therapy for fetal hypothyroidism through maternal supplementation. Goitrogenic agents such as propylthiouracil are transferred across the placenta and may induce fetal hypothyroidism and goiter.

The function of the fetal thyroid hormones appears crucial to somatic growth and for successful neonatal adaptation. Many auditory maturational events may be regulated by thyroid hormones.

Fetal Parathyroid Gland

The fetal parathyroid is capable of synthesizing parathyroid hormone by the end of the first trimester. However, the placenta actively transports calcium into the fetal compartment, and the fetus remains relatively hypercalcemic throughout gestation. This contributes to a suppression of parathyroid hormone, and fetal serum levels in umbilical cord have been reported to be low or undetectable. Fetal serum calcitonin levels are elevated, enhancing bone accretion. Fetal vitamin D levels reflect maternal levels but do not appear to be significant in fetal calcium metabolism.

Fetal Adrenal Cortex

The fetal adrenal differs anatomically and functionally from the adult gland. The cortex is identifiable as early as 4 weeks of fetal age, and by the seventh week, steroidogenic activity can be detected in the inner zone layers.

By 20 weeks, the adrenal cortex has increased to a mass that is considerably larger than its relative postnatal size. During gestation, it occupies as much as 0.5% of total body volume, and most of this tissue is composed of a unique fetal zone that subsequently regresses or is transformed into the definitive (adult) zone during the early neonatal period. The inner fetal zone is responsible for the majority of steroids produced during fetal life and comprises 80% of the mass of the adrenal. During the second trimester, the inner fetal zone continues to grow, while the outer zone remains relatively undifferentiated. At about 25 weeks, the definitive (adult) zone develops more rapidly, ultimately assuming the principal role in steroid synthesis during the early postnatal weeks. This transfer of function is accompanied by involution of the fetal zone, which is completed during the first months of neonatal life.

Fetal Gonads

The testis is a detectable structure by about 6 fetal weeks. The interstitial or Leydig cells, which synthesize fetal testosterone, are functional at this same stage. The maximal production of testosterone coincides with the maximal production of hCG by the placenta; binding of hCG to fetal testes with stimulation of testosterone release has been demonstrated. Other fetal testicular products of importance are the reduced testosterone metabolite dihydrotestosterone and müllerian-inhibiting substance. Dihydrotestosterone is responsible for development of the external genital structures, whereas müllerian-inhibiting substance prevents development of female internal structures.

Little is known about fetal ovarian function. By 7–8 weeks of intrauterine life, the ovaries become recognizable, but their importance in fetal physiology has not been established, and the significance of the steroids produced by the ovaries remains unclear.

ENDOCRINE CONTROL OF PARTURITION

During the last few weeks of normal pregnancy, two processes herald approaching labor. Uterine contractions, usually painless, become increasingly frequent, and the lower uterine segment and cervix become softer and thinner, a process known as effacement, or "ripening." Although false alarms are not uncommon, the onset of true labor is usually fairly abrupt, with the establishment of regular contractions every 2–5 minutes, leading to delivery in less than 24 hours. There is a huge literature describing the physiologic and biochemical events that occur during human labor, but the key inciting event has eluded detection. For sheep, it is the fetus that controls the onset of labor. The initial measurable event is an increase in fetal plasma cortisol, which, in turn, alters placental steroid production, resulting in a drop in progesterone. Cortisol reliably induces labor in sheep, but in humans, glucocorticoids do not induce labor and there is no clear drop in plasma progesterone prior to labor. Furthermore, exogenous progesterone does not prevent labor in humans. Emerging primate data suggest that at the time of parturition, an increase in the ratio of the potent repressor progesterone receptor-A to the active progesterone receptor-B may lead to functional suppression of progesterone action and subsequent parturition.

A role for placental CRH in the regulation of parturition is suspected given the sharp increase in placental CRH mRNA from 28 weeks of gestation until delivery. Three weeks before the onset of labor, the exponential rise in plasma CRH is accompanied by an abrupt fall in CRH-binding protein. Glucocorticoids enhance placental CRH expression—thus, the rise in placental CRH that precedes parturition could result from the rise in fetal glucocorticoids that occurs at this time. The increase in placental CRH may stimulate—via stimulation of fetal pituitary ACTH—a further rise in fetal glucocorticoids, completing a positive feedback loop that would be terminated by delivery. Further evidence for a role of CRH in parturition is seen in studies showing CRH receptors in the myometrium and fetal membranes, CRH-stimulating prostaglandin release from human decidua and amnion, and, finally, the CRH-induced augmentation of oxytocin and prostaglandin F_2 actions.

The difficulty in identifying a single initiating event in human labor suggests that there is more than one. Approaching the matter in a different way, one could ask: What are the factors responsible for maintenance of pregnancy, and how can they fail?

Sex Steroids

Progesterone is essential for maintenance of early pregnancy, and withdrawal of progesterone leads to termination of pregnancy. Progesterone causes hyperpolarization of the myometrium, decreasing the amplitude of action potentials and preventing effective contractions. In various experimental systems, progesterone decreases alpha-adrenergic receptors, stimulates cAMP production, and inhibits oxytocin receptor synthesis. Progesterone also inhibits estrogen receptor synthesis, promotes the storage of prostaglandin precursors in the decidua and fetal membranes, and stabilizes the lysosomes containing prostaglandin-synthesizing enzymes. Estrogen opposes progesterone in these actions and may have an independent role in ripening the uterine cervix and promoting uterine contractility. Thus, the estrogen:progesterone ratio may be an important parameter. In a small series of patients, an increase in the estrogen:progesterone ratio has been shown to precede labor. Thus, for some individuals, a drop in progesterone or an increase in estrogen may initiate labor. The cause of the change in steroids may be placental maturation or a signal from the fetus, but there are no data to support either thesis. It has been shown that an increase in the estrogen:progesterone ratio increases the number of oxytocin receptors and myometrial gap junctions; this finding may explain the coordinated, effective contractions that characterize true labor as opposed to the nonpainful, ineffective contractions of false labor.

Oxytocin

Oxytocin infusion is commonly used to induce or augment labor. Both maternal and fetal oxytocin levels increase spontaneously during labor, but neither has been convincingly shown to increase prior to labor. Data in animals suggest that oxytocin's role in initiation of labor is due to increased sensitivity of the uterus to oxytocin rather than increased plasma concentrations of the hormone. Even women with diabetes insipidus are able to deliver without oxytocin augmentation; thus a maternal source of the hormone is not indispensable.

Prostaglandins

Prostaglandin $F_{2\alpha}$ administered intra-amniotically or intravenously is an effective abortifacient as early as 14 weeks of gestation. Prostaglandin E_2 administered by vagina will induce labor in most women in the third trimester. The amnion and chorion contain high concentrations of arachidonic acid, and the decidua contains active prostaglandin synthetase. Prostaglandins are almost certainly involved in maintenance of labor once it is established. They also probably are important in initiating labor in some circumstances, such as in amnionitis or when the membranes are "stripped" by the physician. They probably are part of the "final common pathway" of labor.

Prostaglandin synthetase inhibitors abolish premature labor, but their clinical usefulness has been restricted by their simultaneous effect of closing the ductus arteriosus, which can lead to fetal pulmonary hypertension.

Catecholamines

Catecholamines with α_2-adrenergic activity cause uterine contractions, whereas β_2-adrenergics inhibit labor. Progesterone increases the ratio of beta receptors to alpha receptors in myometrium, thus favoring continued gestation. There is no evidence that changes in catecholamines or their receptors initiate labor, but it is likely that such changes help sustain labor once initiated. The beta-adrenergic drug ritodrine has proved to be a valuable agent in the management of premature labor. Alpha-adrenergic agents have not been useful in inducing labor, because of their cardiovascular side effects.

Nitric Oxide

Uterine smooth muscle may also be affected by nitric oxide (NO), which may act as a uterine smooth muscle relaxant. Some laboratory findings suggest that uterine NO production decreases at term and that inhibitors of NO synthesis might some day be used to initiate or augment human labor.

ENDOCRINOLOGY OF THE PUERPERIUM

Extirpation of any active endocrine organ leads to compensatory changes in other organs and systems. Delivery of the infant and placenta causes both immediate and long-term adjustment to loss of the pregnancy hormones. The sudden withdrawal of fetal-placental hormones at delivery permits determination of their serum half-lives and some evaluation of their effects on maternal systems.

Physiologic & Anatomic Changes

Some of the physiologic and anatomic adjustments that take place after delivery are hormone-dependent, whereas others are themselves responsible for hormonal changes. For example, major readjustments of the cardiovascular system occur in response to the normal blood losses associated with delivery and to loss of the low-resistance placental shunt. By the third postpartum day, blood volume is estimated to decline to about 84% of predelivery values. These cardiovascular changes influence renal and liver clearance of hormones.

Reproductive Tract Changes

The uterus decreases progressively in size at the rate of about 500 g/wk and continues to be palpable abdominally until about 2 weeks postpartum, when it reoccupies its position entirely within the pelvis. Nonpregnant size and weight (60–70 g) are reached by 6 weeks. The reversal of myometrial hypertrophy occurs with a decrease in size of individual myometrial cells rather than by reduction in number. Uterine discharge also changes progressively during this period, with the mixture of fresh blood and decidua becoming a serous transudate and then ceasing in 3–6 weeks.

The endometrium, which is sloughed at the time of delivery, regenerates rapidly; by the seventh day, there is restoration of surface epithelium, except at the placental site. By the second week after delivery, the endometrium resembles normal proliferative-phase endometrium, except for the characteristic hyalinized decidual areas. The earliest documented appearance of a secretory endometrium occurred on day 44 in one series of daily biopsies. These rapid regenerative changes do not apply to the area of placental implantation, which requires much longer for restoration and retains pathognomonic histologic evidence of placentation indefinitely.

The cervix and vagina also recover rapidly from the effects of pregnancy, labor, and delivery. The cervix regains tone over the first week; by 6 weeks postpartum, it usually exhibits complete healing of trauma sustained at the time of delivery. Histologically, involution may continue beyond 6 weeks, with stromal edema, leukocytic infiltration, and glandular hyperplasia still apparent. Similarly, the vagina regains muscular tone following delivery, and rugae appear as early as 3 weeks. However, in women who nurse, the vaginal mucosa may remain atrophic for months, sometimes resulting in dyspareunia and a watery discharge.

Endocrine Changes

A. Steroids

With expulsion of the placenta, the steroid levels decline precipitously, their half-lives being measured in minutes or hours. As a consequence of continued low-level production by the corpus luteum, progesterone does not reach basal prenatal levels as rapidly as does estradiol. Plasma progesterone falls to luteal-phase levels within 24 hours after delivery but to follicular-phase levels only after several days. Removal of the corpus luteum results in a fall to follicular levels within 24 hours. Estradiol reaches follicular-phase levels within 1–3 days after delivery.

B. Pituitary Hormones

The pituitary gland, which enlarges during pregnancy owing primarily to an increase in lactotrophs, does not diminish in size until after lactation ceases. Secretion of FSH and LH continues to be suppressed during the early weeks of the puerperium, and stimulus with bolus doses of GnRH results in subnormal release of LH and FSH. Over the ensuing weeks, responsiveness to GnRH gradually returns to normal, and most women exhibit follicular-phase serum levels of LH and FSH by the third or fourth postpartum week.

C. Prolactin

Serum prolactin (PRL), which rises throughout pregnancy, falls with the onset of labor and then exhibits variable patterns of secretion depending upon whether breast feeding occurs. Delivery is associated with a surge in PRL, which is followed by a rapid fall in serum concentrations over 7–14 days in the nonlactating mother.

In nonlactating women, the return of normal cyclic function and ovulation may be expected as soon as the second postpartum month, with the initial ovulation occurring at an average of 9–10 weeks postpartum. In lactating women, PRL usually causes a persistence of anovulation. Surges of PRL are believed to act on the hypothalamus to inhibit GnRH secretion. Administration of exogenous GnRH during this time induces normal pituitary responsiveness, and occasional ovulation may occur spontaneously even during lactation. The average time for ovulation in women who have lactated for at least 3 months is about 17 weeks. The percentage of nonlactating women who have resumed menstruation increases linearly up to 12 weeks, by which time 70% will have restored menses. In contrast, the linear increase for lactating women exhibits a much shallower slope, and 70% of lactating women will have menstruated by about 36 weeks.

Lactation

Development of the breast alveolar lobules occurs throughout pregnancy. This period of mammogenesis requires the concerted participation of estrogen, progesterone, PRL, GH, and glucocorticoids. hPL may also play a role but is not indispensable. Milk secretion in the puerperium is associated with further enlargement of the lobules, followed by synthesis of milk constituents such as lactose and casein.

Lactation requires PRL, insulin, and adrenal steroids. It does not occur until unconjugated estrogens fall to nonpregnant levels at about 36–48 hours postpartum.

PRL is essential to milk production. Its action involves induced synthesis of large numbers of PRL receptors; these appear to be autoregulated by PRL, since PRL increases receptor levels in cell culture and since bromocriptine, an inhibitor of PRL release, causes a decrease in both PRL and its receptors. In the absence of PRL, milk secretion does not take place; but even in the presence of high levels of PRL during the third trimester, milk secretion does not take place until after delivery, owing to the blocking effect of high levels of estrogen.

Galactopoiesis, or the process of continued milk secretion, is also dependent upon the function and integration of several hormones. Evidence from GH-deficient dwarfs and hypothyroid patients suggests that GH and thyroid hormone are not required.

Milk secretion requires the additional stimulus of emptying of the breast. A neural arc must be activated for continued milk secretion. Milk ejection occurs in response to a surge of oxytocin, which induces a contractile response in the smooth muscle surrounding the gland ductules. Oxytocin release is occasioned by stimuli of a visual, psychologic, or physical nature that prepare the mother for suckling, while PRL release is limited to the suckling reflex arc.

ENDOCRINE DISORDERS & PREGNANCY

PITUITARY DISORDERS

In women of reproductive age, small tumors of the anterior pituitary are not uncommon (see also Chapter 5). While most are nonfunctional and asymptomatic, the most common symptom of pituitary microadenomas is amenorrhea, frequently accompanied by galactorrhea. In the past, few affected women became pregnant, but now most can be made to ovulate and to conceive with the aid of clomiphene citrate, menotropins and hCG, or bromocriptine. Before ovulation is induced in any patient, serum PRL should be determined. Modest elevations of PRL warrant checking IGF-I levels, since hyperprolactinemia occurs in 25% of patients with GH-producing adenomas. If it is elevated, the sella turcica should be evaluated by magnetic resonance imaging (MRI) or by high-resolution CT scanning with contrast. About 10% of women with secondary amenorrhea will be found to have adenomas, while 20–50% of women with amenorrhea and galactorrhea will have detectable tumors.

The effect of pregnancy on pituitary adenomas depends on the size of the adenoma. Among 216 women with microadenomas (< 10 mm in diameter), fewer than 1% developed progressive visual field defects, 5% developed headaches, and none experienced more serious neurologic sequelae. Of 60 patients who had macroadenomas and became pregnant, 20% developed abnormal changes in their visual fields or other neurologic signs, usually in the first half of their pregnancies. Many of these required therapy. Monitoring of patients with known PRL-secreting adenomas during pregnancy is primarily based on clinical examination. The normal gestational increase in PRL may obscure the increase attributable to the adenoma, and radiographic procedures are undesirable in pregnancy.

Visual disturbances are usually experienced as "clumsiness" and are objectively found to be due to visual field changes. The most frequent finding is bitemporal hemianopia, but in advanced cases the defect can progress to concentric contraction of fields and enlargement of the blind spot.

Since the pituitary normally increases in size during pregnancy, headaches are common and bitemporal hemianopia not uncommon in patients with adenomas. These changes almost always revert to normal after delivery, so that aggressive therapy for known pituitary adenomas is not indicated except in cases of rapidly progressive visual loss.

Management

Management of the pregnant woman with a small pituitary adenoma includes early ophthalmologic consultation for formal visual field mapping and repeat examinations once a month or every other month throughout pregnancy.

If visual field disturbances are minimal, pregnancy may be allowed to proceed to term. If symptoms become progressively more severe and the fetus is mature, labor should be induced. If symptoms are severe and the fetus is immature, management may consist of transsphenoidal resection of the adenoma or medical treatment with bromocriptine. While bromocriptine inhibits both fetal and maternal pituitary PRL secretion, it does not affect decidual PRL secretion. Bromocriptine appears not to be teratogenic, and no adverse fetal effects have been reported. In most cases it is probably preferable to surgery. The newer, selective dopamine D_2 receptor agonist cabergoline has given excellent results in normalizing PRL levels, inducing tumor shrinkage, and minimizing side effects. The data available on pregnancies in which cabergoline was used do not show adverse effects; however, since the data are limited compared with the large numbers for bromocriptine safety, the latter is recommended during pregnancy. Radiation therapy should not be used in pregnancy.

Management of PRL-secreting tumors in women who want to become pregnant is controversial. Surgical resection by surgeons with experience in transsphenoidal procedures results in reduction of PRL levels and resumption of normal ovulation in 60–80% of women with microadenomas and 30–50% of women with macroadenomas. The incidence of recurrence is at least 10–16% and will probably increase with further follow-up. Bromocriptine is usually well tolerated and is successful in achieving normal menstrual cycles and lowering PRL levels in 40–80% of patients. Bromocriptine also causes a marked decrease in tumor size, but the original size of the tumor is usually regained within days or weeks after discontinuing therapy. In the case of large tumors, combined medical and surgical management may often be appropriate. Radiation therapy has an important role in arresting growth of tumors that are resistant to other management, particularly large tumors that involve the cavernous sinuses and tumors that secrete both GH and PRL (see Chapter 5).

Lymphocytic adenohypophysitis is an enigmatic autoimmune inflammation of the pituitary that classically occurs in women in late pregnancy or during the puerperium. The clinical presentation is difficult to distinguish from that of a large prolactin-secreting adenoma. Expectant conservative medical management with corticosteroids is sometimes possible, with vigilant postpartum observation to prevent consequences of pituitary insufficiency.

Prognosis & Follow-Up

There appears to be no increase in obstetric complications associated with pituitary adenomas, and no fetal jeopardy. The rate of prematurity increases in women with tumors requiring therapy, but this is probably due to aggressive intervention rather than to spontaneous premature labor.

The postpartum period is characterized by rapid relief of even severe symptoms, with less than 4% of untreated tumors developing permanent sequelae. In some cases, tumors improve following pregnancy, with normalization or lowering of PRL relative to prepregnancy values. Management should include radiography and assessment of PRL levels 4–6 weeks after delivery. There are no contraindications to breast-feeding.

Sheehan's Syndrome

Postpartum pituitary necrosis, or Sheehan's syndrome, is preceded by obstetric hemorrhage leading to severe circulatory collapse. Theoretically, severe hypotension predisposes the enlarged pituitary to ischemia. The posterior pituitary is usually spared, and the most common clinical feature is inability to lactate as a result of deficient PRL production. Loss of axillary and pubic hair is also a common sign. Other manifestations include hypothyroidism and hypocortisolism. Damage is variable, and in some instances there is return to normal fertility.

PREGNANCY & BREAST CANCER

Breast cancer complicates one in 1600–5000 pregnancies. Only one-sixth of breast cancers occur in women of reproductive age, but of these, one in seven is diagnosed during pregnancy or the puerperium. Pregnancy and breast cancer have long been considered such an ominous combination that only one in 20 young women who have had breast cancer have later become pregnant. It now appears, however, that pregnancy has little effect on growth of breast cancer, though it presents problems of detection and management of the cancer.

Influence of Pregnancy on Breast Cancer

Pregnancy is not an etiologic factor in breast cancer. Indeed, there is good evidence that pregnancy at an early age actually reduces the risk of developing mammary cancer, and multiple pregnancies may also make the disease less likely. Moreover, contemporary concepts of the rate of tumor growth suggest that a tumor becomes clinically evident only 8–10 years after its inception. Thus, a tumor cannot arise and be discovered during the same pregnancy. In view of the increased glandular proliferation and blood flow and marked increase in lymph flow that occur during pregnancy, it could be argued that pregnancy accelerates the appearance of previously subclinical diseases, but this has not been demonstrated.

Probably the most important influence of pregnancy on breast cancer is the delay it may cause in making the diagnosis and starting therapy. In some series, the interval between initial symptoms and treatment was 6–7 months longer than in the absence of pregnancy. Larger tumors may be misdiagnosed as galactoceles, and inflammatory carcinoma in the puerperium is liable to be misdiagnosed as mastitis.

At the time of diagnosis, 60% of pregnancy-associated breast cancers have metastasized to regional lymph nodes, and an additional 20% have distant metastases. Stage for stage, however, survival rates following appropriate therapy are comparable to those achieved in nonpregnant patients. Termination of pregnancy, either by abortion or by early delivery, does not influence maternal survival.

Pregnancy After Treatment for Cancer

Pregnancy following definitive treatment of breast cancer has no adverse effect on survival. Indeed, women who become pregnant following stage I or stage II breast cancer have a somewhat better 5-year survival rate than matched controls who did not become pregnant but who survived at least as long as their match before becoming pregnant.

Women who have had breast cancer are frequently advised to avoid pregnancy for 5 years. Because most fertile women with breast cancer are in their mid 30s, such a plan virtually precludes pregnancy. Because pregnancy is not known to influence the rate of cancer recurrence, the only reasons for proscribing pregnancy are to avoid the possibility that management of a recurrence will be complicated by the pregnancy or to avoid the problem of producing motherless children. For a couple strongly desiring pregnancy, these risks may become acceptable in a much shorter time than 5 years, especially if the original lesion was small and the spread of disease minimal.

Estrogen Receptors in Breast Cancer

Determinations of soluble estrogen and progesterone receptors are frequently used in breast cancer to predict whether the tumor is likely to respond to endocrine therapy. There is also evidence that the presence of estrogen receptor-positive tumors is correlated with a lower risk of early recurrence. In the pregnant patient, however, high progesterone levels inhibit estrogen and progesterone receptor synthesis, and high levels of both hormones cause their receptors to become tightly associated with the nuclear fraction. Thus, when soluble receptors are quantified, all breast cancers arising in pregnancy appear to be receptor-negative, making such measurements in pregnancy at best worthless and at worst dangerously misleading. The introduction of immunohistochemical assays, which allow identification of occupied nuclear receptors, provides a more reliable assessment.

Treatment of Breast Cancer in Pregnancy

Once the diagnosis of cancer is made, the patient must be treated surgically without delay. In view of the large percentage of patients with positive nodes, the procedure should be one that provides adequate sampling of the axillary nodes, such as modified radical mastectomy. Simple mastectomy with axillary irradiation should be avoided. Therapeutic abortion is not routinely indicated. If, on the basis of surgical staging, adjuvant therapy is considered advisable, the decision must be made either to terminate the pregnancy by abortion or early delivery or to postpone chemotherapy to the second or third trimester. Since delay in treatment is the principal known reason for the poorer prognosis of breast cancer in pregnancy, delivery should be accomplished as soon as there is a substantial probability of good fetal outcome—usually at 32–34 weeks. Many of the drugs used in cytotoxic therapy of breast carcinoma are contraindicated in pregnancy. Radiation can be given with appropriate shielding, but the dose to the fetus will not be negligible.

HYPERTENSIVE DISORDERS OF PREGNANCY

Hypertension associated with pregnancy is generally categorized as chronic, in which elevated blood pressures antedate the pregnancy or are clinically recognized prior to the 20th week, or gestational, when the onset is beyond 20 weeks of gestation. If the latter is complicated by proteinuria and generalized edema, the triad is referred to as preeclampsia. When seizures accompany this syndrome, the condition is termed eclampsia. The incidence of preeclampsia is about 7%. Women at highest risk include primigravidas under 18 years old, multiparous women over 35 years old, and women with twin gestations, diabetes, hydramnios, pregnancy obesity, or prepregnancy hypertension. As many as half of women with prepregnancy hypertension develop exacerbations of hypertension in the third trimester.

Course of Hypertension in Pregnancy

In normal pregnancies, as well as those complicated by mild essential hypertension, diastolic blood pressure decreases 10–16 mm Hg in the second trimester. Hypertensive patients first seen at that time may be mistakenly identified as having preeclampsia when the blood pressure again increases in the third trimester. Clinically, preeclampsia usually appears after the 32nd week of gestation and, most frequently, during labor. In severe cases, especially those complicated by essential hypertension, acute rises in blood pressure may occur as early as 26 weeks. If hypertension appears in the first or early second trimester, it is associated either with gestational trophoblastic disease or an underlying disorder such as an acute flare-up of lupus nephritis. Occasionally, the onset of hypertension is recognized during the 24 hours following delivery.

In normal pregnancies, all of the components of the renin-angiotensin-aldosterone system are markedly elevated. In pregnancies complicated by chronic hypertension or preeclampsia, these components are slightly reduced toward normal nonpregnant levels, suggesting an appropriate feedback response. The most consistent finding in women with preeclampsia is the increased sensitivity to vasopressor agents compared to women with normal pregnancy. In pregnancies destined to be complicated by preeclampsia, an increase in arteriolar response to angiotensin that becomes statistically significant by 18–22 weeks of gestation–long before changes in blood pressure are detectable. The cause of this increase in vascular sensitivity to angiotensin is not known. Considerable evidence suggests that dyslipidemia, oxidative stress, and endothelial cell dysfunction may explain many of the pathophysiologic features of preeclampsia.

Treatment of Chronic Hypertension

Women with chronic hypertension who become pregnant require special management. Roberts's recommendations are probably the best:

(1) Diastolic pressures under 100 mm Hg should not be treated. However, if a woman is receiving antihypertensive therapy when first seen in pregnancy, therapy should be continued. If she is taking propranolol, consideration may be given to switching to a more specific β_1-antagonist such as metoprolol or atenolol. The rare patient who has been taking ganglionic blockers should receive another form of therapy instead. Owing to a transient decrease in blood volume and placental perfusion associated with thiazide diuretics, use of these agents should usually not be initiated during pregnancy; however, if a woman is already receiving such therapy, it may be continued. Angiotensin-converting enzyme inhibitors may be associated with adverse fetal and neonatal effects, including death.

(2) Diastolic pressures above 100 mm Hg discovered during pregnancy call for antihypertensive management. Initial therapy should be with methyldopa, 250 mg orally at bedtime. This may be increased 1 g twice daily as required. If unacceptable drowsiness lasting more than 2–3 days occurs, the dosage may be reduced, and hydralazine, beginning at 10 mg orally twice daily and increasing up to 100 mg twice daily, may be added. If hydralazine is not tolerated, prazosin may be gradually added to the methyldopa therapy.

(3) Accelerated hypertension at any stage of gestation should be managed with bed rest and, if necessary, intravenous hydralazine. Unless diastolic pressure can be reduced to 110 mm Hg promptly, delivery should be performed regardless of gestational age.

Symptoms & Signs of Preeclampsia

Signs of preeclampsia include sustained blood pressure increase to levels of 140 mm Hg systolic or 90 mm Hg diastolic and proteinuria exceeding 300 mg daily. Symptoms include headaches, visual disturbances, and epigastric pain. Eclampsia may occur even with mild elevation of blood pressure and is associated with a maternal mortality rate as high as 10%. Deaths occur most frequently from cerebral hemorrhage, renal failure, disseminated intravascular coagulopathy, acute pulmonary edema, or hepatic failure. The fetal perinatal mortality rate is in excess of 30%, and the risk of perinatal morbidity due to hypoxia is even higher.

Treatment of Preeclampsia

The only definitive therapy for preeclampsia is delivery. If a modest increase in blood pressure first occurs in association with proteinuria at 32–36 weeks of gestation, bed rest, preferably in the left lateral decubitus position, is frequently effective in temporarily inducing diuresis and controlling progression of the disease, thus gaining time for the developing fetus. If labor occurs or induction of labor is attempted, parenteral magnesium sulfate should be used to prevent seizures and should be continued for 24 hours following delivery. Moderate hypertension need not be treated with antihypertensive agents; however, diastolic blood pressure above 110 mm Hg must be controlled to reduce the risk of intracranial hemorrhage. The agent of choice is hydralazine, 5 mg intravenously at 16- to 20-minute intervals, until the diastolic pressure is approximately 100 mm Hg. If hydralazine is unsuccessful, labetalol, verapamil, or nifedipine, may be used, but these agents are rarely required. Recent trials using low-dose aspirin revealed minimal to no benefit in preventing the development of preeclampsia.

Prognosis

Both preeclampsia and transient hypertension (late-gestation hypertension without proteinuria) are associated with an increased risk of chronic hypertension in later life.

HYPERTHYROIDISM IN PREGNANCY

Pregnancy mimics hyperthyroidism. There is thyroid enlargement, increased cardiac output, and peripheral vasodilation. Owing to the increase in thyroid hormone-binding globulin (TBG), total serum thyroxine is in the range expected for hyperthyroidism. Free thyroxine, the free thyroxine index, and TSH levels, however, remain in the normal range (see Chapter 7).

True hyperthyroidism complicates one or two per 1000 pregnancies. The most common form of hyperthyroidism during pregnancy is Graves' disease. Hyperthyroidism is associated with an increased risk of premature delivery (11–25%) and may modestly increase the risk of early abortion. In Graves' disease, thyroid-stimulating immunoglobulin (TSI), a 7S immune gamma globulin, crosses the placenta and may cause fetal goiter and transient neonatal hyperthyroidism, but these effects rarely jeopardize the fetus.

Treatment

The treatment of maternal hyperthyroidism is complicated by pregnancy. Radioiodides are strictly contraindicated. Iodide therapy can lead to huge fetal goiter and is contraindicated except as acute therapy to prevent thyroid storm before thyroid surgery. All antithyroid drugs cross the placenta and may cause fetal hypothyroidism and goiter or cretinism in the newborn. However, propylthiouracil in doses of 300 mg/d or less has been shown to be reasonably safe, although even at low doses about 10% of newborns will have a detectable goiter. Propranolol has been used to control maternal cardiovascular symptoms but may result in fetal bradycardia, growth retardation, premature labor, and neonatal respiratory depression. Partial or total thyroidectomy, especially in the second trimester, is a reasonably safe procedure except for the risk of premature labor.

A. PROPYLTHIOURACIL

A reasonable plan of management is to begin therapy with propylthiouracil in doses high enough to bring the free T_4 index into the mildly hyperthyroid range and then to taper the dose gradually. Giving thyroxine along with propylthiouracil in the hope that it will cross the placenta in sufficient quantities to prevent fetal hypothyroidism is not effective and serves only to increase the amount of propylthiouracil required. If the maintenance dose of propylthiouracil is above 300 mg/d, serious consideration should be given to partial thyroidectomy.

B. PROPRANOLOL

Propranolol may be used transiently to ameliorate cardiovascular symptoms while control is being achieved.

Management of Newborn

Newborns should be observed carefully. In infants of mothers given propylthiouracil, even equivocal evidence of hypothyroidism is an indication for thyroxine replacement therapy. Neonatal Graves' disease, which may present as late as 2 weeks after delivery, requires intensive therapy (see Chapter 7).

HYPOTHYROIDISM IN PREGNANCY

Hypothyroidism is uncommon in pregnancy, since most women with the untreated disorder are oligo-ovulatory. As a practical matter, women taking thyroid medication at the time of conception should be maintained on the same or a slightly larger dose throughout pregnancy, whether or not the obstetrician believes thyroid replacement was originally indicated. Physiologic doses of thyroid are innocuous, but maternal hypothyroidism is hazardous to the developing fetus. Women with a personal or family history of thyroid disease or with symptoms suggestive of hypothyroidism should be tested for TSH prior to conception. The correlation between maternal and fetal thyroid status is poor, and hypothyroid mothers frequently deliver euthyroid infants. The strongest correlation between maternal and newborn hypothyroidism occurs in areas where endemic goiter due to iodide deficiency is common. In these regions, dietary iodide supplementation in addition to thyroid hormone treatment of the mother may be of the greatest importance in preventing cretinism.

REFERENCES

General

Burrow GN, Duffy TP (editors): *Medical Complications During Pregnancy,* 5th ed. Saunders, 1999.

Haig D: Genetic conflicts in human pregnancy. Q Rev Biol 1995; 68:495.

Jaffe RB: Endocrine-metabolic alterations induced by pregnancy. In: *Reproductive Endocrinology: Physiology, Pathophysiology, and Clinical Management,* 4th ed. Yen SSC, Jaffe RB, Barbieri RL (editors). Saunders, 1999.

Norwitz ER, Schust DJ, Fisher SJ: Implantation and the survival of early pregnancy. N Engl J Med 2001;345:1400. [PMID: 11794174]

Chorionic Proteins and Pregnancy Tests

Lessey BA: Endometrial integrins and the establishment of uterine receptivity. Hum Reprod 1998;13(Suppl 3):247. [PMID: 9755427]

Lin LS, Roberts VJ, Yen SS: Expression of human gonadotropin-releasing hormone receptor gene in the placenta and its functional relationship to human chorionic gonadotropin secretion. J Clin Endocrinol Metab 1995;80:580. [PMID: 7852524]

Meuris S et al: Temporal relationship between the human chorionic gonadotrophin peak and the establishment of intervillous blood flow in early pregnancy. Hum Reprod 1995;10: 947. [PMID: 7650149]

O'Connor JF et al: Recent advances in the chemistry and immunochemistry of human chorionic gonadotropin: Impact on clinical measurements. Endocr Rev 1994;15:650. [PMID: 7843071]

Wilcox AJ, Baird DD, Weinberg CR: Time of implantation of the conceptus and loss of pregnancy. N Engl J Med 1999; 340:1796. [PMID: 10362823]

Ovarian Proteins

Bani D: Relaxin: a pleiotropic hormone. Gen Pharmacol 1997; 28:13. [PMID: 9112071]

Steroid Hormones

Couse JF, Korach KS: Estrogen receptor null mice: what have we learned and where will they lead us? Endocr Rev 1999; 20:358. [PMID: 10368776]

Mesiano S, Jaffe RB: Human fetal adrenal cortical function in pregnancy and parturition. Curr Probl Obstet Gynecol Fertil 1999;22:195.

Miller WL: Steroid hormone biosynthesis and actions in the materno-feto-placental unit. Clin Perinatol 1998;25:799. [PMID: 9891616]

Pepe GJ, Albrecht ED: Actions of placental and fetal adrenal steroid hormones in primate pregnancy. Endocr Rev 1995; 16:608. [PMID: 8529574]

Strauss JF 3rd, Martinez F, Kiriakidou M: Placental steroid hormone synthesis: unique features and unanswered questions. Biol Reprod 1996;54:303. [PMID: 8788180]

Fetal Endocrinology

Fisher DA: Fetal thyroid function: diagnosis and management of fetal thyroid disorders. Clin Obstet Gynecol 1997;40:16. [PMID: 91039477]

Gluckman PD: The endocrine regulation of fetal growth in late gestation: The role of insulin-like growth factors. J Clin Endocrinol Metab 1995;80:1047. [PMID: 7714063]

Haddow JE et al: Maternal thyroid deficiency during pregnancy and subsequent neuropsychological development of the child. N Engl J Med 1999;341:549. [PMID: 10451459]

Rabinovici J, Jaffe RB: Development and regulation of growth and differentiated function in human and subhuman primate fetal gonads. Endocr Rev 1990;11:532. [PMID: 2292242]

Sinclair AH et al: A gene from the human sex-determining region encodes a protein with homology to a conserved DNA-binding motif. Nature 1990;346:240. [PMID: 1695712]

Wald NJ, Watt HC, Hackshaw AK: Integrated screening for Down's syndrome on the basis of tests performed during the first and second trimesters. N Engl J Med 1999;341:461. [PMID: 10441601]

Parturition

Chwalisz K, Garfield RE: Antiprogestins in the induction of labor. Ann N Y Acad Sci 1994;734:387. [PMID: 7978941]

Haluska GJ et al: Progesterone receptor localization and isoforms in myometrium, decidua, and fetal membranes from rhesus macaques: evidence for functional progesterone withdrawal at parturition. J Soc Gynecol Investig 2002;9:125. [PMID: 12009386]

Weiss G: The role of the time of labor is complex and involves interactions of the mother, the fetus and the placenta, plus membranes. J Clin Endocrinol Metab 2000;854421. [PMID: 11134087]

Puerperium and Lactation

Crowley WR, Armstrong WE: Neurochemical regulation of oxytocin secretion in lactation. Endocr Rev 1992;13:33. [PMID: 1348224]

McNeilly AS, Tay CC, Glasier A: Physiological mechanisms underlying lactational amenorrhea. Ann N Y Acad Sci 1994;709: 145. [PMID: 8154698]

Pituitary Adenomas

Colao A, Lombardi G: Prolactinomas resistant to standard dopamine agonists respond to chronic cabergoline treatment. J Clin Endocrinol Metab 1997;82:876. [PMID: 9253368]

Molitch ME: Disorders of prolactin secretion. Endocrinol Metab Clin North Am 2001;30:585. [PMID: 11571932]

Molitch ME: Pituitary disease in pregnancy. Semin Perinatol 1998;22:457. [PMID: 9880116]

Breast Cancer and Pregnancy

Bernik SF et al: Carcinoma of the breast during pregnancy: a review and update on treatment options. Surg Oncol 1998;7:45. [PMID: 10421505]

Berry DL et al: Management of breast cancer during pregnancy using a standardized protocol. J Clin Oncol 1999;17:855. [PMID: 10071276]

Berry DL et al: Influence of pregnancy on the outcome of breast cancer: a case-control study. Société Française de Sérologie et de Pathologie Mammaire Study Group. Int J Cancer 1997; 4:720.

Hypertensive Disorders

Dekker GA, Sibai BM: Etiology and pathogenesis of preeclampsia: current concepts. Am J Obstet Gynecol 1998;179:1359. [PMID:]

Hubel CA: Oxidative stress in the pathogenesis of preeclampsia. Proc Soc Exp Biol Med 1999;222:222. Review. [PMID: 10601881]

Roberts JM: Pregnancy-related hypertension. In: *Maternal-Fetal Medicine: Principles and Practice,* 4th ed. Creasy RK, Resnick R (editors). Saunders, 1998.

Hyperthyroidism in Pregnancy

Burrow GN, Fisher DA, Larsen PR: Maternal and fetal thyroid function. N Engl J Med 1994;331:1072. [PMID: 8090169]

Foulk RA et al: Does human chorionic gonadotropin have human thyrotropic activity in vivo? Gynecol Endocrinol 1997;11:195. [PMID: 9209900]

Haddow JE et al: Maternal thyroid deficiency during pregnancy and subsequent neuropsychological development of the child. N Engl J Med 1999;341:549. [PMID: 10451459]

Pancreatic Hormones & Diabetes Mellitus

17

Umesh Masharani, MRCP(UK), John H. Karam, MD, & Michael S. German, MD

ADA	American Diabetes Association	**GLP-2**	Glucagon-like peptide 2
ADH	Antidiuretic hormone (vasopressin)	**HDL**	High-density lipoprotein(s)
ATP	Adenosine triphosphate	**HLA**	Human leukocyte antigen
cAMP	Cyclic adenosine monophosphate	**IRS-1**	Insulin receptor substrate-1
CBMW	Capillary basement membrane width	**MODY**	Maturity-onset diabetes of the young
CCK	Cholecystokinin	**NPH**	Neutral protamine Hagedorn
DID-MOAD	Diabetes insipidus, diabetes mellitus, optic atrophy, and neural deafness (Wolfram's syndrome)	**PP**	Pancreatic polypeptide
		RNA	Ribonucleic acid
DNA	Deoxyribonucleic acid	**SSTR**	Somatostatin receptor
FDA	Food and Drug Administration	**UGDP**	University Group Diabetes Program
GAD	Glutamic acid decarboxylase	**UKPDS**	United Kingdom Prospective Diabetic Study
GH	Growth hormone		
GI	Glycemic index	**VLDL**	Very low density lipoprotein(s)
GIP	Gastric inhibitory polypeptide	**VNTR**	Variable number of tandem repeats
GLP-1	Glucagon-like peptide 1		

■ I. THE ENDOCRINE PANCREAS

The pancreas is made up of two functionally different organs: the **exocrine pancreas,** the major digestive gland of the body; and the **endocrine pancreas,** the source of insulin, glucagon, somatostatin, and pancreatic polypeptide. Whereas the major role of the products of the exocrine pancreas (the digestive enzymes) is the processing of ingested foodstuffs so that they become available for absorption, the hormones of the endocrine pancreas modulate every other aspect of cellular nutrition from rate of adsorption of foodstuffs to cellular storage or metabolism of nutrients. Dysfunction of the endocrine pancreas or abnormal responses to its hormones by target tissues result in serious disturbances in nutrient homeostasis, including the important clinical syndromes grouped under the name of **diabetes mellitus.**

ANATOMY & HISTOLOGY

The endocrine pancreas consists of 0.7–1 million small endocrine glands—the islets of Langerhans—scattered within the glandular substance of the exocrine pancreas. The islet volume comprises 1–1.5% of the total mass of the pancreas and weighs about 1–2 g in adult humans.

At least four cell types—A, B, D, and PP (also called α, β, δ, and F)—have been identified in the islets (Table 17–1). These cell types are not distributed uniformly throughout the pancreas. The PP cell, which secretes pancreatic polypeptide (PP), has been found primarily in islets in the posterior portion (posterior lobe) of the head, a discrete lobe of the pancreas separated from the anterior portion by a fascial partition. This lobe originates in the primordial ventral bud as opposed to the dorsal bud. The posterior lobe receives its blood supply from the superior mesenteric artery; the remainder of the pancreas derives most of its blood flow from the celiac artery.

Table 17–1. Cell types in pancreatic islets of Langerhans.

Cell types	Approximate Percentage of Islet Volume		Secretory Products
	Dorsally Derived (Anterior Head, Body, Tail)	Ventrally Derived (Posterior Portion of Head)	
A cell (α)	10%	< 0.5%	Glucagon, proglucagon, glucagon-like peptides (GLP-1 and GLP-2)
B cell (β)	70–80%	15–20%	Insulin, C peptide, proinsulin, amylin, γ-aminobutyric acid (GABA)
D cell (δ)	3–5%	< 1%	Somatostatin
PP cell (F cell)	< 2%	80–85%	Pancreatic polypeptide

Islets in the posterior lobe area consist of 80–85% F cells, 15–20% B cells, and less than 0.5% glucagon-producing A cells. The PP cell volume varies with age and sex—the volume tends to be larger in men and in older persons. In contrast to the posterior lobe, the PP-poor islets located in the tail, body, and *anterior* portion of the head of the pancreas, arising from the embryonic dorsal bud, contain predominantly insulin-secreting B cells (70–80% of the islet cells), with approximately 20% of the cells being glucagon-secreting A cells and about 3–5% D cells that produce somatostatin. A typical islet from this part of the pancreas is depicted in Figure 17–1.

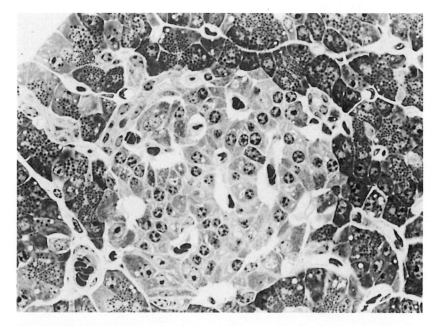

Figure 17–1. Photomicrograph of a section of the pancreas. In the islet of Langerhans, A cells appear mainly in the periphery as large cells with dark cytoplasm. Some D cells are also present in the periphery, while the central core is composed chiefly of B cells. (Reproduced, with permission, from Junqueira LC, Carneiro J, Long JA: *Basic Histology,* 7th ed. McGraw-Hill, 1992.)

Islet Vascularization

The islets are richly vascularized, receiving five to ten times the blood flow of a comparable portion of exocrine pancreatic tissues. The direction of the blood flow within the islet has been postulated to play a role in carrying insulin secreted from the central region of an islet to its peripheral zone—where the insulin modulates and decreases glucagon release from A cells, which are mainly located in the periphery of islets.

HORMONES OF THE ENDOCRINE PANCREAS

1. Insulin

Biosynthesis

The human insulin gene is located on the short arm of chromosome 11. A precursor molecule, **preproinsulin,** a peptide of MW 11,500, is translated from the preproinsulin messenger RNA in the rough endoplasmic reticulum of pancreatic B cells (Figure 17– 2). Microso-

mal enzymes cleave preproinsulin to **proinsulin** (MW about 9000) almost immediately after synthesis. Proinsulin (Figure 17–3) is transported to the Golgi apparatus, where packaging into clathrin-coated secretory granules takes place. Maturation of the secretory granule is associated with loss of the clathrin coating and conversion of proinsulin into **insulin** and a smaller connecting peptide, or **C peptide,** by proteolytic cleavage at two sites along the peptide chain. Normal mature (uncoated) secretory granules contain insulin and C peptide in equimolar amounts and only small quantities of proinsulin, a small portion of which consists of partially cleaved intermediates.

Biochemistry

Proinsulin (Figure 17–3) consists of a single chain of 86 amino acids, which includes the A and B chains of the insulin molecule plus a connecting segment of 35 amino acids. Two proteins—the prohormone-converting enzymes PC1/3 and PC2—are packaged with proinsulin in the immature secretory granules. These enzymes recog-

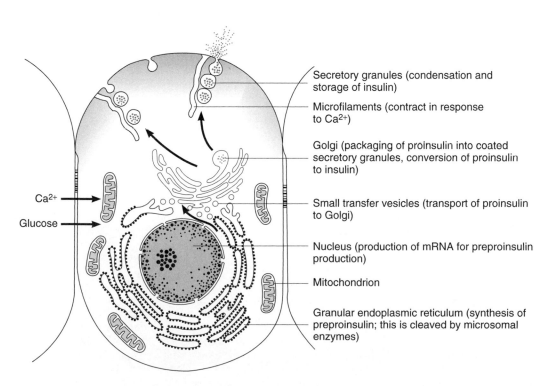

Figure 17–2. Structural components of the pancreatic B cell involved in glucose-induced biosynthesis and release. Schematic representation of secretory granular alignment on microfilament "tracks" that contract in response to calcium. (Based on data presented by Orci L: A portrait of the pancreatic B cell. Diabetologia 1974;10:163.) (Modified and reproduced, with permission, from Junqueira LC, Carneiro J, Long JA: *Basic Histology,* 5th ed. McGraw-Hill, 1986.)

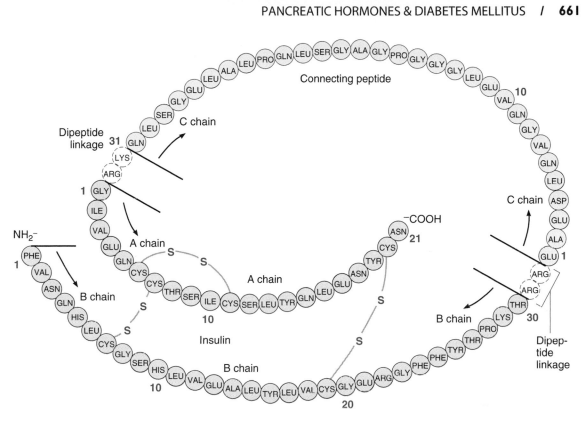

Figure 17–3. Structure of human proinsulin C peptides and insulin molecules connected at two sites by dipeptide links.

nize and cut at pairs of basic amino acids, thereby removing the intervening sequence. After the two pairs of basic amino acids are removed by carboxypeptidase E, the result is a 51-amino-acid insulin molecule and a 31-amino-acid residue, the C peptide, as shown in Figure 17–3.

A small amount of proinsulin produced by the pancreas escapes cleavage and is secreted intact into the bloodstream, along with insulin and C peptide. Most anti-insulin sera used in the standard immunoassay for insulin cross-react with proinsulin; about 3–5% of immunoreactive insulin extracted from human pancreas is actually proinsulin. Because proinsulin is not removed by the liver, it has a half-life three to four times that of insulin. This allows proinsulin to accumulate in the blood, where it accounts for 12–20% of the circulating immunoreactive "insulin" in the basal state in humans. Human proinsulin has about 7–8% of the biologic activity of insulin. The kidney is the principal site of proinsulin degradation.

Of the two major split proinsulin products present in plasma, the one split at arginine 32–33 far exceeds in amount the barely detectable 65–66 split product. In control subjects, concentrations of proinsulin and 32–33 split proinsulin after an overnight fast averaged 2.3 and 2.2 pmol/L, respectively, with corresponding postprandial rises to 10 and 20 pmol/L.

C peptide, the 31-amino-acid residue (MW 3000) formed during cleavage of insulin from proinsulin, has no known biologic activity. It is released from the B cells in equimolar amounts with insulin. It is not removed by the liver but is degraded or excreted chiefly by the kidney. It has a half-life three to four times that of insulin. In the basal state after an overnight fast, the average concentration of C peptide may be as high as 1000 pmol/L.

Insulin is a protein consisting of 51 amino acids contained within two peptide chains: an A chain, with 21 amino acids; and a B chain, with 30 amino acids. The chains are connected by two disulfide bridges as shown in Figure 17–3. In addition, there is an intrachain disulfide bridge that links positions 6 and 11 in the A chain. The molecular weight of human insulin is 5808.

Human insulin differs only slightly in amino acid composition from the two mammalian insulins that have been used for therapeutic insulin replacement. Pork insulin differs from human by only one amino acid—alanine instead of threonine at the carboxyl terminus of the B chain (position B 30). Beef insulin differs by three amino acids—alanine instead of threonine at A 8 as well as the B 30 position and valine instead of isoleucine at A 10.

Endogenous insulin has a circulatory half-life of 3–5 minutes. It is catabolized chiefly by insulinases in liver, kidney, and placenta. Approximately 50% of insulin is removed in a single pass through the liver.

Secretion

The human pancreas secretes about 40–50 units of insulin per day in normal adults. The basal concentration of insulin in the blood of fasting humans averages 10 μU/mL (0.4 ng/mL, or 61 pmol/L). In normal control subjects, insulin seldom rises above 100 μU/mL (610 pmol/L) after standard meals. There is an increase in peripheral insulin concentration beginning 8–10 minutes after ingestion of food and reaching peak concentration in peripheral blood by 30–45 minutes. This is followed by a rapid decline in postprandial plasma glucose concentration, which returns to baseline values by 90–120 minutes.

Basal insulin secretion, which occurs in the absence of exogenous stimuli, is the quantity of insulin secreted in the fasting state. Although it is known that plasma glucose levels below 80–100 mg/dL (4.4–5.6 mmol/L) do not stimulate insulin release, it has also been demonstrated that the presence of glucose is necessary (in in vitro systems) for most other known regulators of insulin secretion to be effective.

Stimulated insulin secretion is that which occurs in response to exogenous stimuli. In vivo, this is the response of the B cell to ingested meals. Glucose is the most potent stimulant of insulin release. The perfused rat pancreas has demonstrated a biphasic release of insulin in response to glucose (Figure 17–4). When the glucose concentration in the system is increased suddenly, an initial short-lived burst of insulin release occurs (the **first phase**); if the glucose concentration is held at this level, the insulin release gradually falls off and then begins to rise again to a steady level (the **second phase**). However, sustained levels of high glucose stimulation (≥ 4 hours in vitro or > 24 hours in vivo) results in a reversible desensitization of the B cell response to glucose but not to other stimuli.

Glucose is known to enter the pancreatic B cell by passive diffusion, which is facilitated by a specific membrane protein termed glucose transporters. Because the transporters function in both directions and the B cell has an excess of glucose transporters, the glucose con-

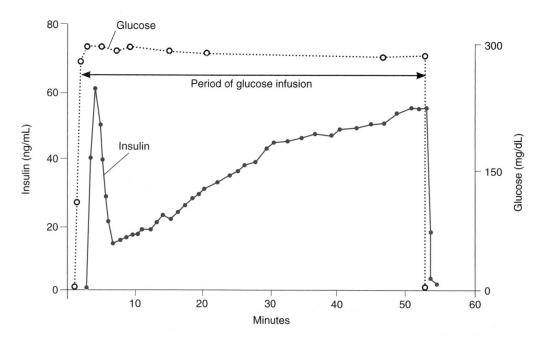

Figure 17–4. Multiphasic response of the in vitro perfused pancreas during constant stimulation with glucose. (Modified from Grodsky GM et al: Further studies on the dynamic aspects of insulin release in vitro with evidence for a two-compartmental storage system. Acta Diabetol Lat 1969;6[Suppl 1]:554.)

centration inside the B cell is in equilibrium with the extracellular glucose concentration. There is a body of data suggesting that *metabolism* of glucose is essential in stimulating insulin release. Indeed, agents such as 2-deoxyglucose that inhibit the metabolism of glucose interfere with release of insulin. The rate-limiting step in glucose metabolism by the pancreatic B cell appears to be the phosphorylation of glucose by the low-affinity enzyme glucokinase. The catabolism of glucose in the B cell results in a rise in the intracellular ATP/ADP ratio. This rise causes the ATP-sensitive potassium channels on the surface of the B cell to close, thereby depolarizing the cell and activating the voltage-sensitive calcium channel.

Insulin release has been shown to require calcium. The following effects of glucose on calcium ion movement have been demonstrated: (1) Calcium uptake is increased by glucose stimulation of the B cell. (2) Calcium efflux from the cell is retarded by some action of glucose. (3) Mobilization of calcium from mitochondrial compartments occurs secondary to cAMP induction by glucose.

cAMP is another important modulator of insulin release. As mentioned above, glucose has been shown to directly induce cAMP formation. Furthermore, many nonglucose stimuli to insulin release are known to increase intracellular cAMP. Elevations of cAMP, however, will not stimulate insulin release in the absence of glucose.

Other factors involved in the regulation of insulin secretion are summarized in Table 17–2. These factors can be divided into three categories: **direct stimulants,** which are known to stimulate insulin release directly;

Table 17–2. Regulation of insulin release in humans.

Stimulants of insulin release
Glucose, mannose
Leucine
Vagal stimulation
Sulfonylureas
Amplifiers of glucose-induced insulin release
1. Enteric hormones:
Glucagon-like peptide I (7–37)
Gastric inhibitory peptide
Cholecystokinin
Secretin, gastrin
2. Neural amplifiers: beta-adrenergic stimulation
3. Amino acids: arginine
Inhibitors of insulin release
Neural: alpha-adrenergic effect of catecholamines
Humoral: somatostatin
Drugs: diazoxide, phenytoin, vinblastine, colchicine

amplifiers, which appear to potentiate the response of the B cell to glucose; and **inhibitors.** The action of the amplifier substances, many of which are gastrointestinal hormones stimulated by ingestion of meals, explains the observation that insulin response to an ingested meal is greater than the response to intravenously administered substrates.

Insulin Receptors & Insulin Action

Insulin action begins with binding of insulin to a receptor on the surface of the target cell membrane. Most cells of the body have specific cell surface insulin receptors. In fat, liver, and muscle cells, binding of insulin to these receptors is associated with the biologic response of these tissues to the hormone. These receptors bind insulin rapidly, with high specificity and with an affinity high enough to bind picomolar amounts.

Insulin receptors, members of the growth factor family (see Chapter 3 and Figures 3–7 and 3–8), are membrane glycoproteins composed of two protein subunits encoded by a single gene. The larger alpha subunit (MW 135,000) resides entirely extracellularly, where it binds the insulin molecule. The alpha subunit is tethered by disulfide linkage to the smaller beta subunit (MW 95,000). The beta subunit crosses the membrane, and its cytoplasmic domain contains a tyrosine kinase activity that initiates the intracellular signaling pathways.

Upon binding of insulin to the alpha subunit, the beta subunit activates itself by autophosphorylation. The activated beta subunit then recruits additional proteins to the complex and phosphorylates a network of intracellular substrates, including insulin receptor substrate-1 (IRS-1), insulin receptor substrate-2 (IRS-2), and others (Figure 17–5). These activated substrates each lead to subsequent recruitment and activation of additional kinases, phosphatases, and other signaling molecules in a complex pathway that generally contains two arms: the mitogenic pathway, which mediates the growth effects of insulin; and the metabolic pathway, which regulates nutrient metabolism. In the metabolic signaling pathway, activation of phosphatidylinositol-3-kinase leads to the movement of GLUT 4-containing vesicles to the cell membrane, increased glycogen and lipid synthesis, and stimulation of other metabolic pathways. After insulin is bound to its receptor, a number of insulin-receptor complexes are internalized. However, it remains controversial whether these internalized complexes contribute to further action of insulin or whether they limit continued insulin action by exposing insulin to intracellular scavenger lysosomes.

Abnormalities of insulin receptors—in concentration, affinity, or both—will affect insulin action. **"Down-regulation"** is a phenomenon in which the

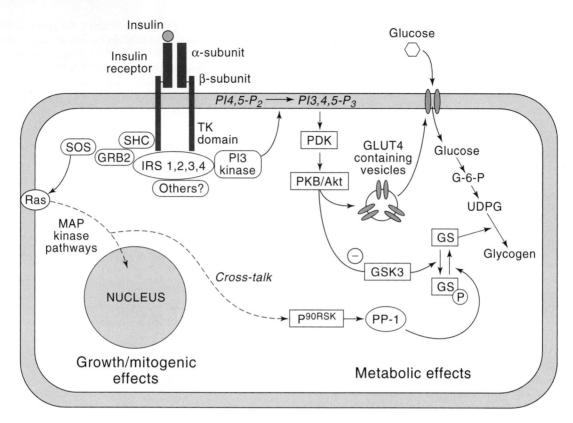

Figure 17–5. A simplified outline of insulin signaling. A minimal diagram of the mitogenic and metabolic arms of the insulin signaling pathway is shown. (GLUT 4, glucose transporter 4; Grb-2, growth factor receptor binding protein 2; GS, glycogen synthase [P indicates the inactive phosphorylated form]; GSK-3, glycogen synthase kinase 3; IRS, insulin receptor substrate [four different proteins]; MAP kinase, mitogen-activated protein kinase; PDK, phospholipid-dependent kinase; PI3 kinase, phosphatidylinositol 3 kinase; PKB, protein kinase B; PP-1, glycogen-associated protein phosphatase-1; Ras, rat sarcoma protein; SHC, Src and collagen homology protein; SOS, son-of-sevenless related protein; TK, tyrosine kinase.)

number of insulin receptors is decreased in response to chronically elevated circulating insulin levels, probably by increased intracellular degradation. When insulin levels are low, on the other hand, receptor binding is up-regulated. Conditions associated with high insulin levels and lowered insulin binding to the receptor include obesity, high intake of carbohydrates, and (perhaps) chronic exogenous overinsulinization. Conditions associated with low insulin levels and increased insulin binding include exercise and fasting. The presence of excess amounts of cortisol decreases insulin binding to the receptor, although it is not clear if this is a direct effect of the hormone itself or one that is mediated through accompanying increases in the insulin level.

The insulin receptor itself is probably not the major determinant of insulin sensitivity under most circum-

stances, however. Clinically relevant insulin resistance most commonly results from defects in postreceptor intracellular signaling pathways, though the exact nature of these defects in most patients remains elusive.

Metabolic Effects of Insulin

The major function of insulin is to promote **storage of ingested nutrients.** Although insulin directly or indirectly affects the function of almost every tissue in the body, the discussion here will be limited to a brief overview of the effects of insulin on the three major tissues specialized for energy storage: liver, muscle, and adipose tissue. In addition, the **paracrine effects** of insulin will be discussed briefly. The section on hormonal control of nutrient metabolism (see below) presents a detailed discussion of the effects of insulin and glucagon on the regulation of intermediary metabolism.

A. PARACRINE EFFECTS

The effects of the products of endocrine cells on surrounding cells are termed "paracrine" effects, in contrast to actions that take place at sites distant from the secreting cells, which are termed "endocrine" effects (Chapter 1). Paracrine effects of the B and D cells on the close-lying A cells (Figure 17–1) are of considerable importance in the endocrine pancreas. The first target cells reached by insulin are the pancreatic A cells at the periphery of the pancreatic islets. In the presence of insulin, A cell secretion of glucagon is reduced. In addition, somatostatin, which is released from D cells in response to most of the same stimuli that provoke insulin release, also acts to inhibit glucagon secretion.

Because glucose stimulates only B and D cells (whose products then inhibit A cells) whereas amino acids stimulate glucagon as well as insulin, the type and amounts of islet hormones released during a meal depend on the ratio of ingested carbohydrate to protein. The higher the carbohydrate content of a meal, the less glucagon will be released by any amino acids absorbed. In contrast, a predominantly protein meal will result in relatively greater glucagon secretion, because amino acids are less effective at stimulating insulin release in the absence of concurrent hyperglycemia but are potent stimulators of A cells.

B. ENDOCRINE EFFECTS

(Table 17–3.)

1. Liver—The first major organ reached by insulin via the bloodstream is the liver. Insulin exerts its action on the liver in two major ways:

a. Insulin promotes anabolism—Insulin promotes glycogen synthesis and storage at the same time it inhibits glycogen breakdown. These effects are mediated by changes in the activity of enzymes in the glycogen synthesis pathway (see below). The liver has a maximum storage capacity of 100–110 g of glycogen, or approximately 440 kcal of energy.

Insulin increases both protein and triglyceride synthesis and VLDL formation by the liver. It also inhibits gluconeogenesis and promotes glycolysis through its effects on enzymes of the glycolytic pathway.

b. Insulin inhibits catabolism—Insulin acts to reverse the catabolic events of the postabsorptive state by inhibiting hepatic glycogenolysis, ketogenesis, and gluconeogenesis.

2. Muscle—Insulin promotes protein synthesis in muscle by increasing amino acid transport as well as by stimulating ribosomal protein synthesis. In addition, insulin promotes glycogen synthesis to replace glycogen

Table 17–3. Endocrine effects of insulin.

Effect on liver:
Reversal of catabolic features of insulin deficiency
  Inhibits glycogenolysis
  Inhibits conversion of fatty acids and amino acids to keto acids
  Inhibits conversion of amino acids to glucose
Anabolic action
  Promotes glucose storage as glycogen (induces glucokinase and glycogen synthase, inhibits phosphorylase)
  Increases triglyceride synthesis and very low density lipoprotein formation

Effect on muscle:
Increased protein synthesis
  Increases amino acid transport
  Increases ribosomal protein synthesis
Increased glycogen synthesis
  Increases glucose transport
  Induces glycogen synthetase and inhibits phosphorylase

Effect on adipose tissue:
Increased triglyceride storage
  Lipoprotein lipase is induced and activated by insulin to hydrolyze triglycerides from lipoproteins
  Glucose transport into cell provides glycerol phosphate to permit esterification of fatty acids supplied by lipoprotein transport
  Intracellular lipase is inhibited by insulin

stores expended by muscle activity. This is accomplished by increasing glucose transport into the muscle cell, enhancing the activity of glycogen synthase, and inhibiting the activity of glycogen phosphorylase. Approximately 500–600 g of glycogen is stored in the muscle tissue of a 70-kg man, but because of the lack of glucose 6-phosphatase in this tissue, it cannot be used as a source of blood glucose. except by indirectly supplying the liver with lactate for conversion to glucose.

3. Adipose tissue—Fat, in the form of triglyceride, is the most efficient means of storing energy. It provides 9 kcal per gram of stored substrate, as opposed to the 4 kcal/g generally provided by protein or carbohydrate. In the typical 70-kg man, the energy content of adipose tissue is about 100,000 kcal.

Insulin acts to promote triglyceride storage in adipocytes by a number of mechanisms: (1) It induces the production of lipoprotein lipase in adipose tissue (this is the lipoprotein lipase that is bound to endothelial cells in adipose tissue and other vascular beds), which leads to hydrolysis of triglycerides from circulating lipoproteins. (2) By increasing glucose transport into fat cells, insulin increases the availability of α-glycerol phosphate, a substance used in the esterification of free fatty acids into triglycerides. (3) Insulin inhibits intracellular lipolysis of stored triglyceride by inhibiting intracellular lipase (also called "hormone-sensitive lipase"). This reduction of fatty acid flux to the liver appears to be a key regulatory factor in the action of insulin to lower hepatic gluconeogenesis and ketogenesis.

Glucose Transporter Proteins

Glucose oxidation is a major source of energy for many cells of the body and is especially essential for brain function. Since cell membranes are impermeable to hydrophilic molecules such as glucose, all cells require carrier proteins to transport glucose across the lipid bilayers into the cytosol. While the intestine and kidney have an energy dependent Na^+-glucose cotransporter, all other cells have non-energy-dependent transporters that facilitate diffusion of glucose from a higher concentration to a lower concentration across cell membranes. Facilitative glucose transporters comprise a large family including at least 13 members, though some of the recently identified members of the family have not yet been shown to transport glucose. The first four members of the family are the ones that have been best-characterized, and they have distinct affinities for glucose and distinct patterns of expression.

GLUT 1 is present in all human tissues. It appears to mediate basal glucose uptake, since it has a very high affinity for glucose and therefore is able to transport glucose at relatively low concentrations as found in the basal state. For this reason, it is an important component of the brain vascular system (blood-brain barrier) to ensure adequate transport of plasma glucose into the central nervous system. GLUT 3, which is also found in all tissues, is the major glucose transporter on the neuronal surface. It also has a very high affinity for glucose and is responsible for transferring glucose into neuronal cells.

In contrast, GLUT 2 has a very low affinity for glucose and seems to act as a transporter only when plasma glucose levels are relatively high, such as postprandially. It is a major transporter of glucose in hepatic, intestinal, and renal tubular cells, so that diffusion of glucose across these cells increases as glucose levels rise. The low affinity of GLUT 2 for glucose reduces hepatic uptake of glucose during the basal state or during fasting. GLUT 2 is also expressed on the surface of the B cells in rodents, but it is not detected at significant levels on human B cells.

GLUT 4 is found in two major insulin target tissues: skeletal muscle and adipose tissue. It appears to be sequestered mainly within an intracellular compartment of these cells and thus is not able to function as a glucose transporter until a signal from insulin results in translocation of GLUT 4 to the cell membrane, where it facilitates glucose entry into these storage tissues after a meal.

Islet Amyloid Polypeptide (IAPP), or Amylin

IAPP, or amylin, is a peptide made up of 37 amino acids that is produced and stored with insulin in the pancreatic B cell, but only in a low ratio of one molecule of amylin to 100 of insulin. It is cosecreted with insulin in response to glucose and other B cell stimulators. Amylin's function has not been determined, but it produces amyloid deposits in pancreatic islets of most patients with type 2 diabetes of long duration. These amyloid deposits are insoluble fibrillar proteins (containing mainly amylin as well as its precursor peptide) that encroach upon and may even occur within pancreatic B cells. Islets of nondiabetic elderly persons may contain less extensive amyloid deposits. Whether amyloid deposition contributes to the islet dysfunction seen in type 2 diabetes or is simply a consequence of disordered and hyperstimulated islet function remains an unresolved question.

2. Glucagon

Biochemistry

Pancreatic glucagon, the gene for which is located on human chromosome 2, is a single-chain polypeptide consisting of 29 amino acids with a molecular weight of 3485 (Figure 17–6). It is synthesized in the A cells in the islets of Langerhans and derived from a much larger 160-amino-acid precursor molecule. Within this proglucagon molecule are several other peptides connected in tandem: glicentin-related peptide, glucagon, glucagon-like peptide 1 (GLP-1), and glucagon-like peptide 2 (GLP-2). The combination of glicentin-related peptide with glucagon consists of 69 amino acids and comprises the hormone glicentin, which is predominantly secreted from the intestine and not the pancreas (Figure 17–6). Both GLP-1 and GLP-2 increase after meals. An endogenous truncated derivative of GLP-1, with the first six of its 37 amino acids absent (GLP-1 [7–37]), is an extremely potent stimulator of pancreatic B cells and is felt to be the major physiologic gut factor ("incretin") that potentiates glucose-induced insulin secretion after meals. It is released by small intestinal L cells of the duodenum during mixed meals and is several times more potent than glucagon itself as an insulinotropic secretagogue, whereas intact GLP-1 (1–37) and GLP-2 do not stimulate insulin secretion. In healthy humans, the average fasting plasma immunoreactive glucagon level is 75 pg/mL (25 pmol/L). Only 30–40% of this is actually pancreatic glucagon, the remainder being a heterogeneous composite of

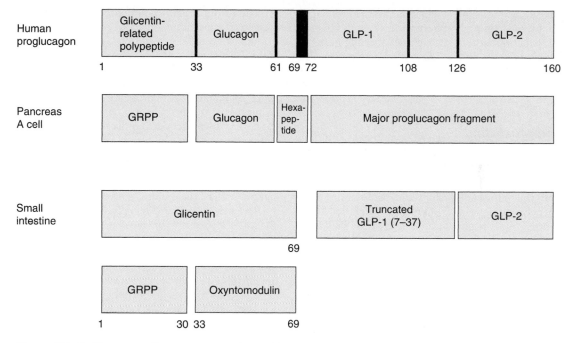

Figure 17–6. Tissue-specific secretory products of human proglucagon. (GLP-1, glucagon-like peptide-1; GLP-2, glucagon-like peptide-2; GRPP, glicentin-related polypeptide.)

higher-molecular-weight molecules with glucagon immunoreactivity such as proglucagon, glicentin, truncated GLP-1, and GLP-2. The circulation half-life of pancreatic glucagon is 3–6 minutes. Glucagon is mainly removed by the liver and kidney.

Secretion

Glucagon secretion is inhibited by glucose—in contrast to the effect of glucose on insulin secretion. There are conflicting data about whether the effect of glucose is a direct one on the A cell or whether it is mediated via release of insulin or somatostatin, both of which are known to inhibit the A cell directly (see above).

In addition, since γ-aminobutyric acid (GABA) is released by B cells and its receptors have recently been detected on A cells, GABA may participate in the inhibition of A cells during B cell stimulation.

Many amino acids stimulate glucagon release, although there are differences in their ability to do so. Some, such as arginine, release both glucagon and insulin; others (eg, alanine) stimulate primarily glucagon release. Leucine, a good stimulant for insulin release, does not stimulate glucagon. Other substances that promote glucagon release are catecholamines, the gastrointestinal hormones (cholecystokinin [CCK], gastrin, and gastric inhibitory polypeptide [GIP]), and glucocorticoids. Both sympathetic and parasympathetic (vagal) stimulation promote glucagon release; this is especially important in augmenting the response of the A cell to hypoglycemia. High levels of circulating fatty acid are associated with suppression of glucagon secretion.

Action of Glucagon

In contrast to insulin, which promotes energy storage in a variety of tissues, glucagon is a humoral mechanism for making energy available to the tissues between meals, when ingested food is not available for absorption. Glucagon stimulates the breakdown of stored glycogen, maintains hepatic output of glucose from amino acid precursors (gluconeogenesis), and promotes hepatic output of ketone bodies from fatty acid precursors (ketogenesis). The liver, because of its geographic proximity to the pancreas, represents the major target organ for glucagon, with portal vein glucagon concentrations reaching as high as 300–500 pg/mL (100–166 pmol/L). Binding of glucagon to its receptor on hepatocytes results in activation of adenylyl cyclase and generation of cAMP, which both promotes glycogenolysis and stimulates gluconeogenesis. Uptake of alanine by liver cells is facilitated by glucagon, and fatty acids are directed away from reesterification to triglycerides and toward ketogenic pathways (see below). It is unclear whether physiologic levels of glucagon affect tissues other than the liver.

The ratio of insulin to glucagon affects key target tissues by mediating phosphorylation or dephosphorylation (either or both) of key enzymes affecting nutrient metabolism. In addition, this ratio increases or decreases actual quantities of certain enzymes, thereby controlling the flux of these nutrients into or out of storage.

3. Somatostatin

The gene for somatostatin is on the long arm of chromosome 3. It codes for a 116-amino-acid peptide, preprosomatostatin, from whose carboxyl terminal is cleaved the hormone somatostatin, a 14-amino-acid cyclic polypeptide with a molecular weight of 1640 (Figure 17–7). It is present in D cells at the periphery of the human islet (Figure 17–1). It was first identified in the hypothalamus and owes its name to its ability to inhibit release of growth hormone (pituitary somatotropin). Since that time, somatostatin has been identified in a number of tissues, including many areas of the brain, the gastrointestinal tract, and the pancreas. In the central nervous system and the pancreas, somatostatin-14 predominates, but approximately 5–10% of the somatostatin-like immunoreactivity in the brain is due to a 28-amino-acid peptide, somatostatin-28. This consists of an amino terminal region of 14 amino acids and a carboxyl terminal segment containing somatostatin-14. In small intestine, the larger molecule is more prevalent, with 70–75% of the hormone having 28 amino acids and only 25–30% being somatostatin-14. In contrast, pancreatic D cells synthesize only somatostatin-14. The larger peptide somatostatin-28 is ten times more potent than somatostatin-14 in inhibiting growth hormone and insulin, whereas somatostatin-14 is more effective in inhibition of glucagon release.

Almost every known stimulator of release of insulin from pancreatic B cells also promotes somatostatin release from D cells. This includes glucose, arginine, gastrointestinal hormones, and tolbutamide. The importance of circulating somatostatin is unclear, since a major role of this peptide may be as a paracrine regulator of the pancreatic islet and the tissues of the gastrointestinal tract. Physiologic levels of somatostatin in humans seldom exceed 80 pg/mL (49 pmol/L). The metabolic clearance of exogenously infused somatostatin in humans is extremely rapid; the half-life of the hormone is less than 3 minutes.

Recently, molecular cloning has demonstrated the existence of at least five somatostatin receptors (SSTR1–5) which are G protein-coupled receptors with seven membrane-spanning domains. They vary in size from 364 to 418 amino acids (with 105 amino acids invariant) and are found in the central nervous system and in a wide variety of peripheral tissues including the pituitary gland, the small intestine, and the pancreas. These receptors activate tyrosine phosphatases that interfere with the secretory process by dephosphorylating proteins. Inhibition of insulin secretion is due to binding of ligand to SSTR5, whereas inhibition of growth hormone release as well as glucagon release by A cells of the pancreas are due to effects of SSTR2. This explains why an analog of somatostatin, octreotide, which has a much greater affinity for SSTR2 than for SSTR5, can be effective in correcting growth hormone excess without much of an effect on carbohydrate tolerance when used to treat acromegaly.

Somatostatin acts in several ways to restrain the movement of nutrients from the intestinal tract into the

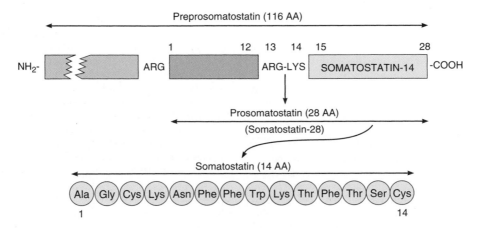

Figure 17–7. Amino acid sequence of somatostatin and its cleavage from dibasic amino acid residue in prosomatostatin and preprosomatostatin.

circulation. It prolongs gastric emptying time, decreases gastric acid and gastrin production, diminishes pancreatic exocrine secretion, decreases splanchnic blood flow, and retards xylose absorption. Neutralization of circulating somatostatin with antisomatostatin serum is associated with enhanced nutrient absorption in dogs. This implies that at least some of the effects of somatostatin are truly endocrine, as opposed to the paracrine effects discussed earlier.

4. Pancreatic Polypeptide

Pancreatic polypeptide (PP) is found in PP cells located chiefly in islets in the posterior portion of the head of the pancreas. PP is a 36-amino-acid peptide with a molecular weight of 4200. Little is known about its biosynthesis. Circulating levels of the peptide increase in response to a mixed meal; however, intravenous infusion of glucose or triglyceride does not produce such a rise, and intravenous amino acids cause only a small increase. Vagotomy abolishes the response to an ingested meal.

In healthy subjects, basal levels of PP average 24 + 4 pmol/L and may become elevated owing to a variety of factors including old age, alcohol abuse, diarrhea, chronic renal failure, hypoglycemia, or inflammatory disorders. Values above 300 pmol/L are found in most patients with pancreatic endocrine tumors such as glucagonoma or VIPoma and in all patients with tumors of the pancreatic PP cell. As many as 20% of patients with insulinoma and one-third of those with gastrinomas also have pancreatic polypeptide plasma concentrations of greater than 300 pmol/L.

The physiologic action of PP is unknown.

■ II. DIABETES MELLITUS

Clinical diabetes mellitus is a syndrome of disordered metabolism with inappropriate hyperglycemia due either to an absolute deficiency of insulin secretion or a reduction in the biologic effectiveness of insulin (or both).

■ CLASSIFICATION

Traditionally, diabetes was classified according to the patient's age at onset of symptoms (juvenile-onset versus adult-onset). In 1979, the NIH Diabetes Data Group proposed a classification that divided diabetes into two main types—insulin-dependent and non-insulin-depen-

dent—but this "therapeutic classification" proved unsatisfactory as more information on the pathogenesis and etiology of diabetes mellitus accumulated. In 1997, an international committee of diabetologists recommended several changes in the classification of diabetes that have been endorsed by the American Diabetes Association and the World Health Organization (Table 17–4). They include the following:

(1) The terms "insulin-independent diabetes mellitus" and "non-insulin-dependent diabetes mellitus" and their acronyms IDDM and NIDDM were eliminated since they are based upon pharmacologic rather than etiologic considerations.

(2) The terms "type 1 diabetes" and "type 2 diabetes" are retained, with arabic rather than roman numerals. Type 1 diabetes is due to pancreatic islet B cell destruction, which in over 95% of cases is caused by an autoimmune process, while in less than 5% the B cell destruction is idiopathic. Patients with type 1 diabetes are generally prone to ketoacidosis and require insulin replacement therapy. Type 2 diabetes, the much more prevalent form, is a heterogeneous disorder encompassing a spectrum of defects consisting in some cases of defects in B cell function alone but most commonly associated with insulin resistance in the presence of an associated impairment in compensatory insulin secretion.

Of the approximately 16 million patients in the United States who have diabetes, about 1.5 million have type 1. The remainder mainly have type 2 diabetes except for a third group ("other specific types") recently defined by the ADA who have rare monogenic defects of either pancreatic B cell function or of insulin action, primary diseases of the endocrine pancreas, or drug-induced diabetes (Table 17–4).

TYPE 1 DIABETES MELLITUS

Type 1 is a severe form of diabetes mellitus and is associated with ketosis in the untreated state. About 9% of diabetics in North America and 20% of diabetics in Scandinavian countries have type 1 diabetes. It is most common in young individuals but occurs occasionally in nonobese adults. It is a catabolic disorder in which circulating insulin is virtually absent, plasma glucagon is elevated, and the pancreatic B cells fail to respond to all known insulinogenic stimuli. In the absence of insulin, the three main target tissues of insulin (liver, muscle, and fat) not only fail to appropriately take up absorbed nutrients but continue to deliver glucose, amino acids, and fatty acids into the bloodstream from their respective storage depots. Furthermore, alterations in fat metabolism lead to the production and accumulation of ketones. This inappropriate persistence of the fasted state postprandially can be reversed by the administration of insulin.

Table 17–4. Etiologic classification of diabetes mellitus.[1]

I. Type 1 diabetes[2] (B cell destruction, usually leading to absolute insulin deficiency)
  A. Immune-mediated
  B. Idiopathic
II. Type 2 diabetes[2] (may range from predominantly insulin resistance with relative insulin deficiency to a predominantly secretory defect with insulin resistance)
III. Other specific types
  A. Genetic defects of B cell function
    1. Chromosome 12, HNF-1α (formerly MODY 3)
    2. Chromosome 7, glucokinase (formerly MODY 2)
    3. Chromosome 20, HNF-4α (formerly MODY 1)
    4. Mitochrondrial DNA
    5. Others
  B. Genetic defects in insulin action
    1. Type A insulin resistance
    2. Leprechaunism
    3. Rabson-Mendenhall syndrome
    4. Lipoatrophic diabetes
    5. Others
  C. Diseases of the exocrine pancreas
    1. Pancreatitis
    2. Trauma, pancreatectomy
    3. Neoplasia
    4. Cystic fibrosis
    5. Hemochromatosis
    6. Fibrocalculous pancreatopathy
    7. Others
  D. Endocrinopathies
    1. Acromegaly
    2. Cushing's syndrome
    3. Glucagonoma
    4. Pheochromocytoma
    5. Hyperthyroidism
    6. Somatostatinoma
    7. Aldosteronoma
    8. Others
	III. Other specific types (cont'd)
	  E. Drug- or chemical-induced
	    1. Vacor
	    2. Pentamidine
	    3. Nicotinic acid
	    4. Glucocorticoids
	    5. Thyroid hormone
	    6. Diazoxide
	    7. Beta-adrenergic agonists
	    8. Thiazides
	    9. Phenytoin
	    10. Alpha-interferon
	    11. Others
	  F. Infections
	    1. Congenital rubella
	    2. Cytomegalovirus
	    3. Others
	  G. Uncommon forms of immune-mediated diabetes
	    1. Stiff-man syndrome
	    2. Anti-insulin receptor antibodies
	    3. Others
	  H. Other genetic syndromes sometimes associated with diabetes
	    1. Down's syndrome
	    2. Klinefelter's syndrome
	    3. Turner's syndrome
	    4. Wolfram's syndrome
	    5. Friedreich's ataxia
	    6. Huntington's chorea
	    7. Laurence-Moon-Biedl syndrome
	    8. Myotonic dystrophy
	    9. Porphyria
	    10. Prader-Willi syndrome
	    11. Others
	IV. Gestational diabetes mellitus (GDM)

[1]Modified from American Diabetes Association: Diabetes Care 1999;22(Suppl 1):1185.
[2]Patients with any form of diabetes may require insulin treatment at some stage of their disease. Such use of insulin does not, of itself, classify the patient.
HNF = hepatic nuclear factor.

Genetics of Type 1 Diabetes

Studies in monozygotic twins suggest that genetic influences are less marked in type 1 diabetes than in type 2 diabetes. Only 30–40% of identical twins of type 1 diabetic patients will develop the disease. This also suggests that an environmental factor is required for induction of diabetes in these cases. In contrast, the identical twin of a type 2 diabetic is much more prone to develop diabetes, often with onset within a year after onset of the disease in the sibling.

Type 1 diabetes is believed to result from an infectious or toxic environmental insult to genetically predisposed persons whose aggressive immune system destroys pancreatic B cells while overcoming the invasive agent. Environmental factors that have been associated with altered pancreatic islet cell function include viruses (mumps, rubella, coxsackievirus B4), toxic chemical agents such as vacor (a nitrophenylurea rat poison), and other destructive cytotoxins such as hydrogen cyanide from spoiled tapioca or cassava root.

At least half of the familial aggregation of type 1 diabetes is accounted for by genes in the major histocompatibility locus on the short arm of chromosome 6. The most important of these are the HLA class II molecules DQ and DR, which code for antigens expressed on the surface of macrophages and B lymphocytes (see Chapter 4 and Figure 4–2). The class II molecules bind to peptide antigens and present them to T cells by binding to the T cell receptor. In contrast to the DR genes, which have polymorphisms only in their beta subunit, the DQ genes have polymorphic alpha and beta subunits, so that in the approved nomenclature a specific DQ allele is identified by an assigned number for each of its A and B subunits. Of approximately 21 known DR genes, only DR3 and DR4 are major susceptibility risk factors for type 1 diabetes. As many as 95% of type 1 diabetic patients have a DR3 or a DR4—or both—compared with 45–50% of Caucasian nondiabetic controls. The highest risk for type 1 diabetes in the United States is borne by individuals who express both a DR3 and a DR4 allele. These are generally in linkage disequilibrium with DQ genes that themselves confer high risk, particularly DQA1*0501, DQB1*0201 (coupled with DR3), and DQA1*0301, DQB1*0302 (coupled with DR4). Only 2% of children born in the United States are DR3 or DR4 heterozygotes, yet they comprise about 40% of all children developing type 1 diabetes.

DQ alleles are associated not only with risk for type 1 diabetes but also with dominant protection, often in linkage with HLA-DR2. The most protective of these—and a quite common allele—is DQA1*0102, DQB1*0602. It occurs in over 20% of individuals but in less than 1% of children developing type 1 diabetes. In fact, in clinical trials for the prevention of type 1 diabetes, subjects with this particular highly protective DQ allele are excluded despite the presence of islet cell antibody-positive first-degree relatives.

It remains a mystery why people with certain HLA types are predisposed to development of type 1 diabetes. The concept of an autoimmune destruction of pancreatic B cells due to selective loss of immune tolerance is supported by evidence that immune suppression therapy interrupts progression to insulin deficiency in a number of newly diagnosed type 1 patients. Moreover, extensive infiltration with both helper and cytotoxic T lymphocytes is present in the islets of children who just developed type 1 diabetes, and their serum contains autoantibodies against structural and secretory proteins of the pancreatic B cells before the onset of type 1 diabetes and for some time after diagnosis.

On the strength of the above evidence, a theory for autoimmune B cell destruction has been proposed based on molecular mimicry, wherein the immune system mistakenly targets B cell proteins that share homologies with certain viral or other foreign peptides (such as partially digested cow's milk dietary proteins). The efficiency of presenting certain proteins depends on the composition of the class II antigens on the surface of the antigen-presenting cells (macrophages). Efficiency of antigen presentation by the class II HLA proteins could play a role during the deletion of self-reactive T cells in the thymus. Failure to properly delete T cells that recognize B cell antigens would predispose to later development of type 1 diabetes. Alternatively, efficiency of antigen presentation could play a role later during the peripheral development of an autoimmune response.

Circulating islet cell autoantibodies, virtually absent in nondiabetics, have been detected in as many as 85% of type 1 diabetics tested in the first few weeks after onset of diabetes. Moreover, when sensitive immunoassays are used, up to 60% of these patients also have detectable antibodies to insulin prior to receiving insulin therapy, and these are especially prevalent with an onset of disease in childhood. The high prevalence of these islet cell and insulin autoantibodies in type 1 diabetes, as well as in certain of their siblings who later develop overt diabetes, supports the concept that autoimmune mechanisms may contribute significantly to progressive B cell destruction.

The most common islet cell antibodies in patients with type 1 diabetes are directed against glutamic acid decarboxylase (GAD), an enzyme localized within pancreatic B cells. This enzyme has isoforms with molecular weights of 65,000 and 67,000 which are also found in central nervous system "inhibitory" neurons that secrete γ-aminobutyric acid. Evidence that a rare neurologic condition, "stiff-man syndrome," was associated with autoimmunity to neurons containing GAD—and that these patients also had islet cell autoantibodies and a high incidence of type 1 diabetes—led to the discovery that antibodies to GAD made up the bulk of antibodies previously described in type 1 diabetes as being against a 64-kDa antigen in pancreatic B cells.

Manifestations of stiff-man syndrome are not seen in the vast majority of patients with type 1 diabetes even though their islet cell antibodies contain a major component that reacts in vitro with GAD-containing neurons. The blood-brain barrier may have some protective effect against neuronal damage of a degree that might cause stiff-man syndrome in type 1 diabetes. Patients with stiff-man syndrome generally have much higher GAD antibody levels than most patients with type 1 diabetes.

A genetic link to chromosome 11 has been identified in type 1 diabetes. Studies of a polymorphic DNA locus flanking the 5′ region of the insulin gene on chromosome 11 revealed a slight but statistically significant linkage between type 1 diabetes and this genetic locus in a Caucasian population of type 1 diabetics. This polymorphic locus, which consists of a variable number of tandem repeats (VNTR) with two common sizes in Caucasians, small (26–63 repeats) or large (140–243 repeats), does not encode a protein. An intriguing proposal to explain how the VNTR might influence susceptibility to type 1 diabetes was based on findings that insulin gene transcription is facilitated in the fetal thymus gland by the presence of the large allele of the VNTR locus flanking the insulin gene. The large VNTR allele might produce a dominant protective effect by promoting negative selection (deletion) by the thymus of insulin-specific T lymphocytes that play a critical role in the immune destruction of their pancreatic B cells.

The established genetic association with the HLA region of chromosome 6 contributes much more (about 50%) to the genetic susceptibility to type 1 diabetes than does this locus flanking the insulin gene on chromosome 11, which contributes about 10%. The recommended nomenclature for these two known susceptibility gene associations are *IDDM1* for the HLA region and *IDDM2* for the insulin gene region. Approximately 16 other genes with lesser degrees of linkage to type 1 diabetes are being investigated.

Immunomodulation in the Treatment & Prevention of Type 1 Diabetes

Since the destruction of B cells in type 1 diabetes is a progressive, immune-mediated process, therapies that block or modulate the immune response should be able to stop the destruction. Unfortunately, trials of immunosuppression therapies have been generally disappointing. Although some reduction or elimination of insulin requirement in patients with new-onset type 1 diabetes has been observed, most subjects manifest continued carbohydrate intolerance while being exposed to considerable risk from the adverse effects of immunosuppressive drugs. Because of its substantial side effects and increased risks of infection and malignancy, broad immunosuppression is not recommended for the treatment of patients with newly diagnosed type 1 diabetes.

More specific strategies for immunosuppression, such as the use of monoclonal antibodies against particular T cell products, may reduce the hazards of long-term immunotherapy. A trial using a humanized monoclonal antibody against CD3, hOKT3γ1(Ala-Ala), showed efficacy in reducing the decline in insulin production in patients newly diagnosed with type 1 diabetes. CD3 is an antigen expressed on the surface of activated T cells, and the hOKT3γ1(Ala-Ala) monoclonal antibody is believed to modulate the autoimmune response by selectively inhibiting the pathogenic T cells or inducing regulatory T cells. Patients were treated for 14

days with the antibody within 6 weeks after diagnosis of type 1 diabetes. One year later, the majority of patients in the treated group had maintained or increased insulin production and improved glycemic control relative to the control group. This and other approaches that selectively modulate the autoimmune T cell response hold the promise that type 1 diabetes may eventually be preventable without prolonged immunosuppression.

A nonimmunosuppressive modality that showed promise in animal models of type 1 diabetes is nicotinamide, an inhibitor of poly(ADP-ribose) synthetase, an enzyme whose repair of DNA injury tends to deplete the cell of its vital supply of NAD. A series of trials of nicotinamide after the onset of type 1 diabetes have generally been disappointing and inconclusive as regards any benefit. A large randomized trial known as the European Nicotinamide Diabetes Intervention Trial (ENDIT) concluded that nicotinamide provides no protection to islet cell antibody-positive first-degree relatives of patients with type 1 diabetes. Daily exposure to insulin antigen has been shown to delay or prevent the onset of type 1 diabetes in animal models of type 1 diabetes as well as in a small pilot study in nondiabetic humans at high risk to develop type 1 diabetes (first-degree relatives of patients with type 1 diabetes, positive islet cell antibodies, and a blunted insulin release to glucose). Because of these encouraging findings, a large-scale randomized multicenter Diabetes Prevention Trial in type 1 diabetes (DPT-1) has begun under the auspices of the National Institutes of Health to test low-dose insulin injections in nondiabetic relatives of people with type 1 diabetes, who are at high risk to develop type 1 diabetes themselves (having islet cell antibodies and a low serum insulin response to a glucose load). Volunteers with *high* risk (antibody titer and a low serum insulin response) will be assigned to a control group or to a group receiving 0.25 units of ultralente insulin per kilogram of body weight given in divided doses. Volunteers at *intermediate* risk, who have islet cell antibodies and also insulin autoantibodies but normal serum insulin responses to glucose loading, will be randomly assigned to a control group or to a group receiving oral insulin. Because of a lower rate of volunteer recruitment and the lower incidence of diabetes in this "intermediate risk" group, this arm of the study had not been completed as of the end of 2002. In addition, intervention trials using other therapies, such as OKT3, are in various stages of development.

TYPE 2 DIABETES

Type 2 diabetes—previously classified as non-insulin-dependent diabetes (NIDDM)—afflicts individuals with insulin resistance who generally have relative rather than absolute insulin deficiency. It accounts for

80–90% of cases of diabetes in the United States. These patients are usually adults over age 40 with some degree of obesity. They do not require insulin to survive, though over time their insulin secretory capacity tends to deteriorate, and many need insulin treatment to achieve optimal glucose control. Ketosis seldom occurs spontaneously, and if present it is a consequence of severe stress from trauma or infection.

The nature of the primary defect in type 2 diabetes is obscure. Tissue insensitivity to insulin has been noted in most type 2 patients irrespective of weight and has been attributed to several interrelated factors (Table 17–5). These include a putative (as yet undefined) genetic factor, which is aggravated in time by further enhancers of insulin resistance such as aging, a sedentary lifestyle, and abdominal visceral obesity. In addition, there is an accompanying deficiency in the response of pancreatic B cells to glucose, a genetic disorder that may be aggravated by gradual displacement of B cells due to deposition of intra-islet amyloid with aging. Furthermore, both the tissue resistance to insulin and the impaired B cell response to glucose appear to be further aggravated by sustained hyperglycemia, which may impede both insulin signaling and B cell function. Treatment that reduces the hyperglycemia toward normal reduces this acquired defect in insulin resistance and also improves to some degree glucose-induced insulin release. Type 2 diabetes frequently goes undiagnosed for many years, since the hyperglycemia develops quite gradually and is generally asymptomatic initially. Despite this mild presentation, these patients are at increased risk of developing macrovascular and microvascular complications.

The genetics of type 2 diabetes is complex and poorly defined despite the strong genetic predisposition in these patients. This is probably because of the heterogeneous nature of this disorder as well as the difficulty in sorting out the contribution of acquired factors affecting insulin action and glycemic control.

Subgroups of Type 2 Diabetes

Two subgroups of patients with type 2 diabetes are currently distinguished by the absence or presence of obesity. It is at present impossible to identify diagnostic characteristics that allow further clear-cut separation into more specific subtypes. Circulating insulin levels vary with the prevailing degree of hyperglycemia and are considered too unreliable to be of use in classifying type 2 diabetes.

A. OBESE TYPE 2 DIABETES

The prevalence of obesity varies among different racial groups. While obesity is apparent in no more than 30% of Chinese and Japanese patients with type 2 diabetes, it is present in 60–80% of North Americans, Europeans, or Africans with type 2 diabetes and approaches 100% of type 2 patients among Pima Indians or Pacific Islanders from Nauru or Samoa. Patients with type 2 diabetes have an insensitivity to endogenous insulin that is correlated with the presence of a predominantly abdominal distribution of fat, producing an abnormally high waist to hip ratio. In addition, distended adipocytes and overnourished liver and muscle cells may also resist the deposition of additional glycogen and triglycerides in their storage depots. Hyperplasia of pancreatic B cells is often present and probably accounts for the normal or exaggerated insulin responses to glucose and other stimuli seen in the milder forms of this disease. In more severe cases, secondary (but potentially reversible) failure of pancreatic B cell secretion may result after exposure to prolonged fasting hyperglycemia. This phenomenon has been called "desensitization" or "glucose toxicity." It is selective for glucose, and the B cell can recover some degree of sensitivity to glucose stimulation once the sustained hyperglycemia is corrected by any form of therapy, including diet therapy, sulfonylureas, and insulin.

Not all patients with obesity and insulin resistance develop hyperglycemia, however. An underlying defect in the ability of the B cells to compensate for the increased demand may determine which patients will develop diabetes in the setting of insulin resistance. Furthermore, as noted above, patients with type 2 diabetes suffer from a progressive decline in B cell function that results in worsening hyperglycemia even when the degree of insulin resistance remains stable.

B. METABOLIC SYNDROME (SYNDROME X)

When type 2 patients predominantly present with insulin resistance, the diabetes may represent only one

---

Table 17–5. Factors reducing response to insulin.

Prereceptor inhibitors: Insulin antibodies
Receptor inhibitors:
  Insulin receptor autoantibodies
  "Down-regulation" of receptors by hyperinsulinism:
    Primary hyperinsulinism (B cell adenoma)
    Hyperinsulinism, secondary to a postreceptor defect
      (obesity, Cushing's syndrome, acromegaly,
      pregnancy) or prolonged hyperglycemia (diabetes
      mellitus, post-glucose tolerance test)
Postreceptor influences:
  Poor responsiveness of principal target organs: obesity,
    hepatic disease, muscle inactivity
  Hormonal excess: glucocorticoids, growth hormone, oral
    contraceptive agents, progesterone, human chorionic
    somatomammotropin, catecholamines, thyroxine

facet of a metabolic syndrome. **Hyperglycemia** in these patients is frequently associated with **hyperinsulinemia, dyslipidemia,** and **hypertension,** which together lead to **coronary artery disease** and **stroke.** It has been suggested that this aggregation results from a genetic defect producing insulin resistance, particularly when obesity aggravates the degree of insulin resistance. In this model, impaired action of insulin predisposes to hyperglycemia, which in turn induces hyperinsulinemia. If this hyperinsulinemia is of insufficient magnitude to correct the hyperglycemia, type 2 diabetes will be manifested. The excessive insulin level could also increase sodium retention by renal tubules, thereby contributing to or causing hypertension. Increased VLDL production in the liver, leading to hypertriglyceridemia (and consequently a low HDL-cholesterol level), has also been attributed to hyperinsulinism. Moreover, it has been proposed that high insulin levels can stimulate endothelial and vascular smooth muscle cell proliferation—by virtue of the hormone's action on growth factor receptors—to initiate atherosclerosis.

While there is full agreement on an association of the above disorders, the mechanism of their interrelationship remains speculative and open to experimental investigation. Controversy persists about whether or not hypertension is caused by hyperinsulinism, since these two manifestations, which often coexist in whites, are not highly associated in American blacks or Pima Indians. Moreover, patients with hyperinsulinism due to an insulinoma are generally normotensive, and there is no reduction of blood pressure after surgical removal of the insulinoma restores normal insulin levels.

An alternative unifying hypothesis could be that visceral obesity directly induces the other components of this syndrome. Visceral obesity is an independent risk factor for all of the other components of metabolic syndrome. In addition to the metabolic effects of visceral obesity, adipocytes produce a number of secreted products including TNFα, leptin, adiponectin, and resistin (see Chapter 20). Although the full details of the role of these molecules in causation of the metabolic syndrome are still under investigation, the adipocyte clearly is not just an innocent bystander but plays an active role in the development of systemic insulin resistance, hypertension, and hyperlipidemia. Furthermore, thrombi in atheromatous vessels may be more hazardous in patients with visceral obesity because they also have an associated increase in plasminogen activator inhibitor-1, a circulating factor produced by omental and visceral adipocytes that inhibits clot lysis. This discussion emphasizes the importance of measures such as diet and exercise that reduce visceral adiposity in the management of patients with metabolic syndrome and obese type 2 diabetes.

Australian epidemiologists prefer to group these disorders together as a syndrome, without necessarily implying that a single cause is responsible for the other components. They suggest the acronym CHAOS to signify coronary artery disease, hypertension, adult-onset diabetes, obesity, and stroke. The main value of grouping these disorders as a syndrome, regardless of its nomenclature, is to remind physicians that the therapeutic goals are not only to correct hyperglycemia but also to manage the elevated blood pressure and hyperlipidemia that result in considerable cardiovascular morbidity as well as cardiovascular deaths in these patients. It also raises awareness that indiscriminate therapeutic use of high doses of exogenous insulin may conceivably have adverse effects on a patient's risk profile for cardiovascular disease if the hypothesis behind the insulin resistance syndrome is substantiated. Finally, it reminds physicians that when choosing antihypertensive agents or lipid-lowering drugs to manage one of the components of this syndrome, their possible untoward effects on other components of the syndrome should be carefully considered. For example, physicians aware of this syndrome are less likely to prescribe antihypertensive drugs that raise lipids (diuretics, beta-blockers) or that raise blood sugar (diuretics). Likewise, they will refrain from prescribing drugs that correct hyperlipidemia but increase insulin resistance with aggravation of hyperglycemia (niacin).

C. NONOBESE TYPE 2 DIABETES

Approximately 20–40% of type 2 diabetic patients are nonobese, though this percentage varies according to the population studied—eg, higher in Asian populations and lower in Pacific Islanders and Pima Indians of the American Southwest and Mexico. Among nonobese type 2 diabetic patients, deficient insulin release by the pancreatic B cell seems to be the major defect, but some insulin resistance may also contribute. However, this degree of insulin resistance does not seem to be clinically relevant to the treatment of most nonobese type 2 patients, who generally respond to appropriate therapeutic supplements of insulin in the absence of rare associated conditions such as lipoatrophy or acanthosis nigricans.

Currently, type 2 diabetes is considered of idiopathic origin. However, with developments in biotechnology, a variety of etiologic genetic abnormalities have been documented within this heterogeneous group, particularly in those presenting with clinical and laboratory manifestations similar to those seen in the nonobese type 2 subgroup. When the genetic defect has been defined, these patients have recently been reclassified within a group designated "other specific types" (Table 17–4). In most of these patients, impaired insulin action at the postreceptor level and an absent or delayed early phase of insulin release in response to glucose can be demonstrated. However, other insulinogenic stimuli, such as acute infusion of amino acids, intravenous tolbutamide, or intramuscular glucagon, often remain partially effective in eliciting acute insulin release.

The hyperglycemia in patients with nonobese type 2 diabetes often responds to dietary therapy or to oral antidiabetic agents. Occasionally, insulin therapy is required to achieve satisfactory glycemic control even though it is not needed to prevent ketoacidosis.

OTHER SPECIFIC TYPES OF DIABETES

Genetic Defects of Pancreatic B Cell Function

This subgroup of monogenic disorders is characterized by a diabetes that occurs in late childhood or before the age of 25 years as a result of a partial defect in glucose-induced insulin release and accounts for up to 5% of diabetes in North American and European populations. A strong family history of early-onset diabetes occurring in one parent and in one-half of the parent's offspring suggests autosomal dominant transmission. These patients are generally nonobese, and because they are not ketosis-prone and may initially achieve good glycemic control without insulin therapy, their disease has been called "maturity-onset diabetes of the young" (MODY). Six types have been described with single-gene defects, and all have been shown to produce a defect in glucose-induced insulin release. MODY 2 results from an abnormal glucokinase enzyme. Other forms of MODY are due to mutations of nuclear transcription factors that regulate B cell gene expression (Table 17–6).

MODY 1 includes 74 members of a pedigree known as the R-W family, descendants of a German couple who immigrated to Michigan in 1861. They have been studied prospectively since 1958, and in 1996 the genetic defect was shown to be a nonsense mutation of a nuclear transcription factor found in liver as well as in pancreatic B cells. This gene has been termed hepatocyte nuclear factor-4α (HNF-4α) and is found on chromosome 20. Mutations of this gene are among the rarest of the MODY groups, with very few other mutations reported in families with other than the Michigan pedigree. Its role in reducing glucose-induced insulin secretion has not yet been clarified. These patients display a progressive decline in B cell function and develop chronic complications of diabetes comparable in degree to those with idiopathic type 2 diabetes. They often fare better with insulin therapy.

MODY 2 was first described in French families but has now been found in racial groups from most parts of the world. At least 26 different mutations of the glucokinase gene on chromosome 7 have been identified

Table 17–6. Genetic defects of pancreatic B cell function.

Syndrome	Mutation	Chromosome
MODY 1	Hepatocyte nuclear factor-4α	20q
MODY 2	Glucokinase gene	7p
MODY 3	Hepatocyte nuclear factor-1α	12q
MODY 4	Insulin promoter factor-1	13q
MODY 5	Hepatocyte nuclear factor-1β	17q
MODY 6	NeuroD1	2q
Mitochondrial dysfunction	Transfer RNAs (leucine or lysine tRNA)	Mitochondrial DNA
Mutant insulin or proinsulin	Insulin gene	11p

and characterized. Reduced sensitivity of pancreatic B cell glucokinase to plasma glucose causes impaired insulin secretion, resulting in fasting hyperglycemia and mild diabetes. A reduction in glucokinase activity within the pancreatic B cell is critical in determining the threshold of plasma glucose at which the B cell secretes insulin, since glucokinase acts as a glucose sensor. While some of these mutations can completely block this enzyme's function, others interfere only slightly with its action. In contrast to all the other forms of MODY, patients with one mutated glucokinase allele (heterozygotes) have a benign course with few or no chronic complications and respond well to diet therapy or oral antidiabetic drugs without the need for insulin treatment. On the other hand, rare individuals who inherit two mutated glucokinase alleles have permanent neonatal diabetes, a nonimmune form of absolute insulin deficiency that presents at birth.

MODY 3 is caused by mutations of hepatocyte nuclear factor-1α (HNF-1α), whose gene is located on chromosome 12. This is the most common form of MODY in European populations, with many different mutations having been reported. Like HNF-4α, the HNF-1α transcription factor is expressed in pancreatic B cells as well as in liver, and its role in glucose-induced insulin secretion has not been clarified. In contrast to most patients with type 2 diabetes, there is no associated insulin resistance, but the clinical course of these two disorders is otherwise similar as to prevalence of microangiopathy and failure to continue to respond to oral agents with time. These patients have been noted to display an exaggerated response to sulfonylureas early in the course of the disease.

MODY 4 results from mutation of a pancreatic nuclear transcription factor known as insulin promoter factor-1 (IPF-1), whose gene is on chromosome 13. It mediates insulin gene transcription and regulates expression of other B cell-specific genes such as glucokinase and glucose transporter-2. When both alleles of this gene are nonfunctioning, agenesis of the entire pancreas results; but in the presence of a heterozygous mutation of IPF-1, a mild form of MODY has been described in which affected individuals developed diabetes at a later age (mean onset at 35 years) than occurs with the other forms of MODY, in whom onset generally occurs before the age of 25 years.

MODY 5 was initially reported in a Japanese family with a mutation of HNF-1β, a hepatic nuclear transcription factor that acts with HNF-1α to regulate gene expression in pancreatic islets. Mutations in this gene cause a moderately severe form of MODY with progression to insulin treatment and severe diabetic complications in those affected. In addition, congenital kidney defects and nephropathy have been reported in affected individuals prior to the onset of diabetes, suggesting that decreased levels of this transcription factor in the kidney, where it is also normally expressed at high levels, may contribute to renal dysfunction.

MODY 6, a milder form of MODY similar to MODY 4, results from mutations in the gene encoding the islet transcription factor neuroD1. Like IPF-1, neuroD1 plays an important role in the expression of insulin and other B cell genes.

The identification of mutations in multiple genes encoding pancreatic transcription factors in patients with MODY has led to the screening of other genes encoding pancreatic transcription factors in patients with diabetes. Heterozygous mutations in genes encoding several factors, including ISL-1, PAX-6, and PAX-4, have been identified in patients with later-onset diabetes. The association of diabetes with heterozygous mutations in so many B cell genes highlights the critical importance of optimal B cell function in metabolic regulation. Even modest defects in glucose-induced insulin secretion can result in hyperglycemia.

Diabetes Mellitus Associated with a Mutation of Mitochondrial DNA

Since sperm do not contain mitochondria, only the mother transmits mitochondrial genes to her offspring. Diabetes due to a mutation of mitochondrial DNA that impairs the transfer of leucine into mitochondrial proteins has been described in 22 Japanese families involving 52 individuals. Most patients have a mild form of maternally transmitted diabetes that responds to oral hypoglycemic agents, although some patients have a nonimmune form of type 1 diabetes. As many as 63% of patients with this subtype of diabetes have a hearing loss, and a smaller proportion (15%) had a syndrome of myopathy, encephalopathy, lactic acidosis, and stroke-like episodes (MELAS).

Mutant Insulins

Despite awareness of this disorder over the past 12 years, only eight families have been identified as having abnormal circulating forms of insulin. In three of these families, there is impaired cleavage of the proinsulin molecule; in the other five families, abnormalities of the insulin molecule itself have been reported (Table 17–7).

Analysis of the insulin gene, circulating insulin, and clinical features of family members in these cases indicates that individuals with mutant insulin are heterozygous for this defect, with both a normal and an abnormal insulin molecule being equally expressed. However, because the abnormal insulin binds to receptors poorly, it has very low biologic activity and accumulates in the blood to exceed the concentration of the normal insulin. This decreased removal rate of mutant insulin results in hyperinsulinemia after overnight fasting and a subnormal molar ratio of C peptide to immunoreactive insulin. A mild form of diabetes mellitus may or may not be present in association with mutant insulin, depending on the concentration and bioactivity of circulating normal and abnormal insulins and on the insulin responsiveness of peripheral tissues. Since there is no obvious resistance to insulin in any of these cases, it appears that abnormal insulin does not interfere with binding of normal insulin to receptors; therefore, a feature of this syndrome is the normal response to exogenously administered insulin.

With improved screening techniques becoming available such as the polymerase chain reaction, more cases of mutation of the insulin gene will undoubtedly be detected. However, from present experience it is unlikely that patients with this defect will make up more than a very small fraction of the diabetic population.

Table 17–7. Mutant insulins and proinsulins.

	Amino Acid Substitution
Insulin Chicago (USA)	B 25 (Phe → Leu)
Insulin Los Angeles (USA)	B 24 (Phe → Ser)
Insulin Wakayama (Japan) I, II, III (three families)	A 3 (Val → Leu)
Proinsulin Tokyo (Japan)	Arg 65 (Arg → His)
Proinsulin Boston (USA)	Arg 65 (Arg → ?)
Proinsulin Providence (USA)	B 10 (His → Asp)

Genetic Defects of Insulin Action

These are rare and unusual causes of diabetes that result from mutations of the insulin receptor (type A insulin resistance) or from other genetically determined postreceptor abnormalities of insulin action. Metabolic abnormalities associated with these disorders may range from hyperinsulinemia and modest hyperglycemia to severe diabetes. Some individuals have acanthosis nigricans, which seems to be a consequence of very high circulating insulin levels that cross over to bind to insulin-like growth factor receptors on epidermal and melanin-containing cutaneous cells. A similar action of extremely high insulin levels on ovarian hilar cells may cause women with these mutations to become virilized and have enlarged cystic ovaries. Leprechaunism and the Rabson-Mendenhall syndrome are two rare pediatric syndromes characterized by extreme insulin resistance due to inheritance of two mutant insulin receptor alleles.

Alterations in the structure and function of the insulin receptor cannot be demonstrated in patients with insulin-resistant lipoatrophic diabetes, suggesting that the defect must reside in postreceptor pathways. Lipoatrophic insulin resistance in animals can be reversed by replacing the adipocyte products leptin and adiponectin, demonstrating the importance of the adipocyte in regulating insulin function.

Diabetes Due to Diseases of the Exocrine Pancreas

Any process that diffusely damages or displaces at least two-thirds of the pancreas can cause diabetes, though individuals with a predisposition to type 2 diabetes are probably more susceptible to developing diabetes with lesser degrees of pancreatic involvement. Acquired causes include pancreatitis, trauma, infection, pancreatic carcinoma, and pancreatectomy. When extensive enough, hemochromatosis and cystic fibrosis can also displace B cells and cause deficiency in insulin secretion. Fibrocalculous involvement of the pancreas may be accompanied by abdominal pain radiating to the back and associated with pancreatic calcifications on x-ray. Since glucagon-secreting A cells are also damaged or removed by these processes, less insulin is usually required for replacement—as compared with most other forms of diabetes, where A cells are intact.

Endocrinopathies

Excess production of certain hormones—growth hormone (acromegaly), glucocorticoids (Cushing's syndrome or disease), catecholamines (pheochromocytoma), thyroid hormone (thyrotoxicosis), glucagon

(glucagonoma), or pancreatic somatostatin (somatostatinoma)—can produce the syndrome of type 2 diabetes by a number of mechanisms. In all but the last instance (somatostatinoma), peripheral responsiveness to insulin is impaired. In addition, excess of catecholamines or somatostatin decreases insulin release from B cells. Diabetes mainly occurs in individuals with preexisting defects in insulin secretion, and hyperglycemia typically resolves when the hormone excess is corrected.

Drug- or Chemical-Induced Diabetes

Many drugs are associated with carbohydrate intolerance or frank diabetes mellitus. Some act by interfering with insulin release from the B cells (thiazides, phenytoin), some by inducing insulin resistance (glucocorticoids, oral contraceptive pills), and some by causing B cell destruction such as vacor (a rat poison) and intravenous pentamidine. Patients receiving alpha interferon have been reported to develop diabetes associated with islet cell antibodies and in certain instances severe insulin deficiency.

While calcium channel blockers as well as clonidine are potent inhibitors of glucose-induced insulin release from in vitro preparations of pancreatic B cells, the inhibitory concentrations required are quite high and are not generally achieved during standard antihypertensive therapy with these agents in humans.

Infections Causing Diabetes

Certain viruses have been associated with direct pancreatic B cell destruction in animals. Diabetes is also known to develop frequently in humans who had congenital rubella, though most of these patients have HLA and immune markers characteristic of type 1 diabetes. In addition, coxsackievirus B, cytomegalovirus, adenovirus, and mumps have been implicated in inducing certain cases of diabetes.

Uncommon Forms of Immune-Mediated Diabetes

These include two rare conditions associated with autoantibodies implicated in causing diabetes.

Stiff-man syndrome is an autoimmune disorder of the central nervous system characterized by stiffness and painful spasm of skeletal muscle. Many patients have high titers of autoantibodies that react with glutamic acid decarboxylase (GAD) in the central nervous system and also in pancreatic B cells. Approximately one-third develop severe B cell destruction and diabetes.

A severe form of insulin resistance has been reported in patients who developed high titers of antibodies that bind to the insulin receptor and block the action of insulin in its target tissues. As in other states of extreme insulin resistance, these patients often have acanthosis nigricans. In the past, this form of immune-mediated diabetes was termed type B insulin resistance.

Other Genetic Syndromes Sometimes Associated with Diabetes

A number of genetic syndromes are accompanied by an increased incidence of diabetes mellitus. These include the chromosomal abnormalities of Down's syndrome, Klinefelter's syndrome, and Turner's syndrome.

Wolfram's syndrome (DIDMOAD syndrome) is a rare autosomal recessive disease which in its complete form includes optic atrophy, diabetes insipidus, neural deafness, and a nonimmune form of pancreatic B cell death resulting in insulin deficiency and diabetes mellitus. It has recently been found to be associated with a genetic mutation on the short arm of chromosome 4 and an increased frequency of HLA-DR2 antigen.

■ CLINICAL FEATURES OF DIABETES MELLITUS

The principal clinical features of the two major types of diabetes mellitus are listed for comparison in Table 17–8.

TYPE 1 DIABETES

Patients with type 1 diabetes present with a characteristic symptom complex, as outlined below. An absolute deficiency of insulin results in excessive accumulation of circulating glucose and fatty acids, with consequent hyperosmolality and hyperketonemia. The severity of

Table 17–8. Clinical features of diabetes at diagnosis.

	Diabetes Type 1	Diabetes Type 2
Polyuria and thirst	++	+
Weakness or fatigue	++	+
Polyphagia with weight loss	++	-
Recurrent blurred vision	+	++
Vulvovaginitis or pruritus	+	++
Peripheral neuropathy	+	++
Nocturnal enuresis	++	-
Often asymptomatic	-	++

the insulin deficiency and the acuteness with which the catabolic state develops determine the intensity of the osmotic and ketotic excess.

Clinical Features

A. SYMPTOMS

Increased urination is a consequence of osmotic diuresis secondary to sustained hyperglycemia. This results in a loss of glucose as well as free water and electrolytes in the urine. Nocturnal enuresis due to polyuria may signal the onset of diabetes in very young children. Thirst is a consequence of the hyperosmolar state, as is blurred vision, which often develops as the lenses and retinas are exposed to hyperosmolar fluids.

Weight loss despite normal or increased appetite is a common feature of type 1 diabetes when it develops subacutely over a period of weeks. The weight loss is initially due to depletion of water, glycogen, and triglyceride stores. Chronic weight loss due to reduced muscle mass occurs as amino acids are diverted to form glucose and ketone bodies.

Lowered plasma volume produces dizziness and weakness due to postural hypotension when sitting or standing. Total body potassium loss and the general catabolism of muscle protein contribute to the weakness.

Paresthesias may be present at the time of diagnosis of type 1 diabetes, particularly when the onset is subacute. They reflect a temporary dysfunction of peripheral sensory nerves and usually clear as insulin replacement restores glycemic levels closer to normal; thus, their presence suggests neurotoxicity from sustained hyperglycemia.

When insulin deficiency is severe and of acute onset, the above symptoms progress in an accelerated manner. Ketoacidosis exacerbates the dehydration and hyperosmolality by producing anorexia, nausea, and vomiting, thus interfering with oral fluid replacement. As plasma osmolality exceeds 330 mosm/kg (normal, 285–295 mosm/kg), impaired consciousness ensues. With progression of acidosis to a pH of 7.1 or less, deep breathing with a rapid ventilatory rate (Kussmaul respiration) occurs as the body attempts to eliminate carbonic acid. With worsening acidosis (to pH 7.0 or less), the cardiovascular system may be unable to maintain compensatory vasoconstriction; severe circulatory collapse may result.

B. SIGNS

The patient's level of consciousness can vary depending on the degree of hyperosmolality. When insulin deficiency develops relatively slowly and sufficient water intake is maintained to permit renal excretion of glucose and appropriate dilution of extracellular sodium chloride concentration, patients remain relatively alert and physical findings may be minimal. When vomiting occurs in response to worsening ketoacidosis, dehydration progresses and compensatory mechanisms become inadequate to keep plasma osmolality below 330 mosm/kg. Under these circumstances, stupor or even coma may occur. Evidence of dehydration in a stuporous patient, with rapid deep breathing and the fruity breath odor of acetone, suggests the diagnosis of diabetic ketoacidosis.

Postural hypotension indicates a depleted plasma volume; hypotension in the recumbent position is a serious prognostic sign. Loss of subcutaneous fat and muscle wasting are features of more slowly developing insulin deficiency. In occasional patients with slow, insidious onset of insulin deficiency, subcutaneous fat may be considerably depleted. An enlarged liver, eruptive xanthomas on the flexor surface of the limbs and on the buttocks, and lipemia retinalis indicate that chronic insulin deficiency has resulted in chylomicronemia, with circulating triglycerides elevated usually to over 2000 mg/dL (Chapter 19).

TYPE 2 DIABETES

Patients with type 2 diabetes also present with characteristic signs and symptoms. The presence of obesity or a strongly positive family history of mild diabetes also suggests a high risk for the development of type 2 diabetes.

Clinical Features

A. SYMPTOMS

The classic symptoms of polyuria, thirst, recurrent blurred vision, paresthesias, and fatigue are manifestations of hyperglycemia and osmotic diuresis and are therefore common to both forms of diabetes. However, many patients with type 2 diabetes have an insidious onset of hyperglycemia and may be relatively asymptomatic initially. This is particularly true in obese patients, whose diabetes may be detected only after glycosuria or hyperglycemia is noted during routine laboratory studies. Chronic skin infections are common. Generalized pruritus and symptoms of vaginitis are frequently the initial complaints of women with type 2 diabetes. Diabetes should be suspected in women with chronic candidal vulvovaginitis as well as in those who have delivered large infants (> 9 lb, or 4.1 kg) or have had polyhydramnios, preeclampsia, or unexplained fetal losses. Occasionally, a man with previously undiagnosed diabetes may present with impotence.

B. SIGNS

Nonobese patients with this mild form of diabetes often have no characteristic physical findings at the time of diagnosis. Obese diabetics may have any variety of fat distribution; however, diabetes seems to be more often associated in both men and women with localization of fat deposits on the upper part of the body (particularly the abdomen, chest, neck, and face) and relatively less fat on the appendages, which may be quite muscular. This centripetal fat distribution has been termed "android" and is characterized by a high waist to hip ratio. It differs from the more centrifugal "gynecoid" form of obesity, in which fat is localized more in the hips and thighs and less in the upper parts of the trunk. Refined radiographic techniques of assessing abdominal fat distribution with CT scans has documented that a "visceral" obesity, due to accumulation of fat in the omental and mesenteric regions, correlates with insulin resistance, whereas fat predominantly in subcutaneous tissues of the abdomen has little, if any, association with insulin insensitivity. Mild hypertension may be present in obese diabetics, particularly when the "android" form of obesity is predominant. In women, candidal vaginitis with a reddened, inflamed vulvar area and a profuse whitish discharge may herald the presence of diabetes.

Laboratory Findings in Diabetes Mellitus

Tests of urine glucose and ketone bodies as well as whole blood or plasma glucose measured in samples obtained under basal conditions and after glucose administration are very important in evaluation of the diabetic patient. Tests for glycosylated hemoglobin have proved useful in both initial evaluation and in assessment of the effectiveness of therapeutic management. In certain circumstances, measurements of insulin or C peptide levels and levels of other hormones involved in carbohydrate homeostasis (eg, glucagon, GH) may be useful. In view of the increased risk of atherosclerosis in diabetics, determination of serum cholesterol (including its beneficial HDL fraction) and triglycerides may be helpful. From these three measurements, an estimate of LDL-cholesterol can be made. (See Chapter 19.)

URINALYSIS

Glycosuria

Several problems are associated with using urine glucose as an index of blood glucose, regardless of the method employed. First of all, the glucose concentration in bladder urine reflects the blood glucose at the time the urine was formed. Therefore, the first voided specimen in the morning contains glucose that was excreted throughout the night and does not reflect the morning blood glucose at all. Some improvement in the correlation of urine glucose to blood glucose can be obtained if the patient "double voids"—that is, empties the bladder completely, discards that sample, and then urinates again about one-half hour later, testing only the second specimen for glucose content. However, difficulty in completely emptying the bladder (large residual volumes), problems in understanding the instructions, and the inconvenience impair the usefulness of this test. Self-monitoring of blood glucose has replaced urine glucose testing in most patients with diabetes (particularly those receiving insulin therapy).

Several commercial products are available for determining the presence and amount of glucose in urine. The older and more cumbersome bedside assessment of glycosuria with Clinitest tablets has generally been replaced by the dipstick method, which is rapid, convenient, and glucose-specific. This method consists of paper strips (Clinistix, Tes-Tape) impregnated with enzymes (glucose oxidase and hydrogen peroxidase) and a chromogenic dye that is colorless in the reduced state. Enzymatic generation of hydrogen peroxide oxidizes the dye to produce colors whose intensity depends on the glucose concentration. These dipsticks are sensitive to as little as 0.1% glucose (100 mg/dL) but do not react with the smaller amounts of glucose normally present in nondiabetic urine. The strips are subject to deterioration if exposed to air, moisture, and extreme heat and must be kept in tightly closed containers except when in use. False-negative results may be obtained in the presence of alkaptonuria and when certain substances such as salicylic acid or ascorbic acid are ingested in excess. All of these false-negative results occur because of the interference of strong reducing agents with oxidation of the chromogen.

Differential Diagnosis of Glycosuria

Although glycosuria reflects hyperglycemia in over 90% of patients, two major classes of nondiabetic glycosuria must be considered:

A. NONDIABETIC GLYCOSURIA DUE TO GLUCOSE

This occurs when glucose appears in the urine despite a normal amount of glucose in the blood. Disorders associated with abnormalities in renal glucose handling include Fanconi's syndrome (an autosomal dominant genetic disorder), dysfunction of the proximal renal tubule, and a benign familial disorder of the renal tubule manifest only by a defect in renal glucose reabsorption (occurs predominantly in males).

In addition, glycosuria is relatively common in pregnancy as a consequence of the increased load of glucose presented to the tubules by the elevated glomerular filtration rate during pregnancy. As many as 50% of pregnant women normally have demonstrable sugar in the urine, especially after the first trimester. This sugar is almost always glucose except during the late weeks of pregnancy, when lactose may be present (see below).

B. NONDIABETIC GLYCOSURIA DUE TO SUGARS OTHER THAN GLUCOSE

Occasionally, a sugar other than glucose is excreted in the urine. Lactosuria during the late stages of pregnancy and the period of lactation is the most common example. Much rarer are other conditions in which inborn errors of metabolism allow fructose, galactose, or a pentose (1-xylose) to be excreted in the urine. Testing the urine with glucose-specific strips will help differentiate true glucosuria from other glycosurias.

Ketonuria

In the absence of adequate insulin, three major "ketone bodies" are formed and excreted into the urine: β-hydroxybutyric acid, acetoacetic acid, and acetone (see also Serum Ketone Determinations, below). Commercial products are available to test for the presence of ketones in the urine. Acetest tablets, Ketostix, and Keto-Diastix utilize a nitroprusside reaction that measures only acetone and acetoacetate. Although these tests do not detect β-hydroxybutyric acid, which lacks a ketone group, the semiquantitative estimation of the other ketone bodies is nonetheless usually adequate for clinical assessment of ketonuria. Ketostix and Keto-Diastix have short shelf-lives once the containers are opened and thus may give false-negative results.

Other conditions besides diabetic ketoacidosis may cause ketone bodies to appear in the urine; these include starvation, high-fat diets, alcoholic ketoacidosis, fever, and other conditions in which metabolic requirements are increased.

Proteinuria

Proteinuria as noted on a routine dipstick examination of the urine is often the first sign of renal complications of diabetes. If proteinuria is detected, a 24-hour urine collection should be analyzed to quantify the degree of proteinuria (normal individuals excrete < 30 mg of protein per day) and the rate of urinary creatinine excretion; at the same time, serum creatinine levels should be determined so that the creatinine clearance (an estimate of the glomerular filtration rate) can be calculated. In some cases, heavy proteinuria (3–5 g/d) develops later, along with other features of the nephrotic syndrome such as edema, hypoalbuminemia, and hypercholesterolemia.

Microalbuminuria

Urinary albumin can now be detected in microgram concentrations using a radioimmunoassay method that is more sensitive than the dipstick method, whose minimal detection limit is 0.3–0.5%. Conventional 24-hour urine collections, in addition to being inconvenient for patients, also show wide variability of albumin excretion, since several factors such as sustained upright posture, dietary protein, and exercise tend to increase albumin excretion rates. For these reasons, many clinics prefer to screen patients by measuring the albumin-creatinine ratio in an early morning spot urine collected upon awakening—prior to breakfast or exercise—and brought in by the patient for laboratory analysis. A ratio of albumin (μg/L) to creatinine (mg/L) of < 30 is normal, and a ratio of 30–300 indicates abnormal microalbuminuria. When this screening test is positive, a timed overnight urine collection is recommended. This begins at bedtime, when the urine is discarded and the time recorded. The collection is ended at the time the bladder is emptied the next morning, and this urine, as well as any other urine voided overnight, is assayed for albumin. Normal subjects excrete less than 15 μg/min during overnight urine collections; values between 20 and 200 μg/min or higher represent abnormal microalbuminuria, which may be an early predictor of the development of diabetic nephropathy.

BLOOD GLUCOSE TESTING

Normal Values

The range of normal fasting plasma or serum glucose is 70–110 mg/dL (3.9–6.1 mmol/L). Plasma or serum from venous blood samples has the advantage over whole blood of providing values for glucose that are independent of hematocrit and reflect levels in the interstitial spaces to which body tissues are exposed. For these reasons—and because plasma and serum lend themselves to automated analytic procedures—they are used in most laboratories. The glucose concentration is 10–15% higher in plasma or serum than in whole blood because structural components of blood cells are absent. Whole blood glucose determinations are seldom used in clinical laboratories but have been used by diabetic patients during self-monitoring of capillary blood glucose, a technique widely accepted in the management of diabetes mellitus (see below). Recently, however, many new reflectance meters have been modified to directly record serum glucose rather than to calculate whole blood glucose concentrations.

Venous Blood Samples

Samples should be collected in tubes containing sodium fluoride, which prevents glycolysis in the blood sample that would artifactually lower the measured glucose level. If such tubes are not available, samples must be centrifuged within 30 minutes of collection and the plasma or serum stored at 4 °C.

The laboratory methods regularly used for determining plasma glucose utilize enzymatic methods (such as glucose oxidase or hexokinase), colorimetric methods (such as o-toluidine), or automated methods. The automated methods utilize reduction of copper or iron compounds by reducing sugars in dialyzed serum. They are convenient but are not specific for glucose, since they react with other reducing substances (which are elevated in azotemia or with high ascorbic acid intake).

Capillary Blood Samples

There are several paper strip methods (glucose oxidase, glucose dehydrogenase or hexokinase) for measuring glucose on capillary blood samples. A reflectance photometer or an amperometric system is then used to measure the reaction that takes place on the reagent strip. The current blood glucose meters require very small volumes of blood (as little as 0.3 μL); automatically time the entire reaction (as short as 5 seconds); do not require wiping off the strip; and store previous values in an electronic memory for downloading onto a personal computer. Very high or very low hematocrit values can lead to inaccuracies in measurements. It is therefore important to refer to the manufacturer's information sheet regarding hematocrit ranges for particular meters. Some meters such as the FreeStyle (Therasense, Inc) have been approved for measuring glucose in blood samples obtained at alternative sites such as the forearm and thigh. There is, however, a 5- to 20-minute lag in the glucose response on the arm with respect to the glucose response on the finger. Forearm blood glucose measurements could therefore result in a delay in the detection of rapidly developing hypoglycemia. To monitor their own blood glucose levels, patients must prick their fingers with a lancet. Thirty-gauge lancets are now available that reduce discomfort while providing an adequate blood drop for measurement. Automatic spring-loaded devices such as the Autolet or SoftClix are useful in simplifying the finger-pricking technique and ensuring an adequate blood sample. Bedside glucose monitoring in a hospital setting requires rigorous quality control programs and certification of personnel to avoid errors. When properly done, these methods are also of great value to health care professionals in the bedside management of seriously ill hospitalized diabetic patients.

Interstitial Fluid Glucose Samples

Two continuous glucose monitoring systems are currently available for clinical use. The system manufactured by MiniMed Medtronic involves inserting a subcutaneous sensor (rather like an insulin pump cannula) that measures glucose concentrations in the interstitial fluid for 72 hours. The glucose values are not available for evaluation at time of measurement—the data are downloaded onto a computer in a physician's office after collection. The other system, Glucowatch, measures glucose in interstitial fluid extracted through intact skin by applying a low electric current (reverse iontophoresis). This process can cause local skin irritation, and sweating invalidates the glucose measurement. Both systems require calibration with finger blood glucose measurements. Their main value appears to be in identifying episodes of asymptomatic hypoglycemia, especially at night.

SERUM KETONE DETERMINATIONS

As noted above in the section on ketonuria, there are three major ketone bodies: β-hydroxybutyrate (often the most prevalent in diabetic ketoacidosis), acetoacetate, and acetone. The same testing materials used for determining urine ketones may be used to measure serum (or plasma) ketones. However, whereas urine readily penetrates "intact" Acetest tablets, more viscous fluids such as serum or plasma do not have access to the bulk of the tablet unless it is first crushed. When a few drops of serum are placed on a crushed Acetest tablet, the appearance of a purple color indicates the presence of ketones. A strongly positive reaction in undiluted serum correlates with a serum ketone concentration of at least 4 mmol/L. It must be kept in mind that Acetest tablets (as well as Ketostix and Keto-Diastix) utilize the nitroprusside reaction, which measures only acetoacetate and acetone. Specific enzymatic techniques are available to quantitate each of the ketone acids, but these techniques are cumbersome and not necessary in most clinical situations.

GLYCATED HEMOGLOBIN ASSAYS

Glycohemoglobin (GHb) is produced by a ketoamine reaction between glucose and the amino terminal amino acid of both beta chains of the hemoglobin molecule. The major form of glycohemoglobin is hemoglobin A_{1c}, which normally comprises only 4–6% of total hemoglobin. The remaining glycohemoglobins (2–4% of total hemoglobin) contain phosphorylated glucose or fructose and are termed hemoglobin A_{1a} and A_{1b}, respectively. The hemoglobin A_{1c} fraction is abnormally elevated in diabetics with chronic hyperglycemia. Specific assays for hemoglobin A_{1c} are technically less convenient than assays for total glycohemoglobin and offer little advantage for clinical purposes. Therefore, many laboratories measure the sum of these three glycohemo-

globins and report it simply as hemoglobin A_1 or "glycohemoglobin."

The glycation of hemoglobin is dependent on the concentration of blood glucose. The reaction is not reversible, so that the half-life of glycated hemoglobin relates to the life span of red cells (which normally circulate for up to 120 days). Thus, glycohemoglobin generally reflects the state of glycemia over the preceding 8–12 weeks, thus providing a method of assessing chronic diabetic control. A hemoglobin A_1 close to the normal range (4.5–6%) or a glycated hemoglobin of 5–7% would reflect good control during the preceding 2–3 months, whereas a hemoglobin A_{1c} > 8% or glycated hemoglobin greater than 8% would reflect poor control during the same period.

Conditions Interfering with Glycohemoglobin Measurements (Table 17–9)

The most common laboratory error in measuring glycohemoglobins occurs when chromatographic methods measure an acutely generated intermediary aldimine in blood (prehemoglobin A_{1c}), which fluctuates directly with the prevailing blood glucose level. This artifact can falsely elevate glycohemoglobin by as much as 1–2% during an episode of acute hyperglycemia. It can be eliminated either by washing the red blood cells with saline prior to assay or by dialyzing the hemolysate prior to chromatography. Other substances that falsely elevate "glycohemoglobin" are carbamoylated hemoglobin and hemoglobin F; the former is seen in association with uremia, and the latter circulates in some adults with genetic or hematologic disorders. In these cases, more intricate methodology such as thiobarbituric acid colorimetry or isoelectric focusing is required to distinguish hemoglobin A_{1c} from the interfering substance.

Table 17–9. Factors interfering with chromatographic measurement of glycohemoglobins.

Substances causing falsely high values:
Prehemoglobin A_{1c} (reversible aldimine intermediate)
Carbamoylated hemoglobin (uremia)
Hemoglobin F
Conditions causing falsely low values:
Hemoglobinopathies (hemoglobins C, D, and S)
Reduced life span of erythrocytes:[1]
Hemorrhage of therapeutic phlebotomies
Hemolytic disorders

[1]This causes falsely low values of *all* methods used to measure HbA_{1c}.

Hemoglobinopathies such as those associated with hemoglobin C, D, and S will cause falsely low values, since their glycosylated products elute only partially from chromatographic columns. In addition, these hemoglobinopathies are often associated with hemolytic anemias that shorten the life span of red blood cells, thereby further lowering glycohemoglobin measurements. Falsely low values are also seen in patients with chronic or acute blood loss from hemorrhage or from phlebotomies in diabetic patients with hemochromatosis; under these conditions, measurements of glycohemoglobin are not valid for assessment of diabetic therapy.

Glycohemoglobin assays suffer from the lack of universally available reference standards. The National Glycohemoglobin Standardization Program, sponsored in part by the American Diabetes Association to standardize GHb determinations, began in mid 1996 and is currently in progress to certify the manufacturers of GHb assays. Clinical laboratories are urged to use only "certified" assays and to participate also in a proficiency testing survey by the College of American Pathologists. However, in a reliable laboratory where reversible aldimines (prehemoglobin A_{1c}) are routinely removed prior to chromatography, they are useful in assessing the effectiveness of diabetic therapy and particularly helpful in evaluating the reliability of a patient's self-monitoring records of urine or blood glucose values. A glycated hemoglobin test is currently not recommended for diagnostic screening purposes since the test is generally too insensitive to rule out impaired glucose tolerance. However, a value above the normal range in a certified laboratory is generally a specific indicator of diabetes mellitus.

When abnormal hemoglobins or hemolytic states affect the interpretation of glycohemoglobin results or when a narrower time frame is required, eg, when ascertaining glycemic control at the time of conception in a diabetic woman who has recently become pregnant, serum fructosamine assays offer some advantage. Serum fructosamine is formed by nonenzymatic glycosylation of serum proteins (predominantly albumin). Since serum albumin has a much shorter half-life (14–21 days) than hemoglobin, serum fructosamine generally reflects the state of glycemic control for only the preceding 2 weeks. In most circumstances, however, glycohemoglobin assays remain the preferred method for assessing long-term glycemic control in diabetic patients.

LIPOPROTEINS IN DIABETES

Levels of circulating lipoprotein are dependent on normal levels and action of insulin, just as is the plasma glucose. In type 1 diabetes, moderately deficient control of hyperglycemia is associated with only a slight elevation of LDL cholesterol and serum triglycerides and little if any changes in HDL cholesterol. Once the hyperglycemia is corrected, lipoprotein levels are generally normal. However, in obese patients with type 2 diabetes, a distinct "diabetic dyslipidemia" is characteristic of the insulin resistance syndrome. Its features are a high serum triglyceride level (300–400 mg/dL), a low HDL cholesterol (less than 30 mg/dL), and a qualitative change in LDL particles producing a smaller dense LDL whose membrane carries supranormal amounts of free cholesterol. Since a *low* HDL cholesterol is a major feature predisposing to macrovascular disease, the term "dyslipidemia" has preempted the previous label of "hyperlipidemia," which mainly described the elevated triglycerides. Measures designed to correct this obesity and hyperglycemia, such as exercise, diet, and hypoglycemic therapy, are the treatment of choice for diabetic dyslipidemia, and in occasional patients in which normal weight was achieved all features of the lipoprotein abnormalities cleared. Since primary disorders of lipid metabolism may coexist with diabetes, persistence of lipid abnormalities after restoration of normal weight and blood glucose should prompt a diagnostic workup and possible pharmacotherapy of the lipid disorder. Chapter 19 discusses these matters in detail.

■ DIAGNOSIS OF DIABETES MELLITUS

Diagnostic Criteria

(1) Symptoms of diabetes (thirst, increased urination, unexplained weight loss) plus a random plasma glucose concentration > 200 mg/dL (11.1 mmol/L).
(2) Fasting plasma glucose > 126 mg/dL (7.0 mmol/L) after an overnight (at least 8-hour) fast.
(3) Two-hour plasma glucose > 200 mg/dL (11.1 mmol/L) during a standard 75 g oral glucose tolerance test (see below).

These three criteria are the most recent recommendations of an international committee of diabetes experts who have revised previous diagnostic criteria. The diagnosis of diabetes can be based on any one of the above criteria but should be confirmed on a later day with one of the three methods listed above.

A major change from previous criteria is the lowering of the cut-off level of fasting plasma glucose from > 140 mg/dL (7.8 mmol/L) to > 126 mg/dL (7.0 mmol/L). A new diagnostic category, impaired fasting glucose (IFG), has been added to impaired glucose tolerance (IGT). Both terms refer to a stage intermediate between normal glucose homeostasis and diabetes. IFG refers to a level of plasma glucose after an overnight fast that is > 110 mg/dL (above the normal upper limit of 110 mg/dL [6.1 mmol/L]) but less than the level of 126 mg/dL (7.0 mmol /L), which indicates diabetes.

The corresponding category for the IGT when the oral glucose tolerance test is used is as follows:

Two-hour plasma glucose > 140 mg/dL (7.8 mmol/L) but less than 200 mg/dL (11.1 mmol/L).

Many individuals with IGT are euglycemic in their daily lives and may have normal or near-normal glycosylated hemoglobin levels. These subjects may also have fasting plasma glucose levels in the normal range (< 110 mg/dL [6.1 mmol/L]) and often manifest their impaired glucose metabolism only when challenged with a standardized oral glucose tolerance test.

ORAL GLUCOSE TOLERANCE TEST

An oral glucose tolerance test is only rarely indicated, as there is a preference in clinical situations to use fasting plasma glucose levels for diagnosis because they are easier and faster to perform, more convenient and acceptable to patients, more reproducible, and less expensive. Recently, an international committee of diabetologists has recommended simplifying the glucose tolerance test to require only an overnight fasting measurement and one 2 hours after a standard 75 g oral glucose load. Samples at 30, 60, and 90 minutes are no longer required.

If the fasting plasma glucose is between 110 and 126 mg/dL ("impaired fasting glucose"), an oral glucose tolerance test may be considered, especially in men with erectile dysfunction or women who have delivered infants above 9 lb (4.1 kg) birth weight or have had recurrent vaginal yeast infections.

Preparation for Test

In order to optimize insulin secretion and effectiveness, especially when patients have been on a low-carbohydrate diet, a minimum of 150–200 g of carbohydrate per day should be included in the diet for 3 days preceding the test. The patient should eat nothing after midnight prior to the test day.

Testing Procedure

Adults are given 75 g of glucose in 300 mL of water; children are given 1.75 g of glucose per kilogram of ideal body weight. The glucose load is consumed within 5 minutes. Blood samples for plasma glucose are obtained at 0 and 120 minutes after ingestion of glucose.

Interpretation (Table 17–10)

An oral glucose tolerance test is normal if the fasting venous plasma glucose value is less than 110 mg/dL (6.1 mmol/L) and the 2-hour value falls below 140 mg/dL (7.8 mmol/L). A fasting value of 126 mg/dL (7 mmol/L) or higher or a 2-hour value of greater than 200 mg/dL (11.1 mmol/L) is diagnostic of diabetes mellitus. The diagnosis of "impaired glucose tolerance" is reserved for values between the upper limits of normal and those values diagnostic of diabetes. False-positive results may occur in patients who are malnourished at test time, bedridden, or afflicted with an infection or severe emotional stress. Diuretics, oral contraceptives, glucocorticoids, excess thyroxine, phenytoin, nicotinic acid and some of the psychotropic drugs may also cause false-positive results.

INSULIN LEVELS

To measure insulin levels during the glucose tolerance test, serum or plasma must be separated within 30 minutes after collection of the specimen and frozen prior to assay. Normal immunoreactive insulin levels range from 5–20 μU/mL in the fasting state, reach 50–130 μU/mL at 1 hour, and usually return to levels below 30 μU/mL by 2 hours. Insulin levels are rarely of clinical

Table 17–10. The Diabetes Expert Committee criteria for evaluating the standard oral glucose tolerance test.[1]

	Normal Glucose Tolerance	Impaired Glucose Tolerance	Diabetes Mellitus[2]
Fasting plasma glucose (mg/dL)	< 110	110–125	≥ 126
Two hours after glucose load (mg/dL)	< 140	≥ 140 but < 200	≥ 200

[1]Give 75 g of glucose dissolved in 300 mL of water after an overnight fast in subjects who have been receiving at least 150–200 g of carbohydrate daily for 3 days before the test.
[2]A fasting plasma glucose > 126 mg/dL is diagnostic of diabetes if confirmed on a subsequent day to be in the diabetic range after either an overnight fast or 2 hours after a standard glucose load.

usefulness during glucose tolerance testing for the following reasons: When fasting glucose levels exceed 120 mg/dL (6.7 mmol/L), B cells generally have reduced responsiveness to further degrees of hyperglycemia regardless of the type of diabetes. When fasting glucose levels are below 120 mg/dL (6.7 mmol/L), late hyperinsulinism may occur as a result of insulin resistance in type 2 diabetes; however, it also may occur even in mild forms or in the early phases of type 1 diabetes when sluggish early insulin release results in late hyperglycemia that may stimulate excessive insulin secretion at 2 hours.

INTRAVENOUS GLUCOSE TOLERANCE TEST

The intravenous glucose tolerance test is performed by giving a rapid infusion of glucose followed by serial plasma glucose measurements to determine the disappearance rate of glucose per minute. The disappearance rate reflects the patient's ability to dispose of a glucose load. Perhaps its most widespread present use is to screen siblings at risk for type 1 diabetes to determine if autoimmune destruction of B cells has reduced peak early insulin responses (at 1–5 minutes after the glucose bolus) to levels below the normal lower limit of 40 μU/mL. It has also been used to evaluate glucose tolerance in patients with gastrointestinal abnormalities (such as malabsorption). Caution should be used in clinical interpretation of the results, because the test bypasses normal glucose absorption and associated changes in gastrointestinal hormones that are important in carbohydrate metabolism. Furthermore, the test is relatively insensitive, and adequate criteria for diagnosis of diabetes have not been established for the various age groups.

Preparation for Test

Preparation is the same as for the oral glucose tolerance test (see above).

Testing Procedure

Intravenous access is established and the patient is given a bolus of 50 g of glucose per 1.7 m^2 body surface area (or 0.5 g/kg of ideal body weight) as a 25% or 50% solution over 2–3 minutes. Timing begins with injection. Samples for plasma glucose determination are obtained from an indwelling needle in the opposite arm at 0, 10, 15, 20, and 30 minutes. The plasma glucose values are plotted on semilogarithmic paper against time. K, a rate constant that reflects the rate of fall of blood glucose in percent per minute, is calculated by determining the time necessary for the glucose concentration to fall by one-half ($t_{1/2}$) and using the following equation:

$$K\ (glucose) = \frac{0.693}{t_{1/2}} \times 100$$

The average K value for a nondiabetic patient is approximately 1.72% per minute; this value declines with age but remains above 1.3% per minute. Diabetic patients almost always have a K value of less than 1% per minute.

Careful attention to venous access is essential, since leakage or infiltration of this hypertonic solution into subcutaneous tissues can cause considerable discomfort which can last for several days.

Clinical Trials in Diabetes

A fundamental controversy regarding whether microangiopathy is related exclusively to the existence and duration of hyperglycemia or whether it reflects a separate genetic disorder has recently been resolved by the findings of the Diabetes Control and Complications Trial (DCCT) and of the United Kingdom Prospective Diabetes Study (UKPDS), which confirmed the beneficial effects of intensive therapy to achieve improved glycemic control in both type 1 and type 2 diabetes, respectively (see below).

With increased understanding of the pathophysiology of both type 1 and type 2 diabetes, large prospective studies have been initiated in attempts to prevent onset of these disorders. Investigators with the Diabetes Prevention Trial 1 (DPT-1) and the Diabetes Prevention Program (DPP) have recently reported their findings (see below).

Clinical Trials in Type 1 Diabetes

A. THE DIABETES CONTROL AND COMPLICATIONS TRIAL (DCCT)

In September 1993, a long-term randomized prospective study involving 1441 type 1 diabetic patients in 29 medical centers reported that "near" normalization of blood glucose resulted in a delay in the onset and a major slowing of the progression of established microvascular and neuropathic complications of diabetes during an up to 10-year follow-up period.

The patients were divided into two study groups with equal numbers of subjects. Approximately half of the total group had no detectable diabetic complications (prevention trial), whereas mild background retinopathy was present in the other half (intervention trial). Some patients in the latter group had slightly elevated microalbuminuria and mild neuropathy, but no one with serious diabetic complications was enrolled in the trial. Multiple insulin injections (66%) or insulin pumps (34%) were used in the intensively treated group, and those subjects were trained to modify their therapy in response to frequent glucose monitoring. The conventionally treated group used no more than two insulin injections, and clinical well-being was the goal with no attempt to modify management based on glycated hemoglobin or glucose results. Patients were between the ages of 13 and 19 years, with an average age of 27 years, and half of the subjects were women.

In the intensively treated subjects, a mean glycated hemoglobin of 7.2% (normal, > 6%) and a mean blood glucose of 155 mg/dL were achieved, whereas in the conventionally treated group glycated hemoglobin averaged 8.9%, with an average blood glucose of 225 mg/dL. Over the study period, which averaged 7 years, there was an approximately 60% reduction in risk of diabetic retinopathy, nephropathy, and neuropathy in the intensively treated group.

Intensively treated patients had a threefold greater risk of serious hypoglycemia as well as a greater tendency toward weight gain. However, there were no deaths from hypoglycemia in any subjects in the DCCT study, and no evidence of posthypoglycemic neurologic damage was detected.

The general consensus of the American Diabetes Association is that intensive insulin therapy associated with comprehensive self-management training should become standard therapy in most type 1 patients after the age of puberty. Exceptions include those with advanced renal disease and the elderly, since in these groups the detrimental risks of hypoglycemia outweigh the benefit of tight glycemic control. In children under age 7 years, the extreme susceptibility of the developing brain to damage from hypoglycemia contraindicates attempts at tight glycemic control, particularly since diabetic complications do not seem to occur until some years after the onset of puberty.

B. THE DIABETES PREVENTION TRIAL-1

This NIH-sponsored multicenter study was designed to determine whether the development of type 1 diabetes could be prevented or delayed by immune intervention therapy. The study recruited 339 first-degree or second-degree relatives of patients with type 1 diabetes who—by genetic, immunologic, and metabolic testing—were deemed to be at high risk of developing diabetes. These subjects lacked a protective HLA haplotype; were islet cell antibody-positive; had impaired first-phase insulin response in an intravenous glucose tolerance test; and had normal or impaired oral glucose tolerance tests.

One hundred and sixty-nine test subjects were assigned to the intervention group and received daily low-dose subcutaneous ultralente insulin plus annual 4-day continuous intravenous infusions of insulin. One hundred and seventy subjects were assigned to an observation group. The primary end point was development of diabetes, and the median follow-up was 3.7 years. Unfortunately, the intervention failed to delay or prevent onset of type 1 diabetes—69 subjects in the intervention group and 70 subjects in the observation group developed diabetes.

Although this trial has been discontinued, a related study is still in progress using oral insulin in lower-risk first-degree relatives who have islet cell antibodies but whose early insulin release remains intact.

C. IMMUNE INTERVENTION TRIALS IN NEW-ONSET TYPE 1 DIABETES

At time of diagnosis of type 1 diabetes, patients still have significant B cell function. This explains why soon after diagnosis patients go into a partial clinical remission ("honeymoon") requiring little or no insulin. This clinical remission is short-lived, however, and eventually patients lose all B cell function and have more labile glucose control. Attempts have been made to prolong this partial clinical remission using drugs such as cyclosporine, azathioprine, prednisone, and antithymocyte globulin. These agents, however, had limited efficacy, and there were concerns about their toxicity and the need for continuous treatment.

Recently, newer agents that may induce immune tolerance and appear to have few side effects have been used in new-onset type 1 patients. Two small studies, one with a heat shock protein peptide (DiaPep277) and another with an anti-CD3 antibody, have demonstrated that these agents can preserve endogenous insulin production. Larger phase 2 clinical trials are currently in progress.

Clinical Trials in Type 2 Diabetes

A. KUMAMOTO STUDY

The Kumamoto study involved a relatively small number of type 2 patients (n = 110) who were nonobese and only slightly insulin-resistant, requiring less than 30 units of insulin per day for intensive therapy. Over a 6-year period it was shown that intensive insulin therapy, achieving a mean HbA_{1c} of 7.1%, significantly reduced microvascular end points compared with conventional insulin therapy, achieving a mean HbA_{1c} of 9.4%. Cardiovascular events were neither worsened nor improved by intensive therapy, and weight changes were likewise not influenced by either form of treatment.

B. Veterans Affairs Cooperative Study

This study involved 153 obese men who were moderately insulin-resistant and were followed for only 27 months. Intensive insulin treatment resulted in mean HbA_{1c} differences from conventional insulin treatment (7.2% versus 9.5%) that were comparable to those reported in the Kumamoto study. However, a difference in cardiovascular outcome in this study has prompted some concern. While conventional insulin therapy resulted in 26 total cardiovascular events, there were 35 total cardiovascular events in the intensively treated group. This difference in this relatively small population was not statistically significant, but when the total events were broken down to major events (myocardial infarction, stroke, cardiovascular death, congestive heart failure, amputation), the 18 major events in the group treated intensively with insulin were reported to be statistically greater ($P = .04$) than the ten major events occurring with conventional treatment. While this difference may be a chance consequence of studying too few patients for too short a time, it raises the possibility that insulin-resistant patients with visceral obesity and long-standing type 2 diabetes may develop a greater risk of a serious cardiovascular event when intensively treated with high doses of insulin. At the end of the study, 64% of the intensively treated group were receiving either (1) an average of 113 units of insulin per day when only two injections per day were used or (2) an average of 133 units per day when multiple injections were given. Unfortunately, the UKPDS (see below), which did not find any effect of intensive therapy on cardiovascular outcomes, does not resolve the concern generated by the Veterans Affairs study, since their patient population consisted of newly diagnosed diabetic patients in whom the obese subgroup seemed to be less insulin-resistant, requiring a median insulin dose for intensive therapy of only 60 units per day by the 12th year of the study.

C. The United Kingdom Prospective Diabetes Study (UKPDS)

This study began in 1977 as a multicenter clinical trial designed to determine in type 2 diabetic patients whether the risk of macrovascular or microvascular complications could be reduced by intensive blood glucose control with oral hypoglycemic agents or insulin and whether any particular therapy was better than the others. Newly diagnosed type 2 diabetic patients aged 25–65 years were recruited between 1977 and 1991, and a total of 3867 were studied over 10 years. Their median age at baseline was 54 years; 44% were overweight (> 20% over ideal weight), and baseline HbA_{1c} was 9.1%. Therapies were randomized to include a control group on diet alone and separate groups intensively treated with either

insulin, chlorpropamide, glyburide, or glipizide. Metformin was included as a randomization option in a subgroup of 342 overweight patients, and—much later in the study—an additional subgroup of both normal-weight and overweight patients who were responding unsatisfactorily to sulfonylurea therapy were randomized to either continue on their sulfonylurea therapy alone or to have metformin combined with it.

In 1987, a further modification was made to evaluate whether tight control of blood pressure with stepwise antihypertensive therapy would prevent macrovascular and microvascular complications in 758 hypertensive patients among this UKPDS population—compared with 390 patients whose blood pressure was treated less intensively. The tight control group were randomly assigned to treatment with either an angiotensin-converting enzyme (ACE) inhibitor (captopril) or a beta-blocker (atenolol). Both drugs were stepped up to maximum doses of 100 mg/d, and then, if blood pressure remained higher than the target level of < 150/85 mm Hg, more drugs were added in the following stepwise sequence—a diuretic, slow-release nifedipine, methyldopa, and prazosin—until the target level of tight control was achieved. In the control group, hypertension was conventionally treated to achieve target levels < 180/105 mm Hg, but these patients were not given either ACE inhibitors or beta-blockers.

1. Results of the UKPDS—Intensive glycemic therapy in the entire group of 3897 newly diagnosed type 2 diabetic patients followed over 10 years showed the following: Intensive treatment with either sulfonylureas, metformin, combinations of these, or insulin achieved mean HbA_{1c} levels of 7.0%. This level of glycemic control decreased the risk of microvascular complications in comparison with conventional therapy (mostly diet alone), which achieved mean levels of HbA_{1c} of 7.9%. Weight gain occurred in intensively treated patients except when metformin was used as monotherapy. No cardiovascular benefits nor adverse cardiovascular outcomes were noted regardless of the therapeutic agent. Hypoglycemic reactions occurred in the intensive treatment groups, but only one death from hypoglycemia was documented out of 27,000 patient-years of intensive therapy.

When therapeutic subgroups were analyzed, some unexpected and paradoxical results were noted. Among the obese patients, intensive treatment with insulin or sulfonylureas did not reduce microvascular complications compared with diet therapy alone. This was in contrast to the significant benefit of intensive therapy with these drugs in the total group. Furthermore, intensive therapy with metformin was more beneficial in obese persons than diet alone with regard to reducing myocardial infarctions, strokes, and diabetes-related deaths, but there was no significant reduction of diabetic microvascular complications with metformin as compared with the diet group. Moreover, in the subgroup of obese and nonobese patients in whom metformin was added to sulfonylurea failures, rather than showing a benefit, there was a 96% increase in diabetes-related deaths compared with the matched cohort of patients with unsatisfactory glycemic control on sulfonylureas who remained on sulfonylurea therapy. Chlorpropamide also came out poorly on subgroup analysis in that those receiving it as intensive therapy did less well as regards progression to retinopathy than those conventionally treated with diet.

Intensive antihypertensive therapy to a mean of 144/82 mm Hg had beneficial effects on microvascular disease as well as on all diabetes-related end points, including virtually all cardiovascular outcomes, in comparison with looser control at a mean of 154/87 mm Hg. In fact, the advantage of reducing hypertension by this amount was substantially more impressive than the benefit which accrued by improving the degree of glycemic control from a mean HbA_{1c} of 7.9% to 7.0%. More than half of the patients needed two or more drugs for adequate therapy of their hypertension, and there was no demonstrable advantage of ACE inhibitor therapy over beta-blockers as regards diabetes end points. Use of a calcium channel blocker added to both treatment groups appeared to be safe over the long term in this diabetic population despite some controversy in the literature about its safety in diabetics.

2. Implications of the UKPDS—It appears that glycemic control to levels of HbA_{1c} to 7.0% shows benefit in reducing total diabetes end points, including a 25% reduction in microvascular disease, as compared with HbA_{1c} levels of 7.9%. This reassures those who have questioned whether the value of intensive therapy, so convincingly shown by the DCCT in type 1 diabetes, can safely be extrapolated to older patients with type 2 diabetes. It also refutes the presence of a "threshold" of glycemic control, since in this group there was a benefit from this modest reduction of HbA_{1c} below 7.9%, whereas in the DCCT a threshold was suggested in that further benefit was less apparent at HbA_{1c} levels below 8%.

Because of the complexity of the overall design in which many of the original therapy groups received additional medications to achieve glycemic goals but remained assigned to their original treatment group, statistical analysis may have been compromised. For instance, in the diet group which was used as a control for all the drug treatment groups, only 58% of their total "patient-years" were actually drug-free, while the remainder consisted of nonintensive therapy with various hypoglycemic drug regimens to avoid unacceptable hyperglycemia. This probably explains in part why the mean HbA_{1c} for this group was only 7.9% on "diet alone" therapy for over 10 years. In view of these crossovers within treatment groups, caution is suggested regarding several subgroup analyses that are controversial. These include the inference that metformin was superior to insulin or sulfonylureas in reducing diabetes-related end points in obese patients compared with diet therapy, even though all three treatment groups achieved the same degree of glycemic control. Conversely, the finding of excess mortality in the subgroup of patients receiving combination therapy with metformin and sulfonylureas need not necessarily preclude this combination in patients doing unsatisfactorily on sulfonylureas alone, though it certainly indicates a need for clarification of this important question.

Probably the most striking and clearest implication of the UKPDS is the remarkable benefit to the hypertensive type 2 diabetic patient of intensive control of blood pressure. Of interest was the observation that there was no demonstrable advantage of ACE-inhibitor therapy on outcome despite a number of short-term reports in smaller populations implying that these drugs have special efficacy in reducing glomerular pressure beyond their general antihypertensive effects. Moreover, slow-release nifedipine showed no evidence of cardiac toxicity in this study despite some previous reports claiming that calcium channel blockers may be hazardous in patients with diabetes. Finally, the greater benefit in diabetes end points from antihypertensive than from antihyperglycemic treatments may be that the difference between the mean blood pressures achieved (144/82 versus 154/87) is therapeutically more influential than the slight difference in HbA_{1c} (7.0% versus 7.9%). Greater hyperglycemia in the control group most likely would have rectified this discrepancy in outcomes. At present, the ADA recommends vigorous treatment of both hyperglycemia and hypertension when they occur, with an expectation that reductions in microvascular and cardiovascular outcomes will be additive.

D. THE DIABETES PREVENTION PROGRAM (DPP)

This was a randomized clinical trial in 3234 overweight men and women, aged 25–85 years, who showed impaired glucose tolerance. Results from this study indicated that intervention with a low-fat diet and 150 minutes of moderate exercise (equivalent to a brisk walk) per week reduces the risk of progression to type 2 diabetes by 58% as compared with a matched control group. Another arm of this trial demonstrated that use of 850 mg of metformin twice daily reduced the risk of developing type 2 diabetes by 31% but was relatively ineffective in those who were either less obese or in the older age group.

■ TREATMENT OF DIABETES MELLITUS

DIET

A proper diet remains a fundamental element of therapy in all patients with diabetes. However, in over half of cases, diabetics fail to follow their diet. The reasons include unnecessary complexity of dietary instructions and poor understanding of the goals of dietary control by the patient and physician.

ADA Recommendations

The American Diabetes Association releases an annual position statement on medical nutrition therapy that replaces the calculated ADA diet formula of the past with suggestions for an individually tailored dietary prescription based on metabolic, nutritional, and lifestyle requirements. They contend that the concept of one diet for "diabetes" and prescription for an "ADA diet" no longer can apply to both major types of diabetes. In their medical nutrition therapy recommendations for persons with type 2 diabetes, the 55–60% carbohydrate content of previous "ADA" diets has been reduced considerably because of the tendency of high carbohydrate intake to cause hyperglycemia, hypertriglyceridemia, and a lowered HDL cholesterol. In obese type 2 patients, glucose and lipid goals join weight loss as the focus for therapy. These patients are advised to limit their carbohydrate intake by substituting noncholesterologenic monounsaturated oils such as olive oil, rapeseed (canola) oil or the oils in nuts and avocados. This maneuver is also indicated in type 1 patients on intensive insulin regimens in whom near-normoglycemic control is less achievable on diets higher in carbohydrate content. In these patients, the ratio of carbohydrate to fat will vary among individuals in relation to their glycemic responses, insulin regimens, and exercise patterns.

The current recommendations for both types of diabetes continue to limit cholesterol to 300 mg daily and advise a daily protein intake of 10–20% total calories. They suggest that saturated fat be no higher than 8–9% of total calories with a similar proportion of polyunsaturated fat and that the remainder of the caloric needs be made up of an individualized ratio of monounsaturated fat and of carbohydrate containing 20–35 g dietary fiber. Previous recommendations of polyunsaturated fat supplements as part of a prudent diabetic diet have been revised because of their potential hazards. Polyunsaturated fatty acids appear to promote oxidation of LDL and lower HDL cholesterol, both of which may contribute to atherogenesis; furthermore, in large quantities during supplementation, they may promote carcinogenesis. Poultry, veal, and fish continue to be recommended as a substitute for red meats for keeping saturated fat content low. Stearic acid is the least cholesterologenic saturated fatty acid, since it is rapidly converted to oleic acid—in contrast to palmitic acid (found in animal fat as well as coconut oil), which is a major substrate for cholesterol formation. In contrast to previous recommendations, the present ADA position statement adduces no evidence that reducing protein intake below 10% of total caloric intake (about 0.8 g/kg/d) is of any benefit in patients with nephropathy with renal impairment, and in fact the investigators feel it may be detrimental.

Exchange lists for meal planning can be obtained from the American Diabetes Association (1660 Duke Street, Alexandria, VA 22314) and its affiliate associations or from the American Dietetic Association (430 North Michigan Avenue, Chicago, IL 60611). Their Internet address is http://www.eatright.org.

Special Considerations in Dietary Control

A. DIETARY FIBER

Plant components such as cellulose, gum, and pectin are indigestible by humans and are termed dietary "fiber." **Insoluble fibers** such as cellulose or hemicellulose, as found in bran, tend to increase intestinal transit time and may have beneficial effects on colonic function. In contrast, **soluble fibers** such as gums and pectins, as found in beans, oatmeal, or apple skin, tend to decrease gastric and intestinal transit so that glucose absorption is slower and hyperglycemia is diminished. Although the ADA diet does not require insoluble fiber supplements such as added bran, it recommends foods such as oatmeal, cereals, and beans with relatively high soluble fiber content as stable components of the diet in diabetics. High soluble fiber content in the diet may also have a favorable effect on blood cholesterol levels.

B. GLYCEMIC INDEX

Quantitation of the relative glycemic contribution of different carbohydrate foods has formed the basis of a "glycemic index" (GI), in which the area of blood glucose (plotted on a graph) generated over a 3-hour period following ingestion of a test food containing 50 g of carbohydrate is compared with the area plotted after giving a similar quantity of reference food such as glucose or white bread:

$$\frac{\text{Blood glucose area of test food}}{\text{Blood glucose area of reference food}} \times 100$$

White bread is preferred to glucose as a reference standard because it is more palatable and has less tendency to slow gastric emptying by high tonicity, as happens when glucose solution is used.

Differences in GI were noted in normal subjects and diabetics when various foods were compared. In comparison to white bread, which was assigned an index of 100, the mean GI for other foods was as follows: baked potato, 135; table sugar (sucrose), 86; spaghetti, 66; kidney beans, 54; ice cream, 52; and lentils, 43. Some investigators have questioned whether the GI for a food ingested alone is meaningful, since the GI may become altered considerably by the presence of fats and protein when the food is consumed in a mixed meal.

Further studies of the reproducibility of the GI in the same person and the relation of a particular food's GI to its insulinotropic action on pancreatic B cells are needed before the utility of the GI in prescribing diabetic diets can be appropriately assessed. At present, however, it appears that small amounts of sucrose—particularly when taken with high-fiber substances such as cereals or whole-grain breads—may have no greater glycemic effects than comparable portions of starch from potatoes, rice, or bread.

C. SWEETENERS

The nonnutritive sweetener **saccharin** is widely used as a sugar substitute (Sweet 'N Low) and continues to be available in certain foods and beverages despite warnings by the FDA about its potential long-term bladder carcinogenicity. The latest position statement of the ADA concludes that all nonnutritive sweeteners which have been approved by the FDA are safe for consumption by all people with diabetes.

Aspartame (NutraSweet) may prove to be the safest sweetener for use in diabetics; it consists of two major amino acids, aspartic acid and phenylalanine, which combine to produce a nutritive sweetener 180 times as sweet as sucrose. A major limitation is its heat lability, which precludes its use in baking or cooking. Sucralose (Splenda) and acesulfame potassium (Sunett, Sweet One, DiabetiSweet) are two other nonnutritive sweeteners approved by the FDA as safe for general use. They are both highly stable and, in contrast to aspartame, can be used in cooking and baking.

Other sweeteners such as sorbitol and fructose have recently gained popularity. Except for acute diarrhea induced by ingestion of large amounts of sorbitol-containing foods, their relative risk has yet to be established. **Fructose** represents a "natural" sugar substance that is a highly effective sweetener which induces only slight increases in plasma glucose levels and does not require insulin for its utilization. However, because of potential adverse effects of large amounts of fructose (up to 20% of total calories) on raising serum cholesterol and LDL cholesterol, the ADA feels it may have no overall advantage as a sweetening agent in the diabetic diet. This does not preclude, however, ingestion of fructose-containing fruits and vegetables or fructose-sweetened foods in moderation.

D. FISH OIL AND OTHER OILS

Omega-3 fatty acids in high doses have been shown to lower plasma triglycerides and VLDL cholesterol. They may also reduce platelet aggregation. In the Lyon Diet Heart Study in nondiabetics, a high intake of α-linolenic acid was beneficial in secondary prevention of coronary heart disease. This diet, which is rich in vegetables and fruits, also supplies a high intake of natural antioxidants. There is limited clinical information on the use of these oils in patients with diabetes.

ORAL AGENTS FOR THE TREATMENT OF HYPERGLYCEMIA

The drugs for treating type 2 diabetes fall into three categories: (1) Drugs that primarily stimulate insulin secretion. Sulfonylureas remain the most widely prescribed drugs for treating hyperglycemia. The meglitinide analog repaglinide and the D-phenylalanine derivative nateglinide also bind the sulfonylurea receptor and stimulate insulin secretion. (2) Drugs that alter insulin action. Metformin works primarily in the liver. The thiazolidinediones appear to have their main effect on skeletal muscle and adipose tissue. (3) Drugs that principally affect absorption of glucose. The α-glucosidase inhibitors acarbose and miglitol are such currently available drugs.

1. Drugs That Stimulate Insulin Secretion

Sulfonylureas

This group of drugs contains a sulfonic acid-urea nucleus that can be modified by chemical substitutions to produce agents that have similar qualitative actions but differ widely in potency. The primary mechanism of action of the sulfonylureas is to stimulate insulin release from pancreatic B cells.

A. MECHANISM OF ACTION

Specific receptors on the surface of pancreatic B cells bind sulfonylureas in the rank order of their insulinotropic potency (glyburide with the greatest affinity and tolbutamide with the least). It has been shown that activation of these receptors closes potassium channels, resulting in depolarization of the B cell. This depolarized state permits calcium to enter the cell and actively promote insulin release (Figure 17–8). These ATP-sensitive K$^+$ channel-specific receptors have been characterized and appear to consist of two proteins: a protein that binds the sulfonylurea—the sulfonylurea receptor (SUR)—and an internal rectifying potassium channel (Kir6.2). Four molecules of Kir6.2 form the pore and are associated with four molecules of the SUR.

There is a family of sulfonylurea receptors. SUR1/Kir6.2 is found in B cells and in the brain; it is activated by diazoxide and is sensitive to inhibition by sulfonylureas at low concentrations (IC$_{50}$ about 1 nm for glyburide). Mutations in SUR1 or Kir6.2 have been

identified that result in persistent hyperinsulinemic hypoglycemia of infancy. SUR2A/Kir6.2 is found in cardiac and skeletal muscle. It is insensitive to diazoxide but sensitive to other potassium channel openers such as pinacidil and cromakalim, and it is a hundredfold less sensitive to glyburide. SUR2B/Kir6.2 appears to be widely distributed in vascular smooth muscle. It has not been established that the difference in affinities of these receptors for sulfonylureas is of clinical relevance. Controversy also persists, however, about whether this well-documented insulinotropic action during acute administration is sufficient to explain adequately the hypoglycemic effect of sulfonylureas during chronic therapy. Additional extrapancreatic effects of sulfonylureas, such as their potentiation of the peripheral effects of insulin

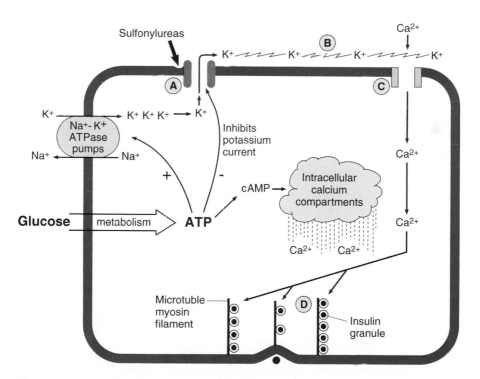

Figure 17–8. Proposed mechanism for sulfonylurea stimulation of insulin release by the pancreatic B cell. Energy-dependent pumps maintain a high intracellular concentration of potassium (K$^+$). In the resting B cell, K$^+$ diffuses from the cell through non-energy-dependent potassium channels (A). This current of potassium ions generates an electrical potential that polarizes the resting cell membrane (B) and closes a voltage-gated calcium channel (C), thereby preventing extracellular calcium from entering the cell. When sulfonylureas bind to a specific receptor on the potassium channel (or when glucose metabolism generates ATP), the potassium channel closes. This depolarizes the cell, allowing calcium to enter and cause microtubules to contract (D), moving insulin granules to the cell surface for emeiocytosis. (Modified and reproduced, with permission, from Karam JH: Type II diabetes and syndrome X. Endocrinol Metab Clin North Am 1992;21:339.)

at the receptor or postreceptor level, have been invoked to account for their continued effectiveness during long-term treatment despite a lack of demonstrable increase in insulin secretion. However, several clinical trials have failed to demonstrate any therapeutic benefit on long-term glycemic control when sulfonylureas are added to insulin therapy in the patient with type 1 diabetes. These observations suggest that in vitro evidence for a potentiation by sulfonylureas of the peripheral effects of insulin may have little clinical relevance.

B. INDICATIONS

Sulfonylureas are not indicated in ketosis-prone type 1 diabetic patients, since these drugs require functioning pancreatic B cells to produce their effect on blood glucose. Moreover, clinical trials show no benefit from the use of sulfonylureas as an adjunct to insulin replacement in type 1 diabetic patients. The sulfonylureas seem most appropriate for use in the nonobese patient with mild maturity-onset diabetes whose hyperglycemia has not responded to diet therapy. In obese patients with mild diabetes and slight to moderate peripheral insensitivity to levels of circulating insulin, the primary emphasis should be on weight reduction. When hyperglycemia in obese diabetics has been more severe, with consequent impairment of pancreatic B cell function, sulfonylureas may improve glycemic control until concurrent measures such as diet, exercise, and weight reduction can sustain the improvement without the need for oral drugs.

C. SULFONYLUREAS CURRENTLY AVAILABLE IN THE USA (TABLE 17–11.)

1. First-generation sulfonylureas (tolbutamide, tolazamide, acetohexamide, and chlorpropamide)—

a. Tolbutamide (Orinase)—Tolbutamide is supplied in tablets of 500 mg. It is rapidly oxidized in the liver to an inactive form. Because its duration of effect is short (6–10 hours), it is usually administered in divided doses (eg, 500 mg before each meal and at bedtime). The usual daily dose is 1.5–3 g; some patients, however, require only 250–500 mg daily. Acute toxic reactions such as skin rashes are rare. Because of its short duration of action, which is independent of renal function, tolbutamide is probably the safest agent to use in elderly patients, in whom hypoglycemia would be a particularly serious risk. Prolonged hypoglycemia has been reported rarely, mainly in patients receiving certain drugs (eg, warfarin, phenylbutazone, or sulfonamides) that compete with sulfonylureas for hepatic oxidation, resulting in maintenance of high levels of unmetabolized active sulfonylureas in the circulation.

b. Tolazamide (Tolinase)—Tolazamide is supplied in tablets of 100, 250, and 500 mg. The average daily dose is 200–1000 mg, given in one or two doses. Tolazamide is comparable to chlorpropamide in potency but is devoid of disulfiram-like or water-retaining effects. Tolazamide is more slowly absorbed than the other sulfonylureas, with effects on blood glucose not appearing for several hours. Its duration of action may last up to 20 hours, with maximal hypoglycemic effect occurring between the fourth and fourteenth hours. Tolazamide is metabolized to several compounds that retain hypoglycemic effects. If more than 500 mg/d is required, the dose should be divided and given twice daily. Doses larger than 1000 mg/d do not improve the degree of glycemic control.

c. Chlorpropamide (Diabinese)—This drug is supplied in tablets of 100 and 250 mg. It has a half-life of 32 hours and a duration of action of up to 60 hours. It is slowly metabolized by the liver, with approximately 20–30% excreted unchanged in the urine. Since the metabolites retain hypoglycemic activity, elimination of the biologic effect is almost completely dependent on renal excretion, so that its use is contraindicated in patients with renal insufficiency. The average maintenance dose is 250 mg daily (range, 100–500 mg), given as a single dose in the morning. Chlorpropamide is a potent agent, and prolonged hypoglycemia can occur as an adverse effect, especially in elderly patients, who may have impaired renal clearance. Doses in excess of 500 mg/d increase the risk of cholestatic jaundice, which does not occur with the usual dose of 250 mg/d or less. About 15% of patients taking chlorpropamide develop a facial flush when they drink alcohol, and occasionally they may develop a full-blown disulfiram-like reaction, with nausea, vomiting, weakness, and even syncope. There appears to be a genetic predisposition to the development of this reaction.

Other side effects of chlorpropamide include water retention and the development of hyponatremia, effects that are mediated through an ADH mechanism. The hyponatremia is generally a benign condition with sodium values between 125 and 130 mEq/L, but occasional cases of symptomatic hyponatremia with sodium concentrations below 125 mEq/L have been reported, particularly when concomitant diuretic therapy is being used. Chlorpropamide stimulates ADH secretion and also potentiates its action at the renal tubule. Its antidiuretic effect is somewhat unusual, since three other sulfonylureas (acetohexamide, tolazamide, and glyburide) appear to facilitate water excretion in humans.

Since other sulfonylureas have now become available with comparable potency but without the disadvan-

Table 17–11. Oral antidiabetic drugs.

Drug	Tablet Size	Daily Dose	Duration of Action
Sulfonylureas			
Tolbutamide (Orinase)	250, 500 mg	0.5–2 g in 2 or 3 divided doses	6–12 hours
Tolazamide (Tolinase)	100, 250, 500 mg	0.1–1 g as single dose or in 2 divided doses	Up to 24 hours
Acetohexamide[1] (Dymelor)	250, 500 mg	0.25–1.5 g as single dose or in 2 divided doses	8–24 hours
Chlorpropamide[1] (Diabinese)	100, 250 mg	0.1–0.5 g as single dose	24–72 hours
Glyburide (DiaβΒeta, Micronase)	1.25, 2.5, 5 mg	1.25–20 mg as single dose or in 2 divided doses	Up to 24 hours
(Glynase)	1.5, 3, 6 mg	1.5–18 mg as single dose or in 2 divided doses	Up to 24 hours
Glipizide (Glucotrol)	5, 10 mg	2.5–40 mg as single dose or in 2 divided doses on an empty stomach.	6–12 hours
(Glucotrol XL)	5, 10 mg	Up to 20 or 30 mg daily as a single dose	Up to 24 hours
Glimeperide (Amaryl)	1, 2, 4 mg	1–4 mg as single dose	Up to 24 hours
Meglitinide analogs Repaglinide (Prandin)	0.5, 1, 2 mg	4 mg in two divided doses given 15 minutes before breakfast and dinner	3 hours
D-Phenylalanine derivative Nateglinide	60, 120 mg	60 or 120 mg 3 times a day before meals	1–5 hours
Biguanides Metformin (Glucophage)	500, 850 mg	1–2.5 g. One tablet with meals 2 or 3 times daily	7–12 hours
Extended-release metformin (Glucophage XR)	500 mg	500–200 mg once a day	Up to 24 hours
Thiazolidinediones Rosiglitazone (Avandia)	2, 4, 8 mg	4–8 mg as single dose or in 2 divided doses	24–30 hours
Pioglitazone (Actos)	15, 30, 45 mg	15–45 mg as single dose	30 hours
Alpha-glucosidase inhibitors Acarbose (Precose)	50, 100 mg	75–300 mg in 3 divided doses with first bite of food	4 hours
Miglitol (Glyset)	25, 50, 100 mg	75–300 mg in 3 divided doses with first bite of food	4 hours

[1]There has been a decline in use of these formulations. In the case of chlorpropamide, the decline is due to its numerous side effects (see text).

tages of depending solely on renal excretion or of causing water retention and alcohol-related flushing, there presently is less need to choose chlorpropamide when prescribing sulfonylurea therapy in type 2 patients.

d. Acetohexamide (Dymelor)—This agent is supplied in tablets of 250 and 500 mg. Its duration of action is about 10–16 hours (intermediate in duration of action between tolbutamide and chlorpropamide).

The usual daily dose is 250–1500 mg given in one or two doses. Liver metabolism is rapid, but an active metabolite is produced and excreted by the kidney.

2. Second-generation sulfonylureas: glyburide, glipizide, and glimepiride—These agents have similar chemical structures, with cyclic carbon rings at each end of the sulfonylurea nucleus; this causes them to be highly potent (100- to 200-fold more so than tolbutamide). The drugs should be used with caution in patients with cardiovascular disease as well as in elderly patients, in whom hypoglycemia would be especially dangerous.

a. Glyburide (glibenclamide)—Glyburide is supplied in tablets containing 1.25, 2.5, and 5 mg. The usual starting dose is 2.5 mg/d, and the average maintenance dose is 5–10 mg/d given as a single morning dose. If patients are going to respond to glyburide, they generally do so at doses of 10 mg/d or less, given once daily. If they fail to respond to 10 mg/d, it is uncommon for an increase in dosage to result in improved glycemic control. Maintenance doses higher than 20 mg/d are not recommended and may even worsen hyperglycemia. Glyburide is metabolized in the liver into products with such low hypoglycemic activity that they are considered clinically unimportant unless renal excretion is compromised. Although assays specific for the unmetabolized compound suggest a plasma half-life of only 1–2 hours, the biologic effects of glyburide clearly persist for 24 hours after a single morning dose in diabetic patients. Glyburide is unique among sulfonylureas in that it not only binds to the pancreatic B cell membrane sulfonylurea receptor but also becomes sequestered within the B cell. This may also contribute to its prolonged biologic effect despite its relatively short circulating half-life.

A formulation of "micronized" glyburide, which apparently increases its bioavailability, is now available in "bent" tablet sizes of 1.5 mg, 3 mg, and 6 mg. These are easy to break in half with very mild pressure at the angle of the bend in the tablet.

Glyburide has few adverse effects other than its potential for causing hypoglycemia. It is particularly hazardous in patients over 65 years of age, in whom serious, protracted, and even fatal hypoglycemia can occur even with relatively small daily doses. Drugs with a shorter half-life, eg, tolbutamide or possibly glipizide, are preferable in the treatment of type 2 diabetes in the elderly patient. Glyburide does not cause water retention, as chlorpropamide does, and even slightly enhances free water clearance.

b. Glipizide (glydiazinamide)—Glipizide is supplied in tablets containing 5 and 10 mg. For maximum effect in reducing postprandial hyperglycemia, this agent should be ingested 30 minutes before breakfast, since rapid absorption is delayed when the drug is taken with food. The recommended starting dose is 5 mg/d, with up to 15 mg/d given as a single daily dose. When higher daily doses are required, they should be divided and given before meals. The maximum recommended dose is 40 mg/d, though doses above 10–15 mg probably provide little additional benefit in poor responders and may even be less effective than smaller doses.

At least 90% of glipizide is metabolized in the liver to inactive products, and only a small fraction is excreted unchanged in the urine. Glipizide therapy is contraindicated in patients who have hepatic or renal impairment and who would therefore be at high risk for hypoglycemia, but because of its lower potency and shorter half-life, it is preferable to glyburide in elderly patients.

Glipizide has been marketed as Glucotrol-XL in 5 mg and 10 mg tablets. The medication is enclosed in a nonabsorbable shell that contains an osmotic compartment which expands slowly, thereby slowly pumping out the glipizide in a sustained manner. It provides extended release during transit through the gastrointestinal tract, with greater effectiveness in lowering of prebreakfast hyperglycemia than the shorter-duration immediate-release standard glipizide tablets. However, this formulation appears to have sacrificed glipizide's reduced propensity for severe hypoglycemia compared with longer-acting glyburide without showing any demonstrable therapeutic advantages over glyburide.

c. Glimepiride—This sulfonylurea is supplied in tablets containing 1, 2, and 4 mg. It has a long duration of effect with a half-life of 5 hours, allowing once-daily administration. Glimepiride achieves blood glucose lowering with the lowest dose of any sulfonylurea compound. A single daily dose of 1 mg/d has been shown to be effective, and the maximal recommended dose is 8 mg. It is completely metabolized by the liver to relatively inactive metabolic products.

Meglitinide Analogs

Repaglinide is supplied as 0.5, 1, and 2 mg tablets. Its structure is similar to that of glyburide but lacks the sulfonic acid-urea moiety. It also acts by binding to the sulfonylurea receptor and closing the ATP-sensitive potassium channel. It is rapidly absorbed from the intestine and then undergoes complete metabolism in the liver to inactive biliary products, giving it a plasma half-life of less than 1 hour. The drug therefore causes a brief but rapid pulse of insulin. The starting dose is 0.5 mg three times a day 15 minutes before each meal. The dose can be titrated to a maximum daily dose of 16 mg. Like the sulfonylureas, repaglinide can be used in combination with metformin. Hypoglycemia is the main side effect. In clinical trials, when the drug was compared with glyburide, a long-acting sulfonylurea, there was a trend toward less hypoglycemia. Like the sulfonylureas, it causes weight gain. Metabolism is by cytochrome P4503A4 isoenzyme, and other drugs that induce or inhibit this isoenzyme may increase or inhibit the metabolism of repaglinide, respectively. The drug may be useful in patients with renal impairment or in the elderly. It remains to be shown whether this drug has significant advantages over short-acting sulfonylureas.

δ-Phenylalanine Derivative

Nateglinide is supplied in tablets of 60 and 120 mg. This drug binds the sulfonylurea receptor and closes the ATP-sensitive potassium channel. The drug is rapidly absorbed from the intestine, reaching peak plasma levels within 1 hour. It is metabolized in the liver and has a plasma half-life of about 1.5 hours. Like repaglinide, it causes a brief rapid pulse of insulin, and when given before a meal it reduces the postprandial rise in blood glucose. The 60 mg dose is used in patients with mild elevations in HbA_{1c}. For most patients, the recommended starting and maintenance dosage is 120 mg three times a day before meals. Like the other insulin secretagogues, its main side effects are hypoglycemia and weight gain.

2. Drugs That Alter Insulin Action

Biguanides

Unlike sulfonylureas, the biguanides (Table 17–11) do not require functioning pancreatic B cells for reduction of hyperglycemia. Use of **phenformin** was discontinued in the USA because of its association with the development of lactic acidosis in patients with coexisting liver or kidney disease. **Metformin,** a biguanide that is much less likely to produce lactic acidosis, has generally replaced phenformin in the treatment of diabetics.

A. CLINICAL PHARMACOLOGY

The exact mechanism of action of metformin (1,1-dimethylbiguanide hydrochloride) remains unclear. It reduces both the fasting level of blood glucose and the degree of postprandial hyperglycemia in patients with type 2 diabetes but has no effect on fasting blood glucose in normal subjects. Metformin does not stimulate insulin action, yet it is particularly effective in reducing hepatic gluconeogenesis. Other proposed mechanisms include a slowing down of gastrointestinal absorption of glucose and increased glucose uptake by skeletal muscle, which have been reported in some but not all clinical studies. Because of its very high concentration in intestinal cells after oral administration, metformin increases glucose-to-lactate turnover in these cells, and this also contributes to its action in reducing hyperglycemia.

Metformin has a half-life of 1.5–3 hours, is not bound to plasma proteins, and is not metabolized in humans, being excreted unchanged by the kidneys.

B. INDICATIONS AND DOSAGE

Metformin may be used as an adjunct to diet for the control of hyperglycemia and its associated symptomatology in patients with type 2 diabetes, particularly those who are obese or are not responding optimally to maximal doses of sulfonylureas. A side benefit of metformin therapy is its tendency to improve both fasting and postprandial hyperglycemia and hypertriglyceridemia in obese diabetics without the weight gain associated with insulin or sulfonylurea therapy. For this reason—and because of its ability to correct hyperglycemia while having an insulin-sparing action—metformin has particular potential in treating patients with the insulin resistance syndrome (syndrome X, or metabolic syndrome). Metformin is not indicated for patients with type 1 diabetes and is contraindicated in diabetics with renal insufficiency, since failure to excrete this drug would produce high blood and tissue levels of metformin that would stimulate lactic acid overproduction. Likewise, patients with hepatic insufficiency or abusers of ethanol should not receive this drug since lactic acid production from the gut and other tissues, which rises during metformin therapy, could result in lactic acidosis when defective hepatocytes cannot remove the lactate or when alcohol-induced reduction of nucleotides interferes with lactate clearance. Finally, metformin is relatively contraindicated in patients with cardiorespiratory insufficiency, since they have a propensity to develop hypoxia which would aggravate the lactic acid production already occurring from metformin therapy. The "age" cutoff for prescribing metformin has not been defined and remains relative to the overall health of the patient, but generally there is concern that after the age of 65–70 years, the potential for progressive impairment of renal function or development of a cardiac event while taking metformin raises the risk enough to outweigh the benefits of prescribing metformin to the elderly patient with type 2 diabetes.

Metformin is dispensed as 500 mg, 850 mg, and 1000 mg tablets. A 500 mg extended-release preparation is also available. The dosage range is from 500 mg to a maximum of 2550 mg daily, with the lowest possible effective dose being recommended. Eighty-five percent of the maximal glucose-lowering effect is achieved by a daily dose of 1500 mg, and there is little benefit from giving more than 2000 mg daily. It is important to begin with a low dose and increase the dosage very gradually in divided doses—taken with meals—to reduce minor gastrointestinal upsets. A common schedule would be one 500 mg tablet three times a day with meals or one 850 mg or 1000 mg tablet twice daily at breakfast and dinner. The maximum recommended dose is 850 mg three time a day. One to four tablets of the extended-release preparation can be given once a day.

C. Adverse Reactions

The most frequent side effects of metformin are gastrointestinal symptoms (anorexia, nausea, vomiting, abdominal discomfort, diarrhea), which occur in up to 20% of patients. These effects are dose-related, tend to occur at onset of therapy, and often are transient. However, in 3–5% of patients, therapy may have to be discontinued because of persistent diarrheal discomfort. Absorption of vitamin B_{12} appears to be reduced during chronic metformin therapy, and annual screening of serum B_{12} levels and red blood cell parameters has been encouraged by the manufacturer.

Hypoglycemia does not occur with therapeutic doses of metformin, which permits its description as a "euglycemic" or "antihyperglycemic" drug rather than an oral hypoglycemic agent. Dermatologic or hematologic toxicity is rare.

Lactic acidosis (see below) has been reported as a side effect but is uncommon with metformin in contrast to phenformin, and almost all reported cases have involved subjects with associated risk factors that should have contraindicated its use (renal, hepatic, or cardiorespiratory insufficiency, alcoholism, advanced age).

Thiazolidinediones

Drugs of this new class of antihyperglycemic agents sensitize peripheral tissues to insulin. They bind to a nuclear receptor called peroxisome proliferator-activated receptor-gamma (PPAR-γ) and affect the expression of a number of genes that regulate the release of adipokines—resistin and adiponectin—from adipocytes. Adiponectin secretion is stimulated, which sensitizes tissues to the effects of insulin; and resistin secretion is inhibited, which reduces insulin resistance. Observed effects of thiazolidinediones include increased glucose transporter expression (GLUT 1 and GLUT 4), decreased free fatty acid levels, decreased hepatic glucose output, and increased differentiation of pre-adipocytes into adipocytes. Like the biguanides, this class of drugs does not cause hypoglycemia.

Troglitazone (Rezulin) was the first drug in this class to go into widespread clinical use. Unfortunately, about 1.9 % of patients taking this drug developed elevations in liver enzymes over three times normal, which resolved when the drug was stopped. Liver failure, however, occurred if the drug was continued—at least 90 cases have been reported, and 63 of these patients have died. The drug has therefore been withdrawn from clinical use.

Two other drugs in the same class are available for clinical use: Rosiglitazone (Avandia) and pioglitazone (Actos). Both of these drugs are effective as monotherapy and in combination with sulfonylureas, metformin, and insulin. When used as monotherapy, these drugs lower HbA_{1c} by about 1 or 2 percentage points. When used in combination with insulin, they can result in a 30–50% reduction in insulin dosage, and some patients can come off insulin completely. Combination therapy with a thiazolidinedione and metformin has the advantage of not causing hypoglycemia. Patients inadequately managed on sulfonylureas can do well on a combination of sulfonylurea with rosiglitazone or pioglitazone. About 25% of patients in clinical trials fail to respond to these drugs, presumably because they are significantly insulinopenic.

Rosiglitazone therapy is associated with increases in total cholesterol, LDL cholesterol (14–18%), and HDL cholesterol (11–14%). There is reduction in free fatty acids of about 8–15%. The changes in triglycerides were generally not different from changes reported with placebo. The increase in the LDL cholesterol need not necessarily be detrimental—studies with troglitazone showed that there is a shift from the atherogenic small dense LDL particles to larger, less dense LDL particles. Pioglitazone in clinical trials lowered triglycerides (9%) and increased HDL cholesterol (12–19%) but did not result in a consistent change in total cholesterol and LDL cholesterol levels. A prospective randomized comparison of the metabolic effects of pioglitazone and rosiglitazone on patients who had previously been on troglitazone showed similar effects on HbA_{1c} and weight gain. Pioglitazone-treated subjects, however, had lower total cholesterol, LDL cholesterol, and triglycerides when compared with rosiglitazone. Anemia occurs in 3–4% of patients treated with these drugs, but this effect may be due to a dilutional effect of increased plasma volume rather than a reduction in red cell mass. Weight gain occurs, especially when the drug is combined with a sulfonylurea or with insulin.

The dosage of rosiglitazone is 4–8 mg daily and of pioglitazone 15–45 mg daily, and the drugs do not have to be taken with food. Rosiglitazone is primarily metabolized by the CYP2C8 isoenzyme, and unlike troglitazone it does not appear to affect CYP3A4 and has no significant effect on oral contraceptives. Pioglitazone is metabolized by CYP2C8 and CYP3A4. The pharmacokinetics of coadministration of pioglitazone and oral contraceptives has not been evaluated.

These two agents in clinical trials did not—unlike troglitazone—show evidence of drug-induced liver function test abnormalities or hepatotoxicity: The FDA has recommended, however, that patients should not initiate drug therapy with these agents if the ALT is 2.5 times greater than the upper limit of normal. Obviously, caution should be used in initiation of therapy in patients with even mild ALT elevations. Liver function tests should be performed once every 2 months for the first year and periodically thereafter.

3. Drugs That Affect Glucose Absorption

Alpha-Glucosidase Inhibitors

Drugs of this family are competitive inhibitors of intestinal brush border alpha-glucosidases. Two of these drugs, acarbose and miglitol, are available for clinical use. Both are potent inhibitors of glucoamylase, α-amylase, and sucrase. They are less effective on isomaltase and are ineffective on trehalase or lactase. Acarbose binds 1000 times more avidly to the intestinal disaccharidases than do products of carbohydrate digestion or sucrose. A fundamental difference exists between acarbose and miglitol in their absorption. Acarbose has the molecular mass and structural features of a tetrasaccharide, and very little (about 2%) crosses the microvillar membrane. Miglitol, however, is structurally similar to glucose and is absorbable. Both drugs delay the absorption of carbohydrates and reduce postprandial glycemic excursion.

A. ACARBOSE

Acarbose is available as 50 and 100 mg tablets. The recommended starting dose is 50 mg twice daily, gradually increasing to 100 mg three times daily. For maximal benefit on postprandial hyperglycemia, acarbose should be given with the first mouthful of food ingested. In diabetic patients it reduces postprandial hyperglycemia by 30–50%, and its overall effect is to lower the HbA_{1c} by 0.5–1%. The principal adverse effect, seen in 20–30% of patients, is flatulence. This is caused by undigested carbohydrate reaching the lower bowel, where gases are produced by bacterial flora. In 3% of cases, troublesome diarrhea occurs. This gastrointestinal discomfort tends to discourage excessive carbohydrate consumption and promotes improved compliance of type 2 diabetes patients with their diet prescriptions. When acarbose is given alone, there is no risk of hypoglycemia. However, if combined with insulin or sulfonylureas, it might increase risk of hypoglycemia from these agents. A slight rise in hepatic aminotransferases has been noted in clinical trials (5% versus 2% in placebo controls, and particularly with doses greater than 300 mg/d). This generally returns to normal on stopping this drug. In the UKPDS, approximately 2000 patients on diet, sulfonylurea, metformin, or insulin therapy were randomized to acarbose or placebo therapy. By 3 years, 60% of the patients had discontinued the drug, mostly because of gastrointestinal symptoms. In the 40% of patients who remained on the drug acarbose was associated with an 0.5% lowering of HbA_{1c} compared with placebo.

B. MIGLITOL

Miglitol is similar to acarbose in terms of its clinical effects. It is indicated for use in diet- or sulfonylurea-treated patients with type 2 diabetes. Therapy is initiated at the lowest effective dosage of 25 mg three times a day. The usual maintenance dose is 50 mg three times a day, though some patients may benefit from increasing the dose to 100 mg three times a day. Gastrointestinal side effects occur as with acarbose. The drug is not metabolized and is excreted unchanged by the kidney. Theoretically, absorbable α-glucosidase inhibitors could induce a deficiency of one or more of the α-glucosidases involved in cellular glycogen metabolism and biosynthesis of glycoproteins. This does not occur in practice because—unlike the intestinal mucosa, which is exposed to a high concentration of the drug—circulating plasma levels are 200-fold to 1000-fold lower than those needed to inhibit intracellular α-glucosidases. Miglitol should not be used in renal failure since its clearance is impaired in this setting.

Drug Combinations

A glyburide and metformin combination (Glucovance) is available in dose forms of 1.25 mg/250 mg, 2.5 mg/500 mg, and 5 mg/500 mg. This combination, however, limits the clinician's ability to optimally adjust dosage of the individual drugs and for that reason is of questionable merit.

Safety of Oral Hypoglycemic Agents

The University Group Diabetes Program (UGDP) reported that the number of deaths due to cardiovascular disease in diabetic patients treated with tolbutamide or phenformin was excessive when compared to either insulin-treated patients or to patients receiving placebos. At present, a warning label outlining their cardiovascular risk is inserted in each packet of sulfonylureas and metformin dispensed. However, the United Kingdom Prospective Diabetes Study of type 2 diabetes has refuted these conclusions regarding sulfonylureas. It did not confirm any cardiovascular hazard among over 1500 patients treated intensively with sulfonylureas for more than 10 years, compared with a comparable number who received either insulin or diet therapy. Analysis of a subgroup of obese patients receiving metformin also showed no hazard—and even a slight reduction in cardiovascular deaths compared with conventional (diet) therapy.

The question of safety of thiazolidinediones (see above) remains to be resolved regarding the frequency of life-threatening hepatic toxicity and whether monthly monitoring during the first 10 months of treatment adequately protects the patient. Lactic acidosis from metformin (see above) is quite rare and probably not a major consideration for its use—in the absence of major risk factors such as impaired renal function or hepatic function or conditions predisposing to hypoxia.

INSULIN

Insulin is indicated for type 1 diabetics as well as for those type 2 diabetics whose hyperglycemia does not respond to diet therapy and oral hypoglycemic drugs.

Insulin replacement in patients with type 1 diabetes has been less than optimal because subcutaneous injections cannot completely reproduce the normal physiologic pattern of insulin secretion into the portal vein. With the help of appropriate modifications of diet and exercise and careful monitoring of capillary blood glucose levels at home, however, it is possible to achieve acceptable control of blood glucose by using multiple injections of ultrashort-, short-, intermediate-, and long-acting insulins. In some patients, a portable insulin infusion pump may be required for optimal control.

With the development of highly purified human insulin preparations, immunogenicity has been markedly reduced, thereby decreasing the incidence of therapeutic complications such as insulin allergy, immune in-

sulin resistance, and localized lipoatrophy at the injection site.

Characteristics of Currently Available Insulin Preparations

Commercial insulin preparations differ with regard to the animal species from which they are obtained; their purity, concentration, and solubility; and their time of onset and duration of biologic action (Figure 17–9; Table 17–12). Eighteen different formulations of insulin are available in the USA (Table 17–14).

A. SPECIES OF INSULIN

Human insulin is now produced by recombinant DNA techniques (biosynthetic human insulin). Eli Lilly and Novo Nordisk dispense human insulin as regular (R), NPH (N), lente (L), or ultralente (U) formulations (Table 17–14). Three analogs of human insulin—two rapidly acting (insulin lispro, insulin aspart) and one very long-acting (insulin glargine) are now available for clinical use. A limited supply of monospecies pork insulin (Iletin II) remains available for use by certain patients who may benefit from the slightly more prolonged and sustained effect of animal insulin compared with human insulin.

B. PURITY OF INSULIN

Improvements in purification techniques for insulins have reduced or eliminated contaminating insulin precursors that were capable of inducing anti-insulin antibodies. "Purified" insulin is defined by the FDA as containing less than 10 ppm of proinsulin, whether

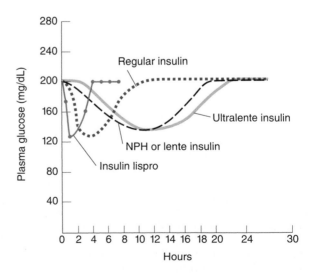

Figure 17–9. Extent and duration of action of various types of insulin (in a fasting diabetic). Duration of action is extended considerably when the dose of a given insulin formulation increases above the average therapeutic doses depicted here. (Modified, with permission, from Katzung BG [editor]: *Basic & Clinical Pharmacology*, 2nd ed. McGraw-Hill, 1985.)

Table 17–12. Summary of bioavailability characteristics of the insulins.

	Insulin Type	Onset	Peak Action	Duration
Ultrashort-acting	Insulin lispro, insulin aspart	5–15 minutes	1–1.5 hours	3–4 hours
Short-acting	Regular, Velosulin	15–30 minutes	1–3 hours	5–7 hours
Intermediate-acting	Lente, NPH	2–4 hours	8–10 hours	18–24 hours
Long-acting	Ultralente	4–5 hours	8–14 hours	25–36 hours
	Insulin glargine	6–8 hours	—	24 hours

extracted from animal pancreas or produced from biosynthetic proinsulin. All human and pork insulins currently available contain less than 10 ppm of proinsulin and are labeled as "purified."

The more highly purified insulins currently in use preserve their potency quite well; therefore, refrigeration while in use is not necessary. During travel, reserve

Table 17–13. Examples of intensive insulin regimens using insulin lispro or insulin aspart and ultralente, NPH, or insulin glargine in a 70 kg man with type 1 diabetes.[1,2,3,4]

	Pre-Breakfast	Pre-Lunch	Pre-Dinner	At Bedtime
Insulin lispro or aspart	5 units	4 units	6 units	—
Ultralente insulin	8 units	—	8 units	—
OR				
Insulin lispro or aspart	5 units	4 units	6 units	—
NPH insulin	3 units	3 units	2 units	8–14 units
Insulin lispro or aspart	5 units	4 units	6 units	—
Insulin glargine	—	—	–	15–16 units

[1]Reproduced, with permission, from Tierney LM Jr, McPhee SJ, Papadakis MA: *Current Medical Diagnosis & Treatment 2003.* McGraw-Hill, 2003.

[2]Assumes that patient is consuming approximately 75 g carbohydrate at breakfast, 60 g at lunch and 90 g at dinner.

[3]The dose of insulin lispro or insulin aspart can be raised by 1 or 2 units if extra carbohydrate (15–30 g) is ingested or if premeal blood glucose is > 170 mg/dL. Insulin lispro or insulin aspart can be mixed in the same syringe with ultralente or NPH insulin.

[4]Insulin glargine cannot be mixed with any of the available insulins and must be given as a separate injection.

supplies of insulin can be readily transported without significant loss of potency provided they are protected from extremes of heat or cold.

Concentrations of Insulins (Table 17–14)

At present, insulins in the USA are available only in a concentration of 100 units/mL (U100); all are dispensed in 10-mL vials. To accommodate children and the occasional adult who may require small quantities of insulin, "low-dose" (0.3 mL) disposable insulin syringes have been introduced so that U100 insulin can now be measured accurately in doses as low as 1 or 2 units. This has eliminated the need for lower concentrations of insulin and has resulted in the phasing out of all U40 insulins in the United States. For use in rare cases of severe insulin resistance in which large quantities of insulin are required, a limited supply of U500 (500 units/mL) regular human insulin is available from Eli Lilly.

Bioavailability Characteristics

Four principal types of insulin are available: (1) ultrashort-acting insulin, with very rapid onset and short duration of action; (2) short-acting insulin, with rapid onset of action; (3) intermediate-acting insulin; and (4) long-acting insulin, with slow onset of action (Table 17–14). Ultrashort-acting and short-acting insulins are dispensed as clear solutions at neutral pH. The long-acting insulin analog insulin glargine is also dispensed as a clear solution but at acidic pH. Other intermediate-acting and long-acting insulins are dispensed as opaque suspensions at neutral pH with either protamine (derived from fish sperm) in phosphate buffer (NPH) or varying concentrations of zinc in acetate buffer (ultralente and lente insulins).

The characteristics of these various insulins are discussed below and summarized in Table 17–12. It is im-

Table 17–14. Some insulin preparations available in the USA.[1]

Preparation	Species Source	Concentration
Ultrashort-acting insulins		
Insulin lispro (Humalog, Lilly)	Human analog (recombinant)	U100
Insulin aspart	Human analog (recombinant)	U100
Short-acting insulins "Purified"[2]		
Regular (Novo Nordisk)[3]	Human	U100
Regular Humulin (Lilly)	Human	U100, U500
Regular Iletin II (Lilly)	Pork	U100
Velosulin (Novo Nordisk)[4]	Human	U100
Intermediate-acting insulins "Purified"[3]		
Lente Humulin (Lilly)	Human	U100
Lente Iletin II (Lilly)	Pork	U100
Lente (Novo Nordisk) Novolin	Human	U100
NPH Humulin (Lilly)	Human	U100
NPH Iletin II (Lilly)	Pork	U100
NPH (Novo Nordisk) Novolin	Human	U100
Premixed insulins % NPH, % regular		
Novolin 70/30 (Novo Nordisk)	Human	U100
Humulin 70/30 and 50/50 (Lilly)	Human	U100
% NPL, % insulin lispro		
Humalog Mix 75/25 (Lilly)	Human analog (recombinant)	U100
% insulin aspart protamine, % insulin aspart		
NovoLogMix 70/30	Human	U100
Long-acting insulins "Purified"[3]		
Ultralente Humulin (Lilly)	Human	U100
Insulin glargine (Lantis, Aventis)	Human analog (recombinant)	U100

[1]All of these agents (except insulin lispro and U500) are available without a prescription.
[2]Less than 10 ppm proinsulin.
[3]Novo Nordisk human insulins are termed Novolin R, L, and N.
[4]Velosulin contains phosphate buffer, which favors its use to prevent insulin aggregation in pump tubing but precludes its being mixed with lente insulin.

portant to recognize that values given for time of onset of action, peak effect, and duration of action are only approximate ones and that there is great variability in these parameters from patient to patient and even in a given patient depending on the size of the dose, the site of injection, the degree of exercise, the avidity of circulating anti-insulin antibodies, and other less well defined variables.

A. ULTRASHORT-ACTING INSULINS

Insulin lispro is an insulin analog wherein two amino acids near the terminal end of the B chain have been reversed in position: the proline at position B28 has been moved to position B29, and the lysine has been moved from B29 to B28. **Insulin aspart** is a single substitution of proline by aspartic acid at position B28. These changes result in these two analogs having less tendency to form hexamers—in contrast to human insulin. When injected subcutaneously, the analogs quickly dissociate into monomers and are absorbed very rapidly, reaching peak serum values as early as 1 hour—in contrast to regular insulin, whose hexamers require considerably more time to dissociate and become absorbed. The amino acid changes in these analogs do not interfere with their binding to the insulin receptor, with its circulating half-life, or with its immunogenicity, which are all identical with that of human regular insulin. The optimal times of preprandial subcutaneous injection of comparable doses of ultrashort-acting analogs and regular human insulin are 20 and 60 minutes before the meal, respectively. Diabetic patients who have had to wait up to an hour after injecting regular human insulin before they can begin a meal appreciate this more rapid onset of action. Patients do need to understand that when using the ultrashort-acting insulins they must ingest adequate absorbable carbohydrate early in the meal to avoid hypoglycemia immediately after a meal. Regular insulin's duration of action is proportionate to the dose, with larger doses lasting much longer. This effect is much less pronounced with insulin lispro and insulin aspart, so that regardless of dose, its duration of action is close to 4 hours, and this reduces the risk of late hypoglycemia. The structural differences between insulin lispro and human insulin may be sufficient to prevent insulin lispro from binding to human insulin antibodies in some patients, and there have been case reports of successful use of insulin lispro in those rare patients who have a generalized allergy to human insulin or who have severe antibody insulin resistance. Unlike the over-the-counter insulins, the analogs do require a physician's prescription.

B. SHORT-ACTING INSULINS

Regular insulin is a short-acting, soluble crystalline zinc insulin whose hypoglycemic effect appears within 15 minutes after subcutaneous injection, peaks at 1–3 hours, and lasts for about 5–7 hours when usual quantities, eg, 5–15 units, are administered. Regular insulin is the only type that can be administered intravenously, and insulin infusions are particularly useful in the treatment of diabetic ketoacidosis and during postoperative management of insulin-requiring diabetics. Because regular insulin when infused intravenously is monomeric and has an immediate effect, there is no advantage to using the more expensive ultrashort-acting insulin analogs for intravenous use.

Regular insulin produced by Novo Nordisk and Eli Lilly is dispensed without a buffer. When it is used in reservoirs or infusion pumps, stability is improved when regular insulin is buffered with disodium phosphate (Velosulin).

C. INTERMEDIATE-ACTING INSULINS

1. Lente insulin—This is a mixture of 30% short-acting semilente with 70% ultralente insulin. Its onset of action is delayed to 2–4 hours, and its peak response is generally reached in about 8–10 hours. Because its duration of action is often less than 24 hours (with a range of 18–24 hours), most patients require at least two injections daily to maintain a sustained insulin effect. The supernatant of the lente suspension contains an excess of zinc ions, which may precipitate regular insulin if it is added to lente.

2. NPH (neutral protamine Hagedorn, or isophane) insulin—This is an intermediate-acting insulin in which the onset of action is delayed by combining two parts of soluble crystalline zinc insulin with one part protamine zinc insulin. The mixture is reported to have equivalent concentrations of protamine and insulin, so that neither is in excess ("isophane"). The peak action and duration of action of NPH insulin are similar to those of lente insulin, however, in contrast to lente insulin, regular insulin retains its solubility and independent rapid action when mixed with NPH.

Flocculation of suspended particles may occasionally "frost" the sides of a bottle of NPH insulin or "clump" within bottles from which multiple small doses are withdrawn over a prolonged period. This instability is a rare phenomenon and might occur less frequently if NPH human insulin were refrigerated when not in use and if bottles were discarded after 1 month of use. Patients should be vigilant for early signs of frosting or clumping of the NPH insulin, because it indicates a pronounced loss of potency. Several cases of diabetic ketoacidosis have been reported in type 1 diabetes patients who had been inadvertently injecting this denatured insulin.

D. LONG-ACTING INSULINS

1. Human ultralente insulin—Ultralente insulin is a relatively insoluble crystal of zinc and insulin suspended in an acetate buffer. Its onset of action is less than that of the previously available beef ultralente. It is generally recommended that the daily dose be split into two equal doses given 12 hours apart. Its peak activity is less than that of NPH insulin, and it is often used to provide basal coverage while the short-acting insulins are used to cover the glucose rise associated with meals.

2. Insulin glargine—Insulin glargine is an insulin analog in which the asparagine at position 21 of the A chain of the human insulin molecule is replaced by glycine and two arginines are added to the carboxyl terminal of the B chain. The arginines raise the isoelectric point of the molecule close to neutral, making it more soluble in an acidic environment. In contrast, human insulin has an isoelectric point of pH 5.4. Insulin glargine is a clear insulin which, when injected into the neutral pH environment of the subcutaneous tissue, forms microprecipitates that slowly release the insulin into the circulation. It lasts for about 24 hours without any pronounced peaks and is given once a day to provide basal coverage. This insulin cannot be mixed with the other insulins because of its acidic pH. When this insulin was given as a single injection at bedtime to type 1 diabetes patients, fasting hyperglycemia was better controlled when compared with bedtime NPH insulin. The clinical trials also suggest that there may be less nocturnal hypoglycemia with this insulin when compared with NPH insulin.

In one clinical trial involving type 2 patients, insulin glargine was associated with a slightly more rapid progression of retinopathy when compared with NPH insulin. The frequency was 7.5% with the analog and 2.7% with the NPH. This finding, however, was not seen in other clinical trials with this analog. In in vitro studies, insulin glargine has a sixfold greater affinity for IGF-I receptor compared with the human insulin. There has also been a report that insulin glargine has increased mitogenicity compared with human insulin in a human osteosarcoma cell line. Circulating levels of insulin glargine, however, are low, and the clinical significance of these observations is not yet clear.

E. INSULIN MIXTURES

Since intermediate insulins require several hours to reach adequate therapeutic levels, their use in type 1 patients requires supplements of regular insulin or insulin lispro or insulin aspart preprandially. It is well established that insulin mixtures containing increased proportions of lente to regular insulins may retard the rapid action of admixed regular insulin. The excess zinc in lente insulin binds the soluble insulin and partially blunts its action, particularly when a relatively small proportion of regular insulin is mixed with lente (eg, 1 part regular to 1.5 or more parts lente). NPH preparations do not contain excess protamine and so do not delay absorption of admixed regular insulin. They are therefore preferable to lente when mixtures of intermediate and regular insulins are prescribed. For convenience, regular or NPH insulin may be mixed together in the same syringe and injected subcutaneously in split dosage before breakfast and supper. It is recommended that the regular insulin be withdrawn first, then the NPH insulin. No attempt should be made to mix the insulins in the syringe, and the injection is preferably given immediately after the syringe is loaded. Stable premixed insulins (70% NPH and 30% regular or 50% of each) are available as a convenience to patients who have difficulty mixing insulin because of visual problems or insufficient manual dexterity. These include Novolin 70:30 (Novo Nordisk) and Humulin 70:30 and 50:50 (Lilly).

With increasing use of ultrashort-acting insulin analogs as a preprandial insulin, it has become evident that combination with an intermediate-acting or long-acting insulin is essential to maintain postabsorptive glycemic control. It has been demonstrated that insulin lispro can be acutely mixed with either NPH or ultralente insulin without affecting its rapid absorption. Premixed preparations of insulin lispro and NPH insulin are unstable because of exchange of insulin lispro with the human insulin in the protamine complex. Consequently, the soluble component becomes over time a mixture of regular and insulin lispro at varying ratios. In an attempt to remedy this, an intermediate insulin composed of isophane complexes of protamine with insulin lispro was developed and given the name NPL (neutral protamine lispro). A premixed combination of NPL (75%) and insulin lispro (25%) is now available for clinical use (Humalog Mix 75/25). This mixture has a more rapid onset of glucose-lowering activity compared with 70% NPH/30% regular human insulin mixture and can be given within 15 minutes before or after starting a meal. Similarly, a 70% insulin aspart protamine/30 insulin aspart (NovoLogMix 70/30) is now available.

G. INSULIN ANALOGS IN CLINICAL TRIALS

Albumin in subcutaneous tissue fluid has a slow disappearance rate, and insulin analogs that bind albumin would have delayed absorption and prolonged action. Insulin analogs with nonesterified fatty acids coupled to B29 Lys bind to albumin, and in clinical trials these fatty acid-acylated insulins show prolonged duration of action without a peak.

Methods of Insulin Administration

A. INSULIN SYRINGES AND NEEDLES

Disposable plastic syringes with needles attached are available in 1-mL, 0.5-mL, and 0.3-mL sizes. Their finely honed 30-gauge attached needles have greatly reduced the pain of injections. They are light, not susceptible to damage, and convenient when traveling. Moreover, their clear markings and tight plungers allow accurate measurement of insulin dosage. The "low-dose" syringes have become increasingly popular, because most patients take less than 30 units at one injection. Two lengths of needles are available: short (8 mm) and long (12.7 mm). Long needles are preferable in obese patients to reduce the variability of insulin absorption. Disposable syringes may be reused until blunting of the needle occurs (usually after three to five injections). Sterility adequate to avoid infection with reuse appears to be maintained by recapping syringes between uses. Cleansing the needle with alcohol may not be desirable, since it can dissolve the silicon coating and increase the pain of skin puncturing.

B. Sites for Injection

Any part of the body covered by loose skin can be used as an injection site, including the abdomen, thighs, upper arms, flanks, and upper outer quadrants of the buttocks. In general, regular insulin is absorbed more rapidly from upper regions of the body such as the deltoid area or the abdomen rather than from the thighs or buttocks. Exercise appears to facilitate insulin absorption when the injection site is adjacent to the exercising muscle. Rotation of sites continues to be recommended to avoid delayed absorption when fibrosis or lipohypertrophy occurs owing to repeated use of a single site. However, considerable variability of absorption rates from different regions, particularly with exercise, may contribute to the instability of glycemic control in certain type 1 patients if injection sites are rotated indiscriminately over different areas of the body. Consequently, diabetologists recommend limiting injection sites to a single region of the body and rotating sites within that region. It is possible that some of the stability of glycemic control achieved by infusion pumps may be related to the constancy of the region of infusion from day to day. For most patients the abdomen is the recommended region for injection, since it provides a considerable area in which to rotate sites and there may be less variability of absorption with exercise than when the thigh or deltoid areas are used. The effect of anatomic regions appears to be much less pronounced with the analogs.

C. Insulin Pumps

Several small portable "open loop" devices for the delivery of insulin are on the market. These devices contain an insulin reservoir and a pump programmed to deliver regular insulin subcutaneously; they do not contain a glucose sensor. With improved methods for self-monitoring of *blood* glucose at home (see below), these pump systems are becoming increasingly popular. In the United States, MiniMed, Disetronic (Deltec), and Animas insulin infusion pumps are available for subcutaneous delivery of insulin. These pumps are small (about the size of a pager) and easy to program. They have many features, including the ability to record a number of different basal rates throughout a 24-hour period and adjust the time over which bolus doses are given. They are able also to detect pressure build-up if the catheter is kinked. Improvements have also been made in the infusion sets. The catheter connecting the insulin reservoir to the subcutaneous cannula can be

disconnected so the patient can remove the pump temporarily (eg, for bathing). The great advantage of **continuous subcutaneous insulin infusion (CSII)** is that it allows for establishment of a basal profile tailored to the patient. The patient therefore is able to eat with less regard to timing because the basal insulin infusion should maintain a constant blood glucose level between meals.

CSII therapy is appropriate for patients who are motivated, mechanically adept, educated about diabetes (diet, insulin action, treatment of hypo- and hyperglycemia), and willing to monitor their blood glucose four to six times a day. Known complications of CSII include ketoacidosis, which can occur when insulin delivery is interrupted, and skin infections. Another major disadvantage is the cost and the time demanded of physicians and staff in initiating therapy. Increasingly, patients are using the ultrashort-acting analogs in the insulin pumps. In a double-blind crossover study comparing insulin lispro with regular insulin in insulin pumps, subjects using insulin lispro had lower HbA$_{1c}$ values and improved postprandial glucose control with the same frequency of hypoglycemia. There does remain a concern that in the event of pump failure, the insulin analogs could result in more rapid onset of hyperglycemia and ketosis.

Implantable insulin pumps delivering insulin into the peritoneum and portal circulation have been examined in clinical trials. The published results suggest that insulin requirements are lower and there is less hypoglycemia with this form of insulin delivery compared with intensive insulin therapy by injections, but safety considerations have not yet been sufficiently resolved to justify FDA approval.

To facilitate treatment of patients who are adhering to a regimen of multiple preprandial injections of regular insulin that supplement a single injection of long-acting insulin delivered by a conventional syringe, portable **pen injectors** have been introduced. Cartridges containing insulin lispro, insulin aspart, regular insulin, and NPH insulin are available for use with these pens. The devices (eg, Novo-Pen, BD pens) eliminate the need to carry an insulin bottle and syringes during the day. Eli Lilly also makes disposable pens containing insulin lispro, NPH, or 70/30 mixtures.

A novel method for delivering preprandial insulin by inhalation is in clinical trials. Several short-term trials have reported that inhaled insulin is as efficacious as subcutaneously delivered insulin in controlling postmeal glucose excursions. The bioavailability of inhaled insulin is about 10%, and so patients would need to inhale about 300–400 units of insulin a day. The current clinical studies excluded patients with pulmonary disorders, and there remain questions about the effects of long-term use on pulmonary tissues.

Pancreas transplantation at the time of renal transplantation is becoming more widely accepted. Patients undergoing simultaneous pancreas and kidney transplantation have an 85% chance of pancreatic graft survival and a 92% chance of renal graft survival after 1 year. Solitary pancreatic transplantation in the absence of a need for renal transplantation should be considered only in those rare patients who fail all other insulin therapeutic approaches and who have life-threatening complications related to lack of metabolic control.

Islet cell transplantation is a minimally invasive procedure, and investigators in Edmonton, Canada, have reported insulin independence in a small number of patients with type 1 diabetes who underwent this procedure. Using islets from multiple donors and steroid-free immunosuppression, over 20 subjects have undergone percutaneous transhepatic portal vein transplantation of islets. All were able to achieve insulin independence, in some cases for more than 2 years of follow-up. All patients had complete correction of severe hypoglycemic reactions, leading to a marked improvement in overall quality of life. All patients continue to have persistent and detectable levels of C-peptide.

Despite these remarkable advances achieved by the Edmonton group, wide application of this procedure for the treatment of type 1 diabetes is limited by the dependence on multiple donors and the requirement for potent long-term immunotherapy.

STEPS IN THE MANAGEMENT OF THE DIABETIC PATIENT

Diagnostic Examination

A. History and Physical Examination

A complete history is taken and physical examination is performed for diagnostic purposes and to rule out the presence of coexisting or complicating disease. Nutritional status should be noted, particularly if catabolic features such as progressive weight loss are present despite a normal or increased food intake. The family history should include not only the incidence but also the age at onset of diabetes in other members of the family, and it should be noted whether affected family members were obese and whether they required insulin. Other factors that increase cardiovascular risk, such as a smoking history, presence of hypertension or hyperlipidemia, or oral contraceptive pill use should be documented.

A careful physical examination should include baseline height and weight, pulse rate, and blood pressure. If obesity is present, it should be characterized as to its distribution and a waist to hip ratio should be recorded. All peripheral arterial pulses should be examined, noting whether bruits or other signs of atherosclerotic disease are present. Neurologic and ophthalmologic examinations should be performed, with emphasis on investigation of abnormalities that may be related to diabetes, such as neovascularization of the retina or stocking/glove sensory loss in the extremities.

B. Laboratory Diagnosis

(See also Laboratory Findings in Diabetes Mellitus, above.) Laboratory diagnosis should include documentation of the presence of fasting hyperglycemia (plasma glucose > 126 mg/dL [7 mmol/L]) or postprandial (post-glucose tolerance test) values consistently above 200 mg/dL (11.1 mmol/L). An attempt should be made to characterize the diabetes as type 1 or type 2, based on the clinical features present and on whether or not ketonuria accompanies the glycosuria. For the occasional patient, measurement of islet cell, glutamic acid decarboxylase (GAD), insulin antibodies, and ICA 512 antibodies can help in distinguishing between type 1 and type 2 diabetes. Many newly diagnosed patients with type 1 diabetes still have significant endogenous insulin production, and C peptide levels may not reliably distinguish between type 1 and type 2 diabetes. With current emphasis on home blood glucose monitoring, laborious attempts to document the renal threshold for glucose are no longer necessary in the initial evaluation of diabetic patients, particularly since "double-voided" urine specimens are difficult to obtain and since acceptable control of glycemia now allows only rare episodes of glycosuria.

Other baseline laboratory measurements that should be made part of the record include either glycohemoglobin or hemoglobin A_{1c}, total and HDL cholesterol, plasma triglycerides, electrocardiogram, chest x-ray, complete blood count, complete urinalysis, and renal function studies (serum creatinine, blood urea nitrogen, and, if necessary, creatinine clearance).

Patient Education & Self-Management Training

Education is the most important task of the physician who provides care to diabetic patients. It must be remembered that education is necessary not only for newly diagnosed diabetic patients and their families but also for patients with diabetes of any duration who may never have been properly educated about their disorder or who may not be aware of advances in diabetes management. The "teaching curriculum" should include explanations of the nature of diabetes, its potential acute and chronic complications, and information on how these complications can be prevented or at least recognized and treated early. The importance of self-monitoring of blood glucose should be emphasized, particularly in all insulin-requiring diabetic patients, and instructions on proper testing and on recording of data should be provided. Patients should be trained in self-management and taught to use algorithms to adjust the timing and quantity of their insulin dose, food, and exercise in response to their recorded blood glucose values, so that optimal blood glucose control is achieved. Patients must be helped to accept the fact that they have diabetes; until this difficult adjustment has been made efforts to cope with the disorder are likely to be futile. Counseling should be directed at avoidance of extremes such as compulsive rigidity or self-destructive neglect. All patients should be made aware of community agencies (Diabetes Association chapters, etc.) that serve as resources for continuing education.

A. Diet Instruction

All diabetic patients should receive individual instruction on diet, as described earlier in this chapter. Unrestricted diets are not advised for insulin requiring diabetics. Until new methods of insulin replacement are available to provide more normal patterns of insulin delivery in response to metabolic demands, multiple small feedings restricted in simple sugars will continue to be recommended.

B. Insulin

Give the patient an understanding of the actions of the various insulins and the methods of administration of insulin. Since infections, particularly pyogenic ones with fever and toxemia, provoke a marked increase in insulin requirements, patients must be taught how to appropriately administer supplemental rapid-acting insulin as needed to correct hyperglycemia during infections. Patients and their families or friends should also be taught to recognize signs and symptoms of hypoglycemia and how to institute appropriate therapy for hypoglycemic reactions (see Acute Complications of Diabetes Mellitus, below).

C. Oral Drugs for Hyperglycemia

Information must be provided on the principles of hypoglycemic therapy (including information about time of onset, peak action, duration of action, and any adverse effects of pharmacologic agents being used). Patients should be made aware of the maximum recommended dose of the oral agent they are taking and should learn to inquire about possible drug interactions whenever any new medications are added to their regimens.

D. Effect of Exercise

Exercise increases the effectiveness of insulin, and regular daily moderate exercise is an excellent means of improving utilization of fats and carbohydrates in diabetic patients. A judicious balance of the size and frequency of meals with moderate regular exercise can often stabilize the insulin dosage in diabetics who tend to slip out of control easily. Strenuous exercise, however, can precipitate hypoglycemia in an unprepared patient, and diabetics must therefore be taught to reduce their insulin dosage or take supplemental carbohydrate in anticipation of strenuous activity. Injection of insulin into a site farthest away from the muscles most involved in exercise may help ameliorate exercise-induced hypoglycemia, since insulin injected into exercising muscle is much more rapidly mobilized. With more knowledge regarding the relationship between caloric intake and expenditure and insulin requirements, the patient can become liberated from much of the regimentation imposed by the disorder.

E. Good Hygiene

All diabetic patients must receive adequate instruction on personal hygiene, especially with regard to care of the feet, skin, and teeth.

F. Infections

Infections with fever and severe illness provoke the release of high levels of insulin antagonists that will bring about a marked increase in insulin requirements. It is essential to limit the period of infection, since infection raises the blood glucose level and this, in turn, can impair the general defense mechanisms that the body uses against bacterial and even viral organisms. Thus, the early and sufficient use of bactericidal antibiotics is imperative. Type 1 diabetics must be taught how to supplement the regimen with regular insulin if persistent glycosuria and ketonuria occur—especially if associated with infection. Patients must understand that insulin therapy should never be withheld in the presence of gastric upset and vomiting if glycosuria with ketonuria is present. When food intake is limited by nausea or vomiting, the patient should take ginger ale, apple juice, or grape juice in small sips and should notify the physician in case supplemental intravenous fluids might be required.

G. Self-Monitoring of Blood Glucose Levels

Patients on insulin therapy and oral agents that can cause hypoglycemia should be instructed in techniques for self-monitoring of blood glucose (see above under blood glucose testing). Self-monitoring is useful in educating patients about the glycemic effects of specific foods in their diet and exercise and reduces the likelihood of unexpected episodes of severe hypoglycemia. Knowledge of the level of blood glucose has been particularly helpful at bedtime in ascertaining the need for supplementary feedings to avoid nocturnal hypoglycemia. Initially, blood glucose levels should be checked at least four times a day in patients taking multiple insulin injections. Generally, these measurements are taken before each meal and at bedtime. In addition, patients should be taught to check their blood glucose level whenever they develop symptoms that could represent a hypoglycemic episode. All blood glucose levels and their timing and corresponding insulin doses should be recorded in an organized fashion and brought with the patient for physician review during regularly scheduled checkups.

H. IDENTIFICATION BRACELET

All patients receiving hypoglycemic therapy should wear a Medic-Alert bracelet or necklace that clearly states that insulin or an oral sulfonylurea drug is being taken. A card in the wallet or purse is less useful, since legal problems may arise if a victim's person and belongings are searched without permission. (Information on how to obtain a Medic-Alert identification device can be obtained from the Medic-Alert Foundation, PO Box 1009, Turlock, CA 95380.)

I. RESTRICTIONS ON OCCUPATION

Certain occupations potentially hazardous to the diabetic patient or others will continue to be prohibited (eg, piloting airplanes, operating cranes).

Avoidance of Stress & Emotional Turmoil

Prevention of psychologic turmoil is of great importance in the control of diabetes, particularly when the disease is difficult to stabilize. One reason blood glucose control in diabetics may be particularly sensitive to emotional upset is that their pancreatic A cells are hyperresponsive to physiologic levels of epinephrine, producing excessive levels of glucagon with consequent hyperglycemia.

Specific Therapy

With the publication of data from the DCCT and the UKPDS, there has been a shift in the guidelines regarding acceptable levels of control. The ADA recommends that for both type 1 and type 2 patients, the goal is to achieve preprandial blood glucose values of 80–120 mg/dL and an average bedtime glucose of 100–140 mg/dL and HbA_{1c} of < 7% (nondiabetic range: 4–6%). Obviously, these goals should be modified taking into account the patient's ability to carry out the treatment regimen, the risk of severe hypoglycemia, and other patient factors that may reduce the benefit of such tight control.

Type 1 Diabetes

Type 1 patients require replacement therapy with exogenous insulin. This should be instituted under conditions of an individualized diabetic diet with multiple feedings and normal daily activities so that an appropriate dosage regimen can be developed.

At the onset of diabetes, many type 1 patients recover some pancreatic B cell function and may temporarily need only low doses of exogenous insulin to supplement their own endogenous insulin secretion. This is known as the "honeymoon period." Within 8 weeks to 2 years, however, most of these patients show either absent or negligible pancreatic B cell function. At this point, these patients should be switched to a more flexible insulin regimen with a combination of short-acting or ultrashort-acting insulin together with intermediate-acting or long-acting insulin. At a minimum, the patient should be on a three-injection regimen, and frequently four or more injections. Twice-daily split-dose insulin mixtures cannot maintain near-normalization of blood glucose without hypoglycemia (particularly at night) and are not recommended. Self-monitoring of blood glucose levels is a requisite for determining the optimal adjustment of insulin dosage and the modulation of food intake and exercise in type 1 diabetes.

A. INSULIN REGIMENS

Certain caveats should be kept in mind regarding insulin treatment. Considerable variations in absorption and bioavailability exist, even when the same dose is injected in the same region on different days in the same individual. Such variation often can be minimized by injecting smaller quantities of insulin at each injection and consequently using multiple injections. Furthermore, a given insulin dosage may demonstrate considerable variability in pharmacokinetics in different individuals, either because of insulin antibodies that bind insulin with different avidity or for other as yet unknown reasons. A properly educated patient should be taught to adjust insulin dosage by observing the pattern of recorded self-monitored blood glucose levels and correlating it with the approximate duration of action and the time to peak effect after injection of the various insulin preparations (Table 17–15). Adjustments should be made gradually—not more often than every 2 or 3 days if possible.

1. Intensive multiple-dose insulin therapy—Small doses of regular insulin injected three times a day before

Table 17–15. Typical patterns of overnight blood glucose levels and serum free immunoreactive insulin levels in prebreakfast hyperglycemia due to various causes in patients with type 1 diabetes.

	Blood Glucose Levels (mg/dL)			Serum Free Immunoreactive Insulin Levels (μU/mL)		
	10 PM	3 AM	7 AM	10 PM	3 AM	7 AM
Somogyi effect	90	40	200	High	Slightly high	Normal
"Dawn phenomenon"	110	110	150	Normal	Normal	Normal
Waning of circulating insulin levels plus "dawn phenomenon"	110	190	220	Normal	Low	Low
Waning of circulating insulin levels plus "dawn phenomenon" plus Somogyi effect	110	40	380	High	Normal	Low

meals with one injection of NPH insulin at bedtime is a commonly used regimen (Table 17–16). The advent of pen injectors has made such multiple injection regimens more convenient.

The ultrashort-acting insulin analogs have been advocated as a safer and much more convenient alternative to regular insulin for preprandial use in regimens of intensive insulin therapy. In clinical studies, combinations of ultrashort-acting insulin analogs (insulin lispro or insulin aspart) with meals together with intermediate-acting (NPH) or longer-acting insulin (ultralente, insulin glargine) for basal coverage have now been shown to have improved HbA$_{1c}$ values with less hypoglycemia when compared with a regimen of regular insulin with meals and NPH at night.

Table 17–13 illustrates some regimens that might be appropriate for a 70 kg person with type 1 diabetes eating meals of standard carbohydrate intake and moderate to low fat content.

2. Intensive insulin therapy using insulin pumps— Continuous subcutaneous insulin infusion (CSII) by portable battery-operated "open loop" devices currently provides the most flexible approach, allowing the setting of different basal rates throughout the 24 hours and permitting patients to delay or skip meals and vary meal size and composition (see Methods of Insulin Administration, above). The dosage is usually based on providing 50% of the estimated insulin dose as basal and the remainder as intermittent boluses prior to meals. For example, a 70-kg man requiring 35 units of insulin per day may require a basal rate of 0.7 units per hour throughout the 24 hours with the exception of 3 AM to 8 AM, when 0.8 units per hour might be appropriate (for the dawn phenomenon). The meal bolus would depend on the carbohydrate content of the meal and the premeal blood glucose value. One unit per 15 g

of carbohydrate plus 1 unit for 50 mg/dL of blood glucose above a target value (eg, 120 mg/dL) is a common starting point. Further adjustments to basal and bolus dosages would depend on the results of blood glucose monitoring. Most patients use the ultrashort-acting insulin analogs in the pumps. Patients using regular insulin should use the buffered insulin preparation (Velosulin) to minimize the risk of precipitation of the insulin in the pump tubing.

3. Selection of patients for intensive insulin therapy—Which regimen and what blood glucose target is appropriate for an individual patient depend on a number of factors such as the stage of the disease, the presence of complications, and the patient's age, motivation, and self-management skills. Patients with autonomic neuropathy and reduced awareness of hypoglycemia might be advised to maintain higher target blood glucose levels. Patients with retinopathy should control blood glucose levels slowly and with careful attention to possible progression of retinal disease (see Ophthalmologic Complications, below).

5. Management of early morning hyperglycemia in type 1 patients—

a. Etiology and diagnosis—One of the more difficult therapeutic problems in managing patients with type 1 diabetes is determining the proper adjustment of insulin dose when the early morning blood glucose level is high before breakfast. Prebreakfast hyperglycemia is sometimes due to the **Somogyi effect,** in which nocturnal hypoglycemia evokes a surge of counterregulatory hormones to produce high blood glucose levels by 7 AM. However, a more common cause of prebreakfast hyperglycemia is the **waning of circulating insulin levels,** which requires use of more (rather than less) intermediate insulin in the evening. These two

Table 17–16. Guidelines for regular and NPH insulin regimens in patients with type 1 diabetes mellitus.

DATE:_____ Type 1 DM patients:_____

YOUR BASIC DAILY DOSE OF INSULIN

Inject regular insulin 30 minutes before meals or as directed by your physician.[1]

INSULIN	BREAKFAST	LUNCH	DINNER	BEDTIME[2]
Regular	_____	_____	_____	_____
NPH	_____	_____	_____	_____

BLOOD GLUCOSE TESTING

The goal of insulin therapy is to lower your blood glucose levels to just above normal values. Here are some acceptable targets to aim for. Keep a daily record of your blood glucose concentrations. Test _4_ times daily.

TEST TIME		ACCEPTABLE BLOOD GLUCOSE TARGET[3]
Fasting (first morning test before breakfast)	95 to 150 mg/dL	_____
Before meals	95 to 140 mg/dL	_____
Two hours after meals	Less than 180 mg/dL	_____

SUPPLEMENTING YOUR BASIC INSULIN DOSE-REGULAR INSULIN

Once your basic dose of insulin has been established, you will learn to adjust your dose based upon blood glucose measurements before meals.

Supplement your basic insulin dose with regular insulin as indicated: If your glucose before the meal is in the following range:

2 units less	70–85 mg/dL[4]
1 unit less	85–95 mg/dL
no change	95–140 mg/dL
1 unit extra	141–180 mg/dL
2 units extra	181–220 mg/dL
3 units extra	221–260 mg/dL
4 units extra[5]	261–300 mg/dL
For glucose greater than 300	Check the urine for ketones. If POSITIVE call physician.

SIGNATURE:_____   DATE:_____

Footnote 1:
Doses depend on body size, exercise patterns, food consumption, and general sensitivity to insulin. This is an example of a regimen for a 70-kg adult type 1 diabetes patient receiving six feedings per day with average carbohydrate intake and limited exercise:

Insulin	Breakfast	Lunch	Dinner	Bedtime
Regular	8 units	7 units	10 units	—
NPH	2 units	—	—	8 units

Footnote 2:
Regular insulin is generally not recommended at bedtime. However, if blood glucose exceeds 300 mg/dL, 2 or 3 units of regular insulin may precede a bedtime snack. Adjustments of bedtime NPH insulin depends on prebreakfast blood glucose values. If they are between 141 and 180 mg/dL for three mornings, add 1 unit NPH to the basic bedtime dose, or if 181–250 mg/dL, add 2 units NPH.

Footnote 3:
In patients with hypoglycemia unawareness, autonomic neuropathy, advanced age, or with cardiac or cerebral atherosclerosis, good glucose targets should be adjusted upward appropriately. Pregnant patients may require downward adjustment of target glucose values (Chapter 16).

Footnote 4:
If blood glucose is less than 70 mg/dL, no insulin is given until 30 minutes after a carbohydrate snack, when blood glucose is checked to ascertain insulin dosage.

Footnote 5:
If extra (or reduced) insulin is consistently needed at a given time period, appropriate adjustments should be made in either the basic insulin dose, food consumption, or exercise during the interval *prior* to the time the unsatisfactory blood glucose measurement was generated.

phenomena are not mutually exclusive and can occur together to produce a greater magnitude of hyperglycemia in affected patients with type 1 diabetes. A third phenomenon—the **"dawn phenomenon"**—has been reported to occur in as many as 75% of type 1 patients and in the majority of type 2 patients and normal subjects as well. It is characterized by a reduced tissue sensitivity to insulin between 5 AM and 8 AM (dawn), and apparently is evoked by spikes of growth hormone released hours before, at onset of sleep. When the "dawn phenomenon" occurs alone, it may produce only mild hyperglycemia in the early morning; however, when it is associated with either or both of the other phenomena, it can further aggravate the hyperglycemia (Table 17–15). Diagnosis of the cause of prebreakfast hyperglycemia can be facilitated by asking the patient to self-monitor blood glucose levels at 3 AM in addition to monitoring at the usual times, bedtime and 7 AM. When this was done, the Somogyi effect was found to be much less prevalent and of lower magnitude as a cause of prebreakfast hyperglycemia than had been previously suspected. In insulin-treated patients, serum levels of free immunoreactive insulin (particularly in the basal or low ranges) are difficult to quantitate accurately because of technical interference from circulating insulin antibodies. In specialized research laboratories, however, free insulin levels have been measured in hospitalized patients with prebreakfast hyperglycemia (Table 17–15).

b. Treatment—When a particular pattern emerges from monitoring blood glucose levels at 10 PM, 3 AM, and 7 AM, appropriate therapeutic measures can be taken. Prebreakfast hyperglycemia due to the Somogyi effect can be treated by either reducing the dose of intermediate insulin at supper, giving a portion of it at bedtime, or supplying more food at bedtime. When the "dawn phenomenon" alone is present, shifting a portion of the intermediate insulin from dinnertime to bedtime often suffices. Insulin glargine given at bedtime results in lower fasting glucose values when compared with bedtime NPH. When insulin pumps are used, the "dawn phenomenon" can be controlled by stepping up the basal infusion rate (eg, from 0.8 unit/h to 1 unit/h) from 6 AM until breakfast. Finally, in cases in which the circulating insulin level is waning, either increasing the evening insulin dose or, preferably, shifting it from dinnertime to bedtime (or both) may be efficacious. Switching to ultralente insulin or insulin glargine or insulin pump administration can also solve this problem.

B. Type 2 Diabetes

The principles of therapy are less well defined in this heterogeneous group of diabetic patients than is the case with type 1 diabetes. Therapeutic recommendations are based upon the relative contributions of B cell insufficiency and insulin insensitivity in individual patients. With prolonged duration of type 2 diabetes, deposits of amyloid accumulate in islets and encroach on pancreatic B cells, resulting in progressive diminution of insulin-secretory capacity.

1. The obese patient—The most common type of patient with type 2 diabetes is obese with insulin insensitivity. Characteristically, obese patients compensate for their insulin resistance with increased basal levels of circulating insulin and are capable of responding to a glucose load with hypersecretion of insulin. However, as hyperglycemia progresses, the insulin response to a glucose load decreases. This refractoriness of the B cell may be partially reversed with therapeutic correction of the hyperglycemia and seems to be selectively related to the hyperglycemic stimulation, since other B cell-stimulating agents such as sulfonylureas, arginine, and glucagon still provoke rapid insulin release.

a. Weight reduction—One of the primary modes of therapy in the obese type 2 diabetic patient is weight reduction. Normalization of glycemia can be achieved by reducing adipose stores, with consequent restoration of tissue sensitivity to insulin. A combination of caloric restriction, increased exercise, modification of behavior, and consistent reinforcement of good eating habits is required if a weight reduction program is to be successful. Knowledge of the symptoms of diabetes and an understanding of the risks and complications of diabetes often increase the patient's motivation for weight reduction. Even so, significant weight loss is seldom achieved and even more difficult to maintain in the morbidly obese patient. Weight control is variable in moderately obese patients depending on the enthusiasm of the therapist and the motivation of the patient. Orlistat is a reversible inhibitor of gastric and pancreatic lipases and prevents the hydrolysis of dietary triglycerides. These triglycerides are then excreted in the feces. In a 1-year study in obese patients with type 2 diabetes, those taking orlistat had lost more weight, had lower HbA$_{1c}$ values, and had improved lipid profiles. The main adverse reactions were gastrointestinal, with oily spotting, oily stool, flatus, and fecal urgency and frequency. Malabsorption of fat-soluble vitamins also occurs, and patients should take a multivitamin tablet containing fat-soluble vitamins at least 2 hours before or 2 hours after the administration of orlistat.

b. Hypoglycemic agents—Hypoglycemic agents, including insulin as well as the oral hypoglycemic drugs are generally *not* indicated for long-term use in the obese patient with mild diabetes. A weight reduction program can be disrupted by real or imagined hypoglycemic reactions when insulin therapy is used, and weight gain is quite common in the insulin-treated obese diabetic patient. Metformin, an insulin-sparing agent and one that does not increase weight or provoke hypoglycemia, offers obvious advantages over insulin or sulfonylureas in treating hyperglycemia in obese patients.

If metformin therapy (combined with a weight reduction regimen) is inadequate in achieving target glucose values, a thiazolidinedione or a sulfonylurea should be added. Some individuals may require metformin, a thiazolidinedione, and a sulfonylurea to achieve adequate glycemic control. Insulin therapy should be instituted if the combination of these three drugs fails to restore euglycemia. Weight-reducing interventions should continue and may allow for simplification of this regimen in the future.

2. The nonobese patient—In the nonobese type 2 diabetic with moderately severe hyperglycemia, pancreatic B cells are refractory to glucose stimulation. Peripheral insulin resistance is also detectable but is considerably less intense than in obese diabetics who have a comparable degree of hyperglycemia; it is also of less therapeutic import, since insulin-treated nonobese patients do not generally need an excessive dosage of insulin.

a. Diet—If hyperglycemia is mild (fasting blood glucose levels of < 200 mg/dL [11.1 mmol/L]), normal metabolic control can occasionally be restored by a diet devoid of simple sugars and with calories calculated to maintain ideal body weight. Restriction of saturated fats and cholesterol is also strongly advised. An individualized diet with a recommended exchange list should be prescribed for these nonobese type 2 patients.

b. Oral agents for hyperglycemia—When diet therapy alone is not sufficient to correct hyperglycemia, a trial of oral antihyperglycemic drugs is indicated to supplement the dietary regimen. In the nonobese type 2 patient, sulfonylureas are generally the first-line oral drug of choice, and metformin or thiazolidinediones (or both) are added later if glycemic control is inadequate. Failing this, these individuals will require insulin.

c. Insulin—When the combination of metformin, a sulfonylurea, and a thiazolidinedione fails and type 2 patients require insulin, various insulin regimens may be effective (Table 17–13). There is no consensus about how insulin therapy should be instituted. One proposed regimen adds a bedtime intermediate-acting insulin to reduce excessive nocturnal hepatic glucose output while continuing daytime sulfonylurea therapy. If the patient remains hyperglycemic during the day, an additional insulin dosage can be added in the morning and the daytime sulfonylurea can be discontinued. The most popular insulin regimen under these circumstances is to use a split dose of a fixed 70:30 mixture of NPH:regular insulin before breakfast and before dinner, and this can be adjusted appropriately depending on premeal and bedtime blood glucose values. If more than 50 units per day does not achieve satisfactory glycemic control, these patients may benefit from more intensive multiple-injection regimens as described for type 1 patients. Metformin principally reduces hepatic glucose output and the thiazolidinediones improve peripheral resistance, and it is a reasonable option to continue these drugs when insulin therapy is instituted because they may permit the use of lower doses of insulin and simpler regimens.

Immunopathology of Insulin Therapy

At least five molecular classes of insulin antibodies are produced during the course of insulin therapy: IgA, IgD, IgE, IgG, and IgM. Human insulin is much less antigenic than the older animal (especially beef) insulins, but because of its hexameric presentation at therapeutic injection doses, it is also treated as a foreign substance by the immune system and results in detectable—albeit low—titers of insulin antibodies in most patients.

A. INSULIN ALLERGY

Insulin allergy, a hypersensitivity reaction of the immediate type, is a rare condition in which local or systemic urticaria occurs immediately after insulin injection. This reaction is due to histamine release from tissue mast cells sensitized by adherence of IgE antibodies to their surface. In severe cases, anaphylaxis can occur. The appearance of a subcutaneous nodule at the site of insulin injection, occurring several hours after the injection and lasting for up to 24 hours, has been attributed to an IgG-mediated complement-binding Arthus reaction. Because sensitivity was often due to noninsulin protein contaminants, the highly purified insulins have markedly reduced the incidence of insulin allergy, especially of the local variety. Antihistamines, corticosteroids, and even desensitization may be required, especially for systemic hypersensitivity in an insulin-dependent patient. A protocol for allergy testing and insulin desensitization is available from the Eli Lilly Company. A trial of insulin analogs should also be considered. There is a case report of successful use of insulin lispro in the face of generalized allergy to human insulin.

B. IMMUNE INSULIN RESISTANCE

All patients who receive insulin (including insulin analogs) develop a low titer of circulating IgG antibodies, and this neutralizes to a small extent the rapid action of insulin. With the old animal insulins, a high titer of circulating antibodies sometimes developed, resulting in extremely high insulin requirements, often to more than 200 units/d. This is now very rarely seen with the switch to the highly purified pork or human insulins and has not been reported with use of the analogs.

C. LIPODYSTROPHY AT INJECTION SITES

Rarely, a disfiguring atrophy of subcutaneous fatty tissue occurs at the site of insulin injection. Although the cause of this complication is obscure, it seems to represent a form of immune reaction, particularly since it occurs predominantly in females and is associated with lymphocyte infiltration in the lipoatrophic area. This complication has become even less common since the development of highly purified insulin preparations of neutral pH. Injection of highly purified preparations of insulin directly into the atrophic area often results in restoration of normal contours.

Lipohypertrophy, on the other hand, is not a consequence of immune responses; rather, it seems to be due to the pharmacologic effects of depositing insulin in the same location repeatedly. It can occur with purified insulins and is best treated with localized liposuction of the hypertrophic areas by an experienced plastic surgeon. It is prevented by rotation of injection sites. There is a case report of a patient who had intractable lipohypertrophy (fatty infiltration of injection site) with human insulin but no longer had the problem when he switched to insulin lispro.

◼ ACUTE COMPLICATIONS OF DIABETES MELLITUS

HYPOGLYCEMIA

Hypoglycemic reactions (see below and Chapter 18) are the most common complications that occur in insulin-treated diabetic patients. They may also occur in patients taking oral sulfonylureas, especially older patients or those with impaired liver or kidney function treated with long-acting and highly potent agents such as chlorpropamide or glyburide. Hypoglycemia may result from delay in taking a meal or from unusual physical exertion without supplemental calories or a decrease in insulin dose.

Clinical Features

Signs and symptoms of hypoglycemia may be divided into those resulting from neuroglycopenia (insufficient glucose for normal central nervous system function leading to confusion and coma) and those resulting from stimulation of the autonomic nervous system. There is great variation in the pattern of hypoglycemic signs and symptoms from patient to patient; however, individual patients tend to experience the same pattern from episode to episode. In older diabetics, in patients with frequent hypoglycemic episodes, and in those with diabetic autonomic neuropathy, autonomic responses may be blunted or absent, so that hypoglycemia may be manifested only by signs and symptoms of neuroglycopenia. The gradual onset of hypoglycemia with intermediate-acting or long-acting insulin also makes recognition more difficult in older patients.

A. NEUROGLYCOPENIA

Signs and symptoms of neuroglycopenia include mental confusion with impaired abstract and, later, concrete thought processes; this may be followed by bizarre antagonistic behavior. Stupor, coma, and even death may occur with profound hypoglycemia. Full recovery of central nervous system function does not always occur if treatment is delayed.

B. AUTONOMIC HYPERACTIVITY

Signs and symptoms of autonomic hyperactivity can be both adrenergic (tachycardia, palpitations, sweating, tremulousness) and parasympathetic (nausea, hunger). Except for sweating, most of the sympathetic symptoms of hypoglycemia are blunted in patients receiving beta-blocking agents for angina or hypertension. Though not absolutely contraindicated, these drugs must be used with great caution in insulin-requiring diabetics.

C. COUNTERREGULATORY RESPONSES TO HYPOGLYCEMIA

(Table 17–17.)

1. Normal counterregulation—When plasma glucose is acutely lowered in normal subjects by intravenous insulin, a rapid surge of both glucagon and epinephrine acts to counterregulate the hypoglycemia. The hormonal responses tend to begin after plasma glucose falls below 70 mg/dL (3.9 mmol/L). If they fail to correct the decline of plasma glucose, symptoms of autonomic hyperactivity usually become apparent once plasma glucose falls below 60 mg/dL (3.3 mmol/L). Plasma glucagon is considered the first line of defense against acute hypoglycemia, while the role of epinephrine and the sympathetic system is to provide a backup system. The latter helps to restore euglycemia and serves as an

Table 17–17. Counterregulatory responses to hypoglycemia.

Normal Counterregulation	Defective Counterregulation in Type 1 Diabetes[1]
Glucagon rises rapidly to three to five times baseline after insulin-induced hypoglycemia, provoking hepatic glycogenolysis.	Glucagon response to insulin-induced hypoglycemia is lost after onset of type 1 diabetes.
Adrenergic discharge (1) raises hepatic glucose output by glycogenolysis and (2) provides warning to subject of impending hypoglycemic crisis.	Blunted or absent adrenergic response may occur as a result of– (1) Neural damage associated with advanced age or autonomic neuropathy (2) Neural dysfunction (iatrogenic) from frequent hypoglycemia or (?) human insulin therapy

[1]Type 2 diabetics are less well characterized as to their defective counterregulation of glucagon loss but appear to have the same frequency and causes of adrenergic loss as do type 1 diabetics.

alarm system to warn the subject of the urgent need for carbohydrate intake in case the counterregulatory response is inadequate to prevent the potentially disastrous consequences of life-threatening neuroglycopenia.

2. Defective counterregulation in diabetes—For unexplained reasons, patients with type 1 diabetes uniformly lose their ability to secrete glucagon in response to acute insulin-induced hypoglycemia (but not in the presence of amino acids in protein-containing meals) within a few years after developing diabetes. After that time, they are solely dependent upon triggered autonomic adrenergic responses to counteract an impending hypoglycemic crisis as well as for early warning. It is well documented that with advanced age these autonomic responses may be blunted considerably, and in diabetic patients with clinical autonomic neuropathy as a complication of diabetes they may be absent. In these circumstances, reduced awareness of hypoglycemia can lead to potentially life-threatening sequelae from neuroglycopenic convulsions or coma.

3. "Iatrogenic" autonomic failure—Cryer has proposed that frequent and recurrent hypoglycemic episodes such as may be encountered in patients receiving intensive insulin therapy to achieve normoglycemia may result in failure of the sympathetic nervous system to respond to hypoglycemia. Adaptation of the central nervous system to recurrent hypoglycemic episodes is associated with increased glucose transport into the brain despite subnormal levels of plasma glucose. This results from up-regulation of glucose transporter 1 at the blood-brain barrier induced by recurrent hypoglycemia. The threshold for recognizing hypoglycemia is thereby altered, so that much lower plasma glucose levels are needed to trigger an autonomic response— and by the time this occurs, cognition may already be impaired in some cases, with onset of neuroglycopenia.

That this adaptation and autonomic failure is a consequence of chronic hypoglycemia and not diabetes is evidenced by reports of patients with insulinomas who had chronic recurrent episodes of hypoglycemia of which they often were unaware. These were patients who had loss of epinephrine responses and symptoms during acute insulin-induced hypoglycemia and whose symptoms and adrenergic responses during repeat testing returned to normal after euglycemia had been restored following resection of the insulinomas. This documented reversibility of the syndrome of hypoglycemia unawareness due to chronic hypoglycemia has exciting implications for therapy of those diabetic patients whose unawareness may be iatrogenic as a result of recurrent hypoglycemia during attempts at normalization of blood glucose with intensive insulin therapy.

4. Human insulin and hypoglycemic unawareness—In 1987, a preliminary report contended that hypoglycemia unawareness became more prevalent in diabetics transferred from beef-pork to human insulin. Although occasional studies gave support to this claim, most investigators failed to find evidence for a detrimental effect of human insulin on recognition of hypoglycemia. There is some evidence that many of the anecdotal reports of loss of hypoglycemic awareness after changing from animal to human insulin may be a consequence of an increased number of hypoglycemic episodes. The latter may occur on switching from animal to human insulin if the switch is made at equivalent or nearly equivalent dosages without taking the precaution of using a lower human insulin dose to compensate for the reduced neutralization of the injected insulin by preexisting anti-beef or anti-pork insulin antibodies. Another possible cause of more frequent hypoglycemic episodes is the inclination of patients and their physicians to attempt tighter glycemic control when switching from animal to human insulin as part of a general upgrading of diabetes care. As evidenced by the results of the Diabetes Control and Complications Trial (DCCT), the risk of frequent hypoglycemic episodes is greatly increased when "normalization" of the blood glucose is attempted with present suboptimal methods of insulin delivery, and this was independent of the species of insulin used in the DCCT. Although the controversy has not been completely resolved, most authorities do not recommend restricting the use of human insulin because of fear of hypoglycemia.

D. MANAGEMENT OF HYPOGLYCEMIC UNAWARENESS

(Table 17–18.) Avoiding recurrent hypoglycemia is the main principle of therapy to restore hypoglycemic awareness. Many insulin-treated diabetics have nocturnal episodes of hypoglycemia of which they are often unaware. These may be detected only with screening by capillary blood testing at least once a week at 2–3 AM. If such episodes do occur, appropriate reduction of evening insulin doses or an increase in the amount of food taken as a snack at bedtime should be advised.

When hypoglycemic unawareness occurs while the patient is awake, two patterns of presentation have been described. In some cases, patients appear perfectly alert with no obvious neuroglycopenia or adrenergic symptoms when a scheduled preprandial capillary blood glucose measurement indicates a level below 40 or 50

Table 17–18. Hypoglycemic "unawareness" in type 1 diabetes mellitus.

I. Sleeping patient (nocturnal hypoglycemia)
II. Hypoglycemia with unawareness while awake—
   A. Manifestations:
      1. Without detectable neuroglycopenia:
         a. Adaptation to chronic hypoglycemia (increased brain glucose transporter I)
      2. With neuroglycopenia:
         a. Maladaptation to hypoglycemia
   B. Mechanisms:
      1. Defective autonomic response:
         a. Due to diabetic autonomic neuropathy
         b. Iatrogenic
            i. Frequent hypoglycemia
            ii. Human insulin therapy (?)
   C. Management:
      1. Identify patients at risk and reevaluate glycemic goals
      2. Advise frequent self-monitoring of blood glucose
      3. Learn to detect subtle symptoms of neuroglycopenia
      4. Avoid recurrent hypoglycemia
      5. Frequent snacks should be prescribed
      6. Multiple small doses of insulin may be needed
      7. Injectable glucagon made available to family

---

mg/dL (2.2 or 2.7 mmol/L). This suggests some degree of adaptation with probable provision of increased glucose transporter-1 proteins among brain capillaries to provide minimum requirements of glucose to the brain despite the hypoglycemia. These patients are at increased risk, however, of developing severe neuroglycopenia if hypoglycemia progresses.

In the second pattern of presentation, patients exhibit neuroglycopenia and progress to require assistance for recovery without having had any awareness of the impending crisis. This form of unawareness is life-threatening and requires immediate measures to prevent recurrences.

When either of these patterns of hypoglycemic unawareness presents while the patient is awake, careful evaluation for autonomic neuropathy with reduced or absent adrenergic responses is indicated. Evidence for this condition consists of orthostatic hypotension or a fixed heart rate measured during a change in position, during respiration, or after a Valsalva maneuver.

If autonomic neuropathy is detected, glycemic target goals should be appropriately raised by lowering the daily insulin dosage and ensuring that it is administered in multiple small doses, which have a more predictable pharmacokinetic pattern than do larger depot injections. To further lower the risk of severe hypoglycemic episodes, the frequency of self-monitoring of blood glucose should be increased to provide awareness of glycemic status at regular intervals, and patients should be trained to detect subtle signs or symptoms of autonomic responses they might otherwise overlook.

In patients without obvious autonomic neuropathy who have lost awareness to hypoglycemia, special efforts should be made to avoid hypoglycemia for weeks or months in order to reverse central nervous system adaptation to recurrent hypoglycemia. This can be done by increasing the frequency of self-monitoring of blood glucose, raising the mean blood glucose level to be targeted, eating frequent small snacks, and reducing the size of insulin doses at any one injection.

Treatment

All of the manifestations of hypoglycemia are rapidly relieved by glucose administration. Because of the danger of insulin reactions, diabetic patients should carry packets of table sugar or a candy roll at all times for use at the onset of hypoglycemic symptoms. Tablets containing 3 g of glucose are available. The educated patient soon learns to take the amount of glucose needed to correct symptoms without ingesting excessive quantities of orange juice or candy, which can provoke very high glycemic levels. Family members or friends of the patient should be provided with a glucagon emergency kit (Lilly), which contains a syringe, diluent, and a 1 mg ampule of glucagon that can be injected intramuscularly if the patient is found unconscious; these kits are available by prescription. Detailed instructions in the use of glucagon are an essential part of the diabetic education program. An identification MedicAlert bracelet, necklace, or card in the wallet or purse should be carried by every diabetic receiving hypoglycemic drug therapy. The telephone number for the Medic-Alert Foundation International in Turlock, California, is 800-ID-ALERT.

A. THE CONSCIOUS PATIENT

Patients with symptoms of hypoglycemia who are conscious and able to swallow should eat or drink orange juice, glucose tablets, or any sugar-containing beverage or food except pure fructose (which does not cross the blood-brain barrier).

B. THE UNCONSCIOUS PATIENT

In general, oral feeding is contraindicated in stuporous or unconscious patients. The preferred treatment is 50 mL of 50% glucose solution given rapidly over 3–5 minutes. If trained personnel are not available to administer intravenous glucose, the treatment of choice is for a family member or friend to administer 1 mg of glucagon intramuscularly (see above), which will usually restore the patient to consciousness within 10–15 minutes; the patient should then be given an oral form of sugar to ingest. If glucagon is not available, small amounts of honey, syrup, or glucose gel can be rubbed into the buccal mucosa. Rectal administration of syrup or honey (30 mL per 500 mL of warm water) has also been used effectively.

COMA

Coma is a *medical emergency* calling for immediate evaluation to determine its cause so that proper therapy can be started. There are several causes of coma that result directly from diabetes mellitus or its treatment. When evaluating a comatose diabetic patient, these must be considered *in addition* to the myriad causes included in the differential diagnosis of coma (cerebrovascular accidents, head trauma, intoxication with alcohol or other drugs, etc).

Etiologic Classification of Diabetic Coma

The causes of coma resulting directly from diabetes mellitus or its treatment include the following:

A. HYPERGLYCEMIC COMA

Hyperglycemic coma may be associated with either severe insulin deficiency (diabetic ketoacidosis) or with mild to moderate insulin deficiency (hyperglycemic, hyperosmolar, nonketotic coma).

B. HYPOGLYCEMIC COMA

This results from excessive doses of insulin or certain oral hypoglycemic agents (see above).

C. LACTIC ACIDOSIS

Lactic acidosis in diabetics is particularly apt to occur in association with severe tissue anoxia, sepsis, or cardiovascular collapse.

Emergency Management of Coma

The standard approach to *any comatose patient* is outlined below. Prompt action is required.

(1) Establish an airway.

(2) Establish intravenous access. About 30 mL of blood should be drawn and sent for complete blood count, serum electrolyte determinations, renal function and liver function tests, and blood glucose measurements.

(3) Administer 50 mL of 50% dextrose in water to all comatose patients, unless bedside monitoring of blood glucose shows hyperglycemia.

(4) Administer 1 ampule (0.4 mg) of naloxone intravenously and 100 mg of thiamine intravenously. (See also Chapter 24.)

Diagnosis of Coma

After emergency measures have been instituted, a careful history (from family, friends, paramedics, etc), physical examination, and laboratory evaluation are required to resolve the differential diagnosis. Patients in deep coma from a hyperosmolar nonketotic state or from hypoglycemia are generally flaccid and have quiet breathing—in contrast to patients with acidosis, whose respirations are rapid and deep if the pH of arterial blood has dropped to 7.1 or below. When hypoglycemia is a cause of the coma, hypothermia is usually present and the state of hydration is usually normal. Although the clinical laboratory remains the final arbiter in confirming the diagnosis, a rapid *estimation* of blood glucose and ketones can be obtained by the use of bedside glucose and ketone meters (see Laboratory Findings in Diabetes Mellitus, above). Table 17–19 is a summary of some laboratory abnormalities found in diabetic patients with coma attributable to diabetes or its treatment. The individual clinical syndromes are discussed in detail on the following pages.

1. Diabetic Ketoacidosis

This acute complication of diabetes mellitus may be the first manifestation of previously undiagnosed type 1 diabetes or may result from increased insulin requirements in type 1 diabetes patients during the course of infection, trauma, myocardial infarction, or surgery. It

Table 17–19. Summary of some laboratory abnormalities in patients with coma directly attributable to diabetes or its treatment.

	Urine			Plasma		
	Glucose	**Acetone**	**Glucose**	**Bicarbonate**	**Acetone**	**Osmolality**
Hyperglycemia, hyperosmolar coma Diabetic ketoacidosis	++ to ++++	++++	High	Low	++++	+++
Hyperglycemic nonketotic coma	++ to ++++	0 or +[1]	High	Normal or slightly low[2]	0	++++
Hypoglycemia	0[3]	0 or +	Low	Normal	0	Normal
Lactic acidosis	0 to +	0 or +	Normal, low, or high	Low	0 or +	Normal

[1] A small degree of ketonuria may be present if the patient is severely stressed or has not been eating because of illness.
[2] A patient may be acidotic if there is severe volume depletion with cardiovascular collapse or if sepsis is present.
[3] Leftover urine in bladder might still contain sugar from earlier hyperglycemia.

is a life-threatening medical emergency with a mortality rate just under 5% in individuals under 40 years of age but with a more ominous prognosis in the elderly, who have mortality rates over 20%. In all cases, precipitating factors such as infection should be searched for and treated appropriately. Poor compliance, either for psychological reasons or because of inadequate patient education, is probably the most common cause of diabetic ketoacidosis, particularly when episodes are recurrent. In adolescents with type 1 diabetes, recurrent episodes of severe ketoacidosis often indicate the need for counseling to alter this behavior.

Diabetic ketoacidosis has been found to be one of the more common serious complications of insulin pump therapy, occurring in approximately one per 80 patient months of treatment. Many patients who monitor capillary blood glucose regularly ignore urine ketone measurements, which would signal the possibility of insulin leakage or pump failure before serious illness develops.

Patients with type 2 diabetes may also develop ketoacidosis under severe stress such as sepsis, trauma, or major surgery.

Pathogenesis

Acute insulin deficiency results in rapid mobilization of energy from stores in muscle and fat depots, leading to an increased flux of amino acids to the liver for conversion to glucose and of fatty acids for conversion to ketones (acetoacetate, β-hydroxybutyrate, and acetone). In addition to this increased availability of precursor, there is a direct effect of the low insulin:glucagon ratio on the liver that promotes increased production of ketones as well as of glucose. In response to both the acute insulin deficiency and the metabolic stress of ketosis, the levels of insulin-antagonistic hormones (corticosteroids, catecholamines, glucagon, and GH) are consistently elevated. Furthermore, in the absence of insulin, peripheral utilization of glucose and ketones is reduced. The combination of increased production and decreased utilization leads to an accumulation of these substances in blood, with plasma glucose levels reaching 500 mg/dL (27.8 mmol/L) or more and plasma ketones reaching levels of 8–15 mmol/L or more.

The hyperglycemia causes osmotic diuresis leading to depletion of intravascular volume. As this progresses, impaired renal blood flow reduces the kidney's ability to excrete glucose, and hyperosmolality is worsened. Severe hyperosmolality (> 330 mosm/kg) correlates closely with central nervous system depression and coma.

In a similar manner, impaired renal excretion of hydrogen ions aggravates the metabolic acidosis that occurs as a result of the accumulation of the ketone acids, β-hydroxybutyrate and acetoacetate. The accumulation of ketones may cause vomiting, which exacerbates the intravascular volume depletion. In addition, prolonged acidosis can compromise cardiac output and reduce vascular tone. The result may be severe cardiovascular collapse with generation of lactic acid, which then adds to the already existent metabolic acidosis.

Clinical Features

A. SYMPTOMS AND SIGNS

As opposed to the acute onset of hypoglycemic coma, the appearance of diabetic ketoacidosis is usually preceded by a day or more of polyuria and polydipsia associated with marked fatigue, nausea, and vomiting.

Eventually, mental stupor ensues and can progress to frank coma. On physical examination, evidence of dehydration in a stuporous patient with rapid and deep respirations and the "fruity" breath odor of acetone would strongly suggest the diagnosis. Postural hypotension with tachycardia indicates profound dehydration and salt depletion. Abdominal pain and even tenderness may be present in the absence of abdominal disease, and mild hypothermia is usually present.

B. LABORATORY FINDINGS

Four-plus glycosuria, strong ketonuria, hyperglycemia, ketonemia, low arterial blood pH, and low plasma bicarbonate (5–15 mEq/L) are typical laboratory findings in diabetic ketoacidosis. Serum potassium is usually normal or slightly elevated (5–8 mEq/L) despite total body potassium depletion, because of the shift of potassium from the intracellular to extracellular spaces that occurs in systemic acidosis. The average total body potassium deficit resulting from osmotic diuresis, acidosis, and gastrointestinal losses is about 5–10 mEq/kg body weight. Similarly, serum phosphate is elevated (6–7 mg/dL), but total body phosphate is generally depleted. Serum sodium is generally reduced (to about 125–130 mEq/L) because severe hyperglycemia pulls intercellular water into the interstitial compartment, thereby diluting the already depleted sodium ions lost by polyuria and vomiting. (For every 100 mg/dL of plasma glucose above normal, serum sodium decreases by 1.6 mEq/L.) Serum osmolality can be directly measured by standard tests of freezing-point depression or can be estimated by calculating the molarity of sodium, chloride, and glucose in the serum. A convenient formula for estimating *effective* serum osmolality is as follows (physiologic values in humans are generally between 280 and 300 mosm/kg):

$$mosm/kg = 2[Na^+] + \frac{Glucose\ (mg/dL)}{18}$$

These calculated estimates are usually 10–20 mosm/kg lower than values recorded by standard cryoscopic techniques. Blood urea nitrogen and serum creatinine are invariably elevated because of dehydration. While urea exerts an effect on freezing point depression as measured in the laboratory, it is freely permeable across cell membranes and therefore not included in calculations of effective serum osmolality. In the presence of keto acids, values from multichannel chemical analysis of serum creatinine may be falsely elevated and therefore quite unreliable. However, most laboratories can correct for these interfering chromogens by using a more specific method if asked to do so.

The nitroprusside reagents (Acetest and Ketostix) used for the bedside assessment of ketoacidemia and ketoaciduria measure only acetoacetate and its by-product, acetone. The sensitivity of these reagents for acetone, however, is quite poor, requiring over 10 mmol/L, which is seldom reached in the plasma of ketoacidotic subjects—although this detectable concentration is readily achieved in urine. Thus, in the plasma of ketotic patients, only acetoacetate is measured by these reagents. The more prevalent β-hydroxybutyrate has no ketone group and is therefore not detected by the conventional nitroprusside tests. This takes on special importance in the presence of circulatory collapse during diabetic ketoacidosis, wherein an increase in lactic acid can shift the redox state to increase β-hydroxybutyrate at the expense of the readily detectable acetoacetate. Bedside diagnostic reagents would then be unreliable, suggesting no ketonemia in cases where β-hydroxybutyric acid is a major factor in producing the acidosis.

In about 90% of cases, serum amylase is elevated. However, this often represents salivary as well as pancreatic amylase and correlates poorly with symptoms of pancreatitis, such as pain and vomiting. Therefore, in patients with diabetic ketoacidosis, an elevated serum amylase does not justify a diagnosis of acute pancreatitis; serum lipase may be useful if the diagnosis of pancreatitis is being seriously considered.

C. DATA RECORDING ON A FLOW SHEET

The need for frequent evaluation of the patient's status cannot be overemphasized. Patients with moderately severe diabetic ketoacidosis (pH < 7.2) are best managed in an intensive care unit. Essential baseline blood chemistries include glucose, ketones, electrolytes, arterial blood gases, blood urea nitrogen, and serum creatinine. Serum osmolality should be estimated and tabulated during the course of therapy.

Typically, the patient with moderately severe diabetic ketoacidosis will have a plasma glucose of 350–900 mg/dL (19.4–50 mmol/L), the presence of serum ketones at a dilution of 1:8 or greater, slight hyponatremia of 130 mEq/L, hyperkalemia of 5–8 mEq/L, hyperphosphatemia of 6–7 mg/dL, and an elevated blood urea nitrogen and creatinine. Acidosis may be severe (pH ranging from 6.9 to 7.2 and bicarbonate ranging from 5 to 15 mEq/L); P_{CO_2} is low (15–20 mm Hg) from hyperventilation.

A comprehensive flow sheet that includes vital signs, serial laboratory data, and therapeutic interventions should be meticulously maintained by the physician responsible for the patient's care (Figure 17–10). Plasma glucose should be recorded hourly and electrolytes and pH at least every 2–3 hours during the initial treatment period. Insulin therapy is greatly facilitated when

DIABETIC KETOACIDOSIS FLOW SHEET

Name _____

Hospital No. _____

Age _____ Initial weight _____

Initial level of consciousness

_____ Alert
_____ Lethargic
_____ Semicomatose
_____ Comatose

DATE									
TIME									
BLOOD PRESSURE									
PULSE									
BLOOD									
Creatinine									
Blood urea nitrogen									
Glucose									
Acetone									
Hematocrit									
pH									
P_{O_2}									
P_{CO_2}									
Na^+									
K^+									
HCO_3^-									
Cl^-									
URINE									
Volume									
Glucose									
Acetone									
REGULAR INSULIN									
Intravenous									
Intramuscular									
Units									
Hours									
INTRAVENOUS FLUIDS									
Type									
Amount									
HCO_3^-									
Phosphate									
OTHER									

Figure 17–10. Flow sheet for treatment of diabetic ketoacidosis.

plasma glucose results are available within a few minutes of sampling. This can be achieved by the use of bedside glucose meters for measurements of capillary blood glucose (see Blood Glucose Testing, above). Fluid intake and output as well as details of insulin therapy and the administration of other medications should also be carefully recorded on the flow sheet.

Treatment

A. IMMEDIATE RESUSCITATION AND EMERGENCY MEASURES

If the patient is stuporous or comatose, immediately institute the emergency measures outlined in the section on coma (see above). Once the diagnosis of diabetic ketoacidosis is established in the emergency room, administration of at least 2 L of isotonic saline (0.9% saline solution) in an adult patient in the first 2–3 hours is necessary to help restore plasma volume and stabilize blood pressure while acutely reducing the hyperosmolar state. In addition, by improving renal plasma flow, fluid replacement also restores the renal capacity to excrete hydrogen ions, thereby ameliorating the acidosis as well. Immediately after the initiation of fluid replacement, a rapid bolus of 0.3 unit of regular insulin per kilogram of body weight should be given intravenously. This will inhibit both gluconeogenesis and ketogenesis while promoting utilization of glucose and keto acids. If arterial blood pH is 7.0 or less, intravenous bicarbonate may be administered (details of administration are outlined below). Gastric intubation is recommended in the comatose patient to prevent vomiting and aspiration that may occur as a result of gastric atony, a common complication of diabetic ketoacidosis. An indwelling bladder catheter is required in all comatose patients but should be avoided, if possible, in a fully cooperative diabetic patient because of the risk of bladder infection. In patients with preexisting cardiac or renal failure or those in severe cardiovascular collapse, a central venous pressure catheter or a Swan-Ganz catheter should be inserted to evaluate the degree of hypovolemia and to monitor subsequent fluid administration.

B. SPECIFIC MEASURES

Each case must be managed individually depending on the specific abnormalities present and subsequent response to initial therapy.

1. Insulin—Only regular insulin, and preferably human insulin, should be used in the management of diabetic ketoacidosis. As noted above, a "loading" dose of 0.3 unit/kg body weight of regular insulin is given initially as an intravenous bolus to prime the tissue insulin receptors. Following the initial bolus, doses of insulin as low as 0.1 unit/kg, given hourly by slow intravenous drip—or even when given intramuscularly—are as effective in most cases as the much higher doses previously recommended, and they appear to be safer. When a continuous infusion of insulin is used, 25 units of regular human insulin should be placed in 250 mL of isotonic saline and the first 50 mL of solution flushed through to saturate the tubing before connecting it to the intravenous line. An I-Vac or Harvard pump provides a reliable infusion rate. The insulin dose should be "piggy-backed" into the fluid line so the rate of fluid replacement can be changed without altering the insulin delivery rate. If the plasma glucose level fails to fall at least 10% in the first hour, a repeat loading dose is recommended. Rarely, a patient with insulin resistance is encountered; this requires doubling the insulin dose every 2–4 hours if severe hyperglycemia does not improve after the first two doses of insulin and fluid replacement.

Insulin therapy, either as a continuous infusion or as injections given every 1–2 hours, should be continued until arterial pH has normalized.

2. Fluid replacement—In most adult patients, the fluid deficit is 4–5 L. Initially, isotonic saline is preferred for restoration of plasma volume and, as noted above, should be infused rapidly to provide 1 L/h over the first 1–2 hours. After the first 2 L of fluid have been given, the fluid should be changed to 0.45% saline solution given at a rate of 300–400 mL/h; this is because water loss exceeds sodium loss in uncontrolled diabetes with osmotic diuresis. Failure to give enough volume replacement (at least 3–4 L in 8 hours) to restore normal perfusion is one of the most serious therapeutic shortcomings affecting satisfactory recovery. In the same way, excessive fluid replacement (more than 5 L in 8 hours) may contribute to acute respiratory distress syndrome or cerebral edema. When blood glucose falls to approximately 250 mg/dL, the fluids should be changed to a 5% glucose solution to maintain plasma glucose in the range of 250–300 mg/dL. This will prevent the development of hypoglycemia and will also reduce the likelihood of cerebral edema, which could result from too rapid decline of blood glucose. Intensive insulin therapy should be continued until the ketoacidosis is corrected.

3. Sodium bicarbonate—The use of sodium bicarbonate in management of diabetic ketoacidosis has been questioned since clinical benefit was not demonstrated in one prospective randomized trial and because of the following potentially harmful consequences: (1) development of hypokalemia from rapid shift of potassium into cells if the acidosis is overcorrected; (2) tissue anoxia from reduced dissociation of oxygen from hemoglobin when acidosis is rapidly reversed (leftward shift of the oxygen dissociation curve); and (3) cerebral acidosis resulting from lowering of cerebrospinal fluid pH. It must be emphasized, however, that these considerations are less important when severe acidosis exists. It is therefore recommended that bicarbonate be administered to diabetic patients in ketoacidosis if the arterial blood pH is 7.0 or less with careful monitoring to prevent overcorrection.

One to two ampules of sodium bicarbonate (one ampule contains 44 mEq/50 mL) should be added to 1 L of 0.45% saline. (**Note:** Addition of sodium bicarbonate to 0.9% saline would produce a markedly hypertonic solution that could aggravate the hyperosmolar state already present.) This should be administered rapidly (over the first hour). It can be repeated until the arterial pH reaches 7.1, but *it should not be given if the pH is 7.1 or greater* since additional bicarbonate would increase the risk of rebound metabolic alkalosis as ketones are metabolized. Alkalosis shifts potassium from serum into cells, which could precipitate a fatal cardiac arrhythmia. As noted earlier, serious consideration should be given to placement of a central venous or Swan-Ganz catheter when administering fluids to severely ill patients with cardiovascular compromise.

4. Potassium—Total body potassium loss from polyuria and vomiting may be as high as 200 mEq. However, because of shifts of potassium from cells into the extracellular space as a consequence of acidosis, serum potassium is usually normal to slightly elevated prior to institution of treatment. As the acidosis is corrected, potassium flows back into the cells, and hypokalemia can develop if potassium replacement is not instituted. If the patient is not uremic and has an adequate urine output, potassium chloride in doses of 10–30 mEq/h should be infused during the second and third hours after beginning therapy as soon as the acidosis starts to resolve. Replacement should be started sooner if the initial serum potassium is inappropriately normal or low and should be delayed if serum potassium fails to respond to initial therapy and remains above 5 mEq/L, as in cases of renal insufficiency. Cooperative patients with only mild ketoacidosis may receive part or all of their potassium replacement orally.

An ECG can be of help in monitoring the patient's potassium status: high peaked T waves are a sign of hyperkalemia, and flattened T waves with U waves are a sign of hypokalemia.

Foods high in potassium content should be prescribed when the patient has recovered sufficiently to take food orally. Tomato juice has 14 mEq of potassium per 240 mL, and a medium-sized banana has about 10 mEq.

5. Phosphate—Phosphate replacement is seldom required in treating diabetic ketoacidosis. However, if severe hypophosphatemia of less than 1 mg/dL (< 0.35 mmol/L) develops during insulin therapy, a small amount of phosphate can be replaced per hour as the potassium salt. Correction of hypophosphatemia helps to restore the buffering capacity of the plasma, thereby facilitating renal excretion of hydrogen. It also corrects the impaired oxygen dissociation from hemoglobin by regenerating 2,3-diphosphoglycerate. However, three randomized studies in which phosphate was replaced in only half of a group of patients with diabetic ketoacidosis did not show any apparent clinical benefit from phosphate administration. Moreover, attempts to use the phosphate salt of potassium as the sole means of replacing potassium have led to a number of reported cases of severe hypocalcemia with tetany. To minimize the risk of inducing tetany from too rapid replacement of phosphate, the average deficit of 40–50 mmol of phosphate should be replaced intravenously at a rate *no greater than 3–4 mmol/h* in a 60- to 70-kg person. A stock solution (Abbott) provides a mixture of 1.12 g KH_2PO_4 and 1.18 g K_2HPO_4 in a 5-mL single-dose vial (this equals 22 mmol of potassium and 15 mmol of phosphate). One-half of this vial (2.5 mL) should be added to 1 L of either 0.45% saline or 5% dextrose in water. Two liters of this solution, infused at a rate of 400 mL/h, will correct the phosphate deficit at the optimal rate of 3 mmol/h while providing 4.4 mEq of potassium per hour. (Additional potassium should be administered as potassium chloride to provide a total of 10–30 mEq of potassium per hour, as noted above.) If the serum phosphate remains below 2.5 mg/dL after this infusion, a repeat 5-hour infusion can be given.

It remains controversial whether phosphate replacement is beneficial. Several clinics prohibit its use in the routine treatment of diabetic ketoacidosis, since the risk of inducing hypocalcemia is thought to outweigh its potential benefits. However, potential hazards of phosphate replacement can be greatly reduced by administering phosphate at a rate no greater than 3–4 mmol/h. To prevent errors of overreplacement, phosphate should be administered separately rather than included as a component of potassium replacement.

6. Hyperchloremic acidosis during therapy—Because of the considerable loss of keto acids in the urine during the initial phase of therapy, substrate for subsequent regeneration of bicarbonate is lost and correction of the total bicarbonate deficit is hampered. A portion of the bicarbonate deficit is replaced with chloride ions infused in large amounts as saline to correct the dehydration. In most patients, as the ketoacidosis clears during insulin replacement, a hyperchloremic, low-bicarbonate pattern emerges with a normal anion gap. This is a relatively benign condition that reverses itself over the subsequent 12–24 hours once intravenous saline is no longer being administered.

Prognosis

Insulin and fluid and electrolyte replacement combined with careful monitoring of patients' clinical and laboratory responses to therapy have dramatically reduced the morbidity and mortality rates of diabetic ketoacidosis. However, this complication still represents a potential threat to survival, especially in older people with cardiovascular disease. Even in specialized centers, the mortality rate may approach 5–10%. Therefore, physicians treating diabetic ketoacidosis must not be lured into adopting "cookbook" approaches that lessen their attentiveness to changes in the patient's condition. Signs to be watched for include failure of improvement in mental status after a period of treatment, continued hypotension with minimal urine flow, or prolonged ileus (which may suggest bowel infarction). Laboratory abnormalities to be watched include failure of blood glucose to fall by 80–100 mg/dL during the first hour of therapy, failure to increase serum bicarbonate or arterial pH appropriately, serum potassium above 6 or below 2.8 mEq/L, and electrocardiographic evidence of cardiac arrhythmias. Any of these signs call for a careful search for the cause of the abnormality and prompt specific therapy.

Disposition

After recovery and stabilization, patients should receive intensive detailed instructions about how to avoid this potentially disastrous complication of diabetes mellitus. They should be taught to recognize the early symptoms and signs of ketoacidosis.

Urine ketones should be measured in patients with signs of infection or in those using an insulin pump when capillary blood glucose is unexpectedly and persistently high. A combined glucose and ketone meter (Precision, Medisense) that is able to measure blood betahydroxybutyrate concentration on capillary blood is available and provides an alternative to monitoring for ketonuria. When heavy ketonuria and glycosuria persist on several successive examinations, supplemental regular insulin should be administered and liquid foods such as lightly salted tomato juice and broth should be ingested to replenish fluids and electrolytes. Patients should be instructed to contact the physician if ketonuria persists, and especially if vomiting develops or if appropriate adjustment of the infusion rate on an insulin pump does not correct the hyperglycemia and ketonuria. In adolescents, recurrent episodes of severe diabetic ketoacidosis often indicate poor compliance with the insulin regimen, and these patients should receive intensive family counseling.

2. Hyperglycemic, Hyperosmolar, Nonketotic State

This form of hyperglycemic coma is characterized by severe hyperglycemia, hyperosmolality, and dehydration in the absence of significant ketosis. It occurs in middle-aged or elderly patients with non-insulin-dependent diabetes which is often mild or occult. Lethargy and confusion develop as serum osmolality exceeds 300 mosm/kg, and coma can occur if osmolality exceeds 330 mosm/kg. Underlying renal insufficiency or congestive heart failure is common, and the presence of either worsens the prognosis. A precipitating event such as pneumonia, cerebrovascular accident, myocardial infarction, burns, or recent operation can often be identified. Certain drugs, such as phenytoin, diazoxide, glucocorticoids, and thiazide diuretics, have been implicated in its development, as have procedures associated with glucose loading, eg, peritoneal dialysis.

Pathogenesis

A partial or relative insulin deficiency may initiate the syndrome by reducing glucose utilization by muscle, fat, and the liver while at the same time inducing hyperglucagonemia and increasing hepatic glucose output. The result is hyperglycemia that leads to glycosuria and osmotic diuresis with obligatory water loss. The presence of even small amounts of insulin is believed to prevent the development of ketosis by inhibiting lipolysis in the adipose stores. Therefore even though a low insulin:glucagon ratio promotes ketogenesis in the liver, the limited availability of precursor free fatty acids from the periphery restricts the rate at which ketones are formed. If a patient is unable to maintain adequate fluid intake because of an associated acute or chronic illness or has suffered excessive fluid loss (eg, from burns or therapy with diuretics), marked dehydration results. As plasma volume contracts, renal insufficiency develops; this, then, limits renal glucose excretion and contributes markedly to the rise in serum glucose and osmolality. As serum osmolality exceeds 320–330 mosm/kg, water is drawn out of cerebral neurons, resulting in mental obtundation and coma.

Clinical Features

A. SYMPTOMS AND SIGNS

The onset of the hyperglycemic, hyperosmolar, nonketotic state may be insidious, preceded for days or weeks by symptoms of weakness, polyuria, and polydipsia. A history of reduced fluid intake is common, whether due to inappropriate absence of thirst, gastrointestinal upset, or, in the case of elderly or bedridden patients, lack of access to water. A history of ingestion of large quantities of glucose-containing fluids, such as soft drinks or orange juice, can occasionally be obtained; these patients are usually less hyperosmolar than those in whom fluid intake was restricted. The absence of toxic features of ketoacidosis may retard recognition of the syndrome and thus delay institution of therapy until dehydration is profound. Because of this delay in diagnosis, the hyperglycemia, hyperosmolality, and dehydration in hyperglycemic, hyperosmolar, nonketotic coma is often more severe than in diabetic ketoacidosis.

Physical examination will reveal the presence of profound dehydration (orthostatic fall in blood pressure and rise in pulse, supine tachycardia or even frank shock, dry mucous membranes, decreased skin turgor). The patient may be lethargic, confused, or comatose. Kussmaul respirations are absent unless the precipitating event for the hyperosmolar state has also led to the development of metabolic acidosis (eg, sepsis or myocardial infarction with shock).

B. Laboratory Findings

Severe hyperglycemia is present, with blood glucose values ranging from 800 to as high as 2400 mg/dL (44.4–133.2 mmol/L). In mild cases, where dehydration is less severe, dilutional hyponatremia as well as urinary sodium losses may reduce serum sodium to about 120–125 mEq/L—this protects, to some extent, against extreme hyperosmolality. Once dehydration progresses further, however, serum sodium can exceed 140 mEq/L, producing serum osmolalities of 330–440 mosm/kg* (normal, 280–295 mosm/kg). Ketosis is usually absent or mild; however, a small degree of ketonuria may be present if the patient has not been eating because of illness. Acidosis is not a part of the hyperglycemic, hyperosmolar state, but it may be present (usually lactic acidosis) because of other acute underlying conditions (sepsis, acute renal failure, myocardial infarction, etc). (See Lactic Acidosis, below.)

Treatment

There are some differences in fluid, insulin, and electrolyte replacement in this disorder, as compared to diabetic ketoacidosis. However, in common with the treatment of ketoacidotic patients, careful monitoring of the patient's clinical and laboratory response to therapy is essential.

A. Fluid Replacement

Fluid replacement is of paramount importance in treating nonketotic hyperglycemic coma. If circulatory collapse is present, fluid therapy should be initiated with isotonic saline. In all other cases, initial replacement with hypotonic (usually 0.45%) saline is preferable, because these patients are hyperosmolar with considerable loss of body water and excess solute in the vascular compartment. As much as 4–6 L of fluid may be required in the first 8–10 hours. Careful monitoring of fluid quantity and type, urine output, blood pressure, and pulse is essential. Placement of a central venous pressure or Swan-Ganz catheter should be strongly considered to guide replacement of fluid, especially if the patient is elderly or has underlying renal or cardiac disease. Because insulin therapy will decrease plasma glucose and therefore serum osmolality, a change to isotonic saline may be necessary at some time during treatment in order to maintain an adequate blood pressure and a urine output of at least 50 mL/h. Once blood glucose reaches 250 mg/dL, 5% dextrose in 0.45% or 0.9% saline solution should be substituted for the sugar-free fluids. When consciousness returns, oral fluids should be encouraged.

B. Electrolyte Replacement

Hyperkalemia is less marked and much less potassium is lost in the urine during the osmotic diuresis of hyperglycemic, hyperosmolar, nonketotic coma than in diabetic ketoacidosis. There is, therefore, less severe total potassium depletion, and less potassium replacement is needed to restore potassium stores to normal. However, because the initial serum potassium usually is not elevated and because it declines rapidly as insulin therapy allows glucose and potassium to enter cells, it is recommended that potassium replacement be initiated earlier than in ketotic patients: 10 mEq of potassium chloride can be added to the *initial* liter of fluid administered if the initial serum potassium is not elevated and if the patient is making urine. When serum phosphate falls below 1 mg/dL during insulin therapy, phosphate replacement can be given intravenously with the same precautions as those outlined for ketoacidotic patients (see above). If the patient is awake and cooperative, part or all of the potassium and phosphate replacement can be given orally.

C. Insulin Therapy

In general, less insulin is required to reduce the hyperglycemia of nonketotic patients than is the case for patients in diabetic ketoacidosis. In fact, fluid replacement alone can decrease glucose levels considerably. An ini-

---

*A convenient method for estimating serum osmolality is provided in the section on diabetic ketoacidosis.

tial dose of 15 units of regular insulin given intravenously and 15 units given intramuscularly is usually quite effective in lowering blood glucose. In most cases, subsequent doses need not be greater than 10–25 units every 4 hours. (Insulin should be given intramuscularly or intravenously until the patient has stabilized; it may then be given subcutaneously.) Some patients—especially those who are severely ill because of other underlying diseases—may require continuous intravenous administration of insulin (in a manner similar to that described for ketoacidosis) with careful monitoring, preferably in an intensive care setting.

D. SEARCH FOR THE PRECIPITATING EVENT

The physician must initiate a careful search for the event that precipitated the episode of hyperglycemic, hyperosmolar, nonketotic coma if it is not obvious after the initial history and physical examination. Chest x-rays and cultures of blood, urine, and other body fluids should be obtained to look for occult sources of sepsis; empiric antibiotic coverage should be considered in the seriously ill patient. Cardiac enzymes and serial ECGs can be ordered to look for evidence of "silent" myocardial infarction.

Prognosis

The overall mortality rate of hyperglycemic, hyperosmolar, nonketotic coma is over ten times that of diabetic ketoacidosis, chiefly because of its higher incidence in older patients, who may have compromised cardiovascular systems or associated major illnesses. (When patients are matched for age, the prognoses of these two forms of hyperosmolar coma are reasonably comparable.)

Disposition

After the patient is stabilized, the appropriate form of long-term management of the diabetes must be determined. This must include patient education on how to recognize situations (gastrointestinal upset, infection) that will predispose to recurrence of hyperglycemic, hyperosmolar, nonketotic coma as well as detailed information on how to prevent the escalating dehydration (small sips of sugar-free liquids, increase in usual hypoglycemic therapy, or early contact with the physician) that culminates in hyperosmolar coma. For a detailed discussion of therapeutic alternatives for type 2 diabetic patients, see Steps in the Management of the Diabetic Patient (above).

3. Hypoglycemic Coma

Hypoglycemia is a common complication of insulin replacement therapy in diabetic patients. In most cases, it is detected and treated by patients or their families before coma results. However, it remains the most frequent cause of coma in the insulin-treated diabetic patient. In addition, it can occur in any patient taking oral agents that stimulate pancreatic B cells (eg, sulfonylureas, meglitinide, D-phenylalanine analog), particularly if the patient is elderly, has renal or liver disease, or is taking certain other medications that alter metabolism of the sulfonylureas (eg, phenylbutazone, sulfonamides, or warfarin). It occurs more frequently with the use of long-acting sulfonylureas than when shorter-acting agents are used.

Clinical Findings & Treatment

The clinical findings and emergency treatment of hypoglycemia are discussed at the beginning of this section.

Prognosis

Most patients who arrive at emergency rooms in hypoglycemic coma appear to recover fully; however, profound hypoglycemia or delays in therapy can result in permanent neurologic deficit or even death. Furthermore, repeated episodes of hypoglycemia may have a cumulative adverse effect on intellectual functioning.

Disposition

The physician should carefully review with the patient the events leading up to the hypoglycemic episode. Associated use of other medications, as well as alcohol or narcotics, should be noted. Careful attention should be paid to diet, exercise pattern, insulin or sulfonylurea dosage, and general compliance with the prescribed diabetes treatment regimen. Any factors thought to have contributed to the development of the episode should be identified and recommendations made in order to prevent recurrences of this potentially disastrous complication of diabetes therapy.

If the patient is hypoglycemic from use of a long-acting oral hypoglycemic agent (eg, chlorpropamide or glyburide) or from high doses of a long-acting insulin, admission to hospital for treatment with continuous intravenous glucose and careful monitoring of blood glucose is indicated.

4. Lactic Acidosis

When severely ill diabetic patients present with profound acidosis and an anion gap over 15 mEq/L but relatively low or undetectable levels of keto acids in plasma, the presence of excessive plasma lactate (> 5 mmol/L) should be considered, especially if other causes of acidosis such as uremia are not present.

Pathogenesis

Lactic acid is the end product of anaerobic metabolism of glucose. Normally, the principal sources of this acid are the erythrocytes (which lack the enzymes for aerobic oxidation), skeletal muscle, skin, and brain. The chief pathway for removal of lactic acid is by hepatic (and to some degree renal) uptake for conversion first to pyruvate and eventually back to glucose, a process that requires oxygen. Lactic acidosis occurs when excess lactic acid accumulates in the blood. This can be the result of overproduction (tissue hypoxia), deficient removal (hepatic failure), or both (circulatory collapse). Lactic acidosis is not uncommon in any severely ill patient suffering from cardiac decompensation, respiratory or hepatic failure, septicemia, or infarction of the bowel or extremities.

With the discontinuance of phenformin therapy in the USA, lactic acidosis in patients with diabetes mellitus has become uncommon, but it still must be considered in the acidotic diabetic if the patient is seriously ill, and especially if the patient is receiving metformin therapy as well.

Clinical Features

A. SYMPTOMS AND SIGNS

The main clinical features of lactic acidosis are marked hyperventilation and mental confusion, which may progress to stupor or coma. When lactic acidosis is secondary to tissue hypoxia or vascular collapse, the clinical presentation is variable, being that of the prevailing catastrophic illness. In the rare instance of idiopathic or spontaneous lactic acidosis, the onset is rapid (usually over a few hours), the cardiopulmonary status is stable, and mentation may be relatively normal.

B. LABORATORY FINDINGS

Plasma glucose can be low, normal, or high in diabetic patients with lactic acidosis, but usually it is moderately elevated. Plasma bicarbonate and arterial pH are quite low. An anion gap will be present (calculated by subtracting the sum of the plasma bicarbonate and chloride from the plasma sodium; normal is 12–15 mEq/L). Ketones are usually absent from plasma, but small amounts may be present in urine if the patient has not been eating recently. Other causes of "anion gap" metabolic acidosis should be excluded—eg, uremia, diabetic or alcoholic ketoacidosis, and salicylate, methanol, ethylene glycol, or paraldehyde intoxication. In the absence of azotemia, hyperphosphatemia may be a clue to the presence of lactic acidosis.

The diagnosis is confirmed by demonstrating, in a sample of blood that is promptly chilled and separated, a plasma lactate concentration of 6 mmol/L or higher (normal is about 1 mmol/L). Failure to rapidly chill the sample and separate the plasma can lead to falsely high plasma lactate values as a result of continued glycolysis by the red blood cells. Frozen plasma remains stable for subsequent assay.

Treatment

The cornerstone of therapy is aggressive treatment of the precipitating cause. An adequate airway and good oxygenation should be ensured. If hypotension is present, fluids and, if appropriate, pressor agents must be given to restore tissue perfusion. Appropriate cultures and empiric antibiotic coverage should be instituted in any seriously ill patient with lactic acidosis in whom the cause is not immediately apparent. Alkalinization with intravenous sodium bicarbonate to keep the pH above 7.2 has been recommended in the emergency treatment of severe lactic acidosis. However, there is no evidence that the mortality rate is favorably affected by administering bicarbonate and the matter is at present controversial, particularly because of the hazards associated with bicarbonate therapy. Hemodialysis may be useful in those cases in which metformin accumulation and the attendant lactic acidosis occurred in patients with renal insufficiency. Dichloroacetate, an anion that facilitates pyruvate removal by activating pyruvate dehydrogenase, reverses certain types of lactic acidosis in animals, but in a prospective controlled clinical trial involving 252 patients with lactic acidosis, dichloroacetate failed to alter either hemodynamics or survival.

■ CHRONIC COMPLICATIONS OF DIABETES MELLITUS (TABLE 17–20)

In most patients with diabetes, a number of pathologic changes occur at variable intervals during the course of the disease. These changes involve the vascular system for the most part; however, they also occur in the nerves, the skin, and the lens.

In addition to the above complications, diabetic patients have an increased incidence of certain types of infections and may handle their infections less well than the general population.

Classifications of Diabetic Vascular Disease

Diabetic vascular disease is conveniently divided into two main categories: microvascular disease and macrovascular disease.

Table 17–20. Chronic complications of diabetes mellitus.

Eyes	**Skin**
Diabetic retinopathy	Diabetic dermopathy (shin spots)
Nonproliferative (background)	Necrobiosis lipoidica diabeticorum
Proliferative	Candidiasis
Cataracts	Foot and leg ulcers
Subcapsular (snowflake)	Neurotropic
Nuclear (senile)	Ischemic
Kidneys	**Cardiovascular system**
Intercapillary glomerulosclerosis	Heart disease
Diffuse	Myocardial infarction
Nodular	Cardiomyopathy
Infection	Gangrene of the feet
Pyelonephritis	Ischemic ulcers
Perinephric abscess	Osteomyelitis
Renal papillary necrosis	**Bones and joints**
Renal tubular necrosis	Diabetic cheirarthropathy
Following dye studies (urograms, arteriograms)	Dupuytren's contracture
Nervous system	Charcot joint
Peripheral neuropathy	**Unusual infections**
Distal, symmetric sensory loss	Necrotizing fasciitis
Motor neuropathy	Necrotizing myositis
Foot drop, wrist drop	*Mucor* meningitis
Mononeuropathy multiplex (diabetic amyotrophy)	Emphysematous cholecystitis
Cranial neuropathy	Malignant otitis externa
Cranial nerves III, IV, VI, VII	
Autonomic neuropathy	
Postural hypotension	
Resting tachycardia	
Loss of sweating	
Gastrointestinal neuropathy	
Gastroparesis	
Diabetic diarrhea	
Urinary bladder atony	
Impotence (may also be secondary to pelvic vascular disease)	

A. MICROVASCULAR DISEASE

Disease of the smallest blood vessels, the capillary and the precapillary arterioles, is manifested mainly by thickening of the capillary basement membrane. Microvascular disease involving the retina leads to diabetic retinopathy, and disease involving the kidney causes diabetic nephropathy. Small vessel disease may also involve the heart, and cardiomegaly with heart failure has been described in diabetic patients with patent coronary arteries.

B. MACROVASCULAR DISEASE

Large vessel disease in diabetes is essentially an accelerated form of atherosclerosis. It accounts for the increased incidence of myocardial infarction, stroke, and peripheral gangrene in diabetic patients. Just as in the case of atherosclerosis in the general population, the exact cause of accelerated atherosclerosis in the diabetic population remains unclear. Abnormalities in vessel walls, platelets and other components of the clotting system, red blood cells, and lipid metabolism have all been postulated to play a role. In addition, there is evidence that coexistent risk factors such as cigarette smoking and hypertension may be important in determining the course of the disease.

Prevalence of Chronic Complications by Type of Diabetes

Although all of the known complications of diabetes can be found in both types of the disease, some are more common in one type than in the other. Renal failure due to severe microvascular nephropathy is the major cause of death in patients with type 1 diabetes, whereas macrovascular disease is the leading cause in type 2. Although blindness occurs in both types, it occurs more commonly as a result of severe proliferative retinopathy, vitreous hemorrhages, and retinal detachment in type 1 disease, whereas macular edema and ischemia are the usual cause in type 2. Similarly, although diabetic neuropathy is common in both type 1 and type 2 diabetes, severe autonomic neuropathy with gastroparesis, diabetic diarrhea, resting tachycardia, and postural hypotension is much more common in type 1.

Relationship of Glycemic Control to Development of Chronic Complications

The cause of chronic microvascular complications in diabetic patients has now been resolved. A compelling argument for its being a consequence of impaired metabolic control was initially made by observations in Korean patients who ingested a B cell-toxic rodenticide, vacor, during a suicide attempt and developed persistent diabetes. As many as 44% of these patients developed retinopathy during a 6- to 7-year follow-up of their acquired diabetes, while 28% had clinical proteinuria and more than half showed significant thickening of their quadriceps capillary basement membrane width.

However, in patients with idiopathic diabetes mellitus, the most compelling argument for the view that chronic diabetic complications relate to poor glycemic control is based on the findings of the Diabetes Control and Complications Trial (discussed above). This study of 1441 type 1 patients over a 7- to 10-year period conclusively demonstrated that near normalization of blood glucose with intensive therapy was able to substantially prevent or delay the development of diabetic retinopathy, nephropathy, and neuropathy.

Genetic Factors in Susceptibility to Development of Chronic Complications of Diabetes

Although no genetic susceptibility genes have been identified as yet, three unrelated observations indicate that roughly 40% of people may be unusually susceptible to the ravages of hyperglycemia or other metabolic sequelae of an inadequate insulin effect.

(1) In one retrospective study of 164 juvenile-onset diabetics with a median age at onset of 9 years, 40% were incapacitated or dead from end-stage renal disease with proliferative retinopathy after a 25-year follow-up, while the remaining subjects were either mildly affected (40%) or had no clinically detected microvascular disease (20%). This study was completed long before the availability of glycemic self-monitoring methodology, so it is unlikely that any of these patients were near optimal glycemic control.

(2) Data from renal transplantation indicate that only about 40% of normal kidneys developed evidence of moderate to severe diabetic nephropathy within 6–14 years of being transplanted into diabetic subjects with end-stage renal failure, whereas as many as 60% were only minimally affected.

(3) Among children under 21 years of age with type 1 diabetes, 40% had thickening of the capillary basement membrane width (CBMW) of the quadriceps muscle, while 60% had vessels within the normal range. This finding was unrelated to the severity or duration of diabetes and is in contrast to results in diabetic adults 21 years of age or older, in whom virtually 100% have thickened CBMWs.

These three observations support the hypothesis that while approximately 60% of people suffer only minimal consequences from hyperglycemia and other metabolic hazards of insulin insufficiency, 40% or so suffer severe, potentially catastrophic microvascular complications if the disease is poorly controlled. The genetic mechanisms for this increased susceptibility are as yet unknown but could relate to overproduction or reduced removal of accelerated glycosylation end products in particular tissues. If further studies indicate that the presence of early thickening of the CBMW—found in 40% of children—represents a marker of this susceptibility gene and a predictor of severe microvascular disease, it could justify more intensive insulin therapy in that group to achieve near-normalization of blood glucose. The remaining 60% of less susceptible individuals might then be spared the inconveniences of strict glycemic control as well as the risks of hypoglycemia inherent in present methods of intensive insulin therapy.

SPECIFIC CHRONIC COMPLICATIONS OF DIABETES MELLITUS (TABLE 17–20)

1. Ophthalmologic Complications

Diabetic Retinopathy

For early detection of diabetic retinopathy, adolescent or adult patients who have had type 1 diabetes for more than 5 years and *all* type 2 diabetic patients should be referred to an ophthalmologist for examination and follow-up. When hypertension is present in a patient with diabetes, it should be treated vigorously, since hypertension is associated with an increased incidence and accelerated progression of diabetic retinopathy.

A. PATHOGENESIS AND CLINICAL FEATURES

Two main categories of diabetic retinopathy exist: nonproliferative and proliferative.

Nonproliferative ("background") retinopathy represents the earliest stage of retinal involvement by diabetes and is characterized by such changes as microaneurysms, dot hemorrhages, exudates, and retinal edema. During this stage, the retinal capillaries leak proteins, lipids, or red cells into the retina. When this process occurs in the macula, the area of greatest concentration of visual cells, there will be interference with visual acuity; this is the most common cause of visual impairment in type 2 diabetes and occurs in up to 18% of these patients over time.

Proliferative retinopathy involves the growth of new capillaries and fibrous tissue within the retina and into the vitreous chamber. It is a consequence of small vessel occlusion, which causes retinal hypoxia; this in turn stimulates new vessel growth. Proliferative retinopathy can occur in both types of diabetes but is more common in type 1, developing about 7–10 years after onset of symptoms, with a prevalence of 25% after 15 years' duration. Prior to proliferation of new capillaries, a preproliferative phase often occurs in which arteriolar ischemia is manifested as cotton-wool spots (small infarcted areas of retina). Vision is usually normal until vitreous hemorrhage or retinal detachment occurs. Proliferative retinopathy is a leading cause of blindness in the USA, particularly since it increases the risk of retinal detachment. After 10 years of diabetes, half of all patients have at least some degree of retinopathy, and this proportion increases to more than 80% after 15 years of diabetes.

B. TREATMENT

Once maculopathy or proliferative changes are detected, panretinal xenon or argon laser photocoagulation therapy is indicated. Destroying retinal tissue with photocoagulation means that surviving tissue receives a greater share of the available oxygen supply, thereby abolishing hypoxic stimulation of new vessel growth. Results of a large-scale clinical trial (the Diabetic Retinopathy Study) have verified the effectiveness of photocoagulation, particularly when recent vitreous hemorrhages have occurred or when extensive new vessels are located near the optic disk.

The best results with photocoagulation are achieved if proliferative retinopathy is detected early. This is best done by obtaining a baseline fluorescein angiogram within 5–10 years after onset of type 1 diabetes and then repeating this study at intervals of 1–5 years, depending on the severity of the retinal involvement found. Prepubertal children do not develop diabetic retinopathy regardless of the duration of their diabetes. They need not be scheduled for routine ophthalmologic examination until several years after the onset of puberty.

Pituitary ablation, which has been associated with delay in progression of severe retinopathy in the past, is rarely used today because photocoagulation therapy is just as effective and avoids the risks associated with destruction of the pituitary. Occasional cases of rapidly progressive ("florid") proliferative retinopathy in type 1 adolescent diabetics have been reported in which photocoagulation was less effective than pituitary ablation in preventing blindness. Clinical trials have shown that aspirin does not influence the course of proliferative retinopathy, and there is no contraindication for its use to achieve cardiovascular benefit in diabetic patients who have proliferative retinopathy.

Cataracts

Two types of cataracts occur in diabetic patients: subcapsular and senile. **Subcapsular cataract** occurs predominantly in type 1 diabetics, may come on fairly rapidly, and has a significant correlation with the hyperglycemia of uncontrolled diabetes. This type of cataract has a flocculent or "snowflake" appearance and develops just below the lens capsule.

Senile cataract represents a sclerotic change of the lens nucleus. It is by far the most common type of cataract found in either diabetic or nondiabetic adults and tends to occur at a younger age in diabetic patients, particularly when glycemic control is poor.

Two separate abnormalities found in diabetic patients, both of which are related to elevated blood glucose levels, may contribute to the formation of cataracts: (1) glycosylation of the lens protein and (2) an excess of sorbitol, which is formed from the increased quantities of glucose found in the insulin-independent lens. Accumulation of sorbitol leads to osmotic changes in the lens that ultimately result in fibrosis and cataract formation.

Glaucoma

Glaucoma occurs in approximately 6% of persons with diabetes. It is generally responsive to the usual therapy for open-angle disease. Closed-angle glaucoma can result from neovascularization of the iris in diabetics, but this is relatively uncommon except after cataract extraction, when accelerated new vessel growth may occur that involves the angle of the iris and obstructs outflow.

2. Renal Complications

Diabetic Nephropathy

A. PATHOGENESIS AND CLINICAL FINDINGS

About 4000 cases of end-stage renal disease due to diabetic nephropathy occur annually among diabetic patients in the USA. This represents about one-third of all patients being treated for renal failure. The cumulative incidence of nephropathy differs between the two major types of diabetes. Patients with type 1 diabetes who have not received intensive insulin therapy and have had only fair to poor glycemic control have a 30–40% chance of having nephropathy after 20 years—in contrast to the much lower frequency in type 2 diabetes patients not receiving intensive therapy, in whom only about 15–20% develop clinical renal disease. However, since so many more individuals are affected with type 2 diabetes, end-stage renal disease is much more prevalent in type 2 diabetes in the United States and especially throughout the rest of the world. There is no question that improved glycemic control and more effective therapeutic measures to correct hypertension can reduce the incidence of end-stage renal disease in both types of diabetes in the future.

Diabetic nephropathy is initially manifested by proteinuria; subsequently, as kidney function declines, urea and creatinine accumulate in the blood. Thickening of capillary basement membranes and of the mesangium of renal glomeruli produces varying degrees of glomerulosclerosis and renal insufficiency. Diffuse glomerulosclerosis is more common than nodular intercapillary glomerulosclerosis (Kimmelstiel-Wilson lesions); both produce heavy proteinuria.

1. Microalbuminuria—New methods of detecting small amounts of urinary albumin have permitted detection of microgram concentrations—in contrast to the less sensitive dipstick strips, whose minimal detection limit is 0.3–0.5% (weight:volume). Conventional 24-hour urine collections, in addition to being inconvenient for patients, also show wide variability of albumin excretion, since several factors such as sustained erect posture, dietary protein, and exercise tend to increase albumin excretion rates. For these reasons, a timed overnight urine collection or albumin-creatinine ratio in early morning spot urine collected upon awakening is preferable. Normal subjects excrete less than 15 μg/min during overnight urine collections; values of 20 μg/min or higher are considered to represent abnormal microalbuminuria. Subsequent renal failure can be predicted by urinary albumin excretion rates exceeding 30 μg/min. In an early morning spot urine, a ratio of albumin (μg/L) to creatinine (mg/L) of < 30 is normal, and a ratio of 30–300 indicates microalbuminuria. At least two of three overnight timed urine specimens or early morning spot urines over a period of 3–6 months should be elevated before a diagnosis of abnormal microalbuminuria can be justified.

Increased microalbuminuria correlates with increased levels of blood pressure, and this may explain why increased proteinuria in diabetic patients is associated with an increase in cardiovascular deaths even in the absence of renal failure. Careful glycemic control as well as a low-protein diet (0.8 g/kg/d) may reduce both the hyperfiltration and the elevated microalbuminuria in patients in the early stages of diabetes and those with incipient diabetic nephropathy. Antihypertensive therapy also decreases microalbuminuria, and clinical trials with inhibitors of angiotensin I converting enzyme (eg, enalapril, 20 mg/d) show a reduction of microalbuminuria in diabetic patients even in the absence of hypertension. Microalbuminuria has recently been shown to correlate with slightly elevated nocturnal systolic blood pressure in "normotensive" diabetic patients, and antihypertensive therapy corrected this rise in blood pressure during sleep. This action, in addition to a reduction in mean arterial blood pressure, may contribute to the reported efficacy of ACE-inhibitors in reducing microalbuminuria in "normotensive" diabetic patients. However, the main action of these agents in reducing microalbuminuria is believed to be from a specific dilation of the glomerular efferent arteriole, thereby further reducing glomerular filtration pressure.

2. Progressive diabetic nephropathy—Progressive diabetic nephropathy consists of proteinuria of varying severity, occasionally leading to nephrotic syndrome with hypoalbuminemia, edema, and an increase in circulating LDL cholesterol as well as progressive azotemia. In contrast to all other renal disorders, the proteinuria associated with diabetic nephropathy does not diminish with progressive renal failure (patients continue to excrete 10–11 g daily as creatinine clearance diminishes). As renal failure progresses, there is an elevation in the renal threshold at which glycosuria appears.

Hypertension develops with progressive renal involvement, and coronary and cerebral atherosclerosis seems to be accelerated. Once diabetic nephropathy has progressed to the stage of hypertension, proteinuria, or early renal failure, glycemic control is not beneficial in influencing its course. In this circumstance, antihypertensive medications, including ACE inhibitors, and restriction of dietary protein to 0.8 g/kg body weight per day are recommended.

When the serum creatinine reaches 3 mg/dL, consultation with a nephrologist is recommended. When the serum creatinine reaches 5 mg/dL, consultation with personnel at a center where renal transplantation is performed is indicated.

B. TREATMENT

Hemodialysis has been of limited success in the treatment of renal failure due to diabetic nephropathy, primarily because of progression of large-vessel disease with resultant death and disability from stroke and myocardial infarction. Growing experience with chronic ambulatory peritoneal dialysis suggests that it may be a more convenient method of providing adequate dialysis with a lower incidence of complications.

Renal transplantation, especially from related donors, is often successful. For patients with compatible donors and no contraindications (such as severe cardiovascular disease), it is the treatment of choice.

Necrotizing Papillitis

This unusual complication of pyelonephritis occurs primarily in diabetic patients. It is characterized by fever, flank pain, pyuria, and sloughing of renal papillae in the urine. It is treated by intravenous administration of appropriate antibiotics.

Renal Decompensation After Radiographic Dyes

The use of radiographic contrast agents in diabetic patients with reduced creatinine clearance has been associated with the development of acute renal failure. Diabetic patients with normal renal function do not appear to be at increased risk for contrast nephropathy. If a contrast study is considered essential, patients with a serum creatinine of 1.5–2.5 mg/dL should be adequately hydrated before the procedure to produce a gentle diuresis of about 75 mL or so per hour. Other nephrotoxic agents such as nonsteroidal anti-inflammatory agents should be avoided. Although it was once believed that newer nonionic contrast agents were less likely to cause acute renal failure in diabetic patients, more recent prospective trials show no difference between these agents and conventional and much less costly ionic radiographic dyes. After the procedure, serum creatinine should be followed closely. Radiographic contrast material should not be given to a patient with a serum creatinine greater than 3 mg/dL unless the potential benefit outweighs the high risk of acute renal failure.

3. Neurologic Complications (Diabetic Neuropathy)

Peripheral and autonomic neuropathy are the two most common complications of both types of diabetes. Their pathogenesis is poorly understood. Some lesions, such as the acute cranial nerve palsies and diabetic amyotrophy, have been attributed to ischemic infarction of the involved peripheral nerve. The much more common symmetric sensory and motor peripheral neuropathies and autonomic neuropathy are felt to be due to metabolic or osmotic toxicity somehow related to hyperglycemia.

Unfortunately, there is no consistently effective treatment for any of the neuropathies. However, several long-term clinical trials have definitively shown that normalization of blood glucose levels can prevent development and progression of this devastating complication.

Peripheral Sensory Neuropathy

A. PATHOGENESIS AND CLINICAL FEATURES

Sensory loss is commonly preceded by months or years of paresthesias such as tingling, itching, and increasing pain. The pains can vary from mild paresthesias to severe shooting pains and may be more severe at night. Discomfort of the lower extremities can be incapacitating at times. Radicular pains in the chest and the abdominal area may be extremely difficult to distinguish from pain due to an intrathoracic or intra-abdominal source. Eventually, patients develop numbness, and tactile sensations decrease. The sensory loss is generally bilateral, symmetric, and associated with dulled perception of vibration, pain, and temperature, particularly in the lower extremities, but also evident in the hands. Sensory nerve conduction is delayed in peripheral nerves, and ankle jerks may be absent. Highly sensitive neurothesiometer devices are being utilized to characterize the threshold levels for pain and touch, so that signs of sensory defects can be detected earlier and patients with higher risk for neuropathic foot ulcers can be identified. Because all of these sensory disturbances are made worse by pressure applied to the involved nerves, symptoms may appear first in nerves that are entrapped, such as the median nerve in carpal tunnel syndrome or the nerves around the ankle.

Characteristic syndromes that develop in diabetic patients with sensory neuropathy and are related to their failure to perceive trauma include osteopathy of the foot with deformity of the ankle (so-called Charcot joint) and neuropathic ulceration of the foot.

B. TREATMENT

Amitriptyline (50–75 mg at bedtime) has produced remarkable improvement in the lower extremity pain in some patients with sensory neuropathy. Dramatic relief has often occurred within 48–72 hours. This rapid response is in contrast to the 2 or 3 weeks required for an antidepressive effect. Patients often attribute benefit to their having a full night's sleep after amitriptyline in contrast to many prior sleepless nights occasioned by neuropathic pain. Mild to moderate morning drowsiness is a side effect that generally improves with time or can be lessened by giving the medication several hours before bedtime. This drug should be discontinued if there is no improvement after 4–5 days. Desipramine in doses of 25–150 mg per day has been reported to have the same efficacy for neuropathic leg pains as amitriptyline. These tricyclic drugs probably act by directly modulating nociceptive C fibers and their receptors. Gabapentin has also been shown to be effective in the treatment of painful neuropathy and should be tried if the tricyclic drugs prove ineffective. Other drugs have been used, including carbamazepine and phenytoin, but these are of questionable benefit for leg pain. Capsaicin, a topical irritant, has relieved local nerve pain in some studies; it is dispensed as a cream to be rubbed into the skin over the painful region.

It is essential that diabetic patients with peripheral neuropathy receive detailed instructions in foot care (see p 626). Special custom-made shoes are usually required to redistribute weight evenly over an insensitive foot, particularly when it has been deformed by surgery, by asymptomatic fractures, or by a Charcot joint.

Motor Neuropathy

Symmetric motor neuropathy occurs much less frequently than sensory neuropathy and is associated with delayed motor nerve conduction and muscle weakness and atrophy. Its pathogenesis is presumed to be similar to that of sensory loss. Mononeuropathy develops when there is vascular occlusion of a specific nerve trunk; if more than one nerve trunk is involved, the syndrome of **mononeuritis multiplex** occurs. Motor neuropathy is manifested by an abrupt onset of weakness in a distribution that reflects the nerve involved (eg, peroneal nerve involvement produces foot drop). A surprising number of these motor neuropathies improve after 6–8 weeks. Reversible **cranial nerve palsies** can occur and may present as lid ptosis and diplopia (cranial nerve III), lateral deviation of the eye (IV), inability to move the eye laterally (VI), or facial paralysis (Bell's palsy) (VII). Acute pain and weakness of thigh muscles bilaterally can occur with progressive wasting and weight loss. This has been termed **diabetic amyotrophy** and is more common in elderly men. Again, the prognosis is good, with recovery of motor function over several months in many cases. In more severe cases with extensive atrophy of limb musculature, this disorder has been termed "malignant cachexia" and mimics the end stages of advanced neoplasia, particularly when depression produces anorexia and weight loss. With this more severe manifestation of diabetic amyotrophy, recovery of muscle function may only be partial.

Autonomic Neuropathy

Neuropathy of the autonomic nervous system is common in patients with diabetes of long duration and can be a very disconcerting clinical problem. It can affect many diverse visceral functions. With autonomic neuropathy, there may be postural hypotension, resting fixed tachycardia, decreased cardiovascular responses to the Valsalva maneuver, gastroparesis, alternating bouts of diarrhea (often nocturnal) and constipation, difficulty in emptying the bladder, and impotence.

Erectile dysfunction due to neuropathy differs from the psychogenic variety in that the latter may be intermittent (erections occur under special circumstances), whereas diabetic erectile dysfunction is usually persistent. To distinguish neuropathic or psychogenic erectile dysfunction from the erectile dysfunction caused by aortoiliac occlusive disease or vasculopathy, papaverine is injected into the corpus cavernosum penis. If the blood supply is competent, a penile erection will occur (Chapter 12). Urinary incontinence, with large volumes of residual urine, and retrograde ejaculation can also result from pelvic neuropathy.

Gastroparesis should be a diagnostic consideration in type 1 diabetic patients who develop unexpected fluctuations and variability in their blood glucose levels after meals. Radiographic studies of the stomach and radioisotopic examination of gastric emptying after liquid and solid meals are of diagnostic value in these patients. Involvement of the gastrointestinal system may be manifested by nausea, vomiting, and postprandial fullness (from gastric atony); symptoms of reflux or dysphagia (from esophageal involvement); constipation and recurrent diarrhea, especially at night (from involvement of the small bowel and colon); and fecal incontinence (from anal sphincter dysfunction). Gallbladder function is altered, and this enhances stone formation.

Therapy is difficult and must be directed specifically at each abnormality. Use of Jobst fitted stockings, tilting the head of the bed, and arising slowly from the supine position are useful in minimizing symptoms of **orthostatic hypotension.** Some patients may require the addition of a mineralocorticoid such as fludrocortisone acetate (0.1–0.2 mg twice daily). Metoclopramide has been of some help in treating diabetic gastroparesis over the short term, but its effectiveness seems to diminish over time. It is a dopamine antagonist with central antiemetic effects as well as cholinergic action to facilitate gastric emptying. It can be given intravenously (10–20 mg) or orally (20 mg of liquid metoclopramide) before breakfast and supper. Drowsiness is its major adverse effect. Erythromycin is a motilin agonist and can be used to treat gastroparesis. Bethanechol has also been used for gastroparesis (as well as for an atonic urinary bladder) because of its cholinergic effect.

Diabetic diarrhea is occasionally aggravated by bacterial overgrowth from stasis in the small intestine, and a trial of broad-spectrum antibiotics may give relief. If this does not help, symptomatic relief can sometimes be achieved with antidiarrheal agents such as diphenoxylate with atropine or loperamide. Clonidine has been reported to lessen diabetic diarrhea, but its tendency to lower blood pressure in those patients who already have some degree of orthostatic hypotension often limits its usefulness. Metamucil and other bulk-providing agents may relieve either the diarrhea or the constipation phases, which often alternate. Beta-lactulose is useful in managing severe constipation. Bethanechol has occasionally improved emptying of the **atonic urinary bladder.** There are medical, mechanical, and surgical treatments available for treatment of **erectile dysfunction.** Penile erection depends on relaxation of the smooth muscle in the arteries of the corpus cavernosum penis, and this is mediated by nitric oxide-induced cyclic 3′, 5′-guanosine monophosphate (cGMP) formation. Sildenafil (Viagra) is a selective inhibitor of cGMP-specific phosphodiesterase type 5. In response to sexual stimulation, there is local release of nitric oxide and cGMP production, and sildenafil, by inhibiting the breakdown of cGMP, improves the ability to achieve and maintain an erection. In a randomized study of patients with diabetes and erectile dysfunction, 56% taking sildenafil reported improved erections compared with 10% on placebo. The reason for lack of response in the other 44% is not known. Phosphodiesterase type 5 is also present in vascular smooth muscle, and sildenafil can lower systolic and diastolic pressure by 7% and 10%, respectively. Patients with cardiovascular disease may be adversely affected by this blood pressure decline, especially at the time of sexual activity. Sildenafil also potentiates the hypotensive effects of nitrates, and its use in patients taking those agents is contraindicated.

Intracorporeal injection of vasoactive drugs causes penile engorgement and erection. Drugs most commonly used include papaverine alone, papaverine with phentolamine, and alprostadil (prostaglandin E$_1$). Alprostadil injections are relatively painless, but careful instruction is essential to prevent local trauma, priapism, and fibrosis. Intraurethral pellets of alprostadil avoid the problem of injection of the drug.

External vacuum therapy (Erec-Aid System) is a nonsurgical treatment that consists of a suction chamber operated by a hand pump that creates a vacuum around the penis. This draws blood into the corpus cavernosum penis to produce an erection which is maintained by a specifically designed tension ring inserted around the base of the penis and which can be kept in place for up to 20–30 minutes.

Surgical implantation of a penile prosthesis should be considered for motivated patients when medical therapies prove to be unsatisfactory. (See Chapter 12.)

Aldose reductase inhibitors have been generally disappointing, with only marginal therapeutic results in either autonomic or peripheral diabetic neuropathy and a relatively high incidence of toxic side effects such as skin rash and neutropenia.

4. Cardiovascular Complications

Heart Disease

Microangiopathy has recently been recognized to occur in the heart and may explain the existence of congestive cardiomyopathies found in diabetic patients without demonstrable coronary artery disease. Much more commonly, however, heart failure in the diabetic is a consequence of coronary atherosclerosis. Myocardial infarction is three to five times more common in diabetic patients than in age-matched controls and is the leading cause of death in patients with type 2 diabetes. A loss of the protection against myocardial infarction usually present in women during the childbearing years is particularly evident in diabetic women. The exact reason for the increased incidence of myocardial infarction in diabetics is not clear. It may reflect the combination of hyperlipidemia, abnormalities of platelet adhesiveness, coagulation factors, hypertension, and oxidative stress and inflammation.

The American Diabetes Association also recommends lowering blood pressure to 130/80 mm Hg or less. The Antihypertensive and Lipid-Lowering Treatment to Prevent Heart Attack Trial (ALLHAT) randomized 33,357 subjects (age 55 years or older) with hypertension and at least one other coronary artery disease risk factor to receive treatment with chlorthalidone, amlodipine, or lisinopril. Chlorthalidone appeared to be superior to amlodipine and lisinopril in lowering blood pressure, in reducing the incidence of cardiovascular events, in tolerability, and in cost. The study included 12,063 individuals with type 2 diabetes. The Heart Outcomes Prevention Evaluation (HOPE) study randomized 9297 high-risk patients who had evidence of vascular disease or diabetes plus one other cardiovascular risk factor to receive ramipril or placebo for a mean period of 5 years. Treatment with ramipril resulted in a 25% reduction of the risk of myocardial infarction, stroke, or death from cardiovascular disease. The mean difference in blood pressure between the placebo and ramipril groups was 2.2 mm Hg systolic and 1.4 mm diastolic, and the reduction in cardiovascular event rate remained significant after adjustment for this small difference in blood pressure. The mechanism underlying this protective effect of ramipril is unknown. Patients with type 2 diabetes who already have cardiovascular disease or microalbuminuria should therefore be considered for treatment with an ACE inhibitor. More clinical studies are needed to address the question of whether patients with type 2 diabetes who do not have cardiovascular disease or microalbuminuria would specifically benefit from ACE inhibitor treatment.

The American Diabetes Association also recommends aspirin, 81–325 mg/d, for primary prevention in

Table 17–21. Guidelines for perioperative diabetes management with an intravenous insulin infusion.[1]

- Insulin: Regular (human) 25 units in 250 mL of normal saline (1 unit/10 mL).
- Intravenous infusions of insulin: Flush 50 mL through line before connecting to patient. Piggyback insulin line to the perioperative maintenance fluid line.
- Perioperative maintenance fluid: Fluids must contain 5% dextrose (rate 100 mL/h).
- Blood glucose: Monitor hourly intraoperatively.[2]

Blood Glucose (mg/dL)	Insulin	
	(units/h)	(mL/h)
< 80	0.0	0.0
81–100	0.5	5.0
101–140	1.0	10
141–180	1.5	15
181–220	2.0	20
221–260	2.5	25
261–300	3.0	30
301–340	4.0	40
> 341	5.0	50

- Blood glucose < 80 mg/dL: Stop insulin and administer intravenous bolus of 50% dextrose in water (25 mL). Once blood glucose > 80 mg/dL, restart insulin infusion. It may be necessary to modify the algorithm.
- Decreased insulin needs: Patients treated with diet or oral agents or < 50 units insulin per day, endocrinologic deficiencies.
- Increased insulin needs: Obesity, sepsis, steroid therapy, renal transplant, coronary artery bypass.

[1]Reproduced, with permission, from Gavin LA: Perioperative management of the diabetic patient. Endocrinol Metab Clin North Am 1992;21:457.
[2]Blood glucose value ÷ 100 gives a reasonable estimate of infusion dosage (units/h).

of insulin and dextrose can be stopped half an hour after the first subcutaneous dose. Insulin needs may vary in the first several days after surgery because of continuing postoperative stresses and because of variable caloric intake. In this situation, multiple doses of regular insulin guided by blood glucose determinations can keep the patient in acceptable metabolic control.

■ DIABETES MELLITUS & PREGNANCY

John L. Kitzmiller, MD

Hormone & Fuel Balance During Pregnancy

Pregnancy is characterized by major changes in the balance of metabolic fuels and hormones which significantly affect the management of diabetes. Basal hepatic glucose production increases as pregnancy progresses in spite of increased basal insulin secretion, demonstrating insulin resistance of the hepatic cells. However, plasma concentrations of glucose in the fasting state decline slightly, associated with increasing fetal-placental utilization of glucose. Although fat deposition is accentuated in early pregnancy, lipolysis is enhanced by human placental lactogen (hPL) later in gestation, and more glycerol and free fatty acids (FFA) are released in the postabsorptive state (distant from meals). The increased FFA contribute to the impaired glucose utilization by skeletal muscle characteristic of advancing pregnancy. Ketogenesis is also accentuated in the postabsorptive state during pregnancy, secondary to hormonal effects on the maternal liver cells and increased provision of substrate FFA.

The balance of metabolic fuels is also different in the fed state during pregnancy. Despite increased insulin secretion after a carbohydrate or amino acid load (or both) in normal pregnancy, there is a striking reduction in insulin-mediated glucose disposal by peripheral tissue (muscle) by the third trimester. The result is somewhat higher maternal blood glucose levels in nondiabetic subjects and severe hyperglycemia in insufficiently treated pregnant diabetic women. This insulin resistance has been related to hPL, progesterone, cortisol, prolactin, and FFA, with defects at the post-insulin receptor level in hepatic and muscle cells. Glucagon is well suppressed by glucose during pregnancy, and secretory responses of glucagon to amino acids are not increased above nonpregnant levels. After meals, more glucose is converted to triglyceride in pregnant compared with nonpregnant subjects, which would tend to conserve calories and enhance fat deposition.

Overview of Diabetes During Pregnancy

In the past, diabetic pregnant women were classified on the basis of duration and severity of diabetes (Table 17–22). The classification system of Priscilla White was originally used to indicate prognosis of perinatal outcome and to determine obstetric management. Because the perinatal mortality rate has declined dramatically for many reasons in women in all classes, the system is now used mainly to describe and compare populations of diabetic pregnant women. However, certain characteristics of patients are still pertinent. The risk of complications is minimal if gestational diabetes is well controlled by diet alone, and these patients may be otherwise managed as normal pregnant women. Class B patients, mainly women with type 2 diabetes with onset less than 10 years previously, will probably have residual islet B cell function, and control of hyperglycemia may be easier than in class C or D patients, who have brittle type 1 diabetes. Finally, the most complicated and difficult pregnancies occur in women with renal, retinal, or cardiovascular disease (classes F, H, and R).

The hormonal and metabolic effects of pregnancy are associated with increased risks of both hypoglycemic insulin reactions and ketoacidosis. Increasing amounts of insulin are usually required to control hyperglycemia throughout gestation.

If diabetes is poorly controlled in the first weeks of pregnancy, the risks of spontaneous abortion and congenital malformation of the infant are increased. Later in pregnancy, polyhydramnios is also common in women with poorly controlled diabetes and may lead to preterm delivery. Fetal hypoxia may develop in the third trimester if blood glucose levels frequently exceed 180 mg/dL (10 mmol/L). In poorly controlled patients, careful fetal monitoring must be used to prevent stillbirth. The high incidence of fetal macrosomia (birth weight > 90th percentile for gestational age) associated with maternal hyperglycemia and fetal hyperinsulinemia increases the potential for traumatic vaginal deliv-

Table 17–22. Classification of diabetes during pregnancy (Priscilla White).

Class	Characteristics	Implications
Gestational diabetes	Abnormal glucose tolerance during pregnancy; postprandial hyperglycemia during pregnancy.	Diagnosis before 30 weeks' gestation important to prevent macrosomia. Treat with diet adequate in calories to prevent maternal weight loss. Goal is postprandial blood glucose < 130 mg/dL (7.2 mmol/L) at 1 hour or < 105 mg/dL (5.8 mmol/L) at 2 hours. If insulin is necessary, manage as in classes B, C, and D.
A	Chemical diabetes diagnosed before pregnancy; managed by diet alone; any age at onset.	Management as for gestational diabetes.
B	Insulin treatment or oral hypoglycemic agent used before pregnancy; onset at age 20 or older; duration < 10 years.	Some endogenous insulin secretion may persist. Fetal and neonatal risks same as in classes C and D, as is management; can be type 1 or 2.
C	Onset at age 10–20, or duration 10–20 years.	Insulin-deficient diabetes of juvenile onset; type 1.
D	Onset before age 10, or duration > 20 years, or chronic hypertension (not preeclampsia), or background retinopathy (tiny hemorrhages).	Fetal macrosomia or intrauterine growth retardation possible. Retinal microaneurysms, dot hemorrhages, and exudates may progress during pregnancy, then regress after delivery.
F	Diabetic nephropathy with proteinuria.	Anemia and hypertension common; proteinuria increases in third trimester, declines after delivery. Fetal intrauterine growth retardation common; perinatal survival about 90% under optimal conditions; bed rest necessary.
H	Coronary artery disease.	Serious maternal risk.
R	Proliferative retinopathy.	Neovascularization, with risk of vitreous hemorrhage or retinal detachment; laser photocoagulation useful; abortion usually not necessary. With active process of neovascularization, prevent bearing-down efforts.

ery; cesarean deliveries are more common in these cases. Fetal intrauterine growth restriction may occur in diabetic women with vascular disease or those with relative hypoglycemia induced by overzealous treatment.

Neonatal risks linked to maternal glycemic control include respiratory distress syndrome, hypoglycemia, hyperbilirubinemia, hypocalcemia, and poor feeding. Although these problems are usually limited to the first days of life, excess maternal glucose and β-hydroxybutyrate levels with the fetus in utero have been related to diminished performance on intelligence and psychomotor testing during subsequent childhood development. However, if diabetic women adhere to a program of careful management and surveillance, they have greater than 95% chance of delivering a healthy child.

In the following sections, the convention used for designating the number of weeks of gestation is the number of weeks from the last menstrual period, confirmed by ultrasound measurements.

Gestational Diabetes

Impaired glucose tolerance develops in 2–8% of pregnant women, usually during the second half of gestation. The frequency depends on ethnic group (highest in Asian-American, Latina, Native American, Polynesian), and is increased in those with central obesity or a family history of diabetes. The mechanism of glucose intolerance in lean women results from sluggish first-phase insulin release coupled with excessive insulin resistance. In overweight women with gestational diabetes, insulin resistance increases more than in overweight controls, despite increased circulating insulin levels, so that insulin secretion is actually inadequate in relation to the hyperglycemia.

Strategies for diagnosis are outlined in Table 17–23. After diagnosis, the patient should be placed on a diabetic meal plan modified for pregnancy: 25–35 kcal/kg ideal weight, 40–55% carbohydrate, 20% protein, and 25–40% fat. Calories are distributed over three meals and three snacks (Table 17–24). Most patients can be taught to count their carbohydrates and to read food labels. The goal of therapy is not weight reduction but prevention of fasting and postprandial hyperglycemia. If fasting capillary blood glucose levels exceed 90–100 mg/dL (5–5.6 mmol/L) or if 1-hour or 2-hour postprandial glucose values are consistently greater (respectively) than 130 or 105 mg/dL (7.2 or 5.8 mmol/L), therapy is begun with human insulin. As an alternative, consider the sulfonylurea glyburide, which crosses the human placenta poorly. Current research is evaluating its efficacy and safety when dietary therapy fails to produce normoglycemia.

Table 17–23. Screening and diagnosis of gestational diabetes.[1]

Risk for gestational diabetes mellitus should be ascertained at the first prenatal visit

Low risk:
  Universal versus selective screening remains controversial; most diabetes organizations state that blood glucose testing is not normally required if all of the following characteristics are present:
    Member of an ethnic group with a low prevalence of gestational diabetes mellitus
    No known diabetes in first-degree relatives
    Age < 25 years
    Weight normal before pregnancy
    No history of abnormal glucose metabolism or poor pregnancy outcome
Average risk:
  Perform blood glucose testing at 24–28 weeks using one of the following
    One-step protocol: 75 g, 2-hour oral glucose tolerance test on all women:
      Fasting: < 95 mg/dL (5.3 mmol/L)
      1 hour: < 180 mg/dL (< 10 mmol/L)
      2 hours: < 155 mg/dL (< 8.6 mmol/L)
    Two-step protocol: 50 g, 1-hour plasma glucose on all women: if test done in fasting state, threshold is > 130 mg/dL (> 7.2 mmol/L); if test done in fed state, threshold is 140 mg/dL (> 7.8 mmol/L). Then test with 100 g, 3 hours, in fasting state:
      Fasting: < 95 mg/dL (< 5.3 mmol/L)
      1 hour: < 180 mg/dL (< 10 mmol/L)
      2 hours: < 155 mg/dL (< 8.6 mmol/L)
      3 hours: < 140 mg/dL (< 7.8 mmol/L)
      If one value is abnormal, repeat test in 4 weeks
High risk:
  Perform testing as soon as feasible. If negative, repeat at 24–28 weeks

[1]Adapted from Summary and Recommendations, Fourth International Workshop-Conference on Gestational Diabetes Mellitus: Diabetes Care 1998;21(Suppl 2):B162.

Progression to type 2 diabetes later in life will occur in 5–50% of women with gestational diabetes. The wide range in incidence is influenced by body weight, family history, glucose levels, and the need for insulin treatment during pregnancy—and the choice of contraception and lifestyle after pregnancy. All patients with gestational diabetes should undergo a 75 g 2-hour glucose tolerance test at 6–10 weeks after delivery to guide future medical management. Follow-up protocols after pregnancy and criteria for the diagnosis of diabetes mellitus in the nonpregnant state are presented in Table 17–25.

Table 17–24. Management of diet for patients with gestational diabetes.

---

(1) Assess present pattern of food consumption.
(2) Balance calories with optimal weight gain.
   (a) Caloric intake: 25–35 kcal/kg ideal weight.
   (b) Weight gain: 0.45 kg (1 lb) per month during the first trimester; 0.2–0.35 kg (0.5–0.75 lb) per week during the second and third trimesters.
(3) Distribute calories and carbohydrates over 3 meals and 3 snacks; evening snack to include complex carbohydrate and at least one meat exchange.
(4) Use food exchanges to assess the amount of carbohydrate, protein, and fat:
   (a) Carbohydrate: 40–55% of calories or ≥ 150 g/d.
   (b) Protein: 20% of calories or ≥ 74 g/d.
   (c) Fat: 25–40% of calories.
(5) Emphasize high-fiber, complex carbohydrate foods.
(6) Identify individual glycemic responses to certain foods.
(7) Tailor eating plans to personal needs.

Glucose Monitoring & Insulin Management

The goal of insulin therapy during pregnancy is to prevent both preprandial and postprandial hyperglycemia, but in type 1 diabetic patients, caution must be used to avoid debilitating hypoglycemic reactions. Perinatal outcome will be optimal if patients aim for fasting plasma glucose levels below 100 mg/dL (5.6 mmol/L) and postprandial levels below 130 mg/dL (7.2 mmol/L). In type 1 patients with hypoglycemia unawareness, somewhat higher blood glucose targets should be selected. Self-monitoring of capillary blood glucose should be done at home and in the workplace several times daily using glucose oxidase strips and portable reflectance colorimeters with memory capacity. Confirmation of long-term control is provided by sequential measurement of glycosylated hemoglobin and fructosamine.

Most pregnant diabetic patients will require at least two daily injections of a mixture of regular and intermediate insulin in order to prevent fasting and postprandial hyperglycemia. Common insulin regimens are outlined in Table 17–26. The usual practice for initiation of insulin therapy in pregnant women with gestational diabetes mellitus or type 2 diabetes is to give two-thirds of the insulin before breakfast and one-third before supper. More stringent regimens of administering short-acting subcutaneous insulin three times a day before meals and intermediate insulin at bedtime to control overnight and fasting glucose—or of continuous subcutaneous insulin infusion with a portable pump—may be necessary to achieve normoglycemia in

Table 17–25. Follow-up (after pregnancy) of patient with gestational diabetes mellitus.

Encourage breast feeding.
Montitor postprandial blood glucose occasionally to be sure it is < 180 mg/dL (< 10 mmol/L).
Perform 75-g 2-hour oral glucose test at 6–12 weeks postpartum.

Diagnosis	Fasting Blood Glucose mg/dL (mmol/L)	Two-Hour Value mg/dL (mmol/L)
Normal	< 100 (< 6.1)	< 140 (< 7.8)
Impaired glucose tolerance	110–125 (6.1–6.9)	140–199 (7.8–11.1)
Diabetes mellitus	> 125 (7.0)	> 199 (> 11.1)

Contraception: Barrier methods, Cu 7 IUD, low-dose birth control pills such as Ovcon 35, Triphasil (which do not affect glucose tolerance or lipid profiles).
Use diet and exercise for women with impaired glucose tolerance and those with central body obesity. Impaired glucose tolerance implies a high risk of development of type 2 diabetes.
Obtain annual blood glucose test of some kind and especially before the next pregnancy.

---

many women, especially those with type 1 diabetes. These women will also benefit from learning to self-adjust their doses of short-acting insulin based on planned carbohydrate load or premeal blood glucose levels. (See previous section: Insulin.)

Hypoglycemic reactions are more frequent and sometimes more severe in early gestation but are a risk at any time during pregnancy. Therefore, insulin-treated patients must use timely between-meal and bedtime snacks to prevent hypoglycemia—and type 1 diabetic patients must keep glucagon on hand, and a member of the household must be instructed in the technique of injection. Hypoglycemic reactions have not been associated with fetal death or congenital anomalies, but they pose a risk to maternal health.

Diabetic Complications & Pregnancy

A. Vomiting of Pregnancy

In early gestation, diabetic gastroparesis or gastropathy can severely exacerbate the nausea and vomiting of pregnancy (hyperemesis gravidarum), which sometimes will continue into the third trimester. Drugs stimulating gastric motility such as erythromycin and cisapride may be useful, but many patients with this complication will require hyperalimentation to achieve nutritional intake adequate for fetal development.

Table 17–26. Illustration of use of home blood glucose monitoring to determine insulin dosage during pregnancy.

Self-Monitored Capillary Blood Glucose		Insulin Doses
Fasting blood glucose	148 mg/dL (8.2 mmol/L)	14 units regular, 28 units intermediate
1 h after breakfast	206 mg/dL (11.4 mmol/L)	
1 h after lunch	152 mg/dL (8.4 mmol/L)	
1 h after supper	198 mg/dL (11.0 mmol/L)	9 units regular, 10 units intermediate
2–4 AM	142 mg/dL (7.9 mmol/L)	

Suggested changes based on pattern of blood glucose values over 2–3 days: slight increases in presupper intermediate insulin to control fasting blood glucose next day, in morning regular insulin to control postbreakfast glucose, and in presupper regular insulin to control postsupper hyperglycemia. Dose of morning intermediate insulin is adequate to control early afternoon blood glucose. When dose of presupper intermediate insulin is increased, patient should test to detect and prevent nocturnal hypoglycemia. One-hour postprandial testing is advised to detect the probable peaks of glycemic excursions. Patient should also test when symptoms of hypoglycemia appear.

B. DIABETIC RETINOPATHY

Pregnancy also affects diabetic retinopathy. Background diabetic retinopathy may develop or progress during pregnancy, but it usually regresses postpartum. If background retinopathy is already present in early pregnancy, the rate of progression to neovascularization (proliferative diabetic retinopathy) will be 6% → 18% → 38%, depending on the extent of background retinopathy from mild to moderate to severe preproliferative changes. The risk factors for progression to proliferative retinopathy include poor glycemic control before and during early pregnancy, rapid improvement in glycemic control during pregnancy, hypertension, and perhaps the many growth factors derived from placental tissue. These risks are an important reason to institute intensified preconception management of diabetes. During pregnancy, sequential ophthalmologic examinations are essential in women with type 1 or type 2 diabetes, and laser photocoagulation treatment of the retina may be necessary.

C. DIABETIC NEPHROPATHY

The risk of worsening of diabetic nephropathy during pregnancy depends on baseline renal function and the degree of hypertension. Total urinary albumin excretion does not increase much in normal pregnancy, but total urinary protein collections, which obstetricians have used to define preeclampsia, may show a twofold increase in uncomplicated gestation. Diabetic women with microalbuminuria (30–299 mg/24 h) may have worsening of the albuminuria during pregnancy with regression postpartum, and 15–45% will develop the preeclamptic syndrome. Based on pooled data from several studies of pregnant diabetic women with a clinical level of proteinuria (24-hour urinary albumin > 300

mg) at the beginning of pregnancy, if initial renal function is preserved (serum creatinine < 1.2 mg/dL [> 106 μmol/L]; creatinine clearance < 80 mL/min with complete collection), then 15–20% are expected to show moderate decline during gestation, and 6% will have renal failure at follow-up several years after pregnancy. The latter figure may not be different from the course of diabetic nephropathy in nonpregnant women with this level of initial renal function. If initial renal function in pregnancy is impaired (serum creatinine > 1.2 mg/dL [> 106 μmol/L]; creatinine clearance < 80 mL/min with complete collection), then 35–40% are expected to show further decline during pregnancy and 45–50% will have renal failure at follow-up. Thus, careful preconception counseling is important for these patients and their family members.

D. DIABETIC NEUROPATHY

The course of diabetic neuropathy is uncertain during pregnancy, and treatment may be relatively ineffective. The agents commonly used (amitriptyline, desipramine) may produce neonatal withdrawal symptoms.

Fetal Development & Growth

A. CONGENITAL ANOMALIES

Major congenital anomalies are those that may affect the life of the individual or require major surgery for correction. The incidence in infants of poorly controlled diabetic mothers is 6–12%, compared with about 2% in infants born to diabetic women who begin pregnancy with normal glycohemoglobin or infants of a nondiabetic population. Since perinatal deaths due to stillbirth and respiratory distress syndrome have declined in pregnancies complicated by diabetes, the proportion of fetal and neonatal deaths ascribed to congenital anomalies has risen to over 50%. The types of anomalies most common in infants of diabetic mothers and their presumed time of occurrence during embryonic development are listed in Table 17–27. It is apparent that any intervention to reduce the incidence of major congenital anomalies must be applied very early in pregnancy. The finding that the excess risk of anomalies is associated with the group of diabetic women with elevated glycosylated hemoglobin early in pregnancy suggests that poor diabetic control is related to the risk of major congenital anomalies in their infants. Protocols of intensive diabetic management instituted

Table 17–27. Congenital malformations in infants of diabetic mothers.[1]

	Ratio of Incidences Diabetic vs Control Group	Latest Gestational Age for Occurrence (Weeks After Menstruation)
Caudal regression	252	5
Anencephaly	3	6
Spina bifida, hydrocephalus, or other central nervous system defects	2	6
Cardiac anomalies	4	
Transposition of great vessels		7
Ventricular septal defect		8
Atrial septal defect		8
Anal/rectal atresia	3	8
Renal anomalies	5	
Agenesis	6	7
Cystic kidney	4	7
Ureter duplex	23	7
Situs inversus	84	6

[1]Modified and reproduced, with permission, from Kucera J: Rate and type of congenital anomalies among offspring of diabetic women. J Reprod Med 1971;7:61; and Mills JL, Baker L, Goldman AS: Malformations in infants of diabetic mothers occur before the seventh gestational week: Implications for treatment. Diabetes 1979;28:292.

prior to conception and continued through early pregnancy have resulted in significant reduction in the frequency of anomalies. Primary care physicians treating diabetic women of reproductive age should counsel them about the possibility and risks of pregnancy and help them achieve good glycemic control if pregnancy is desired.

B. NEURAL TUBE DEFECTS

Ultrasonography in the first half of pregnancy confirms the dating of gestation and may detect neural tube defects (anencephaly, meningomyelocele) that occur with a higher incidence in infants of poorly controlled diabetic mothers. The physician should also screen all insulin-dependent pregnant women at 14–16 weeks of gestation for elevated serum alpha-fetoprotein levels that may suggest less severe cases of neural tube defects, eg, spina bifida. Later in pregnancy, at 18–22 weeks, sophisticated ultrasonographic examinations are used to detect congenital heart defects or other severe anomalies. Subsequent examinations at 26 and 36 weeks measure fetal growth and well-being.

C. MACROSOMIA

Many fetuses of poorly controlled diabetic mothers are macrosomic (large for dates), with increased fat stores, increased length, and increased abdomen-to-head or thorax-to-head ratios. The hypothesis that fetal macrosomia results from the causal chain of maternal hyperglycemia → fetal hyperglycemia → fetal hyperinsulinemia → fetal macrosomia has been confirmed by clinical and experimental studies. Macrosomic infants of diabetic mothers have significantly higher concentrations of C peptide in their cord sera or amniotic fluid (representing endogenous insulin secretion) than do those with birth weights appropriate for gestational age. Monkey fetuses with insulin-releasing pellets implanted in utero become macrosomic. In human pregnancies, the determinants of fetal hyperinsulinemia may be not only maternal hyperglycemia, however. Other metabolic substrates that cross the placenta, such as branched-chain amino acids, are insulinogenic and may play a role in fetal macrosomia, and transplacental lipids could contribute to fat deposition.

The level of maternal glycemia is related to birth weight adjusted for gestational age, and prevention of maternal hyperglycemia throughout pregnancy can reduce the incidence of macrosomia and birth trauma. The glycemic threshold for fetal macrosomia seems to be *postprandial* peak values above 130 mg/dL (7.2 mmol/L). On the other hand, too tight glycemic control (average peak postprandial blood glucose levels below 110 mg/dL [6.1 mmol/L]) can be associated with insufficient fetal growth and small-for-dates infants, which may also induce complications in the neonatal period.

D. POLYHYDRAMNIOS

Polyhydramnios is an excess volume of amniotic fluid (> 1000 mL, often > 3000 mL). It may cause severe discomfort or premature labor and is most often associated with fetal macrosomia. The excess volume of amniotic fluid is not related simply to the concentration of glucose or other solutes in amniotic fluid or to excess fetal urine output as measured by change in bladder size by means of ultrasonography. Other possible factors include decreased fetal swallowing, decidual and amniotic fluid prolactin, and as yet unknown determinants of the complicated multicompartmental intrauterine transfer of water. Polyhydramnios is rare in women with well-controlled diabetes.

E. GROWTH RETARDATION

In contrast to fetal macrosomia, the fetus of a woman with diabetes of long duration and vascular disease may suffer intrauterine fetal growth restriction related to inadequate uteroplacental perfusion. All body diameters may be below normal on ultrasonographic measurements, but the abdominal circumference is especially affected, and oligohydramnios and abnormal doppler flow measurements of the umbilical cord are common. In these patients provision of adequate rest, meticulous control of hypertension (target < 135/85 mm Hg), maintenance of normal blood glucose levels, and intensive fetal surveillance are all essential for success.

F. INTRAUTERINE DEATH

Prior to the 1970s, the incidence of apparently sudden intrauterine fetal demise in the third trimester of diabetic pregnancies was at least 5%. Since the risk increased as pregnancies approached term, iatrogenic preterm delivery was instituted but the incidence of neonatal deaths from respiratory distress syndrome increased. Except for congenital malformations, the cause of stillbirth is often not obvious. The risk is greater with poor diabetic control, and the incidence of fetal death exceeds 50% if ketoacidosis develops in the mother. Some instances of fetal demise are associated with preeclampsia-eclampsia, which is a common complication in diabetic pregnant women. Fetal death has been associated also with pyelonephritis, which is now largely prevented by screening for and treating asymptomatic bacteriuria. Other than these known risk factors, one can presume—based on experimental studies—that the combination of fetal hyperglycemia and hypoxia leads to acidosis and myocardial dysfunction. Good glycemic control in diabetic women greatly reduces the risk of stillbirth.

Obstetric Management

A. MONITORING

(Table 17–28.) Technologic advances have led to techniques for detecting fetal hypoxia and preventing stillbirth. Most simply, the infrequency of fetal movement as noted in regular fetal kick counts (few than four per hour) may indicate fetal jeopardy. More rigorous analysis of fetal activity patterns using ultrasonography is known as the "fetal biophysical profile," which assesses gross body movements, the tone of the limbs, and chest wall motions as well as reactivity of the fetal heart rate and the volume of amniotic fluid. The measurement of maternal estriol levels for fetal evaluation is now of only historical interest. This assay was based on the knowledge that placental production of estriol is dependent on precursors from the fetal adrenals and correlates with the mass and well-being of the fetal-placental unit, but application of the assay was imprecise and was supplanted by antepartum fetal heart rate (FHR) monitoring. The presence of fetal heart rate accelerations and

Table 17–28. Schedule of obstetric tests and procedures.

Procedure	Risk Based on Glycemic Control, Presence of Vascular Disease	
	Low Risk	High Risk
Ultrasound to date gestation	8–12 weeks	8–12 weeks
Prenatal genetic diagnosis	As needed	As needed
Targeted perinatal ultrasound; fetal echocardiography	18–22 weeks	18–22 weeks
Fetal kick counts	28 weeks	28 weeks
Ultrasound for fetal growth	28 and 37 weeks[1]	Every 3–8 weeks
Antepartum FHR monitoring, backup with biophysical profile	36 weeks, weekly	27 weeks, 1–3 per week
Amniocentesis for lung	…	35–38 weeks
Induction of labor	41 weeks[2]	35–38 weeks

[1]Not needed in normoglycemic, diet-treated women with gestational diabetes mellitus.
[2]Earlier for obstetric reasons or for impending fetal macrosomia.

long-range variability on the nonstress test (NST) and the absence of late decelerations (lower FHR persists after the contraction subsides) on the contraction stress test (CST) indicates that the fetus is well oxygenated. However, the predictive value of a normal result is only valid for a short duration in diabetic women with unstable metabolic control or hypertension. These patients may have to be hospitalized for daily fetal testing. Generally, the NST and CST are sensitive screening tests, and abnormal results of FHR monitoring in these tests will overestimate the diagnosis of fetal distress. Therefore, it is wise to obtain additional evidence of fetal jeopardy (by biophysical ultrasonographic assessment) before cesarean delivery is recommended in preterm pregnancies. In term gestation with abnormal fetal testing, there is little to be gained by continuing the pregnancy.

B. Timing of Delivery

Unless maternal or fetal complications arise, the goal for delivery in diabetic women should be 38–41 weeks in order to reduce neonatal morbidity from preterm deliveries. On the other hand, the obstetrician may wish to induce labor before 39 weeks if there is concern about increasing fetal weight. Before a preterm delivery decision (less than 37 weeks) is made—or at 37–38 weeks in women with poor glycemic control—fetal pulmonary maturity should be determined. Tests for maturity using amniocentesis predict a low risk of neonatal respiratory distress syndrome and include the lecithin/sphingomyelin (L/S) ratio, phosphatidylglycerol, and other biochemical or physical assays of surfactant activity. In pregnancies complicated by hyperglycemia, fetal hyperinsulinemia can lead to low pulmonary surfactant apoprotein production. The lowest risk for respiratory distress syndrome is attained by delaying delivery (if possible) until 38–41 weeks and minimizing the need for cesarean sections.

C. Route of Delivery

Once fetal lung maturity is likely, the route of delivery must be selected based on the usual obstetric indications. If the fetus seems large (> 4200 g) on clinical and ultrasonographic examination of diabetic women, cesarean section probably should be performed because of the possibility of shoulder dystocia and birth trauma. Otherwise, induction of labor is reasonable, because maternal and peripartum risks are fewer following vaginal delivery. Once labor is under way, continuous fetal heart rate monitoring is essential. Maternal blood glucose levels > 150 mg/dL (8.3 mmol/L) can be associated with intrapartum fetal hypoxia.

Insulin Management for Labor & Delivery

The diabetic parturient may be unusually sensitive to insulin during active labor and delivery, and severe maternal hypoglycemia is possible if delivery occurs sooner than anticipated and a high dose of subcutaneous intermediate-acting insulin was previously administered. Protocols for continuous low-dose intravenous insulin administration during labor or prior to cesarean delivery are used to achieve stringent control of blood glucose in order to reduce the incidence of intrapartum fetal distress and neonatal metabolic problems (Table 17–29). A cord blood glucose level at delivery correlates positively with the higher maternal levels, and there is no upper limit on placental transfer of glucose. During labor, maternal plasma glucose can usually be kept below 110 mg/dL (6.1 mmol/L) with 1–2 units of regular insulin and 7.5 g of dextrose given intravenously

Table 17–29. Protocol for intrapartum insulin infusion.[1]

Intravenous fluids

If blood glucose is > 130 mg/dL (> 7.2 mmol/L), infuse mainline Ringer's lactate at a rate of 125 mL/h.

If blood glucose is < 130 mg/dL (< 7.2 mmol/L), infuse mainline Ringer's lactate to keep vein open and begin Ringer's lactate and 5% dextrose at a rate of 125 mL/h controlled by infusion pump.

Insulin infusion

Mix 25 units of regular human insulin (U100) in 250 mL NaCl 0.9% and piggyback to mainline. The concentration is 1 unit/10 mL. Adjust intravenous insulin hourly according to the following table when the blood glucose is > 70 mg/dL (> 3.9 mmol/L).

Blood glucose mg/dL (mmol/L)	Insulin (units/h)	Infusion (mL/h)
< 70 (< 3.9)	None	None
71–90 (3.9–5)	0.5	5
91–110 (5.1–6.1)	1	10
111–130 (6.2–7.2)	2	20
131–150 (7.3–8.3)	3	30
151–170 (8.4–9.4)	4	40
171–190 (9.5–10.6)	5	50
> 190 (> 10.6)	Call MD and check urine ketones	

[1]Protocol useful also for diabetic pregnant women who are "NPO" or being treated with beta-adrenergic tocolysis or corticosteroids. The scale dosages may need to be doubled for the latter. Boluses of short-acting insulin must be used to cover meals.

every hour. If cesarean section is necessary, insulin management is similar, and infants do equally well with general, spinal, or epidural anesthesia as long as the diabetic parturient does not receive rapid high-volume loads of glucose-containing intravenous solutions.

Neonatal Morbidity

Planning for the care of the infant should be started prior to delivery, with participation by the pediatrician or neonatologist in decisions about timing and management of delivery. In complicated cases, the pediatrician must be in attendance to learn about antenatal problems, to assess the need for resuscitation, to identify major congenital anomalies, and to plan initial therapy for the sick infant if required.

A. RESPIRATORY DISTRESS SYNDROME

Infants of poorly controlled diabetic mothers have an increased risk of respiratory distress syndrome. Possible reasons include abnormal production of pulmonary surfactant or connective tissue changes leading to decreased pulmonary compliance. However, in recent years, the incidence of respiratory distress syndrome has declined from 24% to 5%, probably related to better maternal glycemic control, selected use of amniotic fluid tests, and delivery of most infants at term (see above). The diagnosis of respiratory distress syndrome is based on clinical signs (grunting, retraction, respiratory rate > 60/min), typical findings on chest x-ray (diffuse reticulogranular pattern and air bronchogram), and an increased oxygen requirement (to maintain the PaO_2 at 50–70 mm Hg) for more than 48 hours with no other identified cause of respiratory difficulty (heart disease, infection). Survival of infants with respiratory distress syndrome has dramatically improved as a result of advances in ventilation therapy and intrapulmonary administration of surfactant.

B. HYPOGLYCEMIA

Hypoglycemia is common in the first 48 hours after delivery of previously hyperglycemic mothers and is defined as blood glucose below 30 mg/dL (1.7 mmol/L) regardless of gestational age. The symptomatic infant may be lethargic rather than jittery, and hypoglycemia may be associated with apnea, tachypnea, cyanosis, or seizures. Hypoglycemia has been related to elevated fetal insulin levels during and after delivery. Infants of diabetic mothers may also have deficient catecholamine and glucagon secretion, and the hypoglycemia may be related to diminished hepatic glucose production and oxidation of free fatty acids. The pediatrician attempts to prevent hypoglycemia in "well" infants with early feedings of 10% dextrose in water by bottle or gavage

by 1 hour of age. If this is not successful, treatment with intravenous dextrose solutions is indicated. There are usually no long-term sequelae of episodes of neonatal hypoglycemia.

Other possible problems in infants of diabetic mothers include hypocalcemia < 7 mg/dL [1.75 mmol/L], hyperbilirubinemia > 15 mg/dL [256 μmol/L], polycythemia (central hematocrit > 70%), and poor feeding. These complications are also somehow related to fetal hyperglycemia and hyperinsulinemia and probably to intermittent low-level fetal hypoxia. Improved control of the maternal diabetic state has reduced their incidence.

◾ PROGNOSIS FOR PATIENTS WITH DIABETES MELLITUS

In patients with type 1 diabetes, the results of the Diabetes Control and Complications Trial have established the benefit of near-normalization of glycemia in preventing or delaying the progression of diabetic microangiopathy. Similar trials of intensive therapy of hypertension as well as control of blood glucose in the United Kingdom indicate that a similar benefit occurs in type 2 diabetes, particularly with regard to macrovascular disease and microangiopathy. Currently, the prospect for retarding the progression of diabetic eye complications in both types of diabetes is good because of benefits derived from laser photocoagulation. Education as to proper foot care has been immensely valuable in reducing morbidity from diabetic foot problems. Management of hypertension, dyslipidemia, and cessation of cigarette smoking have been of great benefit in preventing or reducing the progression of retinopathy, nephropathy, and atherosclerosis. Newer methods for delivering purified insulins and for self-monitoring blood glucose have improved the overall outlook for patients with diabetes mellitus. However, present methods of subcutaneous insulin delivery need much improvement before physiologic insulin secretion is reproduced. Hypoglycemia remains a serious risk in all regimens of intensive insulin therapy attempting normalization of blood glucose. It is clear that the diabetic patient's intelligence, motivation, and awareness of potential complications of the disease are major factors contributing to a successful outcome. In addition, appropriate education of diabetic patients to provide the knowledge, the guidelines, and the tools to help them take charge of their own day-to-day diabetes management is essential to improve the long-term prognosis.

REFERENCES

The Endocrine Pancreas

Aguilar-Bryan L et al: Cloning of the beta cell high-affinity sulfonylurea receptor: a regulator of insulin secretion. Science 1995;268:423.

Atria TE et al: Secretion of pancreatic polypeptide in patients with pancreatic endocrine tumors. N Engl J Med 1986;315:287.

Daniel S et al: Identification of the docked granule pool responsible for the first phase of glucose-stimulated insulin secretion. Diabetes 1999;48:1686.

Duckworth WC, Bennett RG, Hamel FG: Insulin degradation: progress and potential. Endocr Rev 1998;19:608.

Edwards CMB et al: Glucagon-like peptide 1 has a physiological role in the control of postprandial glucose in humans: studies with the antagonist exendin 9-39. Diabetes 1999;48:86.

Eliasson L et al: PKC-dependent stimulation of exocytosis by sulfonylureas in pancreatic beta cells. Science 1996;271:813.

Fehman H-C, Goke R, Goke B: Cell and molecular biology of the incretin hormones glucagon-like peptide I and glucose-dependent insulin releasing polypeptide. Endocr Rev 1995;16:390.

Galloway JA et al: Biosynthetic human proinsulin: Review of chemistry, in vitro and in vivo receptor binding, animal and human pharmacology studies, and clinical trial experience. Diabetes Care 1992;15:666.

Gribble FM et al: Tissue specificity of sulfonylureas: studies on cloned cardiac and beta cell K^+ ATP channels. Diabetes 1998;47:1412.

Holst JJ: Glucagonlike peptide 1: A newly discovered hormone. Gastroenterology 1994;107:1848.

Kahn BB: Facilitative glucose transporters: Regulatory mechanisms and dysregulation in diabetes. J Clin Invest 1992;89:1367.

Kahn SE, Andrikopoulos S, Verchere CB: Islet amyloid: a long-recognized but unappreciated pathological feature of type 2 diabetes. Diabetes 1999;48:241.

Kumar U et al: Subtype-selective expression of the five somatostatin receptors (hSSTR 1-5) in human pancreatic islet cells. Diabetes 1999;48:77.

Lefebvre PJ: Glucagon and its family revisited. Diabetes Care 1995;18:715.

Philippe J: Structure and pancreatic expression of the insulin and glucagon genes. Endocr Rev 1991;12:252.

Polonsky KS: The beta-cell in diabetes: From molecular genetics to clinical research. Diabetes 1995;44:705.

Rehfeld JF: The new biology of gastrointestinal hormones. Physiol Rev 1998;78:1087.

Resine T, Bell GI: Molecular biology of somatostatin receptors. Endocr Rev 1995;16:427.

Stephens JM, Pilch PF: The metabolic regulation and vesicular transport of GLUT 4, the major insulin responsive glucose transporter. Endocr Rev 1995;16:529.

Swenne I: Pancreatic beta-cell growth and diabetes mellitus. Diabetologia 1992;35:193.

Westermark P et al: Islet amyloid polypeptide A novel controversy in diabetes research. Diabetologia 1992;35:297.

Diagnosis, Classification, & Pathophysiology of Diabetes Mellitus

Alberti KGMM et al: Definition, diagnosis and classification of diabetes mellitus and its complications. Diabet Med 1998;15:539.

Atkinson MA, Eisenbarth GS: Type 1 diabetes; new perspectives on disease pathogenesis and treatment. Lancet 2001;358:221. [PMID: 11476858]

Bell GI: Molecular defects in diabetes mellitus. Diabetes 1991;40:413.

Bjorntorp P: Metabolic implications of body fat distribution. Diabetes Care 1991;14:1132.

Cherrington AD: Control of glucose uptake and release by the liver in vivo. Diabetes 1999;48:1198.

Clare-Salzer MJ, Tobin AJ, Kaufman DL: Glutamate decarboxylase: An autoantigen in IDDM. Diabetes Care 1992;15:132.

Cox NJ et al: Loci on chromosome 2 (NIDDM1) and 15 interact to increase susceptibility to diabetes in Mexican Americans. Nat Genet 1999;21:213.

Davies JL et al: A genome-wide search for human type 1 diabetes susceptibility genes. Nature 1994;371:130.

DeFronzo RA, Ferrannini E: Insulin resistance: A multifaceted syndrome responsible for NIDDM, obesity, hypertension, dyslipidemia, and atherosclerotic cardiovascular disease. Diabetes Care 1991;14:173.

Effects of insulin in relatives of patients with type 1 diabetes mellitus. N Engl J Med 2002;346:1685. [PMID: 12037147]

Ferrannini E: Insulin resistance versus insulin deficiency in noninsulin-dependent diabetes mellitus: problems and prospects. Endocr Rev 1998;19:477.

Goodyear LJ, Kahn BB: Exercise, glucose transport, and insulin sensitivity. Annu Rev Med 1998;49:235.

Gottlieb PA, Eisenbarth GS: Diagnosis and treatment of pre-insulin dependent diabetes. Annu Rev Med 1998;49:391.

Herold KC et al: ANTI-CD3 monoclonal antibody in new-onset type 1 diabetes mellitus. N Engl J Med 2002;346:1692. [PMID: 12037148]

Howard BV, Howard WJ: Dyslipidemia in noninsulin-dependent diabetes mellitus. Endocr Rev 1994;15:263.

Hunter SJ, Garvey WT: Insulin action and insulin resistance: Diseases involving defects in insulin receptors, signal transduction, and the glucose transport effector system. Am J Med 1998;105:331.

Jequier E, Tappy L: Regulation of body weight in humans. Physiol Rev 1999;79:451.

Kadowski T et al: A subtype of diabetes mellitus associated with a mutation of mitochondrial DNA. N Engl J Med 1994;330:962.

Karam JH: Type II diabetes and syndrome X: Pathogenesis and glycemic management. Endocrinol Metab Clin North Am 1992;21:329.

Knowler WC et al: Preventing non-insulin-dependent diabetes. Diabetes 1995;44:483.

Knowler WC et al: Reduction in the incidence of type 2 diabetes with lifestyle intervention or metformin. N Engl J Med 2002;346:393. [PMID: 11832527]

Leahy JL, Bonner-Weir S, Weir GC: Beta-cell dysfunction induced by chronic hyperglycemia: Current ideas on mechanism of impaired glucose-induced insulin secretion. Diabetes Care 1992;15:442.

Meyer C, Doston JM, Gerich JE: Role of the human kidney in glucose counterregulation. Diabetes 1999;48:943.

Miller SP et al: Characterization of glucokinase mutations associated with maturity-onset diabetes of the young type 2 (MODY-2): different glucokinase defects lead to a common phenotype. Diabetes 1999;48:1645.

O'Rahilly S, Moller DE: Mutant insulin receptors in syndromes of insulin resistance. Clin Endocrinol 1992;36:121.

Pugliese A et al : The insulin gene is transcribed in the human thymus and transcription levels correlate with allelic variation at the INS VNTR-IDDM2 susceptibility locus for type 1 diabetes. Nat Genet 1997;15:293.

Raz I et al: B-cell function in new-onset type 1 diabetes and immunomodulation with a heat-shock protein peptide (DiaPep277): a randomized, double-blind, phase II trial. Lancet 2001;358:1749. [PMID: 11734230]

Rossini AA et al: Immunopathogenesis of diabetes mellitus. Diabetes Reviews 1993;1:43.

Saltiel AR, Kahn CR: Insulin signalling and the regulation of glucose and lipid metabolism. Nature 2001;414:799. [PMID: 11742412]

Shepherd PR, Kahn BB: Glucose transporters and insulin action: implications for insulin resistance and diabetes mellitus. N Engl J Med 1999;341:248.

Stumvoll M et al: Renal glucose production and utilization: new aspects in humans. Diabetologia 1997;40:749.

UK Prospective Diabetes Study (UKPDS) Group:

Effect of intensive blood-glucose control with metformin on complications in overweight patients with type 2 diabetes (UKPDS 34). Lancet 1998;352:854.

Efficacy of atenolol and captopril in reducing risk of macrovascular and microvascular complications in type 2 diabetes (UKPDS 39.) BMJ 1998;317:713.

Glycemic control with diet, sulfonylurea, metformin, or insulin in patients with type 2 diabetes mellitus: progressive requirement for multiple therapies (UKPDS 49). JAMA 1999; 281:2005.

Intensive blood-glucose control with sulphonylureas or insulin compared with conventional treatment and risk of complications in patients with type 2 diabetes (UKPDS 33). Lancet 1998;352:837.

Tight blood pressure control and risk of macrovascular and microvascular complications in type 2 diabetes (UKPDS 38). BMJ 1998;317:703.

Vafiadis P et al: Insulin expression in human thymus is modulated by INS VNTR alleles at the IDDM2 locus. Nat Genet 1997;15:289.

Virkamaki A, Ueki K, Kahn CR: Protein-protein interaction in insulin signaling and the molecular mechanisms of insulin resistance. J Clin Invest 1999;103:931.

Zawalich WS, Kelley GG: The pathogenesis of NIDDM: The role of the pancreatic beta cell. Diabetologia 1995;38:986.

Treatment of Diabetes Mellitus

American Diabetes Association: Management of dyslipidemia in adults with diabetes. Diabetes Care 1998;21(Suppl 1):S36.

Bode BW, Tamborlane WV, Davidson PC: Insulin pump therapy in the 21st century. Strategies for successful use in adults, adolescents and children with diabetes. Postgrad Med 2002;111:69. [PMID: 12040864]

Bolli GB et al: Glucose counterregulation and waning of insulin in the Somogyi phenomenon (posthypoglycemic hyperglycemia). N Engl J Med 1984;311:1214.

Bolli GB: Physiological insulin replacement in type 1 diabetes mellitus. Exp Clin Endocrinol Diabetes 2001;109(Suppl 2): 5317. [PMID: 11723567]

Boner G, Cao Z, Cooper ME: Combination antihypertensive therapy in the treatment of diabetic nephropathy. Diabetes Technol Ther 2002;4:313. [PMID: 12165170]

Brink SJ, Stewart C: Insulin pump treatment in insulin-dependent diabetes mellitus: Children, adolescents, and young adults. JAMA 1986;255:617]

Clarke WL et al: Multifactorial origin of hypoglycemic symptom unawareness in IDDM. Diabetes 1991;40:680.

Cryer PE: Hypoglycemia is the limiting factor in the management of diabetes. Diabetes Metab Res Rev 1999;15:42. [PMID: 10398545]

Cryer PE: Iatrogenic hypoglyccmia as a cause of hypoglycemia-associated autonomic failure in IDDM: A vicious cycle. Diabetes 1992;41:255.

Cusi K, DeFronzo RA: Metformin: a review of its metabolic effects. Diabetes Rev 1998;6:89.

DCCT Research Group: Epidemiology of severe hypoglycemia in the diabetes control and complications trial. Am J Med 1991;90:450.

DCCT Research Group: The effect of intensive treatment of diabetes on the development and progression of long-term complications in insulin-dependent diabetes mellitus. N Engl J Med 1993;329:977.

De Lorgeril M et al: Mediterranean diet, traditional risk factors and the rate of cardiovascular complications after myocardial infarction: final report of the Lyon Diet Heart Study. Circulation 1999;99:779.

DeFronzo RA: Pharmacologic therapy for type 2 diabetes mellitus. Ann Intern Med 1999;131:281.

Dunn FL: Management of hyperlipidemia in diabetes mellitus. Endocrinol Metab Clin North Am 1992;21:395.

Franz MJ et al: Evidence-based nutrition principles and recommendations for the treatment and prevention of diabetes and related complications. Diabetes Care 2002;25:148. [PMID: 11772915]

Gavin LA: Perioperative management of the diabetic patient. Endocrinol Metab Clin North Am 1992;21:457.

Groop LC et al: Morning or bedtime insulin combined with sulfonylurea in treatment of NIDDM. Diabetes Care 1992; 15:831.

Heine RJ et al: Absorption kinetics and action profiles of mixtures of short- and intermediate-acting insulins. Diabetologia 1984;27:558.

Kang S et al: Subcutaneous insulin absorption explained by insulin's physicochemical properties. Diabetes Care 1991;14:942.

Karam JH: Type II diabetes and syndrome X: Pathogenesis and glycemic management. Endocrinol Metab Clin North Am 1992;21:329.

Kendall DM, Robertson RP: Pancreas and islet transplantation: challenges for the twenty first century. Endocrinol Metab Clin North Am 1997;26:611.

Khan M et al: A prospective, randomized comparison of the metabolic effects of pioglitazone or rosiglitazone in patients with type 2 diabetes who were previously treated with troglitazone. Diabetes Care 2002;25:708. [PMID: 11919129]

Kirpichnikov D et al: Metformin—an update. Ann Intern Med 2002;137:25. [PMID: 12093242]

Lebovitz HE: Oral therapies for diabetic hyperglycemia. Endocrinol Metab Clin North Am 2001;30:909. [PMID: 11727405]

Little RR et al: Relationship of glycosylated hemoglobin to oral glucose tolerance: Implications for diabetes screening. Diabetes 1988;37:60.

Max MB et al: Effects of desipramine, amitriptyline, and fluoxetine on pain in diabetic neuropathy. N Engl J Med 1992;326:1250.

Nathan DM et al: The clinical information value of the glycosylated hemoglobin assay. N Engl J Med 1984;310:341.

Nolte MS: Insulin therapy in insulin-dependent (type I) diabetes mellitus. Endocrinol Metab Clin North Am 1992;21:281.

Owens DR et al: Insulins today and beyond. Lancet 2001;358:739. [PMID: 11551598]

Perriello G, De Feo P, Bolli GB: The dawn phenomenon: Nocturnal blood glucose homeostasis in insulin-dependent diabetes mellitus. Diabetic Med 1988;5:13.

Robertson RP: Pancreas islet transplantation for diabetes: successes, limitations and challenges for the future. Mol Genet Metab 2001;74:200. [PMID: 11592816]

Robertson RP et al: Therapeutic controversy: Pancreas transplantation for type 1 diabetes. J Clin Endocrinol Metab 1998;83:1868. [PMID: 9626111]

Rosskamp RH, Park G: Long acting insulin analogs. Diabetes Care 1999;22(Suppl 2):B109.

Stacher G: Diabetes mellitus and the stomach. Diabetologia 2001;44:1080. [PMID: 11596661]

Yusuf S et al: Effects of an angiotensin-converting enzyme inhibitor, ramipril, on death from cardiovascular causes, myocardial infarction and stroke in high-risk patients. The Heart Outcomes Prevention Evaluation Study Investigators. N Engl J Med 2000;342:145. [PMID: 10639539]

Acute Complications of Diabetes Mellitus

Bell DS, Alele J: Diabetic ketoacidosis. Why early detection and aggressive treatment are crucial. Postgrad Med 1997;101:193,203.

Chan NN, Brain HP, Feher MD: Metformin-associated lactic acidosis: a rare or very rare clinical entity? Diabet Med 1999;16:273.

Cohen RD: Lactic acidosis: New perspectives on origins and treatment. Diabetes Rev 1994;2:86.

Ennis ED, Stahl EJ, Kreisberg RA: The hyperosmolar hyperglycemic syndrome. Diabetes Rev 1994;2:115.

Genuth SM: Diabetic ketoacidosis and hyperglycemic, hyperosmolar coma. Curr Ther Endocrinol Metab 1997;6:438.

Gonzalez-Campoy JM, Robertson RP: Diabetic ketoacidosis and hyperosmolar nonketotic state: gaining control over extreme hyperglycemic complications. Postgrad Med 1996;99:143.

Henderson G: The psychosocial treatment of recurrent diabetic ketoacidosis: An interdisciplinary team approach. Diabetes Educator 1991;17:119.

Kitabchi AE et al: Management of hyperglycemic crises in patients with diabetes. Diabetes Care 2001;24:131. [PMID: 11194218]

Lorber D: Nonketotic hypertonicity in diabetes mellitus. Med Clin North Am 1995;70:39.

Okuda Y et al: Counterproductive effects of sodium bicarbonate in diabetic ketoacidosis. J Clin Endocrinol Metab 1996;81:314.

Singh RK, Perros P, Frier BM: Hospital management of diabetic ketoacidosis: are clinical guidelines implemented effectively? Diabet Med 1997;14:482.

Trence DL, Hirsch IB: Hyperglycemic crises in diabetes mellitus type 2. Endocrinol Metab Clin North Am 2001;30:817. [PMID: 11727401]

Wagner A et al: Therapy of severe diabetic ketoacidosis. Zero mortality under very-low-dose insulin application. Diabetes Care 1999;22:674.

Wiggam MI et al: Treatment of diabetic ketoacidosis using normalization of blood 3-hydroxybutyrate concentration as the endpoint of emergency management. A randomized controlled study. Diabetes Care 1997;20:1347.

Wrenn KD et al: The syndrome of alcoholic ketoacidosis. Am J Med 1991;91:119.

Chronic Complications of Diabetes Mellitus

Aiello LP et al: Diabetic retinopathy. Diabetes Care 1998;21:143.

American Diabetes Association Position Statement: Diabetes nephropathy. Diabetes Care 2002;25(Suppl 1):S85.

Brownlee M: Glycation products and the pathogenesis of diabetic complications. Diabetes Care 1992;15:1835.

Caputo GM et al: Assessment and management of foot disease in patients with diabetes. N Engl J Med 1994;331:854.

Clark CM, Lee DA: Drug Therapy: Prevention and treatment of the complications of diabetes mellitus. N Engl J Med 1995;332:1210.

Cogan DG et al: Aldose reductase and complications of diabetes. Ann Intern Med 1984;101:82.

Deckert T et al: Microalbuminuria: Implications for micro- and macrovascular disease. Diabetes Care 1992;15:1181.

Donahue RP, Orchard TJ: Diabetes mellitus and macrovascular complications: An epidemiological perspective. Diabetes Care 1992;15:1141.

Feingold KR et al: Muscle capillary basement membrane width in patients with vacor-induced diabetes mellitus. J Clin Invest 1986;78:102.

Ferris FL, Davis MD, Aiello LM: Treatment of diabetic retinopathy. N Engl J Med 1999;341:667.

Horowitz M et al: Gastric emptying in diabetes: clinical significance and treatment. Diabet Med 2002;19:177. [PMID; 11918620]

Ibrahim HN, Hostetter TH: Diabetic nephropathy. J Am Soc Nephrol 1997;8:487. [PMID: 9071718]

Klein R, Klein BEK, Moss SE: Epidemiology of proliferative diabetic retinopathy. Diabetes Care 1992;15:1875.

Knowles HC Jr: Long-term juvenile diabetes treated with unmeasured diet. Trans Assoc Am Physicians 1971;84:95.

Lipshultz LI, Kim ED: Treatment of erectile dysfunction in men with diabetes. JAMA 1999;281:465.

Major outcomes in high-risk hypertensive patients randomized to angiotensin-converting enzyme inhibitor or calcium channel blocker vs diuretic: The Antihypertensive and Lipid-Lowering Treatment to Prevent Heart Attack Trial (ALLHAT). JAMA 2002;298:2981. [PMID: 12479763]

Markell MS, Friedman EA: Diabetic nephropathy: Management of the end stage patient. Diabetes Care 1992;15:1226.

Mauer SM et al: Long-term study of normal kidneys transplanted into patients with type I diabetes. Diabetes 1989;38:516.

Mogensen CE: The kidney in diabetes: how to control renal and related cardiovascular complications. Am J Kidney Dis 2001;37(1 Suppl 2):S2. [PMID: 11158852]

Parkhouse N, Le Quesne PM: Impaired neurogenic vascular response in patients with diabetes and neuropathic foot lesions. N Engl J Med 1988;318:1306.

Ramsay RC et al: Progression of diabetic retinopathy after pancreas transplantation for insulin-dependent diabetes mellitus. N Engl J Med 1988;318:208.

Raskin P et al: Capillary basement membrane width in diabetic children. Am J Med 1975;58:365.

Rosenbloom AL et al: Limited joint mobility in childhood diabetes: Family studies. Diabetes Care 1983;6:370.

Viberti G et al: Effect of captopril on progression to clinical proteinuria in patients with insulin-dependent diabetes mellitus and microalbuminuria. JAMA 1994;271:275.

Vinik AI et al: Diabetic neuropathies. Diabetologia 2000;43:957. [PMID: 10990072]

Diabetes Mellitus & Pregnancy

American Diabetes Association: Gestational Diabetes Mellitus. Definition, detection, and diagnosis. Diabetes Care 2002;25 (Suppl 1):S94.

Barbour LA et al: Human placental growth hormone causes severe insulin resistance in transgenic mice. Am J Obst Gynecol 2002;186:512.

Boden G: Fuel metabolism in pregnancy and in gestational diabetes mellitus. Obstet Gynecol Clin North Am 1996;23:1.

Buchanan TA et al: Preservation of pancreatic B-cell function and prevention of type 2 diabetes by pharmacological treatment of insulin resistance in high-risk Hispanic women. Diabetes 2002;51:2796.

Chew EY et al: Metabolic control and progression of retinopathy. Diabetes Care 1995;18:631.

Combs CA et al: Relationship of fetal macrosomia to maternal postprandial glucose control during pregnancy. Diabetes Care 1992;15:1251.

de Veciana M et al: Postprandial versus preprandial blood glucose monitoring in women with gestational diabetes mellitus requiring insulin therapy. N Engl J Med 1995;333:1237.

Diabetes Control and Complications Trial Research Group: Effect of pregnancy on microvascular complications in the Diabetes Control and Complications Trial. Diabetes Care 2000;23: 1084.

Ekbom P et al: Pregnancy outcome in type 1 diabetic women with microalbuminuria. Diabetes Care 2001;24:1739.

Fine EL et al: Evidence that elevated glucose causes altered gene expression, apoptosis, and neural tube defects in a mouse model of diabetic pregnancy. Diabetes 1999;48:2454.

Friedman JE et al: Impaired glucose transport and insulin receptor tyrosine phosphorylation in skeletal muscle from obese women with gestational diabetes. Diabetes 1999;48:1807.

Garcia-Patterson A et al: In pregnancies with gestational diabetes mellitus and intensive therapy, perinatal outcome is worse in small-for-gestational-age newborns. Am J Obstet Gynecol 1998;179:481.

Hemachandra A et al: The influence of pregnancy on IDDM complications. Diabetes Care 1995;18:950.

Illsley NP: Placental glucose transport in diabetic pregnancy. Clinical Obstet Gynecol 2000;43:116.

Jovanovic-Peterson L et al: Maternal postprandial glucose levels and infant birth weight: The diabetes in early pregnancy study. Am J Obstet Gynecol 1991;164:103.

Kautzky-Willer A et al: Pronounced insulin resistance and inadequate beta-cell secretion characterize lean gestational diabetes during and after pregnacy. Diabetes Care 1997;20:1717.

Kirwan JP et al: TNF-alpha is a predictor of insulin resistance in human pregnancy. Diabetes 2002;51:2207.

Kitzmiller JL et al: Preconception management of diabetes continued through early pregnancy prevents the excess frequency of major congenital anomalies in infants of diabetic mothers. JAMA 1991;265:731.

Kitzmiller JL: Sweet success with diabetes: The development of insulin therapy and glycemic control for pregnancy. Diabetes Care 1993;16(Suppl 3):107.

Kitzmiller JL et al: Pre-conception care of diabetes, congenital malformations, and spontaneous abortions. Technical review. Diabetes Care 1996;19:514.

Kitzmiller JL, Combs CA: Diabetic nephropathy and pregnancy. Obstet Gynecol Clin North Am 1996;23:173.

Kjos SL et al: Contraception and the risk of type 2 diabetes mellitus in Latina women with prior gestational diabetes. JAMA 1998;280:533.

Koren G: Glyburide and fetal safety; transplacental pharmacokinetic considerations. Reprod Toxicol 2001;15:227.

Landon MB, Gabbe SG: Fetal surveillance and timing of delivery in pregnancy complicated by diabetes mellitus. Obstet Gynecol Clin North Am 1996;23:109.

Langer O et al: Intensified versus conventional management of gestational diabetes. Am J Obstet Gynecol 1994;170:1036.

Langer O et al: A comparison of glyburide and insulin in women with gestational diabetes. N Engl J Med 2000;343:1134.

Leunda-Casi A et al: Increased cell death in mouse blastocysts exposed to high D-glucose in vitro: implications of an oxidative stress and alterations in glucose metabolism. Diabetologia 2002;45:571.

McIntyre HD et al: Placental growth hormone (GH), GH-binding protein, and insulin-like growth factor axis in normal, growth-retarded, and diabetic pregnancies: correlations with fetal growth. J Clin Endocrinol Metab 2000;85:1143.

Metzger B, Coustan DR, and the Organizing Committee: Summary and recommendations of the Fourth International Workshop-Conference on Gestational Diabetes. Diabetes Care 1998;21(Suppl 2):B162.

Piper JM: Lung maturation in diabetes in pregnancy: If and when to test. Semin Perinatol 2002;26:206.

Sermer MS et al: Impact of increasing carbohydrate intolerance on maternal-fetal outcomes in 3,637 women without gestational diabetes. Am J Obstet Gynecol 1995;173:145.

Sibai BM et al: Risks of preeclampsia and adverse neonatal outcomes among women with pregestational diabetes. Am J Obstet Gynecol 2000;182:364.

Silverman BL et al: Fetal hyperinsulinism and impaired glucose tolerance in adolescent offspring of diabetic mothers. Diabetes Care 1995;18:611.

Silverman BL, Purdy L, Metzger BE: The intrauterine environment: implications for the offspring of diabetic mothers. Diabetes Rev 1996;4:21.

Tomazic M et al: Comparison of alterations in insulin signaling pathway in adipocytes from type II diabetic pregnant women and women with gestational diabetes. Diabetologia 2002; 45:502.

Verma A et al: Insulin resistance syndrome in women with prior history of gestational diabetes mellitus. J Clin Endocrinol Metab 2002;87:3227.

White P: Diabetes mellitus in pregnancy. Clin Perinatol 1974;1: 331.

Winkler G et al: Tumor necrosis factor system in insulin resistance in gestational diabetes. Diab Res Clin Pract 2002;56:93.

Xiang AH et al: Multiple metabolic defects during late pregnancy in women at high risk for Type 2 diabetes. Diabetes 1999; 48:848.

Hypoglycemic Disorders

John H. Karam, MD, & Umesh Masharani, MRCP (UK)

Circulating plasma glucose concentrations are kept within a relatively narrow range by a complex system of interrelated neural, humoral, and cellular controls. Under the usual metabolic conditions, the central nervous system is wholly dependent on plasma glucose and counteracts declining blood glucose concentrations with a carefully programmed response. This is often associated with a sensation of hunger; and, as the brain receives insufficient glucose to meet its metabolic needs (neuroglycopenia), an autonomic response is triggered to mobilize storage depots of glycogen and fat. In the postabsorptive state, hepatic glycogen reserves and gluconeogenesis from the liver and kidney directly supply the central nervous system with glucose, which is carried across the blood-brain barrier by a specific glucose transport system, while the mobilization of fatty acids from triglyceride depots provides energy for the large mass of skeletal and cardiac muscle, renal cortex, liver, and other tissues that utilize fatty acids as their basic fuel, thus sparing glucose for use by the tissues of the central nervous system.

PATHOPHYSIOLOGY OF THE COUNTERREGULATORY RESPONSE TO NEUROGLYCOPENIA

The plasma concentration of glucose that will signal the need by the central nervous system to mobilize energy reserves depends on a number of factors, such as the status of blood flow to the brain, the integrity of cerebral tissue, the prevailing arterial level of plasma glucose, the rapidity with which plasma glucose concentration falls, and the availability of alternative metabolic fuels.

A hierarchy of responses has been shown to occur as plasma glucose falls in healthy young volunteers, with hormonal counterregulatory responses being triggered at glucose levels slightly higher (approximately 67 mg/dL [3.7 mmol/L]) than those which induce symptoms of hypoglycemia (Figure 18–1). The first symptoms to appear in healthy people are mediated by autonomic neurotransmitters and occur at plasma glucose levels below 60 mg/dL (3.3 mmol/L). The symptoms consist of tremor, anxiety, palpitations, and sweating, which result from sympathetic discharge; and hunger, which is a consequence of parasympathetic vagal response. Ganglionic blockade and cervical cord section or sympathectomy—but not adrenalectomy—ameliorate these symptoms, indicating that they are due to the release of autonomic neurotransmitters and not dependent on adrenal hormones. As plasma glucose falls below 50 mg/dL (2.8 mmol/L), cerebral neuroglycopenia ensues, consisting of impaired cognition, along with weakness, lethargy, confusion, incoordination, and blurred vision. If counterregulatory responses are inadequate to reverse this degree of profound hypoglycemia, convulsions or coma may occur. This can result in brain damage or death, particularly in those who have not adapted to repeated episodes of hypoglycemia (see below).

In elderly people, however, with compromised cerebral blood supply, neuroglycopenic manifestations may be provoked at slightly higher plasma glucose levels. Patients with chronic hyperglycemia, eg, those with poorly controlled insulin-treated diabetes mellitus, may experience symptoms of neuroglycopenia at considerably higher plasma glucose concentrations than persons without diabetes. This has been attributed to a "down-regulated" glucose transport system across the blood-brain barrier. Conversely, in patients exposed to chronic hypoglycemia—eg, those with an insulin-secreting tumor or those with diabetes who are receiving excessively "tight" glycemic control with an insulin pump—adaptation to recurrent hypoglycemia occurs by "up-regulation" of the glucose transporters, which results in "hypoglycemic unawareness" whereby they show greater tolerance to hypoglycemia without manifesting symptoms (Figure 18–2).

Restoring and maintaining an adequate supply of glucose for cerebral function proceeds by a series of neurogenic events that act directly to raise the plasma glucose concentration and to stimulate hormonal responses that augment the adrenergic mobilization of energy stores (Table 18–1).

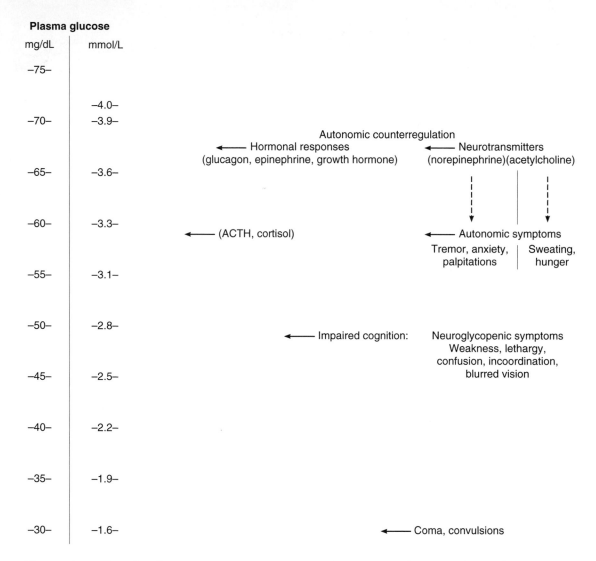

Figure 18–1. Hierarchy of autonomic responses to progressive stepwise reduction in plasma glucose concentration in healthy volunteers. (Adapted from Gerich JE et al: Hypoglycemia unawareness. Endocr Rev 1991;12:356; and from Service FJ: Hypoglycemia disorders. N Engl J Med 1995;332:1144.)

Counterregulatory Response to Hypoglycemia

A. Insulin

Endogenous insulin secretion is *lowered* both by reduced glucose stimulation to the pancreatic B cell and by sympathetic nervous system inhibition from a combination of alpha-adrenergic neural effects and increased circulating catecholamine levels. This reactive insulinopenia appears to be essential for glucose recovery, as it facilitates the mobilization of energy from ex-

isting energy stores (glycogenolysis and lipolysis); increases hepatic enzymes involved in gluconeogenesis and ketogenesis; increases enzymes of the renal cortex, promoting gluconeogenesis; and at the same time prevents muscle tissue from consuming the blood glucose being released from the liver (Chapter 17).

B. Catecholamines

Circulating catecholamines—and norepinephrine produced at sympathetic nerve endings—provide muscle tissue with alternative sources of fuel by activating beta-

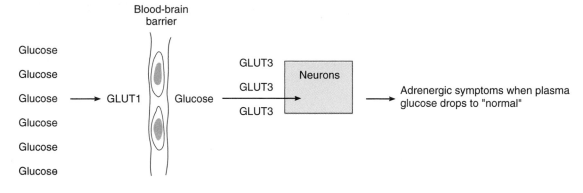

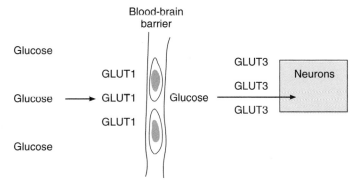

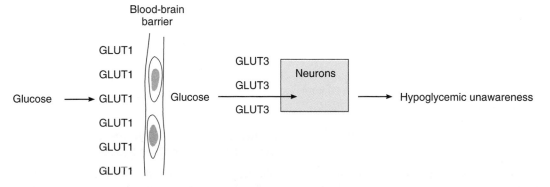

Figure 18–2. Glycemic regulation of glucose transporters. The center panel depicts the normal component of the high-affinity glucose transporter 1 (GLUT1) on the vascular cells of the central nervous system during euglycemia. An appropriate amount of glucose diffuses across the blood-brain barrier and is then transported into the neurons by another high-affinity glucose transporter, GLUT3. The upper and lower panels, respectively, show adaptation by either down-regulation of GLUT1 in the face of chronic hyperglycemia (upper panel) or up-regulation of GLUT1 in the presence of chronic hypoglycemia. (GLUT1, glucose transporter 1; GLUT3, glucose transporter 3.)

Table 18–1. Autonomic nervous system response to hypoglycemia.

Alpha-adrenergic effects
  Inhibition of endogenous insulin release
  Increase in cerebral blood flow (peripheral vasoconstriction)
Beta-adrenergic effects
  Hepatic and muscle glycogenolysis
  Stimulation of plasma glucagon release
  Lipolysis to raise plasma free fatty acids
  Impairment of glucose uptake by muscle tissue
  Increase in cerebral blood flow (increase in cardiac output)
Adrenomedullary discharge of catecholamines
  Augmentation of all of the above alpha- and beta-
    adrenergic effects
Cholinergic effects
  Raises level of pancreatic polypeptide
  Increases motility of stomach
  Produces hunger
  Increases sweating

adrenergic receptors, resulting in mobilization of muscle glycogen, and by providing increased plasma free fatty acids from lipolysis of adipocyte triglyceride. Metabolism of these free fatty acids provides energy to promote gluconeogenesis in the liver and kidney, thereby adding to plasma glucose levels already raised by the glycogenolytic effect of catecholamines on the liver and their direct stimulation of gluconeogenesis by the renal cortex. Their cardiovascular and other side effects provide a signal that diabetic patients learn to recognize as a warning of their need to rapidly ingest absorbable carbohydrate.

C. GLUCAGON

Plasma glucagon is released by the beta-adrenergic effects of both sympathetic innervation and circulating catecholamines on pancreatic A cells as well as by the direct stimulation of A cells by the low plasma glucose concentration itself. Data are available suggesting that a falling-off of intra-islet insulin concentration in subjects with functioning pancreatic B cells can release pancreatic A cells from insulin inhibition and thus augment glucagon release during hypoglycemia. This glucagon release increases hepatic output of glucose by direct glycogenolysis as well as by facilitating the activity of gluconeogenic enzymes in the liver but not in the kidney. As shown in Figure 18–3, plasma glucagon appears to be the key counterregulatory hormone affecting recovery from *acute* hypoglycemia in nondiabetic humans, with the adrenergic-catecholamine response representing a major backup system. However, in most clinical situations, where hypoglycemia develops *more gradually,*

as with inappropriate dosage of insulin or sulfonylureas, or in cases of insulinoma, the role of glucagon may be less influential. When normal volunteers received a prolonged low-dose insulin infusion to produce a gradual decline in plasma glucose levels without waning of insulin levels, the rise of endogenous glucagon contributed much less to counterregulation than after acute hypoglycemia induced by intravenous insulin, which is followed by rapid waning of insulin levels. This finding suggests that glucagon's role in glucose recovery occurs primarily when the level of insulin wanes.

D. CORTICOTROPIN AND HYDROCORTISONE

Pituitary ACTH is released in association with the sympathetic nervous system stimulation by neuroglycopenia. This results in elevation of plasma cortisol levels, which in turn permissively facilitates lipolysis and actively promotes protein catabolism and conversion of amino acids to glucose by the liver and kidney.

E. GROWTH HORMONE

Pituitary growth hormone is also released in response to falling plasma glucose levels. Its role in counteracting hypoglycemia is less well defined, but it is known to antagonize the action of insulin on glucose utilization in muscle cells and to directly activate lipolysis by adipocytes. This increased lipolysis provides fatty acid substrate to the liver and renal cortex which facilitates gluconeogenesis.

F. CHOLINERGIC NEUROTRANSMITTERS

Acetylcholine is released at parasympathetic nerve endings, and its vagal effects induce the sensation of hunger that signals the need for food to counteract the hypoglycemia. In addition, postsynaptic fibers of the sympathetic nervous system that innervate the sweat glands to signal hypoglycemia also release acetylcholine—in contrast to all other sympathetic postsynaptic fibers, which without exception release norepinephrine.

Maintenance of Euglycemia in the Postabsorptive State

Glucose absorption from the gastrointestinal tract ceases by 4–6 hours after a meal. During the "postabsorptive state" immediately following, glucose must be produced endogenously from previously stored nutrients to meet the requirements of the central nervous system and other glucose-dependent tissues. These include 125 mg of glucose per minute required by the brain and spinal cord as well as an additional 25 mg/min by red blood cells and the renal medulla. It was previously thought that the liver is the only organ involved in glucose production during an overnight fast, but recent data indi-

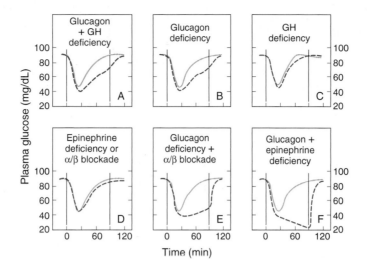

Figure 18–3. Solid lines show changes in plasma glucose that occur in normal subjects in response to acute intravenous insulin administration. Note the rapid recovery of glucose levels mediated by intact counterregulatory mechanisms. The dashed lines show the response to insulin-induced hypoglycemia in patients with deficiencies of the counterregulatory mechanisms induced as follows: **A:** Somatostatin infusion (inhibits both glucagon and growth hormone [GH] release). **B:** Somatostatin infusion plus GH infusion (now with functional isolated glucagon deficiency). **C:** Somatostatin infusion plus glucagon infusion (isolated GH deficiency). Note return of glucose response to normal, implying that glucagon is the main counterregulatory hormone. **D:** Bilateral adrenalectomy, leading to epinephrine deficiency, or infusion of phentolamine plus propranolol (alpha and beta blockers, respectively). Note that such deficiencies cause no major abnormality in response to induced hypoglycemia when glucagon is present. **E and F:** Sympathetic modulation (by phentolamine plus propranolol in **E** and by bilateral adrenalectomy in **F**), which seriously impairs the ability to respond to hypoglycemia in the patient made glucagon-deficient by somatostatin infusion. (Reproduced, with permission, from Cryer PE: Glucose counterregulation in man. Diabetes 1981;30:261.)

cate that the renal cortex also has the requisite enzymes for production and release of glucose.

The liver initially provides glucose by the breakdown of stored hepatic glycogen. However, because these reserves are limited to 80–100 g, they begin to be depleted several hours into the postabsorptive state. Thereafter, hepatic glucose production is augmented by gluconeogenesis—the formation of glucose from amino acids, lactate, and glycerol. These substrates are delivered to the liver and kidney from peripheral stores. Muscle and other structural tissues supply amino acids, mainly alanine; blood cell elements supply lactate, the end product of glycolytic metabolism; and adipose tissue supplies glycerol from lipolysis of triglyceride. In addition, oxidation of the free fatty acids released from adipose cells during lipolysis supplies the energy required for gluconeogenesis and provides ketone bodies, acetoacetate, and β-hydroxybutyrate, which can serve as alternative metabolic fuels for the central nervous system during periods of prolonged fasting. Studies have shown that an insulin infusion does not reduce hepatic glucose production if elevated levels of fatty acids are maintained by intravenous administration of a fat emulsion and heparin, suggesting that fatty acids may be the major mediator of gluconeogenesis.

Role of the Kidney

Although it is generally acknowledged that after fasting for 60 hours the kidney contributes up to 20–25% of endogenous glucose production, its role after an overnight fast remains controversial. One group has found that it produces as much as 25% of the postabsorptive glucose requirement, yet a second group using different methodology found a contribution of no more than 5% in the postabsorptive state. Despite these conflicting findings, it is clear that since the renal medulla removes almost as much glucose as the renal cortex produces, the net renal contribution is minimal in the short-term postabsorptive state as compared to the liver.

The kidney does not have glycogen stores and is dependent on gluconeogenesis as its only source of glucose production. Glutamine—rather than alanine—is the predominant amino acid substrate for renal gluconeogenesis. In addition to its contribution to glucose homeostasis after an overnight fast, the kidney also has been shown to be an important contributor to glucose counterregulation in the event of hypoglycemia. While glucagon does not affect the kidney, the counterregulatory rise in catecholamines has been shown to stimulate gluconeogenesis in the renal cortex. As with the liver, insulin inhibits renal gluconeogenesis and glucose release. Hormonal changes that begin early in the postabsorptive state regulate the enzymatic steps necessary for hepatic glycogenolysis and hepatic and renal gluconeogenesis and ensure the delivery of the necessary substrate (Table 18–2). An appropriate fall in circulating insulin levels with a corresponding rise in glucagon is most important; elevations in the counterregulatory hormones cortisol and growth hormone contribute but are less critical. Thus, numerous endocrine and metabolic events interact to provide a continuous source of fuel for proper functioning of the central nervous system. Malfunction of any of these mechanisms can lead to symptomatic hypoglycemia.

Role of PGC-1 in Regulation of Gluconeogenesis

It has long been known that stress-induced catecholamines as well as glucagon generate cAMP, which promotes gluconeogenesis in the liver. Insulin opposes this action but does not seem to do so by directly reducing cAMP levels, and its mode of action has previously been unexplained. Recently, however, discovery of a new protein expressed in liver **peroxisome proliferator activated receptor-gamma coactivator-1 (PGC-1)**—has provided new insight into the regulation of gluconeogenesis on a cellular level. PGC-1 has been found to act also as a coactivator of gene expression of key gluconeogenic enzymes. It is believed that cAMP increases expression of PGC-1, which acts as a coactivator with glucocorticoids and a hepatic nuclear factor to stimulate expression of key hormones of gluconeogenesis. Insulin inhibits this process by interfering with PGC-1 expression so that gluconeogenic enzymes are not induced.

CLASSIFICATION OF HYPOGLYCEMIC DISORDERS

Symptomatic Hypoglycemia

A clinical classification of the more common causes of symptomatic hypoglycemia in adults is presented in Table 18–3. (Inborn errors of metabolism that produce hypoglycemia in infants and children are not listed and will not be discussed in this chapter.) This classification is useful in directing diagnostic considerations.

Symptomatic fasting hypoglycemia is a serious and potentially life-threatening problem warranting thorough evaluation. Conditions that produce inappropriate fasting hyperinsulinism are the most common cause of fasting hypoglycemia in otherwise healthy adults. These include insulin-secreting pancreatic B cell tumors and iatrogenic or surreptitious administration of insulin

Table 18–2. Hormonal changes to maintain euglycemia in the postabsorptive state.

Decreased insulin secretion
  Increases hepatic glycogenolysis
  Increases lipolysis
  Increases hepatic gluconeogenesis
  Decreases muscle uptake of glucose
Increased glucagon secretion
  Increases hepatic glycogenolysis
  Facilitates hepatic gluconeogenesis
Increased cortisol secretion
  Facilitates lipolysis
  Increases protein catabolism
  Augments hepatic gluconeogenesis

Table 18–3. Common causes of symptomatic hypoglycemia in adults.

Fasting
  With hyperinsulinism
    Insulin reaction
    Sulfonylurea overdose
    Surreptitious insulin or sulfonylurea self-administration
    Autoimmune hypoglycemia (idiopathic insulin antibodies, insulin receptor autoantibodies)
    Pentamidine-induced hypoglycemia
    Pancreatic B cell tumors
  Without hyperinsulinism
    Severe hepatic dysfunction
    Chronic renal insufficiency
    Inanition
    Hypocortisolism
    Alcohol use
    Nonpancreatic tumors
Nonfasting
  Alimentary
  Functional
  Noninsulinoma pancreatogenous hypoglycemic syndrome (NIPHS)
  Occult diabetes
  Ethanol ingestion with sugar mixers

or sulfonylureas. In patients with illnesses that produce symptomatic fasting hypoglycemia despite appropriately suppressed insulin levels, the clinical picture is generally dominated by the signs and symptoms of the primary disease, with hypoglycemia often only a late or associated manifestation. This is in contrast to patients with inappropriate hyperinsulinism, who usually appear healthy between hypoglycemic episodes.

Symptoms of nonfasting hypoglycemia in adults, although distressing to the patient, do not in most cases imply serious illness or warrant extensive evaluation. Overstimulation of the B cells postprandially as a result of accelerated glucose absorption after rapid gastric emptying may result in too rapid disposal of glucose, with resulting symptoms of sympathetic nervous system hyperactivity (alimentary hypoglycemia). Other than in patients who have had gastric surgery, this diagnosis may be difficult to establish. A newly described but quite rare disorder of adult nesidioblastosis called **noninsulinoma pancreatogenous hypoglycemia syndrome** has been found to provoke severe symptoms of hypoglycemia with neuroglycopenia 4–6 hours after meals (see below).

Asymptomatic Hypoglycemia

Hypoglycemia may be seen during prolonged fasting, strenuous exercise, or pregnancy or may occur as a laboratory artifact. In normal men, plasma glucose does not fall below 55 mg/dL (3 mmol/L) during a 72-hour fast. However, for reasons that are not clear, normal women may experience a fall to levels as low as 30 mg/dL (1.7 mmol/L) despite a marked suppression of circulating insulin to less than 5 μU/mL. They remain asymptomatic in spite of this degree of hypoglycemia, presumably because ketogenesis is able to satisfy the energy needs of the central nervous system. Basal plasma glucose declines progressively during normal pregnancy, and hypoglycemic levels may be reached during prolonged fasting. This may be a consequence of a continuous fetal consumption of glucose and diminished availability of the gluconeogenic substrate alanine. The cause of these diminished alanine levels in pregnancy is unclear. The greatly increased glucose consumption by skeletal muscle that occurs during prolonged strenuous exercise may lead to hypoglycemia despite increases in hepatic glucose production. Whether the hypoglycemia in this circumstance contributes to fatigue or other symptoms in distance runners is unknown.

In vitro consumption of glucose by blood cell elements may give rise to laboratory values in the hypoglycemic range. This can be avoided by adding a small amount of the metabolic inhibitor sodium fluoride to collection tubes used for specimens containing in-creased numbers of blood cells (as in leukemia, leukemoid reactions, or polycythemia).

CLINICAL PRESENTATION OF HYPOGLYCEMIA

Regardless of the cause, hypoglycemia presents certain common features characterized by Whipple's triad: (1) symptoms and signs of hypoglycemia, (2) an associated plasma glucose level of 45 mg/dL (2.5 mmol/L) or less, and (3) reversibility of symptoms upon administration of glucose.

The symptoms and signs of hypoglycemia are the consequences of neuroglycopenia. They vary depending on the degree of hypoglycemia, the age of the patient, and the rapidity of the decline. In poorly controlled diabetic patients treated with insulin, a precipitous fall in plasma glucose from hyperglycemia toward euglycemia may produce neuroglycopenic symptoms.

A. ACUTE HYPOGLYCEMIA

A rapid fall in plasma glucose (> 1 mg/dL/min [> 0.06 mmol/L/min]) to low levels often accompanies conditions associated with arterial hyperinsulinism—a condition that leads to increased peripheral glucose uptake and decreased hepatic glucose output. In diabetics, excessive absorption of exogenous insulin either from overtreatment or from rapid mobilization from an injection site during exercise may be responsible. In nondiabetics, reactive hypersecretion of insulin may be the cause, as in postgastrectomy patients with rapid gastric emptying time. The symptoms include anxiety, tremulousness, and feelings of unnaturalness or detachment. These are usually accompanied by palpitations, tachycardia, sweating, and hunger and can progress to neurologic sequelae of ataxia, coma, or convulsions. These warning symptoms of hypoglycemia occur even in the absence of adrenal glands and therefore are due to neurogenic responses to hypoglycemia. The autonomic response has probably evolved as more of an alarm than a counterregulatory mechanism, since glucagon is generally sufficient to provide necessary counterregulation to hypoglycemia once insulin levels wane. In type 1 diabetes, however, the adrenergic system becomes of greater importance since the glucagon response to hypoglycemia is lost in most patients (Chapter 17), and subcutaneous depots of exogenous insulin may prevent inappropriately high levels of insulin from waning.

B. SUBACUTE AND CHRONIC HYPOGLYCEMIA

A relatively slow fall in plasma glucose accompanies conditions caused primarily by a reduction in hepatic glucose output in response to hyperinsulinism (predominantly within the portal vein [insulinoma]), or to the inappropriately sustained effects of long-acting insulin preparations on the liver and kidney in the postabsorptive state, or to metabolic derangements of gluconeogenesis (eg, alcohol hypoglycemia). Symptoms due to hypoglycemia in patients with these conditions may be less apparent, particularly because sympathetic discharge is minimal or delayed until profound hypoglycemia develops. Recurrent hypoglycemic episodes result in hypoglycemic unawareness with impairment of autonomic responses and an increased risk for severe hypoglycemia. These patients develop progressive confusion, inappropriate behavior, lethargy, and drowsiness. If the patient does not eat, seizures or coma may develop—though this is not inevitable, and spontaneous recovery can occur. Because these patients are seldom aware of their degree of functional impairment, a history should be obtained from relatives or friends who have observed the episode. Except for hypothermia (often seen during hypoglycemic coma), there are no identifying characteristics on physical examination. Hypoglycemia will often be misdiagnosed as a seizure disorder, transient ischemic attack, or personality disorder.

Documentation of Low Plasma Glucose Values

With the specific laboratory methods now available, it has been arbitrarily decided that fasting hypoglycemia is present when plasma glucose is 45 mg/dL (2.5 mmol/L) or less after an overnight fast (corresponding to a blood glucose level of 40 mg/dL [2.2 mmol/L] or less). In the fasting state, there is no substantial difference between arterial, venous, or capillary blood samples (in contrast to nonfasting hyperglycemia, in which arteriovenous glucose differences may be considerable because of arterial hyperinsulinism and consequent increases in glucose uptake across capillary beds).

The development of portable blood glucose meters has been of great value for rapid estimation of blood glucose levels, particularly for insulin-treated diabetics undergoing home monitoring. In emergency room or hospital settings, they are helpful in the differential diagnosis of coma, but a sample should also be sent to the laboratory for definitive diagnosis. Although therapeutic decisions to administer glucose can be based on the glucose meter results alone in an emergency situation, such readings are less dependable as the sole laboratory indicator for a definitive diagnosis of hypoglycemia.

Reversibility of Clinical Manifestations of Hypoglycemia with Treatment

Because prolonged hypoglycemia may cause permanent brain damage and death, prompt recognition and treatment are mandatory. (It is prudent to consider the pos-

sibility of hypoglycemic coma in most unconscious patients.)

The goal of therapy is to restore normal levels of plasma glucose as rapidly as possible. If the patient is conscious and able to swallow, glucose-containing foods such as candy, orange juice with added sugar, and cookies should be quickly ingested. Fructose, found in many nutrient low-calorie sweeteners for diabetics, should not be used, because although it can be metabolized by neurons, it is not transported across the blood-brain barrier.

If the patient is unconscious, rapid restoration of plasma glucose must be accomplished by giving 20–50 mL of 50% dextrose intravenously over 1–3 minutes (the treatment of choice) or, when intravenous glucose is not available, 1 mg of glucagon intramuscularly or intravenously. Families or friends of insulin-treated diabetics should be instructed in the administration of glucagon intramuscularly for emergency treatment at home. Attempts to feed the patient or to apply glucose-containing jelly to the oral mucosa should be avoided because of the danger of aspiration.

When consciousness is restored, oral feedings should be started immediately. Periodic blood glucose surveillance after a hypoglycemic episode may be needed for 12–24 hours to ensure maintenance of euglycemia. Prevention of recurrent hypoglycemic attacks depends upon proper diagnosis and management of the specific underlying disorder.

■ SPECIFIC HYPOGLYCEMIC DISORDERS

SYMPTOMATIC FASTING HYPOGLYCEMIA WITH HYPERINSULINISM

1. Insulin Reaction

It is not surprising that insulin-treated diabetics make up the bulk of the patient population with symptomatic hypoglycemia. Present methods of insulin delivery rely upon subcutaneous depots of mixtures of soluble and insoluble insulin whose absorption varies with the site of injection and the degree of exercise in surrounding muscles. Variations in physical and emotional stresses can alter the response of patients to insulin, as can the cyclic hormonal changes relating to menstruation. A deficient glucagon response to hypoglycemia in diabetes compounds the problem, as does the lack of awareness of hypoglycemic symptoms in older patients, in those with neuropathy, and in those with recurrent hypoglycemic episodes, who adapt to lower levels of blood glucose without triggering their autonomic alarm system. (See Figure 18–2 and Chapter 17 for further discussion of hypoglycemic unawareness.)

Once the patient's acute hypoglycemic episode is managed, the physician should carefully examine possible correctable factors that may have contributed to the insulin reaction.

Inadequate Food Intake

An insufficient quantity of food or a missed meal is one of the commonest causes of hypoglycemia in insulin-treated diabetics. Until improved insulin delivery systems are available, patients attempting to achieve satisfactory glycemic control should self-monitor their blood glucose levels and eat three regular meals as well as small mid morning, mid afternoon, and bedtime snacks, particularly when they are receiving multiple injections of insulin daily.

Exercise

The insulin-treated diabetic is especially prone to exercise-induced hypoglycemia. In nondiabetics, the enhancement of skeletal muscle glucose uptake (a 20- to 30-fold increase over basal uptake) is compensated for by enhanced hepatic and renal glucose production. This is mediated primarily by a fall in circulating insulin levels consequent to an exercise-induced catecholamine discharge, which inhibits B cell secretion. Such regulation is impossible in the insulin-treated diabetic, whose subcutaneous depot not only continues to release insulin during exercise but also shows an accelerated absorption rate when the injection site is in close proximity to the muscles being exercised. When this occurs, increased levels of circulating insulin compromise the hepatic and renal output of glucose. To prevent hypoglycemia, insulin-treated diabetics must be advised to avoid injections into areas adjacent to muscles most involved in the particular exercise and either to eat supplementary carbohydrate before exercising or to reduce their insulin dose appropriately.

Impaired Glucose Counterregulation in Diabetes

Most patients with type 1 diabetes have a deficient glucagon response to hypoglycemia. They are thus solely dependent on an adrenergic autonomic response to recover from hypoglycemia and particularly to provide them with symptoms they recognize as a warning of impending hypoglycemia and as a signal to ingest sugar or fruit juice. Some patients, especially those with long-standing diabetes, autonomic neuropathy, or a history of recurrent hypoglycemic episodes, lack both a glucagon and an epinephrine response and are virtually defenseless against insulin-induced hypoglycemia. Insulin infusion tests can be used to identify these alterations in glucose counterregulation; however, at present these tests are cumbersome, and their ability to accurately predict which patients will suffer frequent severe and prolonged hypoglycemic episodes is yet to be established. Easier and more reliable methods of identifying such patients are needed. The ability of a patient to spontaneously recover from hypoglycemia may determine whether or not aggressive attempts to maintain euglycemia are associated with undue risk.

Some patients who originally had a normal counterregulatory response to hypoglycemia (except for glucagon) lose this protective response when insulin therapy is intensified to achieve tight control, which may be associated with frequent hypoglycemic events including nocturnal hypoglycemia. The mechanisms for this reduction of hormonal response are unknown but seem to be related to "up-regulated" mechanisms of glucose transport across the blood-brain barrier induced by relatively low circulating blood glucose levels. However, one study could not confirm an increase in glucose transport across the blood-brain barrier in subjects with hypoglycemic unawareness and suggested that the adaptation to chronic hypoglycemia may be on a neuronal level within the brain. Regardless of the mechanism, this defective counterregulation has been shown to be reversible to a considerable degree by careful monitoring of intensive insulin therapy to avoid any blood glucose measurements below 70 mg/dL for a period of 3 weeks or longer.

Inadvertent or Deliberate Insulin Overdosage in Diabetics

Excessive insulin may be administered inadvertently by patients with poor vision or inadequate instruction or understanding of dosage and injection technique. The widespread use of highly concentrated U100 insulin enhances the likelihood of overdosage with relatively small excesses of administered insulin.

Deliberate overdosage may occur in certain maladjusted patients, particularly adolescents, who wish to gain special attention from their families or escape tensions at school or work.

Miscellaneous Causes of Hypoglycemia in Insulin-Treated Diabetics

A. STRESS

Physical stresses—such as intercurrent illnesses, infection, and surgery—or psychic stresses often require an increased insulin dosage to control hyperglycemia. Reduction to prestress doses is necessary to avoid subsequent hypoglycemia when the stresses have abated.

B. HYPOCORTISOLISM

In patients with type 1 diabetes who have otherwise unexplained hypoglycemic attacks, reduced insulin requirements may indicate unusual causes (eg, Addison's disease).

C. DIABETIC GASTROPARESIS

Unexplained episodes of postprandial hypoglycemia in insulin-treated diabetics may be due to delayed gastric emptying consequent to autonomic neuropathy. This diagnosis can be established by appropriate radiologic studies of gastric motility using liquid or solid test meals containing radioisotopic markers.

D. PREGNANCY

Pregnancy, with high fetal glucose consumption, decreases insulin requirements in the first trimester.

E. RENAL INSUFFICIENCY

Renal insufficiency, through impairment of insulin degradation and renal gluconeogenesis while hepatic gluconeogenesis and food intake are often reduced, also requires a reduction in insulin dosage.

F. DRUGS

Numerous pharmacologic agents may potentiate the effects of insulin and predispose to hypoglycemia. Common offenders include ethanol, salicylates, and beta-adrenergic blocking drugs. Beta blockade inhibits fatty acid and gluconeogenic substrate release and reduces plasma glucagon levels; furthermore, the symptomatic response is altered, because tachycardia is blocked while hazardous elevations of blood pressure may result during hypoglycemia in response to the unopposed alpha-adrenergic stimulation from circulating catecholamines and neurogenic sympathetic discharge. However, symptoms of sweating, hunger, and uneasiness are not masked by beta-blocking drugs and remain indicators of hypoglycemia in the aware patient.

Therapy with angiotensin-converting enzyme (ACE) inhibitors increases the risk of hypoglycemia in diabetic patients who are taking insulin or sulfonylureas, presumably because these drugs increase sensitivity to circulating insulin by increasing blood flow to muscle.

2. Sulfonylurea Overdose

Any of the sulfonylurea drugs may produce hypoglycemia. Chlorpropamide, with its prolonged half-life (35 hours), was a common offender, but its use has been curtailed recently because of its numerous adverse effects. Older patients—especially those with impaired

hepatic or renal function—are particularly susceptible to sulfonylurea-induced hypoglycemia: Liver dysfunction prolongs the hypoglycemic activity of tolbutamide, acetohexamide, and tolazamide, as well as that of the second-generation compounds glyburide and glipizide; renal insufficiency perpetuates the blood glucose-lowering effects of many sulfonylureas, especially chlorpropamide and glyburide. Elderly patients with gradually decreasing creatinine clearance seem to be more at risk for prolonged and severe hypoglycemia when treated with chlorpropamide or glyburide and less so when treated with shorter-acting agents such as tolbutamide or glipizide. In the presence of other pharmacologic agents such as warfarin, phenylbutazone, or certain sulfonamides, the hypoglycemic effects of sulfonylureas may be markedly prolonged.

3. Surreptitious Insulin or Sulfonylurea Administration (Factitious Hypoglycemia)

Factitious hypoglycemia should be suspected in any patient with access to insulin or sulfonylurea drugs. It is most commonly seen in health professionals and diabetic patients or their relatives. The reasons for self-induced hypoglycemia vary, with many patients having severe psychiatric disturbances or a need for attention. Inadvertent ingestion of sulfonylureas resulting in clinical hypoglycemia has also been reported, due either to patient error or to a prescription mishap on the part of a pharmacist.

When insulin is used to induce hypoglycemia, an elevated serum insulin level often raises suspicion of an insulin-producing pancreatic B cell tumor. It may be difficult to prove that the insulin is of exogenous origin. The triad of hypoglycemia, high immunoreactive insulin levels, and *suppressed* plasma C peptide immunoreactivity* is pathognomonic of exogenous insulin administration. The inappropriate presence of circulating antibodies to insulin (usually seen only in insulin-treated individuals), will generally support the diagnosis of factitious hypoglycemia. However, the absence of detectable insulin antibodies does not rule out the possibility of exogenous insulin administration, especially with the advent of human insulins and insulin analogs with low immunogenicity in humans.

When sulfonylurea abuse is suspected, plasma or urine should be screened for its presence. Hypoglycemia with inappropriately elevated levels of serum

---

*C peptide, a major portion of the connecting chain of amino acids in proinsulin, remains intact during the conversion of proinsulin (Chapter 17).

insulin *and* C-peptide along with detectable sulfonylureas in blood or urine are diagnostic of inadvertent or factitious sulfonylurea overdose. While all first- and second-generation sulfonylureas are measureable in standard chromatographic assays, the third-generation drug glimepiride—as well as other insulin secretagogues such as repaglinide and nateglinide—require special methodology.

Treatment of factitious hypoglycemia involves psychiatric therapy and social counseling.

4. Autoimmune Hypoglycemia

In recent years, a rare autoimmune disorder has been reported in which patients have circulating insulin antibodies and the paradoxic feature of hypoglycemia. While some of these patients may be surreptitiously administering insulin, in an increasing number of case reports it has not been possible to document exogenous insulin as the inducer of insulin antibodies. More than 200 cases of insulin-antibody-associated hypoglycemia have been reported since 1970, with 90% of cases reported in Japanese patients. HLA class II alleles—DRB1*0406, DQA1*0301, and DQB1*0302—are associated with this syndrome, and these alleles are ten to thirty times more prevalent in Japanese and Koreans, which may explain the higher prevalence of this syndrome in these populations. Hypoglycemia generally occurs 3–4 hours after a meal and follows an early postprandial hyperglycemia. It is attributed to a dissociation of insulin-antibody immune complexes, releasing free insulin. This autoimmune hypoglycemia, which is due to accumulation of high titers of antibodies capable of reacting with endogenous insulin, has been most commonly reported in methimazole-treated patients with Graves' disease from Japan as well as in patients with various other sulfhydryl-containing medications (captopril, penicillamine) and other drugs such as hydralazine, isoniazid, and procainamide. In addition, it has been reported in patients with autoimmune disorders such as rheumatoid arthritis, systemic lupus erythematosus, and polymyositis as well as in multiple myeloma and other plasma cell dyscrasias where paraproteins or antibodies cross-react with insulin.

In most cases the hypoglycemia is transient and usually resolves spontaneously within 3–6 months of diagnosis, particularly when the offending medications are stopped. The most consistent therapeutic benefit in management of this syndrome has been achieved by dietary treatment with frequent low-carbohydrate small meals; and prednisone therapy (30–60 mg/d) has been used to lower the titer of insulin antibodies.

Hypoglycemia due to insulin receptor autoantibodies is also an extremely rare syndrome; most cases have occurred in women often with a history of autoimmune disease. Almost all of these patients have also had episodes of insulin-resistant diabetes and acanthosis nigricans. Their hypoglycemia may be either fasting or postprandial and is often severe and is attributed to an agonistic action of the antibody on the insulin receptor. Balance between the antagonistic and agonistic effects of the antibody determines whether insulin-resistant diabetes or hypoglycemia occurs. Hypoglycemia was found to respond to glucocorticoid therapy but not to plasmapheresis or immunosuppression.

5. Pentamidine-Induced Hypoglycemia

With the use of intravenous pentamidine for treatment of *Pneumocystis carinii* infection in patients with AIDS, reports of pentamidine-induced hypoglycemia have appeared. The cause of acute hypoglycemia appears to be the drug's lytic effect on B cells, which produces acute hyperinsulinemia in about 10–20% of patients receiving the drug. Physicians treating patients with pentamidine should be aware of the potential complication of acute hypoglycemia, which may be followed later by occasionally persistent insulinopenia and hyperglycemia.

Intravenous glucose should be administered during pentamidine administration and for the period immediately following to prevent or ameliorate hypoglycemic symptoms. Following a complete course of therapy with pentamidine, fasting blood glucose or a subsequent glycohemoglobin should be monitored to assess the extent of pancreatic B cell recovery or residual damage.

Fortunately, with the advent of improved therapies for AIDS, the incidence of pneumocystis pneumonia is decreasing. Moreover, other drugs have been found to be just as effective in treating this pneumonia, so that pentamidine use and its hypoglycemic sequelae have declined in recent years.

6. Pancreatic B Cell Tumors

Spontaneous fasting hypoglycemia in an otherwise healthy adult is most commonly due to insulinoma, an insulin-secreting tumor of the islets of Langerhans. Eighty percent of these tumors are single and benign; 10% are malignant (if metastases are identified); and the remainder are multiple, with scattered micro- or macroadenomas interspersed within normal islet tissue. (As with some other endocrine tumors, histologic differentiation between benign and malignant cells is difficult, and close follow-up is necessary to ensure the absence of metastases.)

These adenomas may be familial and have been found in conjunction with tumors of the parathyroid glands and the pituitary (multiple endocrine neoplasia type 1). (See Chapter 22.) Over 99% of them are located within the pancreas and less than 1% in ectopic pancreatic tissue.

These tumors may appear at any age, though they are most common in the fourth to sixth decades. A slight predominance in women has been reported in some studies, though other ones suggest no sex predilection.

Clinical Findings

The signs and symptoms are chiefly those of subacute neuroglycopenia rather than adrenergic discharge. The typical picture is that of recurrent central nervous system dysfunction at times of exercise or fasting. The preponderance of neuroglycopenic symptoms rather than those more commonly associated with hypoglycemia (adrenergic symptoms) often leads to delayed diagnosis following prolonged psychiatric care or treatment for seizure disorders or transient ischemic attacks. Some patients learn to relieve or prevent their symptoms by taking frequent feedings. Obesity may be the result; however, obesity is seen in less than 30% of patients with insulin-secreting tumors.

Diagnosis of Insulinoma

Experts in this field emphasize that the most important prerequisite to diagnosing an insulinoma is simply to consider it, particularly when facing a clinical presentation of fasting hypoglycemia with symptoms of central nervous system dysfunction such as confusion or abnormal behavior. B cell tumors do not reduce secretion in the presence of hypoglycemia, and a serum insulin level of 5 μU/mL or more with concomitant plasma glucose values below 45 mg/dL (2.5 mmol/L) suggests an insulinoma. Other causes of hyperinsulinemic hypoglycemia must be considered, however, such as surreptitious administration of insulin or sulfonylureas.

A. INSULIN ASSAY

Because the insulin radioimmunoassay is crucial in diagnosing insulin-secreting tumors, it is important to be aware of certain limitations in its use. It detects not only human but also beef and pork insulin as well as newer analogs of insulin such as insulin lispro, insulin aspart, and insulin glargine. Therefore, a high serum level may indicate either endogenous or exogenous insulin. (C peptide measurements are necessary to make this distinction.) In addition, the assay is of no value in patients who have taken insulin in the past year or so, as virtually all will have developed low-titer insulin antibodies that will interfere. Falsely low or elevated values will result depending on the method used. Proper collection of samples is also important: If the serum is not separated and then frozen within 1–2 hours, falsely low values will result, because the insulin molecule will undergo proteolytic digestion.

B. SUPPRESSION TESTS

Failure of endogenous insulin secretion to be suppressed in the presence of hypoglycemia is the hallmark of an insulin-secreting tumor. The most reliable suppression test is the prolonged supervised fast in hospitalized subjects, and this remains the preferred diagnostic maneuver in the workup of suspected insulinomas. A suggested protocol for the supervised fast is set forth in Table 18–4.

In normal men, the blood glucose value will not fall below 55 mg/dL (3.1 mmol/L) during a 72-hour fast, while insulin levels fall below 10 μU/mL; in some normal women, however, plasma glucose may fall below 30 mg/dL (1.7 mmol/L) (lower limits have not been established), while serum insulin levels also fall appropriately to less than 5 μU/mL. (These women remain asymptomatic despite this degree of hypoglycemia, presumably because ketogenesis is able to provide sufficient fuel for the central nervous system.) Calculation of ratios of insulin (in μU/mL) to plasma glucose (in mg/dL) can be useful diagnostically. Nonobese normal subjects maintain a ratio of less than 0.25; obese subjects may have an elevated ratio, but hypoglycemia does not occur with

Table 18–4. Suggested hospital protocol for supervised fast in diagnosis of insulinoma.[1]

(1) Obtain baseline serum glucose, insulin, proinsulin, and C-peptide measurements at onset of fast and initiate reliable intravenous access with normal saline.

(2) Permit only calorie-free and caffeine-free fluids and encourage activity.

(3) Measure all voided urine for acetone.

(4) Obtain capillary glucose measurements with a reflectance meter every 4 hours until values < 60 mg/dL are obtained. Then increase the frequency of fingersticks to each hour, and when capillary glucose value is < 49 mg/dL send a venous blood sample to the laboratory for serum glucose, insulin, proinsulin, and C-peptide measurements. Check frequently for manifestations of neuroglycopenia.

(5) If symptoms of hypoglycemia occur or if a laboratory value of serum glucose is < 45 mg/dL, conclude the fast with a final blood sample for serum glucose, insulin, proinsulin, C-peptide, and sulfonylurea measurements. Intravenous glucose should then be administered (40–50 mL of 50% dextrose in water over 3–5 minutes through the intravenous access line) and administer calorie-containing liquids and food.

[1]Adapted, with permission, from Service FJ: Hypoglycemic disorders. N Engl J Med 1995;332:1144.

fasting. However, most centers no longer calculate this ratio and are relying only on the concentration of insulin being 5 μU/mL or higher in the presence of hypoglycemia. Virtually all patients with insulin-secreting islet cell tumors will fail to suppress their insulin secretion appropriately and will maintain serum insulin concentrations of 5 μU/mL or more despite a fall in plasma glucose below 45 mg/dL. The term "72-hour fast" is actually a misnomer in most cases, since the fast should be immediately terminated as soon as symptoms and laboratory confirmation of hypoglycemia are evident. Most patients with insulinomas will experience progressive and symptomatic fasting hypoglycemia with associated elevated insulin levels within 24–36 hours and no evidence of ketonuria. Consequently, one group recommended reducing the duration of the supervised diagnostic fast to no more than 48 hours for cost considerations as well as patient convenience. However, an occasional patient will not demonstrate hypoglycemia until 72 hours have elapsed, and most centers therefore prefer the fast to be supervised up to 72 hours. Brisk exercise during the fast may help precipitate hypoglycemia. Once symptoms of hypoglycemia occur, plasma glucose should be obtained and the fast immediately terminated if plasma glucose is below 45 mg/dL (2.5 mmol/L).

C. Stimulation Tests

A variety of stimulation tests with intravenous tolbutamide, glucagon, or calcium have been devised to demonstrate exaggerated and prolonged insulin secretion. However, because insulin-secreting tumors have a wide range of granule content and degrees of differentiation, they are variably responsive to these secretagogues. Thus, absence of an excessive insulin secretory response during any of these stimulation tests does not rule out the presence of an insulinoma. In addition, the tolbutamide stimulation test was extremely hazardous to patients with responsive tumors because it induced prolonged and refractory hypoglycemia, and for that reason it is no longer recommended for diagnosis of insulinoma. The glucagon stimulation test is performed as follows: One milligram of glucagon is given intravenously, and serum insulin levels are measured every 5 minutes for 15 minutes. A level exceeding 130 μU/mL suggests an insulin-secreting tumor. However, only about half of patients with insulinomas will demonstrate this hyperinsulinism, and false-positive results may occur. When an exaggerated increase in serum insulin occurs, the hyperglycemic effect of glucagon may be subnormal, and profound hypoglycemia may subsequently develop by 60 minutes. To prevent this, the patient is fed and may also require intravenous glucose after the 15-minute serum sample is obtained. Nausea is an unpleasant side effect, often occurring several minutes after administration of intravenous glucagon.

D. Oral Glucose Tolerance Test

The oral glucose tolerance test is of no value in the diagnosis of insulin-secreting tumors. A common misconception is that patients with insulinomas will have flat glucose tolerance curves, because the tumor will discharge insulin in response to oral glucose. In fact, most insulinomas respond poorly, and curves typical of diabetes are more common. In those rare tumors that do release insulin in response to glucose, a flat curve may result; however, this also can be seen occasionally in normal subjects.

E. Proinsulin Measurements

Insulinoma cells are poorly differentiated, which affects their ability to process insulin and convert it from proinsulin. Thus, in contrast to normal subjects, whose proinsulin concentration is less than 20% of the total immunoreactive insulin, most patients with insulinoma have elevated levels of proinsulin, representing as much as 30–90% of total immunoreactive insulin. While absolute proinsulin measurements may be elevated in other conditions besides insulinoma (such as in insulin-resistant states), an increased percentage of proinsulin-like components in relation to total insulin immunoreactivity is more specific for insulinoma. However, since this assay of the "percent proinsulin" requires laborious methodology with columns to separate serum protein components, its usefulness is limited. *Absolute* serum proinsulin measurements are more readily available in commercial laboratories, and their specificity increases considerably if hypoglycemia is achieved during a prolonged supervised fast. In cases where serum insulin measurements are at borderline levels during a fast in a patient with suspected insulinoma, a serum proinsulin that fails to suppress below 0.2 ng/mL in the presence of hypoglycemia is suggestive of the diagnosis.

F. Glycohemoglobin Measurements

Low glycohemoglobin values have been reported in occasional cases of insulinoma, reflecting the presence of chronic hypoglycemia. However, the diagnostic usefulness of glycohemoglobin measurements is limited by the relatively low sensitivity of this test as well as poor accuracy at the lower range of normal in many of the assays. In addition, it is nonspecific for hypoglycemia, with low levels being found in certain hemoglobinopathies and hemolytic states.

G. Tumor Localization Studies

It is imperative that the surgeon be convinced that the diagnosis of insulinoma has been unequivocally made by clinical and laboratory findings. Only then should surgery be considered, as there is no justification in the use of surgery for exploratory purposes or of localization techniques as a diagnostic tool. The focus of attention should be directed at the pancreas only, since virtually all insulinomas originate from this tissue; ectopic cancers secreting insulin are unknown in the experience of all major centers, with only one published report describing an atypical insulin-producing tumor believed to have originated from a small-cell carcinoma of the cervix.

1. Imaging studies—Prior to surgery, a CT scan of the abdomen should be performed to rule out a large tumor of the pancreas or hepatic metastases from a malignant islet cell tumor. Otherwise, radiographic and arteriographic techniques are seldom helpful in localizing insulinomas preoperatively owing to the small size of most of these tumors (averaging 1.5 cm in diameter in one large series). Standard arteriography has many disadvantages since it is a painful and imprecise procedure that exposes insulinoma patients to hypoglycemia and the discomfort of several hours of invasive and expensive radiography. False-positive or false-negative results are quite common, and in most cases a tumor mass that is large enough to "blush" on arteriography is generally large enough for an experienced surgeon to identify by direct visualization or palpation. Currently there is a growing consensus among experts in this field that present techniques for preoperative localization are of limited usefulness and should be replaced by careful intraoperative ultrasonography and palpation by a surgeon experienced in insulinoma surgery.

Small tumors within the pancreas that are not palpable at laparotomy have been localized using intraoperative ultrasound in which a transducer is wrapped in a sterile rubber glove and passed over the exposed pancreatic surface. This is at present probably the most effective method of localizing insulinomas. Intraoperative ultrasound, combined with careful palpation by a surgeon experienced in insulinoma surgery, has a success rate of up to 97% in recent reports and is the sole localizing approach relied upon at many centers. When the insulinoma is not found at the initial surgery, three localization methods are available prior to reoperation.

2. Localization methods prior to reoperation—

a. Kinetic magnetic resonance imaging—When the insulinoma is not found at the initial surgery, three localization methods are available prior to reoperation:

(1) The least invasive is a kinetic MRI with multiple imaging during gadolinium injection, but its accuracy for small tumors is no better than 40% and its usefulness is therefore limited.

(2) Percutaneous transhepatic pancreatic vein catheterization with insulin assay can also be useful for localizing small insulinomas with about 70% reliability. However, this technique is not widely available, is quite invasive and expensive, and is associated with considerable discomfort and some risk to the patient from intra-abdominal bleeding.

(3) A more acceptable (and the currently favored) localization method correlates imaging from selective arteriography of segments of the pancreas with simultaneous hepatic vein sampling for insulin during a bolus of intra-arterial calcium delivered selectively to these same pancreatic segments. Calcium has been found to be a secretagogue only for neoplastic tissue and not for normal islet tissue, so that a rise in hepatic vein insulin concentration indicates segmental localization of an insulinoma. A step-up of insulin in the hepatic venous effluent regionalizes the hyperinsulinism to the head of the pancreas for the gastroduodenal artery, the uncinate process for the superior mesenteric artery, and the body and tail of the pancreas for the splenic artery. Furthermore, this technique may provide data that are particularly helpful when multiple insulinomas are suspected, as in patients with coexisting pituitary or parathyroid adenomas who develop hypoglycemia, and it has become a major tool in confirming the diagnosis of diffuse islet hyperplasia in the recently described noninsulinoma pancreatogenous hypoglycemia syndrome (NIPHS) (see below). Since diazoxide might interfere with this test, it should be discontinued for at least 48–72 hours before sampling. An infusion of dextrose may be required, therefore, and patients should be closely monitored during the procedure to avoid hypoglycemia (as well as hyperglycemia, which could affect insulin gradients).

Treatment of Insulinoma

The treatment of choice for insulin-secreting tumors is surgical resection.

A. SURGICAL TREATMENT

Tumor resection should be performed only by surgeons with extensive experience with removal of islet cell tumors, since these tumors may be small and difficult to recognize. Success rates as high as 97% have been reported without preoperative localization procedures if surgeons have prior experience with insulinomas and utilize preoperative ultrasonography—although in centers with lower referral rates for this rare disorder (and therefore with less experience with its treatment), success rates are less impressive.

After the pancreas is mobilized, inspected, and palpated, it is imaged to assist in locating the tumor and to reassure the surgeon that no additional tumors exist. An additional benefit of intraoperative ultrasonography is its ability to identify the pancreatic duct and its relationship to the tumor so that the duct can be protected during surgery.

Tumors should be enucleated whenever possible unless they have malignant features (eg, hardness or an appearance of infiltration). When the tumor is in the body or tail of the pancreas and if for some reason enucleation is difficult, a safe and effective alternative is distal resection with preservation of the spleen if possible.

Limited experience with laparoscopy using ultrasound and enucleation suggests that this approach can be successful with a single tumor of the body or tail of the pancreas, but open surgery is required when a tumor is found at the time of laparoscopy to be in the head of the pancreas to ensure that risk of damage to the pancreatic duct is minimized.

1. Preoperative management—Oral diazoxide, a potent inhibitor of insulin secretion, will maintain euglycemia in most patients with insulin-secreting tumors. It acts by opening the ATP-sensitive potassium channel of the pancreatic B cell and hyperpolarizing the cell membrane. This reduces calcium influx through the voltage-gated calcium channel, thereby reducing insulin release. If there is a delay in scheduling surgery once the diagnosis of insulinoma is made, the use of diazoxide is recommended to prevent or reduce the frequency of hypoglycemic episodes. Doses of 300–400 mg/d (divided) will usually suffice, but an occasional patient will require up to 800 mg/d. Side effects include edema due to sodium retention (which generally necessitates concomitant thiazide administration), gastric irritation, and mild hirsutism.

2. Treatment during surgery—

a. Glucose need during surgery—An infusion of 5% or 10% dextrose is needed to maintain euglycemia during the surgical procedure. Careful and frequent blood glucose monitoring is needed to determine the infusion rate required in individual patients to avoid hypoglycemia, especially when the insulinoma is being palpated and manipulated prior to removal.

b. Diazoxide—Diazoxide should be administered preoperatively as well as on the day of surgery in patients who are responsive to it, since the drug greatly reduces the need for glucose supplements and the risk of hypoglycemia during surgery while not masking the glycemic rise indicative of surgical cure.

3. Postoperative hyperglycemia—Postoperatively, several days of hyperglycemia may ensue. A major cause is probably related to edema and inflammation of the pancreas secondary to its mobilization and manipulation during surgical resection of the insulinoma. However, other possible contributing factors include high levels of counterregulatory hormones induced by the procedure, chronic down-regulation of insulin receptors by the previously high circulating insulin levels from the tumor, and perhaps suppression of normal pancreatic B cells by long-standing hypoglycemia. Small subcutaneous doses of regular insulin may be prescribed every 4–6 hours if plasma glucose exceeds 300 mg/dL (16.7 mmol/L), but in most cases pancreatic insulin secretion recovers after 48–72 hours, and very little insulin replacement is required.

4. Failure to find the tumor at operation—In approximately 2–5% of patients with biochemically demonstrated autonomous insulin secretion, no tumor can be found at exploratory laparotomy even with intraoperative ultrasound. The tumor will most likely be in the head of the pancreas, since this is the most difficult area for the surgeon to mobilize and explore; therefore, blind distal two-thirds pancreatectomy is seldom successful and, in contrast to former practice, is no longer recommended by most surgeons in this field. Moreover, complete pancreatectomy is quite hazardous and not a reasonable option. These patients should be maintained on diazoxide and referred to a medical center staffed by people with considerable experience, where a calcium stimulation test during selective arteriography can be scheduled prior to reoperation (see above).

B. MEDICAL TREATMENT

Diazoxide therapy is the treatment of choice in patients with inoperable functioning islet cell carcinomas and in those who are poor candidates for operation. A few patients have been maintained on long-term (over 10 years) diazoxide therapy without apparent ill effects. Hydrochlorothiazide, 25–50 mg daily, should also be prescribed to counteract the edema and hyperkalemia secondary to diazoxide therapy as well as to potentiate its hyperglycemic effect. Frequent carbohydrate feedings (every 2–3 hours) can also be helpful in maintaining euglycemia, though obesity may become a problem.

When patients are unable to tolerate diazoxide because of side effects such as gastrointestinal upset, hirsutism, or edema, a calcium channel blocker such as verapamil (80 mg given orally every 8 hours) may be tried in view of its inhibitory effect on insulin release from insulinoma cells in vitro.

A potent long-acting synthetic octapeptide analog of somatostatin (octreotide) has been used to inhibit release of hormones from a number of endocrine tumors, including inoperable insulinomas, but it has had limited success. Of the five somatostatin receptors (SSTR) that have been identified in humans, SSTR2, which predominates in the anterior pituitary, has a much greater affinity for octreotide than SSTR5, which predominates in the pancreas. This explains why octreotide is much more effective in treating acromegaly than in treating insulinoma, except in the occasional cases where insulinoma cells happen also to express SSTR2. When hypoglycemia persists after attempted surgical removal of the insulinoma and if diazoxide or verapamil is poorly tolerated or ineffective, a trial of 50 μg of octreotide injected subcutaneously twice daily may control the hypoglycemic episodes in conjunction with multiple small carbohydrate feedings.

Streptozocin has proved beneficial in patients with islet cell carcinomas, and with selective arterial administration effective cytotoxic doses have been achieved without the undue renal toxicity that characterized early experience. Benign tumors appear to respond poorly, if at all.

SYMPTOMATIC FASTING HYPOGLYCEMIA WITHOUT HYPERINSULINISM

1. Disorders Associated with Low Hepatic Glucose Output

Reduced hepatic gluconeogenesis can result from a direct loss of hepatic tissue (acute yellow atrophy from fulminating viral or toxic damage); from disorders reducing amino acid supply to hepatic parenchyma (severe muscle wasting and inanition from anorexia nervosa, chronic starvation, uremia, and glucocorticoid deficit from adrenocortical deficiency); or from inborn errors of carbohydrate metabolism affecting glycogenolytic or gluconeogenic enzymes.

2. Ethanol Hypoglycemia

Ethanol impairs gluconeogenesis but has no effect on hepatic glycogenolysis. The metabolism of ethanol has been shown to reduce lactate uptake by gluconeogenic tissues by as much as 60%, thereby depriving these tissues of an important substrate for gluconeogenesis. In the patient who is imbibing ethanol but not eating, fasting hypoglycemia may occur after hepatic glycogen stores have been depleted (within 8–12 hours of a fast). No correlation exists between the blood ethanol levels and the degree of hypoglycemia, which may occur while blood ethanol levels are declining. It should be noted that ethanol-induced fasting hypoglycemia may occur at ethanol levels as low as 45 mg/dL (10 mmol/L)—considerably below most states' legal standards (80 mg/dL [17.4 mmol/L]) for being "under the influence." Most patients present with neuroglycopenic symptoms, which may be difficult to differentiate from the neurotoxic effects of the alcohol. These symptoms in a patient whose breath smells of alcohol may be mistaken for alcoholic stupor. Intravenous dextrose should be administered promptly to all such stuporous or comatose patients. Because hepatic glycogen stores have been depleted by the time hypoglycemia occurs, parenteral glucagon will not be effective. Adequate food intake during alcohol ingestion will prevent this type of hypoglycemia.

3. Nonpancreatic Tumors

A variety of nonpancreatic tumors have been found to cause fasting hypoglycemia. Most are large and mesenchymal in origin, retroperitoneal fibrosarcoma being the classic prototype. However, hepatocellular carcinomas, adrenocortical carcinomas, hypernephromas, gastrointestinal tumors, lymphomas and leukemias, and a variety of other tumors have also been reported.

Laboratory diagnosis depends upon fasting hypoglycemia associated with serum insulin levels below 5 μU/mL. The mechanisms by which these tumors produce hypoglycemia have only recently been elucidated. While very large tumors may metabolize substantial amounts of glucose, this does not explain the increased glucose uptake by muscle and the failure of the liver and kidney to adequately compensate by increasing glucose production. The expression and release of an incompletely processed insulin-like growth factor-II (IGF-II) has provided the best explanation for the clinical manifestations of hypoglycemia in many of these cases.

In normal situations, expression of IGF-II by the liver results in a circulating form of the hormone that is immediately complexed by an IGF-binding protein as well as by an acid-labile protein. This tripartite protein complex is generally inactive in adults since it is unable to properly bind to tissue receptors. However, in patients with nonpancreatic tumors associated with hypoglycemia, a larger, immature form of the IGF-II molecule is released. This incompletely processed molecule can bind to the carrier protein but not to the acid-labile component of serum. It therefore remains active and binds to insulin receptors in muscle to promote glucose transport and to insulin receptors in liver and kidney to reduce glucose output. This immature IGF-II complex also binds to receptors for IGF-I in the pancreatic B cell to inhibit insulin secretion and in the pituitary to suppress growth hormone release. With the reduction of growth hormone, there is a consequent lowering of IGF-I levels as well as IGF-I binding protein 3 and the acid-labile protein. The clinical syndrome of nonpancreatic tumor hypoglycemia, therefore, is supported by laboratory documentation of serum insulin levels below 5 μU/mL with plasma glucose measurements of 45 mg/dL or lower. Values for growth hormone and IGF-I are also decreased. Levels of IGF-II may be increased but often are "normal" in quantity despite the presence of the immature, higher-molecular-weight form of IGF-II, which can only be detected by special laboratory techniques. Treatment is aimed toward the primary tumor, with supportive therapy using frequent feedings. Diazoxide is ineffective in reversing the hypoglycemia caused by these tumors.

NONFASTING HYPOGLYCEMIA (REACTIVE HYPOGLYCEMIA)

Reactive hypoglycemia may be classified as early (within 2–3 hours after a meal) or late (3–5 hours). Early (alimentary) hypoglycemia occurs when there is a rapid discharge of ingested carbohydrate into the small bowel followed by rapid glucose absorption and hyperinsulinism. It may be seen after gastrointestinal surgery and is notably associated with the "dumping syndrome" after gastrectomy; occasionally, it is functional and may result from overactivity of the parasympathetic nervous system mediated via the vagus nerve. Late hypoglycemia (occult diabetes) is caused by a delay in early insulin release, which then results in exaggeration of initial hyperglycemia during a glucose tolerance test. As a consequence, an exaggerated insulin response produces late hypoglycemia. Early or late hypoglycemia may also occur as a consequence of ethanol's potentiation of the insulin-secretory response to glucose, as when sugar-containing soft drinks are used as mixers to dilute alcohol in beverages (gin and tonic, rum and cola).

1. Postgastrectomy Alimentary Hypoglycemia

Reactive hypoglycemia after gastrectomy is a consequence of hyperinsulinism. This results from rapid gastric emptying of ingested food, which produces overstimulation of vagal reflexes and overproduction of beta-cytotropic gastrointestinal hormones, causing arterial hyperinsulinism and consequent acute hypoglycemia. The symptoms are caused by adrenergic hyperactivity in response to the rapidly falling plasma glucose. Treatment is properly directed at avoiding this sequence of events by more frequent feedings with smaller portions of less rapidly assimilated carbohydrate and more slowly absorbed fat or protein. Occasionally, anticholinergic drugs such as propantheline (15 mg orally four times daily) may be useful in reducing vagal overactivity.

2. Functional Alimentary Hypoglycemia

Early alimentary-type reactive hypoglycemia in a patient who has not undergone surgery is classified as functional. It is most often associated with chronic fatigue, anxiety, irritability, weakness, poor concentration, decreased libido, headaches, hunger after meals, and tremulousness. Whether or not hypoglycemia accounts for these symptoms or occurs at all is difficult to prove.

The usual sequence of events is that the patient presents with a number of nonspecific complaints. Normal laboratory findings and a normal physical examination confirm the initial impression that organic disease is not present, and the symptoms are then attributed to the stresses of modern living. The only form of therapy usually given is reassurance or a mild tranquilizer. When this fails to be of benefit, the patient seeks help elsewhere. Inevitably, the question of hypoglycemia is raised—frequently by the patient, who has heard of the diagnosis from friends or relatives with similar symptoms or has read of it in the lay press. The diagnosis is often supported by the demonstration of hypoglycemia with symptoms during a 5-hour oral glucose tolerance test.

Unfortunately, the precipitation of hypoglycemia with or without symptoms during oral glucose tolerance testing does not distinguish between normal and "hypoglycemic" patients. As many as one-third or more of normal subjects who have never had any symptoms will develop hypoglycemia with or without symptoms during a 5-hour glucose tolerance test. In addition, many patients will develop symptoms in the absence of hypoglycemia. Thus, the test's nonspecificity makes it a highly unreliable tool that is no longer recommended for evaluating patients with suspected episodes of postprandial hypoglycemia. Indeed, the ingestion of a mixed meal did not produce hypoglycemia in 33 patients who had been diagnosed as having reactive hypoglycemia on the basis of oral glucose tolerance testing; this attempt to increase specificity for the diagnosis of reactive hypoglycemia may have resulted in loss of sensitivity.

For increased diagnostic reliability, hypoglycemia should be documented during a spontaneous symptomatic episode in routine daily activity. However, attempts to demonstrate this are almost never successful. Patients should be instructed in the proper use of glucose meters with sufficient "memory" capability to bring results to the physician's office for documentation of the episodes. Personality evaluation often discloses hyperkinetic compulsive behavior in thin, anxious patients.

The foregoing discussion should not be taken to imply that functional reactive hypoglycemia does not occur—merely that at present we have no reliable means of diagnosing it. There is no harm (and there is occasional benefit) in reducing or eliminating the content of refined sugars in the patient's diet while increasing the frequency and reducing the size of meals. However, it should not be expected that these maneuvers will cure the asthenia, since the reflex response to hypoglycemia is only a possibly aggravating feature of a generalized primary hyperactivity. Counseling and support and mild sedation should be the mainstays in therapy, with dietary manipulation only an adjunct.

3. Pancreatic Islet Hyperplasia in Adults (Noninsulinoma Pancreatogenous Hypoglycemia Syndrome)

Since 1995, the Mayo Clinic has treated ten adult patients with hyperinsulinemic hypoglycemia who were diagnosed as having generalized islet hyperplasia and nesidioblastosis. Seven of these were men, and hypoglycemia only occurred 2–4 hours after meals and not at all with fasting up to 72 hours. In addition to adrenergic manifestations, the development of severe neuroglycopenic symptoms (including diplopia, dysarthria, confusion, disorientation, and even in some patients convulsions and coma) within 4 hours after meal ingestion distinguishes this syndrome from that of *reactive hypoglycemia*, in which adrenergic symptoms overwhelmingly predominate, and when neuroglycopenic symptoms occasionally occur (usually with postgastrectomy alimentary hypoglycemia) they are generally mild. Furthermore, the absence of hypoglycemia during a fast distinguishes these patients from those with single or multiple insulinoma. Each patient had a positive response to selective arterial calcium stimulation, but localization data with this test were variable among the patients, incriminating only one, two, or all three arteries as perfusing the site of abnormal tissue.

Workers at the Mayo Clinic have called this disorder noninsulinoma pancreatogenous hypoglycemic syndrome (NIPHS). No mutations were detected in the *KIR6.2* and *SUR1* genes, which have been abnormal in some cases of children with a syndrome of familial hyperinsulinemic hypoglycemia and which encode the subunits of the pancreatic ATP-sensitive channel affecting glucose-induced insulin secretion. Following gradient-guided partial pancreatectomy, there was no recurrence of symptoms with up to 4 years of follow-up in all seven of the male patients, but for some unexplained reason the three female patients have had varying degrees of transient or persistent symptom recurrence.

4. Late Hypoglycemia (Occult Diabetes)

This condition is characterized by delay in early insulin release from pancreatic B cells, resulting in initial exaggeration of hyperglycemia during a glucose tolerance test. In response to this hyperglycemia, an exaggerated insulin release produces late hypoglycemia 4–5 hours after ingestion of glucose. These patients are usually quite different from those with early hypoglycemia, being more phlegmatic and often obese and frequently having a family history of diabetes mellitus. In the obese, treatment is directed at reduction to ideal weight. These patients often respond to reduced intake of refined sugars with multiple, spaced small feedings high in dietary fiber. They should be considered early diabetics and advised to have periodic medical evaluations.

REFERENCES

Banarer S, McGregor VP, Cryer PE: Intraislet hyperinsulinemia prevents the glucagon response to hyperglycemia despite an intact autonomic response. Diabetes 2002;51:958. [PMID: 11916913]

Bolli GB, Fanelli CG: Physiology of glucose counterregulation to hypoglycemia. Endocrinol Metab Clin North Am 1999;28: 467. [PMID: 10500926]

Boukhman MP et al: Localization of insulinomas. Arch Surg 1999; 134:818. [PMID: 10443803]

Boyle PJ et al: Adaptation in brain glucose uptake following recurrent hypoglycemia. Proc Natl Acad Sci U S A 1994;91:9352.

Brentjens R, Saltz L: Islet cell tumors of the pancreas: the medical oncologist's perspective. Surg Clin North Am 2001;81:527. [PMID: 11459269]

Cryer PE: Hypoglycemia-associated autonomic failure in diabetes. Am J Physiol Endocrinol Metab 2001;281:E1115. [PMID: 11701423]

Cryer PE: Symptoms of hypoglycemia, thresholds for their occurrence, and hypoglycemic unawareness. Endocrinol Metab Clin North Am 1999;28:495. [PMID: 10500927]

Doppman JL et al: Localization of insulinomas to regions of the pancreas by intra-arterial stimulation with calcium. Ann Intern Med 1995;123:269. [PMID: 7611592]

Ekberg K et al: Contributions by kidney and liver to glucose production in the post-absorptive state and after 60 h of fasting. Diabetes 1999;48:292. [PMID: 10334304]

Fanelli C et al: Long-term recovery from unawareness, deficient counterregulation and lack of cognitive dysfunction during hypoglycemia following institution of rational, intensive insulin therapy in IDDM. Diabetologia 1994;37:1265. [PMID: 7895957]

Fischer KF, Lees JA, Newman JH: Hypoglycemia in hospitalized patients: Causes and outcomes. N Engl J Med 1986;315: 1245. [PMID: 3534567]

Gerich JE et al: Hypoglycemia unawareness. Endocr Rev 1991;12: 356. [PMID: 1760993]

Gorden P et al: Plasma proinsulin-like component in insulinoma: a 25-year experience. J Clin Endocrinol Metab 1995;80:2884. [PMID: 7559869]

Grant CS: Insulinoma. Surg Oncol Clin N Am 1998;7:819. [PMID: 9735136]

Grant CS: Surgical aspects of hyperinsulinemic hypoglycemia. Endocrinol Metab Clin North Am 1999;28:533. [PMID: 10500930]

Hiramoto JS et al: Intraoperative ultrasound and preoperative localization detects all occult insulinomas. Arch Surg 2001;136: 1020. [PMID: 11529824]

Hirshberg B et al: Forty-eight-hour fast: the diagnostic test for insulinoma. J Clin Endocrinol Metab 2000;85:3222. [PMID: 10999812]

Klonoff D et al: Hypoglycemia following inadvertent and factitious sulfonylurea overdosages. Diabetes Care 1995;18:563. [PMID: 7497872]

Kumar U et al: Subtype selective expression of the five somatostatin receptors (hSSTR 1–5) in human pancreatic islet cells. Diabetes 1999;48:77. [PMID: 9892225]

Le Roith D: Tumor-induced hypoglycemia. N Engl J Med 1999; 341:757. [PMID: 10471466]

Marks V, Teale JD: Drug-induced hypoglycemia. Endocrinol Metab Clin North Am 1999;28:555. [PMID: 10500931]

Marks V, Teale JD: Hypoglycemia: factitious and felonious. Endocrinol Metab Clin North Am 1999;28:579. [PMID: 10500932]

Meyer C, Dostou JM, Gerich JE: Role of the human kidney in glucose counterregulation. Diabetes 1999;48:943. [PMID: 10331396]

Mitrakou A et al: Reversibility of unawareness of hypoglycemia in patients with insulinomas. N Engl J Med 1993;329:834. [PMID: 8355741]

Palardy J et al: Blood glucose measurements during symptomatic episodes in patients with suspected postprandial hypoglycemia. N Engl J Med 1989;321:1421. [PMID: 2811957]

Polonsky KS: A practical approach to fasting hypoglycemia. N Engl J Med 1992;326:1020. [PMID: 1545839]

Redmon JB, Nuttal FQ: Autoimmune hypoglycemia. Endocrinol Metab Clin North Am 1999;28:603. [PMID: 10500933]

Seckl MJ et al: Hypoglycemia due to an insulin-secreting small cell carcinoma of the cervix. N Engl J Med 1999;341:733. [PMID: 10471459]

Segel SA et al: Blood-to-brain glucose transport, cerebral glucose metabolism, and cerebral blood flow are not increased after hypoglycemia. Diabetes 2001;50:1911. [PMID: 11473055]

Service FJ: Classification of hypoglycemic disorders. Endocrinol Metab Clin North Am 1999;28:501. [PMID: 10500928]

Service FJ: Diagnostic approach to adults with hypoglycemic disorders. Endocrinol Metab Clin North Am 1999;28:519. [PMID: 10500929]

Service FJ, Natt N: The prolonged fast. J Clin Endocrinol Metab 2000;85:3973. [PMID: 11095416]

Stumvoll M et al: Renal glucose production and utilization: new aspects in humans. Diabetologia 1997;40:749. [PMID: 9243094]

Thompson GB et al: Noninsulinoma pancreatogenous hypoglycemia syndrome: an update in 10 surgically treated patients. Surgery 2000;128:937. [PMID: 11114627]

Witteles RM et al: Adult-onset nesidioblastosis causing hypoglycemia: an important clinical entity and continuing treatment dilemma. Arch Surg 2001;136:656. [PMID: 11387003]

Yoon JC et al: Control of hepatic gluconeogenesis through the transcriptional coactivator PGC-1. Nature 2001;413:131. [PMID: 11557972]

Disorders of Lipoprotein Metabolism

Mary J. Malloy, MD, & John P. Kane, MD, PhD

19

ABCA-1	ATP binding cassette transporter A1	**Lp(a)**	Lipoprotein(a)
ACAT	Acyl-CoA:cholesterol acyltransferase	**LPL**	Lipoprotein lipase
Apo-	Apolipoprotein	**LPR**	LDL receptor-related protein
CETP	Cholesteryl ester transfer protein	**MCP-1**	Monocyte chemoattractant protein-1
FFA	Free fatty acids	**NASH**	Nonalcoholic steatohepatitis
HDL	High-density lipoprotein(s)	**PDGF**	Platelet-derived growth factor
HMG-CoA	Hydroxymethylglutaryl-CoA	**PLTP**	Phospholipid transfer protein
IDL	Intermediate-density lipoprotein(s)	**PPARα**	Peroxisome proliferator activated receptor alpha
LCAT	Lecithin:cholesterol acyltransferase	**SR-BI**	Scavenger receptor, class B, type 1
LDL	Low-density lipoprotein(s)	**VLDL**	Very low density lipoprotein(s)

The clinical importance of hyperlipoproteinemia derives chiefly from the role of lipoproteins in atherogenesis. The greatly increased risk of acute pancreatitis associated with severe hypertriglyceridemia is an additional indication for intervention. Disordered lipid metabolism also underlies the syndrome of nonalcoholic steatohepatitis (NASH). Characterization of hyperlipoproteinemia is important for selection of appropriate treatment and may provide clues to underlying primary clinical disorders.

ATHEROSCLEROSIS

Arteriosclerosis is the leading cause of death in the USA. Abundant epidemiologic evidence establishes its multifactorial character and indicates that the effects of the multiple risk factors are at least additive. Risk factors for atherosclerosis include hyperlipidemia, hypertension, smoking, diabetes, physical inactivity, decreased levels of high-density lipoproteins (HDL), hyperhomocysteinemia, and hypercoagulable states. Certain infectious agents may also be involved. Atheromas are complex lesions containing cellular elements, collagen, and lipids. The progression of the lesion is chiefly attributable to its content of unesterified cholesterol and cholesteryl esters. Cholesterol in the atheroma originates in circulating lipoproteins. Atherogenic lipoproteins include low-density (LDL), intermediate-density (IDL), very low density (VLDL), and Lp(a) species, all of which contain the B-100 apolipoprotein. All the apo B-containing lipoproteins are subject to oxidation by reactive oxygen species in the tissues and also by lipoxygenases secreted by macrophages in atheromas. Oxidized lipoproteins cause impairment of endothelial cell-mediated vasodilation and stimulate endothelium to secrete monocyte chemoattractant protein-1 (MCP-1) and adhesion molecules that recruit monocytes to the lesion. Tocopherols (vitamin E) are natural antioxidants that localize in the surface monolayers of lipoproteins, exerting resistance to oxidation. Increased oxidative stress such as that induced by smoking depletes the tocopherol content. Oxidation of lipoproteins stimulates their endocytosis via scavenger receptors on macrophages and smooth muscle cells, leading to the formation of foam cells. At least four classes of scavenger receptors are recognized. Two are splice variant products of a single gene (class A receptors). Another is a CD36 type protein, and the fourth is an Fc receptor.

Hypertension increases access of lipoproteins to the subintima. Smoking accelerates atherogenesis by reducing HDL and increasing thrombogenesis by platelets—in addition to its pro-oxidant effect. Activated platelets release platelet-derived growth factor (PDGF), stimulating migration and proliferation of cells of smooth muscle origin into the lesion.

Activated macrophages secrete cytokines that drive an inflammatory and proliferative process. Metalloproteases secreted by macrophages weaken the atheroma so that fissuring and rupture can occur. Exposure of blood to subintimal collagen and tissue factor stimulates thrombogenesis, precipitating acute coronary events. Emerging evidence suggests that infectious agents such as *Chlamydia pneumoniae* may contribute to the inflammatory component of atherogenesis in some patients. The inverse relationship between HDL levels and atherogenesis probably reflects the role of certain species of HDL in cholesterol retrieval from the atheroma and in protecting lipoproteins against oxidation.

Reversal of Atherosclerosis

Angiographic intervention trials have shown that regression of atherosclerotic lesions occurs with lipid-lowering therapy. Large trials have demonstrated striking reductions in the incidence of new coronary events in individuals with hyperlipidemia who have had no prior clinical coronary disease (primary prevention) as well as in patients with antecedent clinical coronary disease (secondary prevention). Thus, timely hypolipidemic therapy appropriate to the lipid disorder will decrease the incidence of coronary disease and reduce the need for angioplasty, atherectomy, and bypass surgery. In the intervention trials involving treatment with HMG-CoA reductase inhibitors and with niacin, all-cause mortality was significantly reduced. Side effects of treatment have been minimal in comparison with the magnitude of this benefit.

Average levels of LDL in the United States and northern Europe are higher than in many other nations, where the levels appear to approach the biologic norm for humans. This probably accounts in large part for the higher incidence of coronary disease in industrialized Western nations and suggests that dietary changes that reduce lipoprotein levels would be beneficial.

OVERVIEW OF LIPID TRANSPORT

The Plasma Lipoproteins

Because lipids are relatively insoluble in water, they are transported in association with proteins. The simplest complexes are those formed between unesterified, or free, fatty acids (FFA) and albumin, which serve to carry the FFA from peripheral adipocytes to other tissues.

The remainder of the lipids are transported in spherical lipoprotein complexes (Table 19–1), with core regions containing hydrophobic lipids. The principal core lipids are cholesteryl esters and triglycerides. Triglycerides predominate in the cores of chylomicrons, which transport newly absorbed lipids from the intestine, and in VLDL, which originate in liver. The relative content of cholesteryl ester is increased in the cores of remnants derived from these lipoproteins. Cholesteryl esters are the predominant core lipid in LDL and HDL. Surrounding the core in each lipoprotein is a monolayer containing amphiphilic phospholipids and unesterified (free) cholesterol. Apolipoproteins, noncovalently bound to the lipids, are located on this surface monolayer (Figure 19–1).

Table 19–1. Lipoproteins of human serum.

	Electrophoretic Mobility in Agarose Gel	Density Interval (g/cm³)	Core Lipids	Diameter (nm)	Apolipoproteins in Order of Quantitative Importance
High-density (HDL)	Alpha	1.21–1.063	Cholesteryl ester	7.5–10.5	A-I, A-II, C, E
Low-density (LDL)	Beta	1.063–1.019	Cholesteryl ester	21.5	B-100
Intermediate-density (IDL)	Beta	1.019–1.006	Cholesteryl ester, triglyceride	25–30	B-100, some C and E
Very low density (VLDL)	Prebeta, some "slow prebeta"	< 1.006	Triglyceride	39–100	B-100, C, E
Chylomicrons	Remain at origin	< 1.006	Triglyceride	60–500	B-48, C, E, A-I, A-II, A-IV
Lp(a)	Prebeta	1.04–1.08	Cholesteryl ester	21–30	B-100, Lp(a)

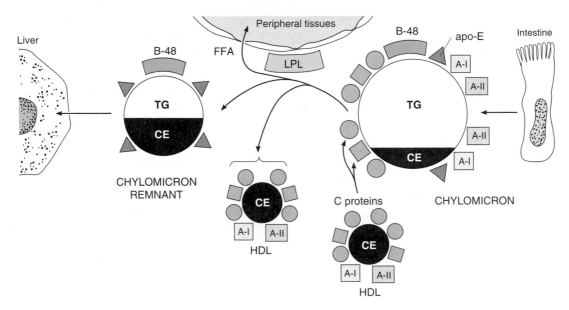

Figure 19–1. Metabolism of chylomicrons. (TG, triglyceride; CE, cholesteryl esters; A-I, A-II, B-48, and C proteins, apolipoproteins.) See text for details.

B Apoproteins

Several lipoproteins contain very high molecular weight B apolipoproteins that behave like intrinsic proteins of cell membranes. Unlike the smaller apoproteins, the B proteins do not migrate from one lipoprotein particle to another. VLDL contain the B-100 protein, which is retained in the formation of LDL from VLDL remnants by liver. The intestinal B protein, B-48, is found only in chylomicrons and their remnants. Apo B-100 has a ligand domain that is conformed as VLDL are transformed into LDL for binding to the LDL receptor.

Other Apoproteins

In addition to the B proteins, the following apoproteins are present in lipoproteins. (The distribution of these proteins is shown in Table 19–1.)

C apoproteins are lower molecular weight proteins that equilibrate rapidly among the lipoproteins. There are four distinct species: C-I, C-II, C-III, and C-IV. Apo C-II is a requisite cofactor for lipoprotein lipase.

Three isoforms of **E apoproteins**—E-2, E-3, and E-4 are the products of allelic genes. Unlike apo E-3 and E-4, apo E-2 does not contain a functional ligand for the LDL receptor. The E-4 alleles are associated with early-onset Alzheimer's disease.

Apoprotein A-I is the major apoprotein of HDL. It is also present in chylomicrons and is the most abundant of the apoproteins of human serum (about 125 mg/dL). It is a cofactor for lecithin:cholesterol acyltransferase (LCAT).

Apoprotein A-II is an important constituent of HDL. It contains cysteine, which permits the formation of disulfide-bridged dimers with apo E.

Apoprotein A-IV is chiefly associated with chylomicrons.

Lp(a) protein is a glycoprotein that has a high degree of sequence homology with plasminogen. It is found as a disulfide-bridged dimer with apo B-100 in LDL-like species of lipoproteins (Lp[a] lipoproteins).

Absorption of Dietary Fat; Secretion of Chylomicrons

Dietary triglycerides are hydrolyzed in the intestine to β-monoglyceride and fatty acids by pancreatic lipase, which is activated by bile acids and a protein cofactor. The partial glycerides and fatty acids form micelles that are absorbed by intestinal epithelium. The fatty acids are reesterified with beta monoglycerides to form triglycerides, and free cholesterol is esterified with fatty acids by acyl-CoA:cholesterol acyltransferase (ACAT). Droplets of triglyceride with small amounts of cholesteryl esters, associated with B-48, acquire a monolayer of phospholipid and free cholesterol. Apo A-I and apo A-II are added, and the nascent chylomicron emerges into the extracellular lymph space (Figure 19–1). The new chylomicron begins to exchange surface components with HDL, acquiring apo C and apo E and losing phospholipids. This process continues as the chylomicron is carried via the intestinal lymphatics to the thoracic duct and thence into the bloodstream.

Formation of Very Low Density Lipoproteins

The liver exports triglycerides to peripheral tissues in the cores of VLDL (Figure 19–2). These triglycerides are synthesized in liver from free fatty acids abstracted from plasma and from fatty acids synthesized de novo. Release of VLDL by liver is augmented by any condition that results in increased flux of FFA to liver in the absence of compensating ketogenesis. Obesity, increased caloric intake, ingestion of ethanol, and estrogens stimulate release of VLDL and are important factors in hypertriglyceridemia.

Metabolism of Triglyceride-Rich Lipoproteins in Plasma

A. Hydrolysis by Lipoprotein Lipase

Fatty acids derived from the triglycerides of chylomicrons and VLDL are delivered to tissues through a common pathway involving hydrolysis by the lipoprotein lipase (LPL) system. Lipoprotein lipase is bound to capillary endothelium in heart, skeletal muscle, adipose tissue, mammary gland, and other tissues.

B. Biologic Regulation of Lipoprotein Lipase

When glucose levels in plasma are elevated and the release of insulin is stimulated, LPL activity in adipose tissue increases, and fatty acids derived from triglycerides of circulating lipoproteins are stored. During prolonged fasting, LPL activity of adipose tissue falls, preventing storage of fatty acids. Heparin is a cofactor for LPL. When it is given intravenously (0.1–0.2 mg/kg), LPL

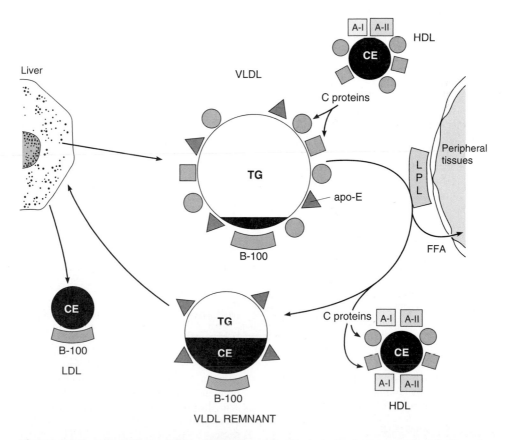

Figure 19–2. Metabolism of VLDL. (TG, triglyceride; CE, cholesteryl esters; A-I, A-II, B-48, and C proteins, apolipoproteins.) See text for details.

activity is displaced into plasma, permitting its measurement. Apo C-II is an obligatory cofactor.

C. Formation of Lipoprotein Remnants

Hydrolysis by LPL results in depletion of triglycerides in the cores of chylomicrons and VLDL, producing progressive decreases in particle diameter. Lipids from the surface and C proteins are transferred to HDL. The "remnant" lipoproteins thus formed contain their original complement of apo B, significant amounts of apo E, and little apo C. They have lost about 70% of their original content of triglyceride and are enriched in cholesteryl esters.

D. Fate of Lipoprotein Remnants

Chylomicron remnants are removed from blood quantitatively by high-affinity, receptor-mediated endocytosis in the liver. The receptors include the LDL (B-100:E) receptors and the related LRP receptors. Endocytosis of chylomicron remnants by both requires the presence of apo E-3 or apo E-4. The lipids enter hepatic pools, and B-48 protein is degraded. Cholesterol derived from chylomicron remnants exerts feedback control of cholesterol biosynthesis in liver. Some VLDL remnants are removed from blood via the B-100:E receptors (see below) and are degraded. Those which escape uptake are transformed into LDL. Thus, the rate of removal of VLDL remnants by liver is a determinant of LDL production. Formation of LDL involves the removal of residual triglycerides by hepatic lipase, facilitated by apo E. LDL contain cholesteryl esters in their cores and retain apo B-100. In normal individuals, a major fraction of VLDL is converted to LDL, and all of the LDL apo B comes from VLDL. In certain hypertriglyceridemic states, conversion of VLDL to LDL is decreased. In the absence of impaired conversion, increased secretion of VLDL results in increased production of LDL. This precursor-product relationship explains the clinical phenomenon referred to as the "beta shift," an increase of LDL (beta-lipoprotein) as hypertriglyceridemia resolves. An example of this occurs temporarily following institution of insulin treatment in uncontrolled diabetes with lipemia. Insulin induces LPL activity, resulting in rapid conversion of VLDL to LDL. Because of its longer half-life, LDL accumulates in plasma. Elevated levels of LDL may persist beyond the time when levels of triglyceride-rich lipoproteins have returned to normal. A similar phenomenon may occur when patients with familial combined hyperlipidemia are treated with fibric acid derivatives.

E. Half-Lives of Lipoproteins

Normally, the half-life of chylomicrons is 5–20 minutes; that of VLDL is 0.5–1 hour; and that of LDL is about 2½ days. At triglyceride levels of 800–1000 mg/dL, LPL is at kinetic saturation. Increased input of triglycerides into plasma at those levels rapidly augments the hypertriglyceridemia.

F. Effect of Dietary Fat Restriction

Individuals consuming a typical North American diet transport 75–100 g or more of triglyceride per day in chylomicrons, whereas the liver exports 10–30 g in VLDL. Thus, the flux of triglyceride into plasma can be influenced most acutely by restriction of dietary fat. When LPL is saturated and triglycerides are measured in thousands of milligrams per deciliter, acute restriction of dietary triglyceride intake will produce a significant reduction in levels. This intervention is especially important in the lipemic patient with impending pancreatitis. If symptoms suggest that pancreatitis is imminent, oral intake should be eliminated, gastric acid should be suppressed with H_2 blockade, and the patient should not be fed by mouth until the symptoms subside and triglycerides decrease to less than 800–1000 mg/dL.

Catabolism of Low-Density Lipoproteins

LDL catabolism is mediated by high-affinity receptors on the cell membranes of virtually all nucleated cells but most importantly hepatocytes. Ligands for these LDL receptors exist in apo B-100 and apo E. After endocytosis, apo B is degraded and the receptor returns to the cell membrane. The cholesteryl esters of LDL are hydrolyzed to free cholesterol for production of cell membrane bilayers. Free cholesterol down-regulates hydroxymethylglutaryl-CoA (HMG-CoA) reductase, a rate-limiting enzyme in the biosynthetic pathway for cholesterol. Cholesterol in excess of need for membrane synthesis is esterified by ACAT for storage. In addition to suppression of cholesterol biosynthesis, the entry of cholesterol via the LDL pathway leads to down-regulation of LDL receptors, an effect also observed with dietary saturated fat.

Metabolism of High-Density Lipoproteins

When isolated by ultracentrifugation, HDL appear to comprise two major classes: HDL_2 and HDL_3. Similar quantities of HDL_3 are isolated from serum of men and women, but about twice as much HDL_2 is found in premenopausal women. Immunochemical studies indicate that there are as many as ten discrete species of HDL that are obscured by ultracentrifugation. One of these, the 67-kDa prebeta-1 HDL, appears to be the primary acquisitor of cholesterol in the retrieval pathway from peripheral tissues.

A. Sources of HDL

Both liver and intestine produce HDL apoproteins, which organize with lipids into the native species of HDL in lymph and plasma. Excess free cholesterol and phospholipids liberated from the surface monolayers of chylomicrons and VLDL as hydrolysis of triglycerides proceeds are transferred to HDL by phospholipid transfer protein (PLTP). Free cholesterol acquired by HDL is esterified by LCAT. This enzyme transfers 1 mol of fatty acid from a lecithin molecule to the hydroxyl group of unesterified cholesterol, forming cholesteryl esters. LCAT is secreted by liver. In severe hepatic parenchymal disease, levels in plasma are low and esterification of cholesterol is impeded, leading to the accumulation of free cholesterol in lipoproteins and in membranes of erythrocytes. This transforms them into the target cells classically associated with hepatic disease.

B. Metabolic Roles for HDL

HDL serve as carriers for the C apoproteins, transferring them to nascent VLDL and chylomicrons. HDL as well as LDL deliver cholesterol to the adrenal cortex and gonads in support of steroidogenesis. HDL play a major role in the centripetal transport of cholesterol. Unesterified cholesterol, exported by the ABCA-1 transporter, is acquired from the membranes of peripheral tissues by prebeta-1 HDL and is esterified by LCAT, passing through other HDL species before the cholesteryl esters are incorporated into HDL of alpha electrophoretic mobility. The cholesteryl esters are then transferred to LDL and to triglyceride-rich lipoproteins mediated by cholesteryl ester transfer protein (CETP). Remnants of chylomicrons and a significant fraction of VLDL remnants and LDL are taken up by liver, providing cholesteryl esters to hepatocytes. Cholesteryl esters are also transferred from HDL to hepatocytes by SR-BI receptors.

C. Catabolism of HDL

The pathways of catabolism of HDL are not yet known. Radiochemical studies indicate that apo A-I and apo A-II are removed from plasma synchronously and that a portion of the degradation occurs in liver and in kidney.

The Cholesterol Economy

Cholesterol is an essential constituent of the plasma membranes of cells and of myelin. It is required for adrenal and gonadal steroidogenesis and for production of bile acids by liver. Cells synthesize cholesterol, commencing with acetyl-CoA. Formation of HMG-CoA is the initial step. The first committed step, mediated by HMG-CoA reductase, is the formation of mevalonic acid, which is then metabolized via a series of isoprenoid intermediaries to squalene. The latter cyclizes to form a series of sterols leading to cholesterol. A small amount of the mevalonate is converted to the isoprenoid substances ubiquinone, dolichol, and isopentenyl pyrophosphate. This pathway also yields the isoprenoid intermediaries geranyl pyrophosphate and farnesyl pyrophosphate that are involved in prenylation of proteins. Prenylation provides an anchor so that proteins such as RAS can bind to membranes. Cholesterol synthesis is tightly regulated by cholesterol or its metabolites, which down-regulate HMG-CoA reductase. Thus, cells can produce cholesterol not provided by circulating lipoproteins. Cholesterol is required for production of cell membranes. Hepatocytes and intestinal epithelial cells use cholesterol for secretion of lipoproteins. In addition, cells constantly transfer cholesterol to circulating lipoproteins, chiefly HDL. Cholesterol is converted to bile acids in liver via a pathway initiated by cholesterol 7α-hydroxylase. Most of the bile acids are reabsorbed from the intestine, but the small amount that is lost in stool provides a means of elimination of cholesterol from the body. Activity of cholesterol 7α-hydroxylase is decreased in hypothyroidism, as are the expression of LDL receptors and hepatic lipase.

Humans do not absorb dietary cholesterol quantitatively. At usual levels of intake, about one-third of the amount ingested is absorbed. Most is transported to liver in chylomicron remnants, leading to suppression of hepatic cholesterogenesis. Individuals may differ substantially in the effect of dietary cholesterol on serum lipoproteins, reflecting differences in the efficiency of absorption.

DIFFERENTIATION OF DISORDERS OF LIPOPROTEIN METABOLISM

Laboratory Analyses of Lipids & Lipoproteins

Because chylomicrons normally may be present in plasma up to 10 hours after a meal, they contribute as much as 600 mg/dL (6.9 mmol/L) to the triglycerides measured during that period. This alimentary lipemia can be prolonged if alcohol is consumed with the meal. Thus, serum lipids and lipoproteins should be measured after a 10-hour fast. If blood glucose is not to be measured, patients may have fruit juice and black coffee with sugar (which provide no triglyceride) for breakfast.

A. Inspection

Much useful information is gained from inspection of the serum, especially before and after overnight refrigeration. Opalescence is due to light scattering by large triglyceride-rich lipoproteins. Serum begins to appear hazy when the level of triglycerides reaches 200 mg/dL (2.3 mmol/L). Chylomicrons are readily detected, because they form a white supernatant layer. Uncommon cases in which binding of immunoglobulins to lipoproteins takes place can be detected by the formation of a curd-like lipoprotein aggregate or a snowy precipitate as serum cools. If one of these disorders is suspected, blood should be kept at 37 °C during the formation of the clot and separation of the serum, because the critical temperatures for precipitation of the cryoglobulin complex may be higher than room temperature.

B. LABORATORY TECHNIQUES

Several chemical techniques provide reliable measures of cholesterol and triglycerides, an essential minimum for differentiation of disorders of lipoproteins. Unesterified and esterified cholesterol are usually measured together, so that the reported value is the total content of cholesterol in serum. A more complete characterization of lipoproteins is achieved by measurement of the cholesterol and triglyceride contents of individual lipoprotein fractions, separated by preparative ultracentrifugation, a technique usually available only in research laboratories. An efficient quantitative method employs vertical rotor ultracentrifugation, affording assessment of lipoprotein particle diameters. LDL particle size can also be assessed by electrophoresis. The content of HDL can be measured using a technique in which they are the only lipoproteins that remain in solution after treatment of the serum with heparin and manganese. Albeit rapid, the results of this technique tend to be unacceptably variable unless rigid quality control is exercised. Prognostic implications of small changes in HDL cholesterol make such controls necessary. An important determinant of the content of cholesteryl esters in HDL is the amount of triglyceride-rich lipoproteins to which the HDL are exposed in plasma. Cholesteryl esters from HDL transfer into triglyceride-rich lipoproteins, leading to an inverse logarithmic dependence of HDL cholesterol upon plasma triglycerides. HDL cholesterol cannot be interpreted without knowledge of the level of serum triglycerides. For example, a level of HDL that would normally contain 45 mg/dL (1.17 mmol/L) of cholesterol would contain 37 mg/dL (0.96 mmol/L) when the triglycerides were 200 mg/dL (2.3 mmol/L) and 30 mg/dL (0.78 mmol/L) when they reach 500 mg/dL (5.7 mmol/L).

More sophisticated tests of composition of isolated lipoprotein fractions are of use in certain instances. The most important of these is analysis of the ratio of cholesterol to triglycerides by chemical techniques and of the apolipoproteins of VLDL by isoelectric focusing. The latter reveals the absence of the normal isoforms of apo E, the underlying molecular defect in familial dysbetalipoproteinemia. In this disorder, there is an unusually high content of cholesterol in VLDL. The apo E genotype can be determined on genomic DNA. Immunoassays are available for a number of apolipoproteins of which apo B and Lp(a) are clinically useful.

Epidemiologic evidence suggests that LDL particles of smaller than normal diameter are associated with an increased risk of atherosclerosis. Small, dense LDL are a constant finding when triglyceride levels are elevated even marginally. Laboratory measurement of LDL diameters is therefore unnecessary in patients with hypertriglyceridemia.

Clinical Differentiation of Abnormal Patterns of Plasma Lipoproteins

A. PRELIMINARY SCREENING

Serum cholesterol and triglyceride levels are both continuously distributed in the population; therefore, some arbitrary levels must be established to define significant hyperlipidemia. Epidemiologic studies in Europe and the USA have shown that there is a progressive increase in risk of coronary artery disease as levels of serum cholesterol increase. Physicians should at least encourage patients at risk to eat diets low in saturated fats and cholesterol to minimize the burden of LDL in plasma.

The National Cholesterol Education Program has developed guidelines for treatment of hypercholesterolemia in adults (Table 19–2). Triglyceride levels above 150 mg/dL (1.7 mmol/L) merit investigation. One abnormality associated with increased risk of coronary artery disease that will not be detected if screening is limited to hyperlipidemia is hypoalphalipoproteinemia, or deficiency of HDL. Many affected individuals

Table 19–2. National Cholesterol Education Program: Adult Treatment Guidelines (2001).

	Desirable	Borderline to High[1]	High
Total cholesterol	< 200 (5.2)[2]	200–239 (5.2–6.2)	> 240 (6.2)
LDL cholesterol	< 130 (3.4)[3]	130–159 (3.4–4.1)	> 160 (4.1)
HDL cholesterol			
Men	> 40 (1.04)		> 60 (1.55)
Women	> 50 (1.30)		
Triglycerides	< 150 (1.7)	150–199 (1.7–2.3)	> 200 (2.3)

[1]Consider as high if coronary disease or more than two risk factors are present.
[2]mg/dL (mmol/L).
[3]Optimal level is < 100 (2.6).

have normal levels of cholesterol and triglycerides and no clinical features to alert the physician. HDL deficiency underscores the importance of controlling other risk factors and avoiding factors that reduce HDL levels, such as smoking, the use of some drugs, and obesity. Niacin can effect major increases in HDL cholesterol in many subjects.

B. IDENTIFICATION OF ABNORMAL PATTERNS

The second step in investigation of hyperlipidemia is determination of the species of lipoproteins that account for the increased content of lipids in serum. In some cases, multiple species may be involved; in others, qualitative properties of the lipoproteins are of diagnostic importance. The physician must search for underlying disorders that cause secondary hyperlipidemias of similar pattern. These may be the sole cause of the lipoprotein abnormality or may aggravate primary disorders of lipoprotein metabolism. The differentiation of specific primary disorders usually requires additional clinical and genetic information.

The following diagnostic protocol, based upon initial measurement of cholesterol, triglycerides, and HDL in serum after a 10-hour fast, supplemented by observation of serum and by additional laboratory measurements where essential, will serve as a guide in identifying abnormal lipoprotein patterns. The term "hyperlipidemia" denotes high levels of any class of lipoprotein; "hyperlipemia" denotes high levels of any of the triglyceride-rich lipoproteins.

Case 1: Serum Cholesterol Levels Increased; Triglycerides Normal

If the serum cholesterol level is modestly elevated (up to 260 mg/dL [6.72 mmol/L]), elevated levels of HDL may account for the observed increase in serum cholesterol. This is usually not associated with disease processes. The LDL cholesterol (in mg/dL) may be estimated by subtracting the HDL cholesterol and the estimated cholesterol contribution of VLDL from the total cholesterol level. The VLDL cholesterol is approximated as one-fifth of the serum triglyceride level.

$$\text{LDL cholesterol} = \text{Total cholesterol} - \left(\frac{\text{TG}}{5} + \text{HDL cholesterol} \right)$$

Calculated values of LDL cholesterol over 130 mg/dL (3.36 mmol/L) are clinically significant. If the patient has atherosclerosis or a family history of premature atherosclerosis, levels in excess of 90–100 mg/dL should be considered significant.

Very high levels of HDL measured by the precipitation technique can signal the presence of the abnormal lipoprotein of cholestasis (Lp-X). This disorder is characterized by elevated alkaline phosphatase activity. Rarely, deficiency of CETP or hepatic lipase can cause high levels of HDL.

Case 2: Predominant Increase of Triglycerides; Moderate Increase in Cholesterol May Be Present

Here it is apparent that the primary abnormality is an increase in triglyceride-rich VLDL (hyperprebeta-lipoproteinemia) or chylomicrons (chylomicronemia), or both (mixed lipemia). Because VLDL and chylomicrons contain free cholesterol in their surface monolayers and a small amount of cholesteryl ester in their cores, the total cholesterol may be increased, though to a much smaller extent than is the triglyceride level. The contribution of cholesterol in these lipoproteins to the total in serum is about 8–25% of the triglyceride content. Low levels of LDL cholesterol often seen in hypertriglyceridemia may offset the increase in cholesterol due to the triglyceride-rich lipoproteins, especially in primary chylomicronemia. Because VLDL and chylomicrons compete as substrates in a common removal pathway, chylomicrons will nearly always be present when triglyceride levels exceed 1000 mg/dL (11.5 mmol/L).

Case 3: Cholesterol & Triglyceride Levels Both Elevated

This pattern can be the result of either of two abnormal lipoprotein distributions. One is a combined increase of VLDL, which provide most of the increase in triglycerides, and LDL, which account for the bulk of the increase in cholesterol. This pattern is termed combined hyperlipidemia and is one of the three phenotypic patterns encountered in kindreds with the disorder termed familial combined hyperlipidemia. The second phenotype is an increase of remnant lipoproteins derived from VLDL and chylomicrons. These lipoprotein particles have been partially depleted of triglyceride by LPL and enriched with cholesteryl esters by the LCAT system, such that the total content of cholesterol in serum is similar to that of triglycerides. This pattern is almost always an expression of familial dysbetalipoproteinemia. Presumptive differentiation can be made with high-quality agarose gel electrophoresis. Diagnosis of this disorder is confirmed by a genotype demonstrating absence of the E-3 and E-4 alleles.

■ I. CLINICAL DESCRIPTIONS OF PRIMARY & SECONDARY DISORDERS OF LIPOPROTEIN METABOLISM

THE HYPERTRIGLYCERIDEMIAS

Atherogenicity

Epidemiologic evidence supports the atherogenicity of VLDL and their remnants. They have been demonstrated in atherosclerotic plaques from humans. Impaired capacity of the VLDL of some individuals to accept cholesteryl esters from the LCAT reaction may also contribute to atherogenesis by impeding centripetal transport of cholesterol.

Cause of Pancreatitis

Very high levels of triglycerides in plasma are associated with a risk of acute pancreatitis, probably from the local release of FFA and lysolecithin from lipoprotein substrates in the pancreatic capillary bed. When the concentrations of these lipids exceed the binding capacity of albumin, they could lyse membranes of parenchymal cells, initiating a chemical pancreatitis. Many patients with lipemia have intermittent episodes of epigastric pain during which serum amylase does not reach levels commonly considered diagnostic for pancreatitis. This is especially true in patients who have had previous attacks. The observation that these episodes frequently evolve into classic pancreatitis suggests that they represent incipient pancreatic inflammation. The progression of pancreatitis can be prevented by rapid reduction of triglycerides, usually accomplished by restriction of all dietary fat. In some cases, parenteral feeding, excluding fat emulsions, may be required for a few days. The clinical course of pancreatitis in patients with lipemia is typical of the general experience with this disease. Fatal hemorrhagic pancreatitis occurs in a few; many develop pseudocysts; and some progress to pancreatic exocrine insufficiency or compromised insulinogenic capacity.

Clinical Signs

When triglyceride levels in serum exceed 3000–4000 mg/dL (34.5–46 mmol/L), light scattering by these particles in the blood lends a whitish cast to the venous vascular bed of the retina, a sign known as **lipemia retinalis.** Markedly elevated levels of VLDL or chylomicrons may be associated with the appearance of **eruptive cutaneous xanthomas** (Figure 19–3E). These lesions, filled with foam cells, appear as yellow morbilliform eruptions 2–5 mm in diameter, often with erythematous areolae. They usually occur in clusters on extensor surfaces such as the elbows, knees, and buttocks. They are transient and disappear within a few weeks after triglyceride levels are reduced below 2000–3000 mg/dL (23–34.5 mmol/L).

Effects of Hypertriglyceridemia on Laboratory Measurements

Very high levels of triglyceride-rich lipoproteins may introduce important errors in clinical laboratory measurements. Light scattering from these large particles can cause erroneous results in most chemical determinations involving photometric measurements in spite of corrections for blank values. Amylase activity in serum may be inhibited by triglyceride-rich lipoproteins; therefore, lipemic specimens should be diluted for measurement of this enzyme. Because the lipoproteins are not permeable to ionic or polar molecules, their core regions constitute a second phase in plasma. When the volume of this phase becomes appreciable, electrolytes and other hydrophilic species will be underestimated with respect to their true concentration in plasma. A practical rule for correcting these values is as follows: For each 1000 mg/dL (11.5 mmol/L) of triglyceride in serum, the measured concentrations of all hydrophilic molecules and ions should be adjusted upward by 1%.

PRIMARY HYPERTRIGLYCERIDEMIA

1. Deficiency of Lipoprotein Lipase or Its Cofactor

Clinical Findings

A. SYMPTOMS AND SIGNS

Because the clinical expressions of these defects are identical, they will be considered together. Both are autosomal recessive traits. On a typical North American diet, lipemia is usually severe (triglyceride levels of 2000–25,000 mg/dL) (23–287.5 mmol/L). Hepatomegaly and splenomegaly are frequently present. Foam cells laden with lipid are found in liver, spleen, and bone marrow. Splenic infarct has been described and may be a source of abdominal pain. Hypersplenism with anemia, granulocytopenia, and thrombocytopenia can occur. Recurrent epigastric pain and overt pancreatitis are frequently encountered. Eruptive xanthomas may be present. These disorders may be recognized in early infancy or may go unnoticed until an attack of acute pancreatitis occurs or lipemic serum is noted on blood sampling as late as middle age. Patients with these disorders are usually not obese and have normal carbohydrate metabolism unless pancreatitis impairs in-

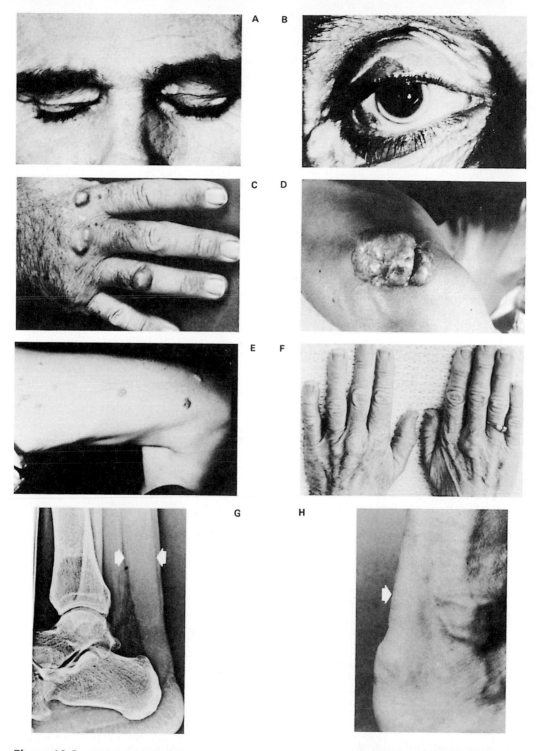

Figure 19-3. Clinical manifestations of hyperlipidemias. **A:** Xanthelasma involving medial and lateral canthi. **B:** Severe xanthelasma and arcus corneae. **C:** Tuberous xanthomas. **D:** Large tuberous xanthoma of elbow. **E:** Eruptive xanthomas, singly and in rosettes. **F:** Xanthomas of extensor tendons of the hands. **G:** Xeroradiogram of Achilles tendon xanthoma. **H:** Xanthoma of Achilles tendon. (Normal Achilles tendons do not exceed 7 mm in diameter in the region between the calcaneus and the point at which the tendon fibers begin to radiate toward their origins.)

sulinogenic capacity. Estrogens intensify the lipemia by stimulating hepatic production of VLDL. Therefore, in pregnancy and lactation or during the administration of estrogenic steroids, the risk of pancreatitis increases.

B. LABORATORY FINDINGS

There is a preponderance of chylomicrons in serum such that the infranatant layer of serum refrigerated overnight may be nearly clear. Many patients have a moderate increase in VLDL, however, and in pregnant women or those receiving estrogens, a pattern of mixed lipemia is usually present. Levels of LDL in serum are decreased, probably representing the predominant catabolism of VLDL by pathways that do not involve the production of LDL. Levels of HDL are also decreased. A presumptive diagnosis of these disorders can be made by restricting oral intake of fat to 10–15 g/d for 3–5 days. Triglycerides drop precipitously, usually reaching 200–600 mg/dL (2.3–6.9 mmol/L) within 3–4 days. Confirmation of deficiency of LPL is obtained by measurement of the lipolytic activity of plasma prepared from blood drawn 10 minutes after heparin, 0.2 mg/kg, is injected intravenously. Analysis of lipolysis is done with and without 0.5 mol/L sodium chloride, which inhibits LPL but does not suppress the activity of other plasma lipases, including hepatic lipase. Absence of the cofactor protein of LPL, apo C-II, can be demonstrated most readily by electrophoresis or isoelectric focusing of the proteins of VLDL.

Treatment

Treatment of primary chylomicronemia is entirely dietary. Intake of fat should be reduced to 10% or less of total calories. In an adult, this represents 15–30 g/d. Because the defect involves lipolysis, both saturated and unsaturated fats must be curtailed. The diet should contain at least 5 g of polyunsaturated fat as a source of essential fatty acids, and fat-soluble vitamins must be provided. Administration of 500 mg daily of marine omega-3 fatty acids is also recommended. Adherence to this diet will invariably maintain triglyceride levels below 1000 mg/dL (11.2 mmol/L) in the absence of pregnancy, lactation, or the administration of exogenous estrogens. Because this is below the level at which pancreatitis usually occurs, compliant patients are at low risk. Pregnant women with these disorders require particularly close monitoring.

2. Endogenous & Mixed Lipemias

Etiology & Pathogenesis

Endogenous lipemia (elevated VLDL) and mixed lipemia probably both result from several genetically determined disorders. Because VLDL and chylomicrons are competing substrates in the intravascular lipolytic pathway, saturating levels of VLDL will cause an impedance in the removal of chylomicrons. Therefore, as the severity of endogenous lipemia increases, a pattern of mixed lipemia may supervene. In other cases, the pattern of mixed lipemia appears to be present continuously. Though specific pathophysiologic mechanisms remain obscure, certain familial patterns are known. In all forms, factors that increase the rate of secretion of VLDL aggravate the hypertriglyceridemia—ie, obesity with insulin resistance, or the appearance of fully developed type 2 diabetes mellitus; alcohol; and exogenous estrogens. Studies of VLDL turnover indicate that either increased production or impaired removal of VLDL may be operative in different individuals. A substantial number of patients with mixed lipemia have partial defects in catabolism of triglyceride-rich lipoproteins, often due to heterozygosity for mutations in lipoprotein lipase. Some patients with mixed lipemia have decreased LPL activity in plasma. Most patients with significant endogenous or mixed lipemia have the hypertrophic form of obesity, in which there is a reduced population of insulin receptors on cell membranes associated with impaired effectiveness of insulin. Mobilization of FFA is maintained at a higher than normal rate, providing an increased flux of fatty acids to the liver, in turn increasing the secretion of triglyceride-rich VLDL.

Clinical Findings

Clinical features of these forms of hypertriglyceridemia depend upon their severity and include eruptive xanthomas, lipemia retinalis, recurrent epigastric pain, and acute pancreatitis. One constellation of clinical features that may be genetically determined is endogenous lipemia with central obesity, insulin resistance, hyperglycemia, and hyperuricemia (metabolic syndrome; syndrome X). There is also a tendency toward the development of hypertension in such patients.

Treatment

The first element of treatment is dietary. In the short term, severe restriction of total fat intake will usually result in a rapid decline of serum triglycerides to 1000–3000 mg/dL (11.2–33.6 mmol/L), averting pancreatitis. The objective of long-term dietary management is reduction to ideal body weight. Because alcohol causes significant augmentation of VLDL production, abstinence is important. If weight loss is achieved, the triglycerides almost always show a marked response, often approaching normal values. When the fall in triglyceride levels is not satisfactory, a fibrate or nicotinic acid (in the absence of insulin resistance), singly or in combination, will usually produce further reductions. When insulin resistance is present, metformin—with or without a thiazolidinedione—may be a useful adjunct. Pioglitazone appears to have more impact on lipids than other agents in this class.

3. Familial Combined Hyperlipidemia

Etiology

Epidemiologic studies of the kindreds of survivors of myocardial infarction revealed this heredofamilial disorder, which is the most common form of hyperlipidemia, occurring in 1–2% of the population. The underlying process involves overproduction of VLDL. Some affected individuals have increased levels of both VLDL and LDL (combined hyperlipidemia); some have increased levels of only VLDL or LDL. The level of apo B-100 is increased. Patterns in the serum of an individual patient may change with time. It is known that mating of an individual having any one of the three phenotypic patterns with a normal individual can result in the appearance of one of the other patterns. Affected children often have hyperlipidemia, but the disorder may not be fully expressed until adulthood.

Clinical Findings

Neither tendinous nor cutaneous xanthomas other than xanthelasma occur. This disorder appears to be inherited as a mendelian dominant trait involving alternative loci. Factors that increase the severity of hypertriglyceridemia in other disorders aggravate the lipemia in this syndrome as well.

Treatment

The risk of coronary disease is significantly increased, and patients should be treated aggressively with diet and drugs. Because LDL often increase with fibrate therapy in these patients and because resins increase triglycerides, the recommended treatment is an HMG-CoA reductase inhibitor. The addition of niacin may be required if triglycerides remain elevated or if HDL deficiency is also present.

4. Familial Dysbetalipoproteinemia (Type III Hyperlipoproteinemia)

Etiology & Pathogenesis

A permissive genetic constitution for this disease occurs commonly, but expression of hyperlipidemia apparently requires additional genetic or environmental determinants. The molecular basis is the presence of iso-forms of apo E that are poor ligands for high-affinity receptors. In its fully expressed form, the lipoprotein pattern is dominated by the accumulation of remnants of VLDL and chylomicrons. Two populations of VLDL are usually present: normal prebetalipoproteins and remnants with beta-electrophoretic mobility. Remnant particles of intermediate density are also present. Levels of LDL are decreased, reflecting interruption of the transformation of VLDL remnants to LDL. The primary defect is impaired hepatic uptake of remnants of triglyceride-rich lipoproteins. The remnant particles are enriched in cholesteryl esters such that the level of cholesterol in serum is often as high as that of triglycerides. Absence of the E-3 and E-4 genes on allele-specific screening of genomic DNA—or of the corresponding proteins on isoelectric focusing of VLDL proteins—confirms the diagnosis. Whereas homozygosity for apo E-2 is present in about 1% of the population, the incidence of clinical hyperlipidemia among these patients is much smaller. Additional mutations of apo E that cannot be distinguished from E-3 by isoelectric focusing are now known to result in dysbetalipoproteinemia. Some of these cause hyperlipidemia in the heterozygous state, a disorder termed dominant dysbetalipoproteinemia.

Clinical Findings

Hyperlipidemia and clinical signs are not usually evident before age 20. In younger patients with hyperlipidemia, hypothyroidism or obesity is likely to be present. Adults frequently have tuberous or tuberoeruptive xanthomas (Figure 19–3C). Both tend to occur on extensor surfaces, especially elbows and knees. Tuberoeruptive xanthomas are pink or yellowish skin nodules 3–8 mm in diameter that often become confluent. Tuberous xanthomas—shiny reddish or orange nodules up to 3 cm or more in diameter—are usually moveable and nontender. Another type, planar xanthomas of the palmar creases, strongly suggests dysbetalipoproteinemia. The skin creases assume an orange color from deposition of carotenoids and other lipids. They occasionally are raised above the level of adjacent skin and are not tender. (Planar xanthomas are also seen in cholestatic disease.)

Some patients have impaired glucose tolerance, which is usually associated with higher levels of blood lipids. Obesity is commonly present and tends to aggravate the lipemia. Patients with the genetic constitution for dysbetalipoproteinemia often develop severe hyperlipidemia if they are hypothyroid.

Atherosclerosis of the coronary and peripheral vessels occurs with increased frequency, and the prevalence of disease of the iliac and femoral vessels is especially high.

Treatment

Management includes a weight reduction diet providing a reduced intake of cholesterol, fat, and alcohol. When the hyperlipidemia does not respond satisfactorily to diet, a fibrate or niacin in low doses (if the patient does not have type 2 diabetes or insulin resistance) is usually effective. These agents can be used together in resistant cases. Some patients respond to the more potent reductase inhibitors alone, and the addition of niacin normalizes the lipid levels in most.

SECONDARY HYPERTRIGLYCERIDEMIA

Diabetes Mellitus

In patients with diabetes, levels of VLDL in plasma are frequently elevated. The severe lipemia associated with absence or marked insufficiency of insulin is attributable to deficiency of LPL activity, because this enzyme is induced by insulin. The administration of insulin usually restores triglyceride levels to normal within a few days. However, if massive fatty liver is present, weeks may be required for the VLDL to return to normal while the liver secretes its triglyceride into plasma. Conversion of massive amounts of VLDL to LDL as the impedance of VLDL catabolism is relieved leads to marked accumulation of LDL that may persist for weeks, leading to a spurious diagnosis of primary hypercholesterolemia.

The moderately elevated VLDL seen in diabetes under average control probably reflects chiefly an increased flux of FFA to liver that stimulates production of triglycerides and their secretion in VLDL. In addition to VLDL, LDL levels are also somewhat increased in diabetics under poor control, probably accounting in part for their increased risk of coronary heart disease. Mild increases in VLDL and in FFA occur in many patients with type 2 diabetes. Some have much higher levels of VLDL, suggesting that an additional genetic factor predisposing to lipemia is present. Still another cause of lipemic diabetes is the compromised insulinogenic capacity that can result from acute pancreatitis in individuals with severe primary lipemias. The deficiency may be severe enough to require exogenous insulin, often only in small doses. In diabetics who develop nephrosis, the secondary lipemia of nephrosis compounds their hypertriglyceridemia. In hyperglycemia, lipoproteins become glycosylated, leading to their uptake by macrophages.

Lipemia may be very severe, with elevated levels of both VLDL and chylomicrons when control is poor. Lipemic patients usually have ketoacidosis when they are insulin-deficient, but lipemia can occur in its absence. Patients with type 1 diabetes who have been chronically undertreated with insulin may have mobilized most of the triglyceride from peripheral adipose tissue, so that they no longer have sufficient substrate for significant ketogenesis. These emaciated individuals may have severe lipemia and striking hepatomegaly.

In type 1 diabetes, the rigid control of blood glucose levels, which can be attained with continuous subcutaneous insulin infusion, is associated with sustained normalization of levels of both LDL and VLDL. The lipemia of type 2 diabetes usually responds well to control of the underlying disorder. In obese insulin-resistant individuals, weight loss is an essential feature of management. Diets containing slowly absorbed carbohydrates are well tolerated, allowing a decrease in the burden of chylomicron triglycerides in plasma (see Chapter 17).

2. Uremia

Uremia is associated with modest isolated increases in VLDL. The most important underlying mechanisms are probably insulin resistance and impairment of catabolism of VLDL. Many uremic patients are also nephrotic. The additional effects of nephrosis upon lipoprotein metabolism may produce a combined hyperlipidemia. Patients who have had renal transplants may be receiving glucocorticoids, which induce elevation of LDL.

3. Human Immunodeficiency Virus Infection

HIV infection per se is associated with hypertriglyceridemia. A syndrome of partial lipodystrophy and insulin resistance, often with marked lipemia, occurs with multidrug treatment that includes inhibitors of viral protease. Acute pancreatitis can ensue. Limited clinical experience suggests that fibric acid derivatives are of some value. Alcohol must be avoided.

4. Corticosteroid Excess

In endogenous Cushing's syndrome, insulin resistance is present and levels of LDL are increased. It appears that the combined hyperlipidemia is primarily due to increased secretion of VLDL, which is then catabolized to LDL. More severe lipemia ensues when steroidogenic diabetes appears, reducing catabolism of triglyceride-rich lipoproteins via the LPL pathway.

5. Exogenous Estrogens

When estrogens are administered to normal women, triglyceride levels may increase by as much as 15%, reflecting increased production of VLDL. Paradoxically, estrogens increase the efficiency of catabolism of triglyceride-rich lipoproteins. Whereas estrogens tend to induce insulin resistance, it is not clear that this is an important mechanism, because certain nortestosterone derivatives decrease plasma triglycerides despite the induction of appreciable insulin resistance.

Certain individuals, usually those with preexisting mild lipemia, develop marked hypertriglyceridemia when receiving estrogens even in relatively small doses. Thus, triglycerides should be monitored in these women. Contraceptive combinations with predominantly progestational effects produce less hypertriglyceridemia than purely estrogenic compounds. Transdermal delivery of estrogen probably results in lesser increases in VLDL secretion because it avoids the hepatic first-pass effect.

6. Alcohol Ingestion

Ingestion of appreciable amounts of alcohol does not necessarily result in significantly elevated levels of triglycerides, but many alcoholics are lipemic. Alcohol profoundly increases triglycerides in patients with primary or secondary hyperlipemias. In **Zieve's syndrome,** the alcohol-induced lipemia is associated with hemolytic anemia and hyperbilirubinemia. Because LCAT originates in liver, severe hepatic parenchymal dysfunction may lead to deficiency in the activity of this enzyme. A resultant accumulation of unesterified cholesterol in erythrocyte membranes may account for the hemolysis seen in Zieve's syndrome.

Alcohol is converted to acetate, exerting a sparing effect on the oxidation of fatty acids. The fatty acids are incorporated into triglyceride in liver, resulting in hepatomegaly due to fatty infiltration and in marked enhancement of secretion of VLDL. In many individuals, there is sufficient adaptive increase in the removal capacity for triglycerides from plasma that levels are normal. In individuals in whom the adaptive response is impaired, marked lipemia may ensue.

7. Nonalcoholic Steatohepatitis (NASH)

This syndrome is characterized by hepatic steatosis and abnormalities of liver enzymes, leading in many cases to cirrhosis in the absence of alcohol ingestion. Many patients have hypertriglyceridemia. The cause is not yet understood, but it is likely that NASH involves misdirection of fatty acids from oxidative pathways to hepatic triglyceride synthesis. Weight reduction in obese patients and treatment of insulin resistance, if present, can mitigate the steatosis and reduce levels of triglycerides.

8. Nephrosis

The hyperlipidemia of nephrosis is biphasic. Before serum albumin levels fall below 2 g/dL, LDL increases selectively. The synthesis and secretion of VLDL appear to be coupled to that of albumin. The increased flux of VLDL from liver increases production of LDL. As albumin levels fall below 1–2 g/dL, lipemia ensues. Impaired hydrolysis of triglycerides by LPL is due to lack of albumin as an FFA receptor. Free fatty acids, which normally circulate complexed to albumin, bind to lipoproteins when albumin levels are low. The ability of these altered lipoproteins to undergo hydrolysis is thus impaired.

Because coronary disease is prevalent in patients with long-standing nephrotic syndrome, treatment of the hyperlipidemia is indicated, though few studies of the effect of treatment have been reported. The hyperlipidemia is resistant to diet. Fibrates may precipitate myopathy even in small doses. Bile acid-binding resins, niacin, and reductase inhibitors are useful.

9. Glycogen Storage Disease

In type I glycogenosis, insulin secretion is decreased. This leads to an increased flux of FFA to the liver, where a substantial fraction is converted to triglycerides, increasing secretion of VLDL. The low levels of insulin in plasma are the probable cause of reduced activity of LPL, which may impair removal of triglycerides. The fatty liver in these patients tends to progress to cirrhosis.

Frequent small feedings help to maintain blood glucose levels and ameliorate the lipemia. Nocturnal nasogastric drip feeding is of considerable benefit. Other forms of hepatic glycogen storage disease may be associated with elevated levels of VLDL and LDL in serum.

10. Hypopituitarism & Acromegaly

Part of the hyperlipidemia of hypopituitarism is attributable to secondary hypothyroidism, but hypertriglyceridemia persists after thyroxine replacement. Deficiency of growth hormone is associated with higher than normal levels of both LDL and VLDL. Decreased insulin levels may be the major underlying defect; however, deficiency of growth hormone may impair the disposal of FFA by oxidation and ketogenesis in the liver, favoring synthesis of triglycerides. Mild hypertriglyceridemia is often associated with acromegaly, probably resulting from insulin resistance. Though growth hormone acutely stimulates lipolysis in adipose tissue, FFA levels are normal in acromegaly.

11. Hypothyroidism

Whereas significant hypothyroidism produces elevated levels of LDL in nearly all individuals, only a few develop hypertriglyceridemia. The increase in LDL results at least in part from decreased conversion of cholesterol to bile acids and down-regulation of LDL receptors. Lipemia, when present, is usually mild, though serum triglycerides in excess of 3000 mg/dL (34.5 mmol/L) can occur in patients with myxedema. It is probable that impaired removal of triglycerides is involved, reflecting decreased activity of hepatic lipase. Increased content of cholesteryl esters and apo E in the triglyceride-rich lipoproteins suggests that accumulation of remnant particles occurs. Hypothyroidism, even of very mild degree, often causes expression of hyperlipidemia in individuals with dysbetalipoproteinemia.

12. Immunoglobulin-Lipoprotein Complex Disorders

Both polyclonal and monoclonal hypergammaglobulinemias may cause hypertriglyceridemia. IgG, IgM, and IgA have each been involved. Of the underlying monoclonal disorders, myeloma and macroglobulinemia are the most important, but lymphomas and lymphocytic leukemias have also been implicated. Lupus erythematosus and other autoimmune disorders have been associated with the polyclonal type. Binding of heparin by immunoglobulin, with resulting inhibition of LPL, can cause severe mixed lipemia. More commonly, the triglyceride-rich lipoproteins have an abnormally high density, probably as a result of bound immunoglobulin, though some may be remnant-like particles. These complexes, which bind lipophilic stains, usually have gamma mobility on electrophoresis.

Xanthomatosis associated with immunoglobulin complex disease includes tuberous and eruptive xanthomas, xanthelasma, and planar xanthomas of large areas of skin. The latter are otherwise seen only in patients with cholestasis. Deposits of lipid-rich hyaline material can occur in the lamina propria of the intestine, causing malabsorption and protein-losing enteropathy. Circulating immunoglobulin-lipoprotein complexes can fix complement, leading to hypocomplementemia. In such patients, administration of whole blood or plasma can cause anaphylaxis. Hence, washed red cells or albumin are recommended when blood volume replacement is required.

Treatment is directed at the underlying disorder. Because the critical temperature of cryoprecipitation of some of these complexes is close to body temperature, plasmapheresis should be done at a temperature above the critical temperature measured in serum.

THE PRIMARY HYPERCHOLESTEROLEMIAS
FAMILIAL HYPERCHOLESTEROLEMIA
Etiology & Pathogenesis

This disorder, which in its heterozygous form occurs in approximately one in 500 individuals, is a codominant trait with high penetrance. Because half of first-degree relatives are affected, all members of a family should be screened. A selective increase in LDL exists from birth. Levels of LDL tend to increase during childhood and adolescence such that serum cholesterol in adult heterozygotes usually varies from about 260 mg/dL to 400 mg/dL (6.7–10.4 mmol/L). Aside from an increase in content of cholesteryl esters, the LDL are normal in structure. Some individuals—especially those in kindreds in which hypertriglyceridemia is present—may have higher than normal levels of VLDL and IDL. In a few patients with familial hypercholesterolemia mutations, the expression is blunted by independent genetic determinants.

The underlying defect is a deficiency of normal LDL receptors on cell membranes. A number of genetic defects affecting the structure, translation, modification, or transport of the receptor protein have been identified.

Some individuals have combined heterozygosity. In cases in which a kinetic mutant is combined with an ablative mutant, the hypercholesterolemia is greater than that seen in simple heterozygosity, usually in the range of 500–800 mg/dL (13–20.8 mmol/L). Those patients who are homozygous for null alleles have extremely severe hypercholesterolemia (approaching 1000 mg/dL [26 mmol/L] or greater) and fulminant arteriosclerosis.

Production rates for LDL are moderately increased in heterozygotes and are higher in homozygotes because of increased conversion of VLDL to LDL. In the heterozygote, a greater fraction of LDL is removed by non-receptor-dependent mechanisms than in normal subjects. In homozygotes, all removal of LDL proceeds through such pathways.

Clinical Findings

A frequent clinical feature is tendinous xanthomatosis. These become more apparent in early adulthood, causing a broadening or fusiform mass in the tendon. They can occur in almost any tendon but are most readily detected in the Achilles and patellar tendons and in the extensor tendons of the hands (Figure 19–3F, G, H). Patients who are physically active may complain of achillodynia. Arcus corneae (Figure 19–3B) may occur as early as the third decade. Xanthelasma (Figure 19–3A) may also be present. Both arcus and xanthelasma are seen in some individuals who do not have hyperlipidemia, however. Coronary atherosclerosis tends to occur prematurely in heterozygotes. It is particularly prominent in individuals who are relatively deficient in HDL. It is probable that this represents a coincident inheritance of both traits. Homozygous familial hypercholesterolemia is catastrophic. Xanthomatosis progresses rapidly. Patients may have tuberous xanthomas (Figure 19–3C and D) and elevated plaque-like xanthomas of the extremities, buttocks, interdigital webs, and aortic valves. Coronary disease may be evident in the first decade of life.

A serum cholesterol in excess of 300 mg/dL (7.8 mmol/L) in the absence of significant hypertriglyceridemia makes the diagnosis of heterozygous familial hypercholesterolemia likely. The presence of affected first-degree relatives is supportive of this diagnosis, especially if no other phenotypes of hyperlipidemia are present in the family that would suggest familial combined hyperlipidemia. The finding of tendon xanthomas is nearly pathognomonic—betasitosterolemia, cerebrotendinous xanthomatosis (cholestanolosis), and ligand-defective apo B excepted. Although the cholesterol content of umbilical cord blood is usually elevated, the diagnosis is most easily established by measuring serum cholesterol after the first year of life.

Treatment

Treatment with HMG-CoA reductase inhibitors may normalize LDL levels. However, achieving optimal levels may require one of the binary combinations involving reductase inhibitors, niacin, bile acid sequestrants, or ezetimibe. Levels of LDL cholesterol less than 100 mg/dL (2.6 mmol/L) can be obtained with combinations of these drugs in most patients. Treatment of homozygotes is extremely difficult. Partial control may be achieved with LDL apheresis in conjunction with niacin and atorvastatin. Striking reduction of LDL levels is observed after liver transplantation, illustrating the important role of hepatic receptors in LDL clearance.

FAMILIAL COMBINED HYPERLIPIDEMIA

In some individuals in kindreds with this disorder (see Primary Hypertriglyceridemia, above), LDL and IDL are the only lipoproteins that are elevated. This pattern may vary in an individual over time, and elevated VLDL alone or combined elevations of LDL and VLDL may be observed in the patient or the patient's relatives. Some affected children express hyperlipi-

demia. In contrast to most cases of familial hypercholesterolemia, the cholesterol level may be as low as 250 mg/dL (6.5 mmol/L) and xanthomas are absent. Studies of kindreds suggest codominant transmission. Coronary atherosclerosis is accelerated, accounting for about 15% of coronary events. The underlying mechanism involves increased secretion of VLDL.

Treatment of the hypercholesterolemia should begin with diet and either niacin or a reductase inhibitor. It may be necessary to use a combination of these agents to normalize levels of LDL and triglycerides.

LP(A) HYPERLIPOPROTEINEMIA

Lp(a) normally comprises a very minor fraction of circulating lipoproteins, but it may be present in high concentrations in some individuals. It contains apo B-100 and the Lp(a) protein, a homolog of plasminogen that can inhibit fibrinolysis. It has been demonstrated in atherosclerotic plaques, and many but not all studies implicate it as an independent risk factor for coronary disease. Plasma levels of Lp(a) can be measured by immunoassay. Whereas most individuals have levels below 10 mg/dL, some may have as much as 200 mg/dL. Levels above 30–50 mg/dL present additional risk of coronary disease. Levels of Lp(a) primarily reflect genetic determinants. Niacin is essentially the only effective treatment, though not all patients respond.

FAMILIAL LIGAND-DEFECTIVE APO B

Mutations involving the ligand domain in apo B-100 impair the ability of LDL to bind to its receptor. Two prevalent mutations at codon 3500 or 3531 occur in about one in 500 individuals and may be found in compound states with familial hypercholesterolemia. The hypercholesterolemia with ligand defects alone is generally less severe than in familial hypercholesterolemia because the removal of VLDL remnants is normal, resulting in a lower production of LDL. Patients may have tendon xanthomas and are at increased risk for coronary disease. Response to reductase inhibitors varies, but many show some resistance because up-regulation of receptors cannot correct the defect completely (though it can decrease LDL production because IDL are endocytosed by liver via interaction of the LDL receptor with apo E).

CHOLESTEROL 7-α-HYDROXYLASE DEFICIENCY

Loss of function mutations in cholesterol 7α-hydroxylase result in diminished catabolism of cholesterol to bile acids and accumulation of cholesterol in hepatocytes. Down-regulation of LDL receptors causes elevated LDL in plasma. VLDL may also be increased. Homozygous patients have marked resistance to reductase inhibitors and may have premature cholesterol gallstone disease. Heterozygous patients have moderately elevated LDL. The hyperlipidemia responds well to niacin.

SECONDARY HYPERCHOLESTEROLEMIA

HYPOTHYROIDISM

In hypothyroidism, LDL and IDL are elevated. Some patients may have lipemia, as described in the section on secondary hyperlipemia. Hyperlipidemia may occur with no overt signs or symptoms of decreased thyroid function. Biliary excretion of cholesterol and bile acids is depressed. Cholesterol stores in tissues appear to be increased, though the number of LDL receptors on cells is decreased. Activity of hepatic lipase is markedly decreased, and atherogenesis is accelerated by myxedema. The hyperlipidemia responds dramatically to treatment with thyroxine.

NEPHROSIS

As described in the section on secondary hypertriglyceridemias, nephrosis produces a biphasic hyperlipoproteinemia. The earliest alteration of lipoproteins in nephrosis is elevation of LDL. Increased secretion of VLDL by liver is probably involved. Because the lipids of the lipoprotein surfaces are altered by enrichment with sphingomyelin, lysolecithin, and FFA, the catabolism of LDL could be impaired. Perhaps the low metabolic rate in affected patients introduces metabolic changes similar to those associated with hypothyroidism. The hyperlipidemia may be an important element in the markedly increased risk of atherosclerosis in these patients. The treatment of choice is a reductase inhibitor or bile acid-binding resin with niacin.

IMMUNOGLOBULIN DISORDERS

One of the lipoprotein abnormalities that can be associated with monoclonal gammopathy is elevation of LDL. A "gamma lipoprotein" that is a stable complex of immunoglobulin and lipoprotein may be observed on electrophoresis. Cryoprecipitation, often in the temperature range encountered in peripheral tissues when the environmental temperature is low, may occur. Patients may have symptoms from the vascular effect of complement fixation resulting from complex formation and may have hyperviscosity syndrome from the elevated immunoglobulins per se. Planar xanthomas may be present.

Treatment is directed at the underlying process. Plasmapheresis is often effective. If cryoprecipitation occurs at critical temperatures near or above room temperature, the procedure must be carried out in a special warm environment. Transfusion of whole blood or serum may be dangerous in these patients because of rapid production of anaphylatoxins from fresh complement in the serum, resulting from interaction with circulating antibody-antigen complexes. This risk can be minimized by the use of packed red blood cells and albumin in place of whole blood.

ANOREXIA NERVOSA

About 40% of patients with anorexia nervosa have elevated LDL, and levels of cholesterol may reach 400–600 mg/dL (10.4–15.6 mmol/L). The hyperlipidemia, which persists despite correction of hypothyroidism, is probably a result of decreased fecal excretion of bile acids and cholesterol. Serum lipoproteins return to normal when proper nutrition is restored.

CHOLESTASIS

The hyperlipidemia associated with obstruction of biliary flow is complex. Levels of cholesterol exceeding 400 mg/dL (10.4 mmol/L) usually are associated with extrahepatic obstruction or with intrahepatic tumor. Several types of abnormal lipoproteins are present. The most abundant, termed Lp-X, is a bilayer vesicle composed of unesterified cholesterol and lecithin, with associated apolipoproteins but no apo B. Lp-X is apparent on electrophoresis as a band of zero to gamma mobility which shows metachromatic staining with Sudan black. It is these vesicular particles that cause the serum phospholipid and unesterified cholesterol content to be extremely high. Another abnormal species, called Lp-Y, contains appreciable amounts of triglycerides and apo B. The LDL in cholestasis also contain an unusually large amount of triglycerides.

Patients may have planar xanthomas, especially at sites of minor trauma, and xanthomas of the palmar creases. Occasionally, eruptive xanthomas are present. Xanthomatous involvement of nerves may lead to symptoms of peripheral neuropathy, and the abnormal lipoproteins may be atherogenic. Whereas bilirubin levels are nearly normal in some patients with chronic cholestasis, all have elevated serum alkaline phosphatase activity.

Neuropathy is the chief indication for treatment of the hyperlipidemia. Bile acid-binding resins are of some value, whereas fibric acid derivatives may cause an increase in cholesterol. Plasmapheresis is the most effective treatment. Large doses of vitamin E are indicated to overcome severe impairment of absorption. Deficiency of other fat-soluble vitamins also occurs.

THE PRIMARY HYPOLIPIDEMIAS

Although the clinician is confronted less frequently by the problem of a striking deficiency in plasma lipids, it is important to recognize the primary and secondary hypolipidemias. A serum cholesterol less than 110 mg/dL (2.9 mmol/L) is noteworthy. Since levels of triglycerides in normal fasting serum may be as low as 25 mg/dL (0.29 mmol/L), significance is limited to cases in which they are virtually absent.

PRIMARY HYPOLIPIDEMIA DUE TO DEFICIENCY OF HIGH-DENSITY LIPOPROTEINS

1. Tangier Disease

Etiology & Pathogenesis

Severe deficiency of HDL occurs in Tangier disease. Heterozygotes lack clinical signs but have about one-half or less of the normal complement of HDL and apo A-I in plasma. Homozygotes lack normal HDL, and apo A-I and apo A-II are present at extremely low levels. Serum cholesterol is usually below 120 mg/dL (3.12 mmol/L) and may be half that value. Mild hypertriglyceridemia is usually present, and LDL are greatly enriched in triglycerides. Mutations in the ATP-dependent transporter ABCA1 underlie this disorder, causing defective efflux of cholesterol from peripheral cells.

Clinical Findings

The clinical features of this rare autosomal-recessive disease include large, orange-colored, lipid-filled tonsils, accumulation of cholesteryl esters in the reticuloendothelial system, and an episodic and recurrent peripheral neuropathy with predominant motor weakness in the later stages. The course of the disease is benign in early childhood, but the neuropathy may appear as early as age 8. Cholesteryl ester accumulates most prominently in peripheral nerve sheaths. Carotenoid pigment may be apparent in pharyngeal and rectal mucous membranes. Splenomegaly and corneal infiltration may also be present. There is some increase in risk of coronary atherosclerosis.

Treatment

Because some of the lamellar lipoprotein material in plasma is believed to originate in chylomicrons, restriction of dietary fats and cholesterol is suggested.

2. Familial Hypoalphalipoproteinemia

Etiology & Pathogenesis

This phenotypic pattern is a partial deficiency of HDL that may involve heterogeneous mechanisms. These presumed constitutional disorders must be differentiated from the condition in which moderately low levels of HDL are seen in individuals consuming a diet very low in fat. White and Asian men on such diets usually have HDL cholesterol levels of 38–42 mg/dL (1–1.1 mmol/L) by ultracentrifugal analysis, in contrast to a median value of 49 mg/dL (1.3 mmol/L) when consuming a typical North American diet. Such levels are common in Asiatic populations and among vegetarians, where the risk of coronary disease is small. HDL cholesterol must also be interpreted in the light of the amount of triglyceride-rich lipoproteins in plasma. Because cholesteryl esters are progressively transferred to the cores of triglyceride-rich lipoproteins as triglyceride levels rise, HDL cholesterol will decrease as an inverse logarithmic function of the triglyceride level.

Etiologic Factor in Coronary Disease

Familial hypoalphalipoproteinemia is fairly common and is an important risk factor in atherosclerosis. This abnormality may be the only apparent risk factor in many cases of premature coronary or peripheral vascular disease and accelerates the appearance of coronary disease in patients with familial hypercholesterolemia or other hyperlipidemias. Hypoalphalipoproteinemia shows a strong familial incidence. Although several mechanisms and modes of transmission may be involved, many kindreds show distributions consistent with autosomal dominance. HDL cholesterol levels are usually below 35 mg/dL (0.9 mmol/L).

Treatment

Increases in HDL cholesterol in several coronary intervention trials have been independently associated with plaque regression. Only limited means of raising HDL levels are at hand. Findings that HDL are composed of ten or more discrete species further complicate this problem. It is not yet known which of these species may be involved in protecting against atherosclerosis or whether their levels can be increased. Though alcohol ingestion can increase total HDL in some individuals, it appears that the effect is primarily on the HDL_3 ultracentrifugal fraction, which correlates poorly with decreased risk. No recommendation for increased alcohol consumption should be made.

Heavy exercise is associated with increases in HDL in some individuals but must be approached with caution in patients who may have coronary disease. Niacin increases total HDL in many subjects, chiefly the HDL_2 ultracentrifugal fraction. Smaller increments in HDL occur with reductase inhibitors and fibric acid derivatives.

The most important reason for measuring HDL cholesterol levels is to identify patients who are at increased risk. Thus, just as with patients who have premature vascular disease or a family history of early arteriosclerosis, patients with low HDL should be treated more aggressively for elevated levels of the atherogenic lipoproteins. Furthermore, vigorous efforts should be directed at the control of other risk factors such as hypertension. Smoking and obesity are known to decrease HDL significantly.

3. Deficiency of LCAT

Another disorder associated with low serum levels of HDL is lecithin-cholesterol acyltransferase deficiency. This rare autosomal recessive disorder is not expressed in clinical or biochemical form in the heterozygote. In the homozygote, clinical characteristics are variable. The diagnosis is usually made in adults, though corneal opacities may begin in childhood. Proteinuria may be an early sign. Deposits of unesterified cholesterol and phospholipid in the renal microvasculature lead to progressive loss of nephrons and ultimate renal failure. Many patients have mild to moderate normochromic anemia with target cells. Hyperbilirubinemia or peripheral neuropathy may be present. Red blood cell lipid composition is abnormal, with increased content of unesterified cholesterol and lecithin. Most have elevated plasma triglycerides (200–1000 mg/dL [2.3–11.2 mmol/L]), and levels of serum cholesterol vary from low normal to 500 mg/dL (13 mmol/L), only a small fraction of which is esterified. The large triglyceride-containing lipoproteins are unusually rich in unesterified cholesterol and appear to have abnormal surface monolayers. LDL are rich in triglycerides, and abnormal vesicular lipoproteins are present in the LDL density interval. Two abnormal HDL species are present:

bilayer disks and small spherical particles. Marked restriction of dietary fat and cholesterol delays the onset of renal disease.

PRIMARY HYPOLIPIDEMIA DUE TO DEFICIENCY OF APO B-CONTAINING LIPOPROTEINS

1. Recessive Abetalipoproteinemia

Etiology & Pathogenesis

This disorder could represent a number of mutations involving the processing of apo B or the secretion of apo B-containing lipoproteins. The predominant cause is mutations involving the microsomal triglyceride transfer protein (MTTP). Heterozygous patients have no abnormalities of lipoproteins or clinical signs. In homozygotes, all forms of apo B are essentially absent. No chylomicrons, VLDL, or LDL are found in plasma, leaving only HDL. Plasma triglycerides are usually less than 10 mg/dL (0.12 mmol/L) and fail to rise after a fat load. Total cholesterol is usually less than 90 mg/dL (2.3 mmol/L). There is a defect in the incorporation of newly synthesized triglycerides into chylomicrons. However, at low levels of fat intake, about 80% of the ingested triglycerides are absorbed, probably by direct absorption of fatty acids via the portal vein.

Clinical Findings

Clinical features include a paucity of adipose tissue associated with malabsorption of long-chain fatty acids due to failure of the intestine to secrete chylomicrons. Red blood cells may be acanthocytic, with a high cholesterol:phospholipid ratio. There may be progressive degeneration of the central nervous system, including cerebellar degeneration and posterior and lateral spinal tract disease. Retinal degeneration may be severe. Levels of fat-soluble vitamins in plasma may be very low. The neurologic defects are due to deficiency of vitamin E (normally transported largely in LDL). Patients are apparently normal at birth and develop steatorrhea with impaired growth in infancy. The neuromuscular disorder often appears in late childhood with ataxia, night blindness, decreased visual acuity, and nystagmus. Cardiomyopathy with arrhythmias has been reported and may be a cause of death.

Treatment

Treatment includes administration of fat-soluble vitamins and essential fatty acids. Very large doses of tocopherol (vitamin E) (1000–10,000 IU/d) limit the progressive central nervous system degeneration. Although vitamin A seems to correct the night blindness, it does not alter the course of retinitis pigmentosa. Vitamins D and K may also be indicated. Restriction of dietary fat minimizes steatorrhea.

2. Familial Hypobetalipoproteinemia

This disorder is usually attributable to defects at the apo B locus, resulting in decreased production of the protein or in the production of truncated gene products. LDL and apo B in heterozygotes are often present at about half of normal levels. If a mutant allele resulting in the complete interdiction of apo B synthesis is present in the homozygous state, the clinical and biochemical features may be indistinguishable from those of recessive abetalipoproteinemia, and treatment is the same as for that disorder. Very short truncations of apo B-100 only allow the formation of abnormally dense, small LDL. Longer truncations permit the formation of larger lipoproteins, even including VLDL-like particles. The latter may be present in the virtual absence of LDL.

Clinical features may be absent in patients who produce at least low levels of LDL-like particles. However, signs and symptoms of tocopherol deficiency may be present. Treatment with tocopherols (800 IU/d) is recommended for all patients.

3. Chylomicron Retention Disease

This disorder presents in the neonate and appears to be based upon the selective inability of intestinal epithelial cells to secrete chylomicrons. Affected individuals have severe malabsorption of triglycerides with steatorrhea. Levels of LDL and VLDL are about half of normal, presumably secondary to malnutrition. Tocopherol levels may be very low and may be associated with neurologic abnormalities. Clinical symptoms diminish somewhat with time if the patient is managed with a low-fat diet and tocopherol supplementation.

SECONDARY HYPOLIPIDEMIA

Hypolipidemia may be secondary to a number of diseases characterized by chronic cachexia, eg, advanced cancer. Myeloproliferative disorders can lead to extremely low levels of LDL, probably owing to increased uptake related to rapid proliferation and membrane synthesis. A wide variety of conditions leading to intestinal malabsorption produce hypolipidemia. In these situations, levels of chylomicrons, VLDL, and LDL in serum are low but never absent. Because most of the lipoprotein mass of fasting serum is of hepatic origin,

massive parenchymal liver failure—eg, in Reye's syndrome—can cause severe hypolipidemia. A precipitous fall in lipoprotein levels during drug treatment of hyperlipidemia can signal hepatic toxicity. Secondary hypobetalipoproteinemia occurs in oroticaciduria.

The hypolipidemias associated with immunoglobulin disorders result from diverse mechanisms. Affected patients usually have myeloma or macroglobulinemia but may have lymphomas or lymphocytic leukemia. Any of the major classes of immunoglobulins may be involved. In many cases, the immunoglobulins are cryoprecipitins; thus, the diagnosis may be missed if blood is not drawn and serum prepared at 37 °C and observed for cryoprecipitation. Immunoglobulin-lipoprotein complexes may precipitate in various tissues. When this occurs in the lamina propria of the intestine, a syndrome of malabsorption and protein-losing enteropathy may result. Monoclonal IgA in myeloma may precipitate with lipoproteins, causing xanthomas of the gingiva and cervix. Lesions in the skin are usually planar and xanthomatous and may involve intracutaneous hemorrhage, producing a classic purple xanthoma. Planar xanthomas occurring in cholestasis may be confused with this condition because the abnormal lipoprotein of cholestasis (Lp-X), like the circulating lipoprotein complex of immunoglobulin and lipoprotein, has gamma mobility on electrophoresis.

OTHER DISORDERS OF LIPOPROTEIN METABOLISM

THE LIPODYSTROPHIES

Classification

Classification of the lipodystrophies is based on their familial or acquired origin and the regional or generalized nature of the fat loss. Insulin resistance is a common feature. Two of these disorders are known to be inherited.

Familial generalized lipodystrophy (Seip-Berardinelli syndrome) is a rare recessive trait associated with mutations in the gene for seipin. It may be diagnosed at birth and is associated with macrosomia. Genital hypertrophy, hypertrichosis, acanthosis nigricans, hepatomegaly, insulin resistance, hypertriglyceridemia, and glucose intolerance are regularly observed.

Familial lipodystrophy of limbs and trunk (Köberling-Dunningan syndrome) appears to be transmitted as a dominant trait associated with mutations in the lamin A gene. Because sequence anomalies in other regions of the gene are associated with muscular dystrophy, cardiac conduction defects, cardiomyopathy, or axonal neuropathies, overlapping phenotypes may occur. It affects women predominantly and is not evident until puberty. The face, neck, and upper trunk are usually spared. Growth is normal, but otherwise this syndrome shares features of the generalized form noted above. It is frequently associated with Stein-Leventhal syndrome and often progresses to fatal cirrhosis.

Acquired forms of lipodystrophy, generalized (Lawrence syndrome) and partial (Barraquer-Simmons syndrome), usually begin in childhood, affect females predominantly, and often follow an acute febrile illness. The generalized type commonly shares the features described above, invariably involving the trunk and extremities but sometimes sparing the face. A sclerosing panniculitis, as seen in Weber-Christian syndrome, may appear at the outset. The partial type usually begins in the face and then involves the neck, upper limbs, and trunk. In this disorder, reduced levels of C3 complement are frequently encountered. Most patients have proteinuria, and some develop overt vascular nephritis.

Associated Disorders

Because a number of patients with disorders resembling both familial and acquired types of lipodystrophy have tumors or other lesions of the hypothalamus, appropriate neurologic evaluation should be obtained. Similarly, the physician should be alert to the association of collagen-vascular disorders, including scleroderma and dermatomyositis, with some cases of acquired lipodystrophy.

RARE DISORDERS

Autosomal Recessive Hypercholesterolemia

In this disorder, LDL are markedly elevated, resulting in total cholesterol levels between 400 and 700 mg/dL (10.4 and 18.1 mmol/L). It is attributed to mutations in the gene for a protein that appears to act as an adaptor with the LDL receptor in liver.

Werner's Syndrome, Progeria, Infantile Hypercalcemia, & Sphingolipidoses

These disorders may be associated with hypercholesterolemia, but levels of triglycerides are usually normal. HDL deficiency is typical of Gaucher's disease, in which hypertriglyceridemia may also occur. Niemann-Pick disease is attributable in most cases to mutations in the *NCP1* gene and may be associated with hypercholesterolemia or hypertriglyceridemia. However, a similar disorder results from mutations in the NCP2 locus. The NCP1 gene product is involved in the postlysosomal transport of lipids.

Wolman's Disease & Cholesteryl Ester Storage Disease

These recessive lipid storage disorders involve the absence and partial deficiency, respectively, of lysosomal acid lipase, resulting in abnormal cholesteryl ester and triglyceride stores in liver, spleen, adrenals, small intestine, and bone marrow. Most patients have elevated levels of both LDL and VLDL. Wolman's disease is fatal in infancy.

Cerebrotendinous Xanthomatosis

In this recessive disorder, impaired synthesis of bile acids due to mutations in the sterol 27-hydroxylase gene results in increased production of cholesterol and cholestanol that accumulate in tissues. Plasma levels of cholesterol and cholestanol are normal or elevated. Cataracts, tendinous xanthomas, progressive neurologic dysfunction, and premature coronary atherosclerosis are hallmarks of this disease. Its central nervous system effects include dementia, spasticity, and ataxia. Death usually ensues before age 50 from neurologic degeneration or coronary disease. Treatment with chenodiol (chenodeoxycholic acid) appears useful. Resins must be avoided because they aggravate the underlying defect.

Phytosterolemia

Mutations in the cassette half transporters ABCG5 or ABCG8 underlie this disorder, which is characterized by normal or elevated plasma cholesterol levels; high concentrations of plant sterol in serum, adipose tissue, and skin; and prominent tendinous and tuberous xanthomas. Substantially larger fractions of phytosterols and cholesterol are absorbed from the intestine than in normal individuals. Serum cholesterol levels may be as high as 700 mg/dL (18.2 mmol/L), reflecting an increase in LDL that contain sitosterol esters in addition to cholesteryl esters. Diagnosis is established by quantitation of phytosterols in plasma by gas-liquid chromatography. Premature coronary atherosclerosis is common, and polyarthritis and leukocytoclastic vasculopathy are frequent. Treatment consists of a diet restricted in plant sterols and cholesterol and the use of bile acid-binding resins, reductase inhibitors, and a selective cholesterol absorption inhibitor (ezetimibe).

Cholesteryl Ester Transfer Protein (CETP) Deficiency

Mutations have been identified that impair the function of CETP, resulting in the retention of cholesteryl esters in HDL. Total HDL cholesterol is increased by 30–50% in heterozygotes and by as much as 200 mg/dL in homozygotes. The risk of atherosclerosis is moderately increased.

■ II. TREATMENT OF HYPERLIPIDEMIA

Initial therapy in all forms of hyperlipidemia is an appropriate diet. In most cases, a "universal" diet (see below) is indicated. In many subjects with lipemia or with mild hypercholesterolemia, compliance with diet is sufficient to control lipoprotein levels. Most patients with severe hypercholesterolemia or lipemia will require drug therapy. Diet must be continued to achieve the full potential of the medications. LDL cholesterol and triglycerides should be below 90 mg/dL (2.3 mmol/L) and 130 mg/dL (1.5 mmol/L), respectively, in patients with known atherosclerosis.

Caution Regarding Drug Therapy

There are insufficient data on which to base an evaluation of the effects on the fetus of drugs used in treatment of hyperlipoproteinemia. Women of childbearing age should be advised of the potential risk and should be given these agents only if pregnancy is being actively avoided. If contraceptives are prescribed, estrogens should be used with caution in patients with hypertriglyceridemia.

In children, hyperlipidemias other than familial hypercholesterolemia rarely require medication. The severity and age at onset of symptomatic coronary disease in the child's family and the presence of other risk factors, especially hypoalphalipoproteinemia and hyper-Lp(a)lipoproteinemia, in the child should be considered in deciding when drug treatment should be started. Dietary treatment is indicated for all children with hyperlipidemia and should be started after the second year. The exception is primary chylomicronemia, in which an appropriate diet should be instituted as soon as the disease is detected.

DIETARY FACTORS IN THE MANAGEMENT OF LIPOPROTEIN DISORDERS

Restriction of Caloric Intake

The secretion of VLDL by liver is greatly stimulated by caloric intake in excess of requirements for physical activity and basal metabolism. Therefore, the total caloric content of the diet is of greater importance than its specific composition in treating endogenous hyperlipemia. There is a positive correlation between serum levels of VLDL triglyceride and various measures of obesity, but many obese patients have normal serum lipids. On the other hand, most patients with hypertriglyceridemia—except those with lipoprotein lipase deficiency—are obese. This association is more consistently observed in persons with centripetal obesity whose weight gain occurred in later childhood or adulthood and who have insulin resistance. As obese patients lose weight, VLDL stabilize at lower levels. There is a modest correlation of LDL levels with body weight in the general population.

Restriction of Fat Intake

In primary chylomicronemia, all types of fats must be restricted rigidly. In the acute management of mixed lipemia with impending pancreatitis, elimination of dietary fat leads to a rapid decrease in triglycerides.

The cholesterol-lowering effect of a significant reduction in total fat is well known. It has also been shown that a 10–15% fall in cholesterol is achieved when individuals who have been consuming a typical North American diet restrict their intake of saturated fats to 8% of total calories. Most saturated and trans fatty acids cause increased levels of LDL cholesterol by down-regulating hepatic LDL receptors. Whereas polyunsaturated fatty acids do not have this effect, they may reduce levels of HDL and are potentially carcinogenic. Monounsaturated fatty acids increase HDL but do not increase LDL. Moderate use of monounsaturated fats such as olive oil, oleic acid-rich safflower oil, or canola oil is indicated.

The omega-3 fatty acids found in fish oils have special properties relevant to the treatment of hypertriglyceridemia and tend to protect against fatal arrhythmias in ischemic myocardium. Substantial decreases in triglyceride levels can be induced in some patients with severe endogenous or mixed lipemia at doses of 3–10 g/d. Certain members of this class of fatty acids, such as eicosapentaenoic acid, are potent inhibitors of platelet reactivity.

Reduction of Cholesterol Intake

The amount of cholesterol in the diet affects serum cholesterol levels, but individual responses vary. Restriction of dietary cholesterol to less than 200 mg/d (5.2 mmol/d) in normal individuals can result in a decrease of up to 10–15% in serum cholesterol, primarily reflecting a decrease in LDL. Dietary cholesterol and saturated fat content have independent effects on levels of serum cholesterol.

Role of Carbohydrate in Diet

When a high-carbohydrate diet is consumed, hypertriglyceridemia often develops within 48–72 hours, and levels of triglycerides rise to a maximum in 1–5 weeks.

Persons with higher basal triglycerides and those consuming hypercaloric diets show the greatest effect. In type 2 diabetics, a high-carbohydrate diet tends to increase insulin resistance. Substitution of monounsaturated fats for the carbohydrate improves insulin resistance and optimizes lipoprotein levels.

Alcohol Ingestion

Ingestion of alcohol is a common cause of secondary hypertriglyceridemia owing to overproduction of VLDL. Some individuals with familial hypertriglyceridemia are particularly sensitive to the effects of alcohol, and abstinence may normalize their triglycerides. Occasionally, chronic alcohol intake may also be associated with hypercholesterolemia. Increased cholesterol synthesis and decreased conversion to bile acids have been observed. Alcohol may account for alimentary lipemia persisting beyond 12–14 hours. This possibility should be excluded by the history or a repeat lipid analysis. A positive correlation has been found between alcohol intake and HDL cholesterol levels; however, increased HDL levels are not observed in all individuals. Because alcohol-induced changes in HDL appear primarily to involve the HDL_3 subfraction, there is no justification for the use of alcohol to increase the "protective effect" of HDL against atherosclerosis. If the low HDL cholesterol is secondary to hypertriglyceridemia, alcohol must be avoided.

Antioxidants

Both alpha and gamma tocopherols (vitamin E) have recognized roles in the elimination of free radicals. Vitamin C assists this activity by restoring the tocopheroxyl radical to active tocopherol. These vitamins have been shown to restore normal vascular reactivity in hyperlipidemic patients, and some epidemiologic evidence suggests that they have an antiatherogenic effect. It is therefore reasonable to include at least 50 IU of mixed tocopherols and 250 mg of vitamin C in the diet each day. Larger doses may partially vitiate the effects of certain hypolipidemic drug regimens and have not been shown to have antiatherogenic potential. Selenium may also be important because it is a cofactor for one species of superoxide dismutase. Diets rich in fruits and vegetables appear to be important, providing isoflavones, quinols, and a number of carotenoid species.

B Vitamins

A significant percentage of Americans carry at least one allele for mutations in the methylene tetrahydrofolate reductase gene that diminishes its efficiency by reducing its affinity for folic acid. This leads to elevated levels of a metabolite of methionine—homocysteine—that has toxic effects on endothelium. Supplementation with 0.8–2 mg of folic acid mitigates this problem. Vitamins B_6 and B_{12} participate in the metabolism of homocysteine. Thus, a B complex supplement should be used. Dietary protein should be restricted to the amount required for replacement of essential amino acids (about 0.5–1 g/kg) in patients with hyperhomocysteinemia.

Other Dietary Substances

Several other nutrients have been studied in relation to atherosclerosis. Caffeine and sucrose have negligible effects on serum lipids, and their statistical relationship to coronary heart disease is generally unimpressive when data are corrected for cigarette smoking. However, when coffee is prepared by protracted boiling of the grounds, a lipid substance (cafestol) is extracted that contributes to hypercholesterolemia. Lecithin has no effect on plasma lipoproteins. A minor reduction in LDL cholesterol is associated with the addition of oat bran and certain other brans to the diet.

The "Universal Diet"

Dietary treatment is an important aspect of the management of all forms of lipoprotein disorders and may in some cases be all that is required. Knowledge of the dietary factors mentioned above allows selection of appropriate modifications for an individual. However, a basic diet is useful in the treatment of most patients, the elements of which are as follows:

(1) A normal BMI should be achieved and maintained.

(2) Fat should provide less than 35% and saturated fat less than 7% of total calories. Monounsaturated oils should predominate and be used for all high-temperature cooking.

(3) Cholesterol should be reduced to less than 200 mg/d.

(4) Complex carbohydrates should predominate among total carbohydrates.

(5) Alcohol should be avoided in patients with hypertriglyceridemia or those requiring weight loss.

(6) Intake of trans fatty acids should be minimized or avoided.

(7) Peroxidized fats resulting from protracted heating should be avoided.

Caloric restriction and reduction of adipose tissue mass are particularly important for patients with increased levels of VLDL and IDL. Levels of VLDL and LDL tend to be lower during periods of substantial weight loss than can be maintained under isocaloric conditions even at ideal body weight.

DRUGS USED IN TREATMENT OF HYPERLIPOPROTEINEMIA (Table 19–3)

BILE ACID SEQUESTRANTS

Mechanism of Action

Cholestyramine, colestipol, and colesevelam are cationic resins that bind bile acids in the intestinal lumen. They are not absorbed and therefore increase the excretion of bile acids in the stool up to tenfold. LDL levels decrease as a consequence of increased expression of high-affinity receptors on hepatic cell membranes. These agents are useful only in disorders involving elevated LDL. Patients who have increased levels of VLDL may have further increases in serum triglycerides during treatment with resins. In combined hyperlipidemia, where the resins may be given to reduce LDL, a second agent such as niacin may be required to control the hypertriglyceridemia. Levels of LDL fall 15–30% in compliant patients with heterozygous familial hypercholesterolemia who are receiving maximal doses of the resins.

Drug Dosage

In disorders involving moderately high levels of LDL, 20 g of cholestyramine or colestipol daily may reduce cholesterol levels effectively. Treatment should commence at one-half this dosage to minimize gastrointestinal side effects. Maximum doses of 30 g of colestipol, 32 g of cholestyramine, or 3.89 g of colesevelam daily are required in more severe cases. These agents are only effective if taken with meals.

Side Effects

Because the resins are not absorbed, systemic side effects are absent. Patients frequently complain of a bloated sensation and constipation, both of which may be relieved by the addition of psyllium to the resin mixture. Malabsorption of fat or fat-soluble vitamins with a daily dose of resin up to 30 g occurs only in individuals with preexisting bowel disease or cholestasis. Hypoprothrombinemia has been observed in patients with malabsorption due to these causes. Cholestyramine and colestipol bind thyroxine, digitalis glycosides, and warfarin and impair the absorption of iron, thiazides, betablockers, and other drugs. Absorption of all these is ensured if they are administered 1 hour before the resin. Colesevelam does not bind digoxin, warfarin, or reductase inhibitors. Because they change the composition of bile micelles, bile acid sequestrants theoretically may increase the risk of cholelithiasis, particularly in obese subjects. In practice, this risk appears to be very small.

The resins should not be used as single agents in patients with hypertriglyceridemia. They should be avoided in those with diverticulitis.

NIACIN (Nicotinic Acid)

Mechanism of Action

Niacin (but not its amide) is able to effect major reductions in LDL and triglyceride-rich lipoproteins. It inhibits secretion of VLDL. It increases sterol excretion acutely, mobilizes cholesterol from tissue pools until a new steady state is established, and decreases cholesterol biosynthesis. That it can cause a continued decrease in hepatic cholesterol production even when given with bile acid-binding resins is probably an important feature of the complementary action of these agents. Levels of HDL, particularly HDL_2, are significantly increased, reflecting a decrease in the fractional catabolic rate of these lipoproteins. Niacin stimulates production of tissue plasminogen activator, an effect that may be of value in preventing thrombotic events. Small, dense LDL are converted to particles of larger diameter during treatment with niacin.

Drug Dosage

The dose of niacin required varies with the diagnosis. Optimal effect on LDL in heterozygous FH is usually only achieved when 4.5–6 g of niacin daily is combined with a resin or reductase inhibitor. For other forms of hypercholesterolemia, dysbetalipoproteinemia, and hypertriglyceridemia, 1.5–3.5 g/d often has a dramatic effect. Because niacin causes cutaneous flushing, it is usually started at a dosage of 100 mg three times daily and increased slowly. Tachyphylaxis to the flushing often occurs within a few days at any dose, allowing stepwise increases. Many patients have no or only occasional flushing when stabilized on a given dose, but most must reach about 3 g/d before flushing ceases. Because the flush is prostaglandin-mediated, 0.3 g of aspirin given 20–30 minutes before each dose when treatment is initiated or the dose increased (or equivalent doses of other cyclooxygenase inhibitors) may mitigate this symptom. It is important to counsel the patient that the flushing is a harmless cutaneous vasodilation and that the drug should be taken with meals two or three times daily. A daily dose of 6.5 g is the maximum under any circumstances.

Side Effects

Some patients have reversible elevations of serum glutamic aminotransferase or alkaline phosphatase activities up to three times the upper limit of normal that do

Table 19–3. Reductase inhibitors.

Drugs (In Increasing Order of Potency)	Dose Range
Fluvastatin	20–80 mg
Pravastatin	10–80 mg
Lovastatin	10–80 mg
Simvastatin	5–80 mg
Atorvastatin	5–80 mg

not appear to be clinically significant. In a group of patients treated continuously for up to 15 years, no significant liver disease developed despite such enzyme abnormalities. Rarely, patients develop a chemical hepatitis signaled by malaise, anorexia, and nausea. Aminotransferase levels are significantly elevated, and levels of lipoproteins may fall precipitously. Treatment should be stopped immediately. About one-fifth of patients have mild hyperuricemia that tends to be asymptomatic unless the patient has had gout. In such cases, allopurinol can be added to the regimen. A few patients will have moderate elevations of blood glucose during treatment. Again, this is reversible except in some patients who have latent type 2 diabetes. Niacin should be avoided in most patients with insulin resistance unless they are receiving insulin. A more common side effect is gastric irritation, which responds well to H_2 blockers and antacids. Antacids that contain aluminum should be avoided. Rarely, patients develop acanthosis nigricans, which clears if the drug is discontinued. Some patients can have cardiac arrhythmias while taking niacin. Reversible macular degeneration has been described rarely.

Niacin should be avoided in patients with peptic ulcer or hepatic parenchymal disease. Liver function, uric acid, and blood glucose should be evaluated before commencing treatment and periodically thereafter.

Most timed-release preparations of niacin should be avoided because of the risk of fulminant hepatic failure. However, if the daily dose is limited to 2 g or less, this rare consequence is unlikely.

FIBRIC ACID DERIVATIVES

Mechanism of Action

These agents—gemfibrozil and fenofibrate—which are ligands for PPARα decrease lipolysis in adipose tissue, reduce levels of circulating triglycerides, and cause modest reductions in LDL. However, in some patients, reductions in VLDL levels are attended by increases in LDL. They cause moderate increases in levels of HDL, including the protein moiety.

Drug Dosage

The fibrates may be useful in the treatment of patients with severe endogenous lipemia, familial dysbetalipoproteinemia, and some patients with combined hyperlipidemia who are intolerant of niacin. The usual dose of gemfibrozil is 600 mg twice daily; that of fenofibrate is one to three 54-mg tablets daily or a single dose of 160 mg.

Side Effects

Skin eruptions, gastrointestinal symptoms, and muscle symptoms have been described as well as blood dyscrasias and elevated levels of aminotransferases and alkaline phosphatase. These drugs enhance the effects of the coumarin and indanedione anticoagulants and increase lithogenicity of bile. Concomitant use of fibrates with reductase inhibitors increases the risk of myopathy. Fibrates should be avoided during pregnancy and lactation and are contraindicated if hepatic or renal disease is present.

HMG-COA REDUCTASE INHIBITORS

Mechanism of Action

Several closely related structural analogs of HMG-CoA act as competitive inhibitors of HMG-CoA reductase, a key enzyme in the cholesterol biosynthetic pathway. Of these, lovastatin, pravastatin, simvastatin, fluvastatin, and atorvastatin are approved for use in the USA. Inhibition of cholesterol biosynthesis induces an increase in high-affinity LDL receptors in the liver, increasing removal of LDL from plasma and decreasing production of LDL. The latter results from increased uptake of lipoprotein precursors of LDL by hepatic receptors. Modest increases in HDL cholesterol and limited decreases in VLDL levels can be achieved. These drugs have no appreciable effect in patients with severe hypertriglyceridemia. Some of the cholesterol-independent effects of reductase inhibitors appear to involve enhanced stability of atherosclerotic lesions and decreased oxidative stress and vascular inflammation, with improved endothelial function. Institution of treatment with a reductase inhibitor should begin immediately in all patients with myocardial infarction regardless of cholesterol level.

Drug Dosage

These drugs are the most effective individual agents for treatment of hypercholesterolemia. Their effects are amplified significantly when combined with niacin or resin. Daily dosage ranges are presented in Table 19–3. Because the rate of cholesterol synthesis is higher at night, reductase inhibitors should be given with the evening meal or at bedtime for greatest effect. Atorvastatin has a longer half life and may be taken at any time. Pravastatin is absorbed optimally when taken more than 3 hours after a meal. At higher doses, a twice-daily regimen is recommended. Patients with heterozygous familial hypercholesterolemia usually require higher doses. Because information on long-term safety is lacking, use of these agents in children should be restricted to those with homozygous familial hypercholesterolemia and selected heterozygotes who are at particularly high risk. Women who are lactating, pregnant, or likely to become pregnant should not be given these drugs.

Side Effects

These agents are generally well tolerated. Side effects, often transient, include changes in bowel function and rashes. Myopathy with markedly elevated creatine kinase levels occurs infrequently. Rarely, myopathy can progress to rhabdomyolysis with myoglobinuria and renal shutdown. There is an increased incidence of myopathy in patients receiving several of the reductase inhibitors with cyclosporine, fibric acid derivatives, macrolides, HIV protease inhibitors, nefazodone, verapamil, and ketoconazole. Other drugs that compete for metabolism by cytochrome P450 3A4 can be expected to have the same effect. Because pravastatin does not compete with these agents for metabolism by cytochrome P450 enzymes, it appears to be compatible at lower dosage with them. Fluvastatin is chiefly metabolized by cytochrome P450 2C9. Thus, competitors for that pathway may cause accumulation of this reductase inhibitor. The myopathy is rapidly reversible upon cessation of therapy. Minor elevations of creatine kinase activity in plasma are noted more frequently, especially with unusual physical activity. Creatine kinase levels should be measured before starting therapy and monitored at regular intervals. Older patients, those taking higher doses and multiple other drugs, those who consume large amounts of alcohol, and diabetics or others with renal insufficiency should be observed more frequently.

Moderate, often intermittent elevations of serum aminotransferases (up to three times normal) occur in some patients. If the patient is asymptomatic, therapy may be continued if activity is measured frequently (at 1- to 2-month intervals) and the levels are stable. In about 2% of patients, some of whom have underlying liver disease or a history of alcohol use, aminotransferase activity may exceed three times the normal limit. This usually occurs after 3–16 months of continuous therapy and may portend more severe hepatic toxicity

such as that described in the section on niacin. The reductase inhibitor should be discontinued promptly in these patients. These agents are contraindicated in the presence of active liver disease and should be used with caution in patients with a history of liver disease. They should be discontinued temporarily during hospitalization for major surgery.

CHOLESTEROL ABSORPTION INHIBITORS

Mechanism of Action

Ezetimibe, the first of this class, inhibits the absorption of cholesterol and phytosterols by enterocytes. By interrupting the enterohepatic circulation of sterols secreted in bile, it increases sterol efflux from the body.

Drug Dosage

Ezetimibe is useful in treating primary hypercholesterolemias and phytosterolemia. Concomitant use of fibric acid derivatives can increase the blood concentration of this drug. Resins can decrease its absorption. It should be avoided in pregnant or lactating women and in patients with liver disease, and used with caution in patients receiving cyclosporine. A single dose of 10 mg daily reduces cholesterol by 15 to 20 percent.

Side Effects

Very few side effects have been reported. The prevalence of elevated liver enzymes may be modestly increased when ezetimibe is given with a reductase inhibitor.

COMBINED DRUG THERAPY (TABLE 19–4)

Combinations of drugs may be useful (1) when LDL and VLDL levels are both elevated; (2) in cases of hypercholesterolemia in which significant increases of VLDL occur during treatment with bile acid-binding resins; and (3) where a complementary effect is required to normalize LDL levels, as in familial hypercholesterolemia or familial combined hyperlipidemia.

Fibric Acid Derivatives with Niacin

The combination of a fibrate with niacin may be more effective than either drug alone in managing marked hypertriglyceridemia.

Niacin & Resins

Niacin usually normalizes triglycerides in individuals who have increased levels of VLDL while taking resins. The combination of niacin and resins is more effective

Table 19–4. The primary hyperlipoproteinemias and their drug treatment.

	Single Drug[1]	Drug Combination
Primary chylomicronemia (familial lipoprotein lipase or cofactor deficiency)		
Chylomicrons, VLDL increased	Dietary management	Niacin plus fibrate[2]
Familial hypertriglyceridemia		
Severe: Chylomicrons, VLDL increased	Niacin, fibrate	Niacin plus fibrate
Moderate: VLDL and perhaps chylomicrons increased	Niacin, fibrate	Niacin plus fibrate
Familial combined hyperlipoproteinemia		
VLDL increased	Niacin, fibrate	
LDL increased	Niacin, reductase inhibitor	Niacin plus resin or reductase inhibitor
VLDL, LDL increased	Niacin, reductase inhibitor	Niacin plus resin or reductase inhibitor
Familial dysbetalipoproteinemia		
VLDL remnants, chylomicron remnants increased	Niacin, fibrate, reductase inhibitor	Fibrate plus niacin or niacin plus reductase inhibitor
Familial hypercholesterolemia		
Heterozygous: LDL increased	Resin, reductase inhibitor, niacin	Two or three of the single drugs
Homozygous: LDL increased	Niacin, atorvastatin	Niacin plus reductase inhibitor
Familial ligand-defective apo B		
LDL increased	Niacin, reductase inhibitor	Niacin plus reductase inhibitor
Lp(a) hyperlipoproteinemia		
Lp(a) increased	Niacin	

[1]Single-drug therapy should be tried before drug combinations are used.
[2]Fibric acid derivative.

than either agent alone in decreasing LDL levels in familial hypercholesterolemia. The combination is also very useful in the treatment of familial combined hyperlipidemia. The absorption of niacin from the intestine is unimpeded by the presence of resin; the two medications may therefore be taken together. Because the resins have potent acid-neutralizing properties, there is further reason to give the two medications together when a patient complains of the gastric irritation that sometimes occurs as an adverse effect of niacin.

HMG-CoA Reductase Inhibitors with Other Agents

The addition of resin or niacin to a reductase inhibitor further decreases plasma levels of LDL in patients with primary hypercholesterolemias. Liver function and plasma creatine kinase activity should be monitored frequently when the combination includes niacin. These three drugs used together are more effective, frequently at lower doses, than any of their binary combinations in reducing LDL. Ezetimibe is synergistic with reductase inhibitors.

POSSIBLE UNTOWARD CONSEQUENCES OF LIPID-LOWERING THERAPY

The risk of coronary heart disease has been found to increase with LDL cholesterol levels in virtually all epidemiologic surveys. Total mortality tends to be slightly higher among individuals with cholesterol levels below 160 mg/dL, however, raising a question about whether very low levels of cholesterol may increase the risk of noncoronary disease. The correlation between deaths from certain digestive and respiratory disorders and low cholesterol levels probably reflect the effect of wasting illnesses on LDL. For instance, the low cholesterol levels seen in hepatic cirrhosis most certainly reflect impaired lipoprotein production by the liver. Increased uptake of LDL by malignant cells is known to decrease LDL in plasma. However, two studies have shown a modest increase in the risk of hemorrhagic stroke at cholesterol levels below 130 mg/dL. In one, the effect was confined to hypertensive patients. In large clinical trials employing niacin or reductase inhibitors, no excess deaths from noncoronary causes occurred in the course of 5 years or more, though impressive reductions in deaths from coronary disease were observed, resulting in significant reduction in all-cause mortality. In a secondary intervention trial (the Four S trial), patients receiving simvastatin had a 37% reduction in new coronary events over a 5- to 6-year period. In the West of Scotland study, treatment with pravastatin resulted in a 22% reduction in all-cause mortality. In the MRFIT study, a proportionate hazards analysis adjusting for covariance demonstrated that the lowest net death rate occurs at a cholesterol level of 122 mg/dL.

Populations in which many individuals have cholesterol levels below 160 mg/dL, such as in Japan, do not have an excess incidence of the noncoronary causes of death. Of great importance in resolving the question of the relative benefit of lipid-lowering therapy is the fact that about 45% of deaths in the USA and Europe are attributable to cardiovascular disease, predominantly coronary disease. Thus, projection of a significant reduction in fatal occlusive coronary events into the age range where coronary disease predominates would be expected to far outweigh the marginal increases that might occur in other causes of death. In the light of the relationship of very low cholesterol levels (< 130 mg/dL) to hemorrhagic stroke, the therapeutic goal for LDL cholesterol in patients with known coronary disease should not be below the 60 mg/dL (1.55 mmol/L) range until that relationship is better understood.

REFERENCES

Mechanisms of Atherogenesis

Libby P: Current concepts of the pathogenesis of the acute coronary syndromes. Circulation 2001;104:365. [PMID: 11457759]

Libby P, Ridker PM, Maseri A: Inflammation and atherosclerosis. Circulation 2002;105:1135. [PMID: 11877368]

Malloy MJ, Kane JP: A risk factor for atherosclerosis: triglyceride-rich lipoproteins. Adv Intern Med 2001;47:111. [PMID: 11795072]

Seman LJ, McNamara JR, Schaefer EJ: Lipoprotein(a), homocysteine, and remnantlike particles: emerging risk factors. Curr Opin Cardiol 1999;14:186. [PMID: 10191979]

Disorders of Lipoprotein Metabolism

Brunzell JD, Deeb SS: Familial lipoprotein lipase deficiency, Apo C II deficiency, and hepatic lipase deficiency. In: *The Metabolic and Molecular Bases of Inherited Disease,* 8th ed. Scriver CR et al (editors). McGraw-Hill, 2001.

Goldstein JL, Hobbs HH, Brown MS: Familial hypercholesterolemia. In: *The Metabolic and Molecular Bases of Inherited Disease,* 8th ed. Scriver CR et al (editors). McGraw-Hill, 2001.

Havel RJ, Kane JP: Introduction: Structure and metabolism of plasma lipoproteins. In: *The Metabolic and Molecular Bases of Inherited Disease,* 8th ed. Scriver CR et al (editors). McGraw-Hill, 2001.

Kane JP, Havel RJ: Disorders of the biogenesis and secretion of lipoproteins containing the B apolipoproteins. In: *The Metabolic and Molecular Bases of Inherited Disease,* 8th ed. Scriver CR et al (editors). McGraw-Hill, 2001.

Mahley RW, Rall SC Jr: Type III hyperlipoproteinemia (dysbetalipoproteinemia): The role of apolipoprotein E in normal and abnormal lipoprotein metabolism. In: *The Metabolic and Molecular Bases of Inherited Disease,* 8th ed. Scriver CR et al (editors). McGraw-Hill, 2001.

Management

Albert CM et al: Blood levels of long-chain n-3 fatty acids and the risk of sudden death. N Engl J Med 2002;346:1113. [PMID: 1948270]

Betteridge DJ: The current management of diabetic dyslipidaemia. Acta Diabetol 2001;38 Suppl 1:S15. [PMID: 11829449]

Executive Summary of the Third Report of The National Cholesterol Education Program (NCEP) Expert Panel on Detection, Evaluation, and Treatment of High Blood Cholesterol in Adults (Adult Treatment Panel III). JAMA 2001;285:2486. [PMID: 11368702]

Kromhout D et al: Prevention of coronary heart disease by diet and lifestyle. Circulation 2002;105:893. [PMID: 11854133]

Schaefer EJ: Lipoproteins, nutrition, and heart disease. Am J Clin Nutr 2002;75:191. [PMID: 11815309]

Stein EA: Managing dyslipidemia in the high risk patient. Am J Cardiol 2002;89:50C. [PMID: 11900720]

Obesity & Overweight

Marc K. Hellerstein, MD, PhD, & Elizabeth J. Parks, PhD

BMI	Body mass index	**REE**	Resting energy expenditure
DRI	Dietary reference intakes	**RQ**	Respiratory quotient
FFM	Fat-free mass	**SNS**	Sympathetic nervous system
LBM	Lean body mass	**TEE**	Total energy expenditure

INTRODUCTION

Obesity is a disorder of body composition defined by a relative or absolute excess of body fat and characterized by several remarkable features. Its prevalence has increased dramatically over the past several decades, both in the industrialized and developing worlds. It is now no exaggeration to state that obesity is an international epidemic. Moreover, obesity is no longer a disorder of adults; prevalence in children has accelerated rapidly, so that 25% of United States children are overweight or obese. At the same time, body fatness has taken on a central—even obsessive—place in popular culture as images and pressures from nonmedical as well as medical sources are ubiquitous and disapproving. This central epidemiologic paradox sets off obesity as occupying a special place among the physical ailments in contemporary society.

Uncertainty about the etiology, pathogenesis, and treatment of obesity is a key element in this paradox. Although the health risks associated with excess body fat are increasingly well documented, therapies remain generally ineffective. Persistent therapeutic failure, accelerating prevalence, and rising morbidity of excess body weight are occurring despite enormous efforts by the medical profession, pharmaceutical industry, and weight-loss industry (in addition to popular culture). This dissonance between therapeutic effort and efficacy represents a second paradox in this area.

The objective of this chapter is to present obesity with a focus on its best-understood aspect—the physiology of energy and fat balance—and to use these physiologic insights as a framework for discussion of current therapies. Because most patients seen by a physician in the United States have probably thought or worried about "getting fat" and typically have a number of questions and misconceptions, many physicians are uneasy about discussing "fatness" with their patients and their patients' children. A central goal here is thus to help health care providers answer questions that may be asked by their patients. Toward this end, what is not known will be directly identified and noted in addition to what is known.

Within this framework, the chapter will focus on the following issues faced by health care providers: (1) Why should obesity be treated, and when? (2) What are the causal factors and pathogenic pathways contributing to overweight, and which of these can be manipulated therapeutically? (3) What specific treatments are available or under investigation, and what are their demonstrated efficacy and risks? (4) Which other medical conditions are affected by body fatness and its treatment? (5) What areas of the field remain controversial or unknown? (6) What are some of the common questions and misconceptions that patients have, and how can we best respond to them?

Definition & Diagnosis of Overweight & Obesity

Obesity is best defined as the presence of an abnormal absolute amount or relative proportion of body fat. The presence of excess body fat usually—not always—results in higher body weight. The criteria for "abnormal" amounts of body fat or body weight can be purely statistical (ie, based on population means) or, more usefully, on epidemiologic associations with adverse health events. The classification criterion used in most large studies has been the body mass index (BMI), derived by dividing the body weight (in kilograms) by the square of the height in meters—or by dividing the weight in pounds by the square of the height in inches and multiplying by 703. Because most of the health outcome data are with BMI, this is at present the recommended basis for classifying overweight and obesity (Table 20–1). The term "morbid obesity" has also been used to emphasize the extreme health risks of body weights above 150 kg.

Although it may be most convenient to use body weight for identification of obese patients, it is important to keep the true definition clear: obesity is a disorder of body fat stores (adiposity). Maintaining this emphasis will help us when thinking about pathogenesis and treatment, wherein body weight and body composition must often be clearly separated.

One important complication regarding diagnosis relates to body fat distribution. All body fat is not created equal. Central or visceral-abdominal obesity ("apple-shaped") is associated with substantially different metabolic profiles and cardiovascular risk factors than gluteal-femoral obesity ("pear-shaped"). Overweight women tend to have different body fat distribution than men, and metabolic and cardiovascular risks vary in parallel. Hypothesized reasons for these differences in risk for adverse health consequences are discussed below. For the clinician, the distinction is extremely important, and overweight patients should be broadly classified as having central or gluteal-femoral types. This can be done quickly and easily by measurement of the waist circumference, using a tape measure. High risk abdominal obesity is defined as waist circumference > 102 cm (> 40 inches) in men and > 88 cm (> 35 inches) in women.

Prevalence of Obesity

The late 20th century has witnessed an extraordinary change in the epidemiology of human body composition. What was in 1950 or 1960 a prevalent condition in the West—particularly the United States and certain Northern European countries—that was observed primarily in older adults has expanded in all respects. The prevalence has reached "epidemic" proportions in the West, increasing even in the past decade in United States adults from 12% obese (defined as BMI > 30) in 1991 to 17.9% in 1998. The prevalence of overweight (defined as BMI > 25) has increased even more, representing more than 60% of men and more than 55% of women in 1994. In some ethnic or racial populations (eg, Mexican-American or African-American women), the prevalence of overweight is greater than 65%. Children are increasingly affected and represent the fastest-growing population group of overweight and obese people in the United States. Children in certain ethnic or racial groups are disproportionately affected. Perhaps most significantly, the rest of the world is catching up to the West. Obesity is now prevalent in regions where it was historically rare, such as South America, Central America, Southeast Asia, Australia, and Africa. This international change is linked to urbanization, with attendant changes in physical activity and a shift away from traditional diets.

The prevalence of obesity is also affected by age. Body composition and the prevalence of obesity vary during the life cycle (Table 20–2). Body weight tends to peak in United States men and women in the sixth and seventh decades, then to fall with further increasing age.

Health Consequences of Overweight & Obesity

Why identify and treat overweight or obesity? Some authors have suggested that body weight should be considered in a manner analogous to characteristics such as height: largely inherited, naturally variable within a population, and best accepted in an individual rather than opposed through interventions. Others have pointed out the considerable social and medical costs of the widespread popular concern about and therapies for perceived excess fatness. These criticisms express considerable truth—the social, psychological and financial costs of both lay and medical approaches to adiposity are indeed great.

The problem is that obesity is not a benign variant. Convincing data exist from a number of studies documenting the substantial disease burden associated with overweight and obesity. In 1991, death and disability attributable to obesity (BMI > 30) has been estimated

Table 20–1. Classification of overweight and obesity based on body mass index (BMI).

	BMI
Underweight	< 18.5
Normal	18.5–24.9
Overweight	25.0–29.9
Obesity	
Class I	30.0–34.9
Class II	35.0–39.9
Class III (extreme)	> 40.0

$$BMI = \frac{Weight\ (kg)}{Height\ (m)^2}$$

Table 20–2. Combined prevalence (%) of overweight (BMI > 25) and obesity (BMI > 30) in United States adults by age, gender, and race or ethnicity (1960–1994).

	NHES I 1960–62 (Ages 20–74)	NHANES I 1971–74 (Ages 20–74)	NHANES II 1976–80 (Ages 20–74)	HHANES 1982–84 (Ages 20–74)	NHANES III 1988–94 (Ages ≥ 20)
AGE- AND GENDER-SPECIFIC CATEGORIES					
Men					
20–29	39.9	38.6	37.0		43.1
30–39	49.6	58.1	52.6		58.1
40–49	53.6	63.6	60.3		65.5
50–59	54.1	58.4	60.8		73.0
60–69	52.9	55.6	57.4		70.3
70–79	36.0	52.7	53.3		63.1
80+	N/A	N/A	N/A		50.6
Women					
20–29	17.0	23.2	25.0		33.1
30–39	32.8	35.0	36.8		47.0
40–49	42.3	44.6	44.4		52.7
50–59	55.0	52.2	52.8		64.4
60–69	63.1	56.2	56.5		64.0
70–79	54.7	55.9	58.2		57.9
80+	N/A	N/A	N/A		50.1
GENDER, RACE OR ETHNICITY, AGE ≥ 20, AGE-ADJUSTED					
Both sexes	43.3	46.1	46.0		54.9
Men	48.2	52.9	51.4		59.9
Women	38.7	39.7	40.8		50.7
White men	48.8	53.7	52.3		61.0
White women	36.1	37.6	38.4		49.2
Black men	43.1	48.9	49.0		56.5
Black women	57.0	57.6	61.0		65.8
White, non-Hispanic men			52.0		60.6
White, non-Hispanic women			37.6		47.4
Black, non-Hispanic men			48.9		56.7
Black, non-Hispanic women			60.6		66.0
Mexican-American men				59.7	63.9
Mexican-American women				60.1	65.9

NHES I = National Health Examination Survey I.
NHANES I = National Health and Nutrition Examination Survey I.
NHANES II = National Health and Nutrition Examination Survey II.
HHANES = Hispanic Health and Nutrition Examination Survey I.
NHANES III= National Health and Nutrition Examination Survey III.
N/A = Not available

at 280,000–325,000 people per year in the United States. Previous studies have given similar estimates. Few factors, with the exception of cigarette smoking, exact as large a public health toll. Excess body fat must be taken seriously from a health perspective.

It is difficult to be certain about the causal link between diseases and body fat. These relationships are confounded by the many metabolic and hormonal alterations that either contribute to or derive from excess adiposity. For example, low cardiorespiratory fitness, though closely linked with body weight, is a strong and *independent* predictor of cardiovascular disease and mortality. In some studies, people in the > 35 BMI category with a good level of fitness have a lower mortality rate than people in the 25–30 BMI category with poor fitness. The specific mechanisms or agencies by which body fat promotes adverse outcomes are not always known. This will be a critical task for future research.

Some of the more serious medical conditions associated with overweight can be listed. Although a number of differences exist among ethnic groups in the United States with regard to prevalence and complications of overweight and obesity, the graded and significant relationship between BMI and prevalence of these health comorbidities applies for all groups.

A. DIABETES MELLITUS TYPE 2

The risk of type 2 diabetes mellitus increases linearly with increasing BMI in the general population. In comparison with a normal-weight individual, BMI > 40 (obesity class 3) in a person under 55 years of age increases the risk of type 2 diabetes mellitus by 18.1-fold in men and 12.9-fold in women. Classification as overweight (BMI 25–30) increases the prevalence of type 2 diabetes mellitus threefold to fourfold in both men and women under 55 years of age. The relative risks associated with excess body weight are less strong in older people but are still present (eg, about twofold for overweight and three- to sixfold for obesity class 3).

One of the most remarkable and worrisome features of the recent change in demographics of obesity is the rapid growth of type 2 ("adult"-type) diabetes in children and teenagers. In many clinics, particularly in urban centers, the majority of new childhood diabetics are overweight, not ketosis-prone, and lacking in immunologic markers of type 1 diabetes. Childhood type 2 diabetes had until the past decade been an extremely unusual condition, often associated with a strong familial component and mendelian inheritance (eg, glucokinase deficiency in some kindreds). The cause and pathogenesis of this extraordinary change in childhood diabetes remain uncertain, but the association with the increasing prevalence of obesity, sedentary lifestyle, or specific dietary factors is difficult to ignore. If this syndrome of childhood obesity and diabetes becomes established as a common consequence of the urbanized industrial world, the long-term health burden may be enormous (eg, for premature heart disease, peripheral vascular disease, renal failure, blindness, and erectile dysfunction).

B. HYPERTENSION

High blood pressure is the most common health condition associated with overweight or obesity in the United States. The relationship between hypertension prevalence and body weight for both men and women under 55 years of age is steeply graded, with relative risk increasing from 1.6 for overweight to 2.5–3.2 for obesity class 1 (BMI 30–35) and 3.9–5.5 for obesity classes 2 and 3 (BMI 35–40 and >40). The prevalence of hypertension is much higher with aging even in normal-weight individuals. The absolute number of persons affected by overweight or obesity is still substantial in those over age 55 despite a less steep relationship with body weight.

C. HYPERLIPIDEMIA AND DYSLIPIDEMIA

The presence of overweight or obesity is associated with high blood cholesterol, but the strength of the relationship is only moderate (less than a twofold relative risk at all weight categories and ages). The relationship to other blood lipid parameters such as hypertriglyceridemia, low HDL cholesterol, and altered composition of lipoprotein particles is much stronger. The difference in serum triglyceride concentrations between individuals with BMI < 21 and those with BMI > 30 is about 65 mg/dL (in women) and 62–118 mg/dL (in men, depending upon age). For HDL cholesterol, each 1-unit BMI change is associated with an HDL-cholesterol decrease of 1.1 mg/dL for young men and 0.7 mg/dL for young women (Figure 20–1).

D. ARTERIOSCLEROTIC HEART DISEASE AND STROKE

The prevalence of coronary artery disease exhibits a significant linear relationship with BMI for both genders and all ages. The relative risk for overweight persons is not statistically significant, but obesity classes 1–3 exhibit relative risks generally between 1.5 and 3.0, with the highest values in obesity class 3. Cerebrovascular accidents are also associated with obesity.

E. GALLBLADDER DISEASE, OSTEOARTHRITIS, CANCER, AND OTHER CONDITIONS

The prevalence of gallbladder disease is strongly associated with higher BMIs. The relative risks with increasing BMI range from fourfold to 21-fold elevated in men and 2.5-fold to 5.2-fold in women under age 55,

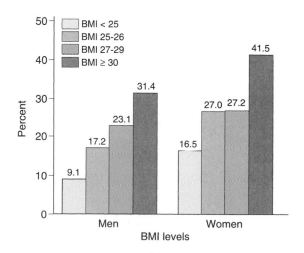

Figure 20–1. NHANES III age-adjusted prevalence of low HDL-cholesterol according to body mass index. Low HDL-cholesterol defined as < 35 mg/dL in men and < 45 mg/dL in women.

Osteoarthritis is also more prevalent in association with higher body weights, and symptoms often improve with weight loss. Several types of cancer are more prevalent in adults who are overweight or obese. Examples include endometrial, breast, prostate, and colon cancer. Sleep apnea is also highly associated with BMI > 30. Menstrual irregularity, infertility, and polycystic ovarian syndrome are more prevalent in premenopausal women with higher BMIs.

Etiology & Pathogenesis

The cause of obesity is multifactorial; that is, a large number of "pathways"—biochemical, dietary, and behavioral—exist that can contribute to the accrual of body fat (Figure 20–2). The nonmendelian (polygenic) inheritance patterns of obesity and body weight are also consistent with the operation of multiple interacting factors.

In a general sense, however, the pathogenesis of obesity (accrual of excess body fat) is simple and clear. There must have been an imbalance between the energy intake and the energy needs of the tissues—or, more specifically, between the intake or synthesis of fat and its oxidation by tissues—at some point in the life of the individual. Moreover, the resulting storage of surplus energy and fat in the only large energy storage depot available in humans (triacylglycerols in adipocytes) has not induced an effective feedback adaptation to dissipate accrued stores.

At its core, then, obesity is a disorder in the operation of a balancing system—ie, an interactive disorder—wherein the system for matching energy intake to expenditure is disrupted. What do we know about energy and nutrient balance systems in humans? Although much is not understood, a number of basic principles have emerged about the operating rules of this system. Understanding these physiologic principles about macronutrient balances is essential for an understanding of the pathogenesis and treatment of obesity.

Some Features of the Macronutrient & Energy Balancing Systems in Humans Can Be Described as Follows

A. INTAKE AND POOL SIZE RELATIONSHIPS

The relationship between daily intake and size of body stores for the different macronutrients (carbohydrates, fats, and proteins) are very different, with important consequences for tissue fuel selection.

The relationship between intake and body stores for each macronutrient (Figure 20–3) shows the unique status of body carbohydrate stores. In addition to the extremely limited storage pool of carbohydrates (< 1000–2000 kcal in the human body), several bio-

chemical facts all lead to the prediction that a system for sensing and preserving body carbohydrate stores over the short term must exist: Fats cannot be converted to carbohydrates in animals; conversion of amino acids to carbohydrates draws upon essential protein stores and is therefore undesirable; and the brain depends almost exclusively on glucose as a fuel under most conditions. Failure to conserve body carbohydrate stores in times of limitation would therefore have predictable adverse phenotypic consequences for the organism (protein wasting or neuroglycopenia), on the one hand. Inability to store excess carbohydrates indefinitely (due to limited whole-body storage capacity for glycogen) in times of surplus is similarly constraining—in the other direction. In contrast, a system for short-term sensing of body fat stores is not likely to be essential, as attested by the great surplus of fat calories relative to daily needs that exists in the body (Figure 20–3).

This quantitative prediction has been strongly supported by experimental data. Dietary carbohydrate intake stimulates its own oxidation, and dietary carbohydrate deprivation reduces whole-body oxidation of carbohydrates. These adaptations in fuel selection of the body to carbohydrate intake occur within a few days. An important feature of this response is that the conversion of surplus dietary carbohydrate to fat through the de novo lipogenesis pathway cannot be a quantitatively important process within this system. If de novo lipogenesis represented a quantitatively significant disposal route, it would act as a safety valve for dietary carbohydrate and obviate the necessity to oxidize surplus carbohydrate stores. Experimental evidence in humans makes it clear that surplus carbohydrate energy is not converted to fat. Instead, when extra carbohydrate calories are added to a mixed diet that includes fats, the oxidation of dietary fat is suppressed. The respiratory quotient (RQ) in this setting increases to 0.98–1.00, reflecting nearly complete replacement of fats by carbohydrate in the whole-body fuel mixture. Stable isotope metabolic measurements have shown that this RQ does not reflect conversion of carbohydrate to fat, followed by direct oxidation of fatty acids in tissues (eg, the former in the daytime, the latter at night). Thus, carbohydrate intake can lead to accrual of body fat, but this occurs by sparing oxidation of dietary fat rather than by conversion of carbohydrate to fat.

B. METABOLIC FACTORS

Short-term metabolic mechanisms have been identified for matching carbohydrate intake and oxidation but not for dietary fats.

The metabolic mechanisms responsible for matching whole-body oxidation of carbohydrates to their dietary intake are shown (Figure 20–4). The major play-

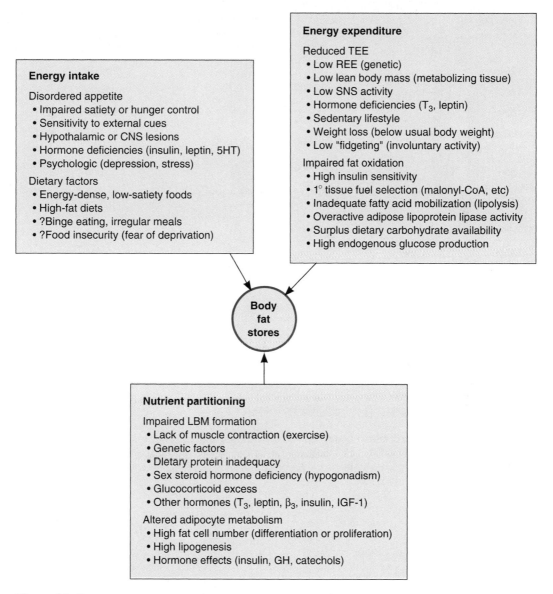

Energy intake

Disordered appetite
- Impaired satiety or hunger control
- Sensitivity to external cues
- Hypothalamic or CNS lesions
- Hormone deficiencies (insulin, leptin, 5HT)
- Psychologic (depression, stress)

Dietary factors
- Energy-dense, low-satiety foods
- High-fat diets
- ?Binge eating, irregular meals
- ?Food insecurity (fear of deprivation)

Energy expenditure

Reduced TEE
- Low REE (genetic)
- Low lean body mass (metabolizing tissue)
- Low SNS activity
- Hormone deficiencies (T_3, leptin)
- Sedentary lifestyle
- Weight loss (below usual body weight)
- Low "fidgeting" (involuntary activity)

Impaired fat oxidation
- High insulin sensitivity
- $1°$ tissue fuel selection (malonyl-CoA, etc)
- Inadequate fatty acid mobilization (lipolysis)
- Overactive adipose lipoprotein lipase activity
- Surplus dietary carbohydrate availability
- High endogenous glucose production

Body fat stores

Nutrient partitioning

Impaired LBM formation
- Lack of muscle contraction (exercise)
- Genetic factors
- Dietary protein inadequacy
- Sex steroid hormone deficiency (hypogonadism)
- Glucocorticoid excess
- Other hormones (T_3, leptin, β_3, insulin, IGF-1)

Altered adipocyte metabolism
- High fat cell number (differentiation or proliferation)
- High lipogenesis
- Hormone effects (insulin, GH, catechols)

Figure 20–2. Biochemical and physiologic pathways to body fat accrual

ers are liver, pancreas, and adipose tissue. Hepatic glucose production closely parallels liver glycogen content. When stores are high, glycogenolysis and glucose production are relatively insensitive to suppression by insulin; when stores are low, the opposite occurs. Expansion of liver glycogen stores therefore leads to increased input of glucose into the circulation. In response, pancreatic insulin secretion increases and serum insulin concentrations rise. As a result, adipocyte lipolysis is inhibited and tissue uptake and oxidation of glucose are stimulated, though glucose production is not sup-

pressed (the liver is insulin-resistant). The net effect is greater oxidation of glucose and less of fat even under postabsorptive conditions (Figure 20–4). Interestingly, increased endogenous glucose production mimics exogenous carbohydrate intake with regard to stimulating whole-body carbohydrate oxidation, suppressing fat oxidation, and accelerating accrual of body fat. Indeed, the best predictor of obesity in Sprague-Dawley rats placed on ad libitum high-fat diets is a high rate of baseline hepatic glucose production and its resistance to suppression by insulin.

A. A lean person

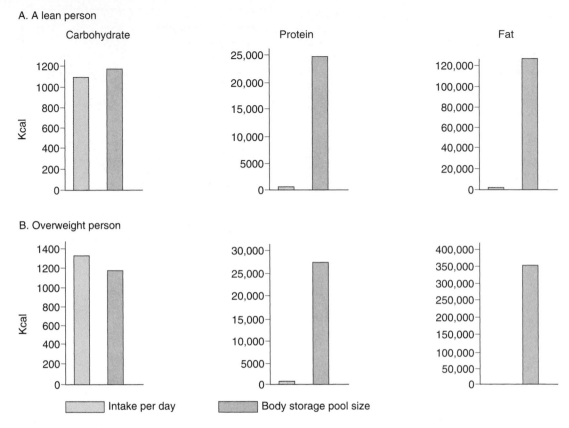

B. Overweight person

Figure 20–3. Comparison of storage pool size and daily throughput for three macronutrients. A typical Western diet is represented (40% fat, 45% carbohydrate, 15% protein; 2400 kcal/d in lean, 3000 kcal/d in obese) and compared for a lean (weight, 70 kg; fat, 20%) and an obese (weight, 100 kg; fat, 45%) man. Note different scales.

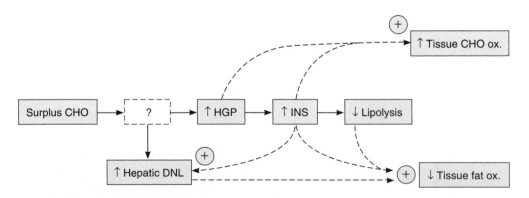

Figure 20–4. Metabolic mechanisms by which surplus carbohydrate intake leads to body fat accrual by suppressing dietary fat oxidation rather than by conversion of carbohydrates into fats. (CHO, carbohydrate; DNL, de novo lipogenesis; HGP, hepatic glucose production; ox, oxidation; INS, insulin.) "?" refers to signal of surplus CHO in organism (not proven, but likely an increase in hepatic glycogen stores).

In contrast, intake of surplus dietary fat has essentially no impact on whole-body fuel selection or almost any other short-term hormonal or metabolic measures. Dietary fat is "invisible" in the short term; there are no metabolic mechanisms for sensing or adjusting expenditures in response to changes in intake of fat. As a result, dietary fat can be stored without inducing any short-term counterresponse in whole-body substrate oxidation.

There is also evidence from animal studies that tissue carbohydrate stores may exert feedback effects on appetite over the short term as part of the mechanism for maintaining whole-body carbohydrate stores. If that is true, factors that promote carbohydrate oxidation will tend to stimulate food intake until tissue glycogen stores are restored. Some investigators have proposed that appetite-modulating effects of tissue carbohydrate stores may explain the lower energy intakes typically observed on high-carbohydrate, low-fat diets (see below).

These fundamental differences in fuel metabolism and storage between carbohydrates and fats may go a long way toward explaining our susceptibility to storage of fat in the body, especially when challenged by increased dietary fat intake. Carbohydrate stores are regulated tightly, while fat stores are not.

C. Oxidation Hierarchy and Competition

Carbohydrates and fats compete for tissue oxidation. Fat oxidation generates products (NADH, acetyl-CoA, ATP) that inhibit glucose uptake, glycolysis, and oxidation of pyruvate in muscle and liver (the Randle effect, or glucose-fatty acid cycle). In the other direction, carbohydrate utilization generates products (malonyl-CoA, α-glycerophosphate, oxaloacetate, citrate) that inhibit fatty acyl-CoA transport into mitochondria, stimulate their reesterification to triglycerides in the cytosol, inhibit ketogenesis from acetyl-CoA, and activate de novo lipogenesis. Carbohydrate utilization thereby inhibits fatty acid oxidation. Interestingly, carbohydrate oxidation tends to win out over fat oxidation; if both fuels are available (with insulin), the carbohydrate is preferentially oxidized. These biochemical observations are congruent with the physiologic model based on macronutrient pool sizes and metabolic fluxes wherein carbohydrates are predicted to have oxidative priority compared with fats (see above).

D. Absence of a Common Energy Currency

Fats (two-carbon precursors) cannot be converted to carbohydrates (three- to six-carbon compounds) because the required enzymes of the glyoxylate shunt do not exist in animals. A functional block also appears to exist under most conditions from carbohydrates to fats (ie, de novo lipogenesis is a pathway only used as a last-resort), as discussed above.

Because metabolic interconversion between energy macronutrients is neither free-flowing nor symmetric, it is therefore misleading to discuss a common "energy" currency. Instead, independent macronutrient systems exist in the body's energy economy, and it is inaccurate to discuss "energy intake" or "energy balance" as though there were a common energy currency in the body. It is more accurate physiologically to consider carbohydrates and fats as independent—though interacting—currencies. These considerations have led to the notion of "macronutrient" balances. According to this model, we should do our accounting of fat and carbohydrate balances separately.

E. Stability Factors

The energy balance equation is dynamic, not static, and this may explain why there is long-term relative stability of body weight and fat stores.

One of the key points about energy balance and weight that is not generally appreciated is that most people do not continuously and relentlessly gain or lose weight. Over the long term, there tends to be relative stability of body weight and body fat stores in most individuals, at least in comparison with the energy throughput of the system. Quantitative estimates make this point clearly. The annual flux of energy through the body (about 1,000,000 kcal/yr) is enormous compared with the typical change in energy content of the body (< 2.5 lb, or 10,000 kcal/yr). This represents an "error" of less than 1% with regard to the balancing of intake and expenditure.

Why is relative weight stability the rule? To answer this question, it is useful to consider what would happen if a person in energy balance simply added a cup of ice cream (500 kcal) every night, and did everything else exactly the same (activity, other food intake). Would the person gain 3500 kcal (almost 0.45 kg) of weight and fat every week for the rest of his life (ie, 227 kg after 10 years)?

The answer is no. The physiologic reason is that weight gain or loss results in increases or decreases, respectively, in total energy expenditure (TEE). Thus, the energy balance system is adaptive (dynamic), not fixed. Moreover, the changes in TEE can be extremely large in response to changes in body weight. It is now well documented that adaptations of TEE to altered body weight are greatly in excess of what would be quantitatively predicted from standard energy costs of tissues calculated in weight-stable humans, whether obese or nonobese. Recent studies in humans by Leibel and colleagues at Rockefeller University make it possible to calculate the consequences on TEE of gaining or losing weight.

If a person gains 10% of body weight by overeating (ie, 7–12 kg in nonobese or obese subjects), about two-thirds of the gain will be as body fat (5–8 kg) and one-third (2–4 kg) as fat-free mass (FFM). FFM is the main determinant of resting energy expenditure (REE; see below) and also affects TEE; the relationship is generally about 45–50 kcal TEE/kg FFM per day both in obese and in nonobese individuals. A 10% weight gain would therefore be expected to increase TEE by 100–200 kcal/d. Conversely, a 10% weight loss consists of about 80% fat and 20% FFM (2–3 kg), so that the expected reduction in TEE would be 100–150 kcal/d (2–3 kg FFM × 50 kcal/kg FFM/d).

But in fact, after stabilization at a 10% weight gain, increases in TEE are much greater than these values. TEE increases by 870 kcal/d (Table 20–3). Accordingly, there is a change in the relationship between TEE and FFM; the ratio increases from 45–50 to 55–60 kcal TEE/kg FFM per d. Carrying the extra weight (or fat) apparently changes the energy costs of all tissues rather than just adding energy costs of new tissue. Change in REE appears to account for only a minority (about 150 kcal/d) of the increased TEE; most of the TEE increase (500–700 kcal/d) relates in some manner to costs of activity.

Conversely, a stable 10% weight loss reduces TEE by 450–550 kcal/d; the relationship between TEE and FFM now falls to about 40 kcal/kg FFM/d (Table 20–3). In this direction, REE accounts for about half of the change in TEE.

The consequences of these changes are profound. If one were to gain 12 kg, he could then eat about 850 kcal/d above his previous intake level and maintain a new stable weight (at the expense of higher weight and fatness). Put differently, if one chose to eat 850 kcal/d above his current intake, he would likely gain about 12 kg and stop there because a new balance between intake and TEE would be reached.

In the other direction, if one were to lose about 17 kg, he then would need to eat about 550 kcal/d less than current intake to maintain this new weight indefinitely. A dieting individual who chooses to reduce the intake by 550 kcal would lose about 17 kg and stop there.

Weight stabilization is therefore reestablished even in the face of permanent changes on the intake side of the balance equation. This has a resemblance to a long feedback loop. An example of this feedback loop has been reported by Ravussin and colleagues, who found that low REE is the best predictor of subsequent long-term weight gain in young Pima Indians. However, REE (and TEE) increase when weight is gained by these individuals, which results in achievement of a new state of energy equilibrium. Thus, the thermogenesis due to weight gain ultimately balances the initial energy surplus relative to TEE.

From this perspective, obesity is the "solution" adopted by the nutrient system for reestablishing balance when faced with surplus fat or energy. Again, weight gain may be seen as a kind of long feedback loop that compensates for baseline deficiencies in TEE or appetite regulation.

Table 20–3. Adaptive nature of energy expenditure in response to weight gain or loss.

Change	Weight (kg)	FFM (kg)	Fat (kg)	kcal TEE ÷ kg FFM	TEE (kcal/d)	Δ TEE (kcal/d)
Weight gain						
Obese						
Basal	131	63	68	51	3160	...
10% gain	143	67	76	59	4030	+870
Nonobese						
Basal	66	54	12	47	2480	...
10% gain	73	56	17	54	3110	+630
Weight loss						
Obese						
Basal	132	64	68	50	3100	...
10% loss	115	60	55	42	2550	−550
Nonobese						
Basal	71	53	18	45	2380	...
10% loss	64	51	13	39	1950	−430

FFM = Fat-free mass.
TEE = Total energy expenditure.

F. FACTORS RELATED TO CONTROL OF BODY FAT STORES

The three determinants of body fat stores—intake, expenditure, and nutrient partitioning—are each under complex control (Figures 20–1, 20–4 and 20–5). A few interesting features are worth emphasizing here.

1. Appetite control pathways—Some of the hypothalamic nuclei involved in control of ingestive behavior are shown in Figure 20–5. Like most complex adaptive networks, interference with one pathway tends to induce compensatory changes in alternative or redundant pathways. This redundancy and network-like structure of the neurobiology of appetite control may in part explain difficulties in maintaining efficacy of some anorexigenic agents over the long term.

2. Nutrient partitioning—Two points that are generally not appreciated regarding the role of macronutrient partitioning deserve to be emphasized. First is the role that muscle protein anabolic capacity can play in determining body fatness. Differences in the capacity to in-

crease the mass of muscle tissue (muscle is normally the largest organ in the mammalian body, representing 40–45% of body weight) may underlie differences in the amount of fat tissue accrued under conditions of nutrient surplus (ie, spillover into fat stores may occur if lean tissue anabolism is blocked). Also, as discussed above, muscle tissue per se represents a calorigenic factor. Genetics, hormones, exercise, and other regulators of muscle metabolism may therefore play an important role in the pathogenesis of obesity.

A second interesting relationship is that observed between insulin resistance and body composition. It is widely appreciated that insulin resistance syndromes generally occur in association with overweight and excess adiposity. The impact of insulin resistance on body weight and macronutrient balance is less often considered. In Pima Indians of the Southwestern United States, resistance of peripheral tissues to insulin-mediated glucose uptake predicts *lower* subsequent body-fat stores and less weight gain. A physiologic explanation is that peripheral insulin resistance increases lipolysis while reduc-

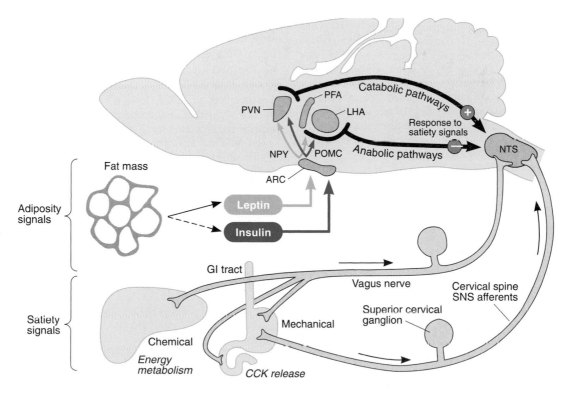

Figure 20–5. Schematic of appetite regulatory pathways in humans. (PVN, paraventricular nucleus; ARC, arcuate nucleus; PFA, prefornical area; LHA, lateral hypothalamic area; NTS, nucleus of tractus solitarius; SNS, sympathetic nervous system; CCK, cholecystokinin; POMC, pro-opiomelanocortin; NPY, neuropeptide Y.)
(Modified, with permission, from Schwartz MW et al: Central nervous system control of food intake. Nature 2000;404:661.)

ing glucose oxidation; the result favors fat oxidation. The interesting implication here is that peripheral insulin resistance, occurring in association with obesity, may represent another long-loop feedback system to allow oxidation of the surplus fat that previously could not be oxidized. Similar to the increases in REE, peripheral insulin resistance may represent a long-term physiologic "solution" to the problem of macronutrient imbalance for fats. As discussed above, both of these long-term adaptations for achieving whole-body fat balance are necessary because no short-term control system exists for dietary or body fat. Of course, the adverse health consequences of insulin resistance (diabetes, hyperlipidemia, etc) may make this adaptation a poor biologic decision—from the health perspective—in modern society.

The consequences of hepatic insulin resistance on body weight are quite different from those of peripheral tissue (muscle and fat) insulin resistance. Increased hepatic glucose production and resulting hyperinsulinemia suppress whole-body fat oxidation and predict weight gain (see above).

3. Energy expenditure—The major determinant of REE is FFM. Thus, "the lean stay lean" on the one hand, and anything that leads to increased metabolically active (lean) tissue will allow equilibration of body weight to be reached at higher levels of energy intake. Moreover, TEE increases out of proportion to changes in FFM when body weight is gained (see above). The net effect is to dampen the effect of any changes in energy intake on body weight, as just discussed.

G. Factors Related to the Organ of Energy Storage

Adipocytes, the storage cells for surplus energy in the body, have their own internal metabolic control systems that can affect the whole-body macronutrient economy.

Body fat stores are influenced by the number and the size (lipid content) of fat cells. Early studies suggested that the number of fat cells was fixed after early childhood and that subsequent gains in adipose mass must reflect increases in fat cell size. This is no longer believed to be true, however; adult humans have preadipocytes and the capacity to form new fat cells. However, the actual extent to which adipocytes differentiate and proliferate from precursors in adults remains unknown. Adipocyte lipogenesis, lipolysis, and avidity for uptake of fatty acids from circulating triglycerides can also influence the systemic availability and balances of lipids. Activity of the intravascular enzyme lipoprotein lipase in adipose tissue relative to muscle also may affect the proportion of fats that are stored or oxidized. The specific effects of these processes on clinical obesity have not been established.

The health risks of obesity are also modulated by the distribution of body fat. Compared with peripheral obesity ("pear-shaped"), midline or truncal obesity ("apple-shaped") is associated with greater health risks. Visceral fat stores are believed to be more lipolytically active and have greater potential to impact liver metabolism given that their venous drainage flows directly to the liver. Visceral obesity is an important predictor of abnormal plasma lipoprotein concentrations; individuals with truncal obesity have higher lipoprotein and triglyceride production rates and elevations in postprandial lipemia. Even a small amount of weight loss may have a dramatic health benefit if it occurs in the abdominal region (see Chapter 19).

CONTROVERSIES & UNCERTAINTIES REGARDING THE PATHOGENESIS OF OBESITY

A number of controversies or unresolved questions pertaining to these matters deserve comment.

Genes Versus Environment

Estimates of genetic heritability have ranged from 20% to as high as 80%. There is no doubt that genetic factors predispose individuals toward different body composition. Many authors have taken this to mean that obesity is a genetic disease and that body fat content is a quantitative genetic trait. Yet the notion that obesity is a genetic disorder—even a complex genetic disorder—is misleading in important ways. This becomes apparent from consideration of a few facts.

(1) The prevalence of obesity has increased markedly worldwide in recent years, yet genes have not changed. Obviously, environmental factors explain population changes that have occurred.

(2) The Pima Indians who live on reservations in Arizona have the highest known prevalence of obesity and diabetes in the world. But their genetic "cousins" living in the mountains of Mexico have almost no obesity.

(3) Variability exists between populations—not only among individuals—and changes occur within populations when migration occurs.

A resolution of these observations is that the phenotypic expression of genes for obesity are environment-specific—ie, obesity is a disorder of the interaction between genes and environment.

Intake Versus Expenditure

The best predictors of future risk for obesity have been on the expenditure side rather than the intake side of the energy balance equation. For example, hours of television watched per day predicts subsequent weight gain in children, and low REE predicts weight gain in Pima Indians. The relation between weight gain and secondary increases in TEE suggests that interventions to increase TEE independent of weight gain could allow energy equilibration on higher caloric intakes at nonobese body weights. Indeed, the more effective weight control strategies have acted to increase TEE (eg, exercise, nicotine, amphetamines; see below). In contrast, most treatment strategies aimed at controlling food intake have proved difficult to sustain. The role of diet in preventing weight gain cannot be ignored, however; in prospective studies, dietary fat intake predicts weight gain in children and adolescents.

Body Fat "Set-Point" Versus "Settling Point"

A subtle but important debate relates to the explanation for the relative weight stability generally present in people. Does this stability imply an active servomechanism (a system that actively resists changes in body weight), or can it be explained on a passive basis? Do the changes in TEE and fat oxidation observed when people gain or lose weight reflect a hormonally or neurally directed response to restore body composition toward a sensed and regulated value? Or do these energetic changes simply reflect intrinsic physiologic costs and efficiencies of the body?

This philosophic debate has importance for the way we think about interventions. If the entire nutrient balance system is fighting our therapeutic attempts at weight loss and avidly defending an overweight person's current body fatness, the situation is indeed bleak. If, on the other hand, all that is needed is a few adjustments in the system parameters (TEE, etc) to achieve a new settling point, the implication is quite different. Unfortunately, the answer remains controversial.

Some authors have questioned whether the assumption of short-term weight stability is accurate in the first place. Many animals exhibit cyclic weight changes in parallel with seasonal availability of food. Under these conditions, the nutrient balance system might well be programmed to alternate between fat anabolic and fat catabolic modes rather than defending a certain body fatness consistently. If humans are like this, then relatively small signals of food availability might induce physiologic programs of weight gain or loss that are currently unrecognized. This interesting perspective deserves further consideration.

New Guidelines (Dietary Reference Intakes)

In 2002, new recommendations were established by the Food and Nutrition Board of the National Academy of Science's Institute of Medicine. The revised guidelines, called the Dietary Reference Intakes (DRIs) for Macronutrients, were designed to promote diets that minimize chronic disease risk. The guidelines state that adults should obtain 45–65% of their daily energy intake (calories) from carbohydrates, 10–35% from protein, and 20–35% from fat. This latter recommendation for fat reflects the changing focus of national dietary advice from previous recommendations of less than 30% of energy from fat to the current recommendations that allow more flexibility in the mix of macronutrients.

The report recommends a minimum intake of carbohydrates (at least 130 g per day, an amount chosen to ensure enough glucose for brain metabolism). The report also advises that "added" sugars (those incorporated into foods and beverages during their production) should not represent more than 25% of total energy. The recommendation of an upper level of intake of sugars is based in part on evidence that people whose diets were high in added sugars had lower intakes of essential nutrients. Moreover, overconsumption of carbohydrates leads to elevations in body weight, though not through fat synthesis (as mentioned above). Rather, overconsumption of carbohydrate can lead to an accumulation of body weight by displacing stored fat that would usually be burned. The new DRIs recognize that overconsumption of carbohydrate, fat, or protein can lead to increased body weight. Diets that focus on delivering the primary source of energy from only one macronutrient therefore have limitations.

Lower-fat, higher-carbohydrate diets have been associated with elevations in blood triglycerides and reductions in HDL cholesterol, typically associated with lower LDL cholesterol levels. Although the atherogenicity of this lipid profile remains uncertain, there is suspicion that these diets will contribute to heart disease development. Furthermore, the consumption of sugars in a single meal may lead to return of hunger sooner than after consumption of a mixed meal. By contrast, the benefits of diets higher in complex carbohydrates may include increased micronutrient intake and an increased fiber intake, the latter of which is associated with several health benefits related to the gastrointestinal tract. Diets high in complex carbohydrates can also provide greater satiety. The vast majority of individuals in the National Weight Control Registry (a national survey of individuals who have lost 30 lb [13.6 kg] and have maintained that loss for at least 1 year) report that they consume low-fat, high-carbohydrate diets to help them manage their weight, in addition to participating in voluntary exercise activities of about 400 kcal/d (3000 kcal/wk; see below).

Diets higher in fat (> 30% energy) are associated with a higher incidence of obesity in many population studies. Furthermore, unless careful attention is paid to the type of fat, higher-fat diets can contain large amounts of saturated and trans fatty acids (the latter found in partially hydrogenated vegetable oils). Because these fats raise blood cholesterol concentrations, the new DRIs continue to focus on the avoidance of saturated fat. On the other hand, some benefits of higher-fat diets have been observed when the primary fats consumed are monounsaturated. LDL cholesterol can be lowered by these diets, while HDL cholesterol is not lowered. For some individuals, higher-fat diets can also be more satisfying even when calories are restricted, thereby helping attempts at weight loss.

Higher-protein diets (> 25% of energy) can also have some undesirable effects. These diets can be virtually devoid of fiber and, with their low content of carbohydrate, are also low in water content, leading to constipation. In addition, higher-protein foods also tend to be high in saturated fat and cholesterol. Lastly, there is some concern that higher-protein diets might increase the filtration load on the kidney and promote the development of renal disease as well as increasing urinary calcium losses and contributing to osteoporosis. The benefits of diets higher in protein have only recently been investigated. It is likely that high-protein diets do result in an increased sense of satiety, thereby leading to a reduction in food intake and to weight loss, perhaps without induction of the hypertriglyceridemia associated with high-carbohydrate and low-fat diets.

The new DRIs recognize that different diet strategies work for different people and are therefore more flexible than previous recommendations regarding macronutrient intake for individuals trying to lose weight and those attempting to maintain their body weight. The new guidelines also focus on the importance of balancing diet with exercise, advocating at least an hour a day of moderate physical activity.

■ SURVEY OF TREATMENT APPROACHES & THEIR EFFICACY

DIETARY THERAPIES

Caloric Intake Restriction

Dietary and behavioral therapy—in particular, the prescription of a hypocaloric diet—has been the mainstay of obesity treatment for the past 40 years. Caloric restriction alone has unfortunately been a generally ineffective approach. The use of very-low-calorie diets (800 kcal/d)

in individuals with BMI > 30 can produce an initial weight loss of about 2 kg/wk, and an average total weight loss of 20 kg after 4 months. However, medical supervision is critical because the loss of electrolytes can be substantial. Intake of at least 1 g/kg of ideal body weight per day of protein of high biologic value is important in preserving lean body mass. After going off the very-low-calorie diet, maintaining the weight loss has proved to be difficult, particularly if patient education has not been incorporated into the therapy. Part of the recidivism may be attributable to the physiologic and behavioral adaptations that occur in response to energy deprivation, including reduced energy expenditure (as discussed above). The behavioral consequences of semistarvation may also play a role in recidivism—eg, fatigue, malaise, and loss of motivation. It simply may not be possible for most people to persist indefinitely in a state of perceived deprivation, particularly when stresses of life arise (as they always do). Programs which are more structured and combine diet (energy restriction to 1200–1800 kcal/d), exercise, and behavioral therapy may have greater success, though the efficacy of these programs is also debated. Programs of this type can produce weight losses in the range of 9–14 kg over 5–6 months, with attrition as low as 20–24%. Average weight losses of 9–10% have been the rule, with about 60–80% maintenance of weight loss after 1 year. Although most participants regain weight after leaving these programs, the amount regained after 1–2 years is frequently less than the original weight loss. The major problem relates to longer-term follow-up. Data are much scarcer for more than 3-year follow-up, but the data that exist suggest almost 100% relapse after 3–5 years. A recent study through the National Weight Control Registry has identified a large number of individuals who have successfully maintained weight loss. The most common features identified among these individuals is voluntary activity of about 3000 kcal per week (ie, 400–450 kcal of daily exercise) and a low-fat diet. It is hoped that the attributes of programs that help individuals lose weight and the characteristics of those who successfully keep weight off will help in the design of future programs incorporating energy restriction. It must be recognized, however, that net benefits to health or longevity have yet to be proved from weight loss diets and that the vast majority of participants regain the great majority of their weight when followed for 3–5 years.

Fat Absorption Inhibitors

Orlistat is a drug that reduces fat absorption by blocking pancreatic lipase in the intestine. In a clinical trial, patients lost 10% of initial body weight after 1 year of use on a 30% fat diet. The major side effect is "intestinal leakage" or fecal fat loss, which can be controlled in patients who combine this drug with the consumption of a reduced fat (35% of energy) diet. The long-term efficacy and safety of fat absorption inhibitors has yet to be determined.

Altered Macronutrient Composition of Diet

A. LOW-FAT DIETS

Interestingly, the one dietary prescription that has most consistently resulted in long-term weight loss is to change the macronutrient composition (to a lower percentage of fat) rather than the total energy content of the diet. Individuals who switch to diets containing less than 25% fat for reasons other than weight loss (eg, to reduce dietary cholesterol and saturated fats or to reduce cancer risk) experience on average a 2–3 kg weight loss over the first 2-month period. For example, in a large study in nurses of the effects of dietary fat restriction on breast cancer risk, randomization into the low-fat arm (without directives to lose weight) resulted in an average > 4 kg weight loss. Many other high-carbohydrate, low-fat diet studies have confirmed these observations. Potential explanations for weight loss include reduced total energy intake due to the feeling of fullness related to the bulk of low-fat, high-fiber diets or due to their lack of palatability; or metabolic explanations related to satiety effects of body glycogen stores. Epidemiologic correlations between fat content of diet and adiposity in populations indirectly support—but do not prove—the importance of macronutrient composition of diet.

B. LOW-CARBOHYDRATE DIETS

Conversely, diets that restrict carbohydrate have enjoyed cyclic popularity according to a variety of theories promoted in the popular weight loss literature. The "Zone diet" and "carbohydrate busters" are examples. The long-term efficacy of these dietary approaches has never been demonstrated. As discussed in detail above, the underlying principle of these diets runs against most of what we know about the physiology and regulation of energy and macronutrient balances. More importantly, numerous studies have shown the opposite effects—namely, that high-carbohydrate, low-fat diets result in weight loss, not weight gain, for most participants. Despite the lack of compelling physiologic or empirical evidence in favor of low-carbohydrate diets, new examples of this class of therapy are continually arising. Some people may achieve at least a temporary weight loss from this (or any) diet due to the motivational effects of participating in a program that is based on a "theory." Also, restriction of carbohydrate and bulk may lessen postprandial lethargy and improve

subjective sense of well-being and alertness in some individuals—or it may simply restrict the universe of food choices available to a person, which may promote compliance with a program of caloric restriction.

SURGICAL TREATMENT OF OBESITY

The surgical management of morbid obesity has continued as a treatment option since jejunoileal bypass was developed in the 1950s. A wide variety of techniques are used, but all impose a risk of serious complications. Intraoperative complications, risks of anesthesia, and postoperative problems (sepsis, bacterial contamination of a blind loop, development of fatty liver and cirrhosis) are all concerns. Both early and long-term weight reductions have generally been satisfactory. The risks associated with these procedures must be balanced in morbid obesity against the limited number of other treatments available and the frequently life-threatening conditions (described above) that may develop in individuals who have suffered with the condition for many years.

PHARMACOLOGIC THERAPIES

Appetite Suppressant Drugs

The most widely prescribed drugs for treatment of obesity have been appetite-suppressant agents. Several classes have been used, including serotonin agonists, sympathomimetics, and, recently, leptin. Studies using these agents have also revealed high recidivism rates after discontinuation of medications. Sibutramine, a serotonin uptake inhibitor, is currently the only drug in this class approved for long-term use. In a recent study, patients who had lost at least 6 kg over a 4-week period on a very-low-calorie diet were then randomized to sibutramine or placebo for 1 year. With continued dietary counseling in both groups, patients who took sibutramine lost significantly more weight (4.9 kg versus 0.45 kg, in the drug-treated and control groups, respectively). At month 12, about 75% of subjects in the sibutramine group maintained at least the same degree of the weight loss achieved with a very-low-calorie diet, compared with 42% in the placebo group.

Because most clinicians are wary of indefinite use of drug therapy in this presumably lifelong disorder, use of anorexiants fell out of favor many years ago in the medical mainstream. A change in philosophy seemed to be evolving in the mid 1990s with the long-term administration of a combination anorexigenic formulation (fenfluramine and phentermine, or "Fen-Phen"). A study of 81 patients treated with this regimen for several years showed long-term efficacy with maintenance of weight loss. Subsequently, the well-publicized reports of a serious adverse effect (heart valve thickening) rapidly led to the withdrawal of fenfluramine from the United States market. Skepticism about use of anorexiants has since resurfaced.

Thermogenic Agents

Thermogenic agents represent a theoretically attractive approach, particularly if low REE predicts subsequent development of obesity and if weight gain itself serves as a way of increasing TEE and fat oxidation to match intake. Several classes of thermogenic agents have been tested.

A. Thyroid Hormone

Thyroid hormone is calorigenic. Indeed, thyroid status used to be assessed (before the development of specific blood assays) longitudinally by following REE. In addition, short-term energy restriction results in striking reductions in serum triiodothyronine (T_3) and thyroid stimulating hormone (TSH)—often called the "euthyroid sick syndrome"—accompanied by reduction in REE of up to 15–20%. Because weight loss tends to slow after the initial days or weeks of energy restriction, preventing this reduced REE by administration of T_3 represented an obvious strategy. Many clinicians and investigators have given T_3 or T_4 as an adjunct to hypocaloric diet therapy. The results are unequivocal and, unfortunately, negative: restoration of serum T_3 to normal or supraphysiologic levels during hypocaloric diets results in no extra loss of fat but greater losses of lean body mass and a more negative nitrogen balance. Thus, the response of the hypothalamic-pituitary-thyroid-tissue axis to energy deficiency is an essential part of the nitrogen preserving response to starvation. Extra weight loss may impress clinicians or patients during coadministration of thyroid hormone, but this in fact is exactly contrary to the goals of obesity therapy. Thyroid replacement therapy is contraindicated in combination with energy-restricted diets.

B. β₃-Adrenergic Receptor Agonists

Adipose tissue expresses an atypical β-adrenergic receptor (ie, in addition to the usual β_1 and β_2 receptors), which has been called the β_3-adrenergic receptor. The tissue distribution of the β_3-adrenergic receptor in humans remains uncertain, but most expression appears to be in adipocytes. Expression is particularly prominent in brown adipose tissue in animals such as rodents that maintain large stores of brown fat, but β_3 receptors are also expressed in white adipose tissue. Interest in the β_3 receptor has focused on its potential role in adrenergic stimulation of lipolysis (in white adipose tissue) and thermogenesis (in brown adipose tissue). Because β_3-selective adrenergic receptor agonists exhibit minimal cross-reactivity with β_1 and β_2 receptors, the β_3 pathway has received considerable attention as a possible therapeutic candidate. Several pharmaceutical companies have developed selective β_3-receptor agonists toward this end. This approach has been further motivated by epidemiologic associations between mutations in the β_3 receptor gene and the development of obesity and diabetes mellitus (eg, in Pima Indians and in populations in Finland and France).

Despite these promising features, there are currently no approved β_3-adrenergic receptor agonists on the market for the treatment of obesity. Clinical trials performed to date have been disappointing. Side effects have been observed in some studies, including tremor and changes in heart rate or blood pressure. There are few reports of clinical trials with β_3 agonists over the past 5–6 years, and no large-scale randomized studies have been conducted.

C. Sympathomimetic Agents

The sympathetic nervous system is involved in all aspects of the macronutrient economy (see above): food intake (suppressive effect), energy expenditure (increase), and nutrient partitioning (favoring of lean body mass [LBM] over fat stores). Although adrenergic agonists such as amphetamines remain in use for weight loss both over the counter and by prescription, these agents are properly looked at with extreme caution by responsible clinicians. The psychoactive side-effects are significant and not dissociable from peripheral effects; the addictive potential and possibility of abuse cannot be ignored; weight recidivism occurs after cessation of therapy; and adverse medical effects include worsening of hypertension, diabetes, and coronary insufficiency.

It is nevertheless of interest that several of the most common addictive drugs of abuse in the Western world are sympathomimetic agents and, indeed, are associated with lower body weight, lower body fat, and increased REE. By far the most important of these in public health terms is nicotine, the active agent in cigarette smoke. Cigarette smoking is associated with lower body weight (3–5 kg) despite similar or higher food intake and higher REE compared with matched nonsmokers. Cessation of smoking leads to an average 3 kg weight gain, and approximately 10–13% of smokers who quit gain over 13 kg. Metabolic ward studies have confirmed the thermogenic effect of cigarette smoking (about 10–15% increased REE), quantitatively consistent with the relationship described between energy expenditure and body in Table 20–3. Pharmacologic studies have shown that this thermogenic effect operates via nicotine, can be reproduced by administration of nicotine, and depends upon release of adrenal catecholamines (epinephrine) into the circulation. The evidence that nicotine increases REE and effectively lowers body weight in cigarette smokers is convincing.

Though of great interest from the perspective of the macronutrient economy, these actions of nicotine and cigarette smoking have devastating public health consequences. Many smokers maintain the habit because of fear of weight gain after cessation. This is particularly so for young women, nowadays the fastest-growing group of cigarette smokers. The marked increases in lung cancer already reported in women over the past generation will undoubtedly accelerate, along with other correlates of cigarette smoking (eg, coronary artery disease), as an unintended consequence of this widely used over-the-counter weight-managing strategy. Indeed, the strongest health argument against the contemporary obsession about slimness, particularly in women, may well be the high rates of cigarette smoking that it promotes.

Another addictive drug with sympathomimetic actions and profound weight-reducing actions is cocaine. Inhaled crack cocaine has unmistakable weight reducing effects.

D. Leptin

Administration of recombinant leptin (the ob gene product) increases TEE and activates the sympathetic nervous system in ob/ob mice—in addition to reducing food intake. The net effect of leptin administration is reduction of adiposity in this leptin-deficient animal model. Clinical trials with recombinant leptin in humans have been equivocal. Administration of extremely high doses of leptin subcutaneously in combination with dietary energy restriction resulted in 7.3 kg lost after 6 months of treatment, compared with 1.4 kg weight loss in the placebo plus energy restriction group. Weight loss was greater than in the placebo group only for the highest dose of leptin (0.3 mg/kg/d), however, which resulted in serum leptin concentrations of 500–600 ng/mL—compared with baseline values in the range of 15–20 ng/mL. Weight loss in the group treated with 0.1 mg leptin/kg/d was not significantly different from placebo despite serum leptin levels in the 200–250 ng/mL range. The long-term metabolic and general health consequences of activation of the sympathetic nervous system by massively supraphysiologic leptin levels remains unknown. Experience with other sympathetic nervous system activators (discussed above) provides ample reason for caution.

The most useful setting for leptin therapy may not prove to be conditions of idiopathic obesity but states of frank leptin deficiency due either to inadequate fat stores or genetic defects in leptin production. Lipoatrophic states such as occur genetically or in HIV/AIDS may benefit from leptin administration by improving insulin sensitivity and lipoprotein concentrations. Ex-

tremely rare individuals with congenital leptin deficiency (who present clinically with massive obesity and hyperphagia in early childhood) also benefit from administration of recombinant leptin.

E. Exercise

Though strictly speaking not a pharmacologic intervention, exercise may be the most effective prescription for weight loss. Meta-analysis has evaluated the effects of exercise training on FFM preservation during diet-induced weight loss. In individuals whose weight loss regimen included diet only, 28% of the weight lost was made up of FFM, while for those who exercised in addition to dieting, only 13% of the weight lost was made up of FFM. When combined with reduced energy intake, exercise increases the amount of weight loss above that achieved by diet alone—in addition to preserving muscle mass. Most importantly, exercise increases the likelihood of sustaining the weight loss over a longer period of time. For these reasons, programs aimed at reducing body weight must include an exercise component.

An interesting but relatively poorly understood area of energy expenditure relates to involuntary activity, or "fidgeting." Differences in involuntary motor activity clearly exist within populations and could contribute to differences in energy expenditure. Some studies attempting to add up all the recognized components of total energy expenditure (eg, REE, thermic effect of food, measurable activity, thermic effect of exercise) have reported a consistent shortfall compared with measured 24-hour total energy expenditure. This shortfall also differs between lean and obese groups. This unmeasured energy expenditure has been attributed to "fidgeting" by some investigators. It has been difficult to quantify the energy costs of involuntary activity directly, however. The factors potentially controlling involuntary activity (eg, behavioral, hormonal, neuromuscular) are also uncertain. Nevertheless, this area represents a potentially important and generally overlooked aspect of whole-body energetics.

Nutrient Partitioning Agents

Perhaps the least-appreciated treatment strategy for obesity is to change body composition (increase lean tissue) without explicitly attempting to induce negative energy or fat balance. Though counterintuitive on the surface, this strategy has a solid rational basis and may prove an effective general approach.

The rationale is that the major determinant of REE is lean body mass (see above). Accordingly, anything that increases lean tissue will increase REE—by at least 50 kcal/kg/d. Muscle anabolic agents therefore act indirectly as whole body thermogenic agents. Consistent with this model are reports of extremely high TEE in bodybuilders (eg, > 4000 kcal/d) out of proportion to the calculated energy expended during their weight lifting activities per se.

Several agents are known to be anabolic for lean tissue.

A. ANDROGENS

Androgen administration to hypogonadal adult men, prepubertal boys, or women results in nitrogen retention and gains in lean tissue, including muscle. Energy expenditure increases in proportion to lean tissue accrual. Effects on body fat stores are inconsistent; either reductions or increases (with android or abdominal distribution) may be observed depending upon energy intake.

B. GROWTH HORMONE

Growth hormone administration at pharmacologic doses to adults increases LBM, stimulates lipolysis and fat oxidation, and reduces body fat stores. These effects have been reported for recombinant growth hormone in a variety of clinical settings, including wasting disorders such as AIDS and in the elderly. REE increases in proportion to FFM. Some investigators in Europe have reported that recombinant-growth hormone reduces abdominal obesity when given for 6–12 months and improves certain metabolic correlates of visceral adiposity. However, the extremely high cost of recombinant-growth hormone, along with concerns that it might directly worsen insulin resistance and hypertriglyceridemia, have to date held back widespread use of this agent for the treatment of obesity.

C. RESISTANCE EXERCISE

Aerobic, energy-utilizing exercise is usually recommended for therapeutic weight loss. As discussed above, resistance exercise programs (weight lifting) aimed at accrual of muscle (LBM) may also be useful for the indirect stimulation of thermogenesis. Prescription of supervised progressive resistance exercise in AIDS patients, for example, results in considerable gains in LBM with proportionate increases in REE and some loss (2 kg) of body fat. Combination of resistance exercise with modestly supraphysiologic androgen therapy further increases LBM gains and REE but worsens HDL cholesterol and may have other adverse effects.

"Alternative" Therapies

Some therapies reported in the lay press have achieved widespread use and therefore deserve comment.

A. CHROMIUM SUPPLEMENTATION

Chromium is the second most widely used mineral supplement in the United States (after calcium). The claims for chromium have included "fat burning," "muscle building," and antihyperglycemic and hypolipidemic actions. Although some evidence exists suggesting a beneficial effect of chromium picolinate on hyperglycemia in patients with type 2 diabetes mellitus, properly controlled trials of chromium administration have failed to show any reductions in body fat or body weight or any gains in LBM. Nor does there exist any solid biochemical or endocrinologic rationale why chromium might promote fat loss or fat oxidation. Use of chromium supplements to alter body composition currently has no evidentiary basis.

B. HERBAL EPHEDRINE

The use of a Chinese "herbal fen/phen" has come into practice. These products, which contain ephedra, are marketed as "natural" tonics for weight loss, muscle building, and energy enhancement. Ephedrine alkaloids are powerful stimulants of the heart and nervous system and may be even more dangerous because the herbals can be impure. Medical complications of herbal ephedrine use are well documented.

■ OTHER CONDITIONS AFFECTED BY TREATMENT OF OBESITY OR OVERWEIGHT

TYPE 2 DIABETES MELLITUS

Diet therapy, consisting primarily of weight loss prescription (hypocaloric diet) plus counting of "carbohydrate exchanges," is widely considered to be first-line therapy for type 2 diabetes mellitus. Remarkably, most clinical and experimental data suggest that neither weight loss itself nor changes in body composition are the agents by which energy-restricted diets lower blood glucose in this disease. Short-term severe caloric restriction (to 600–800 kcal/d for 2–5 days) effectively reduces hyperglycemia (as well as hyperlipidemia) in obese type 2 diabetic patients, with only minor changes in body composition. Most of the response to weight loss diets in type 2 diabetes occurs within the first 2.3 kg; indeed, if glycemia has not improved within 2.3–4.6 kg, there is unlikely to be a response to further weight loss (a useful fact when managing diabetic patients). The short-term response to severe caloric restriction is initially mediated by reduced hepatic glucose production, which appears to be due entirely to a reduced glycogenolytic contribution. Thus, most of the beneficial effects on glycemia of hypocaloric diets appear to be attributable to a starvation effect (ie, liver glycogen depletion) rather than to a reduction in body

Table 20–4. Pathways to fat accrual as guide to therapeutic interventions.

Pathway	Intervention	Comments
Altered energy expenditure		
Low TEE		
Sedentary lifestyle	↑ Voluntary activity (exercise, daily life activities)	Best correlate of weight maintenance; only way to "eat again"
Low FFM (metabolizing tissue)	↑ Lean tissue anabolism (resistance exercise, hormones)	Not systematically tested; improved fitness as an independent health benefit?
Low sympathetic nervous system activity	Sympathomimetic drugs (β_3-adrenergic receptor agonists, leptin, nicotine?)	Basis of most therapeutic agents (prescription and OTC, including nicotine, amphetamines)
Thyroid or leptin deficiency	Replacement therapy	Rare (but effective if truly replacement therapy)
Low "fidgeting" factor	??	Unexplored etiologic factor
Impaired fat oxidation		
Dietary carbohydrate surplus	Carbohydrate restriction (especially energy-dense sweets)	Two-edged sword (if increased fat intake takes its place)
Primary high respiratory quotient (impaired fat oxidization)	Prolongation of overnight fast with or without exercise to burn fat	Strong predictor, but an unexplored therapeutic option
Endogenous carbohydrate availability (↑ HGP)	?Inhibitors of HGP (metformin)	Effective in certain conditions (type 2 diabetes mellitus, HIV-related lipodystrophy)
Altered nutrient partitioning		
Impaired muscle anabolism		
Lack of muscle contraction (exercise)	Resistance exercise	Effective (↑ FFM, ↑ REE, ↓ fat)
Androgen deficiency	Replacement therapy	Effective (↑ FFM, ↑ REE, ↓ fat)
Glucocorticoid excess (endogenous, exogenous)	Normalize	Effective (improves FFM:fat)
Altered adipocyte metabolism		
Impaired fat mobilization (lipolysis)	?Lipolytic agents (rGH, β_3, nicotine?)	Unclear role or effect on fuel selection
Increased de novo lipogenesis	Hydroxycitrate (inhibitor of lipogenesis)	Doubtful in theory (insignificant role of de novo lipogenesis) and practice (toxicities)
Excess energy intake		
Disordered appetite system		
Primary alteration in satiety or hunger	Diet therapy and training?; change in macronutrient selection	Generally ineffective (except if it reduces dietary fat content)
Depression or anxiety	Psychologic or pharmacologic therapy	Some antidepressant drugs reduce weight, some increase weight
Sensitivity to food cues	Diet training; less exposure (eg, to television)	Efficacy unproven
Dietary factors		
High-fat, low-satiety diets	Reduce fat, increase bulk, etc	Effective in population studies (reduces weight)
High sweet, energy-dense diets	Reduce simple sugars	?Efficacy (often replaced with fat)

TEE = Total energy expenditure.
HGP = Hepatic glucose production.
β_3 = β_3-adrenergic receptor agonists.
rGH = Recombinant growth hormone.
FFM = Fat-free mass.
REE = Resting energy expenditure.
OTC = Over-the-counter.

fat stores. The clinical implications of these remarkable physiologic observations have not been fully explored. Some clinicians have considered alternative diet strategies (eg, fasting 1 day per week), but published studies showing efficacy of such an approach are lacking.

Similarly, glycemic improvements in response to exercise programs have been reported without weight loss in type 2 diabetic patients. The implication here, as well, is that body weight and body fat are not the true outcome measures or treatment goals of diet therapy for obese type 2 diabetic patients.

HYPERLIPIDEMIA

Low-fat diets are a cornerstone of treatment for most forms of hyperlipidemia. A tension may sometimes arise, however, between optimal prescriptions for reduction of body weight and serum lipids. Low-fat, high-carbohydrate diets tend to promote weight loss (see above), but they also exacerbate hypertriglyceridemia and low-HDL syndromes. Substitution of monounsaturated fats (eg, olive oil) for carbohydrate has been recommended as a way of preventing hypertriglyceridemia on low saturated fat diets but may interfere with the weight-reducing effects of these diets.

POLYCYSTIC OVARIAN SYNDROME

Obesity and insulin resistance are typically present in the chronic estrus or polycystic ovarian syndrome. One hypothesis concerning the connection is that hyperinsulinemia stimulates thecal cell proliferation in the ovary, which results in constitutive steroid hormone synthesis and a loss of menstrual periodicity. Aromatization of adrenal androgens in adipose tissue also represents a postulated mechanism of altered hormone production. Treatments that improve insulin sensitivity—particularly metformin, which acts primarily on the liver to reduce endogenous glucose production and thereby lessens hepatic insulin resistance; or thiazolidinediones, which act on adipose tissue and muscle to stimulate peripheral glucose uptake—have now been shown to improve signs and symptoms of polycystic ovarian syndrome (see Chapter 13).

HYPERTENSION

A close relationship exists between obesity and hypertension, but the mechanisms are unknown. Prescription of a weight loss diet is as effective as prescription of salt-restriction for the long-term management of essential hypertension. More specific guidelines for dietary control of hypertension are needed.

GALLSTONES

Weight loss (or weight gain) can alter the cholesterol saturation and lithogenicity of bile and thereby provoke gallstone formation. Gallstones are common side effects of weight loss programs. Clinicians should be alert to the possibility of biliary tract disease in patients undergoing therapeutic weight loss.

OSTEOARTHRITIS & OTHER WEIGHT-SENSITIVE STATES

There are several conditions for which body weight has strictly mechanical—as opposed to metabolic—conse-

---

Table 20–5. Some unanswered questions regarding body composition and health.

(1) Reasons for increasing prevalence of overweight and obesity?
   Mostly lower TEE? Role of diet composition or total energy intake?
(2) Metabolic mechanisms of adverse health consequences of obesity?
   Fatness versus fitness? Direct consequence of adipose tissue or its products?
(3) Failure to maintain weight loss long-term?
   True "set-point"? Role of leptin? Efficacy of exercise?
(4) Role of long-term drug therapy for weight control?
   Risks and toxicities vs benefits? Long-term efficacy?
(5) Mediators of beneficial response to diet in diabetes, hypertension, hyperlipidemia, etc?
   Reduced adipose mass versus negative energy balance? Other factors, such as leptin?
(6) Role of adipocyte biology in systemic macronutrient balances?
   Role of proliferation, differentiation, and death of adipocytes in adults? Fat cell size versus number? Intrinsic lipolysis and lipogenesis?
(7) Health risks associated with societal obsession with thinness?
   Anorexia nervosa, impaired growth in children, and other syndromes of underweight? Reliance on cigarette smoking and other unhealthy behaviors? Failure to emphasize fitness? Chronic symptoms of semi-starvation? Adverse psychologic and self-image effects?

TEE = Total energy expenditure.

quences (osteoarthritis, low back pain, pulmonary insufficiency, etc). In these states, it is the excess weight itself that must be the treatment goal; metabolic correlates cannot substitute.

■ A SYSTEMATIC APPROACH TO THE TREATMENT OF OBESITY

Systematic consideration of the number of pathways leading to obesity (ie, factors predisposing to body fat accrual; Figure 20–2) represents a useful exercise. Table 20–4 provides a summary of interventions tried—and their efficacy—in response to these different causes. Under the category of reduced TEE, for example, we see that increased voluntary activity has proved effective for weight loss, as have sympathomimetic agents, whereas "fidgeting" remains an unexplored treatment approach. Perusal of the other major categories similarly reveals areas of success, failure, and unexplored approaches.

It is important to recognize areas of uncertainty or ignorance regarding the control of body composition and the treatment of obesity. A number of fundamental questions remain unanswered (Table 20–5).

REFERENCES

Bouchard C, Perusse L: Genetics of obesity. Annu Rev Nutr 1993;13:337. [PMID: 8369150]

Brownell KD, Kramer FM: Behavioral management of obesity. Med Clin North Am 1989;73:185. [PMID: 2643003]

Christiansen MP et al: Effect of dietary energy restriction on glucose production and substrate utilization in type 2 diabetes. Diabetes 2000;49:1691. [PMID: 11016453]

Flatt JP: Dietary fat, carbohydrate balance, and weight maintenance: effects of exercise. Am J Clin Nutr 1987;45(1 Suppl): 296. [PMID: 3799520]

Hellerstein MK: De novo lipogenesis in humans: metabolic and regulatory aspects. Eur J Clin Nutr 1999;53(Suppl 1):S53. [PMID: 10365981]

Klem ML et al: A descriptive study of individuals successful at long-term maintenance of substantial weight loss. Am J Clin Nutr 1997;66:239. [PMID: 9250100]

Leibel RLM et al: Changes in energy expenditure resulting from altered body weight. N Engl J Med 1995;332:621. [PMID: 7632212]

Miller WC: How effective are traditional dietary and exercise interventions for weight loss? Med Sci Sports Exerc 1999;31. 1129. [PMID: 10449014]

Mokdad AH et al: The spread of the obesity epidemic in the United States, 1991-1998. JAMA 1999;282:1519. [PMID: 10546690]

Must AJ et al: The disease burden associated with overweight and obesity. JAMA 1999;282:1523. [PMID: 10546691]

Parks EJ, Hellerstein MK: Carbohydrate-induced hypertriacylglycerolemia: historical perspective and review of biological mechanisms. Am J Clin Nutr 2000;71:412. [PMID: 10648253]

Pi-Sunyer X et al: Executive summary of the clinical guidelines on the identification, evaluation, and treatment of overweight and obesity in adults. Arch Intern Med 1998;71;412. [PMID: 9759681]

Ravussin E, Gautier JF: Metabolic predictors of weight gain. Int J Obes Relat Metab Disord 1999;23(Suppl 1):37. [PMID: 10193860]

Schwarz J-M et al: Short-term alterations in carbohydrate energy intake in humans. Striking effects on hepatic glucose production, de novo lipogenesis, lipolysis, and whole-body fuel selection. J Clin Invest 1995;96:2735. [PMID: 8675642]

Wei M et al: Relationship between low cardiorespiratory fitness and mortality in normal-weight, overweight, and obese men. JAMA 1999;282:1547. [PMID: 10546694]

Weintraub M et al: A double-blind clinical trial in weight control. Use of fenfluramine and phentermine alone and in combination. Arch Intern Med 1984;144:1143. [PMID: 6375610]

Wing RR et al: Caloric restriction per se is a significant factor in improvements in glycemic control and insulin sensitivity during weight loss in obese NIDDM patients. Diabetes Care 1994;17:30. [PMID: 8112186]

Humoral Manifestations of Malignancy

21

Dolores Shoback, MD, & Janet Funk, MD

APUD	Amine precursor uptake and decarboxylation (cell)	**HTLV-1**	Human T cell leukemia virus type 1
CRH	Corticotropin-releasing hormone	**IGF**	Insulin-like growth factor
FGF	Fibroblast growth factor	**POMC**	Proopiomelanocortin
GHRH	Growth hormone-releasing hormone	**PTH**	Parathyroid hormone
hCG	Human chorionic gonadotropin	**PTHrP**	Parathyroid hormone-related protein
		VIP	Vasoactive intestinal peptide

ECTOPIC HORMONE & RECEPTOR SYNDROMES

Some of the most challenging endocrine problems occur in patients with malignancies of diverse cell-types. This is because both endocrine and nonendocrine tumors secrete polypeptide hormones. As it became recognized that a polypeptide hormone could be produced by tumor cells derived from a tissue that normally did not secrete the hormone, the notion of ectopic hormone production developed. Most tumors associated with ectopic hormone syndromes are derived from cells that are normally capable of producing peptide hormones. Initially, it was thought that ectopic hormone production by tumor cells was a rare event. Interestingly, both the frequency and the original conception of this syndrome have been redefined over the last few decades. It has come to be appreciated—through the use of modern biochemical and molecular biologic techniques—that the synthesis of peptide hormones and the transcription of their genes by tumor cells are in fact quite common occurrences. Tumor cells may differ from normal cells in their ability or inability to process precursor molecules, which may account for the presence or absence of hormone excess states and for the profile of peptide hormone forms and fragments present in the circulation and in tumor cell extracts. However, tumor production of hormone fragments or precursors is much more common than the clinical syndromes of hormone excess.

The classic criteria used to confirm that a tumor is the source of a hormone excess state include the following: (1) evidence of an endocrinopathy in a patient with a tumor; (2) remission of the endocrinopathy after tumor resection; (3) detection of an arteriovenous gradient across the tumor; and (4) documentation of hormone protein and messenger RNA production in the tumor tissue.

In addition to classic hormone excess states resulting from the ectopic or inappropriate secretion of a hormone by an endocrine or nonendocrine tumor, endocrinopathies can result from the ectopic expression of a hormone's receptor. This is well illustrated, for example, by the occurrence of Cushing's syndrome in pregnancy or in relation to meals, due to the ectopic expression of luteinizing hormone or gastric inhibitory polypeptide receptors in adrenal tissue, respectively. Several other examples of ectopic receptor syndromes have been documented. Some of these will be discussed below, particularly as a cause for unusual forms of ACTH-independent Cushing's syndrome.

A variety of peptides are produced by both benign and malignant tumors as listed in Table 21–1. The biochemical pathways and machinery leading to the synthesis, processing, and secretion into the circulation of a peptide hormone are present in all cells. In contrast, the multiple enzymatic steps that lead to the production of a highly active steroid hormone (eg, cortisol or 1,25-dihydroxyvitamin D) are restricted, with rare exceptions, to steroid-producing cells or their precursor cells. Hence, the occurrence of 1,25-dihydroxyvitamin D excess caused by a tumor is distinctly unusual, being observed infrequently in hematologic malignancies and only in those with the ability to 1-hydroxylate 25-hydroxyvitamin D, the immediate precursor of 1,25-dihydroxyvitamin D. Ectopic hormone syndromes—the

Table 21–1. Polypeptide hormones produced ectopically by benign and malignant tumors and their associated endocrinopathies.

Hormone	Syndrome
Parathyroid hormone related protein (PTHrP)	Hypercalcemia
Parathyroid hormone (rare)	Hypercalcemia
Antidiuretic hormone	Hyponatremia
Adrenocorticotropin	Cushing's syndrome
Corticotropin-releasing hormone	Cushing's syndrome
Calcitonin	*No specific syndrome*
Growth hormone-releasing hormone	Acromegaly
Somatostatin	*No specific syndrome*
Pancreatic polypeptide	Diarrhea, electrolyte disturbances
Insulin and insulin-like growth factors	Hypoglycemia
Vasoactive intestinal peptide	Diarrhea
Human chorionic gonadotropin	Children: precocious puberty Men: erectile dysfunction, gynecomastia Women: dysfunctional uterine bleeding
FGF-23	Oncogenic osteomalacia

most common of the paraneoplastic syndromes—thus predominantly reflect peptide hormone excess states. The most common ectopic peptide hormone syndromes are described in greater detail in subsequent sections of this chapter.

APUD Concept of Neuroendocrine Cell Tumors

Over the years since the initial recognition that nonendocrine tumors were the source of the ectopic hormones produced in these endocrine syndromes, the notion developed that the hormones originated from highly specialized neuroendocrine cells in tumors. These cells were thought to derive from the neural crest and were postulated to be able to synthesize and store biogenic amines and were thus designated amine precursor uptake and decarboxylation (APUD) cells. Neuroendocrine cells, like calcitonin-secreting C cells and adrenal chromaffin cells, clearly had these properties, and tissues giving rise

to ectopic hormone syndromes (eg, lung and gastrointestinal tract) also had APUD cells scattered throughout them. It was originally thought that the tumor cells producing excessive amounts of polypeptide hormones were derived exclusively from APUD cells in the tissue of origin (eg, ACTH-producing cells of the lung).

Newer insights into tumor cell biology have led to a better understanding of the pathogenesis and etiology of the ectopic hormone production states. Studies have shown that not all APUD cells are derived from the neural crest. Some of these cells are of endodermal origin. Furthermore, with careful examination of tumors, it has become clear that peptide hormones are often produced by non-APUD cells. It has, however, been appreciated that the clinically evident hormone hypersecretion states are typically caused by tumors that are in fact derived from APUD cells. These cells are the ones with the full capacity to produce and store peptide hormones efficiently in dense secretory granules and then release biologically significant quantities of active hormones in circulating plasma.

HYPERCALCEMIA OF MALIGNANCY

Hypercalcemia, the most common paraneoplastic endocrine syndrome, occurs in 10–15% of malignancies. In the majority of patients (98%), the identity of the tumor is apparent at the time of presentation, and the prognosis is very poor as most patients with hypercalcemia of malignancy do not survive beyond 6 months.

Pathogenesis

Enhanced bone resorption is the primary cause of hypercalcemia of malignancy. Tumor-derived factors induce this increase in osteoclast-mediated resorption via two distinct mechanisms: (1) humoral effects of systemically elevated tumor-derived factors and (2) local autocrine or paracrine effects of factors produced by tumor cells that have metastasized to bone and induce localized osteolysis (Figure 21–1). While the latter mechanism was thought to be the primary cause of hypercalcemia of malignancy when it was initially described in the 1920s, work within the last 2 decades has in fact identified a humoral basis as the most frequent (80%) cause even in settings, such as breast cancer, where lytic bone metastases are present. Decreased renal calcium excretion may also contribute to the pathogenesis, either because of the hypocalciuric effects of certain humoral mediators of hypercalcemia, such as PTH-related protein (discussed below), or because of the decreased glomerular flow that occurs with hypercalcemia-induced nephrogenic diabetes insipidus.

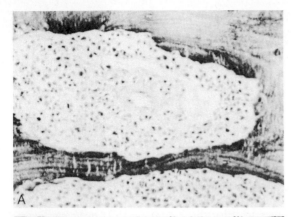

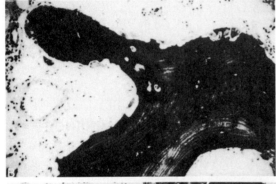

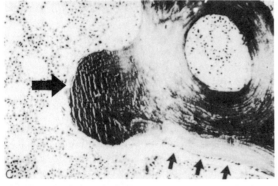

Figure 21–1. Bone histology in hypercalcemia of malignancy versus primary hyperparathyroidism. **A:** Local osteolytic hypercalcemia due to leukemia. Note the presence of tumor cells in marrow spaces and numerous bone-resorbing osteoclasts lining the trabecular surface. **B:** Humoral hypercalcemia due to squamous cell carcinoma. Note the absence of tumor cells in marrow spaces but the presence of numerous active osteoclasts on the trabecular surface. Note also the absence of bone-forming osteoblasts, consistent with uncoupling of bone formation and resorption. **C:** Hyperparathyroidism. Note abundant osteoblasts (small arrows), osteoclasts (large arrow), and osteoid. (Panel A is reproduced, with permission, from Stewart AF, Insogna KL, and Broadus AE: Malignancy-associated hypercalcemia. In: Endocrinology, 3rd ed. DeGroot LJ [editor]. Saunders, 1995. Panels B and C are reprinted, with permission, from Stewart AF, Vignery A, Silverglate A, Ravin ND, LiVolsi V, Broadus AE: Quantitative bone histomorphometry in humoral hypercalcemia of malignancy: uncoupling of bone cell activity. J Clin Endocrinol Metab 1982;55:219. Copyright © 1982 by The Endocrine Society.)

Humoral Mediators

In the 1940s, Fuller Albright, in describing a case of hypercalcemia of malignancy occurring in the absence of significant bone metastases, was the first to propose the existence of a humoral cause of this syndrome. It was not until the late 1980s, however, that this humoral factor was identified. Unlike most other paraneoplastic endocrine syndromes which are due to the ectopic production of well-described hormones with known physiologic functions, the vast majority of cases of humoral hypercalcemia of malignancy are due to the overexpression of PTH-related protein (PTHrP) (Figure 21–2). PTHrP is a peptide that had not previously been identified until it was isolated simultaneously by several independent groups in 1987 from tumors commonly associated with humoral hypercalcemia of malignancy—squamous cell carcinoma of the lung, breast carcinoma, and renal carcinoma.

The amino terminal portion of PTHrP bears strong homology to PTH and binds with equal affinity to PTH receptors (now known as the PTH/PTHrP-1 receptor subtype) in bone and kidney. Therefore, the biochemical markers of PTHrP-mediated hypercalcemia in

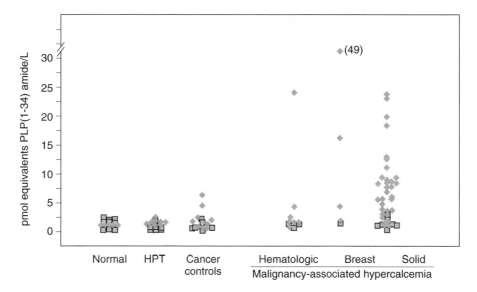

Figure 21–2. Serum levels of amino terminal PTHrP (iPLP[1–34]) in normal subjects, patients with hyperparathyroidism, normocalcemic patients with malignancy, and hypercalcemic patients with malignancy. In this series, 55% of the patients with malignancy-associated hypercalcemia had serum PTHrP levels that exceeded the upper limits of normal, including patients with solid tumors, breast carcinoma, and hematologic malignancies. HPT = hyperparathyroidism; open squares = undetectable PTHrP plotted at detection limit. (Reprinted, with permission, from Budayr AA et al: Increased serum levels of a parathyroid hormone-like protein in malignancy-associated hypercalcemia. Ann Intern Med 1989:111:807.)

vivo are similar to those of hyperparathyroidism and include a decrease in serum phosphate and an increase in nephrogenous cAMP. Some unexplained differences, however, are seen in PTHrP-mediated hypercalcemia of malignancy (versus primary hyperparathyroidism), including normal or suppressed 1,25-dihydroxyvitamin D levels and an uncoupling of bone resorption and formation that results in severe bone loss (Figure 21–1). The reasons for these differences are not yet known but may include the ability of chronic PTHrP (versus intermittent PTH) stimulation or profound hypercalcemia per se to suppress 1,25-dihydroxyvitamin D levels and, the contributions of additional tumor-derived cytokines, such as interleukin-1α or interleukin-6, to the process of bone resorption.

Normal physiologic functions of PTHrP are still being investigated. PTH-related peptide and PTH are ancestrally related genes that have evolved separately. Consistent with this, while PTH is produced primarily at one site, the parathyroid gland, and acts as a calciotropic hormone, PTHrP is produced by a wide variety of cell types and exhibits diverse functions, most of which are unrelated to calcium homeostasis. The normal actions of PTHrP are autocrine or paracrine, rather

than humoral, as both PTHrP and the PTH-PTHrP receptor are now known to be expressed in numerous organs where PTHrP is thought to act locally. Known functions of PTHrP include (1) regulation of endochondral bone formation during development; (2) growth and differentiation of mammary gland, skin, and pancreatic islets; (3) relaxation of vascular and nonvascular smooth muscle; (4) cytokine-like effects during the inflammatory response; (5) neuroprotective effects during aging; and (6) transepithelial calcium transport in the placenta.

While PTHrP is by far the most common mediator of hypercalcemia of malignancy, other calciotropic hormones can also cause the syndrome. To date, ectopic production of PTH has been reported as a cause of hypercalcemia of malignancy only in seven isolated cases, including several neuroendocrine tumors and small cell carcinomas. Additionally, elevated circulating levels of 1,25-dihydroxyvitamin D levels, thought to be due to increased 1α-hydroxylase activity in lymphoproliferative cells, can cause humoral hypercalcemia of malignancy in various types of lymphoma, including Hodgkin's disease, B cell lymphomas, T cell lymphomas, and Burkitt's lymphoma. Other tumor-derived bone-resorbing factors, such as prostaglandins, may also contribute to hypercalcemia of malignancy in certain cases.

Tumors Associated with Hypercalcemia of Malignancy

Hypercalcemia of malignancy occurs frequently with certain common tumors, including squamous cell carcinoma of the lung and breast carcinoma. In contrast, hypercalcemia is rarely seen in other commonly occurring cancers (eg, colon, gastric, thyroid, and oat cell carcinomas), including tumors such as prostate carcinoma that are frequently metastatic to bone.

A. SQUAMOUS CELL CARCINOMAS

Squamous cell carcinomas account for over one-third of all cases of hypercalcemia of malignancy. Humoral effects of tumor-derived PTHrP account for most cases of hypercalcemia in this setting. Twenty-five percent of patients with squamous cell lung carcinomas develop PTHrP-mediated hypercalcemia, while other sites of squamous cell carcinoma (head, neck, esophagus, cervix, vulva, and skin) are similarly associated with a high incidence of hypercalcemia.

B. RENAL CELL CARCINOMA

Renal cell carcinoma is another solid tumor that is frequently associated with hypercalcemia. As with squamous cell carcinomas, humoral effects of tumor-derived PTHrP are causative. While 100% of renal cell tumors in some series have been reported to stain positively for immunoreactive PTHrP, hypercalcemia is only seen in 8% of cases.

C. BREAST CARCINOMA

Hypercalcemia occurs in 20% of patients with advanced-stage breast carcinoma and is only rarely seen in the absence of bone metastases. However, the majority of patients with bone metastases (ie, 70% of those with advanced disease) do not have hypercalcemia. Despite the frequent presence of bone metastases in patients with hypercalcemia, their hypercalcemia is in fact (and paradoxically) mostly humorally mediated. Humoral effects of PTHrP have been shown to be responsible for up to 65% of cases of breast carcinoma-associated hypercalcemia, as evidenced by elevated circulating levels of PTHrP occurring in association with increased levels of nephrogenous cAMP. In the remainder of cases, localized osteolysis, induced by factors produced by tumor cells metastatic to bone, is the cause of hypercalcemia. Even in this setting, however, PTHrP contributes to the etiology of hypercalcemia, as 97% of breast carcinoma bone metastases have been shown to be PTHrP-positive. Evidence obtained from an elegant series of studies using an animal model of metastatic breast cancer now suggests that (1) local bone factors, such as TGF-β, may enhance PTHrP expression in tumor cells metastatic to bone, even when the primary tumor is PTHrP-negative; and (2) this local increase in PTHrP production enhances osteoclast-mediated destruction of adjacent bone. Additional, locally produced bone cytokines such as interleukin-1α, interleukin-6, and tumor necrosis factor-α probably act in concert with PTHrP at sites of bone metastases to enhance osteoclast-mediated lytic bone destruction and thus contribute to hypercalcemia. While the hypercalcemia seen in late stages of cancer is usually unremitting and associated with a survival time of weeks to months, hypercalcemia in breast cancer can be episodic. For example, hypercalcemia often occurs transiently in response to treatment with estrogens or antiestrogens and is associated with a beneficial response to therapy. Recent demonstrations of enhanced PTHrP expression in breast carcinoma cells in response to estrogen or tamoxifen suggests that these episodes of transient hypercalcemia may also be PTHrP-mediated.

D. OTHER SOLID TUMORS

Hypercalcemia is also associated with other solid tumors, though less frequently. In most of these cases, humoral effects of PTHrP are causative. PTHrP-mediated hypercalcemia has been reported for ovarian carcinoma, a tumor type for which one case of tumor-derived, PTH-mediated hypercalcemia has also been reported; bladder carcinoma; large cell and adenocarcinoma of the lung; and endocrine tumors, including islet cell tumors, pheochromocytoma, and carcinoid tumors.

E. MULTIPLE MYELOMA

Most patients with multiple myeloma have extensive bone destruction. However, only 30% of patients develop hypercalcemia, which can be remitting. Although systemic increases in circulating PTHrP have been reported in some cases, locally produced osteolytic factors—rather than humoral mediators—are thought to be responsible for most cases of hypercalcemia in this hematologic malignancy. While the factor or factors stimulating osteoclast activity in this disease have not yet been identified, studies suggest that myeloma cells in the marrow express cytokine-like factors such as TNF-α, TNF-β, IL-1α, IL-1β, IL-6, and PTHrP, which act locally to stimulate the bone-resorbing activity of adjacent osteoclasts. Because renal disease occurs frequently in myeloma due to the filtration of Bence Jones proteins (light chain fragments of IgG), it is hypothesized that patients with renal impairment may be predisposed to development of hypercalcemia in this setting of increased bone resorption.

F. LYMPHOMAS

Hypercalcemia occurs in association with 1–2% of lymphomas and leukemias, is seen primarily in patients with bone involvement, and can occur with a variety of cell types. With the exception of human T cell leukemia virus (HTLV-1)-induced adult T cell leukemia or lymphoma, which will be discussed below, approximately half of the cases of lymphoma-associated hypercalcemia are thought to be due to the local lytic effects of tumor-derived factors, as was discussed for myeloma. The remainder appear to be mediated by a mechanism unique to lymphoma—ie, humoral effects of tumor-derived 1,25-dihydroxyvitamin D. The mechanism leading to increased circulating 1,25-dihydroxyvitamin D in lymphoma is believed to be the same as that seen in hypercalcemic granulomatous disorders, ie, increased production of 1,25-dihydroxyvitamin D by the involved hematopoietic cells due to 1α-hydroxylation of circulating epidermal- and diet-derived 25-hydroxyvitamin D. Both increased intestinal calcium absorption and increased bone resorption are thought to contribute to hypercalcemia in this setting. HTLV-1-induced adult T cell leukemia or lymphoma must be considered separately when evaluating possible causes of hypercalcemia. In this subset of patients, hypercalcemia occurs in two-thirds of cases, responds poorly to treatment, and is due to the humoral effects of tumor-derived PTHrP which is induced by a viral transactivating factor (Tax).

Diagnosis

The diagnosis of hypercalcemia is discussed in detail in Chapter 8. Primary hyperparathyroidism and hypercalcemia of malignancy account for over 90% of all causes of hypercalcemia. Because the incidence of primary hyperparathyroidism is twice that of hypercalcemia of malignancy, primary hyperparathyroidism must also be considered as a potential cause of hypercalcemia in patients with malignancy and can be simply evaluated with current methods by determination of intact PTH levels using a standard two-site immunoradiometric assay. In the setting of hypercalcemia of malignancy and normal renal function, PTH will be suppressed. Further evaluation can be guided, in part, by the tumor type. Elevated PTHrP will be detected in a majority of cases of hypercalcemia of malignancy associated with solid tumors, including breast carcinoma, and in HTLV-1-induced T cell lymphomas. Measurement of 1,25-dihydroxyvitamin D should be considered in all cases of lymphoma-associated hypercalcemia. Lytic bone lesions are usually identified during tumor staging.

Treatment

The treatment of hypercalcemia is discussed in detail in Chapter 8. Because bone resorption is central to all causes of hypercalcemia of malignancy, bisphosphonates are a mainstay of treatment. Moreover, recent evidence suggests that these agents, in addition to reversing hypercalcemia due to both humoral and local lytic factors, may also prevent the progression of bone metastases, particularly in multiple myeloma. Glucocorticoids can be used with some success in the treatment of all causes of hypercalcemia of malignancy but may be particularly efficacious when hypercalcemia is due either to the local lytic effects of neoplastic plasma cells in multiple myeloma or to the increased production of 1,25-dihydroxyvitamin D in lymphoma.

ECTOPIC CUSHING'S SYNDROME

Many tumors produce the ACTH precursor proopiomelanocortin (POMC), and only a fraction of such tumors release sufficient ACTH to cause Cushing's syndrome. Initially, the tumors recognized to cause this syndrome were of nonpituitary origin but were endocrine tumors, such as islet cell carcinomas and pheochromocytomas. Subsequently, a wide variety of different tumor cell types, both endocrine and nonendocrine, have been associated with the "ectopic" ACTH syndrome.

The classic description of the ectopic ACTH syndrome was made by Grant Liddle and coworkers in the early 1960s and was based on a series of patients who mostly had highly malignant tumors (eg, oat cell or small cell carcinoma of the lung). More recently, the ectopic ACTH syndrome has been recognized with increasing frequency with benign tumors, specifically carcinoids. Benign (versus malignant) lesions typically present in a more subtle clinical manner, often over months to years before the tumor is identified. The more gradual development of the clinical syndrome plus the more subtle biochemistry have led to a considerable challenge in distinguishing this form of the ectopic ACTH syndrome from pituitary tumors causing Cushing's disease. This subtle variant of tumor-induced ACTH excess has been dubbed the "occult" ectopic ACTH syndrome. In addition, it is now recognized that tumors can cause an ectopic ACTH-like syndrome through production of corticotropin-releasing hormone (CRH). Indeed, some of the tumors that make the latter cosecrete ACTH as well. Ectopic CRH production has been seen in bronchial carcinoids, medullary thyroid carcinoma, and metastatic prostatic cancer.

Differential Diagnosis

Cushing's syndrome—signs and symptoms resulting from unregulated production of glucocorticoids—is caused by a number of underlying disturbances. These must be differentiated to ensure successful treatment. Causes include pituitary ACTH-dependent Cushing's disease, adrenal tumors or ACTH-independent Cushing's syndrome, and the ectopic ACTH syndrome. In several large series, it has been reported that in 50–80% of patients with Cushing's syndrome there is a pituitary cause. Adrenal adenomas (and very rarely carcinomas) account for 5–30% of cases of Cushing's syndrome. The ectopic ACTH syndrome comprises approximately 10–20% of cases of Cushing's syndrome from referral center populations.

A wide variety of tumors cause ectopic ACTH syndrome (Table 21–2). In the classic and initial descriptions of this syndrome, there was a preponderance of malignant tumors, particularly small cell carcinomas of the lung. It is now clear that most cases of ectopic ACTH syndrome are due to benign tumors. Most recently, microscopic carcinoid "tumorlets," particularly in the lung, have been recognized to cause occult ectopic ACTH syndrome. These tumors may be exceptionally difficult to diagnose by standard techniques.

The diagnosis of Cushing's syndrome requires a rigorous approach. Cushing's syndrome should be suspected first on solid clinical grounds and then established biochemically. This is accomplished by demonstrating the presence of hypercortisolism—a

Table 21–2. Tumors responsible for the ectopic ACTH syndrome.[1]

Lung
  Carcinoma of the lung especially small cell carcinoma, bronchial adenoma, or carcinoid
Pancreas
  Cystadenoma, carcinoma, carcinoid, islet cell adenoma, and carcinoma
Thymus
  Carcinoma, carcinoid
  Pheochromocytoma
  Medullary thyroid carcinoma
  Gastrointestinal carcinoid tumors
  Adenocarcinoma of undetermined origin
Miscellaneous
  Hematologic malignancy
  Carcinomas of the liver, prostate, breast; melanoma, plasmacytoma

[1]Modified, with permission, from The Endocrine Society. Wajchentberg BL et al: Ectopic adrenocorticotropic hormone syndrome. Endocr Rev 1994;15:752.

frankly elevated 24-hour urinary free cortisol level or the lack of suppression of plasma cortisol levels after a 1 mg overnight dexamethasone suppression test (see Chapter 9). In Cushing's syndrome due to any cause and often in ectopic ACTH syndrome, random cortisol levels are elevated. Once hypercortisolism is established, plasma ACTH levels are measured. These levels are markedly elevated in classic forms of the ectopic ACTH syndrome, typically secondary to malignant lung neoplasms. There is, however, considerable overlap between the milder cases of the ectopic ACTH syndrome, caused by benign and slowly growing tumors, and Cushing's disease due to a pituitary tumor. In the former case, the tumors are often small and clinically silent—hence the descriptor "occult" ectopic ACTH syndrome. For these reasons, rigorous biochemical criteria must be applied in appropriate clinical situations to make certain that the correct diagnosis is made. Plasma ACTH levels in patients with clinically evident tumors are often strikingly elevated (390–2300 pg/mL [87–511 pmol/L] by radioimmunoassay). Individuals with ectopic ACTH syndrome due to occult tumors have ACTH levels that overlap with pituitary-dependent Cushing's disease (42–428 pg/mL [9.3–95 pmol/L]). It is said that patients with plasma ACTH levels greater than 200 pg/mL [44.4 pmol/L] typically have the ectopic ACTH syndrome, though further testing must be done to prove this and to localize the tumor.

After hypercortisolism and ACTH excess are established, the degree of suppressibility of ACTH with exogenous glucocorticoid is determined. In classic Cushing's disease due to a pituitary tumor, supraphysiologic doses of dexamethasone usually suppress the elevated plasma ACTH and cortisol levels. Tumors responsible for the ectopic ACTH syndrome are, however, classically unresponsive to these doses of dexamethasone. High-dose dexamethasone suppression testing, as this diagnostic maneuver is called, is accomplished (1) by administering 2 mg of dexamethasone every 6 hours for 2 days and measuring urinary free cortisol or plasma cortisol on the second day, or (2) by administering 8 mg of dexamethasone the night before obtaining an 8 AM plasma cortisol level. In both tests, the expected suppression of baseline urinary free cortisol and plasma cortisol should be 50% or greater if the Cushing's syndrome is due to a pituitary adenoma (ie, Cushing's disease). However, between 15% and 33% of patients with ectopic ACTH syndrome will also meet these suppression criteria (false positives), mimicking Cushing's disease. In addition, 10–25% of patients with Cushing's disease fail to suppress with high-dose dexamethasone (false negatives). The overnight test probably has greater sensitivity and accuracy than the classic 2-day test and is preferred.

Two additional tests have been developed to improve the diagnostic discrimination between Cushing's disease and ectopic ACTH syndrome. The first is CRH testing. Pituitary corticotrophs are normally responsive to CRH in Cushing's disease and unresponsive when ectopic ACTH production or an adrenal lesion is responsible for the cortisol excess. A positive response to CRH is defined as a 50% or greater increase in plasma ACTH and a 20% or greater increase in the plasma cortisol concentrations. An increase in ACTH of 100% and in cortisol of over 50% greatly reduces the likelihood of ectopic ACTH syndrome; however, false-positive and false-negative tests (up to 10%) have been reported. Moreover, in the rare instance of ectopic production of CRH (without concomitant ACTH) by a tumor, a false-positive result may be seen, leading to the erroneous diagnosis of pituitary-dependent Cushing's disease. For these reasons, many clinicians sample the inferior petrosal sinuses for plasma ACTH levels both before and after the injection of CRH to assist with the differential diagnosis. These sinuses drain the pituitary gland. Concomitant peripheral and petrosal sinus samples are obtained, and the central:peripheral ACTH ratio is calculated. In Cushing's disease, the ratio should be ± 2.0 in the basal state. After CRH administration, this ratio should be ± 3.0 in pituitary-dependent Cushing's disease. In the ectopic ACTH syndrome, this ratio should not rise after the CRH. In rare instances of ectopic CRH syndrome, the basal ratio may be 2.0. The stimulation by CRH gives close to 100% discrimination between ectopic ACTH production and a pituitary tumor secreting ACTH. Generally, a combination of tests is performed to reach a biochemical diagnosis before extensive radiologic studies are undertaken.

The majority of patients (70% or more) with ectopic ACTH syndrome will also cosecrete other hormones or tumor marker peptides, among them carcinoembryonic antigen, somatostatin, calcitonin, gastrin, glucagon, vasoactive intestinal peptide, bombesin, pancreatic polypeptide, alpha-fetoprotein, and many others. The presence and secretion of these other hormones (in addition to ACTH) suggests that the source of ACTH is nonpituitary in these patients. Given the variety of peptides and the expense inherent in any screening paradigm, measuring a panel of these hormones in patients suspected of ectopic ACTH syndrome is not recommended.

The path to localization of the tumor responsible for ectopic ACTH production generally starts with a chest radiograph. Most tumors are in the chest or abdomen. Small cell carcinomas of the lung are usually visible on chest x-ray, while bronchial carcinoids are often difficult to detect by plain radiographs. In some situations, these tumors may require a long period (as many as 4 or 5 years) of close follow-up before the tumors are detected. Chest CT scanning should be employed in all subjects with ectopic ACTH to rule out a chest or mediastinal lesion (such as a thymic carcinoid). Abdominal CT scanning is also performed in these patients to confirm the presence of bilateral adrenal enlargement, a sine qua non of the ectopic ACTH syndrome, and to screen for other possible abdominal tumors responsible for the syndrome (pheochromocytoma, islet cell tumor, etc.). In the radiologic evaluation of Cushing's syndrome, it is always important to bear in mind that the presence of a pituitary microadenoma on MRI does very little to support the diagnosis of pituitary-dependent Cushing's disease—as opposed to an ectopic tumor producing ACTH—because of the great numbers (10–20%) of normal individuals with incidental pituitary microadenomas (see Chapter 5).

Octreotide scanning, another important diagnostic technique, can successfully localize tumors responsible for ectopic ACTH production. It relies on the expression of somatostatin or octreotide receptors in neuroendocrine cells. Iodinated or, more recently, indium-111-labeled octreotide scanning has demonstrated medullary carcinomas of the thyroid, small cell lung cancers, islet cell tumors, pheochromocytomas, and other tumors. There remains controversy among experts about whether this form of scanning exceeds the sensitivity and specificity of thin-cut CT-MR scans of the chest and abdomen reviewed by expert radiologists. Octreotide therapy has been used to lower ACTH levels and relieve symptoms of cortisol excess in many of these tumors.

Clinical Features

Cushing's syndrome causes truncal obesity, violaceous striae, hypertension, fatigue, glucose intolerance, osteopenia, muscle weakness, moon facies, easy bruisability, buffalo hump, depression, hirsutism, and edema. Patients with ectopic ACTH syndrome may show some, all, or none of these features depending on the underlying tumor. It has been appreciated from the initial descriptions of this syndrome that these patients typically present with myopathy, weight loss, and electrolyte and metabolic disturbances more commonly than with the classic features of slowly developing Cushing's disease. Hyperpigmentation is also recognized as more common in the ectopic ACTH syndrome than in Cushing's disease. Cortisol excess in older men, especially those at risk for lung tumors, is most commonly due to ectopic ACTH production, whereas ACTH-producing pituitary tumors predominate in young and middle-aged women. Glucose intolerance or frank diabetes and hypokalemic alkalosis are typical metabolic disturbances of the ectopic ACTH syndrome. Because of the extreme elevation in plasma cortisol levels in many of these patients, they are at considerable risk for and often succumb to overwhelming opportunistic infections, often with fungal pathogens.

A critical caveat to remember in the clinical evaluation of patients with ACTH-dependent Cushing's disease is that slowly growing and occult tumors producing ACTH may present in exactly the same way as classic Cushing's disease due to a pituitary tumor. Therefore, both the clinical findings and the laboratory studies summarized above show considerable overlap and may engender confusion in distinguishing these occult tumors from a pituitary lesion.

Increasing numbers of patients who have classic features of Cushing's syndrome have been shown to have adrenal expression of ectopic receptors as the cause of their hypercortisolism. The pathophysiology of this form of Cushing's syndrome is ACTH-independent since other hormones are driving the glucocorticoid hypersecretion. Ectopic expression of receptors for gastric inhibitory peptide, vasopressin, serotonin, β-adrenergic agonists, luteinizing hormone (LH), and interleukin-1 have been reported. In the case of gastric inhibitory peptide, food-stimulated cortisol hypersecretion has been described. In a case report of ectopic LH receptor expression in the adrenals associated with macronodular adrenal hyperplasia, the patient had mild cushingoid features with pregnancy and the gradual development of full-blown Cushing's syndrome with menopause. Thus, it has become increasingly evident that ectopic receptors as well as hormones can be responsible for hypercortisolemic states.

SYNDROME OF INAPPROPRIATE ADH (SIADH) SECRETION

This syndrome is characterized by inappropriate retention of water such that hypertonic or inappropriately concentrated urine is excreted in the presence of hyponatremia. There are many well-recognized causes of this syndrome (Table 21–3).

Etiology & Pathogenesis

Tumors are a common cause of SIADH (see Table 21–3). Bronchogenic carcinoma, particularly small cell carcinoma, has been associated with this syndrome since its initial description in 1957. Small cell carcinoma accounts for 80% of cases of SIADH, but only 3–15% of patients with this tumor have SIADH. Most of these tumors, even from patients without the clinical syndrome, contain ADH by immunostaining. Other tumors that cause the syndrome include breast, pancre-

Table 21–3. Causes of SIADH.[1]

Tumors
  Small cell carcinoma of lung
  Squamous cell carcinoma of lung
  Cancers of the head and neck
  Carcinoma of the duodenum, pancreas, ureter, prostate, uterus, and nasopharynx
  Mesothelioma
  Thymoma
  Hodgkin's lymphoma
  Leukemia
Central nervous system disorders
  Brain tumors (primary and metastatic)
  Brain abscess
  Subdural hematoma, subarachnoid hemorrhage
  Meningitis, encephalitis
  Systemic lupus erythematosus
  Demyelinative disorders
  Head trauma
Drugs
  Nicotine, phenothiazines, tricyclic antidepressants, nonsteroidal antiinflammatory agents, cyclophosphamide, vincristine, chlorpropamide, colchicine, selective serotonin reuptake inhibitors (sertraline, fluoxetine), azithromycin, thiazide diuretics
Pulmonary disorders
  Tuberculosis
  Fungal, bacterial, viral, mycoplasmal pneumonia
  Empyema, lung abscess
  Chronic obstructive pulmonary disease

[1]Modified, with permission, from Verbalis JG: Inappropriate antidiuresis and other hypoosmolar states. In: *Principles and Practice of Endocrinology and Metabolism,* 3rd ed. Becker KL (editor). Lippincott, 2001.

atic, and thymic carcinomas in addition to those listed in Table 21–3. These tumors typically produce AVP, oxytocin, and the carrier protein neurophysin.

Excessive production of vasopressin by tumors leads to an inability to excrete free water. This is due to the fact that tumors release vasopressin independent of serum osmolality. In addition to the production of vasopressin, many tumors also contain the mRNA for the hormone atrial natriuretic peptide (ANP). This has suggested that hyponatremia in these patients may be due to the natriuretic effects of ANP rather than the antidiuretic effects of vasopressin.

Clinical & Laboratory Features

SIADH is the most common cause of hyponatremia in hospitalized patients. It may present with symptoms due to water intoxication and hyponatremia. Although many patients are asymptomatic, depending on the magnitude and chronicity of their hyponatremia, symptomatic individuals usually have fatigue, headache, nausea, and anorexia initially which can progress to altered mental status, seizures, coma, and even death. Most patients will experience weight gain due to water retention but will not have edema. Significant clinical symptoms usually do not develop unless the serum sodium is 125 mEq/mL or less, and there is usually a correlation between the level of symptomatology in these patients and their serum sodium values.

Patients with SIADH exhibit hyponatremia, serum hypoosmolality, a less than maximally dilute urine, and the presence of sodium in the urine. Clinically, the diagnosis of SIADH cannot be made unless there is euvolemia with intact renal, adrenal, and thyroid function. Cirrhosis, nephrosis, and congestive heart failure must be excluded. Generally, the diagnosis is made by the presence of hyponatremia, low serum osmolality, and urine osmolality that is less than maximally dilute. Urinary sodium levels are usually high, and urea nitrogen levels are typically low, as are serum uric acid levels. Rarely is it necessary to measure vasopressin levels to make this diagnosis, although these determinations are now widely available. It is rarely if ever necessary to perform a water-loading test, which can be dangerous in these patients because of their impaired ability to excrete a free water load and their propensity to become water-intoxicated. Once the diagnosis of SIADH is made, all possible causes should be considered (see Table 21–3). Water restriction and demeclocycline are the mainstays of treatment. In an acutely symptomatic patient or when the serum sodium is reduced to dangerously low levels, infusion of hypertonic saline and administration of loop diuretics (eg, furosemide) are the treatments of choice. Many patients with SIADH due to neoplasms will improve and even remit with effective therapy for their underlying cancer.

NON-ISLET CELL TUMORS & HYPOGLYCEMIA

Tumors that cause hypoglycemia are quite rare—especially those derived from tissues other than the pancreatic islets. These tumors are usually large mesenchymal lesions in the chest or abdomen and can be benign or malignant. They include fibromas, fibrosarcomas, mesotheliomas, hemangiopericytomas, lymphomas, hepatomas, hypernephromas, and adrenocortical carcinomas. The hallmark of this clinical syndrome is fasting hypoglycemia. Its differential diagnosis and clinical presentation are discussed more fully in Chapter 18.

The pathogenesis of the hypoglycemia in these cases may involve a variety of mechanisms, including excessive consumption of glucose by what is typically a large tumor; ectopic or abnormal secretion of insulin or insulin-like growth factor-II (IGF-II) and IGF-binding proteins; or inadequate production of counterregulatory hormones such as growth hormone. Examples of all of the above mechanisms in relation to specific tumors have been described. The typical clinical presentation of these patients is the occurrence of increased levels of IGF-II; suppressed levels of insulin, C-peptide, proinsulin, and IGF-I; and lower than expected levels of growth hormone. It is very uncommon to find a non-islet cell tumor that can produce authentic insulin—only rarely has this been well-documented. Patients with tumor-induced hypoglycemia can manifest all the signs and symptoms of fasting hypoglycemia: sweating, intense hunger, anxiety, altered consciousness, and visual and behavioral changes. The presenting symptoms may be subtle, and rarely is the underlying diagnosis suspected at initial presentation.

Several cases of non-islet cell tumors causing hypoglycemia have been carefully studied and reported in the literature. Daughaday and coworkers reported in 1981 that the causative hormone in these cases was probably IGF-II. Subsequently, further work in his laboratory and in others has shown that the IGF-II produced is generally of a higher molecular weight than normal IGF-II—so-called "big IGF-II" with a molecular weight of 11–18 kDa (normal MW of IGF-II is 7.5 kDa). It has been hypothesized that "big" IGF-II is present in excess in these patients because the tumor fails to process IGF-II appropriately. Normally, IGF-II is produced by the liver and circulates bound mainly to IGF binding protein-3 and an acid-labile subunit in a heterotrimeric complex. Fully processed IGF-II from hepatic sources does not cause hypoglycemia because it is sequestered in this complex and is unavailable to interact with receptors. "Big" IGF-II causes hypoglycemia by one of two mechanisms: (1) It does not readily associate into this ternary complex and has greater access to insulin receptors and hence greater biologic activity, or (2) it is produced in excess and can readily bind up all available IGF-BP3 but there is sufficient unbound ("free") IGF-II to interact with insulin receptors and cause hypoglycemia. In tumors causing hypoglycemia, it is estimated that as much as 80% of the circulating IGF-II is free. Increased free IGF-II may also alter the levels of binding proteins, among them IGF binding protein-3 and the acid-labile subunit. Thus, there are a number of possible explanations for this clinical syndrome.

Treatment of this paraneoplastic syndrome usually involves surgery to debulk the tumor. If the lesion is benign, this usually brings relief of the hypoglycemia or even definitive cure. Radiotherapy may also be employed adjunctively. These patients often require continuous glucose infusions to control their symptoms prior to surgery, and glucagon can be used acutely to raise blood glucose levels. In occasional patients, diazoxide therapy has been useful. In one study of a small number of patients, glucocorticoids reduced IGF-II levels, thereby restoring a more normal IGF and IGF-binding protein profile. Owing to the size and advanced stage of clinical progression of these tumors at the time of diagnosis, the outcome is often poor.

OTHER HORMONES SECRETED BY TUMORS

1. Growth Hormone-Releasing Hormone & Growth Hormone

It was recognized in the 1960s that carcinoid tumors are associated with acromegaly. This led to the idea that these tumors could secrete a growth hormone-releasing factor. In 1982, two laboratories reported the purification of the hypothalamic peptide growth hormone-releasing hormone (GHRH). Several biologically active forms of the 44-amino-acid peptide GHRH are typically present in extracts from tumors responsible for ectopic GHRH production. Patients whose tumors release excessive quantities of this peptide develop acromegaly. This classic disorder is characterized by acral enlargement, coarsened facies, soft tissue overgrowth, excessive sweating, arthropathy, and other manifestations (see Chapter 5). Most cases of acromegaly, however—over 90%—are due to pituitary tumors secreting excess GH. Patients with acromegaly due to the ectopic production of GHRH will manifest increases in serum growth hormone (GH) and insulin-like growth factor-I (IGF-I) levels. Circulating levels of GHRH are also elevated, and this is an absolutely critical measurement to make. Evaluation of the pituitary gland typically shows no tumor. The pituitary pathology in patients with ectopic GHRH secretion is usually somatotroph hyperplasia.

In rare instances, hypothalamic tumors such as hamartomas, ganglioneuromas, and gangliocytomas produce excessive GHRH and acromegaly. Since the site of GHRH production is within the hypothalamus, this is not considered ectopic GHRH secretion. The syndrome of ectopic GHRH secretion has been recognized in patients with tumors outside the hypothalamus, most frequently carcinoid tumors of the lung and gastrointestinal tract and islet cell tumors. Other tumors associated with this syndrome include pheochromocytoma, paraganglioma and adenocarcinoma of the lung, hepatic neuroendocrine tumors, and pituitary adenoma. In the latter case, adenoma cells stained positively for both GH and GHRH by immunocytochemistry, and plasma GHRH levels were elevated. Thus, in this situation, there was both autocrine and paracrine regulation of GH secretion and possibly tumor progression.

Because of the nonmalignant nature of most of the tumors responsible for the ectopic GHRH syndrome, the presence of a tumor outside the pituitary or hypothalamus is often not suspected for many years. Symptoms due to the presence of a tumor outside the pituitary gland (such as gastrointestinal or pulmonary complaints) may be the first clue that the acromegaly is due to a nonpituitary tumor. Dynamic testing can also provide a clue that classic pituitary-dependent acromegaly is not the cause of the GH excess. Tumors releasing excessive GHRH may exhibit a GH increase with thyrotropin-releasing hormone (TRH) or with glucose administration and are more likely to have elevated prolactin levels—compared with classic pituitary tumors secreting GH. None of these features allow definitive diagnosis of the ectopic GHRH syndrome, since they are also observed with GH-secreting pituitary tumors. As a group, however, these features can increase the suspicion that one is confronted with an ectopic source of GHRH.

Tumors responsible for the ectopic GHRH syndrome in the chest or mediastinum can often be localized by chest x-ray and CT scanning. In the case of abdominal tumors, endoscopic ultrasound or abdominal CT scanning or MRI may be necessary. Since somatostatin receptors are often present in these tumors, octreotide scanning may also be helpful. Given the low prevalence of the ectopic GHRH syndrome among patients with acromegaly, it is not recommended to screen all acromegalic patients for this possible cause. Rather, it is advised that GHRH levels be measured in patients with any atypical features of acromegaly. If elevated GHRH is established, careful investigation to determine its source is indicated.

There are rare reports of ectopic production of GH by malignant tumors outside the pituitary-hypothalamic region. Acromegaly has been reported due to GH overproduction by a pancreatic islet cell tumor or by a non-Hodgkin lymphoma.

2. Calcitonin

Calcitonin is one of the hormones produced most commonly by tumors. Estimates indicate that 10–30% of malignancies actually make calcitonin or its precursor form procalcitonin. Since calcitonin excess does not produce a clinically evident ectopic hormone syndrome, these patients rarely come to medical attention for their excessive calcitonin secretion. Calcitonin levels have been used as a tumor marker in following responses to treatment.

In addition to medullary carcinoma of the thyroid (discussed in Chapters 7 and 24), in which calcitonin hypersecretion is eutopic (not ectopic), the commonest tumors in which excessive calcitonin is produced include small cell cancers of the lung and pulmonary carcinoids. In studies of the lung malignancies that synthesize calcitonin, it has become clear that pulmonary neuroendocrine cells contain large amounts of calcitonin. These cells are thought to be the cells of origin for lung carcinoid tumors and small cell cancers. In other primary lung cancers (non-small cell), it has been observed that there is often accompanying pulmonary neuroendocrine cell hyperplasia (perhaps secondary to chronic smoking) that may account for the calcitonin hypersecretion. In other tumors not derived from the lung, the cell which is the source of the calcitonin has not been fully elucidated. In addition, in many tumors, the larger forms of calcitonin—a hormone that has complex transcriptional and posttranscriptional mechanisms governing its expression and processing—are made preferentially by these tumors. Such cancers are thought to lack the specialized enzymes required for the final processing of calcitonin.

3. Gonadotropins

Gonadotropins are glycoprotein hormones composed of two subunits: alpha and beta. The alpha subunit is shared by thyrotropin, follicle-stimulating hormone, luteinizing hormone, and chorionic gonadotropin (hCG). The first three hormones are pituitary products, while the latter is a product of the syncytiotrophoblast of the placenta. Although hCG is expressed in nearly all normal tissues, it does not circulate to any appreciable extent except in pregnancy. Trophoblastic tumors like hydatidiform mole and gonadal and nongonadal choriocarcinoma often secrete excessive hCG, which thus is a useful tumor marker in these conditions. Trophoblastic tumors are derived from tissues that have the capacity to make hCG normally; therefore, their production of this hormone is not usually considered as "ectopic." Tumors that do make sufficient quantities of hCG ectopically to raise circulating levels of the hormone include ovarian, prostatic, and testicular tumors (such as seminomas), pinealomas, lung cancers (particularly large cell cancers), gastrointestinal cancers (colon, pancreas, esophagus), breast cancers, melanomas, and hepatoblastomas. Recently, histologic analysis of a spectrum of primary lung neoplasms showed that those of a more differentiated neuroendocrine cell type (eg, small cell lung cancer and carcinoid tumors) were more likely to produce the hCG-α subunit. In contrast, hCG-β subunit expression in trophoblastic and nontrophoblastic tumors typically correlated with a less well differentiated tumor cell phenotype.

Depending on the age and gender of the patient, the clinical signs and symptoms may vary. Importantly not all patients manifest signs of their hCG excess. In susceptible individuals, however, clinical findings may be clearly due to the elevated hCG. Children, for example, with malignant hepatoblastoma can present with precocious puberty. Women may have dysfunctional uterine bleeding. Men with high hCG levels may have signs of hypogonadism with impotence and gynecomastia. Because of the thyroid-stimulating effects of high hCG levels, these patients occasionally demonstrate hyperthyroidism.

Since the beta subunit is unique to each of the glycoprotein hormones, the best means of detecting excessive production of hCG is by measuring the beta hCG subunit by a highly specific radioimmunoassay or immunofluorometric assay. Since hCG can serve as an important tumor marker for initial diagnosis and for recurrence, this value can be followed as an indicator of tumor activity. In contrast to hCG, ectopic production of the gonadotropins FSH and LH is extremely rare.

ONCOGENIC OSTEOMALACIA

Etiology & Clinical Features

Oncogenic osteomalacia is a syndrome seen in association with unusual mesenchymal tumors and rarely with prostate cancer. These patients have hypophosphatemia, renal phosphate wasting, and low serum levels of 1,25-dihydroxyvitamin D. Alkaline phosphatase activity, reflecting bone turnover, is often elevated. Levels of calcium and parathyroid hormone are typically normal. Hypophosphatemia in this syndrome is due to reduced renal phosphate reabsorption. The defect in phosphate reabsorption is due to proximal tubular dysfunction and may be accompanied by glucosuria and aminoaciduria. Clinical symptoms include bone pain, muscle weakness, fractures, back pain, waddling gait, and progressive debility. The syndrome often poses a significant diagnostic dilemma to clinicians since the tumors responsible for it may be very small, obscurely situated, and difficult to identify. Phosphate depletion and low 1,25-dihydroxyvitamin D levels lead to poor bone mineralization and osteomalacia. Typically, the diagnosis of osteomalacia is often not even suspected for years despite the presence of classic symptoms. The humoral basis for the syndrome is supported by the observation that the attendant biochemical abnormalities remit and the rickets heals when the responsible tumor is removed.

Pathology & Pathogenesis

Tumors responsible for this form of acquired osteomalacia are usually small and grow slowly. Because the histology of these tumors is unusual and their locations often unanticipated, this syndrome has been dubbed "strange tumours in strange places" by Weiss and colleagues. The range of locations for these tumors includes the lower extremities (45%), head and neck (27%), and upper extremities (17%). In a review of head and neck tumors that cause oncogenic osteomalacia, Gonzalez-Compta and coworkers noted that in 57% and 20% of cases, respectively, tumors were in the sinonasal and mandibular areas. Because these tumors are often small and in obscure locations, careful physical examination combined with cranial, chest, and abdominal CT scanning are usually needed for diagnosis. In several instances, MRI skeletal surveys—and in some instances indium-111 pentreotide scanning—have been instrumental in localizing the tumors at skeletal sites.

Most tumors causing this syndrome are benign, but malignant lesions have also been reported. The histologic spectrum of tumors has included hemangiomas, hemangiopericytomas, angiosarcomas, chondrosarcomas, prostate cancer, schwannomas, neuroendocrine lesions, and mesenchymal tumors. Many of these tumors have been classified pathologically as mixed connective tissue tumors. They are often located in bone. Osteoclast-like giant cells and stromal cells as well as highly vascular features characterize these tumors. On microscopic analysis, these tumors do not commonly demonstrate neurosecretory granules. As evidence of the slow growth of these tumors, delays in diagnosis of as long as 19 years have been reported.

Most tumors responsible for this syndrome overproduce fibroblast growth factor (FGF) 23, a protein implicated in phosphate wasting. FGF-23 is mutated in cases of autosomal dominant hypophosphatemic rickets. These mutations appear to render the mutant protein less susceptible to proteolytic cleavage and inactivation. Whether FGF-23 is responsible for the changes in vitamin D hydroxylation in oncogenic osteomalacia and whether the osteomalacia is secondary to problems in vitamin D availability or phosphate wasting is unknown. Investigators in the field have noted common features between tumor-induced osteomalacia and X-linked hypophosphatemic rickets. The latter condition is a dominant disorder characterized by rickets or osteomalacia, hypophosphatemia, and low 1,25-dihydroxyvitamin vitamin D levels. Despite these similarities, there are several unresolved differences between the two syndromes. One is that levels of 1,25-dihydroxyvitamin D are inappropriately normal in patients with X-linked hypophosphatemic rickets and frankly low in oncogenic osteomalacia. In addition, patients with X-linked hypophosphatemic rickets demonstrate osteosclerosis and enthesopathy (calcification of tendons and ligaments).

X-linked hypophosphatemic rickets is probably due to defective functioning or synthesis of the *PEX* gene product, or PHEX, a protein that is homologous to neutral, membrane-bound endopeptidases. PHEX is thought to activate or inactivate a circulating factor involved in phosphate metabolism, which was classically termed "phosphatonin" by investigators in this field. It has long been proposed that the normal function of phosphatonin was to block renal phosphate reabsorption. It has been shown that FGF-23, the product of tumors that cause oncogenic osteomalacia, inhibits phosphate uptake in kidney cells. PHEX, the endopeptidase product of the *PEX* gene, can degrade wild-type FGF-23 but not mutant FGF-23 such as is found in autosomal dominant hypophosphatemic rickets.

GUT HORMONES

Vasoactive intestinal peptide (VIP) is a peptide hormone with a number of important functions in the regulation of neuronal activity, differentiation, and survival, particularly in the sympathetic nervous system. A variety of neuroendocrine tumors express and release VIP. Pancreatic islet cell tumors that make VIP are quite rare. They can cause voluminous secretory diarrhea, achlorhydria, and hypokalemia. Other tumors, including small cell carcinomas of the lung, carcinoids, pheochromocytoma, medullary carcinomas of the thyroid, and some colonic adenocarcinomas, also produce VIP which may or may not be responsible for related symptoms. VIP is also made in non-small cell lung carcinomas and may function as an autocrine regulator of cell growth based on in vitro studies.

REFERENCES

Hypercalcemia of Malignancy

Finley RS: Bisphosphonates in the treatment of bone metastases. Semin Oncol 2002;29(Suppl 4):132. [PMID: 21891339]

Hofbauer LC et al: Receptor activation of nuclear factor-kappaB ligand and osteoprotegerin: potential implications for the pathogenesis and treatment of malignant bone diseases. Cancer 2001;92:460. [PMID: 21395914]

Levine PH et al: A study of adult T-cell leukemia/lymphoma incidence in central Brooklyn. Int J Cancer 1999;80:5662. [PMID: 99140392]

Strewler GJ: The parathyroid hormone-related protein. Endocrinol Metab Clin North Am 2000;29:529. [PMID: 11033764]

Syndrome of Inappropriate Secretion of ADH

Adrogue HJ, Madias NE: Hyponatremia. N Engl J Med 2000;342:1581. [PMID: 11001689]

Ferlito A, Rinaldo A, Devaney KO: Syndrome of inappropriate antidiuretic hormone secretion associated with head neck cancers: review of the literature. Ann Otol Rhinol Laryngol 1997;106:878. [PMID: 9342988]

Hirshberg B, Ben-Yehuda A: The syndrome of inappropriate anti-diuretic hormone secretion in the elderly. Am J Med 1997; 103:270. [PMID: 9382118]

Kamoi K et al: Osmoregulation of vasopressin secretion in patients with the syndrome of inappropriate antidiuresis associated with central nervous system disorders. Endocr J 1999;46:269. [PMID: 10460011]

Vanhees SL, Paridaens R, Vansteenkiste JF: Syndrome of inappropriate antidiuretic hormone associated with chemotherapy-induced tumour lysis in small-cell lung cancer: case report and literature review. Ann Oncol 2000;11:1061. [PMID: 11038047]

Cushing's Syndrome

Kaltsas GA et al: A critical analysis of the value of simultaneous inferior petrosal sinus sampling in Cushing's disease and the occult ectopic adrenocorticotropin syndrome. J Clin Endocrinol Metab 1999;84:487. [PMID: 10022405]

Tabarin A et al: Usefulness of somatostatin receptor scintigraphy in patients with occult ectopic adrenocorticotropin syndrome. J Clin Endocrinol Metab 1999;84:1193. [PMID: 10199752]

Hypoglycemia

Baxter RC: The role of insulin-like growth factors and their binding proteins in tumor hypoglycemia. Horm Res 1996;46: 195. [PMID: 8950621]

Furrer J et al: Carcinoid syndrome, acromegaly, and hypoglycemia due to an insulin-secreting neuroendocrine tumor of the liver. J Clin Endocrinol Metab 2001;86:2227. [PMID: 11344231]

Hizuka N et al: Serum high molecular weight form of insulin-like growth factor II from patients with non-islet cell tumor hypoglycemia is O-glycosylated. J Clin Endocrinol Metab 1998; 83:2875. [PMID: 9709962]

Hoekman K et al: Hypoglycaemia associated with the production of insulin-like growth factor II and insulin-like growth factor binding protein 6 by a hemangiopericytoma. Clin Endocrinol (Oxf) 1999;51:247. [PMID: 10468998]

Le Roith D: Tumor-induced hypoglycemia. N Engl J Med 1999; 341:757. [PMID: 10471466]

Mizuta Y et al: Acinar cell carcinoma of the pancreas associated with hypoglycemia: involvement of "big" insulin-like growth factor-II. J Gastroenterol 1998;33:761. [PMID: 9473947]

Seckl MJ et al: Hypoglycemia due to an insulin-secreting small-cell carcinoma of the cervix. N Engl J Med 1999;341:733. [PMID: 10471459]

Teale JD, Marks V: Glucocorticoid therapy suppresses abnormal secretion of big IGF-II by non-islet cell tumours inducing hypoglycaemia (NICTH). Clin Endocrinol (Oxf) 1998;49:491. [PMID: 9876347]

Gonadotropins

Dirnhofer S et al: Selective expression of trophoblastic hormones by lung carcinoma: neurendocrine tumors exclusively produce human chorionic gonadotropin alpha-subunit (hCG alpha). Hum Pathol 2000;31:966. [PMID: 10987258]

Lundin M et al: Tissue expression of human chorionic gonadotropin beta predicts outcome in colorectal cancer: a comparison with serum expression. Int J Cancer 2001;95:18. [PMID: 11241305]

Syrigos KN et al: Beta human chorionic gonadotropin concentrations in serum of patients with pancreatic adenocarcinoma. Gut 1998;42:88. [PMID: 9505891]

Vartiainen J et al: Preoperative serum concentration of hCGbeta as a prognostic factor in ovarian cancer. Int J Cancer 2001;95: 313. [PMID: 11494231]

GHRH and Growth Hormone

Beuschlein F et al: Acromegaly caused by secretion of growth hormone by a non-Hodgkin's lymphoma. N Engl J Med 2000; 342:1871. [PMID: 10861322]

Doga M et al: Ectopic secretion of growth hormone-releasing hormone (GHRH) in neuroendocrine tumors: relevant clinical aspects. Ann Oncol 2001;12(Suppl 2):S89. [PMID: 11762359]

Drange MR, Melmed S: Long acting lanreotide induces clinical and biochemical remission of acromegaly caused by disseminated growth hormone-releasing hormone-secreting carcinoid. J Clin Endocrinol Metab 1998;83:3104. [PMID: 9745411]

Matsuno A: Pituitary somatotroph adenoma producing growth hormone (GH)-releasing hormone (GHRH) with an elevated plasma GHRH concentration: a model case for autocrine and paracrine regulation of GH secretion by GHRH. J Clin Endocrinol Metab 1999;84:3241. [PMID: 10487694]

Othman NH et al: Growth hormone-releasing hormone (GHRH) and GHRH receptor (GHRH-R) isoform expression in ectopic acromegaly. Clin Endocrinol (Oxf) 2001;55:135. [PMID: 11453963]

Calcitonin

Kelley MJ et al: Calcitonin elevation in small cell lung cancer without ectopic production. Am J Respir Crit Care Med 1994; 149:183. [PMID: 8111580]

Ghillani PP et al: Identification and measurement of calcitonin precursors in serum of patients with malignant diseases. Cancer Res 1989;49:6845. [PMID: 2555054]

Oncogenic Osteomalacia

Bowe AE et al: FGF-23 inhibits renal tubular phosphate transport and is a PHEX substrate. Biochem Biophys Res Commun 2001;284:977. [PMID: 11409890]

DiMeglio LA, Econs MJ: Hypophosphatemic rickets. Rev Endocr Metab Disord 2001;2:165. [PMID: 11705322]

Econs MJ: New insights into the pathogenesis of inherited phosphate wasting disorders. Bone 1999;25:131. [PMID: 10423038]

Fukumoto S et al: Diagnostic utility of magnetic resonance imaging skeletal survey in a patient with oncogenic osteomalcia. Bone 1999;25:375. [PMID: 10495143]

Gonzalez-Compta X et al: Oncogenic osteomalacia: case report and review of head and neck associated tumours. J Laryngol Otol 1998;112:389. [PMID: 9659507]

Jan de Beur SM et al: Localisation of mesenchymal tumors by somatostatin receptor imaging. Lancet 2002;359:761. [PMID: 11888589]

Rowe PSN: The role of the PHEX gene (PEX) in families with X-linked hypophosphataemic rickets. Curr Opin Nephrol Hypertens 1998;7:367. [PMID: 9690034]

Weiss D et al: Oncogenic osteomalacia: strange tumours in strange places. Postgrad Med J 1985;61:349. [PMID: 4022870]

White KE et al: Autosomal-dominant hypophosphatemic rickets (ADHR) mutations stabilize FGF-23. Kidney Int 2001;60:2079. [PMID: 11737582]

Gut Hormones

Hejna M et al: Serum levels of vasoactive intestinal peptide (VIP) in patients with adenocarcinomas of the gastrointestinal tract. Anticancer Res 2001;21:1183. [PMID: 11396161]

Smith SL et al: Vasoactive intestinal polypeptide secreting islet cell tumors: a 15-year experience and review of the literature. Surgery 1998;124:1050. [PMID: 9854582]

Multiple Endocrine Neoplasia

22

David G. Gardner, MD

ACTH	Adrenocorticotropic hormone	**MRI**	Magnetic resonance imaging
CT	Computed tomography	**PI-3′K**	Phosphatidyl inositol 3′-kinase
GDNF	Glial cell line-derived neurotrophic factor	**PTH**	Parathyroid hormone
		SMAD	Vertebrate homologs to C elegans Sma and drosophila Mad proteins
GDNFR	Glial cell line-derived neurotrophic factor receptor	**TGFβ**	Transforming growth factor beta
MCT	Medullary carcinoma of thyroid	**ZES**	Zollinger-Ellison syndrome
MEN	Multiple endocrine neoplasia		

A group of heritable syndromes characterized by aberrant growth of benign or malignant tumors in a subset of endocrine tissues have been given the collective term multiple endocrine neoplasia (MEN). The tumors may be functional (ie, capable of elaborating hormonal products that result in specific clinical findings characteristic of the hormone excess state) or nonfunctional. There are three major syndromes: MEN 1 is characterized by tumors involving the parathyroid glands, the endocrine pancreas, and the pituitary; MEN 2A includes medullary carcinoma of the thyroid gland, pheochromocytoma, and hyperparathyroidism; and MEN 2B, like MEN 2A, includes medullary carcinoma of the thyroid, multiple neuromas, and pheochromocytoma, but hyperparathyroidism is typically absent.

MULTIPLE ENDOCRINE NEOPLASIA TYPE 1 (MEN 1)

MEN 1, also known as Wermer's syndrome, is inherited as an autosomal dominant trait with an estimated prevalence of 2–20 per 100,000 in the general population. Approximately 10% of MEN 1 mutations arise de novo. The term "sporadic MEN 1" has been applied to this group. MEN 1 has a number of unusual clinical manifestations (Table 22–1) that occur with variable frequency among individuals within affected kindreds.

Hyperparathyroidism is the most common feature of MEN 1, with an estimated penetrance of 95–100% over the lifetime of an individual harboring the MEN 1 gene. The diagnosis of hyperparathyroidism is usually made through a combination of clinical and laboratory criteria similar to those used in the identification of sporadic disease (see Chapter 8). It is typically the first clinical manifestation of MEN 1, though this varies as a function of the patient population being examined. Hyperparathyroidism in MEN 1 is due to hyperplasia of all four parathyroid glands (or more, if supernumerary glands are present). However, involved glands may undergo metachronous enlargement, and selective resection of these glands often results in sustained clinical remissions. MEN 1 is a rare cause of hyperparathyroidism, accounting for only 2–4% of cases in the general population.

Enteropancreatic tumors in MEN 1 can be either functional (ie, capable of producing a secreted product with biologic activity) or nonfunctional. Gastrinomas, frequently associated with Zollinger-Ellison syndrome, represent approximately 40–60% of the enteropancreatic tumors associated with this syndrome. Of equal importance, roughly 25% of patients with Zollinger-Ellison syndrome are found in MEN 1 kindreds. Insulinomas constitute approximately 20% of the islet cell tumors while the remainder represent a collection of functional (eg, glucagon- or vasoactive intestinal peptide-producing tumors) and nonfunctional tumors. It is noteworthy that the gastrinomas of MEN 1 are often small, multicentric, and ectopically located outside the pancreatic bed, most often in the duodenal submucosa. This latter feature can have a major impact on the ther-

Table 22–1. Clinical manifestations of MEN 1.

Manifestation	(%)
Hyperparathyroidism	95
Enteropancreatic tumors	30–80
Pituitary adenomas	20–25
Carcinoid tumors	10–20
Adrenal adenomas	25–40
Subcutaneous lipomas	30
Facial angiofibromas	85
Collagenomas	70

apeutic approach to these patients (see below). Gastrinomas in MEN 1 are frequently malignant, as are their sporadic counterparts; however, for reasons that are only poorly understood, the biologic behavior of these tumors is less aggressive than that found in sporadic disease.

The diagnosis of gastrinomas is based on demonstration of hypergastrinemia in the presence of gastric acid hypersecretion. This latter criterion excludes other more common causes of hypergastrinemia (eg, achlorhydria). When the diagnosis is in question, the secretin stimulation test, which stimulates gastrin secretion from gastrinomas but not from normal tissue, may be employed. (***Note:*** The availability of secretin for parenteral administration is now quite limited.) Others have advocated measurements of multiple gastrointestinal hormones following a standardized mixed meal as the most efficient means of detecting the presence of neuroendocrine tumors in MEN 1.

Owing to their small size, gastrinomas can be difficult to localize in MEN 1. Computed tomography and MRI may be useful in identifying larger lesions but are typically not helpful in identifying smaller ones. These imaging procedures are useful, however, in demonstrating hepatic metastases when present. The most promising localization techniques studied to date include endoscopic and intraoperative ultrasound, selective arterial secretin injection (followed by hepatic vein sampling for gastrin), and radiolabeled octreotide scanning. Each of these has been employed successfully to identify tumors in studies involving small groups of patients. It is important to recognize, however, that almost half of gastrinomas are not found with preoperative localization studies.

Insulinomas in MEN 1 are detected using conventional biochemical testing (see Chapter 18). They can also be difficult to localize given their potential for multicentricity. Endoscopic ultrasound and selective arterial infusions of calcium with hepatic vein sampling (for insulin) have been used successfully to identify lesions in small groups of patients.

Pituitary adenomas occur in approximately 25% of patients harboring the MEN 1 gene. The majority secrete prolactin, with or without secretion of excess growth hormone, followed by those secreting growth hormone alone, nonfunctional tumors, and those secreting excessive amounts of ACTH (Cushing's disease). A prolactinoma variant of MEN 1 has been described (Burin variant). This variant is characterized by an increased frequency of prolactinomas, carcinoids, and hyperparathyroidism and infrequent appearance of gastrinomas in affected kindreds. It does not appear to be associated with a specific mutation of the MEN 1 gene. Pituitary tumors in MEN 1 are rarely malignant, but recent studies suggest that they may be larger and more aggressive than their sporadic counterparts. Diagnosis and management are similar to that of their sporadic counterparts (see Chapter 5).

Adrenal adenomas, including cortisol-producing adenomas, are seen in MEN 1, theoretically making the differential diagnosis of Cushing's syndrome in this setting complex (ie, adrenal adenoma versus basophilic adenoma of the pituitary gland versus ectopic ACTH secretion from a carcinoid tumor, which is also commonly associated with this syndrome). Empirically, most hypercortisolemia in this setting is due to pituitary disease. Adrenal adenomas are often found together with islet cell tumors in affected patients, and at least in some series they appear to lack the MEN 1 genetic defect. This has led to the suggestion that they represent a secondary rather than a primary manifestation of the underlying genetic defect. This, however, remains controversial. Thyroid disease has been said to be more common in MEN 1; however, with the possible exception of thyroid adenomas, this link remains obscure. Subcutaneous lipomas, skin collagenomas, and multiple facial angiofibromas are seen in 30–90% of family members in affected kindreds. Though clinically of little importance, when present, they may prove useful in identifying affected individuals within a kindred and lead to more effective screening (see below). Carcinoid tumors are seen with increased frequency in MEN 1. They are almost exclusively foregut carcinoids and may be found in the thymus, in the lung (bronchial carcinoids), or in the gastric mucosa. For unclear reasons, thymic carcinoids appear more commonly in males, bronchial carcinoids in females. They occasionally secrete hormonal products (eg, ectopic ACTH), are often malignant, and may behave aggressively. Leiomyomas and, rarely, pheochromocytomas have also been described in MEN 1.

Pathogenesis

MEN 1 is inherited as an autosomal dominant trait. Traditional linkage studies localized the defective gene to the long arm of chromosome 11q13. Parallel analyses of DNA from endocrine tumors taken from MEN 1 patients demonstrated allelic loss in this area, frequently resulting from large DNA deletions. This raised the possibility that the defective gene was a tumor suppressor gene involved in the control of cellular growth. In this paradigm (Figure 22–1), the inherited defective allele is silent in the presence of a normal, functioning allele on the second chromosome. A subsequent somatic mutation (often a deletion that removes the normal allele) results in a null genotype in which the suppressor gene locus is either absent or defective on both alleles. The high frequency with which such deletions occur is thought to account for the dominant nature of this particular genetic defect. Release of the tumor suppressor gene's growth regulatory activity results in a hyperplastic growth response in cells harboring the somatic mutation. This promitogenic state probably provides the substrate for subsequent somatic mutations that result

in acquisition of a true malignant phenotype, as occurs in gastrinomas associated with Zollinger-Ellison syndrome. Recent studies have succeeded in identifying the gene, termed the *menin* gene, which appears to be responsible for MEN 1 (Figure 22–2). Mutations have been identified throughout the entire 610-amino-acid length of the *menin* coding sequence and include nonsense mutations, missense mutations, and deletions. Almost 300 independent mutations have been described in MEN 1 kindreds to date. Menin is a nuclear protein whose precise cellular function has yet to be determined. It has been shown to interact with JunD, a constitutively expressed member of the extended *jun/fos* gene family. Menin suppresses JunD-dependent transcriptional activation in the intact cell, though it is unclear if and how this accounts for its growth regulatory activity since JunD is typically associated with inhibition of cell growth. It is of note that menin does not interact with other members of the Jun/Fos family.

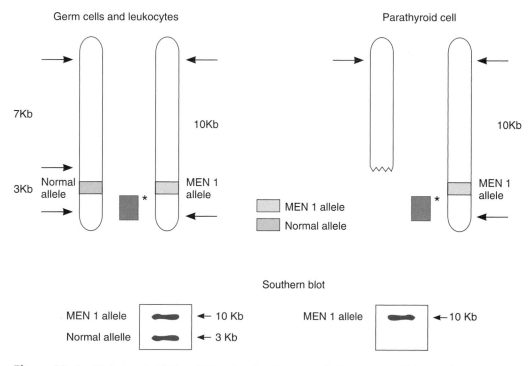

Figure 22–1. Allelic loss in MEN 1. Afflicted patient's germ cells (shown on left) harbor both a normal and defective gene at the MEN 1 locus. Each of these is detected using selective restriction enzyme digestion and Southern blot analysis of the genomic DNA. Affected somatic cells (eg, parathyroid chief cells) undergo a second mutation, typically a deletion of the normal allele, resulting in detection of only the mutant allele by Southern analysis. Sporadic disease is thought to follow sequential mutation or deletion of each MEN 1 allele in the somatic cell. Solid bar (dark blue) with asterisk represents radiolabeled probe used in Southern analysis.

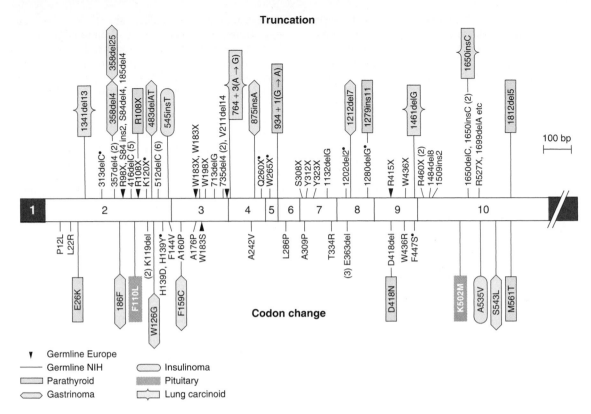

Figure 22–2. Some of the more common germline menin mutations from fifty-six MEN 1 kindreds and somatic mutations from twenty-four endocrine tumors. Mutations above the bar cause protein truncations through stop codons or frameshifts leading to premature stop codons; two cause splice errors. Mutations below the bar cause missense or single-amino-acid codon changes. (Reproduced, with permission, from Marx S et al: Multiple endocrine neoplasia type 1: Clinical and genetic topics. Ann Intern Med 1998;129:484.)

Menin also interacts with SMAD 3, a transcription factor involved in the TGF-β signaling pathway.

The *MEN1* gene is also the gene most frequently mutated in a variety of sporadic endocrine tumors. Parathyroid adenomas (21%), gastrinomas (33%), insulinomas (17%), bronchial carcinoids (36%) and pituitary tumors (5%) often harbor somatic mutations at the *MEN1* locus. It is important to note that screening for germline mutations at the menin locus fails to detect mutations 10–20% of the time despite evidence for loss of heterozygosity at 11q13. It is thought that the relevant mutations may be in regulatory regions surrounding the menin gene. Haplotype testing or genetic linkage analysis can be useful in these cases to identify relevant MEN 1 carriers. Unlike MEN 2 (see below), there is no clear association between specific menin gene mutations and the nature or extent of endocrine gland involvement.

Treatment

Therapy of hyperparathyroidism in MEN 1 is directed toward surgical extirpation of hyperplastic parathyroid tissue, typically with resection of three and one-half glands. This leaves one-half gland in situ in an attempt to preserve residual parathyroid function and avoid hypoparathyroidism. Alternatively, patients may be subjected to total parathyroidectomy with transplantation of the "most normal-appearing" tissue to the nondominant forearm. Prophylactic near-total thymectomy is typically performed at the time of neck exploration to cover the possibility of intrathymic parathyroid glands as well as thymic carcinoid tumors.

Both persistence and recurrence of hyperparathyroidism occur more frequently in MEN 1 than in sporadic disease. Persistence of hyperparathyroidism, defined as a failure to normalize serum calcium and parathyroid hormone (PTH) levels following the initial surgery, occurs in 38% of cases of MEN 1. Recurrent disease, defined as reappearance of hyperparathyroidism following at least 3 months of normocalcemia, is seen in 16% of cases, and this may rise to 50% 8–12 years following surgery. The high frequency of persistent hyperparathyroidism in MEN 1 probably reflects the high frequency of supernumerary glands and ectopically located parathyroid tissue in patients carrying this gene. The increased frequency of recurrent disease is thought to result from the continued presence of the underlying mitogenic stimulus that drives parathyroid gland growth in this syndrome.

Therapy of gastrinomas in MEN 1 remains controversial. Suppression of gastric acid production with proton pump inhibitors (eg, omeprazole) remains a mainstay of therapy. Conservative medical management of these tumors has been predicated on their assumed low-grade malignant behavior, the dominance of complications related to gastric acid hypersecretion in contributing to morbidity and mortality, and the failure of most attempts at surgical resection to alter the natural course of the disease. More recently, recognition of the potential for more aggressive behavior in some of these tumors—in a recent study, 14% of these tumors demonstrated aggressive growth—and the fact that many of these tumors are "ectopically" located in duodenal submucosa rather than the pancreatic bed has renewed interest in the possibility of surgical cure. A number of small studies have reported encouraging results when measures to both localize and remove gastrinoma tissue in the pancreas and duodenum have been used. While the nature of the underlying genetic lesion and the multicentricity of these tumors may place limits on the prospects for cure of this disease in most patients, the slow growth characteristics of these tumors permit long periods of symptom-free survival following reduction of the tumor burden. For patients with liver or other metastatic disease, symptoms related to hypergastrinemia may be controlled with the proton pump antagonists, as described above. More conventional cancer therapy (eg, systemic chemotherapy, radiation therapy, or selective chemoembolization of hepatic metastases) is palliative and reserved for advanced stages of the disease.

It is important to remember that calcium stimulates gastric acid secretion. This may occur through gastrin-dependent and gastrin-independent pathways. In MEN 1 patients with both hyperparathyroidism and Zollinger-Ellison syndrome, correction of the hyperparathyroidism and attendant hypercalcemia frequently results in a reduction in both basal and maximal acid output and a decline in serum gastrin levels. Secretin stimulation tests often normalize following parathyroidectomy. More importantly, there is a reduction in the dose of medication (eg, H_2 blocker) required to control symptoms of Zollinger-Ellison syndrome following parathyroid surgery in approximately 60% of patients.

Unlike gastrinomas, insulinomas are rarely localized outside the pancreatic bed. Therefore, a more aggressive approach can be directed toward the pancreas in planning surgical resection. Enucleation of the identifiable lesions in the pancreatic head and blind resection of the pancreatic body and tail are often more successful in correcting hyperinsulinemia than in restoring normal gastrin levels in patients with Zollinger-Ellison syndrome. Nonsurgical candidates (eg, those with serious coexisting disease or those in whom candidate tumors cannot be identified) can be managed with conventional medical therapy (eg, diazoxide or verapamil). (See Chapter 18.)

Screening

MEN 1 accounts for less than 1% of all pituitary tumors, 2–4% of cases of primary hyperparathyroidism, and about 25% of all gastrinomas. Thus, while routine screening for *menin* gene mutations is not indicated for sporadic cases of hyperparathyroidism or patients with pituitary tumors, screening of all cases of Zollinger-Ellison syndrome is likely to be cost-effective in identifying carriers. The frequency of germline mutations in the *menin* gene in patients with tumors thought to be sporadic based on family analysis is abut 5% for gastrinomas and 1–2% for other manifestations (hyperparathyroidism, prolactinomas, etc). Screening for MEN 1 within affected kindreds should be limited to those individuals for whom the index of suspicion for the syndrome is high (eg, familial history of endocrine tumors or hypersecretory states; history of multiple endocrine tumors or multigland involvement in the propositus). Identification of the carrier state should be done with the intent of acquiring information that will allow the clinician to focus screening on the relevant patient population (eg, members of an affected kindred who do not share the *menin* gene mutation need not be subjected to follow-up screening). Unlike the situation in MEN 2 (see below), carrier analysis should not be used to support a major therapeutic intervention. Such interventions (eg, pancreatic exploration) may be associated with significant morbidity, and there is no evidence that they prolong patient survival. Patients with hyperparathyroidism should be screened for MEN 1—even in the absence of a positive family history or any history of multiple endocrine tumors—if parathyroid hyperplasia is identified at the time of parathyroidectomy or if there is a history of recurrent hyperparathyroidism following parathyroidectomy. Patients with Zollinger-Ellison syndrome should be screened for MEN 1 given its high frequency (about 25%) in such individuals. Patients with isolated pituitary lesions have a low probability of having coexistent MEN 1 and probably do not require screening unless there are other clinical features suggesting the syndrome.

While most clinicians agree that screening for MEN 1 in high-risk groups is worthwhile, details of the individual screening protocols vary considerably—from more focused, cost effective approaches to broad-based screening designed to detect occult disease. One example of a more cost-effective protocol is presented in Figure 22–3. In individuals within affected kindreds, ionized (or albumin-corrected) calcium and parathyroid hormone levels should be checked at yearly intervals. Serum gastrin levels should also be determined annually—or more frequently if Zollinger-Ellison syndrome is a prominent component of the phenotype in the affected kindred. In kindreds in whom disease is particularly aggressive, the secretin stimulation test (if available) can lend additional diagnostic sensitivity. Determination of fasting glucose, insulin, and proinsulin levels may prove useful, particularly if symptoms of hypoglycemia are present. Routine screening for other functional or nonfunctional islet cell tumors is probably not justified without clinical findings (eg, watery diarrhea, hypokalemia). As noted above, these lesions are typically multifocal and may be very small, which makes detection difficult even with sophisticated imaging studies. The same holds true for the pituitary lesions. In the absence of obvious clinical findings (eg, evidence of a hyper- or hyposecretory state or symptoms referable to a mass lesion in the sella turcica), routine screening should be confined to periodic measurements of serum prolactin and perhaps IGF-I. The former has been found to be useful in identifying pituitary disease in females harboring the MEN 1 gene defect. Imaging studies (eg, MRI of the pituitary and CT scan of the abdomen) should be performed at presentation and repeated at 3-year intervals.

Penetrance of MEN 1 is greater than 95% by age 45. Screening should be continued at periodic intervals at least to age 45. If there is no evidence of typical endocrine organ involvement by that age, screening frequency might be reduced. It is important to note, however, that the risk is not reduced to zero at age 45. A minority of patients will present with their first manifestation of the syndrome well after age 45. Surgical resection of diseased tissue (eg, parathyroidectomy) should be followed with continued screening looking both for recurrent disease and involvement of other organ systems.

MULTIPLE ENDOCRINE NEOPLASIA TYPE 2 (MEN 2)

MEN 2 is an autosomal dominant disorder with an estimated prevalence of 1–10 per 100,000 in the general population. It can be subdivided into two independent syndromes: MEN 2A (Sipple's syndrome) and MEN 2B. Manifestations of MEN 2A include medullary carcinoma of the thyroid, pheochromocytoma, and hyperparathyroidism. MEN 2B includes medullary carcinoma of the thyroid, pheochromocytoma, and a number of somatic manifestations (Table 22–2; Figure 22–4), but hyperparathyroidism is rare. Penetrance of MEN 2 is greater than 80% in individuals harboring the defective gene.

Medullary carcinoma of the thyroid is the most common manifestation of MEN 2 and often represents the first clinical presentation in individuals with multiorgan involvement. It also dominates the clinical course of patients affected with the disease. Eighty to 100 percent of individuals at risk will develop medullary carcinoma of the thyroid at some point during their lifetime. The classic thyroid lesion of MEN 2 is hyperplasia of the calcitonin-producing parafollicular cells, which typically serves as the precursor of medullary thyroid carcinoma. These tumors in MEN 2 patients tend to be multicentric and concentrated in the upper third of the thyroid gland, reflecting the normal distribution of parafollicular cells.

As much as one-fourth of all medullary carcinoma of the thyroid is genetic in origin. Roughly 45% of the heritable fraction is attributable to MEN 2A; 50% occurs as an isolated entity (isolated familial medullary carcinoma of the thyroid), and 5% is found in MEN 2B kindreds. The disease tends to behave more aggressively in MEN 2B than with either MEN 2A or familial medullary carcinoma, with earlier presentation (often before age 5) and more rapid progression.

Biochemical diagnosis depends heavily on the calcitonin-producing properties of the hyperplastic parafollicular cells or MCT. These lesions respond to pentagastrin or calcium infusions with significant increments in plasma calcitonin levels (see Chapter 7). Occasionally, immunohistochemical staining of poorly differentiated thyroid tumors for calcitonin will reveal the identity of the malignancy. The presence of extracellular amyloid is also one of the identifying features of these tumors. This material reacts with anti-calcitonin antisera, suggesting that it includes aggregated hormone released from neighboring tumor cells. MCT spreads initially within the thyroid bed and to regional lymph nodes. Distant metastases to liver, lung, and bone occur late in the course of the disease.

Pheochromocytomas develop in approximately 50% of individuals harboring the MEN 2 gene. They are usually located in the adrenal bed, often are bilateral, and are rarely malignant. Diagnosis is based on standard clinical criteria (eg, hypertension, presence of headaches, palpitations, diaphoresis), elevations in plasma or urine catecholamines or catecholamine metabolites (eg, urinary or plasma metanephrine or

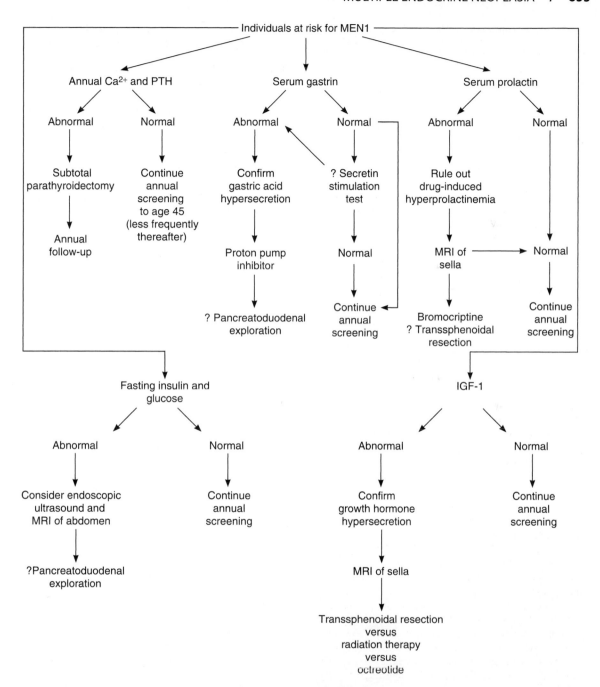

Figure 22–3. Screening for MEN 1. Testing is targeted to individuals with a high probability of harboring the MEN 1 gene (eg, first-degree relatives of affected kindred members). If genetic testing is available and specific mutation is defined, screening might be limited to those individuals harboring the defective gene. Extension of screening to other pancreatic (eg, insulinomas) or pituitary tumors (eg, somatotroph adenomas) is based on the prevalence of the specific lesion in the affected kindred or the presence of signs or symptoms suggesting a particular lesion.

Table 22–2. Clinical manifestations of MEN 2.

Manifestation	(%)
MEN 2A	
Medullary carcinoma of thyroid	80–100
Pheochromocytoma	40
Hyperparathyroidism	25
MEN 2B	
Medullary carcinoma of thyroid	100
Pheochromocytoma	50
Marfanoid habitus	75
Mucosal neuromas	100
Ganglioneuromatosis of bowel	> 40

normetanephrine) and demonstration of an adrenal mass on conventional abdominal imaging. As noted above for medullary carcinoma of the thyroid, pheochromocytomas in MEN 2 are preceded by a hyperplastic phase (adrenal medullary hyperplasia), although, unlike parafollicular cell hyperplasia, the adrenal precursor lesion can be difficult to detect with conventional biochemical testing.

As in MEN 1, hyperparathyroidism in MEN 2 is due to hyperplasia of the parathyroid glands. It is seen in about 25% of patients harboring the MEN 2A gene and is rarely seen as part of MEN 2B. The disease is usually less aggressive than its counterpart in MEN 1 and approximates more closely the behavior of sporadic disease. It responds well to surgical management.

There are a number of other phenotypic features associated with the MEN 2 syndromes. Cutaneous lichen amyloidosis is a pruritic erythematous skin lesion that is seen coincident with or often preceding the development of medullary carcinoma of the thyroid in MEN 2. Amyloid in these lesions is composed of keratin rather than calcitonin, as seen in medullary carcinoma. While the origin of the skin lesion is unknown, it has been noted more frequently in association with specific mutations of the MEN 2 gene (specifically Cys^{634} to Tyr^{634}). In a second variant, MEN 2A or familial MCT is associated with Hirschsprung's disease (congenital megacolon; see below). This is most frequently found with *RET* mutations involving Cys^{609}, Cys^{615}, and Cys^{620}. The intestinal ganglioneuromatosis, the presence of mucosal neuromas, marfanoid habitus and medullated corneal nerves seen in MEN 2B appear to be related to the underlying genetic defect (Figure 22–5). The intestinal lesions can disrupt gut motility, resulting in periods of severe constipation or diarrhea.

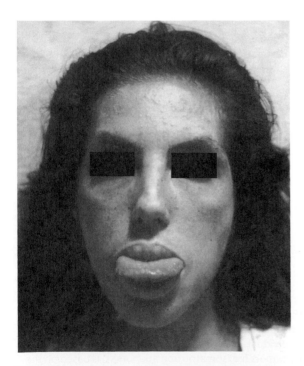

Figure 22–4. Patient with MEN 2B syndrome. Note the multiple neuromas on the lips and tongue and the marfanoid facies.

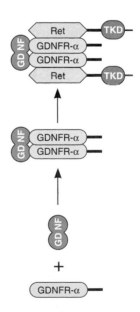

Figure 22–5. Structure of GDNFR-α/RET receptor complex. GDNF identifies the ligand, glial cell line-derived neurotrophic factor, and GDNFR-α the GDNF receptor. TKD, tyrosine kinase domain.

Pathogenesis

The pathogenesis of the MEN 2 syndromes has been worked out in elegant detail. Traditional genetic linkage studies localized the defective genes in MEN 2A, MEN 2B, and familial medullary carcinoma of the thyroid to the pericentromeric region of chromosome 10. Subsequent refinement in these analyses indicated that the defective gene was either closely linked to or identical with the *ret* proto-oncogene. RET is a single transmembrane domain, tyrosine kinase-linked protein which forms part of the receptor for the glial cell line-derived neurotrophic factor (GDNF) (Figure 22–5). This receptor, GDNFα-1, is a glycosyl phosphatidyl inositol-linked cell surface protein that has also been shown to bind additional ligands, neurturin and artemin. As depicted schematically in Figure 22–6, its most striking structural feature is a series of cysteine residues clustered just outside the membrane-spanning segment. These cysteine residues are thought to exert a tonic inhibitory control on RET activity in the normal cell. RET also has a cadherin-like domain in that portion of the molecule projecting into the extracellular space and a tyrosine kinase-like domain in the intracellular portion of the molecule. RET is expressed endogenously in a variety of cells of neural crest origin, and it appears to play an important role in development. Knockout of the *RET* gene locus in mice results in the absence of myenteric ganglia in the submucosa of the small and large intestine and a variety of genitourinary anomalies, implying an important role in renal development.

Characterization of the *RET* gene in patients with MEN 2A demonstrated a number of mutations in affected kindred members which were not present in their normal counterparts. The mutations were clustered in the cysteines located in RET's extracellular, juxtamembrane domain (Figure 22–6). Structurally, these cysteines are encoded by nucleotides in exons 10 and 11 of the *RET* gene. A number of these mutations were simple missense mutations, while others involved deletion or insertion of small segments of DNA, but in each case one of the aforementioned cysteines proved to be involved. Selective mutation of one of these six cysteines has now been shown to account for more than 97% of all *RET* mutations associated with MEN 2A. The most frequently mutated residue is Cys[634]. This amino acid is mutated to arginine (Arg), phenylalanine (Phe), serine (Ser), glycine (Gly), tyrosine (Tyr), or tryptophan (Trp) in approximately 84% of affected MEN 2A kindreds. It has been suggested that mutation of Cys[634] to Arg[634] is associated with the phenotypic expression of hyperparathyroidism, while mutation of Cys[634] to any of the amino acids indicated above is linked to pheochromocytoma. It should be noted that

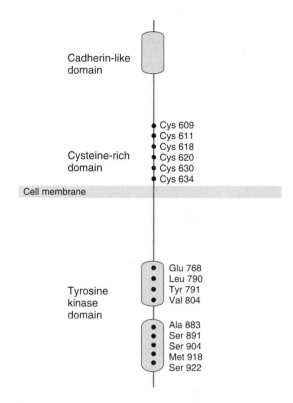

Figure 22–6. Structural schematic of wild type RET, including amino acids that have been shown to be mutated in different disease states. MEN 2A is associated with mutations of Cys[609], Cys[611], Cys[618], Cys[620], Cys[630], Cys[634], and, rarely, Leu[790] and Tyr[791]. Familial medullary carcinoma of the thyroid is frequently associated with mutations at the same Cys residues with the exception of Cys[634], as well as mutations at Glu[768], Leu[790], Tyr[791], Val[804], and Ser[891]. MEN 2B mutations typically involve Met[918] or, more rarely, Ala[883], Ser[922], or Val[804]/Ser[904]. Hirschsprung's disease is associated with multiple mutations or deletions extending over the full length of the RET molecule.

the Cys-to-Arg mutation at position 634 is also the most common mutation at this position, accounting for about 64% of all codon changes at this location. Interestingly, a rare but unique mutation involving a four-amino-acid insertion between Cys[634] and Arg[635] has been described that results in MCT and a high incidence of hyperparathyroidism but not pheochromocytoma.

Ironically, patients with familial medullary carcinoma of the thyroid display many of the same cysteine mutations identified in MEN 2A, implying the existence of independent modulatory genomic factors which restrict the effects of the *RET* mutation to the parafollicular cells of the thyroid in familial medullary carcinoma of the thyroid. The exception is the mutation of Cys[634] to Arg[634], which is almost uniformly associated with MEN 2A. Several additional mutations have been identified that may be more specific for familial medullary carcinoma (Figure 22–6). The observation that mutations of Cys[634] have higher transforming potential than mutations at these other residues has led to the suggestion that MEN 2A represents the more severe phenotype (versus familial MCT) along a spectrum of disease resulting from RET activation. In fact, the noncysteine mutations, which are more common in familial MCT (as high as 60% of familial MCT in one series), are associated with delayed onset of parafollicular C cell disease, but other clinical features (tumor size, bilaterality, the presence of nodal metastases) were not different in patients harboring cysteine versus noncysteine mutations.

Interestingly, patients with MEN 2B do not harbor mutations in the cysteine residues affected in MEN 2A and familial medullary thyroid carcinoma. Instead, the majority possess a single-point mutation involving conversion of Met[918] to Thr[918]. This mutation is found in more than 95% of cases of MEN 2B. A minority of patients have been shown to harbor an independent mutation of Ala[883] to Phe[883], Ser[922] to Tyr[922], or a monoallelic combination of Val[804] to Met[804] plus Ser[904] to Cys[904]. MEN 2B arises from spontaneous de novo mutations in as many as 50% of affected individuals. For unknown reasons, these mutations are found almost exclusively on the paternal allele.

A number of the germline mutations identified in MEN 2A and familial medullary carcinoma of the thyroid and the Met[918] mutation in MEN 2B have been demonstrated as somatic mutations in sporadic medullary carcinoma of the thyroid (about 30–40%) and pheochromocytoma (less than 10%). Sporadic parathyroid disease due to these mutations appears to be rare if it occurs at all. The presence of the Met[918] mutation, in particular, is associated with a less favorable clinical outcome in sporadic medullary carcinoma.

Independent studies have shown a close linkage between the *RET* gene locus and Hirschsprung's disease, a disorder characterized by failure of myenteric ganglia to develop normally in the hindgut of affected individuals. This leads to impaired gut motility and, in severe cases, megacolon (a phenotype similar to that reported for the *RET* knockout mice). Examination of *RET* coding sequence in Hirschsprung kindreds revealed a variety of mutations in both the intracellular and extracellular domains, some of which (eg, deletions) would be predicted to eliminate normal expression of the *RET* gene. This, together with the findings in the *RET*, GDNF, and GDNFR$_\alpha$-1 knockout mice alluded to above, suggests that Hirschsprung's disease represents the null phenotype for the *RET* locus. Interestingly, several patients have been described who possess features of both MEN 2 and Hirschsprung's disease. The *RET* mutations in these cases have involved conversion of Cys[609], Cys[618], or Cys[620] to Arg. These mutations, while promoting dimerization and increasing tyrosine kinase activity in the RET protein (see below), also appear to have difficulty trafficking to and accumulating in the plasma membrane at the cell surface. It is conceivable that predominance of one or the other of these mechanisms in different cell types could result in a phenotype characterized by both activation (eg, MEN 2) and suppression (eg, Hirschsprung's disease) of RET activity in the same individual.

By inference, the defect in RET function in MEN 2 or familial medullary thyroid carcinoma arises from increased or altered activity of the RET tyrosine kinase. In the case of RET$_{MEN}$2A, the increase in activity appears to arise from interference with the tonic inhibition of RET tyrosine kinase activity by the clustered cysteine residues in the extracellular domain. This leads to increased dimer formation, autophosphorylation, and tyrosine kinase activity in the mutant RET molecules. In the case of RET$_{MEN}$2B, there appears to be a change in substrate specificity of the tyrosine kinase that contributes to the phenotype. The activity of RET$_{MEN}$2B—rather than being restricted to conventional RET substrates (RET substrates are similar to those recognized by the epidermal growth factor receptor)—is capable of phosphorylating substrates normally recognized by members of the Src and Abl families of cytoplasmic tyrosine kinases, signaling pathways which are closely identified with the regulation of cell growth. Thus, it appears that RET$_{MEN}$2B has acquired the capacity for activation of a potent mitogenic pathway in the expressing endocrine cells merely by altering its selection of substrates for phosphorylation. RET$_{MEN}$2B also potentiates phosphorylation of Tyr[1062] more effectively than RET$_{MEN}$2A. This tyrosine serves as a docking site for multiple effector proteins, including Shc and PI-3K, implying that RET$_{MEN}$2B may be more effective in triggering downstream signaling pathways.

Treatment

Treatment of heritable medullary carcinoma of the thyroid should include total thyroidectomy with at least central lymph node dissection. Given the multicentric nature of the disease, subtotal thyroidectomy predictably results in recurrent disease. Basal or stimulated calcitonin levels are used in the postoperative setting to evaluate the presence of residual disease. The precise timing of surgery in patients with subclinical disease—

ie, positive by genetic testing but without clinical or laboratory abnormalities—is controversial (see below), but most clinicians would agree that in kindreds with MEN 2B or clinically aggressive medullary thyroid carcinoma, patients should undergo surgery as soon as the genetic defect is demonstrated. Typically, this is before age 6 months in MEN 2B and before 5 years in MEN 2A. Foci of microscopic MCT are common, and metastatic disease has been described in the first year of life in patients with MEN 2B. Patients should always be screened for the presence of pheochromocytoma before undergoing neck exploration. Surgery for metastatic disease is palliative and targeted at reducing tumor burden rather than cure. Localization techniques (eg, MRI or selective venous sampling for calcitonin) can be helpful in identifying foci of malignant tissue. Radiation and chemotherapy are of limited utility and are largely confined to later stages of the disease.

Treatment of pheochromocytomas in MEN 2 is similar to that for sporadic pheochromocytomas (see Chapter 11). Alpha- and (occasionally) beta-adrenergic blockade is used to control blood pressure and associated hyperadrenergic symptoms and to restore normal intravascular volume in preparation for surgical resection of the tumor. Given the propensity for bilaterality of pheochromocytomas in this disorder, some have favored bilateral adrenalectomy at the time of initial surgery. However, since the incidence of bilaterality is well under 100% and because these tumors are rarely malignant, the most prudent strategy in the face of unilateral adrenal enlargement would appear to be unilateral adrenalectomy at the initial surgery with careful attention at follow-up looking for the presence of disease in the contralateral adrenal gland. This vigilant approach has the advantage of minimizing morbidity from recurrent pheochromocytoma while sparing the patient the risks associated with lifelong adrenal insufficiency.

Screening

Genetic screening for MEN 2A, MEN 2B, or familial medullary carcinoma of the thyroid is routinely carried out using polymerase chain reaction (PCR)-based tests designed to identify specific mutations in the *RET* coding sequence (Figure 22–7). Known *RET* mutations account for more than 95% of all instances of multiple endocrine neoplasia, and selected mutations (eg, Cys[634] to Arg[634] in MEN 2A) account for a disproportionate number of affected individuals. Individuals lacking any of the known *RET* mutations can be tested using conventional haplotype analysis if informative genetic markers and affected family members are available. Biochemical testing using basal or stimulated plasma calcitonin levels has been largely supplanted by

genetic screens. The biochemical tests remain useful, however, in identifying residual disease after thyroidectomy.

In view of the fact that a high proportion of cases of MCT are familial to begin with and as much as 6% of patients with apparently sporadic MCT harbor germline *RET* mutations, genetic testing for *RET* germline mutations is probably indicated for all patients presenting with MCT. Controversy persists, however, in terms of what should be done for patients once the mutation has been identified. Some investigators citing incomplete "clinical" penetrance (according to published data, 40% of gene carriers do not present symptomatically prior to age 70) have argued that employing solely genetic criteria in making the decision for operative intervention subjects a small minority of patients to premature thyroidectomy. They argue that genetic testing should be used to identify those patients who require close clinical and biochemical surveillance to assist with the timing of surgery. Ideally, such biochemical testing (eg, pentagastrin stimulation) should be performed on an annual basis. Exceptions to this general approach might include patients with MEN 2B or a particularly aggressive form of familial medullary carcinoma of the thyroid where the potential for significant morbidity and mortality would justify operation in any patient harboring the genetic defect regardless of the physical or biochemical manifestations of the disease.

The more widely shared view is that the true penetrance of medullary carcinoma of the thyroid—combined clinical and preclinical disease—in MEN 2A is closer to 100%. This, when coupled with the high degree of sensitivity and specificity of the PCR-based genetic screens, difficulties encountered in obtaining adequate long-term patient follow-up and biochemical screening, and the potential for false-positive pentagastrin stimulation tests—even within MEN 2 kindreds—has led to the recommendation that total thyroidectomy should be performed in all individuals harboring an MEN 2-associated *RET* mutation. This argument has now been supported by several clinical studies in which parafollicular cell hyperplasia as well as early medullary carcinoma of the thyroid have been identified in operative specimens taken from genetically affected individuals despite normal pentagastrin stimulation tests. False-positive biochemical tests are also a concern. There are several reports in the literature of patients in affected kindreds who have undergone total thyroidectomy following positive pentagastrin stimulation tests but did not, in fact, harbor the MEN 2 gene mutation. Histologic examination of excised tissues revealed parafollicular cell hyperplasia, presumably unrelated to MEN 2, but no medullary thyroid carcinoma. Collectively, these findings point out the relative defi-

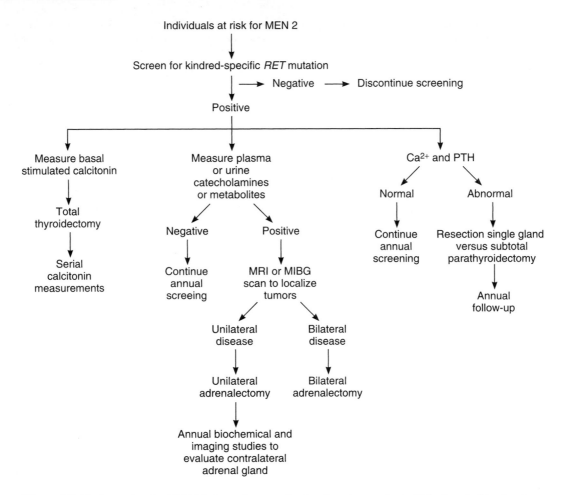

Figure 22–7. Screening for MEN 2A. Genetic screening has largely supplanted biochemical testing in identifying individuals at risk. Details of decisions regarding treatment are discussed in the text. Preoperative plasma calcitonin levels are potentially useful for follow-up but should not supplant genetic testing in assessing the need for surgery. (See also Figure 7–56.)

ciencies of biochemical versus genetic testing and offer a compelling argument for early operation as a means of reliably eradicating the disease.

OTHER DISORDERS CHARACTERIZED BY MULTIPLE ENDOCRINE ORGAN INVOLVEMENT

Carney Complex

Carney complex is an autosomal dominant disorder characterized by cardiac, endocrine, cutaneous, and neural tumors. Myxomas of the heart, breast, and skin are seen frequently in this disorder, as is spotty pigmentation of the skin (lentiginosis). Endocrine tumors include primary pigmented micronodular adrenocortical hyperplasia (an ACTH-independent form of Cushing's syndrome), follicular thyroid carcinomas, adrenocortical carcinoma, somatotroph adenomas of the pituitary gland, and large-cell calcifying Sertoli cell tumors of the testes. In approximately half of the known Carney complex kindreds, the genetic lesion maps to 17q22–24, a locus that harbors the type 1 regulatory subunit of protein kinase A (PKA). This gene functions as a classic tumor suppressor, and loss of heterozygosity at this locus is associated with the Carney phenotype. A second locus, presumably accounting for the remaining approximately half of Carney complex kindreds, is located at 2p16. The nature of the genetic lesion at this locus remains unknown at present; however, the phenotype is indistinguishable from that found with the 17q22–24 mutations alluded to above.

Neurofibromatosis Type 1

Neurofibromatosis type 1 (Recklinghausen's disease) is an autosomal dominant genetic disorder characterized by a variety of skin manifestations, including café au lait spots, subcutaneous neurofibromas, and axillary and inguinal freckles as well as neural gliomas (eg, optic nerve) and hamartomas of the iris (Lisch nodules). In addition, patients may have a number of endocrine neoplasias, including pheochromocytoma, hyperparathyroidism, medullary carcinoma of the thyroid, and somatostatin-producing carcinoid tumors of the duodenal wall. The genetic lesion in neurofibromatosis type 1 is located at 17q11.2, a locus that harbors the neurofibromin gene. Neurofibromin is a homolog of the p21 Ras-dependent GTPase-activating proteins and is thought to function in a tumor suppressor mode through regulation of Ras-dependent signaling activity.

Von Hippel-Lindau Disease

Von Hippel-Lindau disease is a heritable autosomal dominant disorder characterized by retinal and cerebellar hemangioblastomas, renal cell carcinoma, islet cell tumors, pheochromocytomas, and renal, pancreatic, and epididymal cysts. The presence of pheochromocytomas and most of the islet cell tumors is confined to the type 2 variant of the disease, which accounts for 25–35% of affected kindreds. The genetic lesion has been localized to 3p25. The VHL protein, which is normally encoded by this locus, participates in the formation of a multiprotein complex involved in the regulation of hypoxia-induced genes, transcriptional regulation, fibronectin matrix assembly, and ubiquitin ligases.

REFERENCES

MEN 1

Chandrasekharappa SC et al: Positional cloning of the gene for multiple endocrine neoplasia—type 1. Science 1997;276: 404. [PMID: 9103196]

Guo SS, Sawicki MP: Molecular and genetic mechanisms of tumorigenesis in multiple endocrine neoplasia type-1. Mol Endocrinol 2001;15:1653. [PMID: 11579199]

Marx S et al: Multiple endocrine neoplasia type 1: Clinical and genetic topics. Ann Intern Med 1998;129:484. [PMID: 9735087]

Pipeleers-Marichal M et al: Gastrinomas in the duodenums of patients with multiple endocrine neoplasia type 1 and the Zollinger-Ellison syndrome. N Engl J Med 1990;322:723. [PMID: 1968616]

Schussheim DH et al: Multiple endocrine neoplasia type 1: new clinical and basic findings. Trends Endocrinol Metab 2001;12:173. [PMID: 11295574]

Thompson NW: The surgical management of hyperparathyroidism and endocrine disease of the pancreas in the multiple endocrine neoplasia 1 patient. J Intern Med 1995;238:269. [PMID: 8673858]

MEN 2

Brandi ML et al: Consensus guidelines for diagnosis and therapy of MEN type 1 and type 2. J Clin Endocrinol Metab 2001;86: 5658. [PMID: 11739416]

Donis-Keller H et al: Mutations in the RET proto-oncogene are associated with MEN 2A and FMTC. Hum Mol Genet 1993;2:851. [PMID: 8103403]

Hoff AO et al: Multiple endocrine neoplasias. Annu Rev Physiol 2000;62:377. [PMID: 10845096]

Ledger GA et al: Genetic testing in the diagnosis and management of multiple endocrine neoplasia type II. Ann Intern Med 1995;122:118. [PMID: 7992986]

Mulligan LM et al: Specific mutations of the RET proto-oncogene are related to disease phenotype in MEN 2A and FMTC. Nat Genet 1994;6:70. [PMID: 7907913]

Mulligan LM, Ponder BAJ: Genetic basis of endocrine disease: Multiple endocrine neoplasia type 2. J Clin Endocrinol Metab 1995;80:1989. [PMID: 7608246]

Wells SA et al: Predictive DNA testing and prophylactic thyroidectomy in patients at risk for multiple endocrine neoplasia type 2A. Ann Surg 1994;3:237. [PMID: 7916559]

Other Disorders

Stratakis CA et al: Clinical and molecular features of the Carney complex: diagnostic criteria and recommendations for patient evaluation. J Clin Endocrinol Metab 2001;86:4041. [PMID: 11549623]

Geriatric Endocrinology

Susan L. Greenspan, MD, & Neil M. Resnick, MD

ACTH	Adrenocorticotropic hormone	**LHRH**	Luteinizing hormone-releasing hormone
AVP	Arginine vasopressin	**NPH**	Neutral protamine Hagedorn
BMD	Bone mineral density	**PSA**	Prostate-specific antigen
cAMP	Cyclic adenosine monophosphate	**PTH**	Parathyroid hormone
CRH	Corticotropin-releasing hormone	**SERMS**	Selective estrogen receptor modulators
DHEA	Dehydroepiandrosterone	**SIADH**	Syndrome of inappropriate secretion of antidiuretic hormone
DHEAS	Dehydroepiandrosterone sulfate		
FSH	Follicle-stimulating hormone	**TRH**	Thyrotropin-releasing hormone
hCG	Human chorionic gonadotropin	**TSH**	Thyroid-stimulating hormone (thyrotropin)
HPA	Hypothalamic-pituitary-adrenal		
LH	Luteinizing hormone		

Individuals over age 65 comprise the fastest-growing segment of the United States population; each day this group increases by over 1000 people. This increase has led to a remarkable situation—of all the people who have ever lived to the age of 65, more than two-thirds are still alive. Thus, it is becoming increasingly important for the endocrinologist to understand how endocrine physiology and disease may differ in the elderly.

Before considering specific endocrinologic conditions in the elderly, however, it is worthwhile to review some general principles that account for many of the age-related changes in disease presentation in the elderly. First, aging itself—in the absence of disease—is associated with only a gradual and linear decline in the physiologic reserve of each organ system (Figure 23–1). Since the reserve capacity of each system is substantial, age-related declines have little effect on baseline function and do not significantly interfere with the individual's response to stress until the eighth or ninth decade. Second, because each organ system's function declines at a different physiologic rate and because 75% of the elderly have at least one disease, endocrine dysfunction in the elderly often presents disparately, with initial symptoms derived from the most compromised organ

system. For example, hyperthyroidism in an elderly patient with preexisting coronary and conduction system disease may present with atrial fibrillation and a slow ventricular response, while in another equally hyperthyroid patient with a prior stroke it may present with confusion or depression; neither patient may tolerate hyperthyroidism long enough for the classic thyroid-related manifestations (eg, goiter) to become apparent. Third, elderly patients often have multiple diseases and take many medications that may mimic or mask the usual presentation of endocrine disease.

THYROID FUNCTION & DISEASE

The prevalence of thyroid disease in the elderly is approximately twice that in younger individuals, with hypothyroidism ranging from 2% to 7% and hyperthyroidism affecting up to 2% of older individuals (Figure 23–2). The Whickham Survey of 21,000 adults in Great Britain and its follow-up study, conducted between 1972 and 1993, reported that the incidence of overt hypothyroidism increased tenfold when its incidence in women in their twenties was compared with that in women age 75 and older. In addition, some

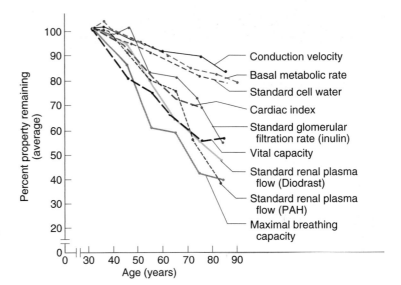

Figure 23–1. Influence of age on physiologic function in humans. (Reproduced, with permission, from Shock NW: Discussion on mortality and measurement. In: *The Biology of Aging: A Symposium.* Strehler BL et al [editors]. American Institute of Biological Sciences, 1960.)

studies suggest that up to 9% of hospitalized elderly patients have overt thyroid disease. Furthermore, "subclinical hypothyroidism"—normal serum levels of thyroid hormones (thyroxine, T_4; triiodothyronine, T_3) but an elevated level of thyrotropin (TSH)—is more prevalent, with estimates of 4–14% in the elderly, and is higher in women than in men. In the elderly, the progression from subclinical to overt hypothyroidism is roughly 2–3% per year. "Subclinical hyperthyroidism"—normal serum thyroxine with suppressed serum TSH levels—may be found in 2% of elderly subjects. The rate of progression to overt hyperthyroidism is less clear. Finally, the overall prevalence of thyroid hormone use in older adults is approximately 7% (10% in women and 2% in men).

There are few major age-related changes in the physiology of the hypothalamic-pituitary-thyroid axis (Chapter 7). Serum TSH levels remain constant, and TSH release remains pulsatile, though the nocturnal rise in serum TSH appears to be blunted with age. Balanced decreases in T_4 secretion and clearance result in no change in serum T_4; T_3 resin uptake, free T_4, and the free T_4 index are also unchanged. There is a slight age-related decline in serum T_3, but values usually remain within normal limits. The effect of age on the release of TSH by thyrotropin-releasing hormone (TRH) is less clear, but most recent studies show little clinically relevant change in either sex. The 24-hour radioiodine uptake is also not significantly altered with age. Thyroid antibodies are common in older women (prevalence up to 32%), but their presence does not serve as a specific screening test for thyroid disease.

DISORDERS OF THE THYROID GLAND

Although the United States Preventive Services Task Force and other cost-benefit analyses recommend annual screening thyroid function tests for older women, there is still no consensus among thyroidologists regarding the utility of screening for thyroid dysfunction in the absence of symptoms. The American Thyroid Association recommends that adults be screened by serum TSH determination every 5 years. However, it is reasonable to measure TSH at any time in older individuals who present with "atypical" symptoms of thyroid disease such as exacerbation of cardiac symptoms, change in mental status, falling, or onset of depression. Despite the sensitivity of the TSH assay, further evaluation with a free T_4 or free T_4 index is often required because up to 98% of elderly subjects with mildly suppressed TSH levels do not have thyrotoxicosis.

1. Hyperthyroidism

Clinical Features

With age, the prevalence of Graves' disease decreases (though it remains the most common cause of hyperthyroidism), and the prevalence of multinodular goiter and toxic nodules increases. Elderly hyperthyroid patients tend to present with symptoms or complications related to the most vulnerable organ system—usually the cardiovascular system (atrial fibrillation, congestive heart failure, angina, and acute myocardial infarction) or the central nervous system (apathy, depression, con-

A. Percentage with high serum TSH (> 4.5 mIU/L)

B. Percentage with low serum TSH (< 0.4 mIU/L)

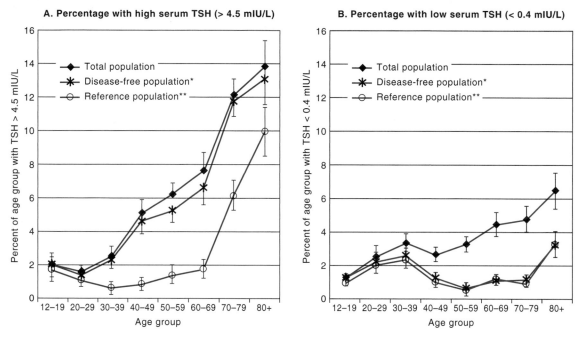

Figure 23–2. Percentage with high or low serum TSH in the total United States population, the disease-free (excludes those people who have reported having thyroid disease, goiter, or taking thyroid medications*) and reference population (excludes those people who reported having thyroid disease, goiter, or taking thyroid medications and those who do not have risk factors such as pregnancy or taking estrogen, androgens, or lithium and who are without the presence of thyroid antibodies or biochemical evidence of hypothyroidism or hyperthyroidism**) by age. **A:** High serum TSH. In the disease-free population, the percentage of people with high serum TSH concentration (> 4.85 μIU/mL; > 4.85 mIU/L) is slightly lower than that of the total population but significantly higher than the percentage in the reference population. **B:** Low serum TSH. The percentage of people with low serum TSH in the disease-free population, on the other hand, is significantly lower than the percentage in the total population and similar to the pattern seen in the reference population. Note the elevated prevalence of low TSH in the populations without thyroid disease or risk factors at ages 20–39 years and again after age 79 years. The higher prevalence of individuals with low TSH or high TSH in the total population is related directly to the people reporting thyroid disease, goiter, or taking thyroid medication and probably reflects inadequate management of clinical thyroid disease. (Reproduced, with permission, from Hollowell JG et al: Serum TSH, T₄, and thyroid antibodies in the United States population [1988 to 1994]: National Health and Nutrition Examination Survey [NHANES III]. J Clin Endocrinol Metab 2002;87:489. Copyright © 2002 by The Endocrine Society).

fusion, or lassitude). The hypercatabolic state also causes muscle wasting, particularly of the quadriceps, thereby increasing the risk of falls. Occasionally, they present with gastrointestinal symptoms, but these differ from those seen in younger patients because they include constipation, failure to thrive, and anorexia and weight loss. Because of degeneration of the sinus node and fibrotic changes in the cardiac conduction system, older patients are less likely than younger ones to present with palpitations (Table 23–1). However, a very low serum TSH concentration is associated with a threefold higher risk of atrial fibrillation in the subse-

quent decade. Hyperthyroidism is also associated with bone loss and fractures.

The physical signs of hyperthyroidism also differ in the elderly (Table 23–1). Sinus tachycardia is less frequent; the thyroid feels normal in size or is not palpable in two-thirds of patients; and lid lag is uncommon. Ophthalmopathy is less common, not only because Graves' disease occurs less often, but also because even with Graves' disease ophthalmopathy occurs less frequently in the elderly. However, although they are less common in the elderly, some findings appear to be highly suggestive of hyperthyroidism. These include in-

Table 23–1. Percentages of patients with symptoms and physical findings attributable to thyrotoxicosis.[1]

	Old₁	Old₂	Young
Number	25	85	247
Mean age	81.5	68.6	40[2]
Range	75–95	60–82	5–73
Symptoms (%)			
Weight loss	44	35	85
Palpitations	36	42	89
Weakness	32	28	70
Dizziness, syncope	20	…	…
Nervousness	20	38	99
No symptoms	8	…	…
Memory loss	8	…	…
Tremor	8	…	…
Local symptoms[3]	8	11	…
Pruritus	4	4	…
Heat intolerance	4	63	89
Physical Findings			
Pulse > 100/min	28[4]	58	100
Atrial fibrillation	32	39	10
New-onset atrial fibrillation	20[5]	…	…
Lid lag	12	35	71
Exophthalmos	8	8	…
Fine skin	40	81	97
Tremor	36	89	97
Myopathy	8	39	…
Hyperactive reflexes	24	26	…
Gynecomastia	(1 male)	1	10
None	8	…	…
Thyroid Examination (%)			
Impalpable or normal	68	37	…
Diffusely enlarged	12	22	100
Multinodular goiter	12	20	…
Isolated nodule	8	21	…

[1]Modified and reproduced, with permission, from Tibaldi JM et al: Thyrotoxicosis in the very old. Am J Med 1986;81:619.
[2]Approximated from graph of patients' ages.
[3]Dysphagia, enlarging neck mass, etc.
[4]Includes five patients with normal sinus rhythm and two who had atrial fibrillation.
[5]This was transient in four of five patients with conversion to normal sinus rhythm.

Note:
Old₁ = Tibaldi JM et al: Thyrotoxicosis in the very old. Am J Med 1986;81:619.
Old₂ = Davis PJ, Davis FB: Hyperthyroidism in patients over the age of 60 years. Clinical features in 85 patients. Medicine (Baltimore) 1974;53:161.
Young = Ingbar SH et al: The thyroid gland. In: *Williams Textbook of Endocrinology.* Williams RH (editor). Saunders, 1981.

creased frequency of bowel movements, weight loss despite increased appetite, fine finger tremor, eyelid retraction, and increased perspiration.

Diagnosis

As in younger patients (Chapter 7), the diagnosis is usually confirmed by standard thyroid function tests, beginning with a depressed TSH level as measured by a sensitive immunoradiometric or chemiluminescent assay. A TRH test is rarely required. There are potential pitfalls, however. Hospitalized elderly patients who are acutely ill (but euthyroid) may have a suppressed serum TSH. Further evaluation of other thyroid function tests should help rule out hyperthyroidism. T_3 toxicosis may be more difficult to diagnose because concomitant nonthyroidal illness is common and can depress serum T_3. Euthyroid hyperthyroxinemia (also due to nonthyroidal illness) may also cause confusion. Elderly patients may also be taking medications such as propranolol, which may elevate levels of serum T_4. Furthermore, iodide-induced hyperthyroidism, known also as the jodbasedow effect, is becoming more common in elderly patients with multinodular goiter because of increased exposure to radiocontrast studies; the resultant hyperthyroidism is generally transient.

Finally, because of screening tests with sensitive TSH assays, "subclinical hyperthyroidism" (normal T_4, T_3, free T_4 with a suppressed TSH) is being recognized more commonly. This is often found in older subjects with autonomous function of a multinodular goiter or nodule. Osteoporosis and atrial fibrillation are complications of subclinical hyperthyroidism that may be an indication for treatment. Recent studies suggest an increase in cognitive impairment and all-cause mortality (especially cardiovascular disease) in patients with subclinical hyperthyroidism. If patients are not treated, careful follow-up is recommended.

Treatment

Beta-blocking agents are useful in alleviating symptoms, but radioactive iodine is the therapy of choice in elderly patients because it is efficient, uncomplicated, and inexpensive. Antithyroid drugs can be used prior to radioactive iodine treatment to render the patient euthyroid and to avoid radiation-induced thyroiditis, but they are not definitive treatment and are more toxic in this age group. Surgery has a more limited role because of its increased morbidity risk.

Following radioactive iodine treatment, patients become euthyroid over a period of 6–12 weeks. They should receive careful follow-up, because hypothyroidism develops in 80% or more of patients who have been adequately treated. Once hyperthyroidism has abated, the metabolic clearance rate of other medications may decrease, and doses may require readjustment. Older patients with subclinical hyperthyroidism require follow-up, especially if presented with an iodine load.

2. Hypothyroidism

Hypothyroidism in the elderly is most often due to Hashimoto's thyroiditis or prior radioactive iodine ablative therapy. The risk for developing hypothyroidism is significantly increased in older women when serum antithyroid antibodies or serum TSH is elevated.

Clinical Features

It is easy to overlook hypothyroidism in an older person, because many euthyroid elderly patients have the same symptoms. Moreover, elderly patients with hypothyroidism are more likely than younger patients to present with cardiovascular symptoms (eg, congestive heart failure or angina) or neurologic findings (eg, cognitive impairment, confusion, depression, paresthesias, deafness, psychosis, or coma). Finally, in the older hypothyroid patient, the physical findings are frequently nonspecific, though puffy face, delayed deep tendon reflexes, and myoedema support the diagnosis.

Diagnosis

Serum TSH is the most sensitive indicator of primary hypothyroidism and should be checked first. The diagnosis should then be confirmed with a low serum T_4 or free T_4. Measurement of serum T_3 is unnecessary and potentially misleading, because T_3 is the form of thyroid hormone most likely to decrease in nonthyroidal illness. Serum TSH should not be used alone to diagnose hypothyroidism because it will not always differentiate symptomatic from "subclinical" hypothyroidism. Furthermore, levels of TSH may be higher at night as a result of the nocturnal rise in serum TSH. Moreover, the pulsatile nature of TSH, resulting in serum TSH slightly above the normal ranges, may lead to a diagnosis of subclinical hypothyroidism in a euthyroid subject. Finally, in hypothyroid patients, serum TSH levels can be reduced to within the normal range by treatment with dopaminergic drugs and corticosteroids. In such patients, determination of free T_4 and reverse T_3 may help to differentiate those with true hypothyroidism from those with nonthyroidal illness (Chapter 7).

Treatment

The doses of thyroid hormone required for adequate replacement decrease with age. Elderly patients should be started on approximately 25–50 μg of levothyroxine, and the dose should be increased by approximately 25 μg every 4–6 weeks until the serum TSH comes into the normal range. In patients with cardiovascular disease, even lower initial doses can be used (12.5 μg) and increased at a slower rate. Desiccated thyroid hormone and preparations containing T_3 should be avoided because T_3 is rapidly absorbed and cleared. The metabolic clearance of other drugs will change as hypothyroidism is corrected, and their dosages may require readjustment. On average, the dose of levothyroxine in the elderly is roughly 1 μg/kg/d compared with 1.7 μg/kg/d in young adults. Overtreatment documented by a suppressed serum TSH should be avoided because of the potential adverse effects to the skeleton and cardiovascular system.

It is still not known whether treating "subclinical hypothyroidism" is beneficial for all patients. However, two-thirds of these patients will remain chemically euthyroid for at least 4 years, and absence of antimicrosomal antibodies may identify patients at lowest risk for progression. One cost-benefit analysis reported that it was worthwhile to screen elderly women for subclinical hypothyroidism with serum TSH measurements and that treatment led to symptomatic improvement and decreased cholesterol levels. Recent guidelines from the American Thyroid Association agree with these recommendations. Elderly patients previously treated with radioactive iodine are more likely to progress to overt hypothyroidism.

3. Multinodular Goiter

The prevalence of multinodular goiter increases with age. However, if swallowing and breathing are not compromised and thyroid function tests are normal, the goiter can be observed without treatment. Levothyroxine therapy rarely shrinks the gland, and although it may prevent further enlargement, the risk of inducing hyperthyroidism is significant because multinodular goiters may develop areas of autonomous function.

4. Thyroid Nodules & Cancer

Thyroid nodules are more common in the elderly. The prevalence of nodules increases with age and is generally higher in women than in men. Furthermore, the prevalence of thyroid nodules detected by ultrasound may be as high as 40% in older women. Ninety percent of these nodules are benign, but the prognosis for elderly patients with malignant nodules may be worse than that for younger patients with malignant nodules. The approach is similar to the workup in a younger patient. The prognosis correlates with the size of the tumor. The outcome in elderly patients may therefore be substantially improved by early evaluation of nodules in patients who are good surgical candidates.

Papillary carcinoma is more common in young and middle-aged patients. However, it has a poorer prognosis in the elderly, possibly because it is detected at a more advanced stage. Follicular carcinoma accounts for 15% of thyroid cancers and usually occurs in middle-aged and older patients. Anaplastic thyroid carcinoma is found almost exclusively in middle-aged and older patients. It presents as a rapidly growing hard mass which is locally invasive, often associated with metastatic lesions, and has a very poor prognosis (Chapter 7).

■ CARBOHYDRATE INTOLERANCE & DIABETES MELLITUS

AGING & THE PHYSIOLOGY OF CARBOHYDRATE INTOLERANCE

Even healthy elderly individuals demonstrate an age-related increase in fasting blood glucose (1 mg/dL [0.6 mmol/L] per decade) and a more significant increase in blood glucose (5 mg/dL [0.28 mmol/L] per decade) in response to a standard glucose tolerance test. According to the criteria of the National Diabetes Data Group, nearly 10% of the elderly have some degree of glucose intolerance. The possible causes of this intolerance include changes in body composition, diet, physical activity, insulin secretion, and insulin action.

With aging, lean body mass decreases and body fat increases. The percentage of body fat correlates positively with fasting levels of serum glucose, insulin, and glucagon. When obesity (or the percentage of body fat) is taken into account, the basal levels of glucose, insulin, and glucagon are not influenced by age. However, older individuals have impaired glucose counterregulation to hypoglycemia, associated with higher plasma insulin levels and reduced levels of glucagon.

Decreased physical activity and a low-carbohydrate diet impair glucose tolerance. Patients who have type 2 diabetes mellitus may have a combination of insulin resistance, decreased insulin secretion, and increased hepatic glucose production. Lean elderly patients with type 2 diabetes mellitus have a profound impairment in insulin release and a mild resistance to insulin-mediated glucose disposal. In contrast, obese elderly patients with type 2 diabetes mellitus have a significant resistance to insulin-mediated glucose disposal but adequate circulating insulin. In both groups, hepatic glucose output does not appear to be increased (Figure 23–3). Furthermore, there may be gender-related changes in glucose metabolism with age; healthy older men have an impairment in nonoxidative glucose metabolism, but women do not. However, much of the carbohydrate intolerance found in average elderly individuals is caused by diet, drugs, lack of exercise, or environmental factors that may be correctable.

DIABETES MELLITUS

Clinical Features

The prevalence of diabetes mellitus increases with age, affecting 16% of persons over age 65 (Figure 23–4). Most diabetes in the elderly is type 2 diabetes. Diabetes may be difficult to diagnose in the elderly because of its often atypical and asymptomatic presentation. For example, polyuria and polydipsia are not present in many elderly patients, because the glomerular filtration rate and thirst threshold decline with age, while the renal threshold for glycosuria increases. Instead, symptoms in these individuals are usually nonspecific (eg, weakness, fatigue, weight loss, or frequent minor infections). These patients may also present with neurologic findings such as cognitive impairment, acute confusion, or depression. Diabetes in the elderly can also predispose to pressure ulcers, falls, incontinence, and a decreased pain threshold.

The American Diabetes Association's Clinical Practice Recommendations for 1998 base the diagnosis of diabetes on a fasting blood glucose greater than 126 mg/dL on two occasions (in the absence of acute illness). A 2-hour glucose tolerance test is needed rarely, if ever. Symptoms of polyuria, polydipsia, and unexplained weight loss and a plasma glucose ≥ 200 mg/dL also are consistent with the diagnosis of diabetes. The ADA also recommends screening adults age 45 and older every 3 years, with more frequent screening for subjects at high risk (family history of coronary heart disease, cigarette smoking, hypertension, obesity, kidney disease, and dyslipidemia). Because the renal threshold for glycosuria increases in the elderly, the diagnosis should not be based on the presence of glycosuria. Increased blood levels of glycosylated hemoglobin or fructosamine support the diagnosis, but these tests are more useful in monitoring treatment.

Since the complications of diabetes mellitus are related to the duration of disease, elderly patients who live long enough will suffer the same complications of nephropathy, neuropathy, and retinopathy as their younger counterparts. The United Kingdom Prospective Diabetes Study (UKPDS) examined the relationship between improved glycemic control and the prevention of complications. Three-thousand and sixty-seven patients with type 2 diabetes mellitus (mean age 54 years) were assigned to intensive therapy (goal of fasting blood glucose < 108 mg/dL) with a sulfonylurea or insulin versus conventional diet therapy. After a me-

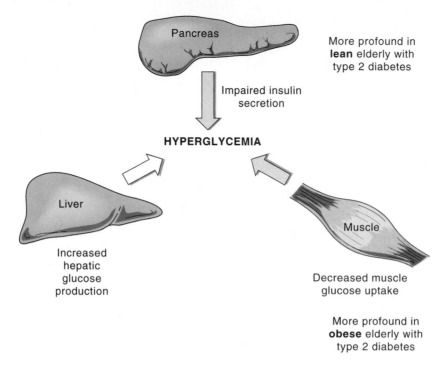

Figure 23–3. The pathogenesis of type 2 diabetes mellitus in obese elderly and lean elderly.

dian follow-up of 10 years, they reported that microvascular complications (retinopathy, neuropathy, and nephropathy) were reduced by 25% with intensive treatment. Treatment with insulin and sulfonylureas gave similar results. There was no difference in the incidence of macrovascular complications, but there was a tendency for fewer myocardial infarctions in the intensive therapy group.

Hypoglycemia in the elderly is associated with important sequelae. Sulfonylureas and insulin should not be withheld for fear of hypoglycemia, but patients need to be monitored carefully. Elderly diabetic patients have an impaired counterregulatory response to hypoglycemia. More importantly, the ability to sense hypoglycemia declines, as does the ability to take corrective action. Coupled with the diminished cortical reserve due to the higher prevalence of age-associated conditions such as stroke, lacunes, amyloid angiopathy, and Alzheimer's disease, the older brain is less able to fully recover from hypoglycemic insult.

Treatment

A reasonable treatment goal in the elderly patient with diabetes mellitus is to maintain the fasting blood glucose below 150 mg/dL (8.3 mmol/L) and the postprandial blood glucose below 220 mg/dL (12.2 mmol/L). Achieving this goal is often difficult and complicated by other medications commonly prescribed for the elderly, eg, thiazide diuretics, phenytoin, and glucocorticoids, which have hyperglycemic effects. Therapy should decrease hyperglycemic symptoms and prevent infections and the potential progression to nonketotic hyperosmolar coma.

Similar to the strategy used in younger patients (Chapter 17), initial therapy should include dietary manipulation, weight reduction for the overweight patient, and an exercise program tailored to the individual's capabilities. If mild to moderate hyperglycemia persists (fasting blood glucose 150–300 mg/dL [8.3–16.7 mmol/L]), an oral hypoglycemic agent should be tried. Chlorpropamide should be avoided because of its long half-life and its propensity to induce both hyponatremia and hypoglycemia. Because of their convenience and potency, second-generation sulfonylureas such as glipizide and glyburide are often used; these drugs increase insulin secretion and the number of insulin receptors and reduce hepatic glucose production. Both have been shown to be well tolerated in short-term trials. Glipizide, which has a shorter half-life

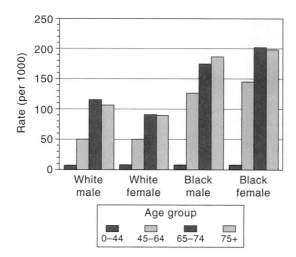

Figure 23–4. Age-specific prevalence of diagnosed diabetes, by race and sex, United States, 1994–1996. (Source: Centers for Disease Control and Prevention, National Center for Health Statistics, Division of Health Interview Statistics, data from the National Health Interview Survey. United States Bureau of the Census, census of the population and population estimates. Data computed by the Division of Diabetes Translation, National Center for Chronic Disease Prevention and Health Promotion, Centers for Disease Control and Prevention.)

than glyburide, is less likely to cause prolonged hypoglycemia in the elderly, which is poorly tolerated. Glimepiride is approved for use with insulin. It has a rapid onset of action and a more prolonged duration of action. Meglitinides are nonsulfonylurea agents that also increase insulin secretion and may be useful in patients with sulfonamide allergy. However, because of their short half-life, hypoglycemia is less common, but they must be given before each meal. Biguanides (eg, metformin) primarily reduce hepatic glucose production and do not have an effect on insulin secretion. In addition, metformin may decrease peripheral insulin resistance and improve the lipoprotein profile. However, metformin should not be used in patients with renal insufficiency (plasma creatinine ± 1.5 mg/dL [132 μmol/L] for men, ≥ 1.4 mg/dL [124 μmol/L] for women), thereby making it an undesirable choice in the elderly. Hypoglycemia is not common. The improvement in glucose control is similar to that achieved with sulfonylureas, but combination therapy with a sulfonylurea may improve glucose control. The side effects of diarrhea, nausea, and anorexia often limit use in the elderly. Alpha-glucosidase inhibitors (acarbose and miglitol) block intestinal α-glucosidase, resulting in a decrease in postprandial hyperglycemia. These agents can

be used alone or in combination with sulfonylureas. However, when used alone they are approximately half as efficacious as sulfonylureas in reducing glucose levels. Side effects in the elderly include abdominal discomfort and flatulence. Thiazolidinediones reduce hepatic glucose production and increase peripheral glucose uptake. Data on pioglitazone and rosiglitazone in the elderly are limited. However, since thiazolidinediones can cause fluid retention and exacerbate congestive heart failure, other oral agents are preferable. In summary, there are now several oral agents that can be used alone or in combination in the elderly, but few data are available for these agents in this age group. Side effects, including hypoglycemia, and cost need to be factored into the choice of therapy.

If the fasting blood glucose remains above 150 mg/dL (8.3 mmol/L) on diet, exercise, and oral agent therapy, insulin should be started in combination with oral agents or by itself. If given alone, the usual initial dose is 15–30 units of NPH (neutral protamine Hagedorn, or isophane insulin) or another intermediate-acting insulin. One daily injection is usually sufficient. Since elderly patients often lack symptoms of hypoglycemia, the fasting, postprandial, and bedtime blood glucose levels must be checked initially even if symptoms are absent. Finally, as in younger patients, it is important to control other adverse factors such as hypertension and smoking, which can contribute to vascular complications associated with diabetes. In addition, the ADA recommends aspirin therapy (81–325 mg/d) for primary prevention in high-risk patients and for secondary prevention in patients with macrovascular disease (eg, history of myocardial infarction, angina, stroke, transient ischemic attack, or peripheral vascular disease). A comprehensive eye examination with yearly follow-ups and preventive foot care are also recommended.

Diabetic ketoacidosis is rarely seen in the elderly. It should be treated cautiously, following a strategy similar to one used in younger patients (Chapters 17 and 24), with particular attention to the correction of electrolytes and water balance.

NONKETOTIC HYPEROSMOLAR COMA

Clinical Features

Nonketotic hyperosmolar coma, also known as nonketotic hypertonicity, occurs almost exclusively in the elderly. Predisposing factors include inadequate insulin secretion in response to hyperglycemia and a reduction in the peripheral effectiveness of insulin. Both factors lead to a progressive increase in serum glucose concentrations. The age-related increased renal threshold prevents osmotic diuresis until significant hyperglycemia is present, while an age-related decline in thirst predisposes to dehydration. Blood glucose concentrations often exceed 1000 mg/dL (55.5 mmol/L) and are coupled with marked elevation of plasma osmolality without ketosis.

This syndrome is frequently seen in elderly patients with type 2 diabetes who are in nursing homes and have limited access to water. However, one-third of such patients have no previous history of diabetes. The most common precipitating event is infection (32–60% of cases); the most common infection is pneumonia. Medications (eg, thiazides, furosemide, phenytoin, glucocorticoids) or other acute medical illnesses can also precipitate this condition. Patients present with an acute confusional state, lethargy, weakness, and occasionally coma. Neurologic findings can be generalized or focal and can mimic an acute cerebrovascular event. Marked volume depletion, orthostatic hypotension, and prerenal azotemia are also usually present.

Treatment

The average extracellular fluid volume deficit is 9 L. It should be replaced initially with normal saline, especially when significant orthostatic hypotension is present. After 1–3 L of isotonic saline has been administered, fluids can be changed to half-normal (0.45%) saline. Half of the fluid and ion deficits should be replaced in the first 24 hours and the remainder over the next 48 hours.

Intravenous insulin in small doses (10–15 units) should be given initially, followed by a drip infusion of 1–3 units/h. Insulin therapy should not be used in lieu of fluids because it will exacerbate intravascular fluid depletion and further compromise renal function as it shifts glucose intracellularly. Potassium deficits should be corrected when the patient is producing urine. Possible precipitating events—such as acute myocardial infarction, pneumonia, or administration of a medication—must be investigated and treated. Although metabolic abnormalities may improve in 1–2 days, mental status deterioration and confusion may persist for a week or more. Over one-third of patients can be discharged without insulin treatment, but they are at significant risk for recurrence and should be monitored carefully (Chapters 17 and 24).

■ OSTEOPOROSIS & CALCIUM HOMEOSTASIS

OSTEOPOROSIS

Despite the high prevalence, severe morbidity, and expense of osteoporosis, until recently most of our knowledge was derived from studies of perimenopausal

women. Yet it is the older woman who typically experiences the ravages of the disease. Twenty-five percent of women have vertebral fractures by age 70; by age 80, the figure is closer to 50%. Over 90% of hip fractures occur in patients over age 70, and by age 90, one woman in three will have sustained such a fracture. Hip fractures are associated with significant morbidity, an increased risk of institutionalization, and an up to 20% increase in mortality rates. Despite the significant differences between perimenopausal and older women, diagnostic and therapeutic approaches for older women are derived largely from studies of perimenopausal or newly postmenopausal women. The relevance of such studies for older women has only recently been questioned.

Definition

The definition of osteoporosis has changed over the years. In 1991, a consensus development conference defined osteoporosis as "a disease characterized by low bone mass and microarchitectural deterioration of bone tissue, leading to enhanced bone fragility and a consequent increase in fracture risk." The World Health Organization issued diagnostic criteria for postmenopausal women based on measurements of bone mineral density or bone mineral content. Osteoporosis is defined as a value of bone mineral density −2.5 SD and below the young adult mean value (Table 23–2). This permits numerical standardization of the definition and establishes criteria for treatment before a fracture takes place.

Factors Affecting Bone Physiology

There are significant physiologic differences between perimenopausal and older women with respect to maintenance of skeletal integrity. While calcium intake is often inadequate in both age groups, calcium absorption declines with age despite an age-related increase in serum levels of parathyroid hormone (PTH). This increase is not due solely to a decrease in renal clearance but may represent secondary hyperparathyroidism from vitamin D insufficiency. When PTH levels are assessed in elderly subjects with normal vitamin D levels, PTH levels are significantly lower than in vitamin D-deficient patients (Figure 23–5).

A. VITAMIN D

Vitamin D deficiency is common in the elderly, and vitamin D metabolism changes with age. Up to 15% of healthy elderly residents of communities in the sunny southwestern USA have frank vitamin D deficiency; still more have subclinical vitamin D deficiency; and up to 50% of elderly nursing home residents are deficient in vitamin D. This occurs because elderly individuals have decreased sun exposure and an impaired ability to

Table 23–2. World Health Organization diagnostic criteria for osteoporosis.[1]

Diagnosis	Criteria
Normal	Bone mineral density or content –1 SD and above the young adult mean value
Osteopenia (low bone mass)	Bone mineral density or content between –1 SD and –2.5 SD of the young adult mean value (includes individuals in whom prevention of bone loss would be most useful)
Osteoporosis	Bone mineral density or content –2.5 SD and below the young adult mean value
Severe osteoporosis (established osteoporosis)	Bone mineral density or content –2.5 SD and below the young adult mean value in the presence of one or more fragility fractures

[1]Modified and reproduced, with permission, from Kanis JA: The diagnosis of osteoporosis. J Bone Miner Res 1994;9:1137.

form vitamin D precursors in the skin, a decreased dietary intake of vitamin D, and (possibly) an age-related decline in vitamin D receptors in the duodenum. In addition, the ability to convert vitamin D to its active moiety ($1,25[OH]_2$-D_3) is impaired with age. Finally, certain vitamin D receptor alleles have been associated with lower bone density and bone loss in some populations, though further investigations of vitamin D metabolism are needed in the elderly in the United States.

B. Bone Loss and Architectural Changes

The rate of bone loss also differs between perimenopausal and older women. Cortical and trabecular bone are lost rapidly at menopause. Older longitudinal studies suggested that bone loss ceased or slowed in older women. However, longitudinal studies suggest that older women lose an average of 0.7–1% per year at the hip, and femoral bone loss increases with age (Figure 23–6). Vertebral bone density changes assessed by anteroposterior measurements can give a misleading assessment of bone mass as a consequence of nonspecific calcifications from osteoarthritis, sclerosis, aortic calcifications, and osteophytes that interfere with and falsely elevate the measurement. Therefore, measurement of femoral bone density is more reliable in the elderly.

In addition, there are changes in bone geometry; cortical bone remodeling in older women is insufficient to compensate for the loss of bone mineral content (Figure 23–7). There are also qualitative changes in trabecular bone, since an age-related reduction in trabecular bone jeopardizes plate integrity or "connectivity";

trabecular plates not only become perforated and disconnected, but with aging they continue to thin, causing further loss of bone strength and compromising the bone's ability to regain structural integrity with conventional therapy (Figure 23–8).

C. Risk Factors

Risk factors for fracture differ in perimenopausal and older women. By age 70, approximately 80% of women have a hip bone density that is osteopenic or osteoporotic, compared with 40% of women in their fifties (Figure 23–9). However, there is significant overlap in bone density between older patients who fall and fracture and those who fall and do not fracture (Figure 23–10). Falling is often cited as a major risk factor for hip fracture in older women. Although more than one-third of elderly women fall annually, however, fewer than 5% of falls result in fracture. A fall to the side, a low hip bone mineral density, low body mass index (lean body habitus), and high fall energy have been shown to be significant independent risk factors for hip fracture in community-dwelling elderly (Table 23–3). In nursing home subjects, a fall to the side, low hip bone mineral density, and impaired mobility were independent risk factors. Other factors, including a maternal history of hip fracture, previous hyperthyroidism, inability to rise from a chair, poor depth perception, poor contrast vision, and use of anticonvulsants or long-acting benzodiazepines are also associated with hip fractures in elderly women. Furthermore, with multiple risk factors, the risk of hip fracture increases significantly.

Evaluation

Screening older patients by obtaining a bone mineral density measurement is a comfortable, painless, noninvasive, rapid technique for determining an individual's bone mass and relative fracture risk. In general, the relative risk of spine or hip fracture roughly doubles for every standard deviation decrease in bone mineral density below the mean. Patients may remain dressed and lie on a padded table. Although several methods are available, currently the best technique uses dual-energy x-ray absorptiometry (DXA) of the hip or spine (Figures 23–11 and 23–12). The National Osteoporosis Foundation guidelines suggest obtaining a bone mass assessment in all women age 65 or older regardless of risk factors. For most elderly women, the hip is the single most useful measurement because nonspecific calcifications can lead to falsely elevated measurements in the posteroanterior view of spine.

Similar to the evaluation in a younger individual who presents with bone loss or a fracture, the workup

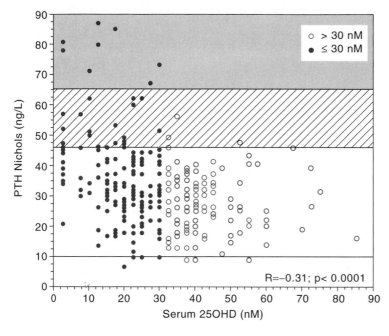

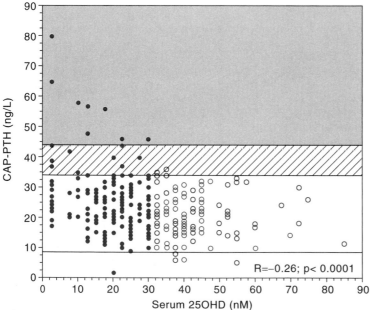

Figure 23–5. Relationship between serum 25OHD and PTH measured with the Allegro assay **(top)** and with the CAP assay **(bottom)**. On both figures, the gray area represents the above-normal PTH values with a reference range obtained in the entire group of 280 subjects, whereas the hatched area represents the additional zone of high PTH values with a reference range obtained in the 113 subjects with a serum 25OHD level above 30 nmol/L. The horizontal line is the low level of the reference range (subjects with 25OHD > 30 nmol/L). (Reproduced with permission from Souberbielle J-C et al: Vitamin D status and redefining serum parathyroid hormone reference range in the elderly. J Clin Endocrinol Metab 2001;86:3086. Copyright © 2001 by The Endocrine Society.)

in an older patient can be designed to exclude secondary causes of osteoporosis. Hyperthyroidism and hyperparathyroidism are both more common in older women, can cause bone loss, and can be clinically silent in older individuals. Because 10% of women over age 65 are receiving thyroid hormone replacement therapy and since thyroid hormone overreplacement results in

bone loss in postmenopausal women, true physiologic replacement with a normal serum TSH (if possible) should be the goal of treatment. Osteomalacia may present as nonspecific muscle or skeletal discomfort and is more common in the elderly. In addition, metastatic carcinoma, multiple myeloma, hepatic and renal disease, and malabsorption (especially secondary to gas-

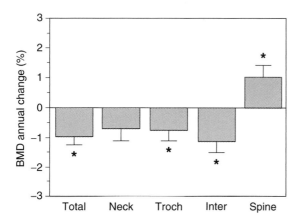

Figure 23–6. Longitudinal annual percentage change in bone mineral density (BMD) (g/cm², mean ± standard error of the mean) of the total hip, femoral neck, trochanter, intertrochanter, and spine in 85 healthy women over age 65 (mean age 77 years) followed for 1 year. (*, $p < 0.05$ difference from zero.) (Modified, with permission, from Greenspan SL et al: Femoral bone loss progresses with age: A longitudinal study in women over age 65. J Bone Min Res 1994;9:1959.)

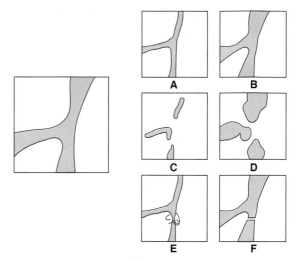

Figure 23–8. Possible effects of osteoporotic treatment regimens on trabecular bone. Left panel: Normal trabecular bone mass and architecture. Treatment resulting in anabolic effects on bone volume may restore normal bone volume and architecture in thin trabeculae (A, B). If trabecular integrity is disrupted before treatment, similar effects on bone volume may not reverse architectural abnormalities (C, D), particularly if treatment impairs the repair of microfractures (E, F). (Modified and reproduced, with permission, from Kanis JA: Treatment of osteoporotic fracture. Lancet 1984;1:27.)

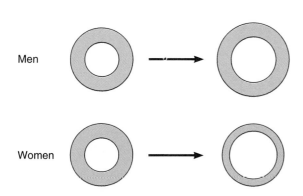

Figure 23–7. Schematic representation of cortical bone remodeling with age in males and females. Note that with age-related bone loss, bone is remodeled in men to increase its diameter and partially offset the loss of strength. In women, bone diameter changes little with age, so that bone strength decreases proportionately more than in men. (Reproduced, with permission, from Ruff CB, Hayes WC: Sex differences in age-related remodeling of the femur and tibia. J Orthop Res 1988;6:886.)

trectomy) should be excluded. Glucocorticoid use and antiseizure medications also can cause significant bone loss in the elderly. Biochemical markers of bone turnover reflect bone formation and resorption. Although these markers are associated with the rate of bone turnover even in elderly women, they cannot be used in lieu of a bone mineral density measurement to assess bone mass. Because factors outside the skeleton contribute to fracture risk in the elderly, however, the search for correctable factors must extend beyond those that affect bone density. Particular attention should be devoted to the patient's local environment and medication use.

Older patients presenting with skeletal discomfort should be evaluated by radiography to rule out a fracture. Vertebral osteoporosis usually presents with anterior wedging, involvement of more than one vertebra, prominent vertebral trabeculae, and vertebral deformities usually occurring below T6 (Figure 23–13). Worrisome signs suggesting that skeletal involvement is not due to osteoporosis alone include nerve root compression, posterior wedging, isolated vertebral involvement (especially above T4), and pedicle destruction. Further-

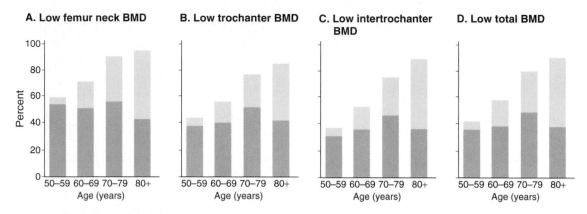

Figure 23–9. Prevalence of low femur bone mineral density (BMD) by age for non-Hispanic white women: light color, osteopenia; dark color, osteoporosis. (Source: CDC/NCHS III, phase 1, 1988–91.)

more, older individuals may complain of persistent groin pain with weight-bearing, while plain radiographs of the hip reveal no fracture. A bone scan may be necessary to confirm the diagnosis of hip fracture.

Treatment

Because the factors that affect bone physiology—the rate of bone loss, the structure of remaining bone, and the risk of fracture—are substantially different in perimenopausal and elderly women, interventions appropriate for perimenopausal women may be inappropriate for older women. Studies of older individuals that use bone density—or preferably fracture—as an end point provide the best data.

A. CALCIUM

Controversy surrounds the use of calcium supplementation in perimenopausal women, and few data are available regarding its use in older women. Theoretically, calcium supplementation seems appropriate because calcium intake in the elderly is low and the ability to adapt to a low-calcium diet declines with age. The National Academy of Sciences recommends 1200 mg per day of elemental calcium in divided doses. A reduction in hip fractures and improvement in bone density has been demonstrated in very elderly women (mean age 84) treated with vitamin D, 800 IU, and calcium, 1200 mg daily. Calcium carbonate supplements should be given in divided doses with meals to improve absorp-

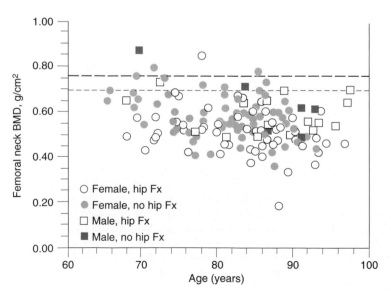

Figure 23–10. Femoral neck bone mineral density (BMD) (g/cm²) versus age (years) in fallers with and without hip fracture (Fx). The lines represent 2 SD less than peak bone mass (theoretical fracture threshold) for women (dots and lower dashed line) and men (boxes and upper dashed line). Mean (± SD) femoral neck peak bone mass for women, 0.895 (± 0.100) and for men, 0.979 (± 0.110) g/cm². (Reproduced, with permission, from Greenspan SL et al: Fall severity and bone mineral density as risk factors for hip fractures in ambulatory elderly. JAMA 1994;271:128.)

Table 23–3. Multiple logistic regression of factors associated with hip fracture in ambulatory elderly individuals.[1]

Factor	Adjusted Odds Ratio	95% Confidence Interval	p Value
Fall to side	5.7	2.3–14	< .001
Femoral neck bone mineral density (g/cm²)[2]	2.7	1.6–4.6	< .001
Fall energy (J)[3]	2.8	1.5–5.2	≤ .001
Body mass index[2] (kg/m²)*	2.2	1.2–3.8	.003

[1]Modified and reproduced, with permission, from Greenspan SL: Fall severity and bone mineral density as risk factors for hip fracture in ambulatory elderly. JAMA 1994;271:128.
[2]Calculated for a decrease of 1 SD.
[3]Calculated for an increase of 1 SD.

tion in the elderly, who may suffer from achlorhydria. Calcium citrate can be used as an alternative in such patients. A potential problem with prescribing high doses of calcium in the elderly includes inducing or exacerbating constipation. In addition, since compliance with other drug regimens decreases as the number of drugs increases, calcium tablets may be taken at the therapeutic expense of more important medications. Finally, because supplementary calcium does interfere with absorption of zinc, elderly patients receiving calcium supplementation should be encouraged to take a multivitamin containing zinc. Calcium absorption is not impaired by psyllium.

B. Vitamin D

There are few data to support the use of vitamin D or its metabolites in the treatment of osteoporosis, and results are equivocal. There is a small therapeutic ratio for vitamin D; toxicity from hypercalcemia can occur with doses as low as 50 µg (2000 IU), especially in individuals who are also taking a thiazide diuretic and calcium supplementation. However, because vitamin D deficiency is common in the elderly and vitamin D is needed for calcium absorption and mineralization of bone and also improves muscle strength, a single daily multivitamin which contains 400 IU is beneficial and will provide a normal vitamin D level even in institutionalized elderly persons. The current recommendation from the National Academy of Sciences is 400–800 IU/d (10–20 µg/d). Clinical trials utilizing calcitriol (1,25-dihydroxy vitamin D₃) as a therapeutic option for osteoporosis have reported conflicting results, though one trial found a threefold reduction in

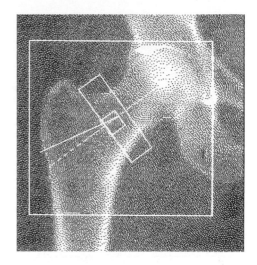

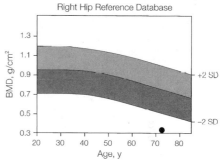

Right Hip Reference Database

Region	BMD, g/cm²	Peak BMD-Matched T Score	% of Mean	Age-Matched Z Score	% of M
Neck	0.328	−4.69	39	−2.75	52
Trochanter	0.176	−5.22	25	−3.77	32
Intertrochanteric	0.428	−4.34	39	−2.93	49
Total	0.330	−5.02	35	−3.37	45
Ward Triangle	0.180	−4.74	24	−2.04	43

Figure 23–11. This patient has a total hip bone mineral density (BMD) of 0.330 g/cm² (black circle on the reference database graph) as measured by dual-energy x-ray absorptiometry, a femoral neck T score of −4.69 and a total hip T score of −5.02. The reference database graph displays age- and sex-matched mean BMD levels ± 2 SD (shaded areas) derived from the third National Health and Nutrition Examination Survey. T score indicates the difference in SD between the subject's BMD and the predicted sex-matched mean peak young adult BMD; Z score, the difference in SD between the subject's BMD and the sex- and age-matched mean BMD; and % of mean, the subject's BMD as a percentage of the mean peak young adult BMD- or age-matched BMD level. (Adapted from bone densitometry report, QDR-4500C bone densitometer, Hologic Inc, Waltham, Massachusetts.)

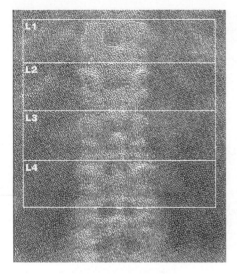

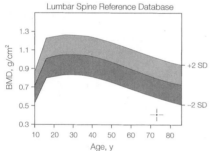

Region	BMD, g/cm²	Peak BMD-Matched		Age-Matched	
		T Score	% of Mean	Z Score	% of Mean
L1	0.305	−5.63	33	−3.62	43
L2	0.406	−5.66	39	−3.42	52
L3	0.382	−6.38	35	−4.03	46
L4	0.495	−5.65	44	−3.23	58
L1-L4	0.410	−5.79	39	−3.53	51

Figure 23–12. This patient has a lumbar spine (L1–L4) bone mineral density (BMD) of 0.410 g/cm² (cross on the reference database graph) measured by dual-energy x-ray absorptiometry and a T score of −5.79. The reference database graph displays age-and sex-matched mean BMD levels ± 2 SDs (shaded areas) derived from a normative database from the manufacturer, Hologic Inc, Waltham, Massachusetts. T score indicates the difference in SD between the subject's BMD and the predicted sex-matched mean peak young adult BMD; Z score, the difference in SD between the subject's BMD and the sex- and age-matched BMD level; and % of mean, the subject's BMD as a percentage of the mean peak young adult BMD- or age-matched BMD level. (Adapted from bone densitometry report, QDR-4500C bone densitometer; Hologic Inc, Waltham, Massachusetts.)

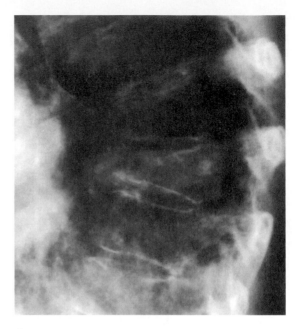

Figure 23–13. Lateral thoracic radiograph demonstrating a thoracic anterior wedge fracture. (Reproduced, with permission, from Clinical Crossroads: A 73-year-old woman with osteoporosis. JAMA 1999;281:1531.)

vertebral compression fractures. The potential for complications such as hypercalcemia, nephrolithiasis, and nephrocalcinosis are unknown, and this therapy is currently still under investigation.

C. Exercise

Although the rationale for exercise therapy is sound, few data are available on results of exercise in elderly women. One study prescribed exercise for older women and found that forearm bone mineral content increased in those who continued exercising during a 3-year trial. Middle-aged women (mean age 60) participating in high-intensity strength training for 1 year had improvements in femoral bone mass, muscle strength, balance, and activity level compared with controls. Walking—generally 30 minutes three times a week—is often suggested for frail individuals.

D. Estrogen and Selective Estrogen Receptor Modulators

There is considerable evidence that estrogen therapy, if initiated at menopause, slows bone loss, temporarily increases bone mass, and may prevent osteoporotic vertebral and hip fractures. If therapy is continued, its efficacy is sustained at least until age 70. In addition, some studies have shown that estrogen will increase femoral bone mass. Fewer data are available about elderly persons taking newly prescribed estrogen. Four studies have reported a positive effect of estrogen on bone mass in older women. The observational study of osteoporotic fractures noted a 50% reduction of hip fractures in older women who were currently taking estrogens and had been doing so for a mean period of 14.5 years. Administration of conjugated estrogens at a dose of 0.625 mg daily (or the equivalent synthetic estrogen dose) has been the standard recommendation to maintain bone mass. However, in older women, doses as low as 0.3 mg/d may be beneficial to skeletal health while minimizing adverse effects such as mastalgia or the return of uterine bleeding.

For women with an intact uterus, combined cyclic regimens with estrogen and progesterone may provoke return of menses and are less well tolerated. Despite the need for gynecologic surveillance and possible endometrial sampling to prevent uterine cancer, older women are more tolerant of combined continuous therapy regimens with estrogen and progesterone, which generally provide an atrophic endometrium within 1 year. Similar to younger women, older women receiving estrogen therapy require annual mammograms (Chapter 13).

Estrogen's protective effect against cardiovascular disease is in doubt. There are few data to support the suggestion that a cardiovascular benefit will accrue when estrogen is newly prescribed to elderly women, in whom the prevalence of heart disease is already high. Moreover, the Heart and Estrogen/Progestin Replacement Study (HERS) and the Women's Health Initiative (WHI) raised doubts about the cardiovascular benefit to women with established heart disease. And furthermore, because of the possible increased relative risk of breast cancer in older women who have taken estrogen for more than 5 years, physicians must assess all the individual risks and benefits for each patient (see Chapter 13).

Selective estrogen receptor modulators (SERMs) have estrogen agonist and antagonist actions. Raloxifene has been approved for the prevention and treatment of postmenopausal osteoporosis. Although improvements in bone mineral density are less with raloxifene than estrogen replacement therapy, studies demonstrate a reduction of approximately 50% in vertebral fractures with no mastalgia, vaginal bleeding, or increased endometrial thickness. Early studies demonstrated a reduction in cholesterol and protection against breast cancer. Raloxifene has not been shown to reduce nonvertebral or hip fractures.

E. OTHER THERAPEUTIC OPTIONS

Bisphosphonates—nonhormonal agents that inhibit bone resorption—effectively prevent osteoporosis. The aminobisphosphonate alendronate has been shown to increase bone mass at the spine (10%) and hip (6–8%) over 3 years in prospective clinical trials in postmenopausal women. Fractures of the spine, forearm, and hip were reduced by approximately 50%. Improvements have also been demonstrated in older women residing in long-term care facilities. Risedronate, another bisphosphonate, has been shown to improve bone mass and reduce vertebral and hip fractures. When taken properly, these medications are well-tolerated—an important factor in choosing therapeutic alternatives for the elderly. Furthermore, alendronate and risedronate can be administered once per week. Prospective studies with etidronate showed a benefit for the spine, but results were not consistent for the hip. Although calcitonin is an approved therapy for osteoporosis, few data are available about its effect on the incidence of fractures. It is expensive and when given by injection is poorly tolerated by the elderly. Nasal calcitonin has been shown to reduce fractures of the spine—but not of the hip—with no improvement in hip bone density. Fluoride therapy causes significant toxicity in one-third of patients and has been associated with an increase in nonvertebral fractures. Although thiazide diuretics have been associated with decreased hip fracture risk in several cross-sectional epidemiologic studies, the results are inconsistent, and the optimal dose and duration are unclear. However, a slight increase in both falls and fractures was noted in the only randomized study of thiazide use, the SHEP trial for hypertension in the elderly. For glucocorticoid-induced bone loss, alendronate and risedronate are the only approved bisphosphonates, but other agents are under investigation.

Parathyroid hormone (1–34), the first anabolic agent, has been shown to significantly increase bone density (9.7% for spine bone density in 18 months) and reduce vertebral and nonvertebral fractures in postmenopausal osteoporotic women. This is given as a subcutaneous daily injection and can be combined with antiresorptive agents. Vertebroplasty and kyphoplasty are interventions in which polymethylmethacrylate (vertebroplasty) or polymethylmethacrylate in a balloon (kyphoplasty) are placed in compressed vertebrae for patients with intractable pain from vertebral fractures. There are no controlled trials with these interventions, and it is not known if the procedures will strengthen or weaken adjacent vertebrae.

Summary of Management Recommendations

In summary, there is ample reason to question the validity of extrapolating data from studies of perimenopausal women when formulating a treatment plan for older women. However, given the prevalence of the problem, it is reasonable to recommend an adequate daily intake of vitamin D (10 μg, or 400 IU) contained in one multivitamin tablet), an adequate daily intake of calcium (totaling 1200 mg), and judicious participation in an individually tailored exercise program. The use of bisphosphonates, estrogen replacement therapy, SERMs, parathyroid hormone, or other treatment needs to be individually considered.

Perhaps more importantly, the risk of falls should be addressed. The risk can be reduced by reviewing medications (including nonprescription agents) and discontinuing (when possible) those with adverse effects on cognition, balance, or blood pressure. Common offenders include long-acting benzodiazepines, tricyclic antidepressants, antipsychotics, antihypertensives, and agents with anticholinergic side effects. It is also important to correct reversible sensory losses and medical conditions and to educate patients about hazards in their environment, such as throw rugs, extension cords, and poorly illuminated stairways, that could lead to falls and fractures. For patients with gait disorders, physical therapy should be considered.

Patients who have recently sustained a hip fracture should receive the same evaluation and consideration as those without a fracture. Because there is a significant overlap in bone density measurements between those that fracture and those that do not (Figure 23–10), a hip fracture should not serve as a reason to omit evaluation or treatment (see also Chapter 8).

HYPERPARATHYROIDISM

Clinical Features

The prevalence of hyperparathyroidism increases with age. While its incidence is less than 10 per 100,000 in women under age 40, the incidence increases to 190 per 100,000 in women over age 60. As a result, over half of all cases of hyperparathyroidism occur in individuals over the age of 65. Most cases are mild. Detection is by routine screening of serum calcium, and few or no symptoms are present. However, with relatively minor elevations of serum calcium (up to 11–12 mg/dL [2.8–3 mmol/L]), some elderly subjects may experience weakness, fatigue, depression, and confusion. Failure to thrive and constipation are commonly seen; renal, gastrointestinal, and skeletal complications occur less often. Other causes of hypercalcemia in the elderly—especially multiple myeloma, malignancy, vitamin D intoxication, and thiazide diuretics—must be considered in the differential diagnosis.

Treatment

For symptomatic patients with serum calcium levels above 12 mg/dL (3 mmol/L) and elevated serum parathyroid hormone levels, parathyroidectomy is well tolerated and is the treatment of choice. For those with more modest elevations, treatment recommendations are less simply stated because it is difficult to differentiate symptoms and signs due to the disease from those seen in older individuals without hyperparathyroidism. Moreover, asymptomatic individuals—especially those with levels of serum calcium under 11 mg/dL (2.8 mmol/L)—have been known to remain asymptomatic for over a decade. Until more data become available, the decision to treat asymptomatic individuals surgically should be made on an individual basis.

In patients whose symptoms may be due to hyperparathyroidism, it is worthwhile to observe the response to medical therapy before considering surgery. In women, a course of estrogen may be effective. Ethinyl estradiol (30–50 μg/d) or conjugated estrogens (0.625–1.25 mg/d) reduce serum calcium by an average of 0.8 mg/dL (0.2 mmol/L), diminish urinary calcium excretion, and antagonize the skeletal effect of PTH. In men and in women with higher elevations of serum calcium, oral phosphates can be used, but they are less well tolerated in the elderly because of their gastrointestinal side effects and the potential for ectopic calcification. Furosemide is a less satisfactory alternative in frail elderly patients because it increases the risk of dehydration and resultant hypercalcemia. On the other hand, parathyroidectomy procedures in elderly patients have similar outcomes compared with younger patients with respect to cure rate, morbidity, mortality, and patient satisfaction. A more recent option for geriatric patients includes a limited or targeted parathyroidectomy and uses preoperative localization and intraoperative measurement of parathyroid hormone rather than the conventional approach of visualization of all glands. This not only improves the success rate but simplifies the surgical procedure as well.

■ CHANGES IN WATER BALANCE

With age, major changes in renal function and homeostatic mechanisms result in significant changes in water balance. Renal blood flow, cortical mass, the number of glomeruli, and tubular function all decline with age, though medullary mass is preserved. Clinically, however, the most relevant change is the age-related decline in creatinine clearance, which is largely due to relative hypertension in the elderly. Because of the decrease in muscle mass associated with aging, however, serum creatinine levels are unchanged and may not accurately reflect the extent of renal functional impairment.

Extrarenal modulators of water balance also change significantly with age. Although there are no changes in the basal level, half-life, volume of distribution, or metabolic clearance of vasopressin, the stimulated responses of vasopressin are significantly altered. Hyperosmolar stimuli increase serum vasopressin levels in older subjects to five times those achieved in younger subjects. On the other hand, the normal vasopressin increase observed in response to overnight dehydration and postural change is impaired in the elderly. Additionally, basal and stimulated levels of serum renin and aldosterone decline with age. In contrast, basal levels of atrial natriuretic factor are three times higher in healthy elderly individuals than in young controls. These elevated levels of atrial natriuretic factor may help identify patients at risk for the development of congestive heart failure. Finally, the thirst sensation appears to be somewhat impaired in healthy elderly individuals and is more impaired in those who are frail.

In addition to physiologic changes, many diseases and drugs further increase the vulnerability of the elderly to changes in water balance. These include kidney disease, hypertension, and congestive heart failure as well as medications that alter water balance (eg, narcotics, diuretics, lithium, chlorpropamide, carbamazepine, amphotericin B, intravenous hypotonic fluids, and hypertonic contrast agents).

HYPERNATREMIA

Clinical Features

The incidence of hypernatremia in elderly patients admitted to the hospital ranges from 1% to 3% and is higher for institutionalized elderly patients. Signs and symptoms are usually nonspecific, eg, lethargy, weakness, confusion, depression, and failure to thrive. The cause is usually multifactorial, including impaired thirst mechanism, renal disease, sedative-induced confusion, use of restraints, reduced access to free water intake, excess water loss due to fever, and decreased response to vasopressin.

Treatment

As in younger patients, initial therapy involves correcting the volume deficit with isotonic saline and then correcting the water deficit with half-normal (0.45%) saline. Roughly 30% of the deficit should be corrected within 24 hours and the remainder within the next 24–48 hours.

HYPONATREMIA

Clinical Features

The prevalence of hyponatremia is approximately 2.5% in the general hospital setting—higher in geriatric units—and rises to 25% in nursing home settings. Presenting symptoms and signs are often nonspecific and include lethargy, weakness, and confusion. The mechanisms predisposing to hyponatremia include the exuberant response of vasopressin to osmolar stimuli, a decreased ability to excrete a water load, and the sodium-wasting tendency of the older kidney. Furthermore, elderly patients often use medications and have diseases that impair free water excretion. Common hyponatremic syndromes in the elderly include the syndrome of inappropriate antidiuretic hormone secretion (SIADH) and thiazide-induced hyponatremia. In the geriatric rehabilitation hospital, approximately half of patients with hyponatremia have SIADH. Furthermore, hyponatremia has been reported with selective serotonin reuptake inhibitors in the elderly.

Treatment

The treatment of hyponatremia in the elderly does not differ from that in younger patients (Chapters 5 and 24).

HYPORENINEMIC HYPOALDOSTERONISM

Hyporeninemic hypoaldosteronism usually occurs in elderly patients with diabetes and mild renal insufficiency. Patients are usually asymptomatic, and hyperkalemia and acidosis are found on routine screening. On the other hand, symptoms of hyperkalemia (eg, heart block) may be provoked by administration of a beta-adrenergic blocking agent, which further compromises extrarenal regulation of potassium homeostasis. After other causes of persistent hyperkalemia are ruled out, patients respond well to administration of small doses of fludrocortisone (0.05 mg/d) or furosemide combined with restriction of potassium.

■ GLUCOCORTICOIDS & STRESS

Cortisol levels increase 20–50% with age. There is an increase in the nocturnal level of cortisol, an age-related morning increase in cortisol in women (not men), and an advancement in the circadian rhythm (Figure 23–14).

In healthy elderly individuals, dynamic testing of the hypothalamic-pituitary-adrenal axis is normal; expected responses to insulin-induced hypoglycemia, metyrapone, dexamethasone, ACTH, and CRH are preserved (Figure 23–15).

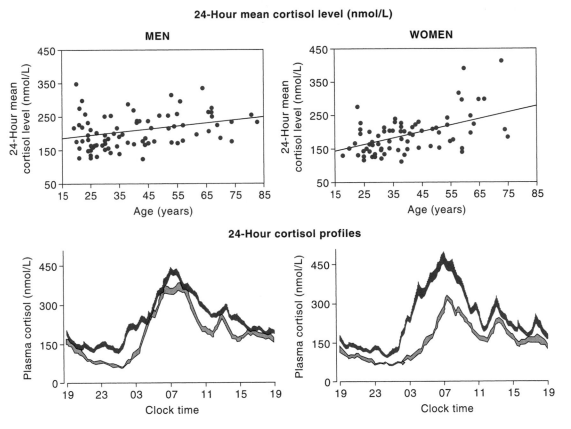

24-Hour mean cortisol level (nmol/L)

Figure 23–14. Upper panels: Age-related changes in 24-hour mean cortisol levels in men and women. The coefficient of correlation for the linear regression was r = 0.29 in men (*P* < .002) and r = 0.50 in women (*P* < .0001). Sex differences in the slope of the regression failed to reach significance. Lower panels: Mean 24-hour cortisol profiles in men and women 50 years of age and older (n = 25 and n = 22, respectively; blue lines) compared with those in 20- to 29-year-old subjects (n = 29 and n = 20, respectively; gray lines). The shading at each time point represents the SEM. (Reproduced, with permission, by van Cauter E, Leproult R, Kupfer DJ: Effects of gender and age on the levels and circadian rhythmicity of plasma cortisol. J Clin Endocrinol Metab 1996;81:2468. Copyright © 1996 by The Endocrine Society.)

DISORDERS OF THE HYPOTHALAMIC-PITUITARY-ADRENAL AXIS

1. Abnormal Response to Stress

In contrast to the normal responses in the elderly to dynamic testing of the hypothalamic-pituitary-adrenal axis, increased stress elicits abnormal responses. For example, although serum cortisol levels increase to the same extent in young and old patients undergoing elective surgery, the increase may be protracted in the elderly. Patients with diabetes mellitus and hypertension have also been found to have an exaggerated and prolonged response to CRH stimulation. Older patients with Alzheimer's disease may also have a delayed and prolonged response to

CRH stimulation. It is not known if these elevated cortisol levels contribute to the increased hypertension, glucose intolerance, muscle atrophy, and impaired immune function observed in the elderly. However, an elevated urinary cortisol level is an independent predictor of osteoporotic fractures in the elderly.

2. Adrenal Hypersecretion

While adrenal hypersecretion (Cushing's syndrome) is uncommon in the elderly, it is easily overlooked because it mimics normal aging processes. Signs such as hypertension, glucose intolerance, weight gain, and osteoporosis are less specific in elderly than in younger patients, but as in younger patients the diagnosis is

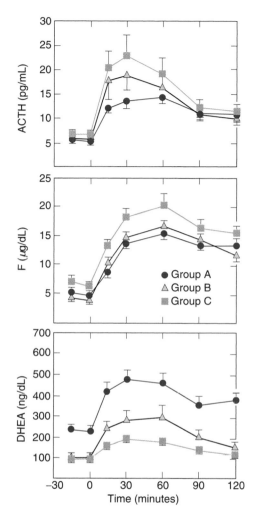

Figure 23–15. Mean values for groups A, B, and C of plasma ACTH *(upper panel),* F or cortisol *(middle panel),* and DHEA (lower panel) before and up to 120 minutes after bolus intravenous injection of ovine CRH (1 μg/kg). Group A, 21–49 years, mean age 35.2 years, n = 19. Group B, 50–69 years, mean age 60.7 years, n = 15. Group C, 70–86 years, mean age 77.1 years, n = 15. (Reproduced, with permission, from Pavlov EP et al: Responses of plasma adrenocorticotropin, cortisol, and dehydroepiandrosterone to ovine corticotropin-releasing hormone in healthy aging men. J Clin Endocrinol Metab 1986;62:767.)

established or excluded using the usual criteria (Chapter 9).

3. Adrenal Insufficiency

Symptoms of adrenal insufficiency in younger patients—eg, failure to thrive, weakness, weight loss, confusion, and arthralgias—are common complaints in adrenally intact elderly patients; the most specific sign of adrenal insufficiency in the elderly is hyperpigmentation. The laboratory findings of adrenal insufficiency are similar to those found in younger patients and include azotemia, hypoglycemia, hyponatremia, hyperkalemia, and eosinophilia. Because the metabolic clearance rate of cortisol decreases with age, older patients generally require lower replacement doses of cortisol (Chapter 9).

■ CHANGES IN REPRODUCTIVE FUNCTION IN MEN

Overall, while sexual activity decreases with age, there are conflicting reports about the physiologic changes in the hypothalamic-pituitary-testicular axis. Longitudinal studies demonstrate an age-related decrease in testosterone and free testosterone and a higher frequency of hypogonadal values (Figures 23–16 and 23–17). Some studies suggest that circulating testosterone and bioavailable testosterone fall with age by 40–65% and are even lower in institutionalized elderly. A decrease in the number or responsiveness of testicular Leydig cells is likely because serum FSH and LH increase with age, and the testosterone response to human chorionic gonadotropin (hCG) decreases. On the other hand, with age there is probably a decrease in the ratio of circulating bioactive to immunoreactive LH. Finally, pituitary changes are suggested by a decreased gonadotropic response to luteinizing hormone-releasing hormone (LHRH) stimulation.

The clinical relevance of these changes is not clear. The correlation between sexual activity and the age-related hormonal changes described is weak. There are decreased concentrations of spermatozoa in the ejaculate of older men, sperm motility and the volume of ejaculate decrease with age, and the proportion of abnormal spermatozoa also increases. Dehydroepiandrosterone (DHEA) and DHEA-sulfate (DHEA-S) are steroids of adrenal origin that decrease with age. Levels do not correlate with cognitive function or decline, and DHEA supplementation has not been shown to be beneficial. However, studies in the elderly are ongoing.

Erectile dysfunction (impotence) becomes more prevalent with age, but an endocrinologic cause be-

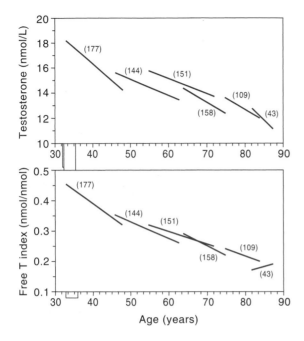

Figure 23–16. Longitudinal effects of aging on date-adjusted testosterone (T) and free testosterone index (free T index). Linear segment plots for total T and free T index versus age are shown for men with T and sex hormone-binding globulin (SHBG) values on at least two visits. Each linear segment has a slope equal to the mean of the individual longitudinal slopes in each decade, and is centered on the median age, for each cohort of men from the second to the ninth decade. Numbers in parentheses represent the number of men in each cohort. With the exception of free T index in the ninth decade, segments show significant downward progression at every age, with no significant change in slopes for T or free T index over the entire age range. (T, testosterone; SHBG, sex hormone binding globulin; T/SHBG, free T index.) (Reproduced, with permission, from Harman SM et al: Longitudinal effects of aging on serum total and free testosterone levels in healthy men. J Clin Endocrinol Metab 2001;86:724. Copyright © 2001 by The Endocrine Society.)

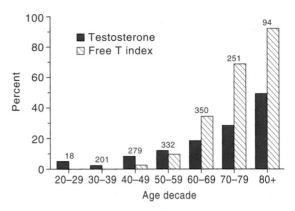

Figure 23–17. Hypogonadism in aging men. Bar height indicates the percentage of men in each 10-year interval, from the third to the ninth decades, with at least one testosterone (T) value in the hypogonadal range, by the criteria of total T < 11.3 nmol/L (325 ng/dL) (shaded bars), or T/SHBG (free T index) < 0.153 nmol/nmol (striped bars). Numbers above each pair of bars indicate the number of men studied in the corresponding decade. The fraction of men who are hypogonadal increases progressively after age 50 by either criterion. More men are hypogonadal by free T index than by total T after age 50, and there seems to be a progressively greater difference, with increasing age, between the two criteria. (T, testosterone; SHBG, sex hormone binding globulin; T/SHBG, free T index.) (Reproduced, with permission, from Harman SM et al: Longitudinal effects of aging on serum total and free testosterone levels in healthy men. J Clin Endocrinol Metab 2001;86:724. Copyright © 2001 by The Endocrine Society.)

comes less likely. The prevalence of erectile dysfunction in men under age 45 is 5%; the prevalence in men over age 75 is 50%. However, over 90% of men in the latter group have coexistent medical conditions or are taking medications that contribute to the problem. Furthermore, up to 30% of men over age 76 develop erectile dysfunction following prostatectomy, compared with 3–11% in younger age groups. Often there are multiple overlapping causes of erectile dysfunction—psychoso-

cial, neurovascular, metabolic (diabetes mellitus), medication-related, and vascular—in the same individual.

The evaluation of erectile dysfunction in the elderly is similar to that in younger individuals (Chapter 12), though more emphasis must be placed on the effects of drugs (both prescribed and nonprescribed) and vascular causes, and a search for multiple causative factors should be undertaken.

■ BENIGN PROSTATIC HYPERPLASIA

Although the pathogenesis of benign prostatic hyperplasia is incompletely understood, testicular androgens are believed to play a permissive role in the development of prostatic adenomas. This mechanism provides the rationale for the use of antiandrogens in the treatment of benign prostatic hypertrophy. Antiandrogen treatment has been investigated using luteinizing hormone releasing hormone (LHRH) agonists (nafarelin, leuprolide, buserelin), androgen receptor inhibitors (cyproterone acetate, flutamide), and 5α-reductase inhibitors (finasteride). Overall, these agents result in a 25–30% reduction in prostate size, but their effects on the voiding symptoms associated with benign prostatic hypertrophy have been modest, variable, and less immediate and substantial than observed with alpha-adrenergic blockers. For instance, finasteride reduces symptoms by half in only one-third of men, and statistically significant effects in the largest trial occurred only after 11 months. One trial showed that finasteride reduced the incidence of both urinary retention and surgery, but 15 men would need to take finasteride for 4 years to prevent such an event in just one of them. Moreover, each of these agents must be continued indefinitely to maintain prostate size reduction, yet many men may find such therapy difficult and undesirable as well as expensive, and the long-term side effects are largely unknown. The LHRH agonists and cyproterone acetate cause impotence; androgen deprivation therapy results in bone loss; flutamide induces gynecomastia, and one report describes serologic as well as histologic evidence of flutamide-induced hepatotoxicity in a small number of patients. Since finasteride decreases dihydrotestosterone while maintaining the circulating levels of testosterone, undesirable antiandrogenic side effects are lower. Finasteride causes a significant decrease in the level of prostate-specific antigen, a serum marker increasingly used for the clinical detection of prostate adenocarcinoma, the most common cancer in men. Thus, if PSA levels fail to decline in a man compliant with therapy, investigation for prostate cancer should be initiated. Since the effect of finasteride on prostate cancer development and progression is unknown, it is unclear whether any antitumor benefit will mitigate finasteride's interference with the use of PSA as a tumor marker.

REFERENCES

Thyroid Function and Disease

Bagchi N, Brown TR, Parish RF: Thyroid dysfunction in adults over age 55 years: A study in an urban US community. Arch Intern Med 1995;150:785. [PMID: 2109585]

Cooper DS: Clinical practice. Subclinical hypothyroidism. N Engl J Med 2001;345:260. [PMID: 11474665]

DeFronzo R: Pharmacologic therapy for type 2 diabetes mellitus. Ann Intern Med 1999;131:281. [PMID: 10877745]

Danese MD et al: Screening for mild thyroid failure at the periodic health examination: A decision and cost-effectiveness analysis. JAMA 1996;276:285. [PMID: 8656540]

Davis PJ, Davis FB: Hyperthyroidism in patients over the age of 60 years: clinical features in 85 patients. Medicine 1974;53:161. [PMID: 4133091]

Greenspan SL et al: Age-related alterations in pulsatile secretion of TSH: Role of dopaminergic regulation. Am J Physiol 1991; 260(3 Part 1):E486. [PMID: 1900670]

Greenspan SL, Greenspan FS: The effect of thyroid hormone on skeletal integrity. Ann Intern Med 1999;130:750. [PMID: 10357695]

Hershman JM et al: Serum thyrotropin and thyroid hormone levels in elderly and middle-aged euthyroid persons. J Am Geriatr Soc 1993;41:823. [PMID: 8340560]

Hollowell JG et al: Serum TSH, T$_4$, and thyroid antibodies in the United States population (1988 to 1994): National Health and Nutrition Examination Survey (NHANES III). J Clin Endocrinol Metab 2002;87:489. [PMID: 11836274]

Ladenson PW et al: American Thyroid Association guidelines for detection of thyroid dysfunction. Arch Intern Med 2000;160: 1573. [PMID: 10847249]

Parle JV et al: Prediction of all-cause and cardiovascular mortality in elderly people from one low serum thyrotropin result: A 10-year cohort study. Lancet 2001;358:861. [PMID: 11567699]

Rosenthal MJ et al: Thyroid failure in the elderly: Microsomal antibodies as discriminant for therapy. JAMA 1987;258:209. [PMID: 3599304]

Samuels ME: Subclinical thyroid disease in the elderly. Thyroid 1998;8:803. [PMID: 9772803]

Sawin CT et al: Low serum thyrotropin (thyroid-stimulating hormone) in older persons without hyperthyroidism. Arch Intern Med 1991;151:165. [PMID: 1985591]

Sawin CT et al: Low serum thyrotropin concentrations as a risk factor for atrial fibrillation in older persons. N Engl J Med 1994; 331:1249. [PMID: 7935681]

Sawin CT et al: The aging thyroid: The use of thyroid hormone in older persons. JAMA 1989;261:2653. [PMID: 2709545]

Sawin CT et al: The aging thyroid: Thyroid deficiency in the Framingham study. Arch Intern Med 1985;145:1386. [PMID: 4026469]

Sawin CT: Subclinical hypothyroidism in older persons. Clin Geriatr Med 1995;11:231. [PMID: 7606692]

Sawin CT: Thyroid dysfunction in older persons. Adv Intern Med 1991;37:223. [PMID: 1373029]

Tibaldi JM et al: Thyrotoxicosis in the very old. Am J Med 1986; 81:619. [PMID: 3766592]

Toft AD. Clinical practice. Subclinical hyperthyroidism. N Engl J Med 2001;345:512. [PMID: 11519506]

U.S. Preventive Services Task Force: Screening for thyroid disease. In: Guiseppi CD, Atkins D, Woolf SH (editors): *Guide to Clinical Preventive Services,* 2d ed. Williams & Wilkins, 1996.

Wang C, Crapo LM: The epidemiology of thyroid disease and implications for screening. Endocrinol Metab Clin North Am 1997;26:189. [PMID: 9074859]

Carbohydrate Intolerance and Diabetes Mellitus

Burge MR et al: A prospective trial of risk factors for sulfonylurea-induced hypoglycemia in type 2 diabetes mellitus. JAMA 1998;279:137. [PMID: 9440664]

Butler RN et al: Type 2 diabetes: Causes, complications, and new screening recommendations. Geriatrics 1998;53:47. [PMID: 9511774]

Cahill GF: Hyperglycemic hyperosmolar coma: A syndrome almost unique in the elderly. J Am Geriatr Soc 1983;31:103. [PMID: 6337203]

Diabetes Control and Complications Trial Research Group: The effect of intensive treatment of diabetes on the development and progression of long-term complications in insulin-dependent diabetes mellitus. N Engl J Med 1993;329:977. [PMID: 8366922]

Elahi D et al: Effect of age and obesity on fasting levels of glucose, insulin, growth hormone and glucagon in man. J Gerontol 1982;37:385. [PMID: 7045192]

Franssila-Kallunki A, Schalin-Jantti C, Groop L: Effect of gender on insulin resistance associated with aging. Am J Physiol 1992;263:E780. [PMID: 1415700]

Johnson KC et al: Prevalence of undiagnosed non-insulin-dependent diabetes mellitus and impaired glucose tolerance in a cohort of older persons with hypertension. J Am Geriatr Soc 1997;45:695. [PMID: 9185690]

Lardinois CK: Type 2 diabetes: Glycemic targets and oral therapies for older patients. Geriatrics 1998;53:22. [PMID: 9824974]

Lorber D: Nonketotic hypertonicity in diabetes mellitus. Med Clin North Am 1995;79:39. [PMID: 7808094]

Meigs JB et al: Metabolic control and prevalent cardiovascular disease in non-insulin-dependent diabetes mellitus (NIDDM): The NIDDM Patient Outcomes Research Team. Am J Med 1997;102:38. [PMID: 9209199]

Meneilly GS, Cheung E, Tuokko H: Counterregulatory hormone responses to hypoglycemia in the elderly patient with diabetes. Diabetes 1994;43:403. [PMID: 8314012]

Meneilly GS et al: NIDDM in the elderly. Diabetes Care 1999;22:1225. [PMID: 8941457]

Morisaki N et al: Diabetic control and progression of retinopathy in elderly patients: Five-year follow-up study. J Am Geriatr Soc 1994;42:142. [PMID: 8126325]

Samos LF, Roos BA: Diabetes mellitus in older persons. Med Clin North Am 1998;82:791. [PMID: 9706121]

Scott RD et al: The association of non-insulin-dependent diabetes mellitus and cognitive function in an older cohort. J Am Geriatr Soc 1998;46:1217. [PMID: 9777902]

Turner RC et al for the UK Prospective Diabetes Study Group: Intensive blood-glucose control with sulphonylureas or insulin compared with conventional treatment and risk of complications in patients with type 2 diabetes (UKPDS 33). Lancet 1998;352:837. [PMID: 9742976]

Warrain JH et al: Epidemiology of non-insulin-dependent diabetes mellitus and its macrovascular complications: A basis for the development of cost-effective programs. Endocrinol Metab Clin North Am 1997;26:165. [PMID: 9074858]

Osteoporosis and Calcium Homeostasis

Black DM et al: Randomised trial of effect of alendronate on risk of fracture in women with existing vertebral fractures. Lancet 1996;348:1535. [PMID: 8950879]

Cauley JA, Seeley DG, Ensrud K: Estrogen replacement therapy and fractures in older women. Ann Intern Med 1995;122:9. [PMID: 7985914]

Chandler JM et al: Low bone mineral density and risk of fracture in white female nursing home residents. JAMA 2000;284:972. [PMID: 10944642]

Chapuy MC et al: Vitamin D_3 and calcium to prevent hip fractures in elderly women. N Engl J Med 1992;327:1637. [PMID: 1331788]

Chen H, Parkerson S, Udelsman R: Parathyroidectomy in the elderly: Do the benefits outweigh the risks? World J Surg 1998; 22:531. [PMID: 9597924]

Chesnut CH III et al: A randomized trial of nasal spray salmon calcitonin in postmenopausal women with established osteoporosis: The Prevent Recurrence of Osteoporotic Fractures Study. Am J Med 2000;109:267. [PMID: 10996576]

Chigot J-P, Menegaux F, Achrafi H: Should primary hyperparathyroidism be treated surgically in elderly patients older than 75 years? Surgery 1995;117:397. [PMID: 7716721]

Col NF et al: Patient-specific decisions about hormone replacement therapy in postmenopausal women. JAMA 1997;277:1140. [PMID: 9087469]

Cummings SR et al: Risk factors for hip fracture in white women. Study of Osteoporotic Fractures Research Group. N Engl J Med 1995;332:767. [PMID: 7862179]

Dawson-Hughes B et al: Effect of calcium and vitamin D supplementation on bone density in men and women 65 years of age or older. N Engl J Med 1997;337:670. [PMID: 9278463]

Ebeling PR et al: Influence of age on effects of endogenous 1,25-dihydroxyvitamin D on calcium absorption in normal women. Calcif Tissue Int 1994;55:330. [PMID: 7866911]

Ettinger B et al: Reduction of vertebral fracture risk in postmenopausal women with osteoporosis treated with raloxifene: Results from a 3-year randomized clinical trial. JAMA 1999; 282:637. [PMID: 10517716]

Genant HK et al for the Estratab/Osteoporosis Study Group: Low-dose esterified estrogen therapy: Effects on bone, plasma estradiol concentrations, endometrium, and lipid levels. Arch Intern Med 1997;157:2609. [PMID: 9531230]

Greenspan SL et al: Alendronate improves bone mineral density in elderly female long-term care facility residents with osteoporosis. A double-blind, placebo-controlled, randomized trial. Ann Intern Med 2002 (in press).

Greenspan SL et al: Fall direction, bone mineral density, and function: Risk factors for hip fracture in frail nursing home elderly. Am J Med 1998;104:539. [PMID: 9674716]

Greenspan SL et al: Femoral bone loss progresses with age: A longitudinal study in women over age 65. J Bone Miner Res 1994; 9:1959. [PMID: 7872062]

Greenspan SL, Greenspan FS: The effect of thyroid hormone on skeletal integrity. Ann Intern Med 1999;130:750. [PMID: 10357695]

Greenspan SL, Myers ER, Maitland LA: Fall severity and bone mineral density as risk factors for hip fracture in ambulatory elderly. JAMA 1994;271:128. [PMID: 8264067]

Halley S et al for the Heart and Estrogen/Progestin Replacement Study (HERS) Research Group: Randomized trial of estrogen plus progestin for secondary prevention of coronary heart disease in postmenopausal women. JAMA 1998;280:605. [PMID: 9718051]

Irvin GL III, Carneiro DM: "Limited" parathyroidectomy in geriatric patients. Ann Surg 2001;233:612. [PMID: 11360891]

Jones G et al: Thiazide diuretics and fractures: Can meta-analysis help? J Bone Miner Res 1995;10:106. [PMID: 7747616]

Lips P: Vitamin D deficiency and secondary hyperparathyroidism in the elderly: Consequences for bone loss and fractures and therapeutic implications. Endocr Rev 2001;22:477. [PMID: 11493580]

Looker AC et al: Prevalence of low femoral bone density in older U.S. women from NHANES III. J Bone Miner Res 1995; 10:796. [PMID: 9383679]

Marshall D, Johnell O, Wedel H: Meta-analysis of how well measures of bone mineral density predict occurrence of osteoporotic fractures. BMJ 1996;312:1254. [PMID: 8634613]

McClung MR et al: Effect of risedronate on the risk of hip fracture in elderly women. N Engl J Med 2001;344:333. [PMID: 11386284]

Neer RM et al: Effect of parathyroid hormone (1-34) on fractures and bone mineral density in postmenopausal women with osteoporosis. N Engl J Med 2001;344:1434. [PMID: 11346808]

Physician's Guide to Prevention and Treatment of Osteoporosis: National Osteoporosis Foundation, 1998.

Rossouw JE et al: Risks and benefits of estrogen plus progestin in healthy postmenopausal women: Principal results from the Womens Health Initiative randomized controlled trial. JAMA 2002;288:321. [PMID: 12117397].

Ruff CB, Hayes WC: Sex differences in age-related remodeling of the femur and tibia. J Orthop Res 1988;6:886. [PMID: 3171769]

Souberbielle J-C et al: Vitamin D status and redefining serum parathyroid hormone reference range in the elderly. J Clin Endocrinol Metab 2001;86:3086. [PMID: 11443171]

Standing Committee on the Scientific Evaluation of Dietary Reference Intakes, Food and Nutrition Board, Institute of Medicine: *Dietary Reference Intakes for Calcium, Phosphorus, Magnesium, Vitamin D, and Fluoride.* National Academy Press, 1997.

Thomas MK et al: Hypovitaminosis D in medical inpatients. N Engl J Med 1998;338:777. [PMID: 9504937]

Tinetti ME et al: A multifactorial intervention to reduce the risk of falling among elderly people living in the community. N Engl J Med 1994;331:821. [PMID: 8078528]

Changes in Water Balance

Anpalahan M: Chronic idiopathic hyponatremia in older people due to syndrome of inappropriate antidiuretic hormone secretion (SIADH) possibly related to aging. J Am Geriatr Soc 2001;49:788. [PMID: 11454119]

Anderson RJ et al: Hyponatremia: A prospective analysis of its epidemiology and the pathogenetic role of vasopressin. Ann Intern Med 1985;102:164. [PMID: 3966753]

Borra SI, Beredo R, Kleinfeld M: Hypernatremia in the aging: Causes, manifestations, and outcome. J Natl Med Assoc 1995;87:220. [PMID: 7731073]

Cyus JC, Krothapalli RK, Arieff AL: Treatment of symptomatic hyponatremia and its relation to brain damage. N Engl J Med 1987;317:1190. [PMID: 3309659]

Davis KM et al: Atrial natriuretic peptide levels in the prediction of congestive heart failure risk in frail elderly JAMA 1992; 267:2625. [PMID: 1533427]

Miller M: Hyponatremia: Age-related risk factors and therapy decisions. Geriatrics 1998;53:32. [PMID: 9672496]

Palevsky PM: Hypernatremia. Semin Nephrol 1998;18:20. [PMID: 9459286]

Terzian C, Frye EB, Piotrowski ZH: Admission hyponatremia in the elderly: Factors influencing prognosis. J Gen Intern Med 1994;9:89. [PMID: 8164083]

Glucocorticoids and Stress

Greendale GA et al: The relation between cortisol excretion and fractures in healthy older people: Results from the MacArthur Studies–Mac. J Am Geriatr Soc 1999;47:799. [PMID: 10404922]

Greenspan SL et al: The pituitary-adrenal glucocorticoid response is altered by gender and disease. J Gerontol 1993;48:M72. [PMID: 8387077]

Pavlov EP et al: Responses of plasma adrenocorticotropin, cortisol and dehydro-epiandrosterone to ovine corticotropin-releasing hormone in healthy aging men. J Clin Endocrinol Metab 1986;62:767. [PMID: 3005357]

Sherman B, Wysham C, Pfohl B: Age-related changes in the circadian rhythm of plasma cortisol in man. J Clin Endocrinol Metab 1985;61:439. [PMID: 4019712]

van Cauter E, Leproult R, Kupfer DJ: Effects of gender and age on the levels and circadian rhythmicity of plasma cortisol. J Clin Endocrinol Metab 1996;81:2468. [PMID: 8675562]

Reproductive Function in Men

Abbasi AA et al: Low circulating levels of insulin-like growth factors and testosterone in chronically institutionalized elderly men. J Am Geriatr Soc 1993;41:975. [PMID: 8409184]

Arlt W et al: Dehydroepiandrosterone supplementation in healthy men with an age-related decline of dehydroepiandrosterone secretion. J Clin Endocrinol Metab 2001;86:4686. [PMID: 11600526]

Bortz WM 2nd, Wallace DH, Wiley D: Sexual function in 1,202 aging males: differentiating aspects. J Gerontol A Biol Sci Med Sci 1999;54:M237. [PMID: 10362006]

DuBeau CE, Mesnick NM: Controversies in the diagnosis and management of benign prostatic hyperplasia. Adv Intern Med 1992;37:55. [PMID: 1373030]

Gormley GJ et al: Effect of finasteride on prostate-specific antigen density. Urology 1994;43:53. [PMID: 7506854]

Harman SM et al: Longitudinal effects of aging on serum total and free testosterone levels in healthy men. J Clin Endocrinol Metab 2001;86:724. [PMID: 11158037]

Harman SM et al: Reproductive hormones in aging men. 2. Basal pituitary gonadotropins and gonadotropin responses to luteinizing hormone-releasing hormone. J Clin Endocrinol Metab 1982;54:547. [PMID: 6799540]

Korenman SG, Morley JE, Morradian AD: Secondary hypogonadism in older men: its relationship to impotence. J Clin Endocrinol Metab 1990;71:963. [PMID: 2205629]

Lepor H et al: The efficacy of terazosin, finasteride, or both in benign prostatic hyperplasia. N Engl J Med 1996;335:533. [PMID: 8684407]

McConnell JD et al: The effect of finasteride on the risk of acute urinary retention and the need for surgical treatment among men with benign prostatic hyperplasia. N Engl J Med 1998; 338:557. [PMID: 9475762]

Tsitouras PD, Martin CE, Harman SM: Relationship of serum testosterone to sexual activity in healthy elderly men. J Gerontol 1982;37:288. [PMID: 7069152]

van den Beld AW et al: Luteinizing hormone and different genetic variants, as indicators of frailty in healthy elderly men. J Clin Endocrinol Metab 1999;84:1334. [PMID: 10199775]

Endocrine Emergencies

David G. Gardner, MD, & Francis S. Greenspan, MD

ACTH	Adrenocorticotropic hormone	PTH	Parathyroid hormone
ADH	Antidiuretic hormone (vasopressin)	PTHrP	Parathyroid hormone-related
ARDS	Adult respiratory distress syndrome		protein
DIDMOAD	Diabetes insipidus, diabetes	SIADH	Syndrome of inappropriate antidi-
	mellitus, opticatrophy deafness		uretic hormone secretion
GFR	Glomerular filtration rate	TSH	Thyroid stimulating hormone

Acute or chronic failure of an endocrine gland can occasionally result in catastrophic illness and even death. Thus, it is important to recognize and appropriately manage these endocrine emergencies. In this chapter we shall discuss crises involving the thyroid, anterior pituitary or adrenal glands; diabetes mellitus, and abnormalities in calcium, sodium, and water balance.

MYXEDEMA COMA

Clinical Setting

Myxedema coma is the end stage of untreated or inadequately treated hypothyroidism. The clinical picture is often that of an elderly obese female who has become increasingly withdrawn, lethargic, sleepy, and confused and then slips into a comatose state. The history from the patient may be inadequate, but the family may report that the patient had thyroid surgery or radioiodine in the past or that she has previously been receiving thyroid hormone therapy. Coma may be precipitated by an illness such a cerebrovascular accident, myocardial infarction, or an infection such as a urinary tract infection or pneumonia. Other precipitating factors include gastrointestinal hemorrhage, acute trauma, excessive hydration, or administration of a sedative, narcotic, or potent diuretic drug. However, myxedema coma is most frequently associated with discontinuation of thyroid hormone therapy by the patient.

Diagnosis

The physical findings are not very specific. The patient may be semicomatose or comatose with dry, coarse skin, hoarse voice, thin head and eyebrow hair, possibly a scar on the neck, and slow reflex relaxation time. There is marked hypothermia, with body temperature sometimes falling to as low as 24 °C (75 °F). It is important to look for complicating factors such as pneumonia, urinary tract infection, ileus, anemia, hypoglycemia, or seizures. Often there are pericardial, pleural, or peritoneal effusions. The key laboratory tests are a low free thyroxine (FT_4) and elevated TSH. Note that in an emergency situation, serum TSH can be done in 1 hour. If the FT_4 is low and the TSH is low-normal, consider central or pituitary hypothyroidism. Pituitary insufficiency can be confirmed with a low serum cortisol, impaired response to the cosyntropin stimulation test, and low FSH and LH. It is essential to check blood gasses, electrolytes, creatinine and an electrocardiogram, in evaluating pulmonary, renal, cardiac and central nervous system status. It may be necessary to differentiate myxedema coma from the "euthyroid sick" syndrome associated with coma due to other causes. These patients may present with a low T_3, normal or low TSH, but the free T_4 (by dialysis) is normal.

Myxedema coma is a complex problem involving a number or organ systems. The pathogenesis is presented in Figure 24–1. The decrease in serum T_4 results in a lowering of intracellular T_3. This can directly affect central nervous system function with altered mental status. The decrease in intracellular T_3 causes decreased thermogenesis, resulting in hypothermia, which in turn causes decreased central nervous system sensitivity to hypercapnia and hypoxia. The resulting respiratory insufficiency induces cerebral anoxia and coma. At the same time the decreased intracellular T_3 results in de-

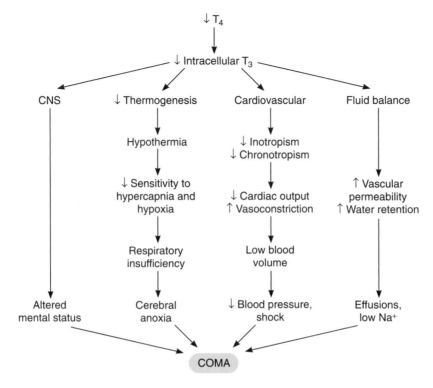

Figure 24–1. Pathogenesis of myxedema coma. (See text for details.)

creased cardiac inotropism and chronotropism, decreased sensitivity to adrenergic stimuli, decreased cardiac output, and generalized vasoconstriction. This results in a low-output state which, if untreated, culminates in hypovolemia, decreased blood pressure, and eventually shock and death. Finally, there is a change in fluid balance with increased water retention due to impaired renal perfusion as well as increased vascular permeability. These changes result in effusions and hyponatremia which in turn contribute to the coma.

Management

Management of myxedema coma involves much more than simply replacing T_4 (Table 24–1). The patient is severely ill and usually is admitted to the ICU for intubation and ventilatory support. Oral medications are poorly absorbed (due to ileus), and all medications should be given intravenously. A loading dose of 300–400 μg of T_4 intravenously is given initially to saturate T_4 binding sites in plasma binding proteins. The patient is then maintained on 50 μg of T_4 intravenously daily. In addition, small doses of T_3 (eg, 10 μg intravenously every 8 hours) may be given over the first 48 hours, but this is usually not necessary. Water re-

striction is necessary to correct the hyponatremia, and intravenous glucose will counteract the tendency to hypoglycemia. It is essential to treat precipitating disease, eg, pneumonia or urinary tract infection. The routine use of hydrocortisone is controversial, but it is necessary in patients with hypopituitarism or multiple endocrine gland failure. If the initial serum cortisol is more than

Table 24–1. Management of myxedema coma.

---

(1) Admit to ICU for ventilatory support and for intravenous medications.

(2) Parenteral thyroxine: Give a loading dose of 300–400 μg IV, then 50 μg IV daily. (May also give liothyronine sodium, 10 μg IV every 8 hours for the first 48 hours.)

(3) Electrolytes: Water restriction for hyponatremia. Avoid fluid overload.

(4) Limit sedation. Appropriate reduction in drug dosage.

(5) Glucocorticoids: Controversial but necessary in hypopituitarism or multiple endocrine failure. Dosage: Hydrocortisone sodium phosphate or sodium succinate, 40–100 mg every 6 hours initially and taper downward over 1 week. (If initial serum cortisol was > 30 μg/dL, corticosteroids are unnecessary.)

---

30 µg/dL, steroid support is probably unnecessary. However, if serum cortisol is less than 30 µg/dL, cortisol should be given intravenously in a dosage of 50–100 mg every 6 hours for the first 48 hours and the dose then tapered over the next week while the pituitary-adrenal axis undergoes formal testing.

Prior to the recognition of the need for intravenous T_4 and for respiratory support, the mortality from myxedema coma was about 80%. Currently, the mortality is about 20% and is mostly due to the underlying or precipitating illness.

THYROID STORM

Clinical Setting

Thyroid storm, or thyrotoxic crisis, is an acute life-threatening exacerbation of thyrotoxicosis. It may occur in a patient with a history of Graves' disease who has discontinued antithyroid medication or in a patient with previously undiagnosed hyperthyroidism. The clinical picture is that of an acute onset of hyperpyrexia (with temperature over 40 °C [104 °F]), sweating, marked tachycardia often with atrial fibrillation, nausea, vomiting, diarrhea, agitation, tremulousness, and delirium. Occasionally, the presentation will be "apathetic" without the restlessness and agitation but with symptoms of weakness, confusion, cardiovascular dysfunction, gastrointestinal upset, and hyperpyrexia. Some of the factors that may precipitate thyroid storm are listed in Table 24–2.

Diagnosis

The diagnosis is largely based in the clinical findings. Serum T_4, free T_4, T_3, and free T_3 are all elevated, and TSH is suppressed. These findings are not different from what is seen in other patients with hyperthy-

roidism, but the difference is in the setting. It is thought that the pathogenesis of thyroid storm is an exacerbation of thyrotoxicosis due to decreased binding of T_4 (associated with saturation of binding sites on thyroxine-binding proteins) with an increase in free T_3 and T_4, as well as an exaggerated response to a surge of catecholamines that results from the stress of the precipitating event. The cause of death is usually cardiac arrhythmia and failure.

Management

The management of thyroid storm is summarized in Table 24–3. Initially it is important to block further synthesis and secretion of thyroid hormone, first with antithyroid drugs and then with iodide. One may give propylthiouracil, 150 mg every 6 hours orally or per rectum, or methimazole, 20 mg every 8 hours orally or per rectum. A few hours after initiation of antithyroid drug therapy, iodides may be started. Traditionally, saturated solution of potassium iodide, 5 drops twice daily, has been used, but currently iopanoic acid in a dose of 0.5 g twice daily orally or intravenously or iohexol 0.6 g (2 mL of Omnipaque 300) intravenously twice daily is the treatment of choice. These drugs will not only inhibit thyroid hormone synthesis but also block the conversion of T_4 to T_3, lowering the thyroid hormone level in the blood. Additional specific therapy includes β-adrenergic blockade with propranolol, 40–80 mg orally every 6 hours or 0.5–1 mg intravenously every 3 hours, monitoring its effect on cardiac rate. In patients with asthma or heart failure, propra-

Table 24–2. Thyroid storm—precipitating factors.

Withdrawal of antithyroid drugs
Severe infection
Diabetic ketoacidosis
Myocardial infarction
Cerebrovascular accident
Cardiac failure
Surgery
Parturition
Trauma (eg, hip fracture)
Radioiodine (rare)
Drug reaction
Iodinated contrast medium

Table 24–3. Management of thyroid storm.

Supportive care
Fluids
Oxygen
Cooling blanket
Acetaminophen
Phenobarbital
Multivitamins
If indicated: antibiotics, digoxin
Specific measures
Propranolol, 40–80 mg orally every 6 hours
Propylthiouracil, 150 mg every 6 hours, or methimazole, 20 mg every 6 hours. May be administered per rectum if oral route is unavailable.
Saturated solution of potassium iodide, 5 drops (250 mg) orally twice daily; or iopanoic acid, 0.5 g IV or orally twice daily; or iohexol, 0.6 g (2 mL of Omnipaque 300) IV twice daily
Dexamethasone, 2 mg every 6 hours
Cholestyramine or colestipol, 20–30 g/d

nolol may be contraindicated, but calcium channel blockade with diltiazem may be very helpful. The half-life of glucocorticoids is markedly reduced in severe thyrotoxicosis, so that adrenal support may be very useful. For this purpose, dexamethasone is given in a dosage of 2 mg every 6 hours for 48 hours, followed by tapering of the dose. Finally, cholestyramine or colestipol will bind T_4 in the gut during its enterohepatic circulation and may help to bring the circulating level of T_4 down more quickly. Supportive therapy includes adequate fluids, oxygen, digoxin for atrial fibrillation or heart failure, parenteral water-soluble vitamins, and a cooling blanket and acetaminophen for hyperpyrexia. Aspirin should be avoided since it will displace T_4 from TBG, resulting in an increase in FT_4. Phenobarbital may be a useful sedative since it stimulates T_4 metabolism via the hepatic microsomal enzyme system. Plasmapheresis or dialysis to remove FT_4 has been reported to be useful in nonresponders, but this is rarely necessary.

Therapy for thyroid storm has improved markedly, so that the mortality has dropped from 100% in the 1920s to about 20–30% in recent series. However, since storm is often associated with other underlying medical problems, it still represents a serious medical complication.

THYROTOXIC PERIODIC PARALYSIS

Clinical Setting

Thyrotoxic periodic paralysis is a rare but frightening thyroid emergency. The usually clinical presentation is of an Asian male with symptoms of untreated hyperthyroidism who awakens at night or in the morning with flaccid paralysis of the lower limbs. Further history reveals that he exercised vigorously or had a large high-carbohydrate meal before retiring. There is no family history of periodic paralysis, but there may be a family history of autoimmune thyroid disease. The paralysis usually involves the lower portion of the body but may involve the arms also. Facial or respiratory muscles are rarely involved. The acute episode may be complicated by extensive paralysis and arrhythmias due to the hypokalemia. The illness has also been reported to occur in Native Americans and patients of Mexican or South American descent.

Diagnosis

The diagnosis is based on the absence of a family history of periodic paralysis, the characteristic presentation, the presence of hyperthyroidism due either to Graves' disease or toxic nodular goiter, and usually a low serum potassium level.

The pathogenesis is summarized in Figure 24–2. Thyrotoxicosis, increased β-adrenergic activity, and an assumed genetic predisposition result in increased Na^+-K^+ ATPase activity with increased intracellular transport of K^+. A high-carbohydrate meal with increased insulin secretion, glycogen deposition, vigorous exercise, a high salt intake, and the normal nocturnal potassium flux then drive serum potassium levels even lower, resulting in flaccid neuromuscular paralysis. Note that there is no loss of total body potassium, merely a shift from extracellular to intracellular space.

Management

The management of this problem is presented in Table 24–4. Supplemental potassium should be given orally in a dose of 2 g potassium chloride every 2 hours while monitoring serum K^+. Propranolol in doses of 60 mg every 6 hours will block the β-adrenergic stimulation of Na^+-K^+ ATPase. Antithyroid drug therapy should be started immediately even though it will take time to bring the patient into a euthyroid state. It is particularly important to avoid intravenous potassium, which may

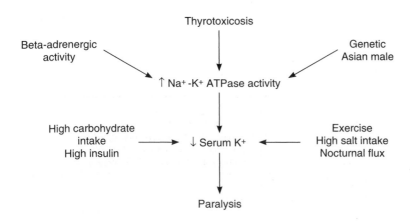

Figure 24–2. Pathogenesis of thyrotoxic periodic paralysis. (See text for details.)

Table 24–4. Management of thyrotoxic periodic paralysis.

---

(1) Oral potassium supplement (potassium chloride, 2 g every 2 hours); monitor serum K+
(2) Large doses of oral propranolol (60 mg every 6 hours)
(3) Antithyroid drug therapy

Avoid:
  IV potassium
  IV glucose
  β-Adrenergic agonists (eg, isoproterenol)

---

raise total body potassium to toxic levels; intravenous glucose, which will stimulate more insulin secretion and hypokalemia; and β-adrenergic agonists such as isoproterenol, which will promote movement of K+ into the intracellular compartment and exacerbate the problem. With appropriate treatment, the recovery is rapid, and once the thyrotoxicosis is controlled the paralysis will not recur.

AMIODARONE INDUCED THYROTOXICOSIS

Clinical Setting

Amiodarone is a benzofuran derivative that is widely used in the treatment of cardiac arrhythmias. It contains two atoms of iodine per molecule, which represents 37.5% iodine by weight. The compound is stored in adipose tissue and has a half-life in the body of 2–3 months, with gradual and continuous release of iodide. The usual daily maintenance dose of amiodarone of 200–400 mg/d will release 6,000–12,000 μg of iodine daily, which when compared to the normal daily requirement of about 150 μg of iodide represents an enormous iodide load.

The structure of amiodarone resembles that of T_3, and it is thought that part of the cardiac depressant effect of amiodarone may be due to binding to and blocking the T_3 receptor in cardiac muscle. However, the effect of amiodarone on the thyroid gland is different and is due in part to a direct effect of iodine on the thyroid cell—to inhibit or stimulate hormone synthesis—and a cytotoxic effect of amiodarone on the follicular cell—inducing destruction of the cell and release of stored hormone. Thus, the drug may induce hypothyroidism, which is easily managed by thyroxine replacement, or hyperthyroidism, which, because of the underlying heart disease, is much more difficult to manage and represents a true thyroid emergency. Two mechanisms have been suggested to explain the development of hyperthyroidism: (1) The high iodine level in a multinodular gland, or in the gland of a patient with la-

tent Graves' disease, or even in a previously normal gland, can induce hyperthyroidism if the gland fails to develop the Wolff-Chaikoff block. This is the jodbasedow effect (see Chapter 7). (2) The toxic effect of amiodarone itself may cause acute and chronic thyroiditis with release of T_4 and T_3 into the circulation and severe thyrotoxicosis.

The patient with amiodarone-induced thyrotoxicosis may have been on the drug for months or years. The underlying heart disease gradually worsens with increasingly frequent episodes of arrhythmia and heart failure. At the same time there may be weight loss, heat intolerance, increased nervousness, and marked muscle weakness. On physical examination, one may find nontender nodular or diffuse thyroid enlargement, tachycardia with or without atrial fibrillation, tremor, hyperreflexia, and, occasionally, lid lag and stare. Laboratory findings are unique because amiodarone inhibits the conversion of T_4 to T_3. Thus, even in the euthyroid patient taking amiodarone, total T_4 may be elevated while FT_4 and TSH will be normal. In the hyperthyroid patient, the FT_4 will be markedly elevated and TSH will be less than 0.03 mU/L. Radioiodine uptake in the iodide-loaded patient will be low. It has been difficult to distinguish thyrotoxicosis due to follicular cell hyperfunction from that due to follicular cell destruction. Thyroid ultrasound with color Doppler studies may show increased circulation with hyperfunction and decreased blood flow with thyroiditis. Also, the cytokine IL-6 is low in patients with hyperfunction, whereas it is markedly elevated in patients with thyroiditis.

Management

Management of amiodarone-induced hyperthyroidism is difficult (Table 24–5). Ideally, amiodarone should be discontinued, but often it cannot be stopped because of the underlying heart disease, and even if it is discontinued the iodine load will persist for several months. Further synthesis of T_4 should be blocked with methima-

Table 24–5. Management of amiodarone-induced hyperthyroidism.

---

(1) Stop amiodarone if possible
(2) Institute β-blocker therapy if possible
(3) Antithyroid drugs: Tapazole, 40–60 mg/d
(4) Potassium perchlorate, 200 mg every 6 hours
(5) Cholestyramine or colestipol, 20–30 g/d
(6) Prednisone, 40 mg/d, for acute thyroiditis. (?Monitor IL-6 levels.)
(7) Thyroidectomy

---

zole in a dosage of 40–60 mg/d. Beta-adrenergic blockade should be instituted with propranolol or a similar drug if cardiac status will permit it. Potassium perchlorate in a dosage of 250 mg every 6 hours will block further iodine uptake and lower intrathyroidal iodide content. Aplastic anemia has occurred in patients on high-dose or long-term potassium perchlorate therapy, so that use of this medication has usually been limited to 1 month. Cholestyramine or colestipol in a dosage of 20–30 g/d will bind T_4 and T_3 in the gut and bring blood levels down more quickly. If there is reason to suspect thyroiditis (elevated serum IL-6, or decreased blood flow on ultrasound), corticosteroid therapy will often yield dramatic results. Prednisone is given in a dosage of 40 mg/d for 1 month, gradually tapering the dose over the following 2 months. If medical therapy is unable to control the disease, thyroidectomy effects a permanent cure and may be used as a last resort.

ACUTE ADRENAL INSUFFICIENCY

Clinical Setting

Acute adrenal insufficiency usually occurs as an acute illness in a patient with chronic adrenal insufficiency. The chronic adrenal insufficiency may be primary, due to destruction of the adrenal glands associated with autoimmune adrenalitis or, rarely, tuberculosis or metastatic malignancy. Chronic adrenal insufficiency may also be secondary to pituitary or hypothalamic disease. However, acute adrenal insufficiency may occur with bilateral adrenal hemorrhage in a previously healthy individual during the course of septicemia with diffuse intravascular coagulopathy or in a patient receiving anticoagulant therapy. In the patient with known adrenal insufficiency, an acute crisis may be precipitated by inadvertent omission of medication or by the concurrent development of a precipitating illness such as severe infection, acute myocardial infarction, cerebrovascular hemorrhage or infarction, surgery without adrenal support, or severe acute trauma. Acute adrenal insufficiency may also be precipitated by the sudden withdrawal of steroid therapy in a patient previously on long-term steroid therapy with associated adrenal atrophy (ie, secondary adrenal insufficiency). Finally, administration of drugs impairing adrenal hormone synthesis such as ketoconazole or mitotane—or drugs increasing steroid metabolism such as phenytoin or rifampin—may precipitate an adrenal crisis.

The patient presents with an acute onset of nausea, vomiting, hyperpyrexia, abdominal pain, dehydration, hypotension and shock. A clue to the diagnosis of primary adrenal insufficiency is the presence of pigmentation in unexposed areas of the skin, particularly in the creases of the palms and in the buccal mucosa. The differential diagnosis includes consideration of other causes of cardiovascular collapse, sepsis and intra-abdominal abscess. Failure of the hypotension to respond to pressors is suggestive of adrenal insufficiency and is an indication for a trial of glucocorticoid therapy.

Diagnosis

Primary adrenal insufficiency is characterized by hyponatremia and hyperkalemia. However, in situations of adrenal crisis, the hyponatremia may be obscured by dehydration. Random serum cortisol determinations are not helpful unless the levels are very low (< 5 µg/dL [138 nmol/L]) during a period of great stress. The key diagnostic test is failure of serum cortisol to rise above 20 µg/dL (552 nmol/L) 30 minutes after intravenous injection of 0.25 mg synthetic ACTH (cosyntropin) (see Chapter 9 for details). Basal serum ACTH will be elevated (> 52 pg/mL [> 11 pmol/L]) in patients with primary adrenal insufficiency but not in patients with secondary adrenal insufficiency due to pituitary or hypothalamic disease. CT scan or sonogram of the abdomen will reveal adrenal enlargement in patients with adrenal hemorrhage, active tuberculosis, or metastatic malignancy.

Management

The management of adrenal crisis is outlined in Table 24–6. Hydrocortisone should be administered in a dosage of 100 mg intravenously followed by 50 mg every 4 hours thereafter. Fluids and Na^+ should be replaced with several liters of 5% glucose in normal saline. After the first 24 hours, the dose of intravenous hydrocortisone can be slowly reduced, but intravenous doses should be given at least every 6 hours because of the short half-life (1 hour) of hydrocortisone in the circulation. When the patient can tolerate oral feedings,

Table 24–6. Management of adrenal crisis.

(1) Hydrocortisone sodium phosphate or sodium succinate, 100 mg IV stat and then 50 mg IV every 4 hours for 24 hours. Then taper slowly downward over the next 72 hours, giving the drug every 4–6 hours IV. When patient is tolerating oral feedings, shift to oral replacement therapy, overlapping the first oral and last intravenous doses.

(2) Replace salt and fluid losses with several liters of 5% glucose in normal saline IV.

(3) Patients with primary adrenal insufficiency may require mineralocorticoid (fludrocortisone) when shifted to oral hydrocortisone maintenance therapy.

(4) Diagnose and treat the illness that precipitated the acute crisis.

hydrocortisone can be given orally, but the first oral dose should overlap the last intravenous dose. Alternatively, hydrocortisone can be administered as a continuous infusion at the rate of 10 mg/h for the first 24 hours, followed by a gradual decrease in the dose. Mineralocorticoid is not necessary during the acute replacement period since enough salt and glucocorticoid are being administered to accommodate the mineralocorticoid deficiency. However, in patients with chronic primary adrenal insufficiency, mineralocorticoid supplementation is necessary when shifting to an oral maintenance program (see Chapter 9). After steroid therapy has been instituted, it is extremely important to evaluate and treat the illness that may have precipitated the acute crisis—infection, myocardial infarction, etc.

Prevention of acute adrenal insufficiency in patients with chronic adrenal insufficiency exposed to stress (eg, severe infection) can be achieved using intravenous hydrocortisone in dosages as outlined above or by administration of dexamethasone sodium phosphate, 4 mg intramuscularly every 24 hours for two doses. Dexamethasone would replace glucocorticoids but not mineralocorticoid and would not be adequate in the presence of severe dehydration and hyponatremia.

PITUITARY APOPLEXY

Pituitary apoplexy is a rare but frightening syndrome of violent headache, visual and cranial nerve disturbances, and mental confusion, resulting from hemorrhage or infarction of the pituitary gland.

Clinical Setting

Pituitary apoplexy usually occurs as a sudden crisis in a patient with a known or previously unrecognized pituitary tumor. However, it may occur in a normal gland during or after parturition or associated with head trauma or anticoagulation therapy. The patient presents with severe headache and visual disturbances, often a bitemporal hemianopia due to compression of the optic chiasm. There may be oculomotor defects, either bilateral or unilateral. Often there are meningeal symptoms with stiff neck and mental confusion, so that the differential diagnosis includes subarachnoid hemorrhage, meningitis, or brain tumor. Finally there may be symptoms of acute secondary adrenal insufficiency with nausea, vomiting, hypotension, and collapse.

Diagnosis

The neurologic problem is best approached with a CT scan of the head, including the anterior pituitary gland. Pituitary enlargement and signs of hemorrhage are diagnostic. Hormonal studies are of academic interest only since therapy would include glucocorticoid support regardless of the acute findings. After appropriate acute therapy, evaluation of anterior and posterior pituitary function may be indicated because of the possibility of permanent pituitary destruction.

Management

Management involves both hormonal and neurosurgical therapy. High-dose dexamethasone, 4 mg twice daily, will provide both glucocorticoid support and relief of cerebral edema. Transsphenoidal pituitary decompression will provide dramatic relief and often preserves some normal pituitary function. After the acute episode has subsided, the patient must be evaluated for the possibility of multiple pituitary deficiencies (see Chapter 5).

DIABETIC KETOACIDOSIS

Clinical Setting

Diabetic ketoacidosis occurs in a setting of absolute or relative insulin deficiency. Specific clinical settings should generate a high index of suspicion for the disorder. Interruptions of normal insulin delivery due to purposeful reduction in insulin dosage or interference with the delivery system (eg, kinking in pump tubing) are frequent precipitating events, as are reduced insulin sensitivity in the setting of systemic infection, myocardial infarction, burns, trauma, or pregnancy. In a significant percentage of patients, diabetic ketoacidosis is the presenting feature of diabetes. In these instances, clinical suspicion and accurate interpretation of the initial laboratory studies will usually lead to the correct diagnosis.

Diagnosis

Diabetic ketoacidosis is characterized metabolically by two prominent features: hyperglycemia and ketoacidosis (see Chapter 17). Patients with diabetic ketoacidosis present with evidence of volume contraction (eg, dry mucous membranes, thirst, orthostatic hypotension) and labored breathing (Kussmaul respiration) related to the underlying acidosis. The breath often has a fruity odor, reflecting the presence of acetone. Patients may have abdominal pain mimicking an acute abdomen, nausea, and vomiting. The latter symptoms may be related to elevated prostaglandins that accrue in the presence of insulin deficiency. Presentation may be dominated by symptoms of the precipitating illness (eg, urinary tract infection, pneumonia, or myocardial infarction).

Plasma glucose levels are elevated, usually to over 250 mg/dL. This reflects impairment in glucose utilization (see above), increased gluconeogenesis and glycogenolysis, and reduced renal clearance of glucose in the setting of decreased glomerular filtration rate (GFR). Osmotic diuresis related to glucose filtration results in reduction in intravascular volume and depletion of total body water, sodium, potassium, phosphate, and magnesium. In general, the relative depletion of water is roughly twice that of the solutes it contains. Hypertonicity in the extracellular fluid compartment, while typically not as severe as that seen in hyperosmotic nonketotic coma (see below), can be significant. Calculated plasma osmolalities greater than 340 mosm/kg are associated with coma. Plasma osmolality—rather than acidemia—correlates most closely with mortality in diabetic ketoacidosis (Figure 24–3).

Arterial blood pH is low and, in the absence of coexistent respiratory disease, is partially compensated by a reduction in PCO_2. The acidosis is metabolic in origin and accompanied by an anion gap which is calculated by subtracting the combined concentrations of chloride and bicarbonate from serum sodium concentration.

Anion gaps greater than 12 mEq/L are considered abnormal. Keto acids account for most of the unmeasured anions that generate the abnormal gap, though under conditions of extreme volume contraction and hypoperfusion lactate accumulation may also contribute. Levels of serum and urinary ketones (measured using the nitroprusside reagent) are typically high in diabetic ketoacidosis. It should be recalled, however, that this reagent reacts strongly only with acetoacetate, less strongly with acetone (which is not a keto acid and does not contribute to the anion gap), and not at all with β-hydroxybutyrate. Thus, paradoxically, the most extreme levels of ketoacidosis may be accompanied by relatively modest levels of ketones measured by this method. As a corollary of this, resolution of severe diabetic ketoacidosis may be linked to transient increases in measurable ketone levels as β-hydroxybutyrate is converted to the more readily detectable acetoacetate.

Serum sodium levels may be high, normal, or low, but in all instances total body sodium is depressed. Esti-

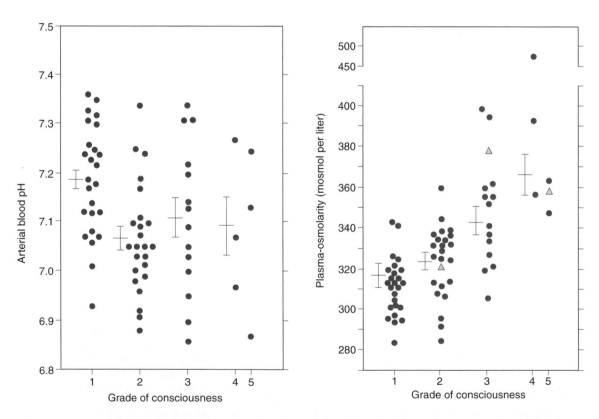

Figure 24–3. **A:** Relationship between state of consciousness and blood pH in patients with diabetic ketoacidosis. **B:** Relationship between state of consciousness and plasma osmolality in diabetic ketoacidosis. Note that the state of consciousness correlates with plasma osmolality rather than blood pH. (Reproduced, with permission, from Fulop M et al: Ketotic hyperosmolar coma. Lancet 1973;2:635.)

mates of depletion range from 7 mEq to 10 mEq/kg body weight. As blood glucose levels rise in diabetic ketoacidosis, they create an osmotic gradient that draws water, as well as intracellular solutes, into the extracellular space. This results in moderate hyponatremia, which can be corrected to account for the dilutional effect of the transmembrane flux of water by adding 1.6 mEq/L to the sodium concentration for every 100 mg/dL increment in plasma glucose above a basal concentration of 100 mg/dL (see below). The decrease in serum sodium partially offsets the increase in tonicity that accompanies the elevation in serum glucose. This results in a net increase in plasma osmolality of 2 mosm/kg H_2O per 100 mg/dL elevation in serum glucose.

$$\text{Corrected Na}^+ = \text{Measured Na}^+ + 1.6\left(\frac{\text{Plasma glucose} - 100}{100}\right)$$

Total body potassium levels are also severely depleted in diabetic ketoacidosis to an average of 5–7 mEq/kg body weight. This results from a number of factors, including exchange of intracellular potassium for extracellular hydrogen ion, impaired movement of K^+ into cells in the insulinopenic state, and increased urinary potassium excretion secondary to the osmotic diuresis and, in those instances where intravascular volume contraction is present, secondary hyperaldosteronism. Serum potassium levels may be high, normal, or low depending on the severity and duration of diabetic ketoacidosis, the status of extracellular fluid volume, and the adequacy of renal perfusion and excretory function. A low serum potassium at presentation generally indicates severe potassium deficiency and, in the presence of adequate renal function, is an indication for early and aggressive repletion (see below). Potassium depletion can result in muscle weakness and cardiac arrhythmias, including ventricular fibrillation.

The H^+ excess in diabetic ketoacidosis titrates endogenous buffer systems including serum bicarbonate, resulting in reduction in concentrations of the latter. Chloride levels may also be low, reflecting the osmotic diuresis alluded to above. Ketone bodies have been estimated to account for one-third to one-half of the osmotic diuresis seen in diabetic ketoacidosis. Electrolyte depletion is further aggravated by the obligate cation (eg, sodium) excretion required to maintain electrical neutrality. In patients who have maintained adequate hydration during the development of diabetic ketoacidosis or in those who are aggressively resuscitated with normal saline, chloride levels may be elevated and the anion gap narrowed. This reflects the enhanced clearance of the keto anions in the kidney, converting the system from an anion gap acidosis

to a hyperchloremic, nongap acidosis (ie, the hydrogen ion excess persists despite clearance of the anion). Since the excreted keto anions represent a lost source for bicarbonate regeneration, correction of the hyperchloremic acidosis may proceed slowly.

Total body magnesium and phosphate levels are also depleted by the osmotic diuresis in diabetic ketoacidosis. Phosphate depletion is amplified by diffusion of the anion from the intracellular to the extracellular compartment in the absence of insulin. Phosphate depletion can result in muscle weakness, rhabdomyolysis, hemolytic anemia, respiratory distress, and altered tissue oxygenation (due to reduction in 2,3-diphosphoglycerate levels in the red blood cell).

Management

Treatment of diabetic ketoacidosis is focused on two major objectives. The first is restoration of normal tonicity, intravascular volume, and solute homeostasis. The second is correction of the insulinopenic state with suppression of counterregulatory hormone secretion, glucose production, and ketogenesis and improved utilization of glucose in target tissues. The flow outline in Table 24–7 provides a general approach to the management of this disorder.

Because depletion of intracellular and extracellular fluids may be severe in diabetic ketoacidosis (typically in the range of 5–10 L), early and aggressive resuscitation with fluids is mandatory. This is usually initiated with administration of 1–2 L of isotonic normal saline (0.9% NaCl) over the first hour of therapy. As intravascular volume is restored, renal perfusion will increase, with a consequent increase in renal clearance of glucose and a fall in plasma glucose levels. If volume contraction is severe, a second liter of normal saline can be administered. If not, half-normal saline (0.45% NaCl) can be initiated at a rate of 250–500 mL/h depending on intravascular volume status. Since water is typically lost in excess of solute in diabetic ketoacidosis, half-normal saline will address both volume depletion and the hypertonicity. It has been suggested that approximately half of the total fluid deficit should be corrected within the first 5 hours of therapy. Half-normal saline can be continued until intravascular volume has been restored or plasma glucose levels fall to 250 mg/dL, at which point D_5W should be started. The latter maneuver reduces the likelihood of insulin-induced hypoglycemia and avoids the theoretical complication of cerebral edema due to osmotically induced fluid shifts from plasma into the central nervous system. This complication is, in fact, seen rarely in adults and uncommonly in children with diabetic ketoacidosis.

Once fluid resuscitation has been initiated, insulin should be administered. Only short-acting (ie, regular)

Table 24–7. Management of diabetic ketoacidosis.

Fluid administration

1. One to liters of normal saline over the first hour. Repeat if clinically significant volume contraction persists after the first hour.
2. Change to half-normal saline, 500–1000 mL/h, depending on volume status. Continue for about 4 hours. Decrease rate to 250 mL/h as intravascular volume returns to normal.
3. Convert fluids to D_5W when plasma glucose falls to 250 mg/dL.

Insulin

1. Administer 10–20 units of regular insulin IV.
2. Mix 50 units of regular insulin in 500 mL of normal saline (1 U/10 mL). Discard first 50 mL of infusion to accommodate insulin binding to tubing. Administer through "piggyback" line along with parenteral fluids at a rate of 0.1 unit/kg/h.
3. Double the infusion rate after 2 hours if there is no improvement in plasma glucose levels.

Potassium

1. Administer supplemental potassium chloride once renal function is established; provide 20 mEq/L of fluids for patients who are initially normokalemic, 40 mEq/L for those who are hypokalemic at presentation.
2. Gauge subsequent replacement based on serum K^+ measurements at 2-hour intervals.

Bicarbonate

1. Sodium bicarbonate only for patients with blood pH less than 7.0.
2. Add one ampule of sodium bicarbonate (44 mEq) to 500 mL of D_5W or half-normal saline. Administer over 1 hour.

insulins should be used. While a number of different insulin regimens have demonstrated efficacy in the treatment of diabetic ketoacidosis, a commonly used regimen includes a loading dose (10–20 units) of regular insulin intravenously followed by a continuous infusion at a rate of 0.1 unit/kg/h. This regimen provides plasma insulin levels in a physiologic range (100–150 mU/mL) with minimal risk of hypoglycemia or hypokalemia. It restores plasma glucose levels at rates equivalent to those obtained with regimens using higher insulin doses. Plasma glucose levels should fall at a rate of 50–100 mg/dL/h. Failure to achieve this end point over a 2-hour period should lead to doubling of the infusion rate with reevaluation an hour later. When plasma glucose concentrations reach 250 mg/dL, D_5W is begun to prevent hypoglycemia (see above). The insulin infusion is continued to suppress ketogenesis and allow restoration of normal acid-base balance.

As noted above, total body potassium stores are depleted in diabetic ketoacidosis and plasma K^+ levels fall with treatment. Repletion of K^+ is almost always indicated in management of diabetic ketoacidosis (one notable exception being diabetic ketoacidosis that occurs in the setting of chronic renal insufficiency); however, the timing of repletion varies as a function of the plasma K^+ level. If the initial K^+ level is less than 4 mEq/L, K^+ depletion is severe and repletion should begin with the first administration of parenteral fluids if renal function is adequate. Twenty milliequivalents of potassium chloride can be added to the first liter of normal saline if the serum K^+ is in the 3.5–4 mEq/L range; 40 mEq should be added for K^+ levels less than 3.5 mEq/L. Particular attention should be devoted to these latter patients, since K^+ levels may plummet to very low levels with initiation of insulin therapy. The general goal of therapy should be to keep the K^+ in a near-normal range. This may require several hundred milliequivalents of potassium chloride administered over several days.

The administration of bicarbonate in the setting of diabetic ketoacidosis has been controversial. Acidosis, in addition to increasing ventilatory work (Kussmaul's respiration), may also suppress cardiac contractile function. Therefore, restoration of normal pH would seem to make sense in the setting of diabetic ketoacidosis. However, there is considerable risk associated with the use of sodium bicarbonate in this setting, including paradoxical acidification of the central nervous system due to the selective diffusion of CO_2 versus HCO_3^- across the blood-brain barrier and an increase in intracellular acidosis, which may worsen rather than ameliorate cardiac function. Volume overload related to the high tonicity (44.6–50 mEq/50 mL) of the bicarbonate solution, hypokalemia resulting from overly rapid correction of the acidosis, hypernatremia, and rebound alkalosis are also potential complications of bicarbonate therapy. In general, pH of 7.0 or greater is not life-threatening to the average patient with diabetic ketoacidosis and will resolve with appropriate volume expansion and insulin therapy. For pH < 7.0, many clinicians would argue for a limited administration of sodium bicarbonate. If bicarbonate is used, careful patient monitoring looking for alterations in mental status or cardiac decompensation is indicated. The goal of therapy should be to maintain pH > 7.0, not to return pH to normal.

Similarly, phosphate administration, once considered a key component in the management of diabetic ketoacidosis, has come under closer scrutiny. Phosphate depletion definitely occurs in diabetic ketoacidosis for the reasons outlined above, and in the past repletion of phosphate (much of it as potassium phosphate salts) has been advocated to forestall the development of muscle weakness and hemolysis and to promote tissue oxygenation through generation of 2,3-diphosphoglycerate in erythrocytes. However, the administration of phosphate salts has been associated with the development of hypocalcemia and deposition of calcium phosphate precipitates in soft tissues, including the vasculature. Thus, in general, parenteral phosphate repletion is not routinely provided for diabetic ketoacidosis patients unless plasma phosphate falls to very low levels (< 1 mmol/L). In this case, 2 mL of a mixture of KH_2PO_4 and K_2HPO_4 solution, containing 3 mmol of elemental phosphorus and 4 mEq of potassium, may be added to 1 L of fluids and introduced over 6–8 hours. In no instance should all K^+ repletion be in the form of potassium phosphate salts. In general, renewal of food ingestion and insulin therapy will complete restoration of total body phosphate stores and return plasma phosphate levels to normal over a period of several days.

Finally, it is necessary to actively seek out and treat the precipitants of diabetic ketoacidosis when they are identified. This includes appropriate cultures of urine and blood (and cerebrospinal fluid, if indicated) and empiric antibiotic therapy directed against the most likely pathogenic organisms (pending the results of the cultures). The presence of fever is typically a good marker for infection or other inflammatory process since it is not a feature of diabetic ketoacidosis per se. Elevated white blood cell counts, on the other hand, are frequently seen with diabetic ketoacidosis alone. Other precipitants should also be looked for. Myocardial infarction, which is often clinically "silent" in diabetic patients, is an uncommon but life-threatening precipitant of diabetic ketoacidosis in patients with established diabetes.

Complications

Aggressive resuscitation with isotonic or hypotonic fluids is a theoretical but uncommon cause of fluid overload during management of diabetic ketoacidosis. Careful attention to the cardiovascular examination, chest x-ray, and urine output should aid in preventing this complication.

Hypoglycemia is relatively rare in the current era given the low doses of insulin used in management and appropriate initiation of glucose-containing fluids as plasma glucose levels fall below 250 mg/dL.

Cerebral edema due to rapid correction of plasma hypertonicity has usually been reported with plasma glucose levels below 250 mg/dL. Clinically significant cerebral edema is relatively uncommon in adult patients. Milder forms of cerebral edema have been noted in many patients being treated for diabetic ketoacidosis but have not been strongly correlated with changes in extracellular tonicity. At present, in a symptomatic adult patient, it would appear prudent to treat hypertonicity exceeding 340 mosm/kg aggressively with hypotonic fluids to avoid complications related to plasma hyperviscosity. Further correction from that point to normal plasma osmolality (about 285 mosm/kg) can probably be accomplished in slower fashion over several days. Cerebral edema occurs in 1–2% of children with diabetic ketoacidosis, frequently with devastating results. Approximately one-third of children with clinically significant cerebral edema will die during the acute illness, and another third will sustain permanent neurologic impairment. Cerebral edema in children may be associated with high initial rates of fluid resuscitation (> 4 $L/m^2/d$) and rapid falls in plasma sodium (or corrected sodium) concentration, though it can occur in clinical settings without an apparent cause. In the absence of definitive trial data to guide therapy, lower rates of fluid administration (< 2.5 $L/m^2/d$) with volume resuscitation spread over a longer time interval would seem appropriate if the clinical situation permits. When signs of cerebral edema appear—deterioration in level of consciousness, focal neurologic signs, hypotension or bradycardia, sudden decline in urine output after an initial period of apparent recovery following treatment for diabetic ketoacidosis—fluid administration should be reduced and mannitol (0.2–1 g/kg intravenously over 30 minutes) should be administered with repetition at hourly intervals based on response. CT or MRI scan of the brain can be done once therapy has been initiated to confirm the diagnosis. Consideration can also be given to mechanical hyperventilation to reduce PCO_2 and in that way decrease intracranial pressure.

Patients with diabetic ketoacidosis are also prone to develop acute respiratory distress syndrome (ARDS), presumably reflecting the sequelae of a damaged pulmonary endothelium and elevated capillary hydrostatic pressures following fluid resuscitation. Patients who present with rales at the time of initial diagnosis may be at higher risk for the development of this complication. Patients may also be at increased risk for development of pancreatitis as well as systemic infection, including fungal infections (eg, mucormycosis).

Abdominal pain and gastric stasis seen in diabetic ketoacidosis may put a semistuporous patient at risk for aspiration. Patients who are felt to be at risk with regard to airway protection should have a nasogastric tube in place for evacuation of stomach contents.

Finally, patients with diabetic ketoacidosis are at risk for recurrence of the disorder if insulin is withdrawn prematurely. The current infusion protocols, because they raise plasma insulin only to physiologic levels, have a very short half-life for control of blood glucose and ketogenesis. Premature cessation of insulin therapy before depot insulin (eg, NPH) can exert its effect may allow the patient to regress into ketoacidosis. To preclude this possibility, subcutaneous regular and intermediate-acting insulin should be provided on the morning when feeding is to be resumed. The insulin drip should be continued for 1 hour following this injection to provide coverage until the depot insulin effect comes on board.

NONKETOTIC HYPEROSMOLAR COMA

Clinical Setting

Hyperosmolar nonketotic coma, like diabetic ketoacidosis, is a consequence of uncontrolled diabetes mellitus; however, there are a number of features of this disorder which clearly distinguish it from diabetic ketoacidosis. First, plasma glucose levels in ketoacidosis are usually in the 250–400 mg/dL rather than the 700–1000 mg/dL range that can be seen with hyperosmolar nonketotic coma. Second, ketosis is rare in hyperosmolar nonketotic coma. Circulating insulin levels are probably adequate to control ketogenesis in the latter, though they are incapable of establishing euglycemia. Third, hyperosmolar nonketotic coma tends to occur more commonly in the elderly population, often those receiving chronic care who have difficulty reporting symptoms or maintaining adequate hydration. Like diabetic ketoacidosis, hyperosmolar nonketotic coma may present as the first manifestation of diabetes mellitus. Mortality remains high in hyperosmolar nonketotic coma (perhaps as high as 20% versus 1–2% in diabetic ketoacidosis); in both cases, mortality increases with age.

Precipitants of hyperosmolar nonketotic coma include many of the same complicating illnesses that lead to diabetic ketoacidosis. Infections (pneumonias are said to be the most common precipitating infection in 40–60% of cases, with urinary tract infections representing 5–16% of the total), myocardial infarction, cerebrovascular accident, pancreatitis, burns, heat stroke, and endocrine dysfunction (eg, Cushing's syndrome, acromegaly) are frequently associated with hyperosmolar nonketotic coma. Administration of hyperosmolar fluids (eg, tube feedings, total parenteral nutrition, peritoneal dialysis) can precipitate hyperosmolar nonketotic coma, as can medications that impair insulin secretion or action (eg, β-adrenergic blocking agents, phenytoin, corticosteroids, or diazoxide). Diuretics—particularly thiazides—can reduce intravascular volume, reduce glomerular filtration rate (the dominant mechanism for glucose clearance), and activate counterregulatory hormones (eg, catecholamines), all of which promote development of the hyperosmolar state. Finally, limited access to free water intake, particularly in patients who are dependent on others for water consumption, is a major determinant in the progression of the hyperosmolar state.

These factors interact in a highly variable fashion to promote the hyperosmolar state associated with hyperosmolar nonketotic coma. In a typical scenario, poorly controlled diabetes—or undiagnosed diabetes presenting for the first time—is aggravated by coincident infection (or other precipitant). This results in significant hyperglycemia as the balance of counterregulatory hormones versus insulin shifts in favor of the former. Hyperglycemia promotes increased insulin resistance and further elevations in blood glucose levels. This leads to an osmotic diuresis in the kidney as plasma glucose levels exceed the threshold for tubular reabsorption. This threshold typically increases with age, leading to even higher plasma glucose levels in the elderly. The osmotic diuresis results in a progressive loss of water and, to a lesser degree, solutes (eg, Na^+, Cl^-, K^+) in the urine. As with diabetic ketoacidosis, the water loss is "buffered" initially by an osmotically driven movement of water out of the cells into the extracellular compartment. As the diuresis continues, however, contraction of intravascular volume ensues and glomerular filtration falls, shutting off the body's primary mechanism for controlling plasma glucose levels in this setting. Glucose levels increase dramatically, often to extraordinarily high levels (normal renal excretory function generally limits elevations in plasma glucose to 500–600 mg/dL). Nausea and vomiting, related to the infection, uremia or hyperosmolality per se, may further aggravate intravascular volume contraction. Factor into this an elderly patient with age-dependent suppression of the thirst mechanism and difficulty communicating a sense of thirst to caregivers and the stage is set for severe dehydration and the hyperosmolar state of hyperosmolar nonketotic coma.

Diagnosis

The diagnosis is usually based on strong clinical suspicion and laboratory assessments of plasma glucose levels and serum osmolality. The typical patient may be a known type 2 diabetic (often taking an oral hypoglycemic agent) who has shown a subtle but steady deterioration over several days immediately preceding admission. The patient demonstrates significant dehydration, somnolence, stupor, or coma. The course may be marked by a precipitating illness, as described above. Tachycardia and low-grade fever may be present, but blood pressure and respiratory rate are normal. Urine output typically is reduced to low levels as the hyperosmolar state progresses.

The clinical presentation is usually dominated by the central nervous system findings. Patients with hyperosmolar nonketotic coma are lethargic and weak, with an altered sensorium. True coma is less common and usually does not appear until plasma osmolality is significantly elevated (see below). Hallucinations are occasionally present, and seizures may be occur in 25% of patients with hyperosmolar nonketotic coma. Focal findings suggesting cortical ischemia may also be seen. A minority of these reflect true cerebrovascular accidents related to thromboembolic complications (see below). Most represent low-flow states in areas of baseline cerebrovascular ischemia and recover with correction of the metabolic abnormality.

Plasma glucose levels are typically high (occasionally > 1000 mg/dL). Measured plasma osmolality is often > 350 mosm/kg. These measurements usually include the contribution of urea, which may accumulate to significant levels in the setting of volume contraction and prerenal azotemia; however, urea does not contribute to the osmotic force that drives fluid movement across cellular membranes since it is freely permeable in these membranes and distributes itself in equivalent concentrations in the intracellular and extracellular compartments. A more accurate measure of the effective osmolality is obtained from the following formula:

$$\text{Effective osmolality} = 2Na^+ + \frac{\text{Glucose}}{18}$$

where Na^+ and glucose are the concentrations of sodium ion and glucose, respectively. Normal effective osmolalities are in the range of 275–295 mosm/kg. Hyperosmolar nonketotic coma is diagnosed with an effective osmolality > 320 mosm/kg, while coma itself is seen with osmolalities > 340 mosm/kg. Coma at effective osmolalities ≤ 340 mosm/kg suggest some other cause (eg, meningitis, cerebrovascular accident, or other metabolic abnormality).

Anion gap acidosis is usually not a major component of hyperosmolar nonketotic coma since ketogenesis is suppressed (see above). If gap acidosis is present, it may suggest lactate accumulation due to tissue hypoperfusion, low-output state or metformin toxicity, or coexistent renal failure or toxic ingestion. Measurement of serum lactate levels, standard renal function tests, or a screen for toxic substances in blood (if a suggestive history is obtained) should help to discriminate among these possibilities.

Management

Therapy is in some ways similar to that for diabetic ketoacidosis except that there is less concern about correction of the acidosis, which is mild or nonexistent with most conventional cases of hyperosmolar nonketotic coma, and greater emphasis is placed on restoration of intravascular volume and serum osmolality.

Resuscitation of intravascular volume is initiated with parenteral fluids. One to two liters of normal saline are administered over the first hour. If the patient is profoundly hyperosmolar (> 330 mosm/L), half-normal saline (0.45% NaCl) should be substituted for normal saline. Volume status is reassessed based on blood pressure, urine output, central venous pressure, or pulmonary capillary wedge pressure, if available. If volume contractions persist, normal saline (or half-normal saline if hypertonicity persists) can be continued at a rate of 1 L/h. Once blood pressure and urine output have been restored, hypotonic fluids (eg, half-normal saline) can be substituted for isotonic saline at a rate of 250–500 mL/h depending on the need for continued volume resuscitation. The total free water deficit can be approximated using the following formula:

$$\text{Water deficit} = \frac{\text{Plasma osmolality} - 295}{295} \times 0.6 \text{ (Body weight)}$$

where plasma osmolality is in milliosmoles per kilogram, body weight in kilograms, and water deficit in liters. Fluid rates should be adjusted to correct half of the free water deficit in the first 12 hours and the remainder over the ensuing 24–36 hours. As with diabetic ketoacidosis, glucose-containing fluids (eg, D_5W) should be started when plasma glucose levels fall to 250 mg/dL.

Insulin therapy is of secondary importance in the management of hyperosmolar nonketotic coma. It is imperative that insulin therapy not be initiated until volume resuscitation is well under way (eg, following 1–2 L of crystalloid). Insulin will promote movement of glucose, electrolytes, and water into the intravascular compartment. In the absence of adequate volume resuscitation, this can lead to hypotension and cardiovascular collapse. Therapy should be initiated with a loading dose of 10–20 units intravenously followed by a drip delivering 0.1 units/kg/h. Conversion back to the outpatient regimen once the acute event has resolved can be accomplished using a strategy similar to that outlined above for diabetic ketoacidosis.

Electrolytes (ie, Na^+, K^+, Cl^-, PO_4^{3-}, and Mg^{2+}) are significantly depleted in hyperosmolar nonketotic coma due to the osmotic diuresis. These should be repleted as needed (beginning with the first liter of fluids if necessary). Once again, parenteral phosphate should be administered with care, keeping serum phosphate above 1 mg/dL until feeding can reestablish phosphate balance.

Complications

A. THROMBOEMBOLIC EVENTS

Coagulopathies related to increased platelet aggregation, hyperviscosity of circulating blood, or disseminated intravascular coagulation can develop in hyperosmolar nonketotic coma. The most appropriate therapy is resuscitation of intracellular volume and treatment of systemic infections. Focal neurologic findings that fail to improve with fluid resuscitation should be further investigated with appropriate consultation and imaging studies, if indicated. Some investigators have recommended low-dose heparin anticoagulation in patients with hyperosmolar nonketotic coma to guard against thromboembolic sequelae. If such therapy is initiated, patients should be closely monitored for development of gastrointestinal bleeding.

B. CEREBRAL EDEMA

This is a serious—though fortunately uncommon—complication of fluid resuscitation in hyperosmolar nonketotic coma (and diabetic ketoacidosis; see above). It occurs more commonly in children than in adults and frequently follows an overly aggressive management strategy involving administration of large amounts of parenteral fluids. The pathogenesis is not completely defined but probably relates to the increase in cortical capillary hydrostatic pressure and the osmotic gradient engendered by the aggressive use of hypotonic fluids in this setting. Cerebral edema rarely appears with serum glucose levels above 250 mg/dL. Appropriate introductions of glucose-containing fluids into the management strategy when plasma glucose approaches this level is an effective way to guard against this complication.

Clinically, brain edema develops after an initial period of improvement. It is often heralded by the development of headache, altered mental status, and seizure activity. If untreated, this can progress to herniation, with respiratory arrest and death. Recognition of the syndrome and appropriate treatment with mannitol, dexamethasone, and furosemide can be life-saving in this setting.

HYPERCALCEMIC CRISIS

Clinical Setting

Severe hypercalcemia, defined arbitrarily as a total Ca^{2+} > 14 mg/dL, usually occurs in the setting of a known hypercalcemic illness but may represent the initial manifestation of such an illness. Patients present initially with polyuria and polydipsia and, with a more protracted course, develop evidence of intravascular volume contraction with decreased urine output. Alterations in the sensorium dominate the clinical picture and range from behavioral changes and drowsiness to stupor and coma. Bradyarrhythmias and heart block are major cardiac sequelae of hypercalcemia. Hypercalcemia also potentiates digoxin activity, increasing the risk of cardiac glycoside toxicity. Gastrointestinal complaints are prominent. Anorexia, nausea, and vomiting, which further aggravate the volume contraction, are frequently present. Abdominal pain may be of sufficient intensity to mimic an acute abdomen.

Most chronic hypercalcemia is caused by primary hyperparathyroidism and is usually detected as a result of routine laboratory screening. Cancer-related hypercalcemia, most of which is caused by parathyroid hormone-related protein (PTHrP), is a less frequent but important cause of chronic hypercalcemia. In acute hypercalcemic crises, malignancy emerges as the major cause of the elevations in serum calcium. Other causes of hypercalcemia (eg, vitamin D intoxication, thiazides, or Addison's disease) are either too uncommon or cause such small increments in serum calcium that they rarely need to be considered in the differential diagnosis.

Hypercalcemia due to any cause creates a state of nephrogenic diabetes insipidus by uncoupling vasopressin from its receptor-effector system in the kidney (Table 24–8). This results in a water diuresis that eventually promotes intravascular volume contraction and reduced glomerular filtration rate, effectively suppressing the only route of egress for calcium mobilized from bone or transported across the gut lumen. Thus, volume contraction is in large part responsible for the very high levels of serum calcium found in hypercalcemic crisis. By inference, resuscitation of intravascular volume (see below) represents an excellent initial intervention to improve renal perfusion and tubular clearance of Ca^{2+}.

Table 24–8. Pathogenesis of hypercalcemic crisis.

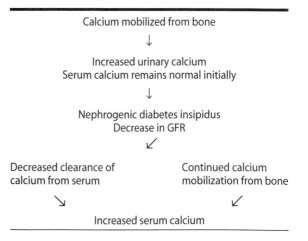

Hypercalcemic crisis should be considered in any patient with disseminated malignancy, particularly epidermoid carcinomas of the head, neck, and lung. This is especially true when there is a change in the patient's mental status or general clinical condition that cannot be explained by tumor progression, infection, or other metabolic abnormality (eg, uremia). It should also be considered in patients with known primary hyperparathyroidism, particularly in a clinical setting characterized by vomiting, diarrhea, or dehydration (eg, due to thiazide therapy).

Diagnosis

The diagnosis is confirmed by measurement of a total or ionized serum calcium level. The latter may be preferable in the presence of low serum albumin, the predominant Ca^{2+}-binding protein in blood, since hypoalbuminemia may mask an elevation in the free fraction if only total calcium levels are assessed. A convenient measure for adjusting total calcium measurements for the presence of hypoalbuminemia is to increase the total calcium by 0.8 mg/dL for each 1 g/dL decrease in serum albumin, based on a normal albumin level of 4 g/dL. The adjusted calcium does not always correlate with the measured ionized calcium, however, and should not be relied upon for more than a rough estimate of the free calcium fraction, particularly if ionized calcium measurements are available.

On the initial presentation with hypercalcemia, plasma samples should be sent for measurement of PTH (preferably using one of the newer immunoradiometric assays that measure only the bioactive, intact hormone), PTHrP, and, if the clinical setting is suggestive, 25-hydroxycholecalciferol or 1,25-dihydroxycholecalciferol levels. Primary hyperparathyroidism is a common disease, and even in a patient with known malignancy it should be excluded as a potentially curable cause of the hypercalcemia.

Management

Intravenous fluids represent the first avenue of approach for management of severe hypercalcemia (Table 24–9). Normalization of intravascular volume will improve GFR and increase renal excretion of calcium. Sodium and calcium handling are closely linked in the distal nephron. Fluid resuscitation with normal saline (0.9% NaCl) both restores GFR and promotes natriuresis and calciuresis by flooding transporter mechanisms responsible for sodium and calcium handling in the distal nephron. Five hundred to 1000 milliliters of normal saline is given over the first hour, with rates of 250–500 mL/h thereafter depending on the state of volume contraction. The latter can be assessed based on

Table 24–9. Therapy for hypercalcemic crisis.

0.9% NaCl (250–500 mL/h) plus furosemide if required

↓

Calcitonin (2–4 mg/kg SC or IM every 8 hours) with or without prednisone

↓

Pamidronate (60–90 mg IV over 12 hours)
or–
Gallium nitrate (200 mg/m² over 5 days)
or–
Plicamycin (25 μg/kg over 4–24 hours)

↓

Evaluate need for retreatment

---

clinical examination, urine output, and assessment of renal function. Several liters of fluid are frequently required before intravascular volume is restored. Continued infusions should be matched with urine outputs to avoid fluid overload. Loop diuretics (eg, furosemide) may be used to accomplish this in patients with an underlying predilection toward fluid retention (eg, congestive heart failure). Saline and loop diuretics can increase urinary calcium excretion by as much as 800 mg/d. This is typically accompanied by a moderate but significant reduction in serum calcium levels (1–3 mg/dL). Careful attention should be devoted to detection of signs of fluid overload. Potassium and magnesium depletion related to the diuresis should be corrected. If loop diuretics are used, it is important that the volume of normal saline administered should at least match urine output. Diuretic-induced volume contraction may lead to reduced GFR and worsening hypercalcemia.

At this point, more definitive and specific therapy should be introduced. Severe hypercalcemia is almost always a result of increased mobilization of calcium from bone. Therefore, most effective therapies for hypercalcemia have been directed against the osteoclasts of bone. Bisphosphonates represent the mainstay of therapy. Pamidronate administered at a dose of 60–90 mg in 250 mL of saline over 24 hours is effective in reducing serum calcium levels, often into the normal range. The effect can take 2–4 days to peak and the duration of the response is variable, lasting from 1 week to several months. Retreatment for recurrent hypercalcemia is usually successful. Side effects of therapy include inflammation at the infusion site, low-grade fever, and transient depression of serum calcium, phosphate, and magnesium. Bisphosphonates derive additional attractiveness from their efficacy in controlling pain and fracture in osteolytic metastases from breast cancer. The mechanism here is not completely understood but may relate to suppression of tumor-induced osteoclastic activity in the neighborhood of the metastases. Etidronate, a first-generation bisphosphonate, has been used parenterally to manage hypercalcemia of malignancy. In general, it is less effective than pamidronate, and it has largely been supplanted by the newer-generation aminobisphosphonates.

Calcitonin has a long history of use in the management of hypercalcemia. It has a direct effect on the osteoclast to suppress bone resorption. It is given either subcutaneously or intramuscularly at a dose of 2–4 units/kg body weight every 6–12 hours after administration of a test dose to exclude hypersensitivity to the drug. In general, the response to calcitonin, which should be noted after 6–12 hours, is modest in magnitude (decrease in serum calcium levels of 1–2 mg/dL) and declines with increasing duration of therapy (tachyphylaxis). Coadministration of glucocorticoids with calcitonin may limit this latter effect and extend the duration of the hypocalcemic effect. Calcitonin is useful largely as adjunctive therapy in controlling hypercalcemia in the acute setting until the effects of more powerful but slower-acting agents (eg, bisphosphonates) become available.

Plicamycin is a tumoricidal antibiotic with pronounced hypocalcemic properties at nontumoricidal doses. It presumably targets the osteoclast and its bone resorptive activity. It is administered as an infusion at a dosage of 15–25 μg/kg body weight over 4–24 hours. Calcium levels fall, often into the normal range, within 24–48 hours in a majority of patients treated. Plicamycin has significant renal and hepatic toxicity, and it induces platelet abnormalities that may result in clinically significant hemorrhage. Toxicity tends to increase with repeated administration, limiting chronic use of the drug. Given the ready availability of less toxic treatment modalities, plicamycin has largely been reduced to second-line status in the management of severe hypercalcemia.

Gallium nitrate has shown efficacy in the management of tumoral hypercalcemia in clinical trials. Like the bisphosphonates and plicamycin, the target of gallium therapy appears to be the osteoclast of bone. Patients are infused with gallium nitrate at a dosage of 200 mg/m^2 over a 5-day period. As with bisphosphonates and plicamycin, normocalcemia is achieved in the majority of patients (about 75% in some studies). In head-to-head comparisons, it appears to be more effective than either etidronate or calcitonin. Its major limitations are the duration of the infusion (often requiring hospitalization) and the potential for significant nephrotoxicity, particularly if it is used in the setting of other nephrotoxic agents.

Other nonselective treatment modalities which are available for management of hypercalcemic crisis include steroids, phosphate, and dialysis. Aside from their potentiation of calcitonin's effects, as described above, steroids are usually effective only in the management of hypercalcemia due to lymphoproliferative disease (eg, multiple myeloma) or vitamin D toxicity (eg, due to ingestion of vitamin D or disseminated granulomatous disease). They are best suited for chronic management of hypercalcemia associated with these disorders. Parenteral phosphate effectively reduces serum calcium levels, though often at the expense of deposition of calcium phosphate salts in parenchymal tissues. Given the availability of the agents described above, it is rarely needed for the management of hypercalcemic crisis. Peritoneal or hemodialysis against a low-calcium bath is also very effective in reducing serum calcium levels and is the treatment of choice for severe hypercalcemia in renal failure patients incapable of tolerating or responding to saline diuresis. In clinically tenuous patients not in renal failure undergoing maximal saline diuresis, persistent hypercalcemia may be an indication for hemodialysis as a tool to bridge the interval until more definitive therapy (eg, bisphosphonates or plicamycin) can achieve its maximal effect.

Finally, some effort should be devoted to addressing the primary cause of the hypercalcemia. In some instances (eg, disseminated malignancy) therapeutic options may be limited and ineffective in controlling serum calcium levels. In other instances (eg, primary hyperparathyroidism), a definitive surgical approach can be curative and limit downstream morbidity. Thus, careful investigation of the source of the hypercalcemia is warranted. Such investigation—even in patients with an obvious potential source of hypercalcemia (eg, malignancy)—may identify correctable problems and, at the very least, assist in the development of long-term management strategies once the acute crisis has resolved.

ACUTE HYPOCALCEMIA

Clinical Setting

Hypocalcemia may be seen in a number of disorders affecting the synthesis or action of parathyroid hormone or vitamin D or following sequestration of calcium into a functionally inaccessible compartment (see Chapter 8). Many of these represent chronic illnesses where hypocalcemic symptoms develop insidiously or where the complication of hypocalcemia is anticipated early and appropriate treatment initiated prior to acute decompensation. However, in selected situations, acute hypocalcemia may dominate the clinical presentation. Appropriate recognition of the high-risk clinical setting should lead to earlier diagnosis and therapeutic intervention with reduced morbidity and mortality.

Probably the most important cause of PTH-deficient hypocalcemia occurs in the postoperative setting following neck surgery for treatment of malignancy or resection of adenomatous or hyperplastic parathyroid glands. This may reflect accidental or purposeful (eg, radical neck dissection) removal of all functioning parathyroid tissue or inadvertent vascular compromise of tissue left in the neck. Residual normal parathyroid tissue can also be functionally atrophied in a patient undergoing surgery for hyperparathyroidism. It can take 1–2 days for PTH secretion and calcium levels to return to normal following resection of the adenoma. Magnesium deficiency can compromise both PTH secretion from the parathyroid gland and PTH action at target tissues in the periphery. Magnesium repletion in patients with low serum magnesium and calcium should be undertaken before launching an exhaustive workup of the hypocalcemia.

Hypocalcemia can be seen in chronic renal insufficiency. Hyperphosphatemia and reduced 1-hydroxylase activity result in deficient 1,25-dihydroxyvitamin D_3 generation and consequent hypocalcemia. Aggressive management of the hyperphosphatemia (eg, with phosphate-binding antacids) and calcitriol are generally useful in promoting normal calcium balance.

Acute sequestration of calcium into bone or nonphysiologic compartments can lead to severe hypocalcemia. Hypocalcemia following removal of a parathyroid adenoma may reflect a hypoparathyroid or aparathyroid state, as discussed above. Alternatively, in patients with severe osteitis fibrosa cystica, the bones, in the absence of PTH-driven bone resorption, serve as a sink for extracellular calcium deposition as previously unmineralized osteoid becomes calcified. This results in the syndrome termed "hungry bones." It is usually distinguished from PTH deficiency by measurements of the hormone (PTH is typically elevated in the hungry bones syndrome). A similar sequestration phenomenon is seen in osteoblastic metastases (eg, in breast or prostatic carcinoma). Typically, osteoclastic activity in these metastases is abrogated through some specific therapeutic intervention, leaving unmineralized matrix to calcify at the expense of extracellular calcium levels.

Sequestration may also occur in nonphysiologic settings such as the peritoneal cavity in acute pancreatitis, where deposition of calcium soaps leads to a subsequent reduction in serum calcium levels. A similar phenomenon occurs in damaged muscle following rhabdomyolysis. Deposition of calcium salts in damaged muscle beds leads to a reduction in serum calcium levels. Interestingly, serum calcium returns to normal or even elevated levels during the recovery phase, reflecting dissolution of the precipitates as the muscle undergoes repair.

Hypocalcemia occurs in the setting of acute systemic illness (eg, toxic shock syndrome), a finding that has been linked to elevated free fatty acids levels in this setting. It has also been associated with specific drugs, including antineoplastic agents such as doxorubicin and cytarabine and other agents such as ketoconazole, pentamidine, and foscarnet.

Diagnosis

Symptomatic hypocalcemia presents with a predictable constellation of signs and symptoms. Most of these findings are related to the increased neuroexcitability that is seen with reductions of extracellular calcium levels (Table 24–10). Symptoms frequently begin as circumoral paresthesias or paresthesias of the fingers or toes. This is followed by increased muscle cramping and spasm (particularly carpopedal spasm) (see Figure 8–17) and diffuse hyperreflexia. The increased propensity for muscle spasm can provoke generalized tetany which if extended to the laryngeal muscles can lead to laryngospasm and respiratory arrest. Increased excitability in the central nervous system can result in seizures, particularly in patients with a history of seizure disorder.

Physical examination looking for evidence of neuromuscular hyperexcitability is often revealing (Table 24–10). Chvostek's sign is evoked by repetitive tapping of the area overlying the facial nerve approximately 2 cm anterior to the ear lobe below the zygomatic arch. A positive test is contraction of musculature innervated by the facial nerve. The extent of the contraction is roughly proportionate to the severity of the hypocalcemia. Trousseau's sign is triggered by inflating a blood pressure cuff on an upper extremity to a level that roughly equates with the systolic blood pressure for 3–5

Table 24–10. Symptoms and signs of acute hypocalcemia.

Symptoms
  Perioral numbness
  Tingling paresthesias in distal extremities
  Hyperreflexia
  Muscle cramps
  Carpopedal spasm
  Laryngospasm
  Seizures
Signs
  Chvostek's sign
  Trousseau's sign
  Hypotension
  Bradycardia
  Prolonged QT interval
  Arrhythmias

minutes. Spasm of the hand musculature (see carpopedal spasm, above) due to transient ischemia of hyperexcitable nerves innervating the hand is regarded as a positive test.

Hypocalcemia can also have significant effects on cardiovascular function, including decreased blood pressure, impaired cardiac contractility, and conduction disturbances. On the electrocardiogram, significant hypocalcemia can manifest as prolongation of the QT interval. Evidence of sequelae of chronic hypocalcemia may also identify individuals who are at risk for acute hypocalcemia. Subcapsular cataracts and basal ganglia calcification are features associated with long-standing hypocalcemia.

Measurement of total serum calcium, albumin, or ionized calcium, if available, leads quickly to the correct diagnosis. Measurement of plasma PTH, 25-hydroxycholecalciferol, and 1,25-dihydroxycholecalciferol will assist in identifying deficiency of PTH secretion, adequacy of vitamin D stores, or impaired synthesis of bioactive vitamin D, respectively. Mg^{2+} levels should be obtained to exclude hypomagnesemia. If present, magnesium repletion should be initiated before additional diagnostic tests are undertaken.

Examination of the medication list looking for drugs with hypocalcemic properties (eg, bisphosphonates, calcitonin, asparaginase, cisplatin, foscarnet) should be performed.

Measurement of serum amylase and lipase should aid in identifying pancreatitis as a source of the hypocalcemia. Creatine kinase and aldolase levels will exclude the presence of rhabdomyolysis.

One area of potential confusion is the evaluation of patients in the immediate postparathyroidectomy period. Differentiating a hypoparathyroid or aparathyroid state from hungry bones syndrome can be difficult acutely. As pointed out above, measurement of plasma PTH levels (high in hungry bones syndrome and low in hypoparathyroidism) provides the most definitive separation of the two but typically takes several days and thus is usually not helpful in the acute setting. Measurement of serum phosphate (elevated in hypoparathyroidism and low-normal or low in hungry bones syndrome) or urinary phosphate (often low or absent in hypoparathyroidism) may be useful in identifying the source of hypocalcemia. Fortunately, the treatment of hypocalcemia in these two conditions is largely the same. Thus, establishment of a definitive diagnosis is important mainly for planning the subacute and long-term management of the patient's disease.

Management

In a life-threatening situation (eg, cardiovascular collapse) or in the setting of frank generalized tetany, 10 mL of calcium gluconate (93 mg of elemental calcium) can be administered intravenously over a 5- to 10-minute period and repeated if necessary. Less acute but recurrent hypocalcemic episodes can be managed with continuous calcium infusions. Nine hundred and thirty milligrams (ten ampules) of calcium gluconate can be mixed in 500 mL of D_5W. Infusion rates are established empirically. The initial infusion rate is typically 0.3 mg/kg/h but may be increased to as much as 2 mg/kg/h in patients with high demands for calcium (eg, hungry bones syndrome).

As the acute situation resolves, selected patients will become candidates for chronic replacement therapy. Those with minor hypocalcemia may be treated with calcium supplements alone. Administration of 1–3 g of elemental calcium (conventional calcium carbonate antacids contain about 40% elemental calcium) may suffice to restore calcium to the low-normal range and eliminate hypocalcemic symptoms. In those with more refractory hypocalcemia—a category that includes most patients with hypoparathyroidism—the addition of some form of vitamin D or a derivative will be required. If cholecalciferol (vitamin D_3) is employed to manage patients with hypoparathyroidism, supraphysiologic doses (50,000 units/d or higher) may be required, reflecting the limited capacity for 1-hydroxylation of the vitamin D prohormone in the hypoparathyroid state. 1,25-Dihydroxycholecalciferol (calcitriol) works faster than vitamin D_3 and circumvents the 1-hydroxylase blockade, but it is more expensive and the risk for acute hypercalcemia may be higher. It is given in a dose of 0.25–1 μg daily.

In all cases the goal of therapy should be to alleviate hypocalcemic symptoms and restore serum calcium levels to the low-normal range. This can usually be accomplished with some combination of vitamin D and supplemental calcium. The latter allows the practitioner additional flexibility in controlling serum calcium levels without requiring frequent dose modification of the longer-acting vitamin D. Efforts to push calcium levels higher may come at the expense of significant hypercalciuria and increased risk for renal stone formation. Difficulty in maintaining calcium even in the low-normal range without unacceptable hypercalciuria may be managed by addition of a thiazide diuretic to the regimen. These agents reduce hypercalciuria and, secondarily, raise serum calcium levels. If thiazides are used, careful follow-up is required to guard against the possibility of iatrogenic hypercalcemia. Efforts should be made to restore calcium to the target range and maintain it at this level indefinitely. Chronic hypocalcemia is associated with development of subcapsular cataracts and basal ganglia calcification which, in some cases, leads to the development of a parkinsonism-like syndrome.

HYPONATREMIA

Clinical Setting

Hyponatremia is the most frequent electrolyte problem observed in hospitalized patients. It is often asymptomatic when mild to moderate in severity and subacute to chronic in its time course of development. However, significant hyponatremia (< 120 mEq/dL) of rapid onset is frequently symptomatic and can be life-threatening.

Hyponatremia typically occurs in one of three clinical settings, each of which is linked to a specific pathophysiologic paradigm (Table 24–11). Hypovolemic hyponatremia is associated with volume contraction. As intravascular volume is reduced by more than about 9%, there is a nonosmotic stimulation of ADH release as the body attempts to retain water to support intravascular volume. Hyponatremia of this type is seen with protracted vomiting, diarrhea, or excessive sweat-

Table 24–11. Classification of hyponatremia.

Hypovolemic
  Extrarenal volume loss
    Excessive perspiration
    Losses due to widespread skin involvement (eg, burns)
    Vomiting
    Diarrhea
  Renal volume loss
    Diuretic use
    Salt-wasting nephropathy
    Cerebral salt-wasting
    Osmotic diuresis with selective repletion of water
Hypervolemic
  Congestive heart failure
  Nephrotic syndrome
  Cirrhosis with ascites
  Chronic renal failure
Normovolemic
  Syndrome of inappropriate antidiuretic hormone secretion
    Intracranial disease
    Pulmonary disease
    Drugs (eg, opioids)
    Severe pain or emotional distress
    Nausea and vomiting
    Postsurgical
    Resetting of the osmostat
  Adrenal insufficiency (may be hypovolemic in presence of severe mineralocorticoid deficiency)
  Hypothyroidism
  Water intoxication
    Psychogenic polydipsia
    Nonpsychogenic polydipsia
    Excessive administration of parenteral hypotonic fluids
    Post transurethral prostatectomy

ing, particularly when fluid loses are replenished with water or hypotonic fluids alone. Volume contraction and hyponatremia may also be seen with disorders of renal sodium handling (eg, diuretic use, mineralocorticoid deficiency, or other salt wasting syndromes). Urinary Na^+ concentration is typically elevated (> 20 mEq/L) in these latter disorders, while in the former urinary Na^+ concentration is low, reflecting aggressive resorption of Na^+ in all tubular segments.

Hypervolemic hyponatremia includes those edematous disorders typified by paradoxical retention of Na^+ and water in the face of a total body excess of each. Specific causes of hyponatremia in this group include congestive heart failure, cirrhosis of the liver with ascites, and nephrotic syndrome. Hyponatremia in this setting presumably results from perceived hypoperfusion by baroreceptors in the arterial circulation. Neural impulses transmitting this information to the hypothalamus trigger an increase in ADH release and net water retention.

Normovolemic hyponatremia is probably the most heterogeneous category and the most difficult to define pathophysiologically. It includes the syndrome of inappropriate ADH (SIADH) secretion, hypothyroidism, glucocorticoid insufficiency (eg, secondary adrenal insufficiency), psychogenic polydipsia, postoperative hyponatremia, and hyponatremia seen following transurethral resection of the prostate (Table 24–11).

Diagnosis

Acute hyponatremia, developing over the course of 24 hours or less, presents with headache, nausea, vomiting, and altered sensorium, which may progress to stupor and coma. These findings are thought to result from cerebral edema as the hypotonic extracellular compartment shifts water into the cerebral cortical cells. Such fluid shifts are opposed early through a reduction in intracellular electrolyte concentration and later by depletion of intracellular solutes (eg, amino acids). This acts to reduce the osmotic gradient and limit the net movement of fluid into brain. With chronicity, such solute shifts can reduce brain water content to near normal. Thus, the acuteness of the reduction in serum Na^+ concentration—as well as the magnitude of the reduction—are important markers of potential morbidity in this disorder. Young menstruating women are particularly susceptible to the deleterious effects of cerebral edema in the postoperative setting. They are 25 times more likely than postmenopausal women or men to die or have permanent brain damage. This increased susceptibility may reflect the effects of estrogen and progesterone to promote solute accumulation in the cells of the central nervous system. Such accumulation would be predicted to increase the osmotic drive that leads to cerebral edema in these patients.

The first step in making the diagnosis is to exclude the presence of pseudohyponatremia. The latter results from high circulating concentrations of triglycerides or osmotically active solutes (eg, glucose or proteins) in circulating plasma. Hypertriglyceridemia artifactually lowers serum sodium by physically excluding it from the sizable nonaqueous phase of the sample being measured. This is usually readily detected in the laboratory (eg, by noting the presence of lactescent serum) and is corrected by centrifuging the sample prior to measuring Na^+ concentration in the aqueous phase. Osmotically active solutes, like glucose, draw water from the intracellular to the extracellular compartment, where it may transiently lower existing electrolyte (eg, Na^+) concentrations (see Diabetic Ketoacidosis, above).

Assuming that the presence of hyponatremia is confirmed, an attempt to examine the different diagnostic possibilities listed above should be initiated. Evidence of congestive heart failure, cirrhosis, or nephrotic syndrome is usually apparent on physical examination and confirmable with standard laboratory or imaging studies. Similarly, renal dysfunction should be excluded using conventional renal function tests. Thiazide diuretic use is a frequent cause of hyponatremia and should be investigated early in the evaluation. A careful history of water consumption should be obtained and measurements of water intake in a monitored setting made to exclude psychogenic polydipsia or dipsogenic diabetes insipidus. Hypothyroidism can be excluded with measurement of plasma TSH and free thyroxine levels and glucocorticoid deficiency through an ACTH stimulation test (see Chapters 7 and 9).

Nonosmotic, non-volume-driven ADH secretion is found in SIADH. This is typically a diagnosis of exclusion in non-volume-contracted individuals without evidence of edema, renal insufficiency, hypothyroidism, or adrenal insufficiency. Serum Na^+ and osmolality are low in the face of a concentrated urine. Urine Na^+ may be modestly elevated (> 20 mEq/L), reflecting activation of natriuretic pathways responding to the increase in total body fluid volume. If findings are equivocal, an abnormal water load test (inability to excrete at least 90% of a 20 mL/kg water load in 4 hours or failure to dilute urine osmolality to below 100 mosm/kg) can be used to confirm the diagnosis. SIADH is seen with a variety of disorders affecting the central nervous system (eg, encephalitis, multiple sclerosis, meningitis, psychosis), the pulmonary system (eg, tuberculosis, pneumonia, aspergillosis), or as a paraneoplastic process associated with a number of solid tumors (eg, small-cell carcinoma of the lung; carcinoma of the pancreas, bladder, or prostate). It may also be seen with certain types of drugs (eg, cyclophosphamide, vinca alkaloids, opioids, prostaglandin synthesis inhibitors, tricyclic antidepressants, carbamazepine, clofibrate, and serotonin reuptake inhibitors).

Some difficulty may be encountered in differentiating SIADH from a second hyponatremic syndrome called cerebral salt wasting. The latter is also associated with central nervous system disease, particularly subarachnoid hemorrhage. It is thought to be due to a centrally mediated renal wasting of sodium with consequent volume contraction, volume-dependent activation of ADH secretion, and hyponatremia. It has been suggested that atrial natriuretic peptide or brain natriuretic peptide may play a central role in mediating the natriuresis associated with this disorder. Comparison of the features of these two disorders (Table 24–12) suggests that clinical or biochemical evidence of volume contraction is the major way to differentiate cerebral salt wasting from the euvolemic hyponatremia of SIADH. This is an important distinction since therapy in the former (ie, cerebral salt wasting) involves intravascular volume repletion while in the latter (ie, SIADH) fluid restriction may represent first line therapy.

Management

When the primary stimulus provoking water retention (eg, diuretic use) or consumption (eg, psychogenic polydipsia) can be identified, specific therapy represents the most rational approach for long-term management.

Table 24–12. Comparison of laboratory findings in syndrome of inappropriate antidiuretic hormone secretion (SIADH) with cerebral salt-wasting (CSW).

	SIADH	CSW
Intravascular volume contraction[1]	No	Yes
Serum sodium	↓	↓
Urine sodium	↑	↑↑
Urine volume	N or ↓	↑
Endocrine		
Plasma ADH	↑	N or ↑
Plasma aldosterone	↓	N or ↑
Plasma renin	↓	N or ↓
Plasma ANP	↑	↑
Urea nitrogen, serum	N or ↓	↑
Serum uric acid	↓	N or ↑

[1]Based on clinical assessment or direct measurement of plasma volume.

N = normal, ANP = atrial natriuretic peptide, BUN = blood urea nitrogen

When the cause of hyponatremia is unclear or unaddressable (eg, SIADH), a more generic approach may be adopted. Patients with asymptomatic (eg, mild or chronic) hyponatremia can be managed with water restriction. Calculations of daily water intake should incorporate that included in nonliquid foods consumed by the patient. For patients who are symptomatic but unable to adhere to water restriction, treatment with demeclocycline (600–1200 mg/d in divided doses), an antibiotic that uncouples ADH from activation of its receptor, may be sufficient to control serum Na⁺ levels. Water restriction is not required with demeclocycline therapy and may even be deleterious. Such therapy should be carefully monitored to guard against precipitous dehydration and renal insufficiency. Alternatively, patients can be managed with regular administration of a loop diuretic (eg, furosemide), which leads to excretion of urine approximately half the toxicity of plasma (loop diuretics disrupt the osmotic gradient required for urine concentration). Loop diuretics should be used concomitantly with NaCl supplementation (2–3 g/d) to increase urinary solute excretion and in that way amplify urinary water loss.

Symptomatic acute hyponatremia is an indication for hypertonic saline (3% NaCl) administration. Estimates of excess total body water can be made using the following equation:

$$\text{Excess water} = \frac{295 - \text{Plasma osmolality}}{295} \times 0.6 \ (\text{Body weight})$$

with plasma osmolality in milliosmoles per kilogram, excess water in liters, and body weight in kilograms.

The rise in serum sodium effected by 1 L of 3% saline infusate can be calculated by the following formula:

$$\Delta Na^+ = \frac{\text{Infusate } Na^+ - \text{Serum } Na^+}{\text{Total body water} + 1}$$

where ΔNa^+ is the change in sodium concentration effected by administration of 1 L of infusate; infusate Na⁺ is the concentration of Na⁺ in the infusion (eg, 513 mmol/L for 3% NaCl); and total body water is body weight (kg) × 0.6 (children or nonelderly men), × 0.5 (nonelderly women and elderly men), or × 0.45 (elderly women). The (+1) in the denominator accounts for the volume of the infusate. Based on the calculated ΔNa^+, one can adjust the infusion rate to provide the desired increase in serum Na⁺ over a fixed time interval.

Calculation of infusion rates can be made using the formula described by Adrogue and Madias: Infusion rates should be adjusted to raise serum Na⁺ levels by no more than 0.5 mEq/h (total < 8–12 mEq/d) to diminish the risk of central demyelination (see below). If necessary, infusion rates can be adjusted to increase serum sodium by 1–2 mEq/h for short periods of time in symptomatic patients; however, the limitation to 8 mEq/d should be adhered to, if possible. Furosemide can be administered, if necessary, to avoid intravascular fluid overload; however, given the ability of this drug to promote excretion of a hypotonic urine, the clinician should be aware that the plasma osmolality may increase faster than predicted by the formula set forth above. Once serum Na⁺ reaches 130 mEq/L, hypertonic saline infusion should be terminated and fluid restriction or normal saline (0.9% NaCl) plus furosemide used for the final correction of serum osmolality.

It is important to mention that interventions directed at the cause of the hyponatremia (versus treatment of the hyponatremia itself) also require close monitoring. Rapid correction of hyponatremia through administration of glucocorticoids in adrenal insufficiency, for example, may be associated with central myelinolysis. Careful monitoring of serum Na⁺ levels in the posttreatment period is mandatory. If Na⁺ appears to be rising too rapidly (> 1 mEq/h), administration of hypotonic fluids or a small dose of desmopressin acetate (0.25–1 μg parenterally) may be indicated.

Complications

Central pontine myelinolysis was first described in alcoholics and malnourished patients. In the original descriptions it was characterized by demyelination confined to the pons, resulting in quadriplegia and, not infrequently, death. Subsequent observational studies linked it to the treatment of hyponatremia. The classic presentation is of a patient who is aggressively treated for hyponatremia with resolution of the presenting findings (ie, those of cerebral edema), only to develop symptoms of mutism, dysphasia, spastic quadriparesis, pseudobulbar palsy, delirium, and, in many cases, death. Surviving patients often have severe neurologic sequelae. More recent studies using CT and MRI indicate that myelinolysis is not confined to the pons but present in many extrapontine locations as well. Lesions are typically symmetrically distributed and clustered in areas where there is close juxtaposition of gray and white matter.

There has been considerable controversy about the prevalence of this particular syndrome and its relationship to the treatment of hyponatremia. However, both animal and human studies are strongly suggestive of a link between this syndrome and rapid, aggressive correction of hyponatremia. Given the imperfect state of our understanding of this disorder, it would seem prudent to approach the correction of chronic hyponatremia, where solute distribution and water content in the brain are undoubtedly altered, cautiously, with rates of correction no greater that 0.5 mEq/h, as indicated above. The risk of solute redistribution in documented acute hyponatremia (ie, duration < 24 hours) is substantially reduced. Clinical signs of cerebral edema in this setting may be approached more aggressively, though repletion rates greater than 1 mEq/h with a maximal correction of 12 mEq over the first 24 hours should be avoided if possible.

DIABETES INSIPIDUS

Clinical Setting

Diabetes insipidus is a disorder due to absolute or relative deficiency in the circulating levels or bioactivity of vasopressin, the antidiuretic hormone (ADH).

ADH release is normally suppressed at plasma osmolalities below 285 mosm/kg, leading to generation of a maximally dilute urine (< 100 mosm/kg). Above 285 mosm/kg, ADH secretion increases linearly with plasma osmolality. At a plasma ADH level of 5 pg/mL, which corresponds to a plasma osmolality of about 295 mosm/kg, the urine is maximally concentrated. Despite the fact that plasma ADH levels continue to rise beyond this point, there is no further concentration of the urine. At 295 mosm/kg, the osmotic threshold for the thirst mechanism is activated. Thirst also rises linearly with increasing plasma osmolality. It provides the body's main defense against hypertonicity, much as suppression of ADH secretion guards against hypotonicity. Provided that the patient remains awake and able to drink and provided that the thirst mechanism remains intact, even complete deficiency of ADH secretion can be adequately compensated by increased water intake.

Defects in ADH secretion (central diabetes insipidus) may occur on a heritable basis, occasionally in association with diabetes mellitus, optic atrophy, and sensorineural deafness (DIDMOAD, or Wolfram's syndrome). It may also be seen as a component of a polyendocrine autoimmune syndrome (see Chapter 4). Secondary causes of central diabetes insipidus include head injury (often with stalk section), pituitary surgery, granulomatous disease (sarcoidosis, tuberculosis, histiocytosis X), infections, vascular aneurysms and thrombosis, and tumors (craniopharyngioma, dysgerminoma, meningioma, metastatic disease from breast, lung, or gastrointestinal tumors). These lesions typically involve large sections of the hypothalamus, sufficient to destroy or functionally impair both the supraoptic and paraventricular nuclei bilaterally.

Osmoreceptors for ADH release are believed to reside in the organum vasculosum of the lamina terminalis, while those controlling thirst are thought to lie in an independent but neighboring location. Thus, those patients with an isolated defect in ADH secretion (either in the osmoreceptors or the secretory nuclei) are protected from severe dehydration by activation of the thirst mechanism. In those with combined involvement of both ADH secretion and the osmoreceptors controlling thirst (hypodipsic or adipsic diabetes insipidus), the risk of volume contraction and severe dehydration is extreme (see below).

Adequacy of the renal response to ADH requires adequate delivery of glomerular filtrate to distal tubular segments, adequacy of tubular function in the ascending limb of the loop of Henle (to establish and maintain the gradient of medullary tonicity and to generate free water for excretion), and a normal response to vasopressin (ie, intact signal transduction mechanism) in the collecting duct. Unresponsiveness to ADH is due to genetic lesions in the V_2 receptor (X-linked recessive diabetes insipidus) or the functionally linked aquaporin-2 water channel (autosomal recessive diabetes insipidus). It may also be seen in an acquired form with hypokalemia or hypercalcemia in various forms of intrinsic renal disease (eg, medullary cystic disease) and following therapy with demeclocycline or lithium.

Diagnosis

The presentation of diabetes insipidus in an alert, conscious patient is typically an abrupt onset of polyuria and polydipsia. Hypertonicity is avoided as long as the thirst mechanism remains intact and water intake is able to keep up with urinary losses. In a patient who is unconscious or otherwise incapable of communicating the need for fluids or in patients with coexistent adipsia, polyuria is transient and quickly followed by evidence of severe dehydration and hyperosmolality. Urine volumes in this setting may be normal or even reduced. The clinical findings in hypernatremia associated with diabetes insipidus are dominated by the effects of cellular dehydration and contraction of intravascular volume. In the brain, this can lead to increased traction on dural veins and venous sinuses. This may result in avulsion of vessels from their cranial attachments and intracranial hemorrhage. Other findings include irritability, lethargy, weakness, muscle twitching, hyperreflexia, seizures, and coma.

The diagnosis of polyuria is usually reserved for urine outputs greater than 2.5 L/d. A careful history should be taken to document oral fluid intake (particularly beer or other hypotonic fluids) or parenteral fluid administration (eg, in a postoperative setting). Neurologic or endocrine symptoms that might suggest either a hypothalamic or intrasellar mass, use of medications that could impair water reabsorption (eg, furosemide, demeclocycline, or lithium) or intercurrent conditions that might mimic diabetes insipidus (eg, osmotic diuresis associated with diabetes mellitus or resolving obstructive uropathy) should also be investigated.

Initial evaluation should include measurement of serum sodium, plasma osmolality, and urine osmolality. Diabetes insipidus is typically associated with normal or elevated serum sodium and osmolality in the face of a submaximally concentrated urine. Plasma glucose measurement and standard renal function tests should help to exclude osmotic diuresis as contributing to the polyuria. Measurement of serum K^+ and Ca^{2+} will assist in excluding polyuria resulting from hypokalemia and hypercalcemia, respectively.

In patients with equivocal initial tests, a water deprivation test may be performed as described in Chapter 5. Patients with diabetes insipidus become progressively more hypertonic with water deprivation but fail to increase urine osmolality. Administration of desmopressin promotes water retention and an increase in urine osmolality in patients with central but not nephrogenic diabetes insipidus. Plasma ADH levels may also be of assistance in defining the nature of the diabetes insipidus. In the presence of high plasma but low urine osmolality, increased plasma ADH levels are associated with nephrogenic diabetes insipidus while subnormal levels are found with central diabetes insipidus.

Coexistence of glucocorticoid deficiency may "mask" the presence of central diabetes insipidus. The development of polyuria with the initiation of glucocorticoid replacement should alert the clinician to the possible presence of diabetes insipidus.

In the 48 hours following pituitary surgery or head trauma, transient diabetes insipidus with polyuria is not uncommon. Over the ensuing 2–14 days, a period of antidiuresis and hyponatremia may dominate the clinical course. This in turn may be followed by persistent polyuria. The first phase is thought to result from transient dysfunction or stunning of the ADH-producing neurons of the hypothalamus; the second from leakage of ADH from damaged or dying neurons; the third by permanent loss of ADH secretory neurons. Not all patients progress through the entire series of events. It is important to recognize the existence of this syndrome and the natural progression of the disorder in evaluating the need for chronic therapeutic intervention.

In pregnancy, there is a resetting of the osmostats controlling both ADH and thirst, resulting in a state of "physiologic" hypoosmolality (about 10 mosm/kg below that seen in the nonpregnant state). In addition, elevations in placental vasopressinase may promote polyuria in patients with otherwise compensated partial central diabetes insipidus. The appropriate treatment for this disorder is desmopressin acetate, an ADH analog that is resistant to degradation by vasopressinase.

Virtually anything that increases the rate of tubular flow (eg, primary polydipsia or central diabetes in-

sipidus) may create a state of functional nephrogenic diabetes insipidus. This is due to washout of the medullary tonicity that is responsible for generating the osmotic gradient which promotes movement of water from the tubular lumen into the medullary interstitium. Primary polydipsia (eg, psychogenic polydipsia or dipsogenic diabetes insipidus) presents with a dilute urine, but plasma osmolality and serum Na^+ levels are typically low or low-normal and ADH levels are low. Moreover, owing to the elevation in tubular flow rates, the response to desmopressin may be limited in magnitude. This may make it difficult to differentiate primary polydipsia from partial forms of nephrogenic diabetes insipidus. Plasma ADH levels may be of assistance in making this distinction.

Management

Acute diabetes insipidus is characterized by polyuria in the presence or absence of plasma hyperosmolality. As noted above, the presence of hyperosmolality is determined by the adequacy of the patient's thirst mechanism. When a hyperosmolar state with clinical evidence of severe dehydration is present, it is necessary to correct intravascular volume. This is accomplished by administering hypotonic fluids (eg, D_5W), which will both restore intravascular volume and move plasma osmolality back toward normal. The rate at which the hyperosmolality is corrected is dictated in part by the severity of the clinical symptoms and by the chronicity of the disorder. Chronic hyperosmolality (> 24 hours) leads to the accumulation of idiogenic osmoles (eg, taurine and myoinositol) in the central nervous system that serve to offset the osmotically driven movement of water out of that compartment. Aggressive correction of the hyperosmolar state can lead to cerebral edema if the rate of hypotonic fluid administration greatly exceeds the rate at which the neurons in the central nervous system eliminate these idiogenic osmoles. Following expansion of intravascular volume with normal saline, correction of plasma osmolality at a rate of 0.5–1 mosm/h—not to exceed 15 mosm within the first 24-hour period—appears to be reasonably effective in reducing plasma tonicity without incurring an increased risk of cerebral edema. Typically, higher infusion rates are used early in the course when serum osmolalities are highest and reduced as osmolality decreases into the range of 330 mosm/kg. Correction of the total free water deficit should be spread over about 48 hours. Total water deficit is defined above in the section dealing with diabetic ketoacidosis. Calculation of hypotonic fluid infusion rates can be made using the formula for change in serum sodium set out in the preceding section, substituting 0 mmol/L for D_5W, 77 mmol/L for 0.45% NaCl, or 154 mmol/L for 0.9% NaCl into the equation, as needed, to calculate the net reduction in serum Na^+. Again, based on the calculated ΔNa^+, one can adjust the rate of delivery of the infusate to provide a specific increment in serum Na^+ concentration over a defined time interval. If signs of cerebral edema (see Hyponatremia, above) appear, hypotonic fluids should be discontinued and appropriate administration of hypertonic fluids (eg, mannitol) initiated.

If the diagnosis of central diabetes insipidus has been established, the patient should receive parenteral desmopressin acetate. The initial dose, in the range of 1–2 μg every 24 hours (administered intravenously or intramuscularly), should be given in the evening with the aim of controlling nocturia and maintaining daily urine output under 2 L. If polyuria returns well before the end of the 24-hour dosing interval, the single dose can be increased or split doses can be administered every 12 hours. Ideally, one would like to see some degree of "breakthrough" polyuria at the end of the dosing interval. This serves to guard against the development of iatrogenic hyponatremia. If this proves difficult to achieve, a dose can be skipped every 48–72 hours. Once the patient has been stabilized on a fixed dose of parenteral desmopressin, conversion to a formulation more suitable for the outpatient setting is indicated. Desmopressin acetate is available in liquid form for insufflation through a nasal cannula or as a fixed-dose (10 μg) nasal spray. The former has the advantage of greater flexibility in adjusting the nasal dose while the latter offers greater convenience for some patients. Parenteral desmopressin is generally about ten times more potent than the nasally administered drug; however, intranasal doses should be titrated for each individual patient. Desmopressin is also available in an oral form. Effective doses can range widely (from 50 μg to 1200 μg/d in divided doses) and should be adjusted for the individual patient.

Treatment of nephrogenic diabetes insipidus is more complex since the problem is one of resistance to—rather than deficiency of—the endogenous hormone. If possible, one should attempt to address the underlying cause of ADH resistance. This can be accomplished by correcting electrolyte abnormalities (eg, hypokalemia or hypercalcemia) or discontinuing medications (eg, demeclocycline, lithium) that are likely to contribute to ADH insensitivity. Failing this, administration of a thiazide diuretic together with salt restriction will often reduce the polyuria. This is assumed to result from contraction of intravascular volume with increased proximal reabsorption of fluids and solutes and, consequently, limited availability of fluid in distal nephron segments for free water generation and excretion. Prostaglandins are endogenous antagonists of ADH activity in the collecting duct. Administration of cyclooxygenase inhibitors (eg, indomethacin, 100 mg/d in divided doses) may improve sensitivity to endogenous ADH and reduce polyuria. If the impairment in ADH responsiveness is mild, higher doses of desmopressin will occasionally prove effective in promoting water retention. Amiloride is the preferred treatment for lithium toxicity. It is thought to prevent the uptake of lithium in collecting duct cells. Lithium-induced diabetes insipidus may not abate following discontinuation of the drug.

Disorders of thirst in the setting of central diabetes insipidus deserve special mention with regard to therapy. Excessive thirst due to altered osmoreceptor function or behavioral conditioning (eg, before desmopressin treatment) may result in severe hyponatremia once desmopressin treatment is initiated. The patient should be cautioned about excessive consumption of water, and fluid must be restricted if necessary.

Adipsic diabetes insipidus is probably one of the most difficult therapeutic problems faced by endocrinologists. These patients have essentially lost all ability to regulate water metabolism on their own. This function must be taken over by the medical team providing their care. Desmopressin is administered in a fixed parenteral dose which is sufficient to reduce urine output to about 1.5–2 L/d with a fluid intake of about 2–2.5 L. The difference here is intended to cover the daily insensible losses (about 500–1000 mL) and may need to be adjusted empirically to maintain normal fluid homeostasis. After plasma osmolality and sodium are in the normal range, fluid intake is balanced against urine output. Any net change in urine output over an 8-hour period (this may be extended as the patient's fluid requirements become more predictable) is accommodated by modifying the fluid orders for the ensuing 8 hours. The patient should also be weighed daily. Any alteration in weight is usually reflective of net changes in water retention and can be corrected through modification of fluid intake. Plasma osmolality and serum sodium should be monitored once or twice weekly and appropriate changes in fluid administration made depending on the direction and magnitude of the shift in osmolality. With this system of redundant monitoring, urine volumes and plasma osmolality can be reasonably well controlled for protracted periods of time.

Complications

If left untreated, polyuria secondary to diabetes insipidus can lead to dilation of the collecting system, hydronephrosis, and renal dysfunction. This is the dominant reason for treating polyuria even in patients with an intact thirst mechanism who are capable of controlling plasma osmolality through water ingestion.

Overly rapid correction of the hyperosmolality can result in cerebral edema. The relative risk of this complication should be minimized by careful attention to the rate at which the water deficit is corrected (see above).

REFERENCES

Myxedema Coma

Pittman CS, Zayed AA: Myxedema coma. Curr Ther Endocrinol Metab 1997;6:98. [PMID: 9174713]

Ringel MD: Management of hypothyroidism and hyperthyroidism in the intensive care unit. Crit Care Clin 2001;17:59. [PMID: 11219235]

Wall CR: Myxedema coma: diagnosis and treatment. Am Fam Physician 2000;62:2485. [PMID: 11130234]

Yamamoto T, Fukuyama J, Fujiyoshi A: Factors associated with mortality of myxedema coma: report of eight cases and literature survey. Thyroid 1999;9:1167. [PMID: 10646654]

Thyroid Storm

Dillmann WH, Thyroid storm. Curr Ther Endocrinol Metab 1997;6:81. [PMID: 9174709]

Jiang YZ et al: Thyroid storm presenting as multiple organ dysfunction syndrome. Chest 2000;118:877. [PMID: 10988222]

Tietgens ST, Leinung MC: Thyroid storm. Med Clin North Am 1995;79:169. [PMID: 7808090]

Yeoung SC, Go R, Balasubramanyam A: Rectal administration of iodide and propylthiouracil in the treatment of thyroid storm. Thyroid 1995;5:403. [PMID: 8563481]

Thyrotoxic Periodic Paralysis

Lin SH, Lin YF: Propanolol rapidly reverses paralysis, hypokalemia and hypophosphatemia in thyrotoxic periodic paralysis. Am J Kidney Dis 2001;37:620. [PMID: 11228188]

Manoukian MA, Foote JA, Crapo LM: Clinical and metabolic features of thyrotoxic periodic paralysis in 24 episodes. Arch Intern Med 1999;159:601. [PMID: 10090117]

Amiodarone-Induced Hyperthyroidism

Burman KD, Wartofsky L: Iodine effects on the thyroid gland: biochemical and clinical aspects. Rev Endocr Metab Disord 2000;1:19. [PMID: 11704988]

Eaton SE et al: Clinical experience of amiodarone-induced thyrotoxicosis over a 3 year period: role of colour-flow Doppler sonography. Clin Endocrinol (Oxf) 2002;56:33. [PMID: 11849244]

Martino E et al: The effects of amiodarone on the thyroid. Endocr Rev 2001;22:240. [PMID: 11294826]

Roti E, Uberti ED: Iodine excess and hyperthyroidism. Thyroid 2001;11:493. [PMID: 11396708]

Acute Adrenal Insufficiency

Oelkers W, Diederich S, Bahr V: Therapeutic strategies in adrenal insufficiency. Ann Endocrinol (Paris) 2001;62:212. [PMID: 11353897]

Perlitz Y et al: Acute adrenal insufficiency during pregnancy and puerperium: case report and literature review. Obstet Gynecol Surv 1999;54:717. [PMID: 10546275]

Rao RH. Bilateral massive adrenal hemorrhage. Med Clin North Am 1995;79:107. [PMID: 7808087]

Sarver RG, Dalkin BL, Ahmann FR: Ketoconazole-induced adrenal crisis in a patient with metastatic prostatic adenocarcinoma: case report and review of the literature. Urology 1997;49:781. [PMID: 9145992]

Pituitary Apoplexy

Biousse V, Newman NJ, Oyesiku NM: Precipitating factors in pituitary apoplexy. J Neurol Neurosurg Psychiatry 2001;71:542. [PMID: 11561045]

da Motta LA et al: Pituitary apoplexy. Clinical course, endocrine evaluations and treatment analysis. J Neurosurg Sci 1999;43:25. [PMID: 10494663]

Lee CC, Cho AS, Carter WA: Emergency department presentation of pituitary apoplexy. Am J Emerg Med 2000;18:328. [PMID: 10830692]

Randeva HS et al: Classical pituitary apoplexy: clinical features, management, and outcome. Clin Endocrinol (Oxf) 1999;51:181. [PMID: 10468988]

Diabetic Ketoacidosis

Bell DS, Alele J: Diabetic ketoacidosis. Why early detection and aggressive treatment are crucial. Postgrad Med 1997;101:193. [PMID: 9126212]

Delaney MF et al: Diabetic ketoacidosis and hyperglycemic hyperosmolar nonketotic coma. Endocrinol Metab Clin North Am 2000;29:683. [PMID: 11149157]

Fleckman AM: Diabetic ketoacidosis. Endocrinol Metab Clin North Am 1993;22:181. [PMID: 8325282]

Kitabchi AE, Wall BM: Diabetic ketoacidosis. Med Clin North Am 1995;79:9. [PMID: 7808097]

White NH: Diabetic ketoacidosis in children. Endocrinol Metab Clin North Am 2000;29,657. [PMID: 11149156]

Hyperosmolar Nonketotic Coma

Lorber D: Nonketotic hypertonicity in diabetes mellitus. Med Clin North Am 1995;79:39. [PMID: 7808094]

Siperstein MD: Diabetic ketoacidosis and hyperosmolar coma. Endocrinol Metab Clin North Am 1992;21:415. [PMID: 1612073]

Hypercalcemic Crisis

Edelson GW, Kleerekoper M: Hypercalcemic crisis. Med Clin North Am 1995;79:79. [PMID: 7808096]

Nussbaum S: Pathophysiology and management of severe hypercalcemia. Endocrinol Metab Clin North Am 1993;22:343. [PMID: 8325291]

Hypocalcemia

Reber PM, Heath H: Hypocalcemic emergencies. Med Clin North Am 1995;79:93. [PMID: 7808098]

Tohme JF, Bilezikian JP: Hypocalcemic emergencies. Endocrinol Metab Clin North Am 1993;22:363. [PMID: 8325292]

Hyponatremia

Adrogue HJ, Madias NE: Hyponatremia. N Engl J Med 2000; 342:1581. [PMID: 10824078]

Kappy MS, Ganong CA: Cerebral salt wasting in children: the role of atrial natriuretic hormone. Adv Pediatr 1996;43:271. [PMID: 8794180]

Kovacs L, Robertson GL: Disorders of water balance—hyponatremia and hypernatremia. Baillieres Clin Endocrinol Metab 1992;6:107. [PMID: 1739390]

Kumar S, Berl T: Sodium. Lancet 1998;352:220. [PMID: 98832227]

Mulloy AL, Caruana RJ: Hyponatremic emergencies. Med Clin North Am 1995;79:155. [PMID: 7808089]

Sahun M et al: Water metabolism disturbances at different stages of primary thyroid failure. J Endocrinol 2001;168:435. [PMID: 11241175]

Diabetes Insipidus

Adrogue HJ, Madias NE: Hypernatremia. N Engl J Med 2000; 342:1493. [PMID: 10816188]

Buonocore CM, Robinson AG: The diagnosis and management of diabetes insipidus during medical emergencies. Endocrinol Metab Clin North Am 1993;22:411. [PMID: 8325295]

Fried LF, Palevsky PM: Hyponatremia and hypernatremia. Med Clin North Am 1997;81:585. [PMID: 9167647]

Morello J-P, Bichet DG: Nephrogenic diabetes insipidus. Annu Rev Physiol 2001;63:607. [PMID: 11181969]

Singer I, Oster JR, Fishman LM: The management of diabetes insipidus in adults. Arch Intern Med 1997;157:1293. [PMID: 92011003]

AIDS Endocrinopathies

25

Grace Lee, MD, & Carl Grunfeld, MD, PhD

ACTH	Adrenocorticotropic hormone	**LDL**	Low-density lipoproteins
AIDS	Acquired immunodeficiency syndrome	**LH**	Luteinizing hormone
CMV	Cytomegalovirus	**PRA**	Plasma renin activity
CRH	Corticotropin-releasing hormone	**PTH**	Parathyroid hormone
DHEA	Dehydroepiandrosterone	T_3	Triiodothyronine
GH	Growth hormone	T_4	Thyroxine
GnRH	Gonadotropin-releasing hormone	**TBG**	Thyroxine-binding globulin
HDL	High-density lipoproteins	**TNF**	Tumor necrosis factor
HIV	Human-immunodeficiency virus	**TRH**	Thyrotropin-releasing hormone
IGF	Insulin-like growth factor	**TSH**	Thyroid-stimulating hormone
IL	Interleukin	**VLDL**	Very low density lipoproteins

Symptoms consistent with endocrine disorders and alterations in endocrine laboratory values are not unusual in individuals infected with the human immunodeficiency virus (HIV). Some of these changes are common to any significant systemic illness; others appear to be more limited to patients with HIV infection or secondary to its therapies. Alterations in endocrine and metabolic function can be associated with HIV infection even before clinically significant immunocompromise occurs. As the infected individual becomes immunocompromised, opportunistic infections and neoplasms—as well as the agents used in the treatment of these disorders—can give rise to further changes in endocrine function. This chapter will discuss alterations in endocrine function that can accompany HIV infection and AIDS, focusing on evaluation and interpretation of clinical and laboratory findings.

THYROID DISORDERS

Opportunistic Infections & Neoplasms

Opportunistic pathogens and neoplasms have been found at autopsy in the thyroid glands of HIV-infected individuals. A few of these pathogens have been associated with clinical thyroid dysfunction. *Pneumocystis carinii* has been associated with inflammatory thyroiditis accompanied by hypothyroidism in seven cases, hyperthyroidism in three cases, and normal thyroid function in one case. Antithyroid antibodies were negative in all six cases in which they were measured. Radionuclide scanning in seven cases revealed poor visualization of the entire thyroid gland in patients with bilateral disease and nonvisualization of the affected lobe in patients with unilateral disease. Two patients with hyperthyroidism had normalization of thyroid function after treatment of the *P carinii* infection. Kaposi's sarcoma has also been reported to infiltrate the thyroid gland, resulting in significant destruction and hypothyroidism in at least one case. In two cases, lymphoma was associated with thyroid infiltration, causing thyroidal enlargement. Thyroid involvement may occur in patients who have disseminated opportunistic infections with *Mycobacterium tuberculosis,* cytomegalovirus, *Cryptococcus neoformans, Aspergillus fumigatus,* and *Rhodococcus equi.* Typically, thyroid function tests in these types of infections are normal or reflect a pattern consistent with nonthyroidal illness (Chapter 7).

Alterations in Thyroid Function Tests

In early studies of thyroid function tests in HIV-infected individuals, some patients were found to have lower thyroxine (T_4) and triiodothyronine (T_3) levels than HIV-negative controls. Patients with low T_3 values in these studies had normal basal and peak TSH levels after TRH stimulation. In most studies, the low T_3 levels were related to severity of disease. When HIV-infected patients were stratified by weight loss and the presence of secondary infection, T_3 levels remained normal during asymptomatic HIV infection, decreased by 19% in AIDS patients who were free of active infection and had stable weight, and decreased by 45% in patients with active secondary infection and weight loss, consistent with the euthyroid sick syndrome. It is notable that even significantly ill HIV-infected patients often do not demonstrate the elevated reverse T_3 (rT_3) levels characteristic of the euthyroid sick syndrome. The significance of this difference, if any, is unknown.

Thyroxine-binding globulin (TBG) is elevated in HIV-infected patients and rises progressively with advancing immunosuppression. This increase does not appear to be due to generalized changes in protein synthesis, increases in sialylation and subsequent clearance of TBG, or changes in estrogen levels. The cause and clinical significance of the increased TBG found in HIV-infected patients are unknown. However, increases in TBG affect total T_4 and T_3 measurements, and this should be considered when interpreting these tests in HIV-infected patients.

Subtle alterations in TSH dynamics have been reported in stable HIV-infected patients. While their TSH and free T_4 levels remain within the normal range, these individuals demonstrate significantly higher TSH values and lower free T_4 values than uninfected controls. In circadian studies, HIV-infected individuals have higher TSH pulse amplitudes with unchanged pulse frequency as well as a higher peak TSH in response to TRH stimulation. These studies are consistent with a subtle state of compensated hypothyroidism in HIV infection; the mechanisms underlying these alterations have not been elucidated.

The typical pattern of alterations in thyroid function tests in HIV-infected patients is outlined in Table 25–1.

Medication Effects

Hepatic microsomal enzymes—and thus thyroid hormone clearance—are increased by rifampin, an agent used for *Mycobacterium avium* prophylaxis. Patients with normal thyroid function should not be clinically affected, though decreases in T_4 may be observed. Patients receiving l-thyroxine may require increased doses, and patients with decreased pituitary or thyroid reserve may develop clinically apparent hypothyroidism when

Table 25–1. Thyroid function tests in HIV-infected patients.

	Basal	After TRH stimulation
T_3	↓	
T_4	Normal	
rT_3	Normal or ↓	
TBG	↑	
TSH	Normal	↑ Pulse amplitude

↓ decreased; ↑ increased

treated with rifampin. Medications used in HIV-infected patients that can affect the endocrine system are listed in Table 25–2.

With the advent of highly active antiretroviral therapy (HAART), there have been reports of newly diagnosed autoimmune diseases such as Graves' disease, Hashimoto's thyroiditis, and alopecia areata. Immune reconstitution with HAART raises the possibility of subsequent induction of autoimmune diseases. One study reported five patients who developed Graves' disease 14–22 months after starting HAART. Prior to starting HAART, none of the patients had thyroid antibodies, but after starting treatment all developed thyroid antibodies and symptoms of hyperthyroidism. Possible theories include thymic regeneration or peripheral T lymphocyte expansion causing irregularities in tolerance, leading to autoimmune dysfunction.

Summary of Thyroid Disorders

In summary, most alterations in thyroid function that occur in HIV infection are similar to those seen in the

Table 25–2. Medications that can affect the endocrine system used in HIV-infected patients.

Thyroid	**Bone, calcium**
Rifampin	Foscarnet
Adrenals, electrolytes	Pentamidine
Ketoconazole	Ketoconazole
Megestrol acetate	Rifampin
Rifampin	**Pancreas, glucose**
Trimethoprim	Pentamidine
Pentamidine	Trimethoprim-sulfameth-
Sulfonamides	oxazole
Amphotericin B	Dideoxyinosine (ddI)
Foscarnet	Dideoxycytosine (ddC)
Gonads	Megestrol acetate
Ketoconazole	Protease inhibitors
Megestrol acetate	**Lipids**
	Protease inhibitors

euthyroid sick syndrome. As with other causes of this syndrome, replacement with thyroid hormone is not warranted at this time. The clinical significance of the changes that appear to be specific to HIV infection, such as elevated TBG, is not certain.

ADRENAL DISORDERS

Opportunistic infections commonly involve the adrenal glands but rarely occupy enough of the gland to cause adrenal insufficiency. Impaired adrenal reserve without overt symptoms of adrenal insufficiency has been described in the HIV population. Those patients with a subnormal response to dynamic testing represent a group for which there is controversy over when to give baseline replacement glucocorticoids and mineralocorticoids and increased doses in stressful situations, especially when baseline levels are normal or elevated. With restoration to health by treatment of opportunistic infections or HIV itself, many of these patients no longer have adrenal insufficiency.

Opportunistic Infections & Neoplasms

Opportunistic organisms are found commonly in the adrenal glands of patients dying of AIDS although they rarely cause clinical adrenal insufficiency. Cytomegalovirus has been associated with significant necrosis of the adrenal gland, though the amount of tissue affected rarely reaches the 90% thought necessary to cause clinical adrenal insufficiency. However, in one preliminary study, the presence of CMV retinitis was associated with an increased rate of adrenal insufficiency compared with AIDS patients without that disorder. Less common opportunistic infections involving the adrenals include *Mycobacterium tuberculosis, Mycobacterium avium-intracellulare, Cryptococcus neoformans, Histoplasma capsulatum, Pneumocystis carinii,* and *Toxoplasma gondii.* In addition, Kaposi's sarcoma and lymphoma can involve the adrenals, but rarely to the extent of inducing adrenal insufficiency.

Glucocorticoids

Classic clinical symptoms of adrenal insufficiency are seldom seen, but some clinicians view the weakness and weight loss seen in patients with AIDS as an indicator of adrenal insufficiency. In addition, subclinical abnormalities in glucocorticoid dynamics are common. HIV-infected patients usually have normal or, even more commonly, elevated basal cortisol levels. ACTH levels in patients with elevated basal cortisol levels have been found to be normal or elevated. Some of these alterations may be mediated by cytokines; both interleukin-1 and TNF can directly stimulate cortisol secretion, while IL-1 and IL-6 can stimulate ACTH and CRH re-

lease. An increase in cortisol levels may also be a direct response to HIV infection itself. An increased cortisol to DHEA ratio has been correlated with body weight loss and HIV-associated malnutrition.

Nearly all HIV-infected patients have a normal cortisol response to high-dose (250 μg) ACTH stimulation testing, but there is some evidence that adrenal reserve may be decreased in as many as half of patients with HIV infection. Recently, two studies have shown that low-dose cosyntropin stimulation (10 μg) resulted in a diagnosis of glucocorticoid insufficiency in 21% of outpatients with HIV and up to 50% of critically ill HIV-infected patients. During CRH stimulation testing, a reduced ACTH or cortisol response was seen in up to 50% of stable HIV-infected patients with CD4 counts less than 500/μL. Thus, HIV-infected patients may have decreased reserve either at the pituitary or at the adrenal level.

Clinically significant abnormalities in glucocorticoid secretion appear to be uncommon in HIV infection; subtle alterations in adrenal biosynthesis may be more common. HIV-infected patients have reduced products of the 17-deoxysteroid pathway (corticosterone, deoxycorticosterone, and 18-hydroxydeoxycorticosterone) with normal or elevated products of the 17-hydroxy pathway (cortisol) before and after ACTH stimulation. It is not known whether this alteration represents an early indication of evolving adrenal insufficiency or is an adaptive response that shifts adrenal synthetic activity to steroids that are crucially needed under conditions such as HIV infection that impose physical stress. Twenty-four hour urine free cortisol levels do not appear to be useful in the evaluation of subtle adrenal alterations in HIV-infected patients.

Glucocorticoid resistance has been described in HIV-infected patients. This syndrome is characterized by symptoms of weakness, fatigue, weight loss, and hyperpigmentation, with elevated cortisol levels and mildly increased ACTH levels. Decreased lymphocyte glucocorticoid receptor affinity for glucocorticoids, resulting in chronic interferon alpha stimulation, has been described in these patients. Partial glucocorticoid resistance could explain the finding of increased basal cortisol in HIV-infected patients; but the prevalence and clinical significance of this syndrome are uncertain.

Adrenal Androgens

HIV-infected patients have decreased basal adrenal androgen levels and impaired adrenal androgen responses to ACTH stimulation. Decreased urinary excretion of adrenal androgens has been seen at all stages of HIV infection as well as in HIV-negative intensive care unit patients. Women with HIV infection also have lower levels compared with women without the infection.

Thus, this change may not be specific to HIV infection but may instead be a feature of the physiologic response to illness. In two studies, a fall in DHEA levels predicted progression to AIDS independent of CD4 cell counts. As DHEA has been shown in vitro to inhibit HIV replication, this raised the possibility that the decreased DHEA levels observed in HIV-infected patients might influence the effects of the HIV infection. The efficacy of DHEA replacement in HIV-infected patients has not been demonstrated.

Mineralocorticoids

Although electrolyte disturbances are not uncommon in HIV-infected patients, provocative testing of the mineralocorticoid axis has revealed few abnormalities. Basal and ACTH-stimulated aldosterone levels have been found to be normal in almost all HIV-infected patients studied, including both outpatients and hospitalized individuals. Longitudinal studies suggest that the aldosterone response to ACTH stimulation may diminish with progression to later stages of HIV infection in up to half of HIV-infected patients; however, basal levels of aldosterone and plasma renin activity remain normal, and clinically significant hypoaldosteronism does not develop.

The usual pattern of alterations in adrenal hormones is shown in Table 25–3.

Medication Effects

Several medications used in the treatment of HIV-related disorders can alter glucocorticoid metabolism. Ketoconazole inhibits the cytochrome P450 enzymes P450scc and P450c11, decreasing cortisol synthesis and leading to adrenal insufficiency in patients with decreased adrenal reserve. Rifampin increases hepatic metabolism of steroids and may lead to adrenal insufficiency in patients with marginal adrenal reserve. Megestrol acetate has intrinsic cortisol-like activity and also decreases serum cortisol and ACTH levels through suppression of the hypothalamic-pituitary-adrenal axis

Table 25–3. Usual pattern of adrenal hormones in HIV infection.

	Basal	After ACTH Stimulation
Glucocorticoids	Normal or ↑ cortisol ↓ 17-Deoxysteroids	Normal cortisol response
Mineralocorticoids	Normal	Normal
Androgens	↓	↓

↓ decreased; ↑ increased

centrally. Patients taking megestrol have decreased cortisol and ACTH levels in response to metyrapone testing. HIV protease inhibitors block the metabolism of the inhaled steroid fluticasone by CYP 3A4 and can lead to Cushing's syndrome even in the absence of systemic steroid use.

Medications used to treat HIV-related illnesses can lead to electrolyte disturbances. Trimethoprim impairs sodium channels in the distal nephron, decreasing potassium secretion, which can result in hyperkalemia. Pentamidine has also been associated with hyperkalemia in rare instances, perhaps through nephrotoxicity. Sulfonamides are associated with interstitial nephritis and hyporeninemic hypoaldosteronism. Finally, amphotericin B causes renal potassium and magnesium wasting. Protease inhibitors do not seem to have an effect on plasma cortisol levels. However, there is debate in the literature about whether these agents increase or decrease urinary free cortisol or 17-hydroxycorticosteroid excretion.

Medications used in HIV-infected patients that can affect the endocrine system are listed in Table 25–2.

Summary of Adrenal Disorders

In summary, there is little evidence for clinically significant impairment of adrenal steroid excretion in HIV infection. The subtle alterations in the glucocorticoid and androgen synthesis pathways may be an adaptive response to physiologic stress and may occur with other illnesses. Patients with HIV infection who exhibit symptoms consistent with adrenal hormone deficiency should undergo provocative testing in the same manner as uninfected individuals. Patients with low baseline and abnormal glucocorticoid or mineralocorticoid responses to provocative testing should be treated with physiologic replacement doses of oral glucocorticoids or mineralocorticoids. These patients should also be covered with high doses of glucocorticoids (usually 150–300 mg of hydrocortisone per day or equivalent) during episodes of severe illness. Electrolyte abnormalities should prompt evaluation for medication effects and the presence of renal disease.

The HIV-infected patient with a minimally elevated or frankly high basal cortisol that does not increase significantly after ACTH stimulation poses a difficult problem. Most of these individuals will have normal responses to prolonged ACTH stimulation, and seronegative patients with significant illness can have similar patterns that revert to normal after treatment of the illness. Chronic glucocorticoid therapy may have significant adverse consequences in these individuals, who are already immunocompromised. Most HIV-infected patients with this pattern and even many with baseline low levels during acute illness do not appear to require long-term glucocorticoid replacement. Consideration could be given to administering short courses of steroid therapy during significant illness for individuals with indeterminate stimulation results.

BONE & MINERAL DISORDERS

Calcium and calciotropic hormone disturbances are associated with several HIV-related illnesses and medications. Hypercalcemia with an elevated 1,25-dihyroxyvitamin D level has been associated with both AIDS-related lymphoma and *Mycobacterium avium* complex infection, suggesting increased conversion of 24-hydroxyvitamin D to 1,25-dihydroxyvitamin D by the infection or tumor.

Histomorphometric analysis of bone biopsies from AIDS patients showed decreased bone formation and bone turnover; these changes were more marked in more severely affected patients. Early studies of patients with HIV did not find decreased bone mineral density. However, more recent studies have found osteopenia or even osteoporosis. There is no agreement yet as to whether osteopenia is the result of HIV infection itself, of prior glucocorticoid use during opportunistic infections, of the use of specific antiretroviral drugs such as protease inhibitors, or nucleoside reverse transcriptase inhibitor (NRTI)-induced hyperprolactinemia. There have been no clinical trials evaluating the efficacy of treatment of HIV associated osteopenia, and no current treatment guidelines exist. There is little evidence for an increase in prevalence of classic pathologic fractures of osteoporosis.

Osteonecrosis of the hip has been reported recently both in adults and in children infected with HIV. It is not known whether this condition is associated with HIV infection itself, with antiretroviral therapy, or with opportunistic infection.

Hypocalcemia has occurred during therapy for CMV retinitis with foscarnet, which can complex ionized calcium and may also have mineral wasting effects at the renal tubule, leading to concurrent hypomagnesemia and hypokalemia. Hypocalcemia and hypomagnesemia have also been reported during pentamidine treatment, and the combination of foscarnet and pentamidine can result in severe, even fatal, hypocalcemia.

AIDS patients may have an impaired ability to respond to drug-induced hypocalcemia. PTH levels both at baseline and during EDTA-induced hypocalcemia are decreased in HIV-infected patients compared with seronegative individuals and seronegative hospitalized patients; all groups had normal magnesium levels. In addition to effects on calcium and magnesium, foscarnet can also cause nephrogenic diabetes insipidus. Ketoconazole and rifampin can alter vitamin D metabolism but may not produce clinically significant effects. Ketoconazole can reduce serum levels of 1,25-dihydroxyvitamin D and lower total—but not ionized—calcium levels; rifampin can decrease 25-hydroxyvitamin D levels but does not appear to change calcium or PTH levels.

Medications used in HIV-infected patients that can affect the endocrine system are listed in Table 27–2.

GONADAL DISORDERS

Testicular Function

Histopathologic changes in the testes of AIDS patients are common; decreased spermatogenesis, thickened basement membrane, and an interstitial infiltrate are often seen in autopsy series. The presence of *Mycobacterium avium-intracellulare,* toxoplasma, and CMV in testicular tissue is not unusual in patients systemically infected with these agents. Kaposi's sarcoma has also been reported in the epididymis of an AIDS patient.

Early in HIV infection, testosterone levels appear to be normal or even elevated. Elevated basal LH levels and an increased LH response to GnRH have been demonstrated in these patients, suggesting pituitary dysfunction. Gonadal function appears to be altered more significantly in the later stages of HIV infection. Low serum testosterone levels, often with symptoms of decreased libido or erectile dysfunction, are not uncommon in men with AIDS. In these hypogonadal men, LH and FSH levels have been found to be low, normal, or high. GnRH testing in hypogonadal men with HIV has been normal in most cases. Sex hormone-binding globulin has been found to be normal in HIV-infected men in all but one study. These results suggest that gonadal dysfunction in men with AIDS is not unusual and can occur at the level of the testis, the pituitary, or the hypothalamus.

The hypogonadism seen in AIDS may not be unique to HIV infection; hypogonadism also occurs with other significant systemic illness. This effect may be cytokine-mediated, since IL-1 and TNF can affect testicular function.

Testosterone replacement therapy in hypogonadal men with HIV results in improved sexual functioning, mood, and energy. Whether testosterone increases lean body mass in AIDS patients is controversial. Testosterone therapy does not appear to exacerbate Kaposi's sarcoma, though the studies of this relationship have been small.

Some medications used in the treatment of HIV-related illness can alter testicular function. Ketoconazole inhibits gonadal steroidogenesis, resulting in lower testosterone levels, oligospermia, and gynecomastia. Megestrol acetate, a progesterone-like agent, can lead to decreases in testosterone in HIV-infected men, perhaps through central feedback on gonadotropins.

Medications used in HIV-infected patients that can affect the endocrine system are listed in Table 27–2.

Ovarian Function

Only recently have issues of ovarian function and fertility been explored in women with HIV infection. HIV can directly infect the female reproductive organs. Involvement of the uterine tubes, uterus, and cervix has been demonstrated, but direct ovarian infection has not yet been assessed.

There is little consensus about whether HIV infection is associated with menstrual irregularities and amenorrhea. Recent studies suggest that HIV infection itself has little impact on the menstrual cycle. However, high viral loads and low CD4 counts are associated with increased cycle variation. It is likely that these women have an increased rate of amenorrhea due to the classic euhormone-sick syndrome or a higher catabolic state. Protease inhibitor therapy has been reported to cause hypermenorrhea in a case series of four women. Similar to men, serum testosterone and adrenal androgen levels appear to be lower in women with advanced HIV disease. Androgen-deficient women may have subtle symptoms of decreased energy, libido, mood, strength, and bone mass. Laboratory diagnosis is difficult in the female population. Total testosterone levels may be increased due to elevations in SHBG in HIV-infected women, and free testosterone levels for women have not been well standardized in clinical laboratories. Thus, diagnosis of androgen deficiency in women has been largely restricted to the research setting. Two small clinical trials have shown that transdermal testosterone increased weight and improved quality of life in HIV-infected women and women with AIDS wasting syndrome. Androgen replacement in women should be approached with caution as certain preparations of androgens such as Estratest (combined estrogen and methyltestosterone) can cause liver dysfunction, and progestin replacement is required to prevent endometrial hyperplasia.

Pregnancy does not seem to affect either the maternal progression of HIV disease or the health status of live newborns at birth. Fertility rates in HIV infected women have been difficult to study because of confounding factors such as sociodemographics, drug use, weight loss, systemic illness, and sexually transmitted diseases. Generally, antiretroviral treatment of pregnant women is recommended because it decreases mother-to-child transmission.

PITUITARY DISORDERS

Opportunistic Infections & Neoplasms

In autopsy series of AIDS patients, nearly 10% of pituitary glands demonstrate some degree of infarction or necrosis; infectious organisms such as cytomegalovirus, *P. carinii*, *Cryptococcus*, *Toxoplasma*, and *Aspergillus*

have been observed. Antemortem pituitary function was not reported in these patients.

Anterior Pituitary Function

Anterior hypopituitarism appears to be rare in AIDS patients; stimulation with TRH, GnRH, or CRH results in normal pituitary responses in almost all patients. Likewise, prolactin levels generally have been found to be normal, with a normal response to TRH stimulation. Some patients have shown a higher maximal pituitary response to stimulation testing compared with uninfected subjects, but the clinical significance of this alteration is not known.

The growth hormone axis has received particular attention in children with HIV who can have poor growth velocity, especially when symptomatically ill. Most of these children demonstrate normal GH levels, though low IGF-I levels can be seen. Low IGF-I in the setting of relatively normal GH is often seen in states of malnutrition, which may partially explain this finding. In adults, IGF-I levels may be low in malnourished or symptomatic HIV-infected patients but are usually normal in clinically stable individuals. Circadian GH secretion does not appear to be altered in adults with HIV infection.

Posterior Pituitary Function

Posterior pituitary function may be altered in HIV infection. Hyponatremia is common in both inpatients and outpatients with HIV. Inappropriately high serum antidiuretic hormone levels have been seen in euvolemic AIDS patients with hyponatremia; however, many of these patients had pulmonary or cerebral infections, which themselves can cause the syndrome of inappropriate antidiuretic hormone secretion. As with any patient, destruction of the posterior pituitary by infection or tumor can lead to neurogenic diabetes insipidus; like anterior pituitary destruction, this appears to be rare in HIV infection.

PANCREATIC DISORDERS

Opportunistic infections and tumors can be seen in the pancreases of AIDS patients at autopsy, though the lesions do not appear extensive enough to cause pancreatic dysfunction routinely.

Glucose homeostasis appears to be altered in divergent ways by HIV infection and its therapies. Early in the epidemic, clinically stable HIV-infected men were found to have higher rates of insulin clearance, increased sensitivity of peripheral tissues to insulin, and an increase in nonoxidative glucose disposal. Hepatic glucose production rates tend to increase, perhaps in response to the increased glucose disposal. In contrast, other infectious states, such as sepsis, are accompanied by insulin resistance and hyperglycemia.

Clinically significant pancreatic dysfunction in HIV-infected patients is often related to medication. With the introduction of HAART, insulin resistance has emerged as a problem. Some of the insulin resistance is attributable to protease inhibitor drugs, which can induce insulin resistance rapidly even in HIV-negative volunteers. However, increased insulin resistance has also been found in HIV-infected subjects on NRTI therapy. Indinavir has been shown to increase insulin resistance in HIV-infected subjects and in non-HIV infected, healthy subjects. In vitro studies suggest that indinavir, ritonavir, and amprenavir cause insulin resistance in part by acutely inhibiting the GLUT4 transporter. However, in one study of HIV-infected patients there was no increase in insulin resistance after 48 weeks of treatment with amprenavir. The effects of other protease inhibitor drugs need to be tested in HIV-infected and HIV-seronegative subjects. Hyperglycemia and diabetes in patients treated with protease inhibitors have been reported. The degree to which the prevalence of diabetes is increased in HIV-infected patients on HAART or protease inhibitors is currently under study, but the degree of insulin resistance seen in HIV-infected patients receiving therapy is of a magnitude that could increase the incidence of diabetes, especially in those with susceptibility, such as genetic background. The effects of protease inhibitor drugs on glucose and lipid metabolism are shown in Table 25–4.

Pentamidine causes pancreatic B cell toxicity, acutely leading to hypoglycemia and, over the long term, to diabetes mellitus. Hypoglycemia during pentamidine treatment is associated with increased length of treatment, higher cumulative doses, and renal insuf-

ficiency. Patients who develop hypoglycemia in association with pentamidine therapy are at increased long-term risk of developing diabetes mellitus. HIV-infected patients who develop diabetes mellitus following pentamidine therapy have low C-peptide levels, suggesting cell destruction. Aerosolized pentamidine therapy has also been reported to cause hypoglycemia and diabetes mellitus. Pentamidine—as well as trimethoprim-sulfamethoxazole and the nucleoside analogs ddI and ddC—have been associated with acute pancreatitis.

Megestrol acetate, which has intrinsic glucocorticoid activity, may be associated with diabetes mellitus in HIV-infected patients, though the rate of hyperglycemia in controlled clinical trials appears to be low.

Medications used in HIV-infected patients that can affect the endocrine system are listed in Table 27–2.

LIPID DISORDERS

Triglyceride levels rise progressively with advancing stages of HIV infection and average twice the normal values in patients with symptomatic AIDS infection. The increase in triglycerides appears to be due to an increase in VLDL. Metabolic changes associated with HIV infection that may contribute to the rise in triglycerides include a decrease in lipoprotein lipase activity, increased hepatic synthesis of free fatty acids, and increased peripheral lipolysis. The increased triglyceride levels correlate strongly with circulating levels of interferon alpha. Both triglyceride and interferon alpha levels fall with antiretroviral therapy, though the role of interferon alpha in triglyceride metabolism has not been fully elucidated.

Plasma cholesterol, HDL, and LDL are decreased in patients at early stages of HIV infection and AIDS. HDL levels tend to decrease first and are often low even before clinically significant immunosuppression occurs. The cause of the low cholesterol levels seen in HIV infection has not been determined. These changes occur early in clinically stable individuals and even before immunosuppression; thus, malabsorption does not appear to play a significant role.

During treatment with HIV protease inhibitor drugs, triglyceride, total cholesterol, and LDL levels increase. Given that earlier studies of antiretroviral therapy were associated with decreased triglyceride levels, it is likely that the increase in triglycerides is a direct effect of protease inhibitors. However, the ability to induce hypertriglyceridemia varies among these drugs. Ritonavir-containing regimens are more likely to induce hypertriglyceridemia. Consistent with these findings, ritonavir—but not indinavir—has been shown to increase triglycerides in HIV-negative volunteers. Therapy for hyperlipidemia is complicated by protease in-

Table 25–4. Effect of protease inhibitors on glucose and lipid metabolism.

	HIV Infection Without Protease Inhibitor	HIV Infection With Protease Inhibitor
Glucose	Normal or ↓	Normal or ↑
Insulin sensitivity	↑	↓
Cholesterol	↓	↑ to normal
Triglycerides	↑	↑
LDL	↓	↑ to normal
HDL	↓	↓

↓ decreased; ↑ increased

hibitor inhibition of CYP 3A4, the enzyme responsible for metabolism of simvastatin and lovastatin; use of pravastatin or atorvastatin is a safer way to prevent rhabdomyolysis.

A series of reports of changes in fat distribution, including loss of peripheral fat (extremities and face) or gain in central fat (abdomen and dorsocervical)—or both effects—has been published in cross-sectional studies of patients treated with highly active antiretroviral therapy. Although initially attributed to HIV protease inhibitors, more recent reports of these changes in patients who have not been treated with protease inhibitors raise the possibility that the changes are related to HAART per se or specific NRTI drugs such as stavudine. Immune reconstitution and restoration to health may also play a role. There are no data supporting a linkage between the findings of fat loss and those of central gain, which must be taken into account when attempting to define the causes and effects of these changes in fat depots. A number of therapeutic interventions attempting to treat the adipose changes seen in HIV have had limited success, including recombinant growth hormone, anabolic steroids, metformin, and thiazolidinediones. Growth hormone treatment shows some decrease in truncal fat and increase in lean body mass at 6 months but is accompanied by significant transient insulin resistance. Metformin and thiazolidinediones reverse some metabolic changes. Metformin reduces visceral fat, but neither drug has significantly increased peripheral fat. Long-term effects on body composition, insulin resistance, lipids, and disease outcomes need to be evaluated.

The relationship between changes in body composition and alterations in metabolism such as hyperlipidemia and insulin resistance is also confounded by the effects of the antiretroviral therapies themselves. As mentioned above, protease inhibitor therapy induces hyperlipidemia and insulin resistance, and this has been shown to be independent of fat distribution. However, it is likely that the development of visceral obesity or severe peripheral fat loss will independently contribute both to hypertriglyceridemia and to insulin resistance.

HAART with a protease inhibitor does not have a major effect on the decreased HDL seen in HIV. Therapy with an NNRTI raises HDL in HIV-infected subjects. Both protease inhibitors and NNRTIs raise LDL.

The effects of HIV protease inhibitors on glucose and lipid metabolism are shown in Table 27–4.

The changes in lipid and glucose metabolism seen in HIV raise the question about whether atherosclerosis will be increased due to HIV or its therapies. Although studies published to date are not large enough for definitive answers, it appears that HIV infection itself is accompanied by increased atherosclerosis and that the use of protease inhibitors will lead to little increase. However, NNRTIs have a better antiatherogenic profile.

Anabolic steroids in experimental use for HIV-associated wasting and lipodystrophy raise LDL and dramatically lower HDL, leading to an atherogenic profile. Medications used in HIV-infected patients that can affect the endocrine system are listed in Table 27–2.

CONCLUSION

Many of the endocrine and metabolic changes that occur in HIV infection and AIDS are similar to the changes associated with any serious illness. The approaches to diagnosis and therapy are therefore the same as in other illnesses. Many of the changes that are unique to HIV infection do not have clear clinical significance. However, drug-induced changes are common and should be searched for.

In the past, the prognosis of AIDS has been poor. Now that highly active antiretroviral therapy is increasing life span, the long-term implications for endocrine and metabolic changes need to be determined.

REFERENCES

General

Sellmeyer DE, Grunfeld C: Endocrine and metabolic disturbances in human immunodeficiency virus infection and the acquired immune deficiency syndrome. Endocr Rev 1996;17:518.

Thyroid

Grunfeld C et al: Indices of thyroid function and weight loss in human immunodeficiency virus infection and the acquired immunodeficiency syndrome. Metabolism 1993;42:1270.

Hommes M et al: Hypothyroid-like regulation of the pituitary-thyroid axis in stable human immunodeficiency virus infection. Metabolism 1993;42:556.

Jubault V et al: Sequential occurrence of thyroid autoantibodies and Graves' disease after immune restoration in severely immunocompromised human immunodeficiency virus-1-infected patients. J Clin Endocrinol Metab 2000;85:4254. [PMID: 11095463]

LoPresti J et al: Unique alterations of thyroid hormone indices in the acquired immunodeficiency syndrome. Ann Intern Med 1989;110:970.

Adrenal

Findling J et al: Longitudinal evaluation of adrenocortical function in patients infected with the human immunodeficiency virus. J Clin Endocrinol Metab 1994;79:1091.

Honour J, Schneider M, Miller R: Low adrenal androgens in men with HIV infection and the acquired immunodeficiency syndrome. Horm Res 1995;44:35.

Jacobson M et al: Decreased serum dehydroepiandrosterone is associated with an increased progression of human immunodeficiency virus infection in men with CD4 cell counts of 200–499. J Infect Dis 1991;164:864.

Mayo J et al: Adrenal function in the human immunodeficiency virus-infected patient. Arch Intern Med 2002;162:1095. [PMID: 12020177]

Membreno L et al: Adrenocortical function in acquired immunodeficiency syndrome. J Clin Endocrinol Metab 1987;65:482.

Norbiato G et al: Glucocorticoid resistance and the immune function in the immunodeficiency syndrome. Ann N Y Acad Sci 1998;840:835.

Bone and Mineral

Aukrust P et al: Decreased bone formative and enhanced resorptive markers in immunodeficiency virus infection: indication of normalization of the bone-remodeling process during highly active antiretroviral therapy. J Clin Endocrinol Metab 1999;84:145. [PMID: 9920075]

Jaeger P et al: Altered parathyroid gland function in severely immunocompromised patients infected with human immunodeficiency virus. J Clin Endocrinol Metab 1994;79:1701.

Paton NIJ et al: Bone mineral density in patients with human immunodeficiency virus infection. Calcif Tissue Int 1997;61:30.

Miller KD et al: High prevalence of osteonecrosis of the femoral head in HIV-infected adults. Ann Intern Med 2002;137:17. [PMID: 12093241]

Serrano S et al: Bone remodeling in human immunodeficiency virus-1-infected patients. A histomorphometric study. Bone 1995;16:185.

Gonads

Chirgwin K et al: Menstrual function in human immunodeficiency virus-infected women without acquired immunodeficiency syndrome. J Acquir Immune Defic Syndr Hum Retrovirol 1996;12:489.

Ellerbrock T et al: Characteristics of menstruation in women infected with human immunodeficiency virus. Obstet Gynecol 1996;87:1030.

Lo JC, Schambelan M. Reproductive function in human immunodeficiency virus infection. J Clin Endocrinol Metab 2001;86:2338. [PMID: 11397819]

Rabkin JG, Wagner GJ, Rabkin R: Testosterone therapy for human immunodeficiency virus-positive men with and without hypogonadism. J Clin Psychopharmacol 1999;19:19. [PMID: 9934939]

Shah PN et al: Menstrual symptoms in women infected by the human immunodeficiency virus. Obstet Gynecol 1994;83:397.

Pituitary

Agarwal A et al: Hyponatremia in patients with the acquired immunodeficiency syndrome. Nephron 1989;53:317.

Dobs A et al: Endocrine disorders in men infected with the human immunodeficiency virus. Am J Med 1988;84:611.

Pancreas

Bouchard P et al: Diabetes mellitus following pentamidine-induced hypoglycemia in humans. Diabetes 1982;31:40.

Carr A et al: Diagnosis, prediction, and natural course of HIV-1 protease-inhibitor-associated lipodystrophy, hyperlipidaemia, and diabetes mellitus: a cohort study. Lancet 1999;353:2093. [PMID: 10382692]

Hadigan C et al: Fasting hyperinsulinemia and changes in regional body composition in human immunodeficiency virus-infected women. J Clin Endocrinol Metab 1999;84:1932.

Heyligenberg R et al: Non-insulin-mediated glucose uptake in human immunodeficiency virus-infected men. Clin Sci 1993;84:209.

Hommes M et al: Insulin sensitivity and insulin clearance in human immunodeficiency virus-infected men. Metabolism 1991;40:651.

Kaufman MB, Simionatto C: A review of protease inhibitor-induced hyperglycemia. Pharmacotherapy 1999;19:114.

Murata H, Hruz PW, Mueckler M: Indinavir inhibits the glucose transporter isoform Glut4 at physiologic concentrations. AIDS 2002;16:859. [PMID: 11919487]

Noor MA et al: Metabolic effects of indinavir in healthy HIV-seronegative men. AIDS 2001;15:F11. [PMID: 11399973]

Osei K et al: Diabetogenic effect of pentamidine: in vitro and in vivo studies in a patient with malignant insulinoma. Am J Med 1984;77:41.

Uzzan B et al: Effects of aerosolized pentamidine on glucose homeostasis and insulin secretion in HIV-positive patients: a controlled study. AIDS 1995;9:901.

Waskin H et al: Risk factors for hypoglycemia associated with pentamidine therapy for *Pneumocystis* pneumonia. JAMA 1988;260:345.

Lipids

Carr A et al: Diagnosis, prediction, and natural course of HIV-1 protease-inhibitor-associated lipodystrophy, hyperlipidaemia, and diabetes mellitus: a cohort study. Lancet 1999;353:2093. [PMID: 10382692]

Dong KL et al: Changes in body habitus and serum lipid abnormalities in HIV-positive women on highly active antiretroviral therapy (HAART). J Acquir Immune Defic Syndr Hum Retrovirol 1999;21:107. [PMID: 10360801]

Gervasoni C et al: Redistribution of body fat in HIV-infected women undergoing combined antiretroviral therapy. AIDS 1999;13:465. [PMID: 10197374]

Grunfeld C et al: Lipids, lipoproteins, triglyceride clearance, and cytokines in human immunodeficiency virus infection and the acquired immunodeficiency syndrome. J Clin Endocrinol Metab 1992;74:1045.

Lo JC et al: The effects of recombinant human growth hormone on body composition and glucose metabolism in HIV-infected patients with fat accumulation. J Clin Endocrinol Metab 2001;86:3480. [PMID: 11502767]

Mulligan K et al: Hyperlipidemia and insulin resistance are induced by protease inhibitors independent of changes in body composition in patients with HIV infection. J Acq Immune Defic Syndr Hum Retrovirol 2000;23:35. [PMID: 10708054]

Safrin S, Grunfeld C: Fat distribution and metabolic changes in patients with HIV infection. AIDS 1999;13:2493. [PMID: 10630518]

Saint-Marc T et al: Fat distribution evaluated by computed tomography and metabolic abnormalities in patients undergoing antiretroviral therapy: preliminary results of the LIPOCO study. AIDS 2000;14:37. [PMID: 10714566]

Endocrine Surgery

26

Geeta Lal, MD, & Orlo H. Clark, MD

INTRODUCTION

Many endocrine diseases are managed by surgical treatment. The details of clinical presentation, diagnosis, and medical management are discussed in other sections of this book. This chapter provides an overview of the principles involved in the surgical therapy for these conditions. The results of endocrine surgical operations are usually most satisfying with removal of the tumor and correction of the metabolic problem it creates.

■ THE THYROID GLAND

EMBRYOLOGY & ANATOMY

The thyroid gland arises in the midline as an endoderm-derived pharyngeal diverticulum at about the third week of gestation. It then descends from its origin at the foramen cecum and ultimately forms a bilobed organ anterolateral to the trachea and larynx. The thyroid lobes are connected just below the cricoid cartilage by an isthmus. The connection to the foramen cecum—the thyroglossal duct—ruptures and is partially resorbed by the sixth week of gestation. Its distal remnant forms the pyramidal lobe. The calcitonin-producing C cells, located posteriorly in the superior gland, arise from the fourth pharyngeal pouch and ultimobranchial bodies.

A number of embryologic or developmental abnormalities of the thyroid have been described and are related to the absence or mutations of thyroid differentiation factors, including thyroid transcription factors 1 and 2 (TTF-1, TTF-2) and transcription factor Pax 8. Thyroglossal duct cysts are usually found in the midline, just inferior to the hyoid bone. A lingual thyroid results from maldescent of the median thyroid anlage and is often accompanied by agenesis of other thyroid tissue. Rests of thyroid tissue may be found in the central compartment of the neck and can be mistaken for metastatic thyroid cancer at operation. Aberrant thyroid tissue, unassociated with lymph nodes, can also be found in the lateral neck or mediastinum. In contrast to the above, thyroid tissue in lymph nodes in the lateral neck (lateral aberrant rests) almost always represents metastatic thyroid cancer and is not a developmental abnormality.

The thyroid gland is supplied by paired superior and inferior thyroid arteries. The former arise from the external carotid artery and the latter from the thyrocervical trunk. Occasionally, a thyroid ima artery arises directly from the aorta or innominate artery and enters the isthmus, replacing an absent inferior artery (see Fig. 7-3).

The thyroid is drained by three sets of veins: the superior, middle, and inferior thyroid veins. The first two drain into the internal jugular vein, whereas the last drains into the innominate veins. Both recurrent laryngeal nerves arise from their respective vagus nerves and enter the larynx at the level of the cricothyroid articulation, posterior to the cricothyroid muscle. The left recurrent laryngeal nerve recurs around the ligamentum arteriosum and ascends to the larynx in the tracheoesophageal groove. The right recurrent laryngeal nerve recurs around the subclavian artery and runs 1–2 cm lateral to the tracheoesophageal groove at the level of the clavicle and courses obliquely to the larynx. The superior laryngeal nerves also arise from corresponding vagus nerves and divide into internal and external branches. The former provides sensation to the larynx and the latter innervates the cricothyroid muscles. A description of parathyroid embryology and anatomy is presented in the next section.

There is considerable controversy in the literature regarding the definitions of various thyroid resections. A description of these terms is presented in Table 26–1.

INDICATIONS FOR SURGERY
DEVELOPMENTAL THYROID ABNORMALITIES

Thyroglossal duct remnants may become symptomatic, forming cysts, abscesses and fistulas. There is also a 1% risk of thyroid cancer development in thyroglossal duct

902

Table 26–1. Definitions of various thyroid resections.

Procedure	Description
Nodulectomy or lumpectomy	Removal of lesion with minimal surrounding tissue
Partial thyroidectomy	Removal of lesion and larger rim of normal tissue
Subtotal thyroidectomy	Bilateral removal of > 50% of each lobe and an isthmusectomy
Lobectomy or hemithyroidectomy	Complete removal of a lobe and isthmus
Near-total thyroidectomy	Complete removal of one lobe and isthmus and all but 1 g (1 cm) of the contralateral lobe (tissue near ligament of Berry)
Total thyroidectomy	Complete removal of both thyroid lobes, isthmus, and pyramidal lobe

cysts. Most are papillary carcinomas, but very rarely a squamous cell carcinoma may develop. Medullary thyroid cancers do not occur at this site.

Treatment consists of the Sistrunk procedure, which involves removal of the cyst and duct up to the foramen cecum. Since the duct may pass anterior to, posterior to, or through the hyoid bone, the mid section of this bone is also resected. Surgery may also be needed for enlarged lingual thyroid tissue causing symptoms such as choking and dysphagia. Prior to resection, care must be taken to determine whether the patient has any other functioning thyroid tissue, usually via a thyroid scan.

HYPERTHYROIDISM

Hyperthyroidism most commonly results from a diffuse toxic goiter (Graves' disease), toxic multinodular goiter, or a single toxic nodule (Plummer's disease). Rarer causes of hyperthyroidism with increased radioactive iodine uptake (RAIU) include a TSH-secreting tumor and a hydatidiform mole. Causes of hyperthyroidism without increased RAIU include subacute thyroiditis, excessive ingestion of medicinal thyroid hormone or cooked thyroid tissue, struma ovarii, and thyroid hormone-secreting metastatic thyroid cancer. These conditions present with the usual symptoms and signs of hyperthyroidism but lack the extrathyroidal manifestations of Graves' disease such as ophthalmopathy, pretibial myxedema, and thyroid acropachy.

Diagnostic Tests

TSH is suppressed and T_3, T_4, free T_4 index, and T_3 uptake are increased. As mentioned, RAIU can be used to distinguish the various causes of hyperthyroidism. Graves' disease is also associated with thyroid-stimulating antibodies.

Management of Hyperthyroidism

Hyperthyroidism may be treated medically with antithyroid medications, but medical treatment is associated with a high failure rate, particularly in patients with large goiters. Destruction of the thyroid gland with radioactive iodine (RAI) is the mainstay of treatment in North America for patients over 30 years of age. However, it is associated with a prolonged latency period before effective action, a slightly increased risk of future benign and malignant thyroid tumors, worsening ophthalmopathy, and unavoidable hypothyroidism (3% per year after the first year, independently of dosage). Furthermore, it is contraindicated in pregnant women, of concern in children, and should be avoided in women wishing to become pregnant for up to 1 year after treatment. Surgery overcomes many of the problems associated with RAI.

Absolute indications for thyroidectomy in patients with Graves' disease include biopsy-proved suspicious or cancerous nodules, local compressive symptoms, reluctance to have RAI, or fear of recurrence after RAI. Women who want to become pregnant after treatment and those who are not controlled or who develop side effects from antithyroid drugs during pregnancy are also candidates for surgery, as are children. Relative indications for thyroidectomy include patients in whom rapid control of the disease is desired, poorly compliant patients, and patients with severe ophthalmopathy, very large goiters, or low RAI uptake.

Preoperative Preparation

Patients are usually treated with antithyroid medications to render them euthyroid and to reduce the risk of thyroid storm. Propylthiouracil (100–200 mg three times daily) or methimazole (10–20 mg three times daily and then once daily) is most often used. In patients who develop agranulocytosis, surgery should be deferred until granulocyte counts reach 1000 cells/μL. In addition, patients are also often treated with propranolol (10–40 mg four times daily) to control the catecholamine response. Relatively large doses may be necessary because of increased catabolism of the drug. Lugol's solution (iodine and potassium iodide) or saturated solution of potassium iodide (3 drops twice daily) is also started about 10 days preoperatively to reduce the vascularity of the gland.

Extent of Surgery

The extent of surgery depends on multiple factors. Patients who have had severe complications with antithyroid drugs, those who want to eliminate the risk of recurrence, and those with carcinoma or severe ophthalmopathy should undergo total or near-total thyroidectomy. The rate of hypothyroidism after surgery ranges from 3% to 48% and is lower than that after RAI therapy. It is primarily determined by the remnant size, the thyroid antibody titer, and whether hypothyroidism was reported to be subclinical or overt. Remnants less than 4 g are associated with an over 50% risk of hypothyroidism, and those greater than 8 g are associated with recurrence rates of 15%. Most surgeons prefer to leave a 4–7 g remnant in adults and a smaller remnant in children. The goal of treatment is usually to make the patient euthyroid while minimizing the risk of recurrence and hypothyroidism. Some surgeons prefer total or near-total thyroidectomy to avoid any chance of recurrence and because it may help patients with Graves' ophthalmopathy. Thyroidectomy can be accomplished safely by bilateral subtotal excision or by the Hartley-Dunhill operation (unilateral lobectomy and isthmusectomy with subtotal contralateral resection). Patients who experience recurrence after surgery are usually treated with RAI.

Patients with hyperthyroidism secondary to toxic multinodular goiter are managed similarly. Those with a solitary toxic nodule are treated by ipsilateral lobectomy and isthmusectomy. Most patients with functioning thyroid nodules and hyperthyroidism have nodules greater than 3 cm.

THYROIDITIS

Acute suppurative thyroiditis is diagnosed by fine-needle aspiration for cytology, smear, Gram stain, and culture and treated by incision and drainage. Thyroidectomy is occasionally needed for clinically co-existent suspicious or cytologically positive thyroid nodules, local compressive symptoms, or persistent infection. Recurrent acute thyroiditis is often due to a fistula from the piriform sinus.

NODULAR GOITER

Thyroidectomy is indicated for multinodular goiters enlarging despite thyroxine suppression, those causing compressive symptoms (choking, dysphagia, hoarseness, positive Pemberton's sign—dilation of neck veins upon elevation of arms), and those containing biopsy-proved suspicious or cancerous nodules. Lobectomy is performed on the side with the concerning nodule, and subtotal thyroidectomy is performed if the contralateral side is abnormal.

THYROID NODULES

Approximately 4% of the North American population develop thyroid nodules. However, the incidence of clinical thyroid cancer is much lower (about 40 patients per million). A thyroid nodule is more likely to be malignant if the patient has a history of therapeutic radiation to the head and neck (6.5–3000 cGy to the thyroid), a family history of thyroid cancer, Cowden's syndrome, or MEN 2, and a history of thyroid cancer. Other features suggesting cancer include male sex, young (under 20) or old (over 70) age; a solitary, "cold" solid (or mixed solid-cystic), hard nodule; the presence of ipsilateral palpable nodes or vocal cord palsy; and a fine-needle aspiration biopsy suspicious of or diagnostic for cancer. About 40% of individuals with a history of therapeutic radiation exposure or a family history of thyroid cancer and a "cold" thyroid nodule will have a thyroid cancer. The cancer is in the index nodule in 60% but may be anywhere in the remaining thyroid in 40% of patients.

Patients with thyroid nodules should be evaluated with TSH measurement and a fine-needle aspiration biopsy. If the biopsy suggests a follicular neoplasm, an RAI scan should be performed to rule out a hot nodule. Most of these patients will have a suppressed serum TSH level.

Nodules with any of the worrisome features mentioned above should be removed with—at minimum—an ipsilateral lobectomy and isthmusectomy.

THYROID CANCER

Malignant thyroid tumors include differentiated lesions (which arise from follicular cells), medullary thyroid cancer (MTC), undifferentiated or anaplastic cancers, and other rare tumors such as lymphomas, squamous cell carcinomas, sarcomas, teratomas, plasmacytomas, paragangliomas, and metastatic thyroid cancers (from melanoma or from breast, kidney, lung, and other head-neck tumors).

1. Differentiated Thyroid Cancer

This group includes papillary, follicular variant of papillary, follicular, and Hürthle cell tumors. Hürthle cell carcinoma has been considered a subtype of follicular carcinoma by some investigators and a unique differentiated thyroid cancer of follicular cell origin by others. The characteristics of these tumors are depicted in Table 26–2. The biologic behavior of the follicular variant is similar to that of papillary carcinoma. In follicular and Hürthle cell tumors, the diagnosis of malig-

Table 26–2. Characteristics of differentiated thyroid cancers.

Feature	Papillary	Follicular	Hürthle
Frequency	80%	10–20%	3–5%
Age group (years)	20–30	40–50	50–60
Multicentric	85%	10%	30%
Lymph node metastases	30–40%	10%	25%
Distant metastases	2–14%	33%	15%
RAI uptake	70%	80%	10%
Prognosis (10-year survival)	95%	85%	65%

nancy can only be made by the presence of capsular, blood vessel, or lymphatic invasion or when lymph node or distant metastases are present. Familial nonmedullary thyroid cancers—especially if there is a family history of more than two affected relatives—are thought to be more aggressive than the sporadic variant.

Surgical Treatment

Occult or minimal papillary carcinomas (< 1 cm) have an excellent prognosis and are adequately treated by lobectomy and isthmusectomy. Patients with high-risk cancers (determined by AGES, AMES, or TNM classification; see Tables 26–3, 26–4, and 26–5) or bilateral cancers are best treated by total or near-total thyroidectomy. Considerable debate exists regarding optimal treatment for low-risk differentiated thyroid cancer.

Proponents of total thyroidectomy argue that this procedure is advantageous for several reasons: RAI can

Table 26–3. AGES system of classifying high-risk patients.[1]

Variable	Description
Age	Women older than 50 years Men older than 40 years
Grade	Poorly differentiated Fibrous stroma Insular, mucoid, and tall cell variants
Extent	Invasive to adjacent tissues or distant metastases
Size	Tumor with a maximum diameter of > 4 cm

[1]Reproduced, with permission, from Clark OH. Papillary thyroid carcinoma: Rationale for total thyroidectomy. In: *Textbook of Endocrine Surgery*. Clark OH, Duh Q-Y (editors). Saunders, 1997

Table 26–4. AMES system for classifying high-risk patients.

Variable	Description
Age	Men > 40 years, women > 50 years
Metastases	Distant metastases
Extent	Invasion of adjacent tissues
Size	> 5 cm

be used to diagnose and treat recurrent or metastatic disease; serum thyroglobulin becomes a sensitive indicator of recurrent disease; the procedure eliminates the risk of occult cancer in the contralateral lobe and reduces the risk of recurrence; it decreases the 1% risk of progression to undifferentiated cancer; it improves survival in patients with tumors over 1.5 cm in diameter; and it decreases the risk of reoperation in case of central neck recurrence. On the other hand, those favoring thyroid lobectomy note that total thyroidectomy is associated with a higher complication rate and that 50% of local recurrences can be cured with surgery. Furthermore, it is argued that under 5% of recurrences occur in the thyroid bed; that multicentricity is not clinically significant; and that the prognosis is excellent in low-risk patients undergoing lobectomy.

Retrospective data indicate that the recurrence rate for patients with low-risk differentiated thyroid cancer

Table 26–5. TNM[1] staging system for papillary or follicular thyroid cancer.[2,3]

Stage	Age < 45 years	Age ≥ 45 Years
I	Any T Any N M0	T1 N0 M0
II	Any T Any N M1	T2 N0 M0
III		T3 N0 M0 T1–3 N1a M0
IV		T4 N0 M0 T1–4 N1b M0 Any T Any N M1

[1]TNM: Primary tumor size, nodal status, distant metastasis status. T1: ≤ 2 cm; T2: 2–4 cm; T3: > 4 cm; T4: any size with local extension. N0: no node metastases; N1a: central nodal metastases; N1b: lateral nodal metastases. M0: no distant metastases; M1: distant metastases. See Table 7–16.
[2]Abbreviated and reproduced, with permission, from American Joint Committee on Cancer: *AJCC Cancer Staging Manual*, 6th ed. Greene FL et al (editors). Springer, 2002.
[3]See also Figure 7–16.

is 10% and that the overall mortality rate is about 4% at 10–20 years. However, among patients who have recurrences, 33–50% die from thyroid cancer. These studies also indicate that near-total or total thyroidectomy resulted in a lower incidence of recurrences and improved survival. Since the most important information regarding risk for recurrence is only available postoperatively, the authors recommend near-total or total thyroidectomy for virtually all patients with differentiated thyroid cancer providing that the hospital complication rates are low (< 2%) and comparable to those compiled from experience with lesser procedures.

It is not usually possible to distinguish follicular and Hürthle cell carcinomas from corresponding adenomas preoperatively. If there are no obvious signs of cancer at surgery (lymphadenopathy, extra-thyroidal invasion), a lobectomy is performed since more than 80% of these tumors will be benign. If final pathology confirms cancer, a completion thyroidectomy is usually recommended.

2. Medullary Thyroid Cancer

This tumor comprises 7% of thyroid malignancies but accounts for about 17% of thyroid cancer-related deaths. It arises from the parafollicular (C cells) of the thyroid, which are derived from the neural crest and secrete calcitonin. Medullary thyroid cancers may be sporadic (75%) or may occur in the setting of MEN 2a, MEN 2b, and familial non-MEN medullary thyroid cancer. In the hereditary setting, the tumors are often bilateral and multicentric (90%). About 50% of patients with sporadic or familial disease have nodal metastases in the central or lateral neck at presentation. All patents presenting with medullary thyroid cancer should be screened for pheochromocytomas, hyperparathyroidism, and mutations of the *RET* proto-oncogene.

Pheochromocytomas should be treated prior to thyroidectomy. Total thyroidectomy and bilateral central compartment lymphadenectomy is the treatment of choice.

3. Undifferentiated (Anaplastic) Thyroid Cancer

This tumor type constitutes about 1% of thyroid cancers and is the most aggressive variant. The peak incidence is in the seventh decade of life. Lymph node involvement is early and common (84%), as is local invasion into the larynx, vocal cords, recurrent laryngeal nerve, esophagus, and major vessels. About 75% of patients have distant metastases. The role of surgery is usually limited to palliation of obstruction by tumor debulking and tracheostomy. In patients without advanced disease, total or near-total thyroidectomy can be performed for cure in a minority of cases. External beam radiation and chemotherapy are usually recommended.

4. Management of Lymph Nodes in Thyroid Cancer

Several retrospective studies have suggested that lymph node metastases do not have a significant effect on survival in papillary thyroid cancers. However, some studies report that when patients are matched for age and have matted nodes—or extranodal invasion—the recurrence rate is higher and the prognosis is worse. Routine prophylactic lymph node dissections are not recommended for papillary and follicular thyroid cancers.

The lymph node regions of the neck are depicted in Figure 26–1. Central compartment nodes (medial to the carotid sheath) are removed at the time of thyroidectomy if involved with tumor. Gross nodal disease in the lateral compartments (II, III, IV, and V) is removed via ipsilateral modified radical neck dissection, which removes all the fibrofatty and lymph node tissue while preserving the internal jugular vein, the accessory nerve, the sensory nerves, and the sternocleidomastoid muscle. Since both Hürthle cell and medullary thyroid cancers have a worse prognosis and do not routinely take up RAI, prophylactic central neck lymph node clearance is recommended. An ipsilateral (or bilateral) prophylactic modified radical neck dissection is also recommended for medullary cancers over 1.5 cm in diameter and when the central neck nodes are involved. Contralateral neck nodes are often involved in medullary thyroid cancers. Since thyroid cancers rarely metastasize to compartment I, these nodes are not routinely removed.

5. Recurrent & Metastatic Thyroid Cancer

Thyroid cancers metastasize to the lungs, bone, liver, and brain. In general, patients with macronodular disease (> 1 cm in diameter) should be treated surgically followed by RAI therapy and TSH suppression (see Chapter 7).

CONDUCT OF THYROIDECTOMY

A 4- to 5-cm incision is placed in or parallel to a natural skin crease 1 cm below the cricoid cartilage. The subcutaneous tissue and platysma are divided, and the strap muscles are separated in the midline from the thyroid cartilage to the suprasternal notch. Initial dissection is begun in the midline by identification of delphian

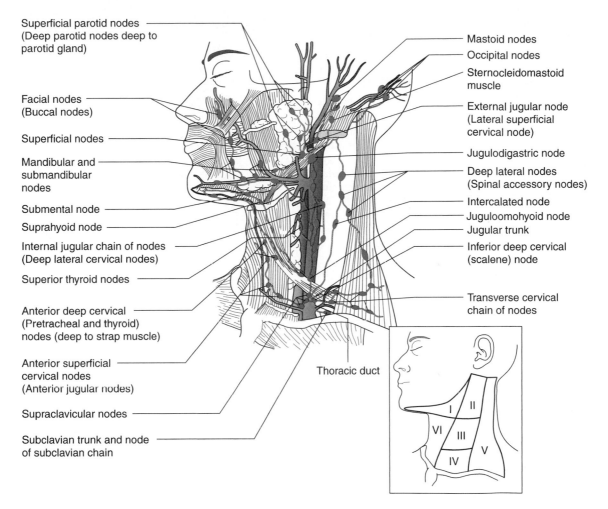

Superficial parotid nodes
(Deep parotid nodes deep to
parotid gland)

Facial nodes
(Buccal nodes)

Superficial nodes

Mandibular and
submandibular
nodes

Submental node

Suprahyoid node

Internal jugular chain of nodes
(Deep lateral cervical nodes)

Superior thyroid nodes

Anterior deep cervical
(Pretracheal and thyroid)
nodes (deep to strap muscle)

Anterior superficial
cervical nodes
(Anterior jugular nodes)

Supraclavicular nodes

Subclavian trunk and node
of subclavian chain

Mastoid nodes

Occipital nodes

Sternocleidomastoid
muscle

External jugular node
(Lateral superficial
cervical node)

Jugulodigastric node

Deep lateral nodes
(Spinal accessory nodes)

Intercalated node

Juguloomohyoid node

Jugular trunk

Inferior deep cervical
(scalene) node

Transverse cervical
chain of nodes

Thoracic duct

Figure 26–1. Lymph node regions of the neck. Level I = submandibular; level II, III, and IV = upper, middle, and lower jugular nodes; level V = posterior triangle nodes; and level VI = central compartment nodes. (Reproduced, with permission, from Roseman BJ, Clark OH: Neck masses. In: *ACS Surgery—Principles and Practice.* Wilmore DW et al [editors]. WebMD Corporation, 2002.)

nodes and the pyramidal lobe, followed by division of the fascia just cephalad to the isthmus. The trachea is then cleared just caudal to the isthmus. The thyrothymic ligaments and the inferior thyroid veins are ligated and divided. The side with the dominant or suspicious mass is approached first. In case of a proposed lobectomy or the absence of cancer, the isthmus is divided. The superior pole vessels are then individually ligated and divided low on the thyroid gland to decrease the risk of injury to the external branch of the superior laryngeal nerve. Tissues are swept lateral to the thyroid by blunt dissection, and the middle thyroid veins are ligated and divided. The recurrent laryngeal

nerve and the superior parathyroid gland are identified at the level of the inferior thyroid artery just caudal to the cricoid cartilage. Once this is accomplished, the ligament of Berry is divided and the thyroid is sharply dissected off the trachea. The same procedure is repeated on the other side for a total thyroidectomy.

Postoperatively, patients are positioned with the back and head elevated 20 degrees. Oral intake is resumed in a few hours, and they are discharged on the first postoperative day.

Several approaches to minimally invasive thyroidectomy such as video-assisted thyroidectomy and endoscopic thyroidectomy via axillary incisions have been proposed. These methods are feasible, but clear benefits over the traditional open approach have not been established.

Complications of Thyroidectomy

General complications after thyroid surgery include bleeding, and wound complications including infection and keloid formation. Specific complications include injury to the recurrent laryngeal nerve (< 1%), or external branch of the superior laryngeal nerve, temporary hypocalcemia (1.6–50%), permanent hypocalcemia (< 2% for total thyroidectomy), and injury to surrounding structures such as the esophagus, major vessels (carotid artery, internal jugular vein), and the cervical sympathetic trunk. Complications increase with tumor stage and decrease with surgeon experience.

■ THE PARATHYROID GLAND

EMBRYOLOGY & ANATOMY

Around the fourth week of gestation, the embryo forms five pairs of endoderm-lined pharyngeal pouches. The inferior parathyroid glands are derived from the third branchial pouch (with the thymus), whereas the superior glands arise from the fourth branchial pouch. Since the inferior glands migrate farther, they are more liable to be found in ectopic locations.

Most individuals have four parathyroid glands that are found as paired structures on the posterior aspect of the thyroid gland. Supernumerary glands occur in up to 22% of people. Fewer than four glands have also been reported in 3–5% of individuals. About 85% of parathyroid glands are found within 1 cm of the point of intersection of the recurrent laryngeal nerve and the inferior thyroid artery. The superior parathyroid glands are usually dorsal to the nerve, whereas the inferior glands are usually ventral to it. The glands may also be found in several ectopic locations (Table 26–6; Figure 26–2). The blood supply to the parathyroid glands is

Table 26–6. Ectopic positions of parathyroid glands.

Superior Glands	Inferior Glands
Tracheoesophageal groove	Thyrothymic ligament
Carotid sheath	Intrathymic
Posterior mediastinum	Carotid sheath
Intrathyroidal	Intrathyroidal
	Anterior mediastinum

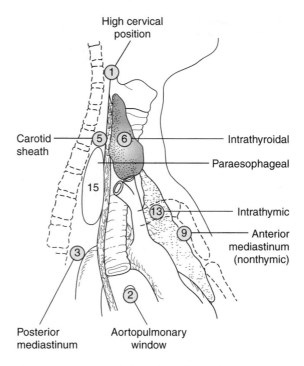

Figure 26–2. Ectopic locations of parathyroid tumors found at reoperation after an initial failed neck exploration. The numbers indicate the actual number of glands found at each location (n = 54). (Reproduced, with permission, from Shen W et al. Reoperation for persistent or recurrent primary hyperparathyroidism. Arch Surg 1996;131:861. Copyright © 1996 by the American Medical Association.)

primarily via the inferior thyroid arteries, but the superior thyroid arteries may also supply both the upper and the lower glands.

INDICATIONS FOR SURGERY

PRIMARY HYPERPARATHYROIDISM

This disorder occurs in 1:500 women and 1:2000 men. It is the most common cause of hypercalcemia in the outpatient population, and along with malignancy-associated hypercalcemia accounts for about 90% of cases of hypercalcemia. It is most often sporadic but may also be inherited as a component of MEN 1 (90–100%), MEN 2a (30%), familial hyperparathyroidism, and familial hyperparathyroidism with jaw tumor syndrome. In sporadic cases, hyperparathyroidism is due to a single enlarged gland (adenoma) in 85% of cases, multiple enlarged glands (hyperplasia) in 11%, double adenomas in 3%, and parathyroid carcinoma in 1%. Parathyroid carcinoma is suspected if patients present with a short history, profound hypercalcemia, and a palpable parathyroid gland. In heritable disorders, hyperparathyroidism is more frequently associated with multiple abnormal parathyroid glands and a higher risk of persistent or recurrent disease. Familial hyperparathyroidism with jaw tumor syndrome is associated with an increased risk of parathyroid cancer.

The classic symptoms of primary hyperparathyroidism include "painful bones, renal stones, abdominal groans, psychic moans, and fatigue overtones." Other symptoms such as polyuria, nocturia, polydipsia, constipation, and musculoskeletal aches and pains may be present. The disorder may also be associated with hypertension, gout, pseudogout, osteopenia, osteoporosis, peptic ulcer disease, and pancreatitis.

Diagnostic Tests

Other causes of hypercalcemia should be excluded. The laboratory tests useful in making the diagnosis are shown in Table 26–7. Primary hyperparathyroidism is characterized by hypercalcemia (95%), hypophosphatemia (50%), hyperchloremia (30%), chloride to phosphate ratio ≥ 33 (95%), elevated 24-hour urinary calcium, and an increased or inappropriately elevated intact parathyroid hormone (PTH). An elevated alkaline phosphatase level suggests bone disease (osteitis fibrosa cystica). Parathyroid tumors are localized using noninvasive means such as Tc-99m sestamibi and ultrasound scanning. MRI scans and invasive localizing studies, including arteriograms, highly selective venous catheterization for PTH, and fine-needle aspiration biopsy of suspected parathyroid masses are only used in cases of recurrent or persistent hyperparathyroidism. Most studies are less sensitive for detecting multiple abnormal glands. Noninvasive localizing studies (Tc-99m sestamibi, ultrasound) are generally used at initial exploration if a focal approach is planned (see Chapter 8).

Table 26–7. Diagnostic tests for primary hyperparathyroidism.

Test	Alteration
Serum tests	
Calcium	Increased
Phosphorus	Decreased
Intact PTH	Increased
Chloride/phosphate ratio	> 33
Alkaline phosphatase	Increased
24-hour urinary calcium	Increased

Surgical Management

A. Asymptomatic Patients

The definition and management of this group of patients are controversial. Most of these patients are diagnosed by screening blood tests performed for other reasons. The 1990 National Institutes of Health consensus conference considered patients to be asymptomatic if they had none of the common symptoms or signs of hyperparathyroidism, including bone, renal, gastrointestinal, or neuromuscular disorders. The consensus guidelines for surgical treatment in this population are outlined in Table 26–8. It was also stated that "medical surveillance may be justified in patients over 50 years old whose renal and bone status are close to normal." This view stemmed from observational studies that suggested stability with respect to serum calcium, stones, and renal function with time. However, more recent investigations suggest that true asymptomatic hyperparathyroidism is rare. Renal function and bone density do improve in this group of patients after surgery, as do neuropsychiatric symptoms and nonspecific symptoms such as fatigue and malaise. Furthermore, parathyroidectomy has also been associated with improved survival (in both asymptomatic and symptomatic patients), is more cost-effective than life-long follow-up, and is successful in 95% of patients with a < 1% complication rate. Therefore, most experienced clinicians recommend parathyroidectomy for "asymptomatic" patients.

Table 26–8. 1990 NIH consensus conference indications for surgery in patients with asymptomatic primary hyperparathyroidism.[1]

Criterion	Description
Serum calcium	> 12 mg/dL
Urinary calcium	> 400 mg/24 h
Creatinine clearance	< 30% of normal age-matched controls in the absence of another identifiable cause
Bone mineral density	< 2 SD below age- and sex-matched normal value
Age	< 50 years
Calciphylaxis	Tissue deposition of calcium
Abdominal x-ray	Presence of renal stones

[1]Data from Consensus Development Conference Panel: Diagnosis and management of asymptomatic primary hyperparathyroidism: Consensus development conference statement. Ann Intern Med 1991;1145:593.

A second meeting was held at the NIH in 2002 to re-evaluate the criteria for parathyroidectomy in asymptomatic patients. The new guidelines are essentially similar to previous recommendations except for the following changes: Surgery is currently recommended if (1) serum calcium is 1 mg/dL above reported normal range, and (2) bone mineral density at any site (forearm, spine, or hip) is 72.5 standard deviations below that of gender and not age-matched controls (T-score rather than Z-score).

B. SYMPTOMATIC PATIENTS

Patients with classic symptoms and metabolic complications are candidates for surgery.

Conduct of Parathyroidectomy

Issues to consider before deciding on the optimal treatment approach are whether one is dealing with sporadic or familial disease and with the initial operation or reexploration. The presence of concurrent thyroid pathology needing surgical treatment must also be taken into account. The positioning, incision, and dissection are as described previously for thyroidectomy.

Bilateral Versus Unilateral Approach

Traditionally, all four parathyroid glands have been explored without preoperative localizing studies, with a 95% success rate in the hands of an experienced surgeon. Investigators in favor of unilateral exploration have suggested decreased recurrent laryngeal nerve injury, less postoperative hypocalcemia, shorter operative time, and early discharge as advantages of this approach. Potential disadvantages of unilateral exploration include the risk of missing multiple abnormal or ectopic parathyroid glands. Neck exploration has been performed in a unilateral or focal approach with localizing studies and intraoperative gamma probe or PTH measurements.

We have found that when two localizing studies—Tc 99m sestamibi and ultrasound—identify the same solitary parathyroid gland in patients with sporadic hyperparathyroidism, this was the only abnormal parathyroid gland in 95% of patients. In these patients, our current approach is to recommend focused parathyroidectomy via a 2.5 cm incision with intraoperative PTH measurement. If the PTH level falls more than 50% within 10 minutes after removal of an abnormal parathyroid gland, the procedure is terminated. If the level does not fall, a PTH measurement is repeated in another 10 minutes as it may fall slowly in some patients. The bilateral approach is used in patients with known familial disease, secondary or tertiary hyperparathyroidism, or a history of lithium treatment—or if the localizing studies are negative or inconsistent. If parathyroid cancer is suspected intraoperatively, it is resected with the ipsilateral thyroid lobe and regional lymph nodes.

Subtotal Parathyroidectomy Versus Total Parathyroidectomy with Autotransplantation

In the latter technique, 12–20 small fragments (1 × 1 mm) of parathyroid tissue are placed into multiple pockets in the forearm muscle of the nondominant arm. The site is marked with silk sutures and is easily accessible under local anesthesia should the patient develop recurrent hypercalcemia. The recurrence rates for hyperparathyroidism appear to be similar after subtotal or total parathyroidectomy. However, a 5% failure rate has been reported after autotransplantation of parathyroid tissue. Therefore, subtotal parathyroidectomy is preferred. The most normal gland is biopsied first, leaving a 50 mg remnant (the size of a normal parathyroid gland); if it appears viable, the remaining glands are excised. Patients undergoing either of these procedures should have tissue cryopreserved. Parathyroid glands should not be routinely biopsied at exploration but rather to confirm parathyroid tissue or help determine if the gland is normal or abnormal. As with thyroid surgery, video-assisted and endoscopic axillary approaches are feasible, but clear benefits compared with the open approach are not apparent.

Kidney stones, bone disease, neuromuscular symptoms, and psychiatric symptoms respond well to surgery, whereas hypertension does not.

PERSISTENT & RECURRENT PRIMARY HYPERPARATHYROIDISM

Persistent hypercalcemia occurs after about 5–10% of explorations. Recurrent hypercalcemia is rare except in patients with familial disease and occurs after an intervening period (over 6 months) of normocalcemia. The most common reasons for persistent hyperparathyroidism are a missed gland in normal or ectopic location, regrowth of hyperplastic tissue, recurrent carcinoma, or parathyromatosis (implantation of tumor broken at the initial procedure). The management of these patients involves confirmation of the diagnosis—in particular, exclusion of familial hypocalciuric hypercalcemia; review of original operative notes and pathology reports; and localization studies, which are a must in this group of patients. The issue of reexploration in mildly symptomatic patients is controversial. The neck is usually reexplored first, and median sternotomy may be needed in 1–2% of patients. Cryopreservation should be performed routinely and autotransplantation selectively. Reexploration by an experienced surgeon is successful in over 90% of patients but is associated with more complications than initial operation.

SECONDARY HYPERPARATHYROIDISM

This disorder occurs most often in individuals with end-stage renal failure but may also occur in other conditions resulting in hypocalcemia such as vitamin D deficiency, idiopathic hypercalciuria, hypermagnesemia, and long-term lithium therapy.

Indications for surgery include situations where the product of serum calcium and phosphate is > 70, renal osteodystrophy with bone pain, severe pruritus, ectopic soft tissue calcifications and tumoral calcinosis, serum calcium > 11 mg/dL with markedly elevated PTH, and calciphylaxis.

These patients should undergo dialysis the day prior to surgery to correct electrolyte (specifically potassium) abnormalities. Patients with this disorder require bilateral exploration and either subtotal parathyroidectomy, leaving a 50–60 mg histologically confirmed well-vascularized remnant of hyperplastic parathyroid distant from the recurrent laryngeal nerve; or total parathyroidectomy with autotransplantation of a similar amount of tissue. The former is usually preferred, as not all autografts function. Upper thymectomy is usually performed in these patients, since up to 15% of patients will have a fifth hyperplastic gland.

SPECIAL CONSIDERATION: FAMILIAL HYPERPARATHYROIDISM

MEN 1 patients should have hyperparathyroidism treated before coexisting gastrinoma. All glands should be identified; ectopic glands should be sought in the neck and upper mediastinum; and bilateral cervical thymectomy should be routinely performed due to the occurrence of thymic carcinoids. All but about 50 mg of the most normal parathyroid gland should be removed. MEN 2a patients should undergo screening for the presence of a pheochromocytoma and *RET* mutation prior to thyroid or parathyroid surgery. Since the parathyroids are at risk during thyroidectomy and central neck node dissection, and hyperparathyroidism is less virulent in these patients, only obviously enlarged glands should be removed. Normal-appearing glands should be marked and parathyroid tissue cryopreserved.

COMPLICATIONS OF PARATHYROID SURGERY

General complications are similar to those associated with thyroidectomy. Specific complications include recurrent laryngeal nerve injury, hypomagnesemia, and hypocalcemia. The latter may arise due to suppressed function of the remaining glands after removal of an adenoma; injury to the parathyroid remnant; or bone hunger, which is the influx of calcium and phosphorus

into metabolically active bones. Bone hunger can be predicted based on the severity of bone disease and the preoperative alkaline phosphatase level and is generally more severe in individuals with secondary hyperparathyroidism. Hypocalcemia can be treated with oral calcium and vitamin D supplementation (calcitriol, 0.25–0.5 μg twice daily). Intravenous calcium is seldom required except in patients with osteitis fibrosa cystica.

■ THE ADRENAL (SUPRARENAL) GLAND

EMBRYOLOGY & ANATOMY

The adrenals are paired structures located superior to the kidneys. The adrenal is divided into an outer cortex and an inner medulla. The cortex originates from mesodermal tissue near the gonads on the adrenogenital ridge at about the fifth week of gestation. Adrenocortical tissue can thus be found in the ovaries, spermatic cord, and testes. The adrenal medulla originates from the neural crest, which is ectodermal in origin.

Each adrenal is supplied by three sets of arteries: the superior adrenal (from the inferior phrenic artery), the middle adrenal (from the aorta), and the inferior adrenal (from the renal artery). These vessels branch into as many as 50 arteries. The left adrenal vein empties into the ipsilateral renal vein, whereas the right adrenal vein drains into the inferior vena cava (see Fig. 9-1).

INDICATIONS FOR SURGERY

PRIMARY HYPERALDOSTERONISM

This disorder accounts for 1% of hypertensive patients and results from an adrenal adenoma (Conn's syndrome, 75%), adrenal hyperplasia (24%), or adrenocortical cancer (1%). Patients present with hypertension, muscular weakness, polydipsia, polyuria, headaches, and fatigue. It is important to distinguish between adenoma and hyperplasia because surgery is virtually always curative for the former (see Chapter 10).

Diagnostic Tests

Plasma electrolyte determinations reveal hypokalemia, hypernatremia, alkalosis, and hypochloremia. Elevated plasma and urine aldosterone levels with suppressed serum renin levels confirm the diagnosis. Tumors are localized with the aid of CT scans, MRI, iodocholesterol scans, or selective venous catheterization for aldosterone and cortisol.

Surgical Management

Patients are prepared for surgery with potassium supplementation, sodium restriction, and treatment with spironolactone (an aldosterone antagonist) or amiloride (a potassium-sparing diuretic). Postoperatively, patients may require saline infusions, fludrocortisone (50–100 μg/d), or, rarely, glucocorticoids if they become addisonian. Patients who respond well to spironolactone also do well after surgery. About 80% experience an improvement in blood pressure, and almost all become normokalemic. Patients with hyperplasia require bilateral adrenalectomy, so that medical therapy is often preferred (see Chapter 10).

HYPERCORTISOLISM

Cushing's syndrome arises from elevated corticosteroid levels resulting from pituitary ACTH secretion leading to bilateral adrenal hyperplasia (Cushing's disease), adrenal adenoma, adrenal carcinoma, ectopic ACTH-secreting tumors (small cell lung cancer; pancreatic, thyroid, thymic, and other cancers), or the exogenous administration of steroids. Patients present with weight gain, muscular weakness, polyuria, emotional lability, moon facies, acne, hirsutism, central obesity, hypertension, diabetes mellitus, and virilization.

Diagnostic Tests

In order to confirm the diagnosis and determine the cause, a low-dose (1 mg) dexamethasone suppression test, urine free-cortisol, plasma ACTH, and high-dose (8 mg) dexamethasone suppression test are performed. Tumors are localized using CT, MRI, or iodocholesterol scans and selective venous catheterization of petrosal veins after corticotropin-releasing factor stimulation (see Chapter 9).

Surgical Management

Cushing's syndrome can be treated with medications that inhibit steroid production (ketoconazole, metyrapone, aminoglutethimide). Cushing's disease is treated with transsphenoidal hypophysectomy and microsurgical excision of the pituitary adenoma. Irradiation may also be used, but the response is delayed and the treatment results in panhypopituitarism. Unilateral adrenalectomy is the treatment of choice in patients with adrenal adenomas or carcinomas, whereas bilateral adrenalectomy is used to treat patients with Cushing's disease who fail to respond to radiation or hypophysec-

tomy and selected patients with Cushing's syndrome secondary to ectopic ACTH production.

Preoperatively, electrolyte abnormalities are corrected and all patients are given exogenous steroids (hydrocortisone, 100 mg intravenously every 8 hours). After unilateral adrenalectomy, steroids are tapered off over months. After bilateral surgery, lifelong treatment with hydrocortisone (20 mg each morning and 10 mg in the evening) is necessary. Fludrocortisone (0.1 mg orally daily) is sometimes needed, and cortisone supplementation must be increased in situations of stress. The prognosis after adrenalectomy for adenoma is excellent. After bilateral adrenalectomy, about 20% of patients develop Nelson's syndrome (hyperpigmentation, headaches, exophthalmos, and blindness) from continuing growth of the pituitary tumor.

SEX STEROID EXCESS

Virilization and feminization can be caused by many disorders including congenital adrenal hyperplasia, adrenal adenomas or carcinomas, ovarian or testicular tumors, hypothalamic or pituitary disease, placental disorders, and exogenous sex steroid administration. Six different variants of congenital adrenal hyperplasia occur, each caused by a specific enzyme defect. Adrenal virilization occurring postnatally usually results from an adenoma or carcinoma. Virilization presents in females with hirsutism, clitoromegaly, alopecia, breast atrophy, and hypomenorrhea. In males, feminizing tumors lead to gynecomastia, testicular atrophy, acne, and hypertension.

Diagnostic Tests

Karyotype analysis; plasma 17-hydroxyprogesterone, 11-deoxycortisol, and testosterone analysis; and urine tests for 17-ketosteroids, pregnanetriol, testosterone, aldosterone, and corticosteroid levels are needed to establish the particular enzyme deficiency. The dexamethasone suppression test (2–4 mg/d in divided doses four times daily for 7 days) can be used to distinguish adrenal hyperplasia from neoplasia. CT, MRI, and iodocholesterol scans are used to localize the tumors.

Surgical Management

Congenital adrenal hyperplasia is generally not amenable to surgical therapy. Adrenalectomy is reserved for treatment of adrenogenital syndrome caused by an adenoma or carcinoma. The perioperative management is similar to that for patients with Cushing's syndrome. Progression of virilization or feminization ceases after adrenalectomy. Adrenal carcinomas have a poor prognosis.

PHEOCHROMOCYTOMA

This catecholamine-secreting tumor of the adrenal medulla and extra-adrenal chromaffin tissue accounts for 0.1–0.2% of all patients with hypertension. It is often called "the 10% tumor" because 10% are bilateral, 10% are malignant, 10% occur in children, 10% are extra-adrenal, and 10% are familial (occurring in association with MEN 2a, MEN 2b, von Hippel-Lindau syndrome, neurofibromatosis, and other neurocutaneous syndromes). Headache, palpitations and diaphoresis constitute the classic triad of pheochromocytoma. Nonspecific symptoms include anxiety, tremulousness, severe headaches, paresthesias, flushing, chest pain, shortness of breath, abdominal pain, nausea, and vomiting as well as others. The most common clinical sign is hypertension, which may be sustained or episodic.

Diagnostic Tests

These should be performed in a nonstressed patient. Twenty-four-hour urine collections should be tested for vanillylmandelic acid, metanephrines, and catecholamines. Plasma catecholamines and chromogranin A levels can also be measured. Provocative tests such as glucagon infusion and clonidine suppression are rarely necessary. Radiologic investigations such as CT scan, MRI scan, and metaiodobenzylguanidine scans are used to localize the tumors and assess for possible extraadrenal tumors (see Chapter 11).

Surgical Treatment

Adrenalectomy is the treatment of choice. Preoperative preparation involves treatment with an alpha-adrenergic blocker such as phenoxybenzamine (10–40 mg four times daily; maximum: 300 mg/d). Beta-blockers such as propranolol (5–40 mg four times daily) are added in patients who have persistent tachycardia and arrhythmias but only after adequate alpha blockade has been established in order to avoid the effects of unopposed alpha stimulation, ie, hypertensive crisis and congestive heart failure. Patients should also be volume-repleted to avoid postoperative hypotension, which ensues with the loss of vasoconstriction after tumor removal. Nitroprusside is the drug of choice for intraoperative blood pressure control. After surgery, 95% of patients with paroxysmal hypertension and 65% with sustained hypertension become normotensive. Malignant pheochromocytoma has a poor prognosis.

ADRENAL CORTICAL CARCINOMA

This rare neoplasm is slightly more common in women than in men and has a bimodal age distribution, occurring more frequently in children under 5 years of age

and in adults in their forties and fifties. About 50% of these tumors are nonfunctioning. The remainder secrete cortisol (30%), androgens (20%), estrogens (10%), aldosterone (2%), or multiple hormones (35%). Adrenocortical cancers are often characterized by the rapid onset of Cushing's syndrome with virilizing features. Nonfunctioning tumors usually present with an enlarging abdominal mass and abdominal pain or, less commonly, with weight loss, hematuria, varicocele, and dyspnea. Most tumors are sporadic, but they can occur within the tumor spectrum of the Li-Fraumeni and MEN 1 syndromes.

Diagnosis

The biochemical workup of a unilateral adrenal mass is outlined in the section on adrenal incidentaloma. CT scan and MRI are the most commonly employed radiologic diagnostic tests. The size of the mass remains the single most reliable indicator of malignancy. Carcinomas are more likely to be present in lesions over 6 cm in diameter. Other features suggesting malignancy on CT include irregular shape and margins, heterogeneity, and hemorrhage. On MRI, carcinomas have a moderate signal intensity on T2-weighted image (adrenal tumor to liver ratio 1.2–2.8). Fine-needle aspiration biopsy is usually performed in patients with an isolated adrenal mass and a history of carcinoma of the lung, breast, stomach, kidney, colon, melanoma, or lymphoma and in those with symptoms and signs of underlying malignancy. Care must be taken to exclude pheochromocytoma prior to biopsy to avoid precipitating a hypertensive crisis (see Chapter 9).

Surgical Treatment

Complete surgical excision offers the only chance of prolonged survival. Transabdominal adrenalectomy with en bloc excision of contiguously involved structures (liver, kidney, spleen, pancreas, or inferior vena cava) is usually recommended. A thoracoabdominal approach may also be used for large (> 10 cm) right-sided tumors. Laparoscopic adrenalectomy is not usually recommended for adrenal cancers. The adrenolytic agent mitotane and other antitumor drugs such as etoposide, cisplatin, and doxorubicin have also been used with partial success for metastatic tumors. Five-year actuarial survival rates of 32–48% have been reported in patients who underwent complete resection. Features predicting poor survival include tumor size over 12 cm, six or more mitoses per high power field, and intratumoral hemorrhage.

ADRENAL INCIDENTALOMA

This entity is defined as an adrenal mass discovered during imaging done for other reasons. Adrenal masses

Table 26–9. Differential diagnosis of the adrenal incidentaloma.

Benign	Malignant

Adrenal cortex
  Functioning adenoma
  Nonfunctioning
    adenoma
	Adrenocortical cancer

Adrenal medulla Pheochromocytoma	Malignant pheochromocytoma

Others
  Cysts
  Myelolipomas
  Ganglioneuroma
  Hematoma
	Metastasis

have been identified in up to 8% of individuals in autopsy series and 4.4% in those undergoing abdominal CT scans. The widespread use of ultrasound, CT, and MRI scans over the last 2 decades has led to the great increase in the number of these lesions identified.

Most of these lesions are benign nonfunctioning adenomas. The differential diagnosis of these lesions is summarized in Table 26–9.

Diagnosis

The workup is used to discern whether the lesion is functional or malignant. Asymptomatic patients with obvious cysts, hemorrhage, myelolipomas, or diffuse metastatic disease do not mandate further testing. All other patients should undergo biochemical testing for hormonally active tumors. At a minimum, this should include serum electrolytes, low-dose (1 mg) dexamethasone suppression testing, and a 24-hour urine collection for catecholamines, metanephrines, vanillylmandelic acid, and 17-ketosteroids. Confirmatory tests can be performed based on the results of these screening tests. Functional tumors and nonfunctional masses over 4 cm (in good-risk patients) are treated by adrenalectomy, as are heterogeneous, irregular or enlarging tumors. Fine-needle aspiratory biopsy should be performed only in patients with a history of carcinoma and a suspected isolated adrenal metastasis (see Chapter 9).

Treatment

Laparoscopic adrenalectomy has become the procedure of choice for most of the lesions described above except those suspected of being or known to be malignant. Patients with nonfunctioning homogeneous lesions less than 4 cm in diameter should be followed with serial examinations and CT or MRI at 3 and 12 months.

Adrenalectomy is indicated for any lesion that grows during the observation period. Patients with stable lesions may be discharged from follow-up.

TECHNIQUE OF ADRENALECTOMY

There are no randomized controlled trials comparing laparoscopic and open adrenalectomies. However, several retrospective studies have shown that the laparoscopic technique is safe and associated with less postoperative pain, shorter mean hospital stay, lower morbidity, and more rapid complete recovery. Laparoscopic adrenalectomy has become the procedure of choice for most adrenal lesions, and the indications are similar to those for open procedure.

Laparoscopic adrenalectomy is contraindicated in patients with adrenocortical cancer or coagulopathy—and relatively contraindicated after previous adrenal surgery. Two approaches have been defined: transperitoneal (lateral and anterior) and posterior retroperitoneal. The former provides a conventional view of anatomy and the anterior approach allows for bilateral procedures without repositioning the patient. The latter approach may be preferable in reoperative cases and obese patients but provides a limited working space.

In general, the adrenal gland is dissected from surrounding tissue using electrocautery or the Harmonic Ultrasonic Scalpel. These methods are also useful for control of the small adrenal arteries, but the adrenal veins need to be clipped. The adrenal is placed in an endocatch bag and morselled prior to extraction.

COMPLICATIONS OF LAPAROSCOPIC ADRENALECTOMY

Specific procedure-related complications include trocar site-associated hematoma and subcutaneous emphysema, injury to surrounding organs such as the spleen, and bleeding from vena caval injury.

■ THE ENDOCRINE PANCREAS

EMBRYOLOGY & ANATOMY

The pancreas is a retroperitoneal organ located at the level of L2. It weighs 75–100 g, is about 15–20 cm in length, and is divided into the head and uncinate process, the neck, the body, and the tail. The uncinate process forms part of the head and surrounds the superior mesenteric vessels. The main pancreatic duct (duct of Wirsung) is 2–3.5 mm wide, runs in the center of the pancreas, and drains the body, tail, and uncinate

Table 26–10. Rare functioning tumors of the endocrine pancreas.[1]

Tumor	Hormone or Candidate	Features
Calcitoninoma	Calcitonin	Secretory diarrhea
Parathyrinoma	PTH-related protein	Hypercalcemia Bone pain Normal serum PTH
GRFoma	Growth hormone-releasing factor	Acromegaly
ACTHoma	Adrenocorticotropic hormone	Cushing's syndrome
Neurotensinoma	Neurotensin	Tachycardia Hypotension Malabsorption

[1]Reproduced, with permission, from Yeo CJ: Neoplasms of the endocrine pancreas. In: *Surgery: Scientific Principles and Practice.* Greenfield LJ (editor). Lippincott-Raven, 1997.

process. The lesser duct (duct of Santorini) usually drains the head, communicates with the duct of Wirsung, and drains separately via a minor papilla located 2 cm proximal to the ampulla of Vater. The common bile duct is found posteriorly in the pancreatic head and joins the main pancreatic duct before draining into the ampulla.

The pancreas originates as dorsal and ventral pancreatic buds from the primitive endoderm around the fifth week of gestation. The former gives rise to the superior head, neck, body, and tail, whereas the later forms the inferior head and the uncinate process. The ventral duct fuses with the dorsal bud to form the duct of Wirsung, and the proximal portion of the dorsal duct forms the duct of Santorini. In 10% of individuals, the ducts fail to communicate, resulting in pancreas divisum, where the entire pancreas is drained by the lesser duct.

INDICATIONS FOR SURGERY

Endocrine pancreatic tumors arise from the islet cells, which are derived from the neural crest.

Common functioning tumors are described below and rare functioning tumors of the endocrine pancreas are described in Table 26–10.

INSULINOMA

This β cell-derived neoplasm is the most common pancreatic endocrine tumor. Insulinomas are evenly distributed throughout the pancreas (one-third each in the head, body, and tail). Most patients (90%) have a benign, solitary lesion. Approximately 10% of patients have malignant insulinomas with metastatic disease to the liver and peripancreatic lymph nodes. The insulinoma syndrome is characterized by the Whipple triad, which includes symptoms of hypoglycemia during fasting, serum glucose < 50 mg/dL, and relief of hypoglycemic symptoms by exogenous glucose. Symptoms arise from neuroglycopenia (confusion, seizures, personality change, coma) or due to a catecholamine surge (tachycardia, diaphoresis, trembling). Other causes of hypoglycemia should be excluded, eg, reactive hypoglycemia, adrenal insufficiency, end-stage liver disease, nonpancreatic tumors (mesothelioma, sarcoma, adrenal carcinoma, carcinoid), and surreptitious administration of oral hypoglycemics or insulin.

Diagnostic Tests

The diagnosis is made if glucose levels fall to < 50 mg/dL while insulin levels are > 20 μU/mL and the insulin to glucose ratio is > 0.4 (normal: < 0.3) during a 72-hour monitored fast. Increased levels of C peptide and proinsulin are also diagnostic, whereas low levels suggest factitious hyperinsulinemia.

Once the diagnosis is confirmed biochemically, noninvasive tests such as double-contrast, fine-cut (5 mm) CT or MRI scan can identify large tumors or liver metastases. Transgastric endoscopic ultrasound is the most successful preoperative localization test (sensitivity 83–93%). Selective arteriography with calcium stimulation of insulin secretion and catheterization of the right hepatic vein (sensitivity 88%) may also be used. Some pancreatic neuroendocrine tumors also express somatostatin receptors and can be imaged using radiolabeled octreotide. Unfortunately, this is only effective in about 30% of patients with insulinomas (see Chapter 18).

Treatment

A. SURGICAL TREATMENT

Operation is the only curative treatment. Prior to surgery, patients are instructed to take several small frequent meals, and diazoxide administration is helpful to avoid hypoglycemic attacks. Glucose levels are monitored perioperatively. The combination of inspection, palpation, and intraoperative ultrasound allows detection of nearly all tumors and their relationship to the pancreatic duct. Small, (< 2 cm) benign tumors in any part of the pancreas not intimately associated with the main pancreatic duct are enucleated. Larger tumors (up to 5 cm) are usually enucleated if in the pancreatic head but are removed by spleen-preserving distal pancreatectomy if located in the tail. Large tumors in the head that appear malignant are usually resected by a Whipple procedure. When a tumor cannot be identified, "blind" distal resections should generally not be performed. However, a small distal pancreatic resection may be sufficient to rule out nesidioblastosis (β-cell hyperplasia). Resection of peripancreatic and duodenal nodes should be performed in patients with probable malignant tumors. Hepatic resection should be attempted for cure or palliation in patients with metastatic tumors. Patients with insulinomas and MEN 1 require distal pancreatectomy and enucleation of tumors from the head of the pancreas. Surgical resection is curative in about 95% of cases. Malignant insulinomas recur in about 33% of cases.

B. MEDICAL TREATMENT

Diazoxide and verapamil are often used to decrease insulin secretion from insulinoma. Combination chemotherapy (streptozocin, fluorouracil, and doxorubicin) has also been used for unresectable insulinomas.

GASTRINOMA
(Zollinger-Ellison Syndrome)

This neoplasm leads to abdominal pain and peptic ulceration of the proximal gastrointestinal tract (90%) and diarrhea (50%). The diagnosis should be suspected in patients with recurrent postoperative and postbulbar ulcers, ulcer associated with diarrhea, a family history of ulcer diathesis or MEN 1, and failure to respond to adequate medical therapy. Up to 75% of gastrinomas occur sporadically. In contrast to insulinomas, 60% of gastrinomas are malignant and present with local invasion and metastases.

Diagnostic Tests

Fasting serum gastrin levels are usually over 200 pg/mL, and values over 1000 pg/mL are diagnostic of gastrinomas unless the patient is hypochlorhydric. Elevated gastrin levels may also be found in several other disease states (Table 26–11), and other tests are therefore necessary. Basal gastric acid output > 15 mEq/h (> 5 mEq/h in patients with previous vagotomy) or a ratio of basal to maximal acid output greater than 0.6 suggests a gastrinoma. An increase of gastrin > 200 pg/mL above the basal level upon stimulation with 2 units/kg secretin confirms the diagnosis.

Radiologic tests used to localize gastrinomas are similar to those used for investigation of insulinomas. However, endoscopic ultrasound and visceral angiograms are less sensitive for gastrinomas. Radiolabeled octreotide scanning is usually positive for tumors larger than 1 cm in diameter. Selective pancreatic angiograms utilizing secretin stimulation for gastrin levels may be helpful. However, about 70% of gastrinomas are in the

Table 26–11. Causes of hypergastrinemia.[1]

A. Hypergastrinemia associated with increased gastric acid
  1. Gastrinoma, sporadic or familial (MEN 1)
  2. Antral G cell hyperfunction (rare)
  3. Retained gastric antrum
  4. Short bowel syndrome
  5. Gastric outlet obstruction
  6. Renal failure (acid can be normal)
  7. *H. pylori* gastritis (acid can be low)
B. Hypergastrinemia associated with little or no gastric acid
  1. Pernicious anema (achlorhydria)
  2. Chronic atrophic gastritis
  3. Vagotomy
  4. Gastric ulcer associated with hypochlorhydria

[1]Reproduced, with permission, from Wilson SD: Gastrinoma. In: *Textbook of Endocrine Surgery.* Clark OH, Duh Q-Y (editors). Saunders, 1997.

duodenum in patients with MEN 1, and 90% are found to the right of the superior mesenteric vessels.

Treatment

A. SURGICAL TREATMENT

Patients are given proton pump inhibitors preoperatively. Most gastrinomas are located in the "gastrinoma triangle," which is bounded by the cystic duct superiorly, the second and third portions of the duodenum inferiorly, and the junction of the neck and body of the pancreas medially. The Whipple procedure is recommended for large (> 6 cm) or clinically malignant tumors in the head of the pancreas. Intraoperative ultrasound, endoscopy with duodenal transillumination, and a longitudinal duodenotomy may be necessary to identify the tumor. All enlarged peripancreatic and periduodenal lymph nodes should be removed. Single hepatic metastases may be resected. Total gastrectomy is rarely indicated today except in noncompliant patients or those refractory to medical therapy when the gastrinoma cannot be identified or completely removed. Most gastrinomas in sporadic disease are solitary, whereas in MEN 1 they are multiple. About 34% of patients with sporadic gastrinomas and 50% with familial gastrinomas remain disease-free at 10 years. Overall survival rates are 94% at 10 years. Patients with radiologically identified recurrent disease may be candidates for repeat resection to avoid obstruction.

B. MEDICAL TREATMENT

Octreotide can be used to decrease gastrin secretion. Hepatic artery embolization of liver metastases may provide palliation.

VIPOMA (VERNER-MORRISON) SYNDROME

This disorder is also known as the WDHA (watery diarrhea, hypokalemia, achlorhydria) or pancreatic cholera syndrome. Patients typically present with high-volume diarrhea (> 5 L/d), muscular weakness and lethargy (due to hypokalemia), hyperglycemia, hypercalcemia, and, rarely, cutaneous flushing. Other common causes of diarrhea should be excluded.

Diagnostic Tests

Since secretion can be episodic, multiple fasting levels of VIP should be measured. Localizing studies should be performed as previously described.

Treatment

A. SURGICAL TREATMENT

Fluid and electrolytes should be aggressively repleted prior to surgery. Diarrhea may be treated with octreotide. Most of these tumors are located in the body and tail and are hence treated by a distal pancreatectomy. Small tumors may be enucleated. If the tumor is not localized, the autonomic chain and adrenals should be examined for extrapancreatic tumors. If no tumor is identified, distal pancreatectomy may be considered. Palliative debulking may be performed for metastatic disease.

B. MEDICAL TREATMENT

Octreotide and hepatic artery embolization may provide palliation of symptoms.

GLUCAGONOMA

Patients with this tumor have mild diabetes, stomatitis, anemia, malnutrition, hypoproteinemia, and a characteristic severe dermatitis (necrolytic migratory erythema). The latter is thought to be secondary to the hypoaminoacidemia.

Diagnostic Tests

The clinical presentation and biopsy of the rash are sufficient for the diagnosis. Hyperglycemia, hypoproteinemia, and an elevated fasting glucagon level (> 150 pg/mL) confirm the diagnosis. Localizing and staging tests described earlier should also be performed.

Treatment

A. SURGICAL TREATMENT

Patients need preoperative octreotide, hyperalimentation, and routine deep venous thrombosis prophylaxis. Up to 70% of these tumors present with metastases, and surgery is the only potentially curable treatment. Most tumors are solitary and located in the tail, where they are amenable to distal pancreatectomy. Palliative debulking in the setting of metastatic disease may help refractory symptoms.

B. MEDICAL TREATMENT

Octreotide and embolization of hepatic metastases may help control symptoms.

SOMATOSTATINOMA

The somatostatinoma syndrome is characterized by steatorrhea, diabetes, hypochlorhydria, and gallstone disease. Most somatostatinomas are malignant (75% have metastases at presentation) and are located in the pancreatic head. The diagnosis is established by fasting somatostatin levels over 100 pg/mL.

Somatostatinoma is usually treated by pancreaticoduodenectomy. Fluid and electrolytes should be repleted preoperatively.

NONFUNCTIONING PANCREATIC TUMORS

About 33% of patients with pancreatic endocrine neoplasms have no evidence of a defined clinical syndrome and are deemed to have nonfunctioning tumors. However, some of these tumors produce pancreatic polypeptide. These tumors usually present with abdominal pain, weight loss, and jaundice—similar to ductal adenocarcinoma of the pancreas. They are most commonly present in the head, neck, and uncinate process. The tumors are localized and staged similar to functional tumors. Endoscopic retrograde cholangiopancreatography and percutaneous transhepatic cholangiography are used for the evaluation of jaundice.

Surgical Treatment

About 50–90% of these tumors are malignant. Surgical resection (pancreaticoduodenectomy—Whipple procedure—or distal pancreatectomy) is the treatment of choice, as these tumors are not amenable to enucleation. Biliary and gastric bypasses may be necessary for palliation. These tumors grow in an indolent fashion. Five-year survival rates after resection are 50%. In patients with unresectable disease, combination chemotherapy (streptozocin and doxorubicin) may provide palliation.

Technique of Pancreatic Resection

Patients are explored through a midline or bilateral subcostal incision. The gastrocolic ligament and the inferior retroperitoneal attachments are divided to permit examination of the body and tail. Kocher's maneuver is performed to facilitate bimanual examination of the head and uncinate process. The duodenum, splenic hilum, small bowel mesentery, gonads (in women), and lymph nodes are assessed for extrapancreatic disease. The liver is examined for metastatic disease. Intraoperative ultrasound may facilitate identification of tumors. Early experience suggests that a laparoscopic approach is also feasible in these tumors when the lesion is identified with localization studies.

Complications of Pancreatic Surgery

The most important complications of pancreatic surgery (tumor enucleation, distal pancreatectomy, or Whipple resection) are pancreatic fistula, pseudocyst, or abscess formation; which may lead to necrotizing retroperitoneal infection; and hemorrhage. Other complications include upper gastrointestinal tract bleeding, marginal ulceration, and biliary fistula formation. The mortality of a Whipple procedure is less than 5% and that of other pancreatic surgical procedures is less than 1%.

REFERENCES

The Thyroid Gland

Alsanea O, Clark OH: Familial thyroid cancer. Curr Opin Oncol 2001;13:44. [PMID 11148685]

Alsanea O, Clark OH: Treatment of Graves' disease: The advantages of surgery. Endocrinol Metab Clin 2000;29:321. [PMID:10874532]

Alsanea O et al: Is familial non-medullary thyroid carcinoma more aggressive than sporadic thyroid cancer? A multicenter series. Surgery 2000;128:1043. [PMID 11114641]

Bergman P, Auldist AW, Cameron F: Review of the outcome of management of Graves' disease in children and adolescents. J Pediatr Child Health 2001;37:176. [PMID 11328475]

Chi DD, Moley JF: Medullary thyroid carcinoma: genetic advances, treatment recommendations, and the approach to the patient with persistent hypercalcitoninemia. Surg Oncol Clin N Am 1998;7:681. [PMID 9735129]

Giuffrida D, Gharib H: Anaplastic thyroid carcinoma: current diagnosis and treatment. Ann Oncol 2000;11:1083. [PMID 11061600]

Kebebew E, Clark OH: Differentiated thyroid cancer: "Complete" rational approach. World J Surg 2000;24:942. [PMID 10865038]

Kebebew E et al: Medullary thyroid carcinoma: clinical characteristics, treatment prognostic factors, and a comparison of staging symptoms. Cancer 2001;88:1139. [PMID 10699905]

Kebebew E et al: Total thyroidectomy or thyroid lobectomy in patients with low-risk differentiated thyroid cancer: Surgical decision analysis of a controversy using a mathematical model. World J Surg 2000;24:1295. [PMID 11038197]

Miccoli P et al: Minimally invasive Video-assisted thyroidectomy: multi-institutional experience. World J Surg 2002;26:972. [PMID 12016476]

Moley JF, DeBenedetti MK: Patterns of nodal metastases in palpable medullary thyroid carcinoma: recommendations for extent of node dissection. Ann Surg 1999;229:880. [PMID 1036393] (Over 75% of patients with palpable medullary thyroid cancer had associated nodal metastases.)

Reeve T, Thomson NW: Complications of thyroid surgery: how to avoid them, how to manage them and observations on their possible effect on the whole patient. World J Surg 2000;24:971. [PMID 10865043] (Common and uncommon complications associated with thyroidectomy.)

Shaha AR: Management of the neck in thyroid cancer. Otolaryngol Clin North Am 1998;31:823. [PMID 9735110] (Treatment of lymph node metastases.)

Witte J et al: Surgery for Graves' disease: Total versus subtotal thyroidectomy—results of a prospective randomized trial. World J Surg 2000;24:1303. [PMID 11038198]

The Parathyroid Gland

Arici C et al: Can localization studies be used to direct focused parathyroid operations? Surgery 2001;129:720. [PMID 11391371]

Bilezikian JP et al: Summary statement from a workshop on asymptomatic primary hyperparathyroidism: A perspective for the 21st century. J Clin Endocrinol Metab 2002;87:5353. [PMID: 12466320]

Brandi ML et al: Guidelines for diagnosis and therapy of MEN type 1 and type 2. J Clin Endocrinol Metab 2001;86:5658. [PMID 11739416]

Consensus Development Conference Panel: Diagnosis and management of asymptomatic primary hyperparathyroidism: Consensus Development Conference statement. Ann Intern Med 1991;114:593.

Eigelberger M, Clark OH: Surgical approaches to primary hyperparathyroidism. Endocrinol Metab Clin North Am 2000; 29:479. [PMID 11033757]

Howe JR: Minimally invasive parathyroid surgery. Surg Clin North Am 2000;80:1399. [PMID 11059711]

Lee PC et al: Parathyromatosis: a cause for recurrent hyperparathyroidism. Endocr Pract 2001;7:189. [PMID 11421566]

Lundgren E et al: Increased cardiovascular mortality and normalized serum calcium in patients with mild hypercalcemia followed for 25 years. Surgery 2001;130:978. [PMID 11742326]

Miccoli P: Minimally invasive surgery for thyroid and parathyroid disease. Surg Endosc 2002;16:3. [PMID 11961594]

Miura D et al: Does intra-operative quick parathyroid hormone assay improve the results of parathyroidectomy? World J Surg 2002;26:926. [PMID 11965444]

Pasieka JL, Parsons LL: Prospective surgical outcome study of relief of symptoms following surgery in patients with primary hyperparathyroidism. World J Surg 1998;22:513. [PMID 9597921]

Perrier ND et al. Parathyroid surgery: Separating promise from reality. J Clin Endocrinol Metab 2002;87:1024. [PMID 11889156]

Shaha AR, Shah JP: Parathyroid carcinoma: a diagnostic and therapeutic challenge. Cancer 1999;86:378. [PMID 10430243]

Silverberg SJ: Natural history of primary hyperparathyroidism. Endocrinol Metabolism Clin North Am 2000;29:451. [PMID 11033755]

Tominaga Y: Surgical management of secondary hyperparathyroidism in uremia. Am J Med Sci 1999;317:390. [PMID 10372839]

The Adrenal Gland

Brunt LM et al: Adrenalectomy for familial pheochromocytoma in the laparoscopic era. Ann Surg 2002;235:713. [PMID 11981218]

Brunt LM, Moley JF: Adrenal incidentaloma. World J Surg 2001; 25:905. [PMID 11572032]

Dackiw APB et al: Adrenal cortical carcinoma. World J Surg 2001; 25:914. [PMID 11572033]

Gordon RD, Stowasser M, Rutherford JC: Primary aldosteronism: are we diagnosing and operating on too few patients? World J Surg 2001;25:941. [PMID 11572036]

Kebebew E, Duh Q-Y: Benign and malignant pheochromocytoma: diagnosis, treatment and follow-up. Surg Oncol Clin N Am 1998;7:765. [PMID 9735133]

Lam KY, Lo CY: Metastatic tumors of the adrenal glands: a 30-year experience in a teaching hospital. Clin Endocrinol 2002;56: 95. [PMID 11849252]

Norton JA et al: Cushing's syndrome. Curr Probl Surg 2001;38: 488. [11427876]

Raeburn CD, McIntyre RC: Laparoscopic approach to adrenal and endocrine pancreatic tumors. Surg Clin N Am 2000;80: 1427. [PMID 11059712]

Reincke M: Subclinical Cushing's syndrome. Endocrinol Metab Clin North Am 2000;29:43. [PMID 10732263]

The Endocrine Pancreas

Akerstrom G, Hessman O, Skogseid B: Timing and extent of surgery in symptomatic and asymptomatic neuroendocrine tumors of the pancreas in MEN 1. Langenbecks Arch Surg 2002;386:558. [PMID 11914931]

Anderson MA et al: Endoscopic ultrasound is highly accurate and directs management in patients with neuroendocrine tumors of the pancreas. Am J Gastroenterol 2000;95:2271. [PMID 11007228]

Azimuddin K, Chamberlain R: The surgical management of pancreatic neuroendocrine tumors. Surg Clin North Am 2001; 81:511. [PMID 11459268]

De Herder WW, Lamberts SW: Somatostatin and somatostatin analogues: diagnostic and therapeutic uses. Curr Opin Oncol 2002;14:53. [PMID 11790981]

Green BT, Rockey DC: Duodenal somatostatinoma presenting with complete somatostatinoma syndrome. J Clin Gastroenterol 2001;33:415. [PMID 11606861]

Norton JA et al: Surgery to cure the Zollinger-Ellison syndrome. N Engl J Med 1999;341:635. [PMID 10460814]

APPENDIX
NORMAL HORMONE REFERENCE RANGES[1,2]

ACTH stimulation test (cosyntropin test): 0.25 mg of synthetic ACTH$_{1-24}$ (cosyntropin) is administered IV or IM, and serum cortisol is measured at 0, 30, and 60 minutes. Normal response: peak cortisol > 20 µg/dL (> 540 nmol/L). A dose of 1 µg of ACTH will give a similar response in the normal individual (see Chapter 9).

Test	Source	Ages, Conditions, Etc	Conventional Units	Conversion Factor	SI Units	Comments
Adrenocorticotropic hormone (ACTH)	Plasma	Basal	9–52 pg/mL	0.222	2–11 pmol/L	Collect in silicone-coated EDTA-containing tubes. Keep iced. Avoid contact with glass during collection and separation. Process immediately. Separate and freeze plasma in plastic tube at –20 °C.
		Dexamethasone suppression	2–5 pg/mL		0.4–1.1 pmol/L	
Aldosterone	Plasma (fasting)	Sodium intake 100–200 mEq/d:		27.7		Levels in pregnant patients are three to four times higher.
		0700, recumbent	3–9 ng/dL		83–250 pmol/L	
		0900, upright	4–30 ng/dL		111–831 pmol/L	
		Adrenal vein	200–400 ng/dL		5540–11,080 pmol/L	
		Sodium intake 10 mEq/d:				
		0700, recumbent	12–36 ng/dL		333–997 pmol/L	
		0900, upright	17–137 ng/dL		471–3795 pmol/L	
Aldosterone-18-glucuronide	Urine	On normal diet (100–200 mEq Na$^+$/d):	5–20 µg/24 h	2.77	14–56 nmol/24 h	Refrigerate during collection.
		On low-sodium diet (< 20 mEq Na$^+$/d):	10–40 µg/24 h		28–112 nmol/24 h	
3α-Androstenediol glucuronide	Serum	Prepubertal children	0.1–0.6 ng/mL	2.14	0.2–1.3 nmol/L	Freeze serum and store at –20 °C.
		Male	2.6–16 ng/mL		5.6–34.2 nmol/L	
		Female	0.6–3.0 ng/mL		1.3–6.4 nmol/L	
Androstenedione	Serum	Male		3.49		
		< 1 year	0.06–0.078 ng/mL		0.2–0.27 nmol/L	
		1–5 years	0.05–0.51 ng/mL		0.17–1.78 nmol/L	
		6–12 years	0.07–0.68 ng/mL		0.24–2.37 nmol/L	
		13–17 years	0.17–1.51 ng/mL		0.59–5.27 nmol/L	
		Adult	0.50–2.50 ng/mL		1.75–8.7 nmol/L	
		Female				
		< 1 year	0.06–0.078 ng/mL		0.20–0.27 nmol/L	
		1–5 years	0.05–0.51 ng/mL		0.17–1.78 nmol/L	
		6–12 years	0.07–0.68 ng/mL		0.24–2.37 nmol/L	
		13–17 years	0.43–2.21 ng/mL		1.50–7.71 nmol/L	
		Adult	0.5–2.50 ng/mL		1.75–8.73 nmol/L	
		Postmenopausal	0.16–1.20 ng/mL		0.56–4.18 nmol/L	

Test	Specimen	Reference value	Conversion factor	SI units	Instructions
Antidiuretic hormone (ADH; vasopressin)	Plasma	If serum osmolality > 290 mosm/kg: 1–13 pg/mL If serum osmolality < 290 mosm/kg: < 2 pg/mL	0.925	0.9–12 pmol/L < 1.85 pmol/L	Collect in EDTA tubes. Keep iced. Centrifuge refrigerated. Store at −70 °C within 2 hours.
C peptide of insulin	Serum	Fasting 0.5–2.0 ng/mL Stimulated 1.5–9.0 ng/mL	0.331	0.17–0.66 nmol/L 0.5–3.0 nmol/L	Freeze serum at −20 °C within 8 hours after collection.
Calcitonin	Serum	Male < 8 ng/L Female < 4 ng/L	0.293	< 2.3 pmol/L < 1.17 pmol/L	Fasting, nonlipemic specimen. Refrigerate, spin down immediately. Store at −20 °C.

Calcitonin stimulation test utilizing calcium infusion: 2 mg/kg of calcium in the form of calcium gluconate is administered IV over 1 minute. Blood samples for calcitonin are obtained at 1, 2, 3, and 5 minutes after the infusion. Normal peak values for calcitonin 2 minutes after calcium infusion: female, < 70 ng/L (< 20.5 pmol/L); male: < 491 ng/L (< 144 pmol/L).

Test	Specimen	Analyte	Reference value	Conversion factor	SI units	Instructions

Catecholamines (fractionated by HPLC)	Plasma	Norepinephrine
		  Supine
		  Ambulatory
			112–658 pg/mL
			212–1109 pg/mL
				0.00591	0.66–3.89 nmol/L
					1.28–6.55 nmol/L
						Collect by intravenous catheter after patient has rested 30 minutes. Collect and centrifuge under refrigeration; freeze in plastic tube at −20 °C.

		Epinephrine
		  Supine
		  Ambulatory
			< 50 pg/mL
			< 95 pg/mL
				0.00546	< 0.27 nmol/L
					< 0.52 nmol/L	

		Dopamine
		  Supine
		  Ambulatory
			< 10 ng/mL
			< 20 ng/mL
				0.00654	< 0.065 nmol/L
					< 0.13 nmol/L	

	Urine	Norepinephrine
		  3–8 years
		  9–12 years
		  13–17 years
		  >17 years
			5–41 µg/24 h
			5–50 µg/24 h
			12–88 µg/24 h
			15–100 µg/24 h
				5.91	29.5–242.3 nmol/24 h
					29.5–295.8 nmol/24 h
					70.9–526 nmol/24 h
					89–591 nmol/24 h
						24-hour urine preservative: 25 mL 6N HCl. Freeze aliquot promptly at −20 °C.

		Epinephrine
		  3–8 years
		  9–12 years
		  13–17 years
		  >17 years
			1–7 µg/24 h
			< 8 µg/24 h
			< 11 µg/24 h
			2–24 µg/24 h
				5.46	5.46–38.2 nmol/24 h
					< 43.7 nmol/24 h
					< 60 nmol/24 h
					11–131 nmol/24 h	

		Dopamine
		  3–8 years
		  9–12 years
		  13–17 years
		  >17 years
			80–378 µg/24 h
			51–474 µg/24 h
			51–645 µg/24 h
			52–480 µg/24 h
				6.54	523–2472 nmol/24 h
					334–3100 nmol/24 h
					334–4218 nmol/24 h
					340–3139 nmol/24 h	

Cholecystokinin	Plasma (fasting)		3.9 ng/mL	0.26	1 pmol/L	

(continued)

NORMAL HORMONE REFERENCE RANGES[1,2] (CONTINUED)

Test	Source	Ages, Conditions, Etc	Conventional Units	Conversion Factor	SI Units	Comments
Chorionic gonadotropin, beta subunit (β-hCG)	Serum	Males and nonpregnant females	Not detectable	1.00	Not detectable	See Chapter 16 for further details and interpretation.
		Females post conception				
		3–4 weeks	9–130 mIU/mL		9–130 IU/L	
		4–5 weeks	75–2600 mIU/mL		75–2600 IU/L	
		5–6 weeks	850–20,800 mIU/mL		850–20,800 IU/L	
		6–7 weeks	4000–100,200 mIU/mL		4000–100,200 IU/L	
		7–12 weeks	11,500–289,000 mIU/mL		11,500–289,000 IU/L	
		12–16 weeks	18,300–137,000 mIU/mL		18,300–137,000 IU/L	
		16–29 weeks	1400–53,000 mIU/mL		1400–53,000 IU/L	
		29–41 weeks	940–60,000 mIU/mL		940–60,000 IU/L	
		Trophoblastic disease:	> 100,000 mIU/mL		> 100,000 IU/L	
Chromogranin A	Serum	Adults	1.6–5.6 ng/mL	1.00	1.6–5.6 µg/L	
Corticotropin-releasing hormone (CRH) test: Ovine CRH in a dose of 1 µg/kg is administered IV. Blood samples for ACTH and cortisol determinations are taken at 15, 30, and 60 minutes. The peak ACTH response of > 10 pg/mL (> 2.2 pmol/L) occurs at 15 minutes. The peak cortisol response of > 10 µg/dL (> 280 nmol/L) occurs at 30–60 minutes (see Chapter 5).						
Corticotropin-releasing hormone	Plasma	Adults (nonpregnant)	24–40 pg/mL	2.0	48–80 pmol/L	Markedly elevated at term pregnancy.
Cortisol	Serum	Total		27.59		Collect and process under refrigeration. Spin down immediately. Salivary cortisol is in equilibrium with free cortisol and may be used as an index to free cortisol. Reference range may vary with method and laboratory.
		AM	3–20 µg/dL		83–552 nmol/L	
		PM	1.5–10 µg/dL		41.4–276 nmol/L	
		Free				
		AM	0.6–1.6 µg/dL		16.5–44.1 nmol/L	
		PM	0.2–0.9 µg/dL		5.5–24.8 nmol/L	

| | | | | | Collect 24-hour specimen with 8 g of boric acid or 10 mL of 6N HCl as preservative. |

Analyte	Specimen	Conventional	Factor	SI Units	Comments
Dehydroepiandrosterone (DHEA)	Urine (free)	24-hour specimen RIA			Collect 24-hour specimen with 8 g of boric acid or 10 mL of 6N HCl as preservative.
		24-hour specimen HPLC			
		AM 1 hour (0700–0800)			
		PM 1 hour (2200–2300)			
		20–90 µg/g Cr	0.312	6.24–28.1 µmol/mol Cr	
		< 50 µg/24 h	2.76	< 138 nmol/24 h	
		50–200 µg/g Cr	0.312	16–62.4 µmol/mol Cr	
		5–45 µg/g Cr	0.312	1.6–14 µmol/mol Cr	
	Serum (fasting preferred)	Male	0.0347		Separate serum immediately and store at −20 °C.
		< 6 years		20–130 ng/dL	0.7–4.5 nmol/L
		6–8 years		20–275 ng/dL	0.7–9.5 nmol/L
		8–10 years		31–345 ng/dL	1.1–12.0 nmol/L
		Pubertal at–			
		Tanner stage II		110–495 ng/dL	3.8–17.2 nmol/L
		Tanner stage III		173–585 ng/dL	5.9–20.3 nmol/L
		Tanner stage IV		160–640 ng/dL	5.6–22.2 nmol/L
		Tanner V		250–900 ng/dL	8.7–31.2 nmol/L
		> 20 years		160–800 ng/dL	5.6–27.8 nmol/L
		Female			
		< 6 years		20–130 ng/dL	0.7–4.5 nmol/L
		6–8 years		20–275 ng/dL	0.7–9.5 nmol/L
		8–10 years		31–345 ng/dL	1.1–12.0 nmol/L
		Pubertal at–			
		Tanner stage II		150–570 ng/dL	5.2–19.8 nmol/L
		Tanner stage III		200–600 ng/dL	6.9–20.8 nmol/L
		Tanner stage IV		200–780 ng/dL	6.9–27.1 nmol/L
		Tanner stage V		215–850 ng/dL	7.5–29.5 nmol/L
		> 20 years		160–800 ng/dL	5.6–27.8 nmol/L
		Postmenopausal		30–450 ng/dL	1.0–15.6 nmol/L
Dehydroepiandrosterone sulfate (DHEAS)	Serum (fasting preferred)	Male	0.0272		Stable 72 hours at 40 °C. Store at −20 °C.
		Cord blood		< 380 µg/dL	< 10.3 µmol/L
		1–5 days		10–250 µg/dL	0.27–6.8 µmol/L
		1–5 months		1–41 µg/dL	0.03–1.1 µmol/L
		6–11 months		5–20 µg/dL	0.14–0.5 µmol/L
		1–5 years		1–40 µg/dL	0.03–1.0 µmol/L
		6–9 years		3–145 µg/dL	0.08–3.9 µmol/L
		10–11 years		15–115 µg/dL	0.41–3.1 µmol/L
		12–14 years		20–500 µg/dL	0.54–13.6 µmol/L
		15–17 years		30–555 µg/dL	0.81–15.1 µmol/L
		18–30 years		125–619 µg/dL	3.4–16.8 µmol/L
		31–50 years		59–452 µg/dL	1.6–12.3 µmol/L
		51–60 years		20–413 µg/dL	0.5–11.2 µmol/L
		61–83 years		10–285 µg/dL	0.27–7.75 µmol/L

(continued)

NORMAL HORMONE REFERENCE RANGES[1,2] (CONTINUED)

Test	Source	Ages, Conditions, Etc	Conventional Units	Conversion Factor	SI Units	Comments
		Female		0.0272		
		Cord blood	<380 μg/dL		<10.3 μmol/L	
		1–5 days	10–250 μg/dL		0.27–6.8 μmol/L	
		1–5 months	5–55 μg/dL		0.14–1 μmol/L	
		6–11 months	5–30 μg/dL		0.14–0.82 μmol/L	
		1–5 years	1–20 μg/dL		0.03–0.54 μmol/L	
		6–9 years	3–140 μg/dL		0.08–3.81 μmol/L	
		10–11 years	15–260 μg/dL		0.40–7.10 μmol/L	
		12–14 years	20–535 μg/dL		0.54–14.6 μmol/L	
		15–17 years	35–535 μg/dL		0.95–14.6 μmol/L	
		18–30 years	45–380 μg/dL1		1.22–10.3 μmol/L	
		31–50 years	12–452 μg/dL		0.33–12.3 μmol/L	
		Postmenopausal	17–77 μg/dL		0.05–2.1 μmol/L	
		Pregnancy (term)	23–177 μg/dL		0.6–3.2 μmol/L	
Deoxycorticosterone (DOC)	Serum (fasting preferred)	Cord blood	111–372 ng/dL	30.26	3359–11,257 pmol/L	Process immediately. Store at –20 °C.
		1 week to 12 months	7–49 ng/dL		212–1483 pmol/L	
		Prepubertal child	2–34 ng/dL		61–1030 pmol/L	
		Adults (0800)	2–19 ng/dL		61–575 pmol/L	
11-Deoxycortisol	Serum	Cord blood	295–554 ng/dL	0.02887	8.52–16.0 nmol/L	Process immediately. Store at –20 °C.
		Premature infants	48–579 ng/dL		1.39–16.7 nmol/L	
		Full-term infants to 3 days	13–147 ng/dL		0.38–4.24 nmol/L	
		1–12 months	<156 ng/dL		<4.5 nmol/L	
		Prepubertal child 1–10 years	20–155 ng/dL		0.58–4.5 nmol/L	
		Adults (0800)	12–158 ng/dL		0.35–4.6 nmol/L	

Dexamethasone suppression test (low dose) for the diagnosis of Cushing syndrome (see Chapter 9): Obtain a baseline serum cortisol at 0700–0800 hours. Administer 1 mg dexamethasone orally at 2300 hours that evening and obtain another serum cortisol at 0700–0800 hours the following morning. **Interpretation:** A normal response (normal suppressibility) is a reduction of the postdexamethasone serum cortisol to < 1.8 μg/dL (< 50 nmol/L).
Dexamethasone suppression test (high dose) for the differential diagnosis of Cushing's syndrome (see Chapter 9): Obtain a baseline serum cortisol at 0700–0800 hours. Administer 8 mg dexamethasone orally at 2300 hours that evening and obtain another serum cortisol at 0700–0800 hours the following morning. **Interpretation:** A reduction of the postdexamethasone serum cortisol to < 50% of the baseline cortisol indicates suppressibility.
Dexamethasone-CRH test: Administer dexamethasone, 0.5 mg every 6 hours orally for eight doses, followed by CRH, 1 μg/kg IV 2 hours after the last dose of dexamethasone. Plasma cortisol is obtained 15 minutes after CRH. Normal: < 1.4 μg/dL (< 38.6 nmol/L). (See Chapter 9.)

	Specimen		Conventional	Factor	SI Units	Comments
Dihydrotestoster-one (male)	Serum	Cord blood	< 2–8 ng/dL	0.0344	< 0.07–0.28 nmol/L	Separate serum within 1 hour after collection and store at –20 °C.
		Premature infants	10–53 ng/dL		0.34–1.82 nmol/L	
		Full-term newborn	5–60 ng/dL		0.17–2.06 nmol/L	
		30–60 days	12–85 ng/dL		0.42–2.92 nmol/L	
		7 months to puberty at–				
		Tanner stage I	< 3 ng/dL		< 0.10 nmol/L	
		Tanner stage II	3–17 ng/dL		0.10–0.58 nmol/L	
		Tanner stage III	8–33 ng/dL		0.28–1.14 nmol/L	
		Tanner stage IV	22–52 ng/dL		0.76–1.79 nmol/L	
		Tanner stage V	24–65 ng/dL		0.83–2.24 nmol/L	
		Adult	30–85 ng/dL		1.03–2.92 nmol/L	
Dihydrotestoster-one (female)	Serum	Cord blood	< 2–8 ng/dL	0.0344	< 0.07–0.28 nmol/L	
		Premature infants	2–13 ng/dL		0.07–0.45 nmol/L	
		Full-term newborn	< 2–15 ng/dL		0.07–0.52 nmol/L	
		30–60 days	< 3 ng/dL		< 0.10 nmol/L	
		7 months to puberty at–				
		Tanner stage I	< 3 ng/dL		< 0.10 nmol/L	
		Tanner stage II	5–12 ng/dL		0.17–0.41 nmol/L	
		Tanner stage III	7–19 ng/dL		0.24–0.65 nmol/L	
		Tanner stage IV	4–13 ng/dL		0.14–0.45 nmol/L	
		Tanner stage V	3–18 ng/dL		0.10–0.62 nmol/L	
		Adult	4–22 ng/dL		0.18–0.76 nmol/L	
Erythropoietin	Serum	Adult	4–26 mIU/mL	1.00	4–26 IU/L	
Estradiol	Serum	Male		3.67		
		1–5 years	3–10 pg/mL		11–37 pmol/L	
		6–9 years	3–10 pg/mL		11–37 pmol/L	
		10–11 years	5–10 pg/mL		18–37 pmol/L	
		12–14 years	5–30 pg/mL		18–110 pmol/L	
		15–17 years	5–45 pg/mL		18–165 pmol/L	
		> 17 years	10–50 pg/mL		37–184 pmol/L	
		Female				
		1–5 years	5–10 pg/mL		18–37 pmol/L	
		6–9 years	5–60 pg/mL		18–220 pmol/L	
		10–11 years	5–300 pg/mL		18–1100 pmol/L	
		12–14 years	25–410 pg/mL		91.8–1505 pmol/L	
		15–17 years	40–410 pg/mL		147–1505 pmol/L	
		Early follicular	20–100 pg/mL		73–367 pmol/L	
		Preovulatory	100–350 pg/mL		367–1285 pmol/L	
		Midcycle peak	150–750 pg/mL		550.5–2753 pmol/L	
		Luteal	100–350 pg/mL		367–1285 pmol/L	
		Postmenopausal	10–30 pg/mL		37–110 pmol/L	

(continued)

NORMAL HORMONE REFERENCE RANGES[1,2] (CONTINUED)

Test	Source	Ages, Conditions, Etc	Conventional Units	Conversion Factor	SI Units	Comments
Estriol (pregnancy)	Serum	Pregnant female		3.47		
		30–32 weeks	2–12 ng/mL		7–42 nmol/L	
		33–35 weeks	3–19 ng/mL		10–66 nmol/L	
		36–38 weeks	5–27 ng/mL		17–94 nmol/L	
		39–40 weeks	10–30 ng/mL		35–104 nmol/L	
		Male and nonpregnant female	< 2 ng/mL		< 7 nmol/L	
Estrone	Serum	Adult male	15–65 ng/L	3.70	55.5–240.5 pmol/L	
		Postpubertal female				
		Early follicular phase	15–150 ng/L		55.5–555 pmol/L	
		Late follicular phase	100–250 ng/L		370–925 pmol/L	
		Luteal phase	15–200 ng/L		55.5–740 pmol/L	
		Postmenopausal	15–55 ng/L		55.5–204 pmol/L	
Follicle-stimulating hormone	Serum or plasma (heparin)	Adult males	1.48–14.26 IU/L	1.00	1.48–14.26 IU/L	
		Adult females				
		Follicular phase	1.37–9.9 IU/L		1.37–9.9 IU/L	
		Midcycle peak	6.17–17.2 IU/L		6.17–17.2 IU/L	
		Luteal phase	1.09–9.2 IU/L		1.09–9.2 IU/L	
		Postmenopausal	14.9–124.3 IU/L		14.9–124.3 IU/L	
		Boys				
		2 weeks	1.22–5.19 IU/L		1.22–5.19 IU/L	
		1–18 months	0.19–2.97 IU/L		0.19–2.97 IU/L	
		19 months–7.9 years	0.25–1.92 IU/L		0.25–1.92 IU/L	
		8.0–9.9 years	0.3–1.67 IU/L		0.2–1.67 IU/L	
		10–11.9 years	0.2–5.79 IU/L		0.2–5.79 IU/L	
		12–14.9 years	0.23–10.37 IU/L		0.23–10.37 IU/L	
		15–18	0.81–8.18 IU/L		0.81–8.18 IU/L	
		Tanner stage		0.22		
		I	0.22–1.92 IU/L		0.22–1.92 IU/L	
		II	0.72–4.60 IU/L		0.72–4.60 IU/L	
		III	1.24–10.37 IU/L		1.24–10.37 IU/L	
		IV	1.70–10.35 IU/L		1.70–10.35 IU/L	
		V	1.54–7.00 IU/L		1.54–7.00 IU/L	

	Specimen	Category	Conventional Value	Conversion Factor	SI Value	Comments
		Girls				Overnight fast required. Store at –20 °C.
		2 weeks	2.09–30.45 IU/L		2.09–30.45 IU/L	
		1–18 months	1.14–14.35 IU/L		1.14–14.35 IU/L	
		19 months–7.9 years	0.70–3.39 IU/L		0.70–3.39 IU/L	
		8.0–9.9 years	0.28–5.64 IU/L		0.28–5.64 IU/L	
		10–11.9 years	0.68–7.26 IU/L		0.68–7.26 IU/L	
		12–14.9 years	1.02–9.24 IU/L		1.02–9.24 IU/L	
		15–18 years	0.33–10.54 IU/L		0.33–10.54 IU/L	
		Tanner stage				
		I	0.50–2.41 IU/L		0.50–2.41 IU/L	
		II	1.73–4.68 IU/L		1.73–4.68 IU/L	
		III	2.53–7.04 IU/L		2.53–7.04 IU/L	
		IV	1.26–7.37 IU/L		1.26–7.37 IU/L	
		V	1.02–9.24 IU/L		1.02–9.24 IU/L	
Gastrin	Serum	Newborn, 1–12 days	69–109 ng/L	0.475	32.8–90.3 pmol/L	Overnight fast required. Store at –20 °C.
		Infants, 1.5–22 months	55–186 ng/L		26.1–88.4 pmol/L	
		Pre- and postpubertal children				
		Fasting 3–4 hours	2–168 ng/L		1.0–80 pmol/L	
		Fasting 5–6 hours	3–117 ng/L		1.4–55.6 pmol/L	
		Fasting > 8 hours	1–125 ng/L		0.5–59.4 pmol/L	
		Adults	< 42 ng/L		< 20 pmol/L	
Glucagon	Plasma	Adults	20–100 pg/mL	0.287	5.7–28.7 pmol/L	Centrifuge immediately under refrigeration. Store in plastic vial at –20 °C. Overnight fast required.
Growth hormone	Serum	Fasting		46.5		Store at –20 °C. **Note:** GH values fluctuate widely, and functional tests must be utilized for diagnosis of GH deficiency or excess. See Chapter 5 for details of suppression and stimulation tests for GH excess or deficiency.
		Children	< 10 ng/mL		< 460 pmol/L	
		Adults	1–5 ng/mL		46–232 pmol/L	
Growth hormone-binding protein	Serum	Males		1.0		Store at –20 °C.
		3–5 years	57–282 pmol/L		57–282 pmol/L	
		6–9 years	60–619 pmol/L		60–619 pmol/L	
		10–15 years	52–783 pmol/L		52–783 pmol/L	
		Adults	66–306 pmol/L		66–306 pmol/L	
		Females				
		3–5 years	62–519 pmol/L		62–519 pmol/L	
		6–9 years	58–572 pmol/L		58–572 pmol/L	
		10–15 years	72–965 pmol/L		72–965 pmol/L	
		Adults	66–306 pmol/L		66–306 pmol/L	

(continued)

NORMAL HORMONE REFERENCE RANGES[1,2] (CONTINUED)

Test	Source	Ages, Conditions, Etc	Conventional Units	Conversion Factor	SI Units	Comments
Growth hormone-releasing hormone	Plasma	Adults	<50 pg/mL	1.0	<50 pg/mL	Store at −20 °C.
Homovanillic acid	Urine	3–8 years 9–12 years 13–17 years >17 years	0.5–6.7 mg/24 h 1.1–6.8 mg/24 h 1.4–7.2 mg/24 h 1.6–7.5 mg/24 h	5.49	2.7–36.8 µmol/24 h 6.0–37.3 µmol/24 h 7.7–39.5 µmol/24 h 8.8–41.2 µmol/24 h	Preservative: 10 mL 6N HCl.
17-Hydroxycorticoids	Urine	Males, age 2–17 years Adult Females, age 2–17 years Adult	1.1–7.5 mg/24 h 0.9–15.3 mg/g creatinine 4–11 mg/24 h 1.9–9.5 mg/g creatinine 1.1–7.5 mg/24 h 0.9–15.3 mg/g creatinine 3–10 mg/24 h 1.9–9.5 mg/g creatinine	2.76	3.0–20.7 µmol/24 h 2.5–42.2 µmol/g creatinine 11.0–30.4 µmol/24 h 5.2–26.2 µmol/g creatinine 3.0–20.7 µmol/24 h 2.4–42.4 µmol/g creatinine 8.3–27.6 µmol/24 h 5.2–26 µmol/g creatinine	Preservative: 10 mL 6N HCl
5-Hydroxyindoleacetic acid	Urine	Age 2–10 years Age > 10 years	<8 mg/24 h <6 mg/24 h	5.23	< 41.8 µmol/24 h < 31.4 µmol/24 h	Preservative: 10 mL 6N HCl. Refrigerate during collection. For 48 hours prior to and during collection, avoid avocados, alcohol, high results).
18-Hydroxycorticosterone	Serum	Supine (8–10 AM) Ambulatory 8–10 AM)	4–37 ng/dL 5–80 ng/dL	27.51	110–1018 pmol/L 138–2201 pmol/L	Refrigerate.
17-Hydroxypregnenolone	Serum	Cord blood Premature infants Full-term infants 3 days 1–6 months 6–12 months Prepubertal child (1–10 years) Pubertal age groups Adults	50–2121 ng/dL 64–2380 ng/dL 10–829 ng/dL 36–763 ng/dL 42–540 ng/dL 15–221 ng/dL 44–235 ng/dL 53–357 ng/dL	0.0307	1.5–65.1 nmol/L 1.9–73.1 nmol/L 0.3–25.5 nmol/L 1.1–23.4 nmol/L 1.3–16.6 nmol/L 0.5–6.7 nmol/L 1.3–7.2 nmol/L 1.6–11.0 nmol/L	Process immediately. Store at −20 °C.

Analyte	Specimen		Conventional value	Factor	SI value
17-Hydroxypro-gesterone	Serum (fasting pre-ferred)	Males		0.0303 →	
		1–5 days	80–420 ng/dL		2.4–12.7 pmol/L
		1–5 months	15–135 ng/dL		0.45–4.1 pmol/L
		6–11 months	25–145 ng/dL		0.75–4.4 pmol/L
		1–5 years	20–80 ng/dL		0.6–2.4 pmol/L
		6–9 years	15–65 ng/dL		0.45–1.97 pmol/L
		10–11 years	15–45 ng/dL		0.45–1.36 pmol/L
		12–14 years	15–180 ng/dL		0.45–5.45 pmol/L
		15–17 years	25–180 ng/dL		0.75–5.45 pmol/L
		Adult	50–250 ng/dL		1.5–7.6 pmol/L
		Tanner stage			
		I	15–65 ng/dL		0.45–1.97 pmol/L
		II	15–120 ng/dL		0.45–3.64 pmol/L
		III	25–130 ng/dL		0.76–3.94 pmol/L
		IV	30–180 ng/dL		0.90–5.45 pmol/L
		V	25–170 ng/dL		0.76–5.15 pmol/L
		Females			
		1–5 days	82–400 ng/dL		2.5–12.1 pmol/L
		1–5 months	20–190 ng/dL		0.6–5.8 pmol/L
		6–11 months	25–155 ng/dL		0.76–4.7 pmol/L
		1–5 years	20–50 ng/dL		0.6–1.5 pmol/L
		6–9 years	20–40 ng/dL		0.6–1.2 pmol/L
		10–11 years	20–70 ng/dL		0.6–2.1 pmol/L
		12–14 years	25–190 ng/dL		0.76–5.8 pmol/L
		15–17 years	35–375 ng/dL		1.1–11.4 pmol/L
		Tanner stage			
		I	20–70 ng/dL		0.6–2.12 pmol/L
		II	20–65 ng/dL		0.6–1.97 pmol/L
		III	30–90 ng/dL		0.9–2.7 pmol/L
		IV	35–235 ng/dL		1.1–7.1 pmol/L
		V	45–375 ng/dL		1.36–11.4 pmol/L
		Follicular	20–100 ng/dL		0.61–3.0 pmol/L
		Midcycle peak	100–250 ng/dL		3.0–7.58 pmol/L
		Luteal	100–500 ng/dL		3.0–15.2 pmol/L
		Postmenopausal	<70 ng/dL		<2.1 pmol/L
Hydroxyproline	Urine	Total		7.62	Preservative: 25 mL 6N HCl. Freeze at –20 °C.
		Males	9–73 mg/24 h		68.6–556.3 µmol/24 h
		Females	7–49 mg/24 h		53.3–373.4 µmol/24 h
		Free	<2.7 mg/24 h		<20.6 µmol/24 h

(continued)

Test	Source	Ages, Conditions, Etc	Conventional Units	Conversion Factor	SI Units	Comments
Insulin	Serum	Fasting	5–20 µU/mL (0.2–0.8 ng/mL)	172.1 (ng/mL → pmol/L)	34.4–137.6 pmol/L	Cold centrifuge. Freeze at –20 °C.
Insulin with oral glucose tolerance test	Serum	1 hour 2 hours	50–130 µU/mL (2–5.2 ng/mL) < 30 µU/mL (< 1.2 ng/mL)	172.1 (ng/mL → pmol/L)	344–895 pmol/L (< 207 pmol/L)	Cold centrifuge. Freeze at –20 °C.
Insulin-like growth factor-I (IGF-I)	Serum	Male 2 months to 5 years 6–8 years 9–11 years 12–15 years 16–24 years 25–39 years Female 2 months to 5 years 6–8 years 9–11 years 12–15 years 16–24 years 25–39 years	 17–248 µg/L 88–474 µg/L 110–565 µg/L 202–957 µg/L 182–780 µg/L 114–492 µg/L 17–248 µg/L 88–474 µg/L 117–771 µg/L 261–1096 µg/L 182–780 µg/L 114–492 µg/L	0.13	 2.2–32.2 nmol/L 11.4–61.6 nmol/L 14.3–73.5 nmol/L 26.3–124.4 nmol/L 23.7–101.4 nmol/L 14.8–64.0 nmol/L 2.2–32.2 nmol/L 11.4–61.6 nmol/L 15.2–100.2 nmol/L 33.9–142.5 nmol/L 23.7–101.4 nmol/L 14.8–64.0 nmol/L	Store refrigerated.
Insulin-like growth-factor-II (IGF-II)	Serum	2 months to 5 years 6–9 years 10–17 years 18–54 years 55–65 years > 65 years	300–860 ng/mL 520–1050 ng/mL 530–1140 ng/mL 405–1005 ng/mL 230–970 ng/mL 210–750 ng/mL	0.134	40.2–115.2 nmol/L 69.7–140.7 nmol/L 71.0–142.8 nmol/L 54.3–145.4 nmol/L 30.8–130.0 nmol/L 28.1–100.5 nmol/L	Store refrigerated.
Insulin-like growth factor binding protein-III (IGFBP III)	Serum	2–23 months 2–7 years 8–11 years 12–18 years 19–55 years 56–82 years	0.7–2.3 ng/mL 0.9–4.1 ng/mL 1.5–4.3 ng/mL 2.2–4.2 ng/mL 2.0–4.0 ng/mL 0.9–3.7 ng/mL	1.0	0.7–2.3 mg/L 0.9–4.1 mg/L 1.5–4.3 mg/L 2.2–4.2 mg/L 2.0–4.0 mg/L 0.9–3.7 mg/L	Separate serum within 1 hour. Free serum in plastic vial at –20 °C.

Test	Specimen	Category	Conventional units	Factor	SI units	Notes
17-Ketosteroids	Urine	Males and females age 2–17 years	0.8–8.1 mg/d	3.47	2.8–28.1 µmol/d	
		Adult males	7–20 mg/d		24.3–69.4 µmol/d	
		Adult females	5–15 mg/d		17.4–52.1 µmol/d	
Luteinizing hormone	Plasma or serum	Males		1.0		Test measures the sum of LH and hCG; high hCG levels in pregnancy or trophoblastic disease cross-react in the assay, giving falsely high LH levels. Freeze specimen at −20°C.
		Cord blood	0.04–2.6 IU/L		0.04–2.6 IU/L	
		2 weeks	4.85–10.02 IU/L		4.85–10.02 IU/L	
		1–18 months	0.04–3.01 IU/L		0.04–3.01 IU/L	
		19 months–7.9 years	0.02–1.03 IU/L		0.02–1.03 IU/L	
		8–9.9 years	0.01–0.78 IU/L		0.01–0.78 IU/L	
		10–11.9 years	0.03–4.44 IU/L		0.03–4.44 IU/L	
		12–14.9 years	0.25–4.84 IU/L		0.25–4.84 IU/L	
		15–18.9 years	0.69–7.15 IU/L		0.69–7.15 IU/L	
		19–70 years	0.95–5.60 IU/L		0.95–5.60 IU/L	
		Tanner stage				
		I	0.02–0.42 IU/L		0.02–0.42 IU/L	
		II	0.26–4.84 IU/L		0.26–4.84 IU/L	
		III	0.64–3.74 IU/L		0.64–3.74 IU/L	
		IV	0.55–7.15 IU/L		0.55–7.15 IU/L	
		V	1.54–7.0 IU/L		1.54–7.0 IU/L	
		Females				
		Cord blood	0.04–2.6 IU/L		0.04–2.6 IU/L	
		2 weeks	0.29–7.91 IU/L		0.29–7.91 IU/L	
		1–18 months	0.02–1.77 IU/L		0.02–1.77 IU/L	
		19 months–7.9 years	0.03–0.55 IU/L		0.03–0.55 IU/L	
		8–9.9 years	0.02–0.24 IU/L		0.02–0.24 IU/L	
		10–11.9 years	0.02–4.12 IU/L		0.02–4.12 IU/L	
		12–14.9 years	0.28–29.38 IU/L		0.28–29.38 IU/L	
		15–18 years	0.11–29.38 IU/L		0.11–29.38 IU/L	
		Follicular phase	1.68–15.0 IU/L		1.68–15.0 IU/L	
		Midcycle peak	21.9–56.6 IU/L		21.9–56.6 IU/L	
		Luteal phase	0.61–16.3 IU/L		0.61–16.3 IU/L	
		Postmenopausal	9.0–52 IU/L		9.0–52 IU/L	
		Tanner stage				
		I	0.01–0.21 IU/L		0.01–0.21 IU/L	
		II	0.27–4.12 IU/L		0.27–4.12 IU/L	
		III	0.17–4.12 IU/L		0.17–4.12 IU/L	
		IV	0.72–15.01 IU/L		0.72–15.01 IU/L	
		V	0.30–29.38 IU/L		0.30–29.38 IU/L	

(continued)

NORMAL HORMONE REFERENCE RANGES[1,2] (CONTINUED)

Test	Source	Ages, Conditions, Etc	Conventional Units	Conversion Factor	SI Units	Comments
Metanephrine	Urine	Metanephrines		5.07		Preservative: 30 mL 3N HCl.
		3–8 years	9–86 µg/d		45.6–436 nmol/d	
		9–12 years	26–156 µg/d		131–790 nmol/d	
		13–17 years	31–156 µg/d		157–790 nmol/d	
		Males > 17 years	26–230 µg/d		132–1166 nmol/d	
		Females > 17 years	19–140 µg/d		96–710 nmol/d	
		Normetanephrines				
		3–8 years	20–186 µg/d		101–943 nmol/d	
		9–12 years	10–319 µg/d		51–1617 nmol/d	
		13–17 years	71–395 µg/d		360–2002 nmol/d	
		Males > 17 years	44–540 µg/d		223–2738 nmol/d	
		Females > 17 years	52–310 µg/d		264–1572 nmol/d	
		Total metanephrine				
		3–8 years	47–260 µg/d		238–1318 nmol/d	
		9–12 years	72–410 µg/d		365–2079 nmol/d	
		13–17 years	130–520 µg/d		659–2636 nmol/d	
		Males > 17 years	90–690 µg/d		456–3498 nmol/d	
		Females > 17 years	95–475 µg/d		482–2408 nmol/d	

Metyrapone stimulation test: Metyrapone in a dose of 30 mg/kg is administered orally at midnight. The 8 AM plasma 11-deoxycortisol is > 7 µg/dL (> 0.2 nmol/L) and plasma ACTH is > 100 pg/mL (22 pmol/L). (See Chapter 5.)

Test	Source	Ages, Conditions, Etc	Conventional Units	Conversion Factor	SI Units	Comments
Osmolality	Serum Urine	Random specimen	285–293 mosm/kg 300–900 mosm/kg	1.00	285–293 mosm/kg 300–900 mosm/kg	
Osteocalcin	Serum	Males and females		1.0		Overnight fast preferred. Store refrigerated.
		2–11 months	27.0–149.0 ng/mL		27.0–149.0 µg/L	
		1–4 years	23.0–105.0 ng/mL		23.0–105.0 µg/L	
		5–9 years	24.0–123.0 ng/mL		24.0–123.0 µg/L	
		Adult males	8.0–52.0 ng/mL		8.0–52.0 µg/L	
		Premenopausal females	5.8–41.0 ng/mL		5.8–41.0 µg/L	
		Postmenopausal females	8.0–56.0 ng/mL		8.0–56.0 µg/L	
		Tanner stage				
		I males and females	20.0–89.0 ng/mL		20.0–89.0 µg/L	
		II males	26.0–91.0 ng/mL		26.0–91.0 µg/L	
		II females	44.0–144.0 ng/mL		44.0–144.0 µg/L	
		III–IV males	48.0–123.0 ng/mL		48.0–123.0 µg/L	
		III–IV females	31.0–90.0 ng/mL		31.0–90.0 µg/L	

Analyte	Specimen	Condition	Conventional Value	Factor	SI Value	Comments
Pancreatic polypeptide	Plasma	20–29 years 30–39 years 40–49 years 50 years and older	26–158 pg/mL 55–284 pg/mL 64–243 pg/mL 51–326 pg/mL	0.246	6.4–38.9 pmol/L 13.5–70.0 pmol/L 15.7–59.8 pmol/L 12.5–80.2 pmol/L	Process immediately and freeze plasma at –60 °C.
Parathyroid hormone	Serum		17–73 pg/mL	0.100	1.8–7.3 pmol/L	Intact hormone assay. Freeze serum at –20 °C.
Parathormone-related protein	Plasma				> 1.3 pmol/L	
Pregnanetriol	24-hour urine	<7 years 7–16 years >16 years	<0.2 mg/d 0.3–1.1 mg/d <2.0 mg/d	2.97	<0.6 µmol/d 0.9–3.3 µmol/d <0.6 µmol/d	Preservative: 20 mL 33% acetic acid.
Pregnenolone	Serum	Adult males Adult females	10–200 ng/dL 10–230 ng/dL	0.0318	0.3–6.4 nmol/L 0.3–7.3 nmol/L	
Progesterone	Serum	Adult males Menstruating females Follicular phase Ovulatory phase Luteal phase Postmenopausal females Pregnant females First trimester Second trimester Third trimester	0.20–1.40 µg/L 0.20–1.50 µg/L 0.80–3.00 µg/L 1.70–27.0 µg/L 0.10–0.80 µg/L 9.0–47.00 µg/L 17.0–146.0 µg/L 5.0–255.0 µg/L	0.0318	0.006–0.045 nmol/L 0.006–0.047 nmol/L 0.025–0.095 nmol/L 0.054–0.086 nmol/L 0.003–0.025 nmol/L 0.29–1.49 nmol/L 0.54–4.64 nmol/L 0.16–8.11 nmol/L	Freeze at –20 °C.
Prolactin	Serum	Adult females Adult males	1.4–24.2 ng/mL 1.6–18.8 ng/mL	0.045	0.06–1.1 nmol/L 0.07–0.85 nmol/L	Freeze serum at –20 °C.
Renin	Plasma	Normal sodium diet (75–150 mmol/d) 0800 recumbent 1200 upright	0.3–3.0 µg/L/h 0.4–8.8 µg/L/h	0.278	0.09–0.9 ng/L/s 0.12–2.7 ng/L/s	Draw in cold tube, separate plasma, and freeze in plastic within 15 minutes after collection.
Secretin	Plasma	Fasting Postprandial	3–15 pg/mL 30 pg/mL	0.33	1–5 pmol/L 10 pmol/L	
Sex hormone-binding globulin	Serum	Males Females	(Not available)		6–44 nmol/L 8–85 nmol/L	Store refrigerated.
Somatostatin	Plasma	Adults	10–22 pg/mL	0.426	4.26–9.37 pmol/L	
Substance P	Serum	Fasting	91 pg/mL	0.77	70 pmol/L	

(continued)

NORMAL HORMONE REFERENCE RANGES[1,2] (CONTINUED)

Test	Source	Ages, Conditions, Etc	Conventional Units	Conversion Factor	SI Units	Comments
Testosterone, total	Serum	Male		0.0347		Freeze at –20°C.
		Newborn	17–61 ng/dL		0.6–2.1 nmol/L	
		1–5 months	1–177 ng/dL		0.03–6.1 nmol/L	
		6–11 months	2–7 ng/dL		0.06–0.24 nmol/L	
		1–5 years	2–25 ng/dL		0.06–0.86 nmol/L	
		6–9 yeras	3–30 ng/dL		0.10–1.0 nmol/L	
		10–11 years	5–50 ng/dL		0.17–1.7 nmol/L	
		12–14 years	10–572 ng/dL		0.30–19.8 nmol/L	
		15–17 years	220–800 ng/dL		7.6–27.8 nmol/L	
		Adult	260–1000 ng/dL		9.0–34.7 nmol/L	
		Tanner stage I	2–23 ng/dL		0.06–0.80 nmol/L	
		Tanner stage II	5–70 ng/dL		0.17–2.4 nmol/L	
		Tanner stage III	15–280 ng/dL		0.52–9.7 nmol/L	
		Tanner stage IV	105–545 ng/dL		3.6–18.9 nmol/L	
		Tanner stage V	265–800 ng/dL		9.2–27.8 nmol/L	
		Female				
		Newborn	16–44 ng/dL		0.55–1.52 nmol/L	
		1–5 months	1–5 ng/dL		0.03–0.17 nmol/L	
		6–11 months	2–5 ng/dL		0.06–0.17 nmol/L	
		1–5 years	2–10 ng/dL		0.06–0.35 nmol/L	
		6–9 years	2–20 ng/dL		0.06–0.69 nmol/L	
		10–11 years	5–25 ng/dL		0.17–0.87 nmol/L	
		12–14 years	10–40 ng/dL		0.34–1.38 nmol/L	
		15–17 years	5–40 ng/dL		0.17–1.38 nmol/L	
		Adult	15–70 ng/dL		0.52–2.43 nmol/L	
		Postmenopausal	5–51 ng/dL		0.17–1.77 nmol/L	
		Tanner stage I	2–10 ng/dL		0.07–0.35 nmol/L	
		Tanner stage II	5–30 ng/dL		0.17–1.04 nmol/L	
		Tanner stage III	10–30 ng/dL		0.35–1.04 nmol/L	
		Tanner stage IV	15–40 ng/dL		0.52–1.39 nmol/L	
		Tanner stage V	10–40 ng/dL		0.35–1.39 nmol/L	
Testosterone, free	Serum	Male		3.47		Freeze at –20 °C.
		Newborn	3.0–19 ng/L		10.4–65.9 pmol/L	
		5–7 months	0.4–4.8 ng/L		1.4–16.6 pmol/L	
		6–9 years	0.1–3.2 ng/L		0.35–11.1 pmol/L	
		10–11 years	0.6–5.7 ng/L		2.08–19.8 pmol/L	
		12–14 years	1.4–156 ng/L		4.9–541 pmol/L	
		15–17 years	80–159 ng/L		278–552 pmol/L	
		Adult	50–210 ng/L		174–729 pmol/L	

Test	Specimen		Reference Range	Factor	SI Units	Comments
Thyroglobulin	Serum	Female		1.00		Freeze at –20°C. The presence of thyroglobulin autoantibodies in the patient's serum may falsely lower the result.
		Newborn	2.0–4.0 ng/L		7.0–13.9 pmol/L	
		5–7 months	0.2–0.6 ng/L		0.7–2.1 pmol/L	
		6–9 years	0.1–0.9 ng/L		0.35–3.12 pmol/L	
		10–11 years	1.0–5.2 ng/L		3.47–18.0 pmol/L	
		12–14 years	1.0–5.2 ng/L		3.47–18.0 pmol/L	
		15–17 years	1.0–5.2 ng/L		3.47–18.0 pmol/L	
		Adult	1.0–8.5 ng/L		3.47–29.5 pmol/L	
		Normal				
		2–16 years	2.3–39.6 ng/mL		2.3–39.6 µg/L	
		Adult	3.5–56 ng/mL		3.5–56 µg/L	
		After total thyroidectomy				
		On T$_4$	<2 ng/mL		<2 µg/L	
		Off T$_4$	<2 ng/mL		<2 µg/L	
Thyroid auto-antibodies	Serum	Thyroperoxidase antibodies	<2 units/mL		<2 units/mL	
		Thyroglobulin antibodies	<2 units/mL		<2 units/mL	
Thyroid-stimulating hormone (TSH)	Serum		0.5–4.7 µIU/mL	1.00	0.5–4.7 mIU/L	Neonatal and cord blood levels are two to four times higher.
Thyroid-stimulating hormone receptor antibody (TSH-R Ab [stim])	Serum		<130% of basal activity			Assay based on cAMP generation in CHO cells transfected with human TSH receptor gene.
Thyroid uptake of radioactive iodine (RAIU)	Activity over thyroid gland	Fractional uptake				Ingestion or administration of iodide will decrease thyroid uptake of RAI.
		2 hours	4–12%			
		6 hours	6–15%			
		24 hours	8–30%			
Thyroxine-binding globulin	Serum		17–36 µg/mL	1.00	17–36 mg/L	
Thyroxine (T$_4$)	Serum	Cord blood	4.6–13 µg/dL	12.87	59.2–167 nmol/L	Refrigerate serum. Fasting preferred. Elevated levels in pregnancy due to increased TBG.
		1–2 days	11.8–23.2 µg/dL		151.9–198.6 nmol/L	
		3–9 days	9.9–21.9 µg/dL		127.4–281.9 nmol/L	
		10–44 days	8.2–16.2 µg/dL		105.5–208.5 nmol/L	
		45–89 days	6.4–14 µg/dL		82.4–180.2 nmol/L	
		3–11 months	7.8–16.5 µg/dL		100.4–212.4 nmol/L	
		1–4 years	7.3–15.0 µg/dL		94.0–193.1 nmol/L	
		5–9 years	6.4–13.3 µg/dL		82.4–171.2 nmol/L	

(continued)

NORMAL HORMONE REFERENCE RANGES[1,2] (CONTINUED)

Test	Source	Ages, Conditions, Etc	Conventional Units	Conversion Factor	SI Units	Comments
		10–14 years	5.6–11.7 µg/dL		72.1–150.5 nmol/L	
		15–19 years	4.2–11.8 µg/dL		54.1–151.9 nmol/L	
		≥20 years	5.0–12.0 µg/dL		64.4–154.4 nmol/L	
Thyroxine, free (FT$_4$)	Serum	0–4 days > 2 weeks	2.2–5.3 ng/dL 0.7–1.9 ng/dL	12.87	28–68 pmol/L 9–24 pmol/L	By dialysis. FT$_4$ by two-step immunoassay is comparable.
Resin T$_4$ uptake (RT$_4$U)	Serum		25–35%	0.01	0.25–0.35	RT$_4$U may be expressed as ratio to normal.
Free thyroxine index	Serum	Product of T$_4$ × RT$_4$U = 1.3–4.2 arbitrary units. (Expressed as T$_4$ adjusted for TBG binding = 5–12 arbitrary units.)			Product of T$_4$ × RT$_4$U = 16–54 arbitrary units or, adjusted: 64–154 arbitrary units.	
Thyroxine: TBG ratio	Serum		T4 (µg/dL) ÷ TBG (µg/mL) = 0.2–0.5		T4 (nmol/L) ÷ TBG (mg/L) = 2.7–6.4	
Triiodothyronine (T$_3$)	Serum	Cord blood 1–2 days 3–9 days 1–11 months 1–4 years 5–9 years 10–14 years 15–19 years ≥20 years	15–75 ng/dL 32–216 ng/dL 50–250 ng/dL 105–280 ng/dL 105–269 ng/dL 94–241 ng/dL 83–213 ng/dL 80–210 ng/dL 70–132 ng/dL	0.0154	0.23–1.2 nmol/L 0.49–3.3 nmol/L 0.77–3.8 nmol/L 1.6–4.3 nmol/L 1.6–4.1 nmol/L 1.4–3.7 nmol/L 1.3–3.3 nmol/L 1.2–3.2 nmol/L 1.1–2.0 nmol/L	Refrigerate serum. Elevated levels in pregnancy due to increased TBG.
Free T$_3$ index	Serum	Expressed as product of T$_3$ × RT$_4$U = 17.5–46 (arbitrary units)			0.275–0.7 (arbitrary units)	
Free T$_3$ (FT$_3$)	Serum		0.23–0.42 ng/dL	15.4	3.5–6.47 pmol/L	
Reverse T$_3$ (RT$_3$)	Serum	Cord blood Children and adults	102–342 ng/dL 10–24 ng/dL	0.0154	1.57–5.27 nmol/L 0.154–0.37 nmol/L	

Vanillylmandelic acid (VMA)	Urine (24-hour)	Newborn Infant Child Adolescent Adult	< 1 mg/d < 2 mg/d 1–3 mg/d 1–5 mg/d 2–7 mg/d	5.88	< 5.8 nmol/d < 11.7 nmol/d 5.8–17.6 nmol/d 5.8–29.4 nmol/d 11.8–41.2 nmol/d	
	Urine (24-hour or "spot")	1–11 months 1–2 years 3–5 years 6–10 years ≥ 10 years	μg VMA/mg Cr < 36 < 31 < 17 < 15 < 11	0.573	mmol VMA/mol Cr < 20.5 < 17.7 < 9.7 < 8.6 < 6.3	
Vasoactive intestinal peptide	Plasma		< 50 ng/mL	0.30	< 15 pmol/L	Freeze at –60 °C.
Vitamin D (25-hydroxy)	Serum	3–17 years > 17 years	13–67 μg/L 9–52 μg/L	2.50	32.5–167 nmol/L 22.5–130 nmol/L	Measures both D_2 and D_3. Freeze serum in plastic tube at –20 °C.
Vitamin D (1,25-dihydroxy)	Serum	3–17 years > 17 years	27–71 ng/L 15–60 ng/L	2.40	64.8–170 pmol/L 36–144 pmol/L	Measures both D_2 and D_3. Freeze serum at –60 °C in plastic tube.

[1] Adapted from the *Clinical Laboratories Manual* of the University of California Hospital and Clinics, San Francisco, California, March 30, 2002; and, with permission, from Quest Diagnostics Nichols Institute normal values for endocrine tests. The factors used in converting conventional units to SI units were derived in part from the *CRC Handbook of Chemistry and Physics*. It is important to emphasize that normal ranges vary among different laboratories, and the clinician must know the normal range for the test of interest in the laboratory performing the test.

[2] Semen analysis is discussed in Chapter 12.

Index

Page numbers followed by the letters f and t indicate figures and tables, respectively.